THE OXFORD HANDBOOK OF

GENETIC COUNSELING

THE OXFORD HANDBOOK OF

GENETIC COUNSELING

Edited by

ROBIN E. GRUBS,

EMILY G. FARROW,

and

MICHAEL J. DEEM

OXFORD
UNIVERSITY PRESS

OXFORD
UNIVERSITY PRESS

Oxford University Press is a department of the University of Oxford.
It furthers the University's objective of excellence in research, scholarship,
and education by publishing worldwide. Oxford is a registered trade mark of
Oxford University Press in the UK and certain other countries.

Published in the United States of America by Oxford University Press
198 Madison Avenue, New York, NY 10016, United States of America.

Library of Congress Cataloging-in-Publication Data
Names: Grubs, Robin E. editor | Farrow, Emily G. editor | Deem, Michael J. editor
Title: The Oxford handbook of genetic counseling / [edited by] Robin E.
Grubs, Emily G. Farrow, and Michael J. Deem.
Other titles: Handbook of genetic counseling | Oxford handbooks
Description: New York, NY : Oxford University Press, [2025] |
Series: Oxford handbooks series |
Includes bibliographical references and index.
Identifiers: LCCN 2025005384 (print) | LCCN 2025005385 (ebook) |
ISBN 9780190069964 hardback | ISBN 9780190069988 epub | ISBN 9780190069995
Subjects: MESH: Genetic Counseling | Genetic Testing
Classification: LCC RB155.7.O84 2025 (print) | LCC RB155.7 (ebook) |
NLM QZ 52 | DDC 616/.042—dc23/eng/20250716
LC record available at https://lccn.loc.gov/2025005384
LC ebook record available at https://lccn.loc.gov/2025005385

DOI: 10.1093/oxfordhb/9780190069964.001.0001

Printed by Marquis Book Printing, Canada

The manufacturer's authorized representative in the EU for product safety is
Oxford University Press España S.A., Parque Empresarial San Fernando de Henares,
Avenida de Castilla, 2 – 28830 Madrid (www.oup.es/en).

FSC www.fsc.org MIX Paper | Supporting responsible forestry FSC® C103567

Contents

PART III CONTEXTS OF GENETIC COUNSELING PRACTICE

PART IV NAVIGATING CONTEMPORARY ISSUES IN GENETIC TESTING AND GENETIC COUNSELING PRACTICE

PART VI CULTURE, DISABILITY, AND THE SOCIAL EFFECTS OF GENETIC COUNSELING

PART VII THE FUTURE OF GENETIC COUNSELING

In bringing together each part, we were mindful of terminology and its relationship to important cultural and social contexts. For example, there is geographic variation in the spelling of "counseling" or "counselling", and "counselor" and "counsellor." While we feel it is important to respect regional conventions in spelling, we utilize "counseling" and "counselor" throughout the volume in order to maintain consistency within chapters and across the volume. We retain, however, "counselling" and "counsellor" when they appear in direct quotations from the literature or wherever appropriate. There has also been discussion within the genetic counseling profession about the word "client" versus "patient" with respect to describing the individual who seeks genetic counseling services. We decided to let contributors choose the terminology that best reflected their views and the topics addressed in the chapters. Some provide the rationale for their choice of terms.

We believe *The Oxford Handbook of Genetic Counseling* will be an invaluable resource for genetic counselors, genetic counseling students and faculty, and bioethicists. Given its scope and diversity of topics, it will also be an important resource for clinical faculty, health researchers, and healthcare providers who are increasingly encountering genetics and genomics in their respective fields.

References

Accreditation Council for Genetic Counseling. (n.d.). *Find an accredited program.* https://www.gceducation.org/students-volunteers/#program

National Society of Genetic Counselors. (n.d.-a). *Genetic counselor workforce.* https://www.nsgc.org/POLICY/Genetic-Counselor-Workforce

National Society of Genetic Counselors. (n.d.-b). *NSGC timeline.* https://www.nsgc.org/About/About-NSGC/Timeline

Stern, A. M. (2009). A quiet revolution: The birth of the genetic counselor at Sarah Lawrence College, 1969. *Journal of Genetic Counseling, 18*(1), 1–11. https://doi.org/10.1007/s10897-008-9186-8

Acknowledgments

We would like to express our immense gratitude to the contributors who have made this volume possible. Constructing the volume in the midst of a pandemic was fraught with difficulties, and we are grateful for our contributors' patience and willingness to persist with us. It has been a privilege to learn from their expertise.

We are indebted to the editorial team at Oxford University Press (OUP). Their support and guidance were instrumental in bringing this volume to completion. Chioma Anomnachi and Zoe Barham assisted as project editors at various stages, and we thank them for their efforts in following up on contractual and editorial matters. We are grateful to Chad Zimmerman, former OUP senior editor, who helped us start this journey, and for his belief from the beginning that this volume would be a valuable contribution to the genetic counseling literature. Finally, we are especially grateful to Marta Moldvai, our current OUP senior editor, whose professionalism, kindness, and assistance enabled us to remain on track throughout the process. Marta never failed to offer help, insight, or encouragement.

Constructing this volume was a labor of love. Many hours were spent on the work necessary to complete it, and, as a result, our families experienced our absences from various events in their lives. We hope they understand and know how much their unwavering support and love mean to us. You are our continual source of inspiration.

Contributors

Bonnie Jeanne Baty, Professor Emerita, Department of Pediatrics, University of Utah Health Sciences Center

Austin Emanuel Bland, Genetic Counselor, Fred Hutchinson Cancer Center

Angus Clarke, Professor in Clinical Genetics, School of Medicine, Cardiff University

Stephanie A. Cohen, Genetic Counselor, Cancer Genetics Risk Assessment Program, Ascension St. Vincent

Debra L. Collins, Genetic Counselor, Hereditary Cancer Clinic; Associate Clinical Professor, University of Kansas Cancer Center

Devin M. Cox, Genetic Counselor, University of Kansas Cancer Center

Deborah Cragun, Director, University of South Florida Genetic Counseling Graduate Program; Associate Professor, College of Public Health

Sandra A. Darilek, Associate Professor, Department of Molecule and Human Genetics & Department of Obstetrics and Gynecology; Chief, Consultagene Clinic, Baylor College of Medicine

Claire Davis, Co-Director, Joan H. Marks Graduate Program in Human Genetics, Sarah Lawrence College

Dena S. Davis, Presidential Endowed Chair in Health, Professor of Bioethics, Lehigh University

Michael J. Deem, Associate Professor, Department of Human Genetics, School of Public Health, Director, Multidisciplinary Master of Public Health Program, Core Faculty, Center for Bioethics & Health Law, University of Pittsburgh

Elizabeth Dietz, Academic Associate, Center for Biology and Society, Arizona State University

Emily G. Farrow, Assistant Clinical Laboratory Director, Clinical Genetics and Genomics Laboratory, Pathology and Laboratory Medicine, Children's Mercy Kansas City; Associate Professor of Pediatrics, University of Missouri—Kansas City School of Medicine

Eleanor Feingold, Dean, College of Science, Professor, Department of Statistics, Oregon State University

Lauren Gallagher, Genetic Counsellor, Newborn Screening Ontario, Children's Hospital of Eastern Ontario

Aaron J. Goldenberg, Professor and Vice Chair, Department of Bioethics; Director, Bioethics Center for Community Health and Genomic Equity, School of Medicine, Case Western Reserve University

Anne E. Greb, Director, Health Education and Outreach, The Anne Wojcicki Foundation

Robin E. Grubs, Associate Professor, Department of Human Genetics, School of Public Health; Affiliate Faculty, Center for Bioethics & Health Law, University of Pittsburgh

Jennifer Hoskovec, Senior Director of Medical Affairs, BillionToOne, Inc.

Edward M. Kloza, Adjunct Professor, Master of Science in Genetic Counseling Program, Bay Path University

Mercy Ygoña Laurino, Director, Cancer Genetics and Prevention, Fred Hutchinson Cancer Center; Clinical Associate Professor, MS Genetic Counseling Program, University of the Philippines-Manila

Samantha J. Leonard, Independent Scholar

Bonnie S. LeRoy, Professor Emerita, Department of Genetics, Cell Biology and Development, University of Minnesota

Elissa Levin, Founder, Precision Medicine Innovation Consulting

Edgar MacBean, Vice President, Business Development and Partnerships, Clint

Gary E. Marchant, Regents Professor and Faculty Director, Center for Law, Science & Innovation, Sandra Day O'Connor College of Law, Arizona State University

Marion McAllister, Professor and Faculty, MSc Genetic & Genomic Counseling, Center for Medical Education, School of Medicine, Cardiff University

Marsha Michie, Associate Professor, Department of Bioethics, Associate Director, Bioethics Center for Community Health and Genomic Equity, School of Medicine, Case Western Reserve University

Melanie F. Myers, Co-Director, Genetic Counseling Graduate Program, Professor, UC Department of Pediatrics, Cincinnati Children's Hospital and University of Cincinnati

Ainsley J. Newson, Professor of Bioethics, Sydney Health Ethics, School of Public Health, Faculty of Medicine and Health, University of Sydney

Hannah M. Oliason, Health Care Attorney, Nilan Johnson Lewis PA

Leslie Ordal, Assistant Program Director, MS in Genetic Counseling, Clinical Assistant Professor, Boise State University

Kelly E. Ormond, Lecturer and ELSI Research Scientist, Health Ethics & Policy Lab, Department of Health Sciences and Technology, ETH Zurich; Clinical Professor, Department of Genetics and Stanford Center for Biomedical Ethics, Stanford University School of Medicine

Lisa S. Parker, Dickie, McCamey & Chilcote Professor of Bioethics, Director, Center for Bioethics & Health Law, University of Pittsburgh

Maria Piantanida, Adjunct Associate Professor, Carlow University; Co-founder, Scholar-Practitioner Nexus; Co-founder, Speaking of Education, podcast

Krista Redlinger-Grosse, Teaching Associate Professor, Director for Fieldwork and Supervisory Training, University of Minnesota Genetic Counseling Program

Robert Resta, Independent Scholar

Joel Michael Reynolds, Associate Professor of Philosophy & Disability Studies, Georgetown University; Senior Research Scholar, Kennedy Institute of Ethics; Senior Bioethics Advisor & Fellow, The Hastings Center; Faculty Scholar, The Greenwall Foundation

Daniel Lee Riconda, Professor, School of Health Professions & Department of Molecular & Human Genetics, Director, Genetic Counseling Program, Baylor College of Medicine

Eric T. Rush, Clinical Geneticist, Division of Clinical Genetics, Underdown/Yeomans Family Endowed Professor in Connective Tissue Disorders Care, Medical Director, Office of Faculty Development, Children's Mercy Kansas City; Professor of Pediatrics, University of Missouri—Kansas City School of Medicine

Carol J. Saunders, Division Director, Clinical Genetics and Genomics Laboratory, Children's Mercy Kansas City; Professor of Pediatrics and Pathology, University of Missouri—Kansas City School of Medicine

Naomi Scheinerman, Assistant Professor of Bioethics, Department of Biomedical Education and Anatomy, The Ohio State University

Tara Schmidlen, Clinical Content Lead, Nest Genomics

Devon Stillwell, Adjunct Graduate Faculty Member and Course Instructor, History Department, Trent University

Isabelle Thiffault, Director of Translational Genetics, Clinical Genetics and Genomics Laboratory, Children's Mercy Kansas City; Associate Professor of Pediatrics and Pathology, University of Missouri—Kansas City School of Medicine

Angela M. Trepanier, Professor of Molecular Medicine and Genetics, Director, Genetic Counseling Graduate Program, Center for Molecular Medicine and Genetics, Wayne State School of Medicine

Megan E. Trinkle-Tucker, Assistant Director and Assistant Professor, Bay Path University

Wendy R. Uhlmann, Clinical Professor, Departments of Internal Medicine and Human Genetics, Senior Genetic Counselor, Medical Genetics Clinic, University of Michigan School of Medicine

Patricia McCarthy Veach, Distinguished Teaching Professor Emerita, Department of Educational Psychology, University of Minnesota

Vickie L. Venne, retired from Genomic Medicine Service, Department of Veterans Affairs

Carol S. Walton, Professor, Department of Pediatrics, Director, Graduate Program in Genetic Counseling, University of Colorado—Anschutz Medical Campus

Nancy Steinberg Warren, Genetic Counseling Education and Training Consultant, Genetic Counseling Toolkit, LLC

Jon Weil, retired from University of California Berkeley

Catherine A. Wicklund, Medical Science Liaison Senior Manager, Clinical Strategy Lead, Myriad Women's Health; Adjunct Professor, Feinberg School of Medicine, Northwestern University

Susan M. Wolf, Regents Professor, McKnight Presidential Professor of Law, Medicine & Public Policy, Faegre Drinker Professor of Law, Professor of Medicine, Chair, Consortium on Law and Values in Health, Environment & the Life Sciences, University of Minnesota

Julia Wynn, Associate Professor of Genetic Counseling, Department of Pediatrics, Columbia University Irving Medical Center

Beverly M. Yashar, Emeritus Professor of Human Genetics, Department of Human Genetics, University of Michigan

Lee A. Zellmer, Supervisor, Laboratory Genetic Counselor, Division of Clinical Laboratory Genetics and Genomics, Children's Mercy Kansas City

PART I

THE EMERGENCE AND ESTABLISHMENT OF THE GENETIC COUNSELING PROFESSION

CHAPTER 1

NEGOTIATING HEREDITY, CHOICE, AND COERCION

A Gendered History of Genetic Counseling and Reproductive Advice, 1910–1960

DEVON STILLWELL

Introduction

In September 1963, physician and clinical geneticist Margery W. Shaw received a letter from a woman whose family suffered from Huntington's disease (HD, also known as Huntington's chorea, or HC). Shaw worked several days a week in the University of Michigan's Heredity Clinic and was consulted frequently (either by mail or in person) by Americans concerned about their family history of hereditary disease. This woman began by outlining her situation:

> It was told to me that you had had a measure of success in treating a woman who was suffering from Huntington's Chorea, a woman who probably has not recovered, but is at least able to function more normally now. My family has a parallel problem. In February my sister in law had a nervous break down [*sic*] which was diagnosed at the U of M to actually be Huntington's Chorea. At this same time we discovered that her mother whom we had been told died from the effects of a brain tumor, had actually had Huntington's Chorea. . . . Since that time I have been trying to find out more about the disease, but my attempts have been fought at every corner. . . . I want to know the truth about this disease, all there is to know. I think I have a right to know, as my husband, children, and future children are directly involved. Boxing with shadows is not in my line, I will not have any peace of mind until I know. (Letter to Margery W. Shaw, 1963)

This woman was desperate to know more about HC since she suspected her husband was showing early symptoms. She told Shaw she understood the basics of HC: that it is inherited, incurable, and managed with tranquilizers or antidepressants. She then pleaded with Shaw to tell her of a cure or at least about new research being conducted, and was especially interested in "the facts concerning the hereditary angle." She concluded, "I've probably trampled all over the medical ethics of this situation, but never the less if you can help me I would appreciate it" (Letter to Margery W. Shaw, 1963). Shaw replied that the woman should come to the clinic in person for a thorough counseling session. Just over 1 month later, the woman visited the clinic and was helped by a female staff member who noted that the woman received a thorough explanation of the 50/50 risk estimate for HC within her family; this staff member also suggested that the woman's husband be examined for signs of the disease. Records for this woman include a detailed family history and a recommendation that all "at risk" family members visit the clinic for an assessment before contemplating marriage and, presumably, procreation ("Comments," 1963).

Counseling for genetic disease within mid-20th-century heredity clinics is one of the most direct and well-known historical precursors to modern genetic counseling. Contemporary genetic counselors will recognize aspects of their practice within the above encounter: taking family histories, calculating risk estimates, and providing genetic information that draws on, and potentially impacts, the health of multiple generations within a single family. Physician-geneticists like Shaw, who performed genetic counseling within heredity clinics first established in the 1940s, were the forerunners to the professional genetic counseling programs that emerged starting in 1969 with the inaugural graduate program at Sarah Lawrence College (SLC). But many were also part of a longer 20th-century tradition of counseling related to genetics and heredity dating back to at least 1910. Indeed, women struggling with the meanings of hereditary disease for their families visited a variety of institutions including marriage and birth control clinics to obtain reproductive counseling and health advice. In other cases, families encountered prototypical counseling practices through engagement with researchers including Eugenics Record Office (ERO) fieldworkers who obtained family histories, documented physical exams, and provided reproductive and family planning information or tools.

This chapter focuses on two specific aspects of this history related to modern genetic counseling as it professionalized starting in the late 1960s. The first emphasis is on gendered aspects of genetic counseling as a profession historically rooted in women counseling women about pregnancy, reproduction, and prenatal and pediatric conditions. Today, 95% of genetic counselors identify as female and, since the initiation of master's-level counseling programs more than five decades ago, only 5% to 10% of program students have been male (National Society of Genetic Counselors, 2020; Stern, 2012). The field was initially conceptualized by psychologist and SLC Dean of Graduate Studies Melissa Richter as a special niche within medical genetics for women interested in social work, psychology, and health with ample room for expanding opportunities as genetic technology revolutionized traditional medical care (Stern, 2009a). Although genetic counselors now see patients for a range of conditions, the field originally focused on providing adoption consultations, evaluating children for pediatric conditions, and acting as something of a gateway between patients and prenatal testing.

Historian Alexandra Minna Stern has suggested that the modern history of genetic counseling is "a herstory whose key protagonists were and continue to be women" (Stern, 2012, p. 103). This chapter pursues this theme by investigating women's roles in counseling American families about health and heredity before the establishment of professional programs, with an eye to women's counseling work as physicians, biologists, social workers, nurses, and activists. The fact that many inquiries, like the one above, also came from women worried about the meanings of genetic disease for their family's health is further evidence of genetic counseling as an enduring "feminized" health space (Stern, 2012; Stillwell, 2014). Genetic counseling, throughout the early 20th century, could be a feminist space as well. Some of the women who performed counseling duties were explicitly feminist in their work and activism (Stern, 2009a, 2012; Stillwell, 2014). Others might be thought of as feminist through their very presence in medicine or related scientific fields where, between 1910 and the 1960s, women's participation was marginalized. Indeed, tracing the feminist leanings and woman-centeredness of individuals performing counseling functions in the early 20th century provides another linkage to the feminism and reproductive rights advocacy of many professional counselors in the 1960s and 1970s, as well as modern-day genetic counselors.

The second emphasis of this chapter is the history of ethics within the evolution of genetic counseling, specifically the ongoing balancing of both choice and potential coercion. The origins of genetic counseling are most often traced to the early 20th-century eugenics movement. Supported by physicians, lawyers, scientists, politicians, and others, the eugenics movement promised "human betterment" through increased knowledge of heredity and more strategic reproductive practices. "Fit" Americans of "good stock" (read: well educated, upper class, and of elite heritage) were encouraged to reproduce, while the "unfit" (read: immigrants, the lower classes, and the "feeble-minded") were discouraged or prohibited from reproduction through institutional segregation and even surgical sterilization (Kevles, 1985; Paul, 1995). Modern genetic counseling sought to distance itself from this legacy through the implementation of professional ethics, specifically the values of "nondirectiveness" and "client-centeredness." These principles, inspired by humanistic psychologist Carl Rogers, became embedded in early genetic counseling graduate programs as a direct effort to preserve patient autonomy and avoid the coercive practices associated with old-fashioned eugenics (Resta, 1997). This chapter explores the early history of genetic counseling with an eye to coercion as many of the figures analyzed here were actively involved in the eugenics movement. I also explore, however, efforts by female counselors to think critically about eugenics and its research methodology, push for a women's rights agenda related to family planning and reproductive control, and shift counseling away from prescriptive practices to a profession built on providing information and education and supporting patient autonomy in decision making. I suggest, then, that this is not a narrative of progress whereby we move, over the 20th century, from coercive practices to unequivocal choice; rather, this is a story of an ongoing negotiation where a range of possibilities and outcomes continue to exist on a spectrum delimited by unequivocal choice or coercion at either end.

This chapter analyzes these two main themes through four case studies: the work of ERO fieldworkers in the 1910s and 1920s; the reproductive and health advice given by birth controller Margaret Sanger and her clinic staff in the 1920s and 1930s; marriage counseling of the 1930s through 1950s as a forum that combined premarital, reproductive, and hereditary advising; and heredity clinics of the 1940s to 1960s. Historical studies of the eugenics movement, marriage counseling, and heredity clinics often focus on well-known, usually male figures, which tends to suggest that hereditary research and advice were primarily the domain of men. This chapter certainly touches on the influence of famous figures in eugenics, genetics, and the science of heredity including Charles B. Davenport, Paul Popenoe, and Sheldon Reed. The main focus here, however, is to uncover the roles of women like Margaret Sanger, as well as lesser known figures like Elizabeth B. Muncey, Hannah Mayer

Stone, Margery W. Shaw, and Estella M. Hughes, in collecting and analyzing hereditary data and offering genetic and reproductive advice.

Through these examples, I suggest that the modern profession of genetic counseling cannot be properly appreciated without a gendered focus on women who have been primarily responsible for on-the-ground engagement with everyday people seeking information about their genetic risks. Moreover, contemporary genetic counselors cannot negotiate current ethical debates surrounding prenatal diagnosis, genetic testing, and the appropriate uses of genetic information without understanding the ongoing struggle to balance individual choice with potential coercion in the decades preceding the professionalization of genetic counseling.

The Eugenics Record Office and Women's Fieldwork

The American eugenics movement is most often associated with Charles B. Davenport, a biologist who founded the ERO in Cold Spring Harbor, New York, in 1910. Davenport acted as director and, alongside Harry Hamilton Laughlin, operated the ERO as the "nerve center" of the national eugenics movement (Allen, 1986, p. 226). The ERO was coordinated by Davenport and Laughlin, but it was staffed by fieldworkers who were responsible for collecting hereditary information in service of eugenic education and research. Many of these fieldworkers were women with scientific and/or medical backgrounds. According to historian Garland Allen, the ERO had trained 156 fieldworkers by 1917 through its intensive summer program. Of these graduates, seven held MDs and eight held PhDs (Allen, 1986). Historian Amy Sue Bix estimates that by 1924, 85% of ERO fieldworkers were women. Davenport specifically recruited intelligent women with backgrounds in biology, psychology, sociology, nursing, or medicine to become fieldworkers (Bix, 1997). The ERO provided scientifically educated women with a place to work in biology at a time when employment opportunities for women in science were scarce (Paul, 1995). Fieldworkers then received additional training in eugenic policies and patterns of genetic inheritance, medical insights on fetal development, and instruction in psychology, intelligence testing, and statistical analysis (Wolff, 2009). The goal of this curriculum was to prepare fieldworkers to travel across the United States to consult, at first, with hospitals, prisons, or psychiatric institutions housing individuals with hereditary diseases; by 1920, however, fieldworkers were visiting families with cancer, HC, and other conditions within their homes (Bix, 1997; Wolff, 2009).

Fieldworkers represented Davenport's key workforce in carrying out the hereditary studies he envisioned; they also represented a significant point of contact between Americans and hereditary science. Davenport sought to train women with scientific backgrounds not only for their academic expertise but also because women seemed uniquely suited to combine the "hard" science of heredity with the "soft" side of family interactions. As historian Diane Paul has noted, women's "natural" nurturance and sympathy were considered useful in cultivating relationships with families the ERO hoped to study (Paul, 1995). Fieldworkers sought out families and sometimes entire communities exhibiting particular traits, investigated official medical records, photographed their subjects, interviewed family members, and recorded pedigrees. According to the records kept by Harry Hamilton Laughlin, these workers conducted 46 interviews per month and collected over 7,600 pages of family case histories and 800 pages of pedigrees just between 1910 and 1913 (Allen, 1986). These records were then stored at the ERO as an archive of genealogical research that the institution's staff could use to support public policy and provide education in hereditary principles. Fieldworkers' use of pedigree charts and written family histories is an important precursor to the methods used by contemporary genetic counselors. That so many fieldworkers were women is also an important indicator of the "feminization" of counseling roles, even in the 1910s and 1920s.

Another goal of the ERO and fieldworkers' research, however, was to provide advice to Americans about the eugenic fitness of a proposed marriage or counsel those concerned about hereditary disease in their families. Whether in person or through correspondence, individuals could take part in a kind of marriage consult with a fieldworker about conditions that may be transmitted intergenerationally in their own family or that of a prospective partner so as to inform a eugenically beneficial mate selection. The ERO received 77 requests for advice by 1913 alone (Allen, 1986). Fieldworkers also performed genetic advising as they interfaced frequently with families in the field. Elizabeth P. Moore, whose involvement at the ERO included the study of hereditary cancers throughout the 1910s, was one such fieldworker. Moore's interest, like many other women in science and medicine, dovetailed at the cross-section between eugenics and child welfare. In addition to being a fieldworker, Moore was involved in organizing baby health conferences and staging child welfare exhibits alongside Fitter Family contests, which assessed the health and heredity of American families at 1920s state fairs (Stern, 2009b). Her interests in health and heredity informed her work at the ERO, which included ascertaining family pedigrees and other information about "cancer families" through interviews and personal correspondence. Americans concerned about hereditary disease also wrote to Moore for information and advice about their chances of inheriting cancer and what this might mean for them as they planned their family lives.

Elizabeth B. Muncey was one of the better known ERO fieldworkers. Muncey was a physician with 14 years of medical experience who carried out longer, more complex studies that involved intense research and lengthy travel across five American states (Wexler, 2008). She was instrumental in producing a study of HC beginning in 1911. For this study, Muncey worked 12-hour days tracking down local records and birth certificates and meeting with physicians and living family members who could provide information on HC. Her written notes are extensive, and her pedigrees included more than 4,500 individuals (Wexler, 2008). Muncey received requests for advice either directly from individuals or through their physicians, and Davenport even relied on her to provide medical diagnoses. Her ability to accurately diagnose the condition was difficult due to inaccurate or incomplete local records, an inability to verify the condition in records related to deceased family members, a lack of cooperation by families under study, and varying terminology for HC (Wexler, 2008). Despite these difficulties, Muncey and other fieldworkers took seriously their contact with American families who acted as important repositories of genetic information but also as subjects in need of education and advice.

Ultimately, Muncey's work on Huntington's formed the basis for Davenport's "Huntington's Chorea in Relation to Heredity and Eugenics" (1915). This text was prescriptive in nature, focused on detailing not just disease transmission but also the medical and policy measures that should be taken to prevent the spread of HC. These measures included suggestions for the surgical sterilization of known choreics, as well as greater attention to heredity in marriage, since "marriage is not solely an affair between two individuals, but means *children*, and the duty of parents to provide them with the best heritage" (Davenport, 1915, p. 211). Importantly, while some fieldworkers avidly pursued their work under the banner of eugenics as a social panacea, others questioned the ethics or morality of the agenda their work supported. As Bix has shown, fieldworkers could be critical of the methodology guiding their work, pointing to problems with obtaining accurate data based on people's memories or issues fitting complex disease experiences into narrowly defined categories. Moreover, they were highly critical of the use of this sometimes unreliable data to shore up eugenic theory and, worse, practical measures like sterilization or segregation (Bix, 1997). This might, then, be considered an early indication that those doing the on-the-ground counseling recognized the importance of accurate genetic information but also noncoercive methods. A focus on ethics in relation to the uses and abuses of hereditary information is an additional connection between modern genetic counselors and (at least some) ERO fieldworkers.

Birth Control Clinics and Reproductive/Health Advice

Birth control activists and clinics are also significant to the early history of genetic counseling. Women sought the advice of birth controllers like Margaret Sanger on how to avoid unwanted pregnancies and exercise a kind of family limitation at a time when the dissemination of contraceptives or contraceptive information was prohibited by the 1873 Comstock Laws. Thousands of women wrote to Sanger or visited the birth control clinics she established or inspired between the 1910s and 1930s for reproductive advice (MacNamara, 2018). Sanger, who coined the term "birth control," opened the first contraceptive clinic in the United States in 1916, followed by the Clinical Research Bureau (CRB) in 1926. She also founded the American Birth Control League (ABCL) in 1921, laying the foundations for what would become the Planned Parenthood Federation of America (PPFA) in 1942. Activism for the legality and availability of birth control had emerged by 1914, and Sanger established herself as one of the movement's most prominent and effective organizers (Gordon, 2002). Trained as a nurse, Sanger moved to New York City in 1911 and was initially involved in socialist activism before turning her attention to birth control. She believed that women's biology and the burden of multiple unplanned or unspaced pregnancies were significant sources of women's subjugation. She pushed for birth control as essential to women's health, their marriages, and their ability to exercise greater gender, class, and sexual equality. Sanger sought to free women from the "bondage of enforced maternity," arguing that "No woman can call herself free who does not own and control her body" nor "until she can choose consciously whether she will or will not be a mother" (Sanger, 1928, p. xi; Sanger, 1920, p. 46). Sanger also earned significant publicity by deliberately violating the Comstock Laws through the establishment of her birth control clinics. In her 1916 trial, she challenged both legal and social perspectives on women's rights to have greater control over their pregnancies.

By the mid-1910s, Sanger had established herself as a leading authority on birth control but also more generally as a women's health advocate. As such, many women, and sometimes men, sought her advice by mail. Historian Trent MacNamara estimates that between 1915 and 1940, Sanger received between 200,000 and 300,000 letters asking for sexual advice or for help finding birth control and accessing abortions (MacNamara, 2018). She received so many requests for advice that, although she had answered letters personally throughout the 1920s, by the 1930s she founded the Margaret Sanger Marriage Advice Bureau to respond to the high volume of requests for counseling and referrals to health services related to women's reproduction (Gordon, 2002). Letter writers sought advice on improving their health and well-being when they contacted Sanger not only about contraception but also about how to have a healthy pregnancy, and especially how to avoid undue pain, disability, or death (MacNamara, 2018). They also wanted information about managing pregnancy-related health conditions and expressed concern about transmitting hereditary diseases. For example, one woman wrote to Sanger:

> I have reasons enough for wanting Birth Control information. The first is because I am not strong and second is: my oldest daughter has convulsions and can't talk. She was in the hospital two months and came out worse than before. She is six years old now and can't talk yet, and we have lots of sickness. My husband is not very healthy and has to work. . . . I am losing my eyesight too. I don't want to bring blind children into this world. . . . Can you help me so not to have any more babies? The doctor said it would be worse every time I would have a baby, so will you help a poor soul? (Sanger, 1928, p. 114)

Sanger herself noted that letter writers demonstrated a "consciousness on the part of many mothers of the disastrous folly of bringing defective children into the world" and an interest in saving "helpless children suffering unto the third and fourth generation 'the sins of the fathers,'" including conditions like Huntington's, epilepsy, tuberculosis, and venereal disease (Sanger, 1928, p. 101).

Birth control clinics provided another resource for women looking for advice on sex, reproduction, and contraception. By 1930, there were 55 clinics located in 23 cities across 12 American states; at the end of that decade, approximately 300,000 women had visited one of several hundred clinics (Gordon, 2002; MacNamara, 2018). Sanger scholar Cathy Moran Hajo has described these clinics as "feminized spaces" due to their clients being overwhelmingly women. Moreover, while men were likely to be involved as advisors, these clinics were also feminized in that Sanger staffed her facilities, when possible, with predominantly female personnel (Hajo, 2010). For example, her first clinic was run by her sister and registered nurse Ethyl Byrne, social worker Elizabeth Stuyvesant, and administrative assistant Fania Mindell (Engleman, 2011). Sanger also sought female physicians to spearhead her clinics, despite women only making up around 5% of medical school students and practicing physicians between the 1920s and 1960s (Morantz-Sanchez, 2000). Dr. Hannah Mayer Stone was particularly important to these efforts. Stone was a pediatrician who was active in the birth control movement in the 1920s and 1930s. She acted as director of the Birth Control Clinical Research Bureau (BCCRB, formerly the CRB) and gave contraceptive advice to more than 1,600 women in just her first year in that position. Stone taught women about their health using anatomical models of the reproductive system and educated women on menstruation, infertility and impotence, and how to plan their pregnancies (Klapper, 2013). Physician involvement in birth control clinics was necessary to make the clinics legal but also to enable clinic personnel to perform physical exams and allow doctors to properly fit women with diaphragms, which accounted for 90% of the contraceptives prescribed there (Hajo, 2010). Female-controlled contraception was a radical and feminist proposal as it promised greater reproductive autonomy for women with no need for male compliance (Engleman, 2011). The activist agendas for enhanced reproductive choice that underlay this clinic work, then, made these spaces not just feminized but feminist in purpose as well.

Clinic visits, while generally hinging on providing women with the tools necessary for informed reproductive planning, varied in their specifics depending on a woman's reason for the consultation. The meeting usually began with an interview with a social worker, who took the patient's health and reproductive histories. Patients then received information about birth control and general sex education, followed by a gynecological and more general physical exam (Hajo, 2010). In addition to providing women with contraception, clinics also offered advice on hygiene, premarital guidance, and infertility counseling for couples finding it difficult to conceive; abortion referrals to safe, professional services were also a key part of the clinics' mandate (Engleman, 2011). The clinics saw predominantly married, working-class women who already had children and who desired to limit their family size for economic and health reasons, as well as to avoid bearing children who would be considered eugenically "unfit." Indeed, clinic visitors, much like the women who corresponded with Sanger, sought birth control and sex education to avoid bearing additional children with cognitive or physical "defects." Clinics offered their services to the "feeble-minded" or "insane," but criminality, promiscuity, and alcoholism were also conditions that clinics sought to prevent in future generations. Clinic personnel often attributed these problems to social environment rather than heredity; at the same time, they drew on eugenic language and classifications as they consulted on diseases often considered hereditary at the time (Hajo, 2010).

Margaret Sanger's activist legacy is significantly complicated by her involvement in eugenics. While Sanger advocated for women's freedom of choice in deciding whether or not to pursue motherhood, she also believed that some women (particularly African American and immigrant women of lower socioeconomic status) were "unfit" for motherhood and could not be trusted to make responsible decisions about their own bodies (Sanger, 1928). She called the alleged overbreeding of the "unfit" the "greatest present menace to civilization" and spoke often of the "quality of the race" and need for "race regeneration" (Sanger, 1921, p. 5). She believed in the surgical sterilization of the "feeble-minded" and argued that birth control was a useful tool to eugenicists by helping "fit" families space their children for the health of both the mother and child. She hoped that such measures would develop "a higher standard of motherhood and family life" that could overcome the social burden of the "unfit" (Sanger, 1919, p. 12). While Sanger's activism was progressive in relation to women's rights to reproductive control, her opinions on race and class were aligned with eugenic values of the period. Indeed, as historian Johanna Schoen has written, birth control services sat at the nexus between eugenic, economic, and humanitarian concerns, and while many activists hoped to improve women's lives, they also believed that poorer Americans should limit their reproduction and that birth control offered a solution to intergenerational poverty and degeneracy (Schoen, 2005). As such, birth control and the counseling offered under that umbrella could be seen as simultaneously empowering and potentially coercive.

Margaret Sanger had tempered her radicalism by 1921 when she founded the ABCL and hoped to attract middle-class women to her cause. By the founding of the PPFA in 1942, both Sanger and the movement for birth control (now called "family planning") had grown considerably more conservative. For Sanger, birth control, though liberating for women's reproductive choices, was always intended to be used within marital relationships to enhance intimacy and promote stability. By the 1940s, she sought to make family planning integral to the health and happiness of a nuclear family centered on traditional gender roles. Nowhere did birth control activism come to serve the status quo more than through its incorporation into marriage counseling of the 1930s through 1950s.

Marriage Counseling, Heredity, and "Nondirectiveness"

Marriage counseling was another forum where birth control and eugenics intertwined and where women had important (although often less visible) roles. One such woman was physician Hannah Stone, who turned to marriage counseling by the 1930s after over a decade of activism and advising in women's health at Margaret Sanger's BCCRB. With her husband, Dr. Abraham Stone, Hannah opened the Marriage Consultation Center in 1931, and the BCCRB referred clients starting in 1932. Beginning in the 1930s, then, women seeking contraceptive advice could also receive counseling related to marital problems, sex education, or premarital consultations (Gordon, 2002). Importantly, the advice couples received in marriage counseling did not support a women's rights agenda; rather, the advice offered by marriage counselors was intended to reinforce a renewed culture of domesticity for women in the mid-20th century, especially traditional gender roles for women as wives and mothers. Counseling related to contraception or reproduction was intended to foster happiness within a conventional marital arrangement and larger sociocultural emphasis on pro-natalism. Many marriage counselors, like birth controllers, also continued to subscribe to eugenic ideals as the movement evolved into the 1930s. Assumptions about the inherent desirability or undesirability of reproduction within certain groups, and the overall importance of heredity to strong marriages and family lines, continued to guide the advice of marriage counselors (Kline, 2005; Ladd-Taylor, 2001; Stern, 2016).

The Stones, like other marriage counselors of the period, had grown their practice and refined their professional philosophies alongside the eugenics movement. They consulted with clients on heredity in relation to sex and reproduction as the goal of marriage counseling was to foster fulfilling marriages but also ensure good matings that would produce healthy offspring (Davis, 2010). At the Marriage Consultation Center, the Stones were particularly interested in performing premarital consults to uncover any hereditary problems that should prevent a marriage and future parenthood (Gordon, 2002). The Stones also reached Americans who were unable to attend their center through *A Marriage Manual* (first published in 1935 and reprinted dozens of times into the 1960s), which took the form of a hypothetical interaction between a physician and couple seeking advice before committing to marriage. The manual gives general advice on "the art of marriage" but is primarily focused on health issues within marriages, the biology of reproduction, and family planning. The manual also touches directly on heredity, including how genetic conditions pass intergenerationally and the role of chromosomes and genes in the inheritance of diseases like epilepsy, tuberculosis, cancer, and venereal disease (Stone, 1952). The Stones addressed the role of "eugenic fitness" in considering a mate, advising that ensuring healthy children means "seek[ing] a person who is both physically and mentally healthy and whose family background is free from any hereditary taints." They counseled:

> The best advice that can be given is to avoid marriage with someone who is afflicted with a serious transmissible defect and refrain from marrying into a family that happens to possess the same kinds of bodily and mental hereditary weaknesses of one's own. (Stone, 1952, p. 20)

Their focus on genetics, the transmission of hereditary conditions, and how to avoid disease links the Stones to both early 20th-century eugenic practices and the goals of early professional genetic counseling.

The Stones were instrumental in professionalizing the field of marriage counseling as a therapeutic specialty, but between 1930 and 1950, Paul Popenoe was widely considered "the man who saves marriages" (Kline, 2005, p. 141). Popenoe is well known for his enthusiasm for sexual sterilization as a solution to the problem of the "unfit" and was a key proponent of California's eugenics program, which sterilized more than 20,000 individuals (Stern, 2016). He focused his interests in heredity and family life on marriage counseling by the 1930s and, in 1932, established the American Institute of Family Relations (AIFR), which would become the largest marriage counseling center in the United States (Davis, 2010). Popenoe offered premarital counseling to Americans experiencing a range of problems from "sexual maladjustment" to how to pick a suitable mate. His writings and his counseling style, however, reveal many affinities with later genetic counseling. Popenoe and other counselors relied on family histories and pedigrees in assessing the risk of potential children for hereditary disease. He performed genetic risk calculations using a Punnett square to provide couples with the chances they might produce offspring with a specific trait or condition. He also wrote extensively about biological issues in reproduction and looked to provide education in hereditary principles (Stern, 2016; Stillwell, 2016). Indeed, as historians Molly-Ladd Taylor and Rebecca Davis have shown, Popenoe expected that AIFR counselors would "[take] heredity into account" while performing premarital counseling and remind couples "that marriage counseling involved essential questions of hereditary fitness" (Davis, 2010, p. 123; Ladd-Taylor, 2001, p. 315).

Despite his notoriety as one of America's leading marriage experts, Popenoe himself did little counseling at the AIFR by the mid-1940s. Instead, couples were referred to an agency counselor, many of whom were women. Counselors like Mrs. Gene Benton and Mary Wilson helped with the AIFR client load and with the correspondence Popenoe received from American women looking for advice about marriage and reproduction. Similarly, much of the counseling performed at the Stones' Marriage Consultation Center was performed by physician Lena Levine, a gynecologist who took over for Hannah Stone and had previously worked with Margaret Sanger. Marriage counseling also occurred in a range of other institutions including family service agencies, where the counseling usually took place between the wife and a female staff member, often a social worker (Davis, 2010). Indeed, other women made significant forays into marriage counseling at this time including Emily Mudd, who had opened the Marriage Counsel of Philadelphia in 1933 and, along with the Stones, created the American Association of Marriage Counselors in 1945 (Dowbiggin, 2008). Mudd, whose professional background was in social work, offered counseling on birth control, pregnancy, abortion, and human anatomy. She strove for a holistic approach to women's health and possessed more of a women's rights agenda than other counselors of the time. Her explicitly feminist counseling agenda placed women's emotional needs at the center of her session. At the same time, she continued to focus on heredity as a key counseling component and counseled from a belief in preventing hereditary defects in subsequent generations (Davis, 2010).

Importantly, as marriage counseling evolved as a therapeutic specialty, it drew on psychological concepts that would become foundational to modern genetic counseling: client-centeredness (or person-centered therapy) and nondirectiveness. Marriage counselors like the Stones and Emily Mudd drew quite explicitly on the principles of Carl Rogers as their counseling evolved into the 1940s. By the mid-20th century, marriage counselors looked to professionalize their field; as popular support for eugenics was on the decline, many sought a reorientation in professional ethics and goals within the client–counselor relationship away from a directive approach. A psychologist and founder of a humanistic approach to counseling, Rogers first discussed his nondirective approach in *Counseling and Psychotherapy* in 1942, in which he outlined that

> Non-directive counseling is based on the assumption that the client has the right to select his own life goals, even though these may be at variance with the goals that the counselor might choose for him. There is also the belief that if the individual has a modicum of insight into himself and his problems, he will be likely to make this choice wisely. (Rogers, 1942, pp. 126–127)

Rogers modified his approach in 1951 to include "client-centeredness" as a key philosophy, which revolved around a counselor's commitment to "genuineness," empathy, and "unconditional positive regard" (Rogers, 1951, pp. 29, 36; Rogers, 1989). Mudd and the Stones pursued Rogers's philosophies as a key component of marriage counseling as they sought to standardize and accredit counseling as a therapeutic profession. Indeed, while they maintained an interest in eugenic values and especially the importance of heredity to marital unions, they also believed in the importance of social, emotional, and psychological considerations in counseling. Popenoe, for his part, also looked to Rogers's principles but was generally less attached to the promise of psychotherapy for the profession of marriage counseling. Popenoe and the AIFR continued to pursue a more directive approach to counseling to ensure successful marriages among their clientele (Davis, 2010; Ladd-Taylor, 2001). As some marriage counselors, then, apparently moved toward a belief in patient autonomy in decision making, there lingered an interest in keeping a more prescriptive approach to advising in hereditary and family matters.

Marriage counseling clinics were prolific between the 1930s and 1960s. While only three marriage counseling centers existed in 1932, by 1968 there were over 1,800. The AIFR, by the 1950s, employed 37 counselors and had allegedly ensured the marital happiness of more than 20,000 people (Ladd-Taylor, 2001). While many Americans received hereditary advice from marriage clinics or through publications by marriage counselors like the Stones, a clinic focused specifically on genetics and reproduction emerged by the 1940s to better predict the traits and diseases of one's offspring: the heredity clinic.

Heredity Clinics, Genetic Research, and an Evolving Ethics

The most recognizable points of origin for modern genetic counseling are the midcentury heredity clinics established at major American universities by physician-geneticists with long-standing interests in genetics and eugenics. In 1941, Lee R. Dice opened the University of Michigan's Heredity Clinic, and William Allan established the Department of Medical Genetics at Wake Forest University (Comfort, 2012; Stern, 2012). While Clarence P. Oliver had opened the Dight Institute for the Promotion of Human Genetics at the University of Minnesota that same year, Sheldon Reed took over in 1947 and developed the clinic's research and counseling activities. Reed coined the term "genetic counseling," defining it as a "kind of genetic social work without eugenic connotations" (Ladd-Taylor, 2003; Stern, 2012, p. 20). Reed's clinic operated similarly to the ERO in its mutual concern with both research and education. He sought to provide couples with "genetic and eugenic interpretations" of their family history and educate the general public in genetic principles. He also collected data from his sessions including pedigree charts and other family health information, which he then used in scientific studies. Before the advent of prenatal technologies, counseling sessions focused on couples with a known history of hereditary disease who were preparing to start a family or who already had a child with a genetic condition. Reed examined their pedigree, calculated the risk of a child inheriting the condition, and provided health information to the (prospective) parents (Stillwell, 2016).

In the 1940s and 1950s, counseling in heredity was most often performed by male physicians or geneticists who ran their clinics as a sideline to (and in service of) their genetic research. Women, however, remained central to the enterprise of genetic counseling as clinic staff and researchers. Between 1943 and 1953, Clarence Oliver, and then Sheldon Reed and J. D. Palm, conducted a study of HC as one of the Dight Institute's longest running projects. Their knowledge of HD drew on the fieldwork of Elizabeth Muncey, whose study was reprinted by Reed to help other clinicians and researchers better advise individuals and couples suffering with, or potentially at risk for, Huntington's (Wexler, 2008). Reed and Palm also based their study on records from University of Minnesota hospitals, the Department of Neuropsychiatry, and the records of the ERO, which, upon the office's closure in 1944, were transferred to the Dight Institute. Reed's study relied on following up with HC families initially identified by the ERO, and to this project he assigned Estella M. Hughes, a psychiatric social worker and expert on Huntington's, having worked on the topic for over two decades. Hughes had worked at the Kalamazoo State Hospital in the early 1920s, and data from this work informed both the ERO Huntington's files and Hughes's oft-cited 1925 report on the disease (Hughes, 1925). For example, in the case of a woman Hughes had interviewed in 1923, Hughes then followed up with her husband and additional family members not originally included in the ERO study to glean further information about the health status of children born since (Hughes, 1952; Palm, 1951b). Hughes performed similar research for a Huntington's study at the University of Michigan alongside Dr. Margery W. Shaw, a heredity counselor, physician-geneticist, and instructor in the university's Department of Human Genetics. As noted above, many questions from American families (and women in particular) about HC were addressed to Shaw into the 1960s.

Reed, Shaw, and others used the data provided by Hughes to inform the advice given in the heredity clinic. Shaw and Palm in particular received letters from Americans who had heard about their studies and were interested in obtaining information and advice. Like other personnel performing a kind of genetic counseling throughout the early 20th century, Reed and his fellow geneticists struggled to balance their eugenic leanings against a belief in choice and autonomy in reproductive decision making. Indeed, the counseling philosophies and values that underlay their practice of genetic counseling were rife with ironies and contradictions. Reed, for example, believed in a kind of nondirective counseling whereby the counselor provided information but had no role in client decision making. He suggested that while parents often asked for direct advice on genetic risk and family planning, the counselor's job was to "explain thoroughly what the genetic situation is, but the decision must be a personal one between the husband and wife, and theirs alone" (Reed, 1955, p. 14). However, despite their apparent support of patient autonomy, physician-geneticists assumed that intelligent people would make rational decisions about mate selection and reproduction that would favor a reduction or elimination of disease and disability within the larger gene pool. When consulting with families about HC, Palm (who conducted much of the clinic's correspondence) believed that greater knowledge of the disease and one's risk of inheritance could help "alleviate some dread of the disorder." In a case where a woman asked Palm about the advisability of castration to prevent the spread of HC, Palm advised against castration or sterilization as too extreme a measure (Palm, 1951a). At the same time, Palm, Reed, and others suggested that family planning was generally desirable when confronting a history of genetic disease, advised premarital consultations, and sought to develop methods of prevention and early detection throughout the 1950s and 1960s.

Into the 1960s and 1970s, geneticists like Margery Shaw continued to ruminate on the question of preserving the autonomy of "counselees" and the ethical complexities inherent in genetic counseling and testing. Shaw advocated the importance of autonomy in counseling but also recognized that more than claiming impartiality, it is the responsibility of the counselor to acknowledge their own perspectives and how they might influence client decisions: "The counselor has freedom to persuade, according to his personal convictions, but he does not have freedom to coerce, based upon his inherent power in the counseling milieu. He must accept the counselee as the ultimate decision-maker" (Shaw, 1974, p. 751). Shaw argued that nondirectiveness was "a backlash to the eugenics movement" and that in her view, "a counselor can't help being involved with the clients" (Check, 1982, p. 2889). Shaw walked back a key feature of nondirectiveness, specifically the notion that counselors can be unbiased and uninvolved with their clients' weighing of genetic information; at the same time, she remained an advocate for client-centered counseling and autonomy in client decision making. She also pushed counselors to address the myriad other social, legal, and ethical issues related to genetic counseling and genetic testing beyond a concern with directiveness. Indeed, she became a leading bioethicist by the 1970s and wrote over 70 papers exploring the complexities of advances in human genetics related to reproductive technologies, legal liabilities in genetic counseling, and other issues related to choice and coercion (Reilly, 2012). For example, she wrote about the importance of preserving *Roe v. Wade* as part of maintaining individual choices in matters of reproduction. She also worked on the topic of personhood, wherein the fetus is legally defined as a person and imbued with the legal rights of any other patient (Check, 1982; Shaw, 1974). Shaw's interest in the ethical and legal dilemmas related to genetics led her to Houston, where she became a professor of medical genetics at the University of Texas Health Sciences Center and took law classes at night, earning her JD degree in 1973.

Heredity counselors then reinforced some aspects of marriage counseling, including a focus on the emotional and psychological relationship between husband and wife, but with even more careful attention to heredity and genetic disease. They sought to distance themselves from earlier models of heredity counseling, especially the field's eugenic origins. While Reed did so by advocating for a kind of nondirective counseling in which the counselor is an impartial educator, Shaw sought to complicate the very notion of "nondirectiveness" and broadened the ethics of genetic counseling to encompass a range of other issues into the 1960s and 1970s. Nondirectiveness and the professional ethics of genetic counselors would become increasingly complex as the field worked to establish itself as a distinct genetics specialty by the late 20th century.

Conclusion

The profession of genetic counseling as we know it today developed from the multiple interwoven strands that make up this history. After the establishment of the SLC program in 1969, a handful of other programs cropped up in the early 1970s at institutions including Rutgers University, the University of California (Irving and Berkeley), and the University of Pittsburgh (Stern, 2012). The (mostly) women who attended these early graduate programs took courses in genetic science, but the curriculum was also framed by a larger interest in reproductive rights and the emerging field of bioethics. Many women within the pioneering cohort of professional genetic counselors were self-described feminists who were active in the reproductive rights movement and fight for access to abortion. They also believed in the importance of a pro-choice position when counseling women about prenatal testing and the possibility of terminating a pregnancy (Stillwell, 2014). Women of the pioneering counseling generation were also committed to the values of nondirectiveness and client-centeredness as they became inculcated in early programs. The field's efforts to distance itself from eugenics by emphasizing patient autonomy through Rogerian principles became more complicated in the 1970s and 1980s with new genetic reproductive technologies. Prenatal diagnostic procedures like amniocentesis brought disability and reproductive rights activists, as well as bioethicists, to the door of genetic counselors from a concern about potential coercion, the uses and abuses of genetic information, and the real possibility of choice in an ever-changing genetic landscape (Stern, 2012). In many cases, genetic counselors and the women they counseled in prenatal and pediatric settings were situated as intermediaries between genetic science and the American public, acting as not only counselors and clients but also ethicists and activists in making personal choices with intensely public and political implications.

Over the last three decades, genetic counseling has evolved and adapted to address new social, ethical, and professional considerations. The field's commitment to nondirectiveness as a core principle has come under revision for many of the reasons Shaw considered in the 1970s and 1980s: that it is overly simplistic, unrealistic, and unhelpful for the complex relationship between counselor and client (Clarke, 1991; Kessler, 1992; Weil, 2003). Moreover, while nondirectiveness was initially helpful in establishing a model of distinctly noncoercive counseling, critics have argued that it has had the undesirable effect of allowing counselors to opt out of nuanced ethical discussions with clients (Stern, 2012).[1] Counselors have continued, however, to pursue client autonomy in decision making as the core of the client–counselor relationship. They have also sought to preserve choice through persistent reproductive rights activism in the face of ongoing attacks on pro-choice politics. While genetic counseling has been continuously dominated by women since the 1970s, the field's client base has become significantly more diverse as genetic counseling expanded to include adult-onset conditions as well. Counselors now consult on all manner of genetic conditions including HD, cancer, Alzheimer's disease, cystic fibrosis, and others. Their contemporary roles also address an increasingly vast array of genetic technologies, including prenatal genetic screening but also predictive genetic testing for HD, in vitro fertilization, and gene editing and therapy.

The SLC program turned 50 years old in 2019 and, indeed, the profession of genetic counseling has evolved significantly since 1969. But in a field that changes rapidly and is often focused on the future, it is beneficial to revisit the past. Thinking through the people and themes that have shaped genetic counseling throughout the 20th century helps us better understand how Americans have encountered hereditary science since the 1910s. It also gives contemporary counselors insight into issues like choice and coercion that continue to impact the profession today.

Acknowledgments

The research presented in this chapter was supported by a Social Sciences and Humanities Research Council (SSHRC) Postdoctoral Fellowship and an Associated Medical Services (AMS) Postdoctoral Fellowship. Archival research was also facilitated by a Bordin-Gillette Researcher Travel Fellowship through the University of Michigan's Bentley Historical Library, and by an American Philosophical Society Library Resident Research Fellowship. The author would like to thank postdoctoral advisors Nathaniel Comfort and Alexandra Minna Stern for their guidance and insight into the history of genetics and genetic counseling.

References

Allen, G. E. (1986). The Eugenics Record Office at Cold Spring Harbor, 1910–1940: An essay in institutional history. *Osiris*, 2, 225–264.

Bix, A. S. (1997). Experiences and voices of eugenics field-workers: "Women's work" in biology. *Social Studies of Science*, 27, 625–668.

Check, W. A. (1982). Margery W. Shaw, MD, JD: Twice a counselor. *Journal of the American Medical Association*, 247(21), 2884–2890.

Clarke, A. (1991). Is non-directive genetic counselling possible? *Lancet* 338(8773), 998–1001.

Comfort, N. C. (2012). *The science of human perfection: How genes became the heart of American medicine*. Yale University Press.

[1] Editors' note: For more on nondirectiveness, see Chapter 23 by Michael J. Deem in this volume.

Comments. (1963, September 16). Box 33, Adult Medical Genetics Clinic Records, University of Michigan Archives, Bentley Historical Library.

Davenport, C. B. (1915). Huntington's chorea in relation to heredity and eugenics. *American Journal of Insanity, 17*, 195–220.

Davis, R. L. (2010). *More perfect unions: The American search for marital bliss*. Harvard University Press.

Dowbiggin, I. (2008). *The sterilization movement and global fertility in the twentieth century*. Oxford University Press.

Engleman, P. C. (2011). *A history of the birth control movement in America*. Praeger.

Gordon, L. (2002). *The moral property of women: A history of birth control politics in America*. University of Illinois Press.

Hajo, C. M. (2010). *Birth control on Main Street: Organizing clinics in the United States, 1916–1939*. University of Illinois Press.

Hughes, E. M. (1925). Social significance of Huntington's chorea. *American Journal of Psychiatry, 81*(3), 537–574.

Hughes, E. M. (1952, June 24). Letter to Sheldon Reed. Dight Institute #1, Box 40, Huntington's Chorea—Correspondence, 1951–1953, Trait Files, Eugenics Record Office Records, American Philosophical Society.

Kessler, S. (1992). Psychological aspects of genetic counseling. VII. Thoughts on directiveness. *Journal of Genetic Counseling, 1*(1), 9–17.

Kevles, D. J. (1985). *In the name of eugenics: Genetics and the uses of human heredity*. University of California Press.

Klapper, M. R. (2013). *Ballots, babies, and banners of peace: American Jewish women's activism, 1890–1940*. New York University Press.

Kline, W. (2005). *Building a better race: Gender, sexuality, and eugenics from the turn of the century to the baby boom*. University of California Press.

Ladd-Taylor, M. (2001). Eugenics, sterilisation, and the strange career of Paul Popenoe. *Gender & History, 13*(2), 298–327.

Ladd-Taylor, M. (2003). "A kind of genetic social work": Sheldon Reed and the origins of genetic counseling. In M. L.-T. Georgina Feldberg (Ed.), *Women, health, and nation: Canada and the United States since 1945* (pp. 67–83). McGill-Queens University Press.

Letter to Margery W. Shaw. (1963, August 1). Box 33, Adult Medical Genetics Clinic Records, University of Michigan Archives, Bentley Historical Library.

MacNamara, T. (2018). *Birth control and American modernity: A history of popular ideas*. Cambridge University Press.

Morantz-Sanchez, R. (2000). *Sympathy and science: Women physicians in American medicine*. University of North Carolina Press.

National Society of Genetic Counselors. (2020). *Professional status survey*.

Palm, J. D. (1951a, December 26). Letter from J.D. Palm. Dight Institute #1, Box 40, Huntington's Chorea—Correspondence, 1951–1953, Trait Files, Eugenics Record Office Records, American Philosophical Society.

Palm, J. D. (1951b, December 26). Letter to Mrs. Estella Hughes. Dight Institute #1, Box 40, Huntington's Chorea—Correspondence, 1951–1953, Trait Files, Eugenics Record Office Records, American Philosophical Society.

Paul, D. B. (1995). *Controlling human heredity: 1865 to the present*. Humanities Press.

Reed, S. C. (1955). *Counseling in medical genetics*. W. B. Saunders.

Reilly, P. R. (2012). Margery Wayne Shaw, MD, JD (1923–2012): A remembrance. *American Journal of Human Genetics, 91*(5), 773–777.

Resta, R. (1997). Eugenics and nondirectiveness in genetic counseling. *Journal of Genetic Counseling, 6*(2), 255–258.

Rogers, C. (1989). A client-centered/person-centered approach to therapy. In H. Herschenbaum & V. Land Hendeson (Eds.), *The Carl Rogers reader: Selections from the lifetime work of America's preeminent psychologist, author of On becoming a person and A way of being* (pp. 135–152). Houghton Mifflin.

Rogers, C. R. (1942). *Counseling and psychotherapy: Newer concepts in practice.* Houghton Mifflin.

Rogers, C. R. (1951). *Client-centered therapy: Its current practice, implications, and theory.* Houghton Mifflin.

Sanger, M. (1919). Birth control and racial betterment. *Birth Control Review, 3*(2), 11–23.

Sanger, M. (1920). *Woman and the new race.* Brentano's.

Sanger, M. (1921). The eugenic value of birth control propanda. *Birth Control Review, 5*(10), 5.

Sanger, M. (1928). *Motherhood in bondage.* Brentano's.

Schoen, J. (2005). *Choice and coercion: Birth control, sterilization, and abortion in public health and welfare.* University of North Carolina Press.

Shaw, M. W. (1974). Genetic counseling. *Science, 184*(4138), 751.

Stern, A. M. (2009a). A quiet revolution: The birth of the genetic counselor at Sarah Lawrence College, 1969. *Journal of Genetic Counseling, 8*(1), 1–11.

Stern, A. M. (2009b). Better babies contests at the Indiana State Fair: Child health, scientific motherhood, and eugenics in the Midwest, 1920–35. In A. Stern & H. Markel (Eds.), *Formative years: Children's health in the United States, 1880–2000* (pp. 121–152). University of Michigan Press.

Stern, A. M. (2012). *Telling genes: The story of genetic counseling in America.* Johns Hopkins University Press.

Stern, A. M. (2016). *Eugenic nation: Faults and frontiers of better breeding in America.* University of California Press.

Stillwell, D. (2014). "Pretty pioneering-spirited people": Genetic counsellors, gender culture, and the professional evolution of a feminised health field, 1947–1980. *Social History of Medicine, 28*(1), 172–193.

Stillwell, D. (2016). Helping couples fulfill "the highest of life's goals": Mate selection, marriage counselling, and genetic counseling in the United States. *Journal of Genetic Counseling, 25*(1), 157–165.

Stone, H. M. (1952). *A marriage manual: A practical guidebook to sex and marriage.* Simon and Schuster.

Weil, J. (2003). Psychosocial genetic counseling in the post-nondirective era: A point of view. *Journal of Genetic Counseling, 12*(3), 199–211.

Wexler, A. (2008). *The woman who walked into the sea: Huntington's and the making of a genetic disease.* Yale University Press.

Wolff, T. (2009). *Mendel's theatre: Heredity, eugenics, and early twentieth-century American drama.* Palgrave MacMillan.

CHAPTER 2

THE DEVELOPMENT OF EDUCATION FOR GENETIC COUNSELORS

BONNIE JEANNE BATY AND CLAIRE DAVIS

Introduction

This chapter focuses on basic and advanced education for certified genetic counselors[1] (CGCs) in the United States and Canada, approaching education from the moment someone enters a genetic counseling program to the end of their career. We examine the history of genetic counseling education, the development of genetic counseling graduate programs, drivers of genetic counseling education, curricular development of genetic counseling graduate education, relevant educational models, and the development of advanced skills by CGCs.

The Development of Genetic Counseling Graduate Programs

The term "genetic counselor" is frequently stated to have been coined by Sheldon Reed in 1948 (Reed, 1975). Early genetic counseling was done by individuals with academic and later medical doctorates. In 1969, the first master's genetic counseling graduate program was started at Sarah Lawrence College, with the first graduates in 1971 (Sarah Lawrence College, 2019). New programs were quickly developed by other institutions in the United States in the early 1970s, so by 1975, there were seven genetic counseling graduate programs.[2]

[1] "Certified genetic counselor" refers to genetic counselors who are certified by the American Board of Genetic Counseling, American Board of Medical Genetics, or Canadian Board of Genetic Counselling.

[2] The genetic counseling graduate programs operating between 1969 and 1975 were at Sarah Lawrence College; the University of Pittsburgh; the University of Colorado; Rutgers University; the University

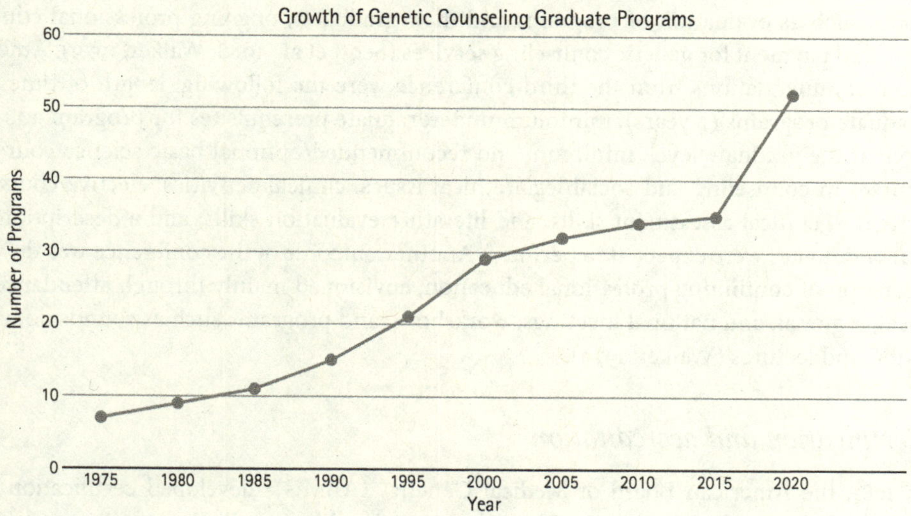

FIGURE 2.1 Growth of genetic counseling graduate programs in the United States and Canada from 1975 to 2020.

(Data abstracted from Stern, 2012; National Society of Genetic Counselors Late Career Special Interest Group [personal communication]; Accreditation Council for Genetic Counseling, 2022)

Figure 2.1 shows genetic counseling program growth, which illustrates an increase in the number of new programs per year between 1975 and 2020.

Drivers of genetic counseling education

We define drivers of genetic counseling education as influences that were both complex and important to shaping genetic counseling education.

Genetic counseling education consensus conferences

Initially, genetic counseling graduate programs individually determined the content of their curricula (Dumars et al., 1978). In an effort to standardize curricula, three consensus conferences were held between 1974 and 1979 to develop recommended content of the didactic portion of genetic counseling graduate programs. The initial meeting was informal and attended by representatives of the few existing programs, while the last two were funded by the March of Dimes and Office of Maternal Child Health, and stakeholders were expanded to include representatives of state, federal, and private agencies; legislators; directors of genetics centers; health insurance representatives; and other healthcare providers providing genetic counseling. These meetings resulted in recommendations for graduate genetic counseling program curricula, as well as other education-related

of California, Berkeley; the University of California, Irvine; and the State University of New York, Stony Brook.

issues such as evaluation of programs and their graduates, ongoing professional education, and payment for genetic counseling services (Scott et al., 1988; Walker, 1979). Among the recommendations from the third conference were the following: length of time for graduate programs (2 years); minimum undergraduate prerequisites for program admission; at the graduate level, minimum and recommended/optional basic science courses, courses in counseling and social/legal/ethical issues, clinical activities, elective courses/activities, clinical assessment skills, and literature evaluation skills; and a description of roles graduates were expected to perform. Another outcome of the conference was the expectation of continuing professional education, envisioned mainly through attendance at local, regional, and national meetings, workshops, and programs such as rounds, journal clubs, and lectures (Walker, 1979).

Certification and accreditation

In 1981, the American Board of Medical Genetics (ABMG)[3] developed certification for six medical genetics specialties: Clinical Geneticist, Medical PhD Geneticist, Clinical Biochemical Geneticist, Clinical Cytogeneticist, Clinical Immunogeneticist, and Genetic Counselor (American Board of Genetics and Genomics, 2019; Smith & Heimler, 1980). A national certification examination was developed, with a common *general exam*, taken by all subspecialties, and a *subspecialty exam*, taken only by practitioners in each subspecialty. Thus, genetic counselors took the same general exam as all doctoral-level geneticists. As a group, genetic counselors were among the highest scoring specialty practitioners (Resta, 2020). Interestingly, the term "geneticist" has sometimes been used to include and sometimes to exclude genetic counselors. We advocate use of the term "geneticist" to include master's-trained genetic counselors, with the history of general exam scores to bolster this claim.

In 1991, clinical geneticists received recognition as a medical specialty from the American Medical Association, which stipulated that all members of a medical specialty must have doctoral degrees to be recognized as a new medical specialty. ABMG members voted to form a new organization to certify genetic counselors in the United States and Canada, to be called the American Board of Genetic Counseling (ABGC), which was established in 1993. Initially, both the ABMG and ABGC collaborated on the certifying exam, but in 1996 the ABGC took control of the genetic counseling exam and eventually changed it from a general and specialty exam to a single exam format (ABGC, 2019a). Canadian genetic counselors also have a certification exam administered by the Canadian Board of Genetic Counselling (CBGC, 2023a).

Initially, the ABMG controlled education of genetics practitioners only through requirements for clinical training sites. The ABGC pioneered a number of practices that ensure quality and consistency of training, including accreditation of genetic counseling training programs, offered for the first time in 1995 (ABGC, 2019a). Thus, genetic counseling training programs had to meet comprehensive requirements for education set by the ABGC to achieve accreditation, further standardizing genetic counselor training.

[3] Editors' note: While at the time of these events the organization was ABMG, it is now the American Board of Medical Genetics and Genomics (ABMGG).

These requirements were in the areas of institutional support, program management, required curriculum content, clinical training, faculty composition, and student policies and procedures, such as evaluation, remediation, and graduation requirements.

In 1996, the ABGC developed practice-based competencies (PBCs) in line with other accrediting organizations and the trend toward competency-based education (CBE). CBE is "oriented to graduate outcome abilities and organized around competencies derived from an analysis of societal and patient needs" (Frank et al., 2010, p. 636) and enhances accountability of training programs to learners (by detailing what will be learned) and the general population (by showing that training gives healthcare professionals the skills necessary to provide appropriate and quality care). To initiate the process of developing PBCs, in 1994 the ABGC sponsored a consensus development conference with stakeholders from the existing genetic counseling graduate programs and board of directors of the ABGC, along with expert consultants in accreditation and education (Fiddler et al., 1996). PBCs were conceptualized as minimum criteria for entry-level genetic counselors and envisioned as outcome-based criteria for accreditation, guides for graduate education, and drivers for continued professional development in the field. Using a case-based narrative approach, attendees identified 27 competencies organized into four domains: communication skills; critical thinking skills; interpersonal, counseling, and psychosocial assessment skills; and professional ethics and values. Development of a competency-based accreditation process moved the emphasis from course content and clinical hours to "an accreditation model that fosters the development of practice-based skills that integrate knowledge from several disciplines" (Fine et al., 1996, p. 118), and this remains the model of accreditation in the field today. The PBCs have been continually updated to reflect current entry-level genetic counselor competencies (Doyle et al., 2016), and they have been critical in not only driving the processes of accreditation and certification but also generally providing the basis for the continued evolution of genetic counseling graduate programs (Riconda et al., 2018). Programs use the competencies to develop curricula, construct student and faculty evaluation tools, and measure student readiness to enter the workforce. The current PBCs list seven competencies and include genetics and genomics expertise, risk assessment, counseling, communication, research, healthcare systems, and professional identity. There are 25 subcompetencies within these seven main competencies (Accreditation Council for Genetic Counseling [ACGC], 2023). European countries (Skirton et al., 2010) and Canada (CBGC, 2023b; Ferrier et al., 2013) have also developed genetic counseling competencies, and other countries have incorporated both the ACGC and European competencies (Ingvoldstat et al., 2016).

Development of accreditation and the PBCs challenged the ABGC to standardize needed outcomes (codified in the PBCs) while allowing programs to decide the best avenues to achieve those outcomes, thus allowing creativity and special strengths of programs while covering the basic knowledge and skills necessary to function as a competent genetic counselor. For example, one program might require students to enroll in a cultural competence course, while another might embed this information and skills training throughout multiple program experiences. The PBCs are now critical in the measurement of genetic counselor competence, as measured by the ABGC certification examination, and "program competence," as measured by the ACGC accreditation process.

After investigating best accreditation and certification practices, the ABGC formed separate accreditation and certification organizations. The ABGC continued to handle certification of individual genetic counselors, while the newly formed ACGC took over the accreditation of genetic counseling graduate programs in the United States and Canada in 2013. Another change inspired by the National Commission for Certifying Agencies (NCCA) requirements was the development of a national practice analysis by the ABGC. The practice analysis describes the job responsibilities of entry-level genetic counselors to identify the knowledge and skills needed to provide effective genetic counseling. A validation survey is conducted every 5 years and used to derive a detailed certification examination content outline reflective of current practice (ABGC, 2020). In 2015 the ABGC received accreditation from the NCCA of its Certified Genetic Counselor certification program (ABGC, 2018). The ACGC joined the Association of Specialized and Professional Accreditors in 2013 and views recognition by the Council for Higher Education Accreditation to be valuable (ACGC, 2013). Recognition by these general accrediting organizations aligns genetic counseling accreditation with broader educational trends in other professions and provides assurance that genetic counseling accreditation is a valid and robust process. These organizations provide guidance about quality process improvement and best practices that will influence the development of certification, accreditation, and genetic counseling graduate education in the future.

ABGC certification expires after 5 years, and CGCs can recertify either through continuing education credit administered through the National Society of Genetic Counselors (NSGC) or sitting for the certification examination again. Similar recertification procedures are available through the CBGC to Canadian genetic counselors (CBGC, 2020a). These requirements are an important driver of postgraduate continuing education, as well as meeting U.S. state licensure requirements for continuing education for licensed genetic counselors.

Licensure, billing, and reimbursement practices

California passed the first genetic counselor licensure law in 2000, and Utah issued the first genetic counselor licenses in 2002. In states with licensure, genetic counseling practice, including the right to use the title "Genetic Counselor," is controlled by licensure requirements. Licensure laws have currently been passed in over half the states in the United States (NSGC, 2020b). Canada does not currently regulate the genetic counseling profession. Licensure affects genetic counseling education through its requirement for board certification and continuing education. Licensure laws also contain scope-of-practice definitions, which delineate professional practice boundaries and influence education. Although the NSGC provides national models for licensure laws and scope of practice (NSGC, 2019), states are free to legislate their own requirements. For example, one controversial component of genetic counselor licensure is whether or not the genetic counselor scope of practice includes the right and responsibility to order genetic tests. States are inconsistent in their licensure bill language, with some allowing genetic test ordering, some not allowing it, and some not addressing the issue one way or the other. The ACGC and ABGC have addressed this issue by requiring programs to include education "related to ordering genetic testing" (ACGC, 2019). Billing and reimbursement practices also affect educational content by requiring knowledge of these practices, which have both legal and patient case management ramifications.

Subspecialty development

The most frequent early subspecialties of genetic counseling were pediatric genetics and perinatal genetics. In the 1990s, cancer and other adult genetic counseling developed, and after 2000, more and more genetic counselors began working in subspecialties such as neurogenetics, cardiovascular genetics, and single disease settings.[4] Because of these subspecialty settings, genetic counselors sought education from nongenetic organizations providing national or regional conferences, lectures, courses, symposia, and workshops on the medical topic most helpful in their specialized setting. Many of these genetic counselors have developed national and international reputations as experts in a specialized area of genetics.

Another effect of subspecialty development is the necessity for genetic counselors to set up a program of self-training when entering into a new subspecialty (Haverbusch et al., 2019). To some degree, this has always been a necessity for genetic counselors. The field has changed so rapidly that education and skills development have always occurred extensively as new scientific discoveries are made and genetic counseling roles are extended. However, the spread of genetic counselors to more and more subspecialty positions has accelerated this trend. Although a solid understanding of the clinical and scientific aspects of a subspecialty is important, it is the core skills of genetic counselors that are often most valued in a subspecialty setting (Hudson et al., 2019). Because of the importance of core genetic counseling skills, the rapidly changing landscape of genetic discoveries in most fields of medicine, the model of multidisciplinary teams providing subspecialty service, and the content limitations of 2-year master's genetic counseling programs, continuing education will likely continue to aid genetic counselors in developing subspecialty clinical and scientific knowledge.

When the number of genetic counseling positions in specific subspecialties increases, this drives genetic counseling programs to incorporate more content related to the subspecialty into genetic counseling core curricula. Cancer genetic counseling started as a subspecialty but is now considered part of the core curriculum. Other subspecialties are in various stages of this transformation (e.g., neurogenetics, cardiovascular genetics, assisted reproductive technology, psychiatric genetics, pediatric oncology). Factors influencing this progression are the frequency of new positions in these subspecialties, the amount of independence as genetics experts in their area of practice, and progression of genetic knowledge in the specialty. In addition to subspecialty development driving genetic counseling graduate program didactic content, skill sets from other specialties may sometimes be introduced into genetic counseling programs. For example, genetic counselors working in the perinatal hospice setting may have learned from general hospice techniques, which are then adopted by genetic counseling programs.

Nondirect patient care

Initially, genetic counselors mainly provided direct patient care, but nondirect patient care positions existed since the early days of the profession and have steadily increased

[4] Editors' note: For further information on subspecialization in genetic counseling, see Chapter 10 by Catherine A. Wicklund and Angela M. Trepanier in this volume.

(NSGC, 2020a). The language of the NSGC Professional Status Survey was changed from "clinical and non-clinical" care to "direct and non-direct" patient care, emphasizing that most genetic counselors provide patient care, either directly or indirectly (NSGC, 2018). Direct patient care is provided to patients in face-to-face or electronic encounters (e.g., phone, telemedicine), while nondirect patient care includes activities such as providing information to other healthcare professionals for their patients, planning patient healthcare in a public health setting, or providing laboratory services used by healthcare providers and their patients. This growth has had a strong influence on core genetic counseling graduate education (McWalter et al., 2018), as well as continuing education (Balkite & Smith, 2009).

Most recently, the vast increase in genetic counseling jobs in the industry has been a driver for genetic counseling education.[5] Currently, 28% of genetic counselors work in jobs classified as noncommercial or commercial laboratory or other biotechnology company (NSGC, 2020a). The increase of jobs in this sector has led to discussions about the obligation of genetic counseling graduate programs to provide education and skills training for industry jobs (McWalter et al., 2018; Swanson et al., 2014; Waltman et al., 2016). Some think that genetic counseling master's programs should do more to teach the skills necessary for industry jobs (e.g., management skills), while others think that genetic counseling programs should continue to focus on core skills useful in any genetic counseling position. Most genetic counselors in industry positions have utilized formal and informal in-house training to attain new skills. ACGC standards state that programs must provide exposure to "the full range of practice settings and full range of PBCs" and mention as examples the industry-related roles of variant interpretation; test development, implementation, and performance; utilization management; customer liaison and support; sales and marketing; and leadership and management (ACGC, 2019, p. 21). This requirement has bolstered incorporation of industry-related knowledge and skills training into coursework, fieldwork placements, and supplemental activities in genetic counseling graduate programs (e.g., Grove et al., 2019).

Another influence of industry on education has been the diversity of roles that genetic counselors have taken on in industry settings, such as direct patient care, education, product development, management, and marketing. An example of how practice influences education is the clinical training task force of the ACGC, which looked at clinical training requirements, with the goal of making them more applicable to the diverse roles that genetic counselors fulfill today.

Consumer self-advocacy

Another driver of genetic counseling education is the rise of consumer advocacy and self-empowerment, both in general and specifically in the realm of genetics, disabilities, and congenital conditions. Consumer influence on healthcare in general has changed our ideas of patient-centered care, the provider–patient/consumer relationship, and self-advocacy. The rise of consumer advocacy groups in the 1980s, often led by consumers, demanded more attention to models of care provision, the needs of consumers with specific conditions,

[5] Editors' note: For further discussion on genetic counseling roles in industry, see Chapter 13 by Elissa Levin and Edgar MacBean in this volume.

and research agendas. These considerations led to a recognition of the need for consumer input into genetic counseling education, opportunities for clinical fieldwork that include exposure to consumer viewpoints and concerns, inclusion of new education content, recognition of ethical/legal/social issues involving consumers, inclusion of disability perspectives throughout the spectrum of genetic counseling, and a continuing but expanding emphasis on the whole family as client. These developments introduced expanded content into genetic counseling programs, encouraged consumer input on advisory committees, and provided opportunities for less traditional learning modes such as community partnerships; use of nonacademic books, movies, and websites; and use of consumers as supplemental instructors. Consumer involvement also influenced the move from a predominantly teaching model of genetic counseling to models that incorporate both education and counseling, including models of shared decision making and the Reciprocal-Engagement Model of genetic counseling.[6]

The most recent trend affecting genetic counseling programs is the advent and popularity of direct-to-consumer (DTC) testing. Although this type of testing usually circumvents the healthcare system, genetic counselors are becoming involved as employees of companies offering DTC testing and as consultants when consumers are deciding about testing or seeking professional help in understanding and/or adjusting to results. Thus, genetic counseling trainees need information about DTC testing procedures, psychosocial implications, and ethical/legal/social ramifications. It is unclear how this consumer-driven and market-driven phenomenon will influence practice and education in the future.[7]

Professionalization

The aforementioned drivers are all part of the professionalization of the field of genetic counseling. These professionalization milestones influence each other and genetic counseling education in an iterative way.[8] For example, licensure and scope of practice were developed as tools to provide safe and effective genetic counseling, but once developed, programs needed to teach about these important components of professional practice. PBCs were developed by the ABGC to inform programs about areas of entry-level competence their students were expected to develop but also influenced the development of scopes of practice, continuing education, and professional development (Fine et al., 1996). A genetic counseling program may develop an emerging strategy for developing practitioner skills (e.g., motivational interviewing), and this may be adopted by other programs and accrediting bodies, thus spreading innovation. The development of practice standards influenced the content of certification examinations, but continuing education influences the development of practice. The development of new job opportunities influences education both directly and indirectly through accreditation.

[6] Editors' note: For further discussion on the Reciprocal-Engagement Model, see Chapter 5 by Patricia McCarthy Veach and Bonnie S. LeRoy in this volume.

[7] Editors' note: Additional information on DTC genetic testing can be found in Chapter 11 by Anne E. Greb in this volume.

[8] Editors' note: For a historical account of the development of genetic counseling as a profession in the United States, see Chapter 3 by Vickie L. Venne and Edward M. Kloza in this volume.

One of the more recent phases of genetic counseling professionalization is the increased growth trajectory of the job market in general.[9] With this rapid expansion has come a parallel expansion of genetic counseling graduate programs and total student slots (ACGC, 2018). The growth illustrated in Figure 2.1 was enabled by several influences. These include promotion of the profession accompanied by vastly increased press coverage, efforts by the ACGC to increase growth-friendly standards, and efforts by genetic counseling programs and the Genetic Counselor Educators Association (GCEA).[10] The NSGC and Canadian Association of Genetic Counsellors (CAGC) have taken the lead in dedicating resources to the promotion and marketing of the profession, but this has been aided by other genetics professional organizations, government, and private industry. Examples are the U.S. Department of Labor workforce projections (Bureau of Labor Statistics, U.S. Department of Labor, 2023), industry scholarships, and NSGC publications and social media initiatives. The ACGC and CBGC have simplified required program documentation and revised their standards to enable more flexibility in training. Genetic counseling programs, aided by the GCEA, have mentored developing programs, developed alternative training models (e.g., distance courses, joint programs), and are developing new admission pipelines.

Growth of genetic counseling internationally

While the focus of this chapter is the development of genetic counseling education in the United States and Canada, where early genetic counseling graduate programs and practices first developed, since the 1990s genetic counseling has developed into an international profession (Abacan et al., 2019; Ormond et al., 2024).[11] Genetic counseling training programs have developed in many other countries, and in 2006 the first international meeting of genetic counseling educators was held in Manchester, England, where 45 established or developing genetic counseling educational programs were represented. At that time, the Transnational Alliance for Genetic Counseling (TAGC) was started, sponsored by a Jane Engelberg Memorial Fellowship grant (Edwards, 2013; TAGC, 2020). The TAGC and the continuing series of international educational conferences have provided a forum for exchanges of information about genetic counseling educational programs, as well as networking that continues to facilitate international educational collaboration (e.g., international clinical student rotations, research, educational strategies, regulatory strategies) that enriches genetic counseling education worldwide. Although genetic counseling has become a worldwide profession, there are differences in healthcare service delivery models, regulatory systems, and educational systems, which have resulted in differences in the professional development of genetic counselors around the world (Abacan et al., 2019). Skirton et al. (2010) developed core curricula for genetic counseling training in Europe,

[9] Editors' note: For further examination of possible growth of the genetic counseling profession, see Chapter 33 by Megan E. Trinkle-Tucker and Beverly M. Yashar in this volume.

[10] Editors' note: The GCEA was previously the Association of Genetic Counseling Program Directors (AGCPD) but officially changed its name in 2023.

[11] Editors' note: For further information on the global expansion of genetic counseling, please see Chapter 34 by Mercy Ygoña Laurino and Austin Emanuel Bland in this volume.

and Ingvoldstat et al. (2016) compared genetic counseling education programs internationally, advocating for international standards for genetic counseling education.

Genetic counseling program curricular development

Drivers of genetic counseling education gave rise and shape to the general structure of graduate training, codified in standards for accreditation. To be accredited, a graduate training program must have didactic coursework (curriculum) covering key content areas; fieldwork and clinical training to develop competencies, particularly in the realm of patient care; research activities to engage with scientific literature and actively contribute to generation of knowledge pertinent to the profession; and supplemental activities (laboratory exposure, teaching opportunities) to complement, extend, and enhance other programmatic elements. Accredited genetic counseling master's-level graduate programs in the United States and Canada all have to meet the accreditation standards of the ACGC, and those accredited programs have a proven track record of graduating competent genetic counselors or a plan that promises such success if they are new programs. It is by enacting accreditation standards in nuanced and varied ways that each program generates its unique culture and contribution to the profession.

As a result of the influences driving genetic counseling graduate education, as well as local resources, program size, and placement within institutions, graduate programs in the United States and Canada have developed both overlapping and unique features. All programs include didactic coursework, but the number of courses, course credit distribution, course content, and mode of delivery vary considerably. For example, all programs need to teach basic genetics concepts used in genetic counseling service delivery, but some utilize courses taken by students in multiple professional disciplines or develop intentional interdisciplinary courses, while others have designed tailored courses for genetic counseling students only. Some programs teach basic subjects through traditional courses, while others utilize hybrid courses that record lectures viewed in advance coupled with sessions designed to incorporate the lecture material, such as mock pedigrees, designing clinic plans, or debates about ethical issues. Some programs have developed distance learning courses, either for a small number of courses or for the majority of their formal courses. These courses may enable expansion of genetic counseling programs, flexibility in clinical placements, and/or reaching a different student demographic (e.g., rural or low-income students). Seminar courses may be most variable, often designed to cover topics not included in traditional courses and utilizing techniques such as discussion of the literature, interactive class exercises, and role-playing.

All programs must develop psychosocial competencies, but how this is done also differs among programs. Some include courses dedicated to psychosocial skills, while others spread psychosocial topics among multiple courses that may include nonpsychosocial objectives. There are also differences in the amount of clinical supervision that focuses on psychosocial topics, both within and between programs, as well as differences in supplemental activities that provide opportunities to develop psychosocial skills. Programs may include creative activities like psychosocial rounds, optional rotations with an emphasis on psychosocial skills (e.g., perinatal hospice, facilitation of bereavement groups, child life team), group therapy for students, or incorporation of psychosocial goals as a consistent part of clinical rotation goals.

All programs also include fieldwork, but the overall plan of student progression through placements varies widely in type of practice setting, roles practiced by students, length and type of placements, and patient and client populations.

Supplemental activities include experiences that are not provided through courses or fieldwork, such as journal clubs, teaching activities, laboratory exposure, and community involvement. Some activities fall into the category of supplemental for some programs, while being covered in fieldwork placements or courses in others. For example, one program might require case conference attendance along with case debriefing as a professional course, while another might require case conference attendance as part of a clinical placement.

Research activities are another required component that might take the shape of a thesis, independent nonthesis research project, or capstone project. Some programs require a formal research course, while others use different strategies to teach or mentor research techniques. Programs may provide faculty-generated research ideas and/or encourage student-generated ideas. In addition to the goal of exposing genetic counseling students to the mechanics of research (e.g., research coordination, obtaining informed consent, data gathering, and research design, analysis, and publication), research activities build scholarly skills in comprehensive literature reviews in both clinical and industry settings. This helps students become critical consumers of scientific literature and nurtures a commitment to evidence-based professional practice.

Accreditation standards specify content areas that must or should be covered, but there is variability according to content area. For example, informal presentations and discussions at GCEA meetings revealed that most programs utilize didactic courses to teach traditional topics such as basic genetics, clinical genetics, cancer genetics, and reproductive genetics. There is more variability in areas such as subspecialties and newer topics (e.g., cardiovascular genetics, neurological genetics, consumer-initiated genetic testing), through inclusion in an array of courses, seminars, and clinical placements, and more utilization of supplementary activities. Even more variability is seen with topics such as professionalism, leadership, teaching, ELSI (ethical, legal, and social issues), public health, and community involvement, which may be covered in formal courses, seminars, fieldwork placements, and supplementary activities, along with more variability in the extent and formality of coverage of these topics. Another area of programmatic individuality is the use of elective experiences such as optional courses, certificate programs, dual degrees, international rotations, fieldwork placements that do not involve direct patient care, work or internship experiences, leadership training, or other types of nonmandatory experiences that enrich student learning and opportunities. The use of PBCs in training and accreditation (discussed above) recognizes and supports this rich variety of training strategies.

The GCEA was formed to promote collaborative interactions among genetic counseling graduate programs and support high standards of practice. The GCEA has multiple initiatives to facilitate recruitment, admissions, education, and guidance for genetic counseling students and programs (Association of Genetic Counseling Program Directors, 2020). This organization has been key in driving educational program quality, consistency, and access. Example initiatives include the introduction of a formal program to match applicants to programs; a workforce task force to examine and make recommendations regarding the applicant pool; recruitment and cultivation of program directors; new program development; clinical training and curriculum development; and an ad hoc committee to examine advanced training for CGCs. With the current explosion of demand for genetic counselors, these activities have enabled genetic counseling programs to streamline activities, rapidly expand both the number of programs and the number of student slots available, and prepare for future changes in the profession.

There are also many challenges to both individual graduate programs and genetic counseling education as a whole. These challenges include teaching to the future (e.g., it is difficult to teach about a role that is just emerging, such as interpretation and counseling about DTC tests), graduating enough genetic counselors to keep up with job demand (e.g., the number of fieldwork placements often limits the number of students a program can accept), newer education models and their regulation (e.g., programs with all online coursework, programs located at multiple institutions), pressure to include more and more content, and alternative training to the master's degree in genetic counseling or its equivalent. The relevant professional genetic counseling organizations concerned with education (ABGC, ACGC, CBGC, NSGC, CAGC, GCEA) in the United States and Canada are engaged in ongoing conversations about these and other issues that will shape the future of genetic counseling education.

One development that exemplifies these challenges and resulting responses is the 2020 global COVID-19 pandemic. In a few short months, the pandemic resulted in catastrophic and unforeseen changes to public life in every part of the world. This included a cessation of all in-person university classes and all opportunities for trainee face-to-face clinical interactions. Programs quickly transitioned from in-person classes to online classes, using tools to maintain real-time classes, breakout groups, role plays, standardized patients, and proctored exams. As the healthcare sector rapidly ramped up telemedicine capabilities and devised the best strategies to mitigate health risks to patients and providers, programs scrambled to devise the best experiential educational strategies, with the help of the relevant professional organizations. Strategies such as vastly increased use of telemedicine visits, distance supervision, virtual research defense presentations, and a national pool of standardized patients and patient scenarios helped students impacted by the sudden and unprecedented restrictions. Programs developed other strategies to help mitigate isolation for students such as online social interactions, counseling of students, and graduation ceremonies and celebrations. Development of these alternative educational strategies have often persisted beyond the pandemic, as many were useful to extend program capacity, particularly the increased use of telemedicine patient encounters, online coursework, and distance clinical supervision.

General Educational Models Influence Genetic Counseling Education

Why use general educational models?

Theory is instrumental in grounding the work of genetic counselors, offering a conceptual framework within which the counselor can think through questions and preferences when considering alternative actions and judgments. Coupled with experimentation, theory enables the examination of genetic counseling practice from multiple angles, fleshing out the beginnings of a new way of doing things and a different way of seeing something. Strengths, weaknesses, and omissions of counselors' own perceptions and practice strategies can be identified through comparing and contrasting them to theoretical approaches. Turning one's attention to specific educational methods in genetic counseling education—the ways in which one goes about training and learning the craft—education theories reveal points of alignment with current approaches and sources of inspiration for further progress. These theories apply equally to master's-level genetic counseling education as well as advanced education.

Experiential learning

That one readily learns from experience is implicit in nearly all of education. In adult learning, theories of experiential learning are grounded in the work of John Dewey, who stipulated that we make meaning from our experience, translating it to knowledge (Dewey, 1938). Adults are acknowledged as bringing extensive life experience to bear on current learning (Knowles, 1980)—connecting previous and new knowledge, refining skills for greater effect in new contexts, and reshaping attitudes through encounters with alternative perspectives. Kolb (1984) described learning as a continuous, cyclical process anchored in experience. In Kolb's view, the process may begin with a *concrete experience* during which one perceives multiple aspects of an event directly through participation or engagement. This is followed by *reflective observation*, which entails remembering the experience, considering it thoroughly, and noting important features or highlights. Reflection on particular aspects of an experience gives way to *abstract conceptualization*, a step characterized by thinking of generalized theories or formulations of specific features; this theorizing is akin to categorizing types or trends and recognizing patterns across similar experiences. Theories are subsequently tested through *active experimentation*, when newly derived knowledge is applied to adjusted actions and behaviors, which in turn creates a new concrete experience, and so on. Though the process can begin at any point, it is most effective when completed in full, "closing the loop."

Experiential learning informs all aspects of genetic counseling education, though its influence is perhaps most noticeable during clinical training and fieldwork, when students are learning directly in the context of future practice. The process of learning clinical skills aptly mirrors Kolb's theory of experiential learning. The patient encounter serves as a *concrete experience* for the genetic counseling student. When practicing genetic counseling skills, the student perceives their thoughts, emotions, and actions through interaction with the client, noting the reactions and responses of the client and supervisor. Following the encounter, the student engages in *reflective observation* by recalling their performance and noting important moments, perhaps enhanced by debriefing the session with their supervisor and documenting participation in the case. These reflections—in company with those related to other encounters, as well as reflections on coursework and past personal and professional experiences—contribute to insights on their performance overall, preferences for particular specialties, deeper awareness of overarching strengths and weaknesses, and comparison of their performance to peers and practicing genetic counselors (an illustration of *abstract conceptualization*). Finally, insights gleaned throughout the process thus far are applied to the next patient encounter when the student *actively experiments* by adjusting techniques or trying alternative approaches.

Experiential learning is most effective when the cycle is completed in full, when engagement in experience, reflection, conceptualization, and experimentation are all accomplished. If any one step is omitted, learning is not maximized. If the student only observes and doesn't actively interact with the patient, their perceptions of the experience will be limited—they'll necessarily garner fewer and less intense impressions, as participation is vicarious rather than direct. If the student doesn't intentionally and deeply reflect, details will be lost or revised, diluting any subsequent examination and synthesis of overall performance or change over time. If the student doesn't proceed from reflection to conceptualization, discrete experiences of learning remain disconnected, and a holistic picture of development and progress will not be constructed. And if the student doesn't have access to repeated opportunities to practice skills, to experiment, or to apply tentative views as an emerging professional, learning momentum will not be obtained or maintained.

Genetic counselors and genetic counseling students are quite familiar with reflection, which is a critical component of experiential learning, featuring prominently in Kolb's and others' theories. Donald Schon (1983) did extensive work on reflection and reflective practice, particularly among professionals. He distinguished between two types of reflection: reflection-on-action and reflection-in-action. Reflection-on-action occurs when a student looks back on an experience to make more sense of it, generating insights that can be applied to similar situations in the future. In genetic counseling education, reflection-on-action is commonly practiced through formalized self-assessment, such as a reflection paper that is rooted in specific examples of past performance, debrief discussions with supervisors regarding specific clinical encounters, or case summaries. Through reflection, the student produces a deep and full account of thoughts and feelings arising during an experience, synthesizes themes of what was learned, and considers alternative interpretations or strategies. In contrast to the retrospective nature of reflection-on-action, reflection-in-action occurs when one analyzes one's actions in real time, making immediate adjustments to better suit the emerging demands of the circumstance; it is more immediate and implicit. Evidence of a student's reflection-in-action includes responding to emerging cues about the effectiveness of their performance by altering a preset agenda during a role play or clinical encounter; adjusting language and descriptions to match another's preferences, needs, and values; and recognizing countertransference and actively mitigating it. Reflection-in-action might enhance one's perception of an experience by increasing awareness of multiple features, reactions, and responses, and thereby further inform reflection-on-action by providing more and specific information for consideration. Schon (1983) characterized reflection-in-action as the more complex capacity, framing it as concurrent reflection and action, with continuous interplay between self and situation.

There are many theories and models of experiential learning, and Fenwick (2000) constructed a useful schema to categorize theories with similar features. She noted Kolb's experiential learning cycle and Schon's reflection-on-action as representative of the most common conception of learning from our experiences through systematic retrospective reflection that constructs new understanding ("constructivist"); in these theories, experience and reflection occur at different points in time. Kolb's experiential learning cycle mirrors Schon's reflection-on-action in that both begin with experience, which is followed by careful thinking about one's responses to that experience; generalizing those responses to themes, principles, and patterns toward a deeper understanding of present self and situation; and ultimately formulating alternative approaches for future use. Learning generated from the cycle is reinforced by repetition—the quality and depth of learning are directly proportional to the number of cycles completed over time. In contrast, Fenwick (2000) differentiates experiential learning theories that couple experience and reflection as occurring simultaneously, with learning "situated" in experience, concurrent in time and space, similar to Schon's reflection-in-action. In these situated theories, one learns *in* rather than *from* experience. This distinction is evident in students' appreciation for the learning they derive during fieldwork (direct participation in clinical care) as compared to the learning from role play and simulation. Fieldwork requires students to learn in real time by actively engaging in the authentic work and practice of genetic counseling; learning and doing occur simultaneously. In role play and simulations, students perform and subsequently assess their performance, learning after doing—that is, from the experience of practicing skills through artificial interactions.

Experiential learning continues to be a central feature of professional development following graduation from a genetic counseling training program as formal education transitions to professional education and learning and "new knowledge structures are created through everyday experience" (Cervero, 1988, p. 41). Genetic counselors learn constantly on the job during their work with patients, clients, and coworkers, and these personal habits of professional learning can be connected to Kolb's theory of experiential learning; each client encounter constitutes a *concrete experience*, the genetic counselor's introspective debriefing of the case serves as *reflective observation*, discussion with colleagues furthers *abstract conceptualization*, and ongoing tweaks to one's unique approach to practice work as *active experimentation*. These experiences of learning are complemented by opportunities for continuing professional education: conferences, workshops, courses, and trainings in person and online. Continuing professional education—as described in both the adult learning and healthcare literatures—has been found to be most effective when practice based, interactive, and ongoing (Bluestone et al., 2013; Robertson et al., 2003; Webster-Wright, 2009), all three features that also can be found in the everyday experiences of professional practice.

Self-directed learning

Knowles defined important differences between the learning of children and adults, perhaps most notably that adults tend to take more initiative and exercise personal preferences in many, if not all, aspects of the learning process, including setting learning goals, choosing learning strategies and activities, and determining how learning will be assessed (Knowles & Associates, 1984). Grow (1991) refined understanding of this overarching trait of self-directedness by delineating a continuum of learner self-directedness consisting of four levels (dependent, interested, involved, and self-directed). Grow (1991) suggested that an educator's approach to teaching (or the level of supervision provided to adult learners) should align with the learner's level of self-directedness and that many difficulties in teaching and learning can be explained by a mismatch between the educator's approach and the learner's level. Complementary to the four levels of learner self-directedness, there are four roles an educator can assume with respect to teaching: authority, guide, facilitator, and consultant. In Grow's (1991) estimation, a dependent learner benefits most from an educator who acts as an authority, whereas a self-directed learner is best served by an educator who consults at the learner's request.

Genetic counseling education reflects appreciation for this kind of alignment when standards for program accreditation stipulate sequencing of courses and graduated levels of supervision appropriate to the student's stage of development. More advanced students are believed to benefit from more independence with limited oversight, whereas beginning students may require direct supervision. Mismatch between student and educator levels may explain why some students respond well to certain instructors or supervisors while others resist (the "strict" instructor or supervisor might inspire a more dependent learner while demotivating a self-directed learner, whereas the "permissive" instructor or supervisor might confuse a dependent learner and encourage a self-directed learner) or why certain groups work more collaboratively than others (similar versus divergent levels of self-directedness).

Variable levels of self-directedness might also be highlighted in students' thesis or research work. Those with higher levels of self-direction would readily assume oversight of a study or project, demonstrating proactive management and participation throughout each phase of the research process. Alternatively, a strong desire for an advisor's guidance would be evident in those with lower levels of self-direction. Grow's (1991) notion of mismatch could here again help to explain why some research proceeds smoothly and some sluggishly based on alignment of the advisor's role and student's self-directedness. The self-directed student researcher would benefit most from an advisor who plans through consultation and is responsive to the student's judgments and emerging concerns. The dependent student researcher would be expected to prefer an advisor who continually directs the research process with clear instructions. Mismatch in styles could contribute to power struggles as the self-directed student resists the authoritative advisor, delays as the consultative advisor awaits questions from a dependent student, and confusion as students and advisors hold discrepant expectations for each other's roles and responsibilities. A strong match in styles would prompt high-efficiency, collaborative, and enjoyable research experiences, such as when an expert advisor coaches an eagerly receptive dependent student or the delegating advisor relishes the creative independence of a self-directed student.

The influence of self-directed learning theory assumes a different shape for practicing genetic counselors who are no longer learning within the framework of formalized graduate study that partners them with instructors or supervisors. Instead, differential levels of self-directedness might be inferred from individuals' choices about strategies for lifelong learning. As Cervero and Daley (2016) note:

> In an evidence-based approach, professionals study the latest research in their professional area, decide how to implement that in their practice, make changes in their performance, and then document the results. . . . [This] could incorporate formal continuing professional education, or it could be a completely self-directed process for the professional. (p. 16)

One genetic counselor might take courses or attend lectures that match a desire for learning dependent on or guided by others, whereas another genetic counselor might craft a unique path of trial and error in keeping with a preference for being fully self-directed. An individual can be consistent in their preferences for self-directedness across all their professional learning activities or may display different levels of self-directedness depending on the context and subject matter of learning. For example, a genetic counselor with years of experience in reproductive genetics might choose a dependent approach to learning about neurogenetics and a self-directed approach to new prenatal testing technologies, or a novice genetic counselor might acquire new knowledge by attending a lecture yet work on skill development by initiating and engaging with a peer supervision group.

Communities of practice

Theories of experiential learning and self-directed learning shed light on instances or discrete processes of learning during a genetic counseling student's time in training or a genetic counselor's professional development. A more global view of genetic counseling education as a dynamic and social system of learning might be better illuminated by exploring the theory of community of practice. Wenger (2011) defined community of practice as "groups of people who share a concern or a passion for something they do and learn how to do it better as they interact regularly" (p. 11). Communities of practice are characterized by a common purpose or goal; engagement, collaboration, and exchange among its members; and a shared collection of resources and practices (Wenger, 1998). Learning within a community of practice has been described as moving from the periphery—imagined as the borders and outer boundaries of the group, partial participation—to the center, where one is embedded in the community by close connections to other members, competently performing pertinent practices and potentially generating new practices. Learning in communities of practice has been compared to an apprenticeship model in trade professions, although the community of practice model is often less hierarchical. Communities of practice may be overlapping, with an individual or group having membership in multiple communities.

A genetic counseling training program operates a community of practice, constituted as a unique group of individuals—students, advisors, supervisors, administrators, instructors, clients, patients, and the encircling healthcare communities. Each program develops its culture, tone, and reputation as the sum total of all interactions of its members, changing and fluctuating over time as members enter and leave (through admissions and graduations, arrival and departure of faculty). Each individual contributes to the collective goal by engaging with other members through interactions that convey and swap knowledge, skills, values, and resources that become shared over time. All members of a training program share the goal of providing quality genetic counseling services, yet each community might pursue that goal with variable emphasis on particular values or aspects of practice. Students move from the periphery to the center of genetic counseling practice, particularly through fieldwork, beginning with observation and increasingly taking on more tasks of the genetic counseling professional until they are acting as the genetic counselor themselves. Their learning is facilitated by interaction with members of the clinical genetics community—their instructors, supervisors, genetic counselors, medical geneticists, patients, peers, and other healthcare professionals—and by the sharing and exchange of resources such as scientific literature, practice guidelines, and useful websites.

That each individual or group is situated in a constellation of communities is illustrated by a student being a member of their cohort as well as a member of their training program. Similarly, practicing genetic counselors hold membership in their respective work environments at multiple levels (team, department, clinic, company, institution), the alumni network of their graduate training program, professional organizations, and the profession generally. While each genetic counseling training program is a community of practice in and of itself, the set of all genetic counseling training programs constitutes an overlay of yet another community of practice; all are accountable to the same accreditation standards and develop the same PBCs in their students. The standards and the PBCs detail the shared understanding of competent practice held by our professional community of practice as a whole.

Genetic Counseling Continuing Education

There is inevitably a difference between posttraining professional practice and the information, skills, and practices learned in training. Graduate genetic counseling training is based on a generalist mindset, but much of practice is subspecialty based, and many genetic counselors work in non-patient-facing areas of practice. There are rapid changes in genetic information and available clinical diagnoses and tests, as well as advances in professional opportunities and counseling strategies. Continuing education in its many forms enables genetic counselors to utilize the most current information and techniques in their service provision, keep current with general topics when they specialize, develop advanced skills and knowledge, and qualify for career-enhancing positions.

Continuing education for practicing genetic counselors: Content and skill-building education

Continuing education for the first graduates of genetic counseling programs was offered by various national and regional genetics organizations. The American Society of Human Genetics (ASHG) is the national professional organization for geneticists. Its emphasis has traditionally been on research, since the vast majority of geneticists were engaged in research. As the field of medical genetics developed, the content of the ASHG meeting contained more clinically relevant information, and most clinical geneticists and genetic counselors attended these meetings. Another important source of continuing education was the annual March of Dimes Birth Defects Meeting, which was primarily clinical in nature, but not focused on genetics. These educational offerings were mainly content oriented, providing excellent information about genetic diseases and techniques (e.g., Bayesian analysis, molecular mechanisms), but also included public health, policy, behavioral science, and psychosocial topics.

In 1979, genetic counselors developed the first professional genetic counseling society, the NSGC. The purpose of the NSGC was to promote the profession, and one of the earliest activities was to develop and host a series of regional and national education meetings that offered continuing education specifically targeted for genetic counselors (Heimler, 1997; National Society of Genetic Counselors, 1981; Rollnick, 1981, 1983). Early national NSGC meetings were held in conjunction with the ASHG or March of Dimes meetings, allowing genetic counselors to attend back-to-back meetings within the logistics of a single trip. In

1998, NSGC members voted to hold a free-standing meeting, as it was difficult to attend two meetings at once and the content of the NSGC meeting had become increasingly scientifically robust (NSGC, 2020c). Beginning in 2000, a separate NSGC conference was convened. Although the need for content-oriented continuing education is ongoing and has expanded into many medical subspecialties, one of the hallmarks of the NSGC educational offerings is the inclusion of information and skill building related to the counseling aspect of practice.

Continuing education is required to maintain ABGC certification and licensure by states with genetic counselor licensure. There is now a wide array of professional educational meetings, workshops, courses, and other professional activities that qualify as approved continuing education. Continuing education activities are measured in continuing education units (CEUs), with Category 1 CEUs awarded for programs preapproved by the NSGC and targeted to genetic counselors, Category 2 CEUs awarded for programs approved by other organizations (e.g., CMEs are eligible if the education is relevant to a genetic counselor's continuing education and approved by the NSGC), and Professional Activity Credits (PACs) awarded for other activities determined by the ABGC to promote professional development (ABGC, 2016). Davis (2018) found that between 2002 and 2015, 86% of genetic counselor CEU activities were Category 1, with the remainder split between Category 2 and PACs (most commonly earned through publication, clinical supervision, teaching, or leadership). CEUs earned online (courses, conference recordings, or literature) steadily increased from 2% in 2005 to 36% in 2015. About two-thirds of CEUs were provided by professional societies: the NSGC (47%), ASHG (14%), and ACMG (7%). In 2019, the ABGC convened the Continued Competence Task Force to reexamine offerings to ensure that continuing education is of relevance to genetic counseling practice, imparts knowledge about current practice and scientific knowledge, and maintains/increases genetic counselor competencies (ABGC, 2019b). In Canada, the CACG has a similar continuing education process (CBGC, 2020b), which requires both continuing practice credits, earned by employment as a genetic counselor, and continuing education credits.

Additional paths to advanced skill development

As robust paths to advanced skill development were enabled by NSGC educational programs and ABGC recertification through CEUs, other diverse avenues emerged that aided genetic counselors in developing advanced skills. In addition to developing advanced skills through sheer experience, genetic counselors were attaining skills through formal and informal paths such as additional academic degrees, certificates, academic courses, other institutional courses and trainings, and on-the-job training (Baty et al., 2016). In 2020, 14% of genetic counselors responding to the NSGC Professional Status Survey reported additional advanced degrees besides master's degrees in genetic counseling or human/medical genetics (NSGC, 2020a). As professionalization of the field of genetic counseling progressed, consideration of advanced degrees in genetic counseling was formally explored (Atzinger et al., 2007; Gaupman et al., 1991; Kloza, 1988; Walker et al., 1990; Wallace et al., 2008).

In 2011 the ABGC convened the Genetic Counseling Advanced Degree Task Force to investigate the possibility of a required, entry-level clinical doctorate. The group scoured the literature, interviewed stakeholders, investigated other healthcare fields that had either developed or decided against clinical doctorates, educated the general membership, and conducted a national survey (Nagy et al., 2014) of genetic counselors and genetic counseling students. The vote was heavily in favor (81%) of maintaining the master's degree as the entry-level education required to become a genetic counselor. The GCEA conducted a survey of genetic counseling programs to assess their ability to transition to a clinical doctorate, which found that 53% of programs would have serious difficulty in making the transition (Reiser et al., 2015), with a projected 26% decrease in student capacity. In 2013, the task force made the recommendation to maintain the master's degree as the entry-level degree in genetic counseling (Canadian Association for Genetic Counselling/Association canadienne de conseil génétique, 2013; Valverde et al., 2016).

In response to the clear interest in advanced skill training and career development, the GCEA convened the Committee on Advanced Training for Certified Genetic Counselors (CATCGC), a national committee with the charge to investigate all paths to advanced skills. The group consisted of both program directors and non–program directors with expertise in genetic counseling education, including advanced education, and general professional educational development. The CATCGC developed the model of advanced training for certified genetic counselors to describe the landscape of advanced genetic counseling skills. The three components of the model, visualized as grids, were domains of advanced skills that genetic counselors developed (e.g., research, education, psychosocial, business, public health), paths to develop those skills (e.g., additional advanced degrees, certificates, CEUs, on-the-job training), and positions that genetic counselors could qualify for due to attainment of advanced skills (e.g., administration positions; Baty et al., 2016). Plans are in progress to develop an interactive web resource that will enable the model to be used for educational planning and career development. Potential advantages of the web resource are the ability to keep the information up to date, interactivity within the model itself as well as between the model and its users, the inclusion of mentoring, and incorporation of skills, paths, and positions that may develop in the future. The CATCGC also conducted an interview study of genetic counselors with advanced skills to see if the model matched their experiences. Overall, the model was found to be useful and adjustments were made from recommendations by the interviewees (Baty et al., 2019).

The interview study also provided information about career trajectories of the interviewees, which led to a framework adapted from the general career development literature. The Career Trajectory Framework is composed of predisposing influences, career change considerations and decisions, and outcomes of career changes (Davis et al., 2019). Cycles of decision making often occur in an iterative manner, together making up a career trajectory. The framework may be used to help plan education and career development during the arc of an individual's career, from the time of considering admission to a genetic counseling training program to legacy plans at career's end. Individual career trajectories may also be visualized as a career lattice, with both horizontal and vertical movement.

The model of advanced training for certified genetic counselors, concept of a genetic counseling career lattice, and Career Trajectory Framework are synergistic with the general educational models discussed in the previous section. *Self-directed learning* is consistent with a preponderance of internally driven motivations to pursue continuing education with the aim of better performing existing professional duties or moving to a new practice setting. Self-directed learning also fits with the choice of many possible paths to multiple advanced skills and career positions. *Experiential learning* coincides with "on the job" paths as well as some aspects of formal academic programs. *Communities of learning* pertain to both cohorts of master's graduate students and continuing education among colleagues and working groups. Implicit in all of these models is the importance of lifelong learning to deepen competence and foster career development.

Conclusion

The development of genetic counseling educational programs has paralleled the growth and professionalization of the field of genetic counseling. In the early 1970s the first graduates of master's genetic counseling programs forged a new profession. The many milestones of professional progress since then influenced genetic counseling education in a reciprocal way, as developments in the field challenged programs to enrich their curricula, and quality education with a focus on core competencies enabled genetic counselors to expand their roles in healthcare. Future developments in genetic counseling education will continue the process of matching education to the expanding requirements of genetic counseling practice while exploring lifelong learning and advanced skill acquisition to create new professional opportunities.

References

Abacan, M., Alsubaie, L., Barlow-Stewart, K., Caanen, B., Cordier, C., Courtney, E., Davoine E., Edwards, J., Elackatt N. J., Gardiner, K., Guan, Y., Huang, L-H., Malmgren, C. I., Kejriwal, S., Kim, H. J., Lambert, D., Lantigua-Cruz, P. A., Lee, J. M. H., Lodahl, M., . . . Wicklund, C. (2019). The global state of the genetic counseling profession. *European Journal of Human Genetics*, 27, 183–197. https://doi.org/10.1038/s41431-018-0252-x

Accreditation Council for Genetic Counseling. (2013). *ACGC is now a proud member of ASPA*. https://www.gceducation.org/acgc-is-now-a-proud-member-of-aspa/

Accreditation Council for Genetic Counseling. (2018). *ACGC annual accreditation report*. https://www.gceducation.org/acgc-annual-accreditation-report/

Accreditation Council for Genetic Counseling. (2019). *Standards of accreditation for graduate programs in genetic counseling*. https://www.gceducation.org/standards-of-accreditation/

Accreditation Council for Genetic Counseling. (2022). *Find an accredited program*. https://www.gceducation.org/students-volunteers/#program

Accreditation Council for Genetic Counseling. (2023). *Practice-based competencies*. https://www.gceducation.org/forms-resources/

American Board of Genetic Counseling. (2016). *Voluntary recertification*. https://www.abgc.net/ABGC/media/Documents/ABGC-Voluntary-Certification-Flyer-9-16_FNL.pdf

American Board of Genetic Counseling. (2018). *ABGC newsletter, Spring 2018*. https://www.abgc.net/ABGC/media/Documents/ABGC_Newsletter_Sp18_webFNL.pdf

American Board of Genetic Counseling. (2019a). *ABGC restructuring committee*. https://www.abgc.net/about-abgc/detailed-history.aspx/

American Board of Genetic Counseling. (2019b). *ABGC newsletter, Spring 2019*. https://www.abgc.net/ABGC/media/Documents/ABGC_Newsletter_Sp19_FNL.pdf

American Board of Genetic Counseling. (2020). *Practice analysis and information*. https://www.abgc.net/for-diplomates/practice-analysis.aspx/

American Board of Genetics and Genomics. (2019). *ABMGG history*. http://www.abmgg.org/pages/history.shtml

Association of Genetic Counseling Program Directors. (2020). Discover GCEA. Educating future genetic counselors. https://educategc.org

Atzinger, C. L., Blough-Pfau, R., Kretschmer, L., Huether, C. A., Johnson, J. A., & Warren, N. S. (2007). Characterization of the practice and attitudes of genetic counselors with doctoral degrees. *Journal of Genetic Counseling*, *16*, 223–239. https://doi.org/10.1007/s10897-006-9062-3

Balkite, B., & Smith, M. (2009). Evolving roles, expanding opportunities. In W. R. Uhlmann, J. L. Schuette, & B. M. Yashar (Eds.), *A guide to genetic counseling* (2nd ed., pp. 523–552). Wiley.

Baty, B. J., Davis, C., Erby, L., Hippman, C., & Trepanier, A. (2019). Genetic counselors with advanced skills: I. Refining a model of advanced training. *Journal of Genetic Counseling*, *29*, 759–770. https://doi.org/10.1002/jgc4.1203

Baty, B. J., Trepanier, A., Bennett, R. L., Davis, C., Erby, L., Hippman, C., Lerner, B., Matthews, A., Myers, M. F., Robbins, C. B., & Singletary, C. N. (2016). Developing a model of advanced training to promote career advancement for certified genetic counselors: An investigation of expanded skills, advanced training paths, and professional opportunities. *Journal of Genetic Counseling*, *25*, 625–634. https://doi.org/10.1007/s10897-015-9916-7

Bluestone, J., Johnson, P., Fullerton, J., Carr, C., Alderman, J., & BonTempo, J. (2013). Effective in-service training design and delivery: Evidence from an integrative literature review. *Human Resources for Health*, *11*, 51.

Bureau of Labor Statistics, U.S. Department of Labor. (2023). *Occupational outlook handbook, genetic counselors*. https://www.bls.gov/ooh/healthcare/genetic-counselors.htm

Canadian Association for Genetic Counselling/Association canadienne de conseil génétique. CAGC-ACCG Annual Newsletter. (2013). https://cagc-accg.ca/doc/CAGC%20Newsletter%20-%20English.pdf/

Canadian Board of Genetic Counselling. (2020a). *Recertification*. https://www.cbgc-cccg.ca/?page=9

Canadian Board of Genetic Counselling. (2020b). *Continuing education credits (CECs)*. https://www.cbgc-cccg.ca/?page=10

Canadian Board of Genetic Counselling. (2023a). *Certification*. https://www.cbgc-cccg.ca/?page=5

Canadian Board of Genetic Counselling. (2023b). *Core competencies*. https://www.cbgc-cccg.ca/?page=40

Cervero, R. M. (1988). *Effective continuing education for professionals*. Jossey-Bass.

Cervero, R. M., & Daley, B. J. (2016). Continuing professional education: A contested space. *New Directions for Adult and Continuing Education*, *2016*, 9–18. https://doi-org/10.1002/ace.20191

Davis, C. R. (2018). *Incorporating innovations into practice: Professional learning of genetic counselors* [Doctoral dissertation, Teachers College, Columbia University].

Davis, C., Baty, B. J., Hippman, C., Trepanier, A., & Erby, L. (2019). Genetic counselors with advanced skills: II. A new career trajectory framework. *Journal of Genetic Counseling*, *29*(5), 771–785. https://doi.org/10.1002/jgc4.1204

Dewey, J. (1938). *Experience and education*. Collier Books.

Doyle, D. L., Awwad, R. I., Austin, J. C., Baty, B. J., Bergner, A. L., Brewster, S. J., Erby, L. A. H., Franklin, C. R., Greb, A. E., Grubs, R. E., Hooker, G. W., Noblin, S. J., Ormond, K. E., Palmer, C. G., Petty, E. M., Singletary, C. N., Thomas, M. J., Walton, C. S., & Uhlmann,

W. R. (2016). 2013 review and update of the genetic counseling practice based competencies by a task force of the accreditation council for Genetic Counseling. *Journal of Genetic Counseling*, 25, 868–879. https://doi.org/10.1007/s10897-016-9984-3

Dumars, K. W. (1978). Genetic associate training program. *Journal of Medical Education*, 53(9), 768–770.

Edwards, J. G. (2013). The transnational alliance for genetic counseling: Promoting international communication and collaboration. *Journal of Genetic Counseling*, 22, 688–689.

Fenwick, T. J. (2000). Expanding conceptions of experiential learning: A review of the five contemporary perspectives on cognition. *Adult Education Quarterly*, 50(4), 243–272.

Ferrier, R. A., Connolly-Wilson, M., Fitzpatrick, J., Grewal, S., Robb, L. Rutberg, J., Lilley, M., & CAGC Core Competencies Working Group. (2013).The establishment of core competencies for Canadian genetic counsellors: Validation of practice based competencies. *Journal of Genetic Counseling*, 22, 690–706. https://doi.org/10.1007/s10897-013-9651-x

Fiddler, M. B., Fine, B. A., & Baker, D. L. (1996). A case-based approach to the development of practice-based competencies for accreditation of and training in graduate programs in genetic counseling. *Journal of Genetic Counseling*, 5, 105–112.

Fine, B. A., Baker, D. L., & Fiddler, M. B. (1996). Practice-based competencies for accreditation of and training in graduate programs in genetic counseling. *Journal of Genetic Counseling*, 5, 113–121.

Frank, J. R., Mungroo, R., Ahmad, Y., Wang, M., De Rossi, S., & Horsley, T. (2010). Toward a definition of competency-based education in medicine: A systematic review of published definitions. *Medical Teacher*, 32, 631–637.

Gaupman, K. M., Edwards, J. E., Brooks, K. A., & Young, S. R. (1991). ASHG/NSGC Activities related to education. The doctoral degree in genetic counseling: Attitudes of genetic counselors. *American Journal of Human Genetics*, 49, 488–493.

Grove, M. E., White, S., Fisk, D. G., Rego, S., Dagan-Rosenfeld, O., Kohler, J. N., Reuter, C. M., Bonner, D., Undiagnosed Diseases Network, Wheeler, M. T., Bernstein, J. A., Ormond, K. E., & Hanson-Kahn, A. K. (2019). Developing a genomics rotation: Practical training around variant interpretation for genetic counseling students. *Journal of Genetic Counseling*, 28, 466–476. https://doi-org/10.1002/jgc4.1094

Grow, G. (1991). Teaching learners to be self-directed: A stage approach. *Adult Education Quarterly*, 41(3), 125–149.

Haverbusch, V. C. E., Heise, E. M., Foreman, A. K. M., & Callanan, N. P. (2019). An examination of the factors contributing to the expansion of subspecialty genetic counseling. *Journal of Genetic Counseling*, 28, 616–625. https://doi-org/10.1002/jgc4.1077

Heimler, A. (1997). An oral history of the National Society of Genetic Counselors. *Journal of Genetic Counseling*, 6, 315–336.

Hudson, P. E., Zajo, K., Gerhardt, C. A., Stanek, J., & Varga, E. (2019). Defining the role of a genetic counselor within pediatric hematology and oncology comprehensive care teams: Perspectives of the provider team and patients. *Journal of Genetic Counseling*, 28, 1139–1147. https://doi-org/10.1002/jgc4.1164

Ingvoldstat, C., Seven, M., Taris, M., Cordier, C., Paneque, M., & Skirton, H. (2016). Components of genetic counsellor education: A systematic review of the peer-reviewed literature. *Journal of Community Genetics*, 7(2), 107–118. https://doi.org/10.1007/s12687-015-0255-z

Kloza, E. (1988). Corner thoughts. *Perspectives in Genetic Counseling*, 10(3), 2.

Knowles, M. S. (1980). *The modern practice of adult education: From pedagogy to andragogy* (2nd ed.). Cambridge Books.

Knowles, M. S., and Associates. (1984). *Andragogy in action: Applying modern principles of adult learning*. Jossey-Bass.

Kolb, D. A. (1984). *Experiential learning: Experience as the source of learning and development*. Prentice Hall.

McWalter, K., Cho, M. T., Hart, T., Nussbaum, R., Sebold, C., Knapke, S., Klein, R., Friedman, B., Willaert, R., Singleton, A., Williams, L., Butler, E., & Juusola, J. (2018). Genetic counseling in industry settings: Opportunities in the era of precision health. *American Journal of Medical Genetics Part C: Seminars in Medical Genetics*, *178C*, 46–53. https://doi.org/10.1002/ajmg.c.31606

Nagy, R., Peay, H., Hicks, M., Kloos, J., Westman, R., Conway, L., Finucane, B., Fitzpatrick, J., Gordon, E., Ramos, E., Sekhon-Warren, J., Silver, J., Walton, C., & Reiser, C. (2014). Genetic counselors' and genetic counseling students' attitudes around the clinical doctorate and other advanced educational options for genetic counselors: A report from the genetic counseling advanced degree task force. *Journal of Genetic Counseling*, *24*, 626–634.

National Society of Genetic Counselors. (1981). *Perspectives in Genetic Counseling*, *3*(3).

National Society of Genetic Counselors. (2018). *Professional status survey 2018: Demographics and methodology*. https://www.nsgc.org/Policy-Research-and-Publications/Professional-Status-Survey

National Society of Genetic Counselors. (2019). *Model legislative provisions*. https://www.nsgc.org/Policy-Research-and-Publications/State-Licensure-for-Genetic-Counselors/Model-Legislative-Provisions

National Society of Genetic Counselors. (2020a). *Professional status survey 2020*. https://www.nsgc.org/Portals/0/Docs/Policy/PSS%20Executive%20Summary%202020%20FINAL%20 05-03-20.pdf

National Society of Genetic Counselors. (2020b). *States issuing licenses for genetic counselors*. https://www.nsgc.org/Policy-Research-and-Publications/State-Licensure-for-Genetic-Cou nselors/States-Issuing-Licenses

National Society of Genetic Counselors. (2020c). *NSGC timeline*. https://www.nsgc.org/About/About-NSGC/Timeline

Ormond, K. E., Abad, P. J., MacLeod, R., Nishigaki, M., & Wessels, T. M. (2024). The global status of genetic counselors in 2023: What has changed in the past 5 years? *Genetics in Medicine Open*, *2*(Suppl 2), 101887. https://doi-org.ezproxy.lib.utah.edu/10.1016/j.gimo.2024.101887

Reed, S. C. (1975). A short history of genetic counseling. *Social Biology*, *21*, 332–339.

Reiser, C., LeRoy, B., Grubs, R., & Walton, C. (2015). Report on an investigation into an entry level clinical doctorate for the genetic counseling profession and a survey of the Association of Genetic Counseling Program Directors. *Genetic Counseling*, *24*(5), 689–701.

Resta, R. (2020). *Why "H.R.3235 The Access to Genetic Counselors Services Act" makes ACMG feel threatened by genetic counselors (again)*. https://thednaexchange.com/2020/03/01/why-h-r-3235-the-access-to-genetic-counselors-services-act-makes-acmg-feel-threatened-by-genetic-counselors-again/

Riconda, D., Grubs, R. E., Campion, M. W., & Cragun, D. (2018). Genetic counselor training for the next generation: Where do we go from here? *American Journal of Medical Genetics*, *178C*, 38–45. https://doi.org/10.1002/ajmg.c.31598

Robertson, M. K., Umble, K. E., & Cervero, R. M. (2003). Impact studies in continuing education for health professions: Update. *Journal of Continuing Education in the Health Professions*, *23*(3), 146–156.

Rollnick, B. R. (1981). Continuing education criteria: A proposal presented to the Annual Membership Meeting of the National Society of Genetic Counselors, Inc. *Perspectives in Genetic Counseling*, *3*(4), 2–4.

Rollnick, B. R. (1983). Continuing education criteria and continuing education units: Policy issues. *Perspectives in Genetic Counseling*, *5*(1), 1.

Sarah Lawrence College. (2019). *History of the Joan H. Marks Graduate Program in Human Genetics*. https://www.sarahlawrence.edu/genetic-counseling/history.html.

Schon. D. A. (1983). *The reflective practitioner: How professionals think in action*. Basic Books.

Scott, J. A., Walker, A. P., Eunpu, D. L., & Djurdjinovic, L. (1988). Genetic counselor training: A review and considerations for the future. *American Journal of Human Genetics*, *42*, 191–199.

Skirton, H., Lewis, C., Kent, A., Coviello, D. A., & Members of Eurogentest Unit 6 and ESHG Education Committee. (2010). Genetic education and the challenge of genomic medicine: Development of core competences to support preparation of health professionals in Europe. *European Journal of Human Genetics*, *18*(9), 972–977.

Smith, A. C. M., & Heimler, A. (1980). Certification of genetic counselors. *Perspectives in Genetic Counseling*, *2*(2), 1,5.

Stern, A. M. (2012). *Telling genetics: The story of genetic counseling in America*. Johns Hopkins University Press.

Swanson, A., Ramos, E., & Snyder, H. (2014). Next generation sequencing is the impetus for the next generation of laboratory-based genetic counselors. *Journal of Genetic Counseling*, *23*, 647–654. https://doi-org/10.1007/s10897-013-9684-1

Transnational Alliance for Genetic Counseling. (2020). *About the TAGC international network*. https://sc.edu/study/colleges_schools/medicine/centers_and_institutes_new/transnational_alliance_for_genetic_counseling/index.php

Valverde, K., Mueller, R., Paciotti, B., & Conway, L. (2016). An exploratory study of employers' attitudes towards a clinical doctorate in genetic counseling. *Journal of Genetic Counseling*, *25*, 179–188.

Walker, A. P. (1979). Asilomar East. *Perspectives in Genetic Counseling*, *1*, 1–4.

Walker, A. P., Scott, J. A., Biesecker, B. B., Conover, B., Blake, W., & Djurdjinovic, L. (1990). Report of the 1989 Asilomar meeting on education in genetic counseling. *American Journal of Human Genetics*, *46*, 1223–1230.

Wallace, J. P., Myers, M. F., Huether, C. A., Bedard, A. C., & Warren, N. S. (2008). Employability of genetic counselors with a PhD in genetic counseling. *Journal of Genetic Counseling*, *17*, 209–219.

Waltman, L., Runke, C., Balcom, J., Riley, J. D., Lilley, M., Christian, S., Zetszche, L., & Goodenberger, M. L. (2016). Further defining the role of the laboratory genetic counselor. *Journal of Genetic Counseling*, *25*, 786–798. https://doi.org/10.1007/s10897-015-9927-4

Webster-Wright, A. (2009). Reframing professional development through understanding authentic professional learning. *Review of Educational Research*, *79*(2), 702–739.

Wenger, E. (1998). *Communities of practice: Learning, meaning, and identity*. Cambridge University Press.

Wenger, E. (2011). *Communities of practice: A brief introduction*. https://scholarsbank.uoregon.edu/xmlui/handle/1794/11736

CHAPTER 3

THE PROFESSIONALIZATION OF GENETIC COUNSELING

VICKIE L. VENNE AND EDWARD M. KLOZA

Introduction: What Is a Profession?

As the field of clinical genetics is relatively new, complex, and yet a common staple of the popular media, the question "What is a genetic counselor?" is one that many, if not most, practitioners of the profession have been asked frequently. While "teacher," "doctor," "nurse," "engineer," "plumber," and even "financial advisor" identify a wide scope with differing expertise within each of those occupations, a mental image of the profession easily comes to mind. To be identified as a profession, the practitioners must exhibit essential, exclusive, and complex skills. And they need to identify a niche that separates themselves from others with similar (and often overlapping) characteristics (Forsyth & Danisiewicz, 1985). In addition, a profession is typically distinguished by a professional association, perhaps a journal, a code of ethics, and, in the healthcare delivery field, accreditation with certification, licensure, and credentialing (Baty, 2018). Genetic counseling, based on these distinguishing features, represents a unique profession.

This chapter describes key milestones in the development of the genetic counseling profession in the United States.[1] It examines the initial efforts to distinguish physician geneticists from genetic counselors as well as current congressional efforts for Centers for Medicare and Medicaid Services (CMS) recognition. The early challenges that culminated in opting for the term "genetic counselor" and the establishment of the National Society of Genetic Counselors (NSGC) are recounted. Major achievements that are discussed include the creation of an executive office, a code of ethics, and publications such as the *Journal of Genetic Counseling* (JOGC), the formation of the American Board of Genetic Counseling, and the process of licensure.

[1] Editors' note: For a global perspective on genetic counseling, see Chapter 34 by Mercy Ygoña Laurino and Austin Emanuel Bland in this volume.

What's in a Name?

Shakespeare asked this long before graduates of the nascent genetic counseling programs began grappling with the question themselves as they struggled with differentiating who they were and what they did on their way to establishing a unique profession. At the time, and given the expanse of other issues these alumnae (as most were women) had to address, the implications of this determination could have been easily underestimated. After all, how much difference could it make whether we called ourselves "counselors," "associates," or "assistants"? As it turned out, these early practitioners recognized that their decision regarding a professional label would have a lasting impact on the development and growth of the profession itself.

Until the mid-1970s, providing genetic information to families was largely the purview of physicians—typically pediatricians or obstetricians—responding to families in which a child had been born with a birth defect or working with couples wondering if their developing baby would be healthy (Reed, 1974). Other than dysmorphology and family history evaluations, physicians had access to relatively few of the resources that they have at their disposal today. Biochemical tests and chromosome analysis (with primitive banding) were the primary laboratory options. Molecular genetics was decades away. Amniocentesis to evaluate fetal chromosomes only became available in 1966, and maternal serum screening for Down syndrome was not offered clinically until 1986 (Golbus et al., 1979; Palomaki, 1986).

When Sarah Lawrence College accepted the first genetic counseling class in 1969 and several other master's-level training programs launched in the 1970s, the clinical experiences offered to their students fell under the umbrella of "genetic counseling." While the term had been coined in 1948 (Reed, 1974), many of the communication responsibilities overlapped with those of medical geneticists once a diagnosis was confirmed. By the mid-1970s, graduates of these programs were actively discussing the formation of a professional society, an important milestone in the development of a burgeoning profession.

What to call themselves was high on the agenda when master's-trained genetics experts first gathered in 1978 to discuss forming a professional organization (Heimler, 1979). They recognized that the name they chose for the profession would determine, to a significant extent, how broad or narrow their perceived scope of activities would be. Too narrow of a focus would possibly create an impediment to filling yet-unseen clinical or administrative gaps in genetic services; too broad of a focus could give the mistaken impression that these new genetic specialists had nothing new or valuable to offer.

While those who trained in master's-level programs typically earned their degree in genetic counseling, job titles varied, as they do now to some degree. Descriptive options at that time included "genetic associate," "genetic assistant," and "genetic counselor." Audrey Heimler (who would become the first president of the new professional organization, the NSGC) recalled spirited discussions among counselors (Heimler, 1997). The By-Laws Committee established to form the organization gave serious consideration to "genetic associates" and liked the flexibility of this title, since not all graduates were providing clinical counseling. Another concern was that "counselor" might suggest to some that their clients/patients were somehow damaged or weak, invoking comparisons to marriage counselors salvaging floundering relationships or substance abuse counselors addressing addiction. Those advocating for genetic "counselor" argued that it validated the training and expertise conferred by the education of the graduates and were concerned that the term "associate" conjured the idea of subordination. There was an expectation that professionals could educate others about the title such that the word "counselor" would be viewed in the intended context—professionals trained to guide families through an ever-changing field unfamiliar to most.

Medical geneticists, who often employed and worked with these new genetic specialists, also had opinions about the name. There was significant disapproval of the term "counselor." It was regarded as encompassing responsibilities that were considered exclusively in the realm of licensed physicians, such as making a diagnosis, documenting a family history, estimating the risk of recurrence, helping the family determine an action to take, and identifying and counseling extended family members (Fraser, 1974). "Practicing medicine without a license" was a common allegation in some conversations, and these early debates prepared master's-trained genetic specialists to defend their role in the genetics community, as they continue to do. As the By-Laws Committee continued to explore the future of this new profession, three meetings convened stakeholders from around the country, in large part to discuss a common educational framework for this new profession. One of the meetings, sponsored by the March of Dimes, specifically considered "the role of the genetics associate in the provision of genetic services and to explore means of supporting the new professional" (Walker, 1979, p. 1). It was at that meeting that the designation of "genetic counselor" was accepted to describe graduates of a master's-level program, signified by the following meeting recommendation: "Efforts should be made to secure general acceptance of the job classification 'genetic counselor' by relevant governmental agencies, hospitals, clinics, and other providers of health services" (Walker, 1979, p. 2). It is interesting to note that the name debate arose again in 2005 (Blumenthal & Biesecker, 2005), and at a plenary session of the NSGC Annual Conference in 2023 (Means et al., 2023). "Genetic counselor" still carried the day.

Forming the National Society of Genetic Counselors

Once the organization's, and with it, the profession's, name was determined, membership criteria for the NSGC needed to be established. The By-Laws Committee was again called upon to deal with the contentious issues of eligibility criteria and membership categories. In addition to medical geneticists (who provided genetic counseling as well as taught and mentored genetic counselors), other allied health professionals such as nurses and social workers were increasingly involved with genetic issues and laid claim to professional counseling skills. Elizabeth Thompson, a nurse with deep roots in clinical genetics, advocated for "full membership status for registered nurses and those with master's degrees in other fields, whose knowledge of genetic disorders and counseling was acquired during training and/or in job settings" (Heimler, 1997, p. 321). Joan Weiss, representing social workers, felt that most of them would identify with their own professional society (social work), so associate membership in the NSGC would be reasonable (Heimler, 1997).

Ultimately, three membership categories were established. *Full membership* was reserved for persons with a master's or PhD in human genetics from a recognized genetic counseling training program or in a related field (nursing, social work, public health) if their primary responsibility was genetic counseling encompassing a broad range of genetic disorders. *Associate membership* was available for those whose interest focused on genetic counseling but who did not desire or qualify for full or student membership. *Student membership* was available for students in a college or master's degree program (NSGC, 2014).

On October 1, 1979, the NSGC was legally incorporated. One of the early actions of this new *national* professional organization involved creating a mechanism to ensure *regional* representation. Six geographic regions were identified, corresponding to service regions established by the Department of Health, Education, and Welfare (currently the Department of Health and Human Services; McInerney, 1979). These regions were already supported by regional genetic programs, and genetic counselors in these regions were, at that time, already coordinating and sharing interests with other professional genetic colleagues in their regions. Prior to the advent of email, listservs, and online meetings, continuing education and communications were more limited, and regional meetings or conferences were convened annually or biennially. The first regional meeting took place in Berkeley, California, on May 19, 1979, and the other five regions had active planning committees in place at that time. The expectation was that the meetings could be used not only to share clinical and counseling advances but also to discuss administrative issues relevant to the profession and the NSGC. Elected representatives for each region would serve on the board of directors, bringing constituents' concerns from regional meetings to the national forum, and vice versa. By July 1980, a relationship with the March of Dimes Birth Defects Foundation was established, which resulted in financial support for several subsequent national NSGC educational meetings.

Publications and the Birth of the *Journal of Genetic Counseling*

Regional representatives were expected to stay in touch with members prior to the availability of email and listservs, and they often communicated by phone or post. A commitment to communicate was met on a society-wide level with a quarterly newsletter that was mailed to each member. The first issue, published in March 1979, was four pages, with no date or title on its masthead (Heimler, 1979). With Deborah Eunpu as the first editor, the newsletter took on a more professional format and included general operational news, updates from leadership, letters from members, case studies, invited discussions about controversial topics, and, most important for many, job postings. Periodically, such as in 1981, a special issue was published to highlight findings from the Professional Status Survey (Begleiter et al., 1981), which is discussed below.

Most genetic counselors in the 1980s were in clinical roles housed in academic settings. As their colleagues were publishing in clinical journals, few genetic counselors had a venue to publish articles related to their practice. As one more step toward professionalization, many felt it was time for genetic counselors to establish a publication that would focus on clinical, educational, ethical, and legal topics specific to genetic counseling. In the late 1980s, an ad hoc committee chaired by Ed Kloza explored the logistics and feasibility of a journal specific to the genetic counseling profession (Kloza, 1989). The committee recognized the need for a journal focused on the scholarly research specific to genetic counseling as well as the responsibility of the profession to encourage it. Thus was born the JOGC in March 1992, published quarterly with Deborah Eunpu serving as the inaugural editor (Eunpu, 1992).

In addition to two to three original articles and letters to the editor, the first few volumes included a "Genetic Library" column, which reviewed articles relevant to the profession (Resta, 1993). Over the next 30 years of publication, the quality of content and professional recognition of the JOGC continued to flourish under the successive editorial leadership of Robert Resta, Allyn McConkie-Rosell, Bonnie LeRoy, Christina Palmer, and Jehannine Austin. By 1998, the journal grew from being a quarterly publication to producing six issues per year (Resta, 1997).

The first "special issue" of JOGC was published in June 1997 (Schneider & Resta, 1997), containing original articles focused on providing cancer genetic counseling. This was followed by a second special issue about cancer counseling nearly a decade later (Venne & Schneider, 2006). During LeRoy's tenure as journal editor, the JOGC was publishing, on average, one special issue annually in addition to regular issues. Due to the growth of article quality, reputation, and global scope of the JOGC throughout the 1990s and to the present, it is now commonly recognized as *the* flagship journal of the genetic counseling profession.

Professional growth is commonly reflected and recognized by the increased quality, utilization, and number of submissions to a professional journal. But professional growth is also reflected through recognition from outside the profession. To that end, when McConkie-Rosell served as journal editor, she worked tirelessly to have the JOGC included in a variety of abstracting and indexing services. Beginning with Volume 18, published in 2009, the JOGC was indexed and abstracted in Science Citation Index Expanded. This meant that the first impact factor—a measure of the average number of citations that articles published in a specific journal have received in the past 2 years—was first available in 2012 (National Center for Biotechnical Information, 2020). Though it is a controversial measure, the impact factor allows a rough comparison of quality among similar journals, and a higher impact factor number generally reflects increasing quality of submissions.

As genetic counselors begin seeking professional recognition in their positions, especially in academia, one common criterion of such recognition includes publication in a journal distinguished by a comparatively high impact factor. Therefore, since many genetic counselors publish in the JOGC, the journal's impact factor typically enhances their opportunities for academic advancement. Thus, the assignment of an impact factor became an important step in the growth of the profession.

Practice Guidelines

Additional documents that enhanced the genetic counseling profession came in the form of position statements and practice guidelines. Position statements are typically the profession's response to social issues and are often grounded in a professional code of ethics; they will be discussed later in the chapter. Practice guidelines are published documents resulting from a committee review of evidence-based clinical data to assist healthcare professionals with clinical challenges or quality improvement in care. The Institute of Medicine (IOM) characterizes guideline recommendations as follows: "Clinical Practice Guidelines are statements that include recommendations intended to optimize patient care that are informed by a systematic review of evidence and an assessment of the benefits and harms of alternative care options" (IOM, 2011, p. 15). Practice guidelines can be published by the organization alone or jointly with other professional organizations. The rigorous process consistent with IOM standards has been adopted by many professional organizations, including the NSGC. Examples of topics covered by NSGC practice guidelines include multiple miscarriage recurrence risk, cancer risks, family history collection, and consanguinity counseling. A key aspect of practice guidelines is that they are evidence based and periodically reviewed. Thus, practice guidelines may be considered as professional standards, deviation from which may raise the specter of legal liability for the practitioner. Clinical guidance documents that can also impact the practice of genetic counseling include practice resources, which can help healthcare professionals deliver consistent and high-quality care, though they do not meet the same evidentiary standards as practice guidelines.

National Conferences

In addition to the aforementioned regional meetings, the first national NSGC conference was held in 1981 in San Diego, California (Rollnick, 1981), and was financially supported by the March of Dimes. The meeting consisted of three invited speakers, five workshops, and seven contributed papers, and the occasion served as an opportunity for the 182 attendees to network. Given the success of the meeting and the corresponding momentum that the NSGC enjoyed, a decision was made to hold annual educational conferences.

During the first 18 years, the NSGC's annual conference was held in conjunction with the American Society of Human Genetics (ASHG) annual meeting in the fall. NSGC membership was still relatively small, and meetings were held in large hotels rather than convention centers. In the early 1990s, the Louisiana legislature's decision to significantly limit access to abortion caused NSGC leadership to reconsider holding its 1993 conference in New Orleans along with the ASHG. Considerations of the value that many genetic counselors place on reproductive freedom resulted in the NSGC Board of Directors boycotting New Orleans and choosing an alternate acceptable venue (Leopold, 1992). While the ASHG, with a larger attendance, was locked into financially restrictive contracts at the convention center, the NSGC was able to pivot to an Atlanta, Georgia, location in 1993. After 1993, the NSGC and ASHG continued to meet jointly until 2000, when the NSGC disengaged its conference from the ASHG to meet in Savannah, Georgia, and it has maintained its independent conference format since then. Because about 50% of the NSGC membership regularly attends the conference, and because of its steady and rapid growth, the NSGC eventually outgrew hotel conference settings. Since 2005, the conferences have moved to cities with conference centers that can accommodate 2,000 to 4,000 or more attendees, with space for associated plenary presentations, workshops/breakout sessions, concurrent platform presentations, posters, special interest group meetings, and vendors.

Creation of an Executive Office

During the first decade of the profession, most of the NSGC's operations were conducted by volunteers, almost all with full-time jobs. Committees, board meetings, planning sessions, publications, and annual conferences were managed by phone, post, and fax machine. In 1981, a membership directory was organized and collated by volunteers before being printed and mailed to all 282 members. The annual conferences were especially time-consuming to organize. In 1984, Deb Eunpu approached the part-time executive director of the local Committee to Combat Huntington Disease, Bea Leopold. They both participated in the Philadelphia Huntington Disease Clinic at that time, with Leopold serving as an advocate for the families. Leopold, who had experience coordinating meetings, was invited to attend the sixth annual education conference (in Philadelphia) and then was hired to plan the conference the following year in San Diego. Her success with that meeting led to an invitation to become the first executive director, a part-time position that she started in 1987.

Leopold was instrumental in growing the NSGC as a profession. Under her guidance, the NSGC moved away from a dining-room-table effort to an independent, cohesive, national organization. Prior to her tenure, the NSGC secretary, treasurer, and annual conference coordinator each kept a separate (and not always similar) database. Leopold combined, computerized, and updated these databases as board leadership changed. This simple but important task signaled the beginning of formal organization of the membership. And the organization grew. Quarterly newsletters, membership management, annual conference logistics, and much more were handled by the executive office. With an executive director (and staff support) to manage operations, the board of directors was able to focus on the NSGC's mission. This led to another legacy Leopold left the organization—the strategic planning process. Beginning in 1988, it became customary for the incoming NSGC president to attend, with the executive director, a management training meeting. That long weekend event was an opportunity to network with other nonprofit organizations, learn association language and processes, and brainstorm the vision that the incoming president would bring to the organization. From those meetings and a close working association with NSGC leadership, Leopold instituted a strategic planning process that continues to drive the NSGC into the future.[2]

The rapid growth of the profession, from about 300 members in 1981 to around 2,000 members in 2005, and the increased demands on the organization to complete its strategic goals prompted the transition to a larger, more experienced executive office (Weiloch, 2005). SmithBucklin, located in Chicago, was at that time the nation's largest association management firm. It had extensive public relations, marketing, fundraising, and lobbying experience and was well staffed and strategically connected. Fundraising became a priority, since the NSGC also created the Genetic Counseling Foundation in 2005 to support research, education, policy development, and collaborative projects within the field of genetic counseling (Allain & Ormond, 2005). Though there was much enthusiasm for the

[2] Details based on personal correspondence between the authors and Bea Leopold.

foundation, financial support never met expectations. A decision was made to fold the foundation in 2007.

By 2020, the SmithBucklin executive office staff included one full-time executive director and 29 part-time employees who work in both Chicago and Washington, DC offices. The partnership between the executive office staff and the NSGC members is a rich one that successfully drives the growing profession. Staff responsibilities include operations as well as education, sales, and government relations. The direction and responsibilities are dictated by the strategic plan, which is evaluated regularly. However, the implementation of the strategic plan and society goals is possible in part because over 1,000 NSGC members volunteer in some way each year. While some of the volunteer activity is highly visible (board of directors, committee chairs, publications, conference committee members), other members volunteer as part of committees and may never directly interact with a staff member.

Professional Status Survey

As the NSGC executive office became the organizing hub for the genetic counseling profession, curiosity arose regarding the demographics of the profession as well as the types of settings in which genetic counselors worked. While these data might prove to be interesting and helpful as the profession examined trends and tried to anticipate needs, perhaps the question whose response was most anticipated was "How much do you earn?" Beginning in 1980, a Professional Status Survey was distributed to all NSGC members, who were encouraged to respond completely and honestly regarding (among many other questions) their educational background and work environment, along with their salary and benefits (Begleiter et al., 1981). Each counselor was then able to evaluate where they stood with respect to other counselors using factors such as region, type of institution, and/or specialty. Armed with this documentation, they were able to petition their employers for salary or benefit increases or revised workloads. Counselors could consider locating to a region that offered better pay or changing their specialty or type of institution (e.g., academic medical center vs. commercial laboratory). Between 1980 and 1989 there were three surveys; afterward, the surveys were conducted every 2 years from 1990 to 2018. The expansion and diversification of the field has resulted in surveys being distributed and published annually since 2019. This detailed profile, which recently began including counselors outside of the United States, is also used by employers, human resource departments, and prospective counseling students to document professional expectations.

The National Society of Genetic Counselors Code of Ethics

The nascent professionals in genetic counseling, already dealing with sensitive issues such as confidentiality in the face of family dynamics, nondirectiveness, patient self-determination, pregnancy termination, and the right to die, had no idea in 1985 that by 2020, they would be faced with quandaries about cloning, gene editing, and in vitro fertilization. Nevertheless, genetic counselors recognized at that time that the profession needed, both for itself and for outsiders—some of whom were critical of the field—an ethical framework that could guide genetic counselors' professional behaviors and obligations. The NSGC leadership asked Judith Benkendorf to chair an ad hoc Committee on Ethical Codes and Principles. The committee first reviewed the codes of ethics of several health professions, such as the American Nurses Association and the American Association for Counseling and Development, deemed similar enough to genetic counseling to provide insight into what a genetic counseling code of ethics should resemble. The committee recommended that the NSGC develop a code of ethics that outlined how counselors should interact with their clients, their colleagues, and society, as well as how they should regard their own position and obligations to self. The NSGC Code of Ethics was first published in 1992 (Benkendorf et al., 1992) and has since been revised three times, the latest amendment occurring in 2017 (Senter et al., 2018).

A code of ethics informs potential members of expectations and, if integrated into their training, can enhance their ability to recognize and resolve ethical challenges and conflicts of interest. Though not stated as such, the NSGC Code of Ethics acknowledges that genetic counselors, by virtue of the arcane and sensitive knowledge they have of genetics and of the patient/family, wield power that should be used for the benefit, not detriment, of the patient. It also protects the genetic counselor if a request is made of them to act in a manner contrary to the NSGC Code of Ethics. This is a professional safeguard that genetic counselors are expected to take seriously.

Producing a code of ethics is a dynamic process that has resulted in thoughtful organizational reflections and actions, one of which was the development of a conflict-of-interest document. In mid-2016, the NSGC chartered a task force to explore this issue on behalf of the membership. That group developed resources to assist NSGC members in identifying and mitigating potential conflicts arising from the practice of their profession (NSGC, 2018; Senter et al., 2018; Stoll et al., 2017).

Another byproduct of the NSGC Code of Ethics was the formation of the NSGC's *position statements*. The final section of the NSGC Code of Ethics speaks to the relationship between genetic counselors and society. To that end, in 2010, the first position statement, addressing reproductive freedom, was published (NSGC, 2020a).[3] Many position statements are suggested by members, and those that are developed are presented to the membership for comment before a final adoption by a majority vote of the board of directors. This mechanism does not preclude the issuing of timely statements in response to unexpected or impactful events affecting the profession, such as the United States Supreme Court's overturning of *Roe v. Wade* and *Planned Parenthood v. Casey* with its 2022 *Dobbs v. Jackson Women's Health Organization* decision. The NSGC's "Statement RE: Supreme Court Decision on *Dobbs v. Jackson Women's Health Organization*" was released jointly with the American College of Genetics and Genomics and the ASHG immediately after the issuing of that decision (NSGC, 2022). The public statement demonstrates the NSGC's shared values with other genetic organizations and reaffirms much of the content of the NSGC's first position statement.

[3] Editors' note: This position statement was revised by the NSGC in 2022.

Departure From the American Board of Medical Genetics

A serious threat to the forward progress of the profession occurred in the early 1990s when the American Board of Medical Genetics (ABMG)[4] applied to the American Board of Medical Specialties (ABMS) to accept medical genetics as a specialty (Kloza, 1992). The ABMS required a description of the ABMG membership, and when it learned that a substantial proportion (~40%) of ABMG members were master's-level genetic counselors, the ABMS would only conditionally recognize the ABMG. As an arm of the American Medical Association, the ABMS wanted to limit membership to physicians. The ABMG also included a significant number of PhDs, but while a precedent existed in radiation medicine for the inclusion of doctoral-level practitioners, no such provision existed for individuals with master's degrees. For the ABMG and medical geneticists to be welcomed into the ABMS, the ABMG would need to divest itself of all nondoctoral members. Genetic counselor members had taken the same exams as MD and PhD members and had earned their ABMG certification. Attempts were made to persuade the ABMS to include genetic counselors, and many avenues of appeal were explored though ultimately rejected. For the ABMG to move forward with their application, its members had to vote out the master's-level counselors by a two-thirds majority. Genetic counselors made up nearly 40% of the ABMG membership, and if they voted as a bloc to oppose separation, then the vote would fail, and genetic counselors would retain their position in the ABMG. However, it was recognized that this action could create significant challenges. For example, genetic counselors might be regarded as the group that prevented (or delayed) the recognition of medical genetics as a medical specialty. This exclusion likely would have resulted in medical geneticists having to piggyback onto recognized specialties such as pediatrics and obstetrics, within which many of them practiced, for professional standing and financial reimbursement in practice.

Discussion and debate between genetic counselors and medical geneticists sometimes deteriorated into divisive confrontation. Even within the genetic counseling community itself, relationships were strained as it became clear that this issue posed an existential threat to the profession—both sides thinking that their position was the only one with a future.

The ABMG did not intend to set counselors adrift. The organization arranged financial support for the creation of the American Board of Genetic Counseling (ABGC). It also supported a restructuring committee of counselors to create the infrastructure upon which the ABGC would be built. The understanding was that genetic counselors who were ABMG certified would retain their certification but would no longer be considered ABMG "members." Furthermore, these ABMG-certified counselors could be grandparented into the newly formed ABGC. Going forward, it would be the ABGC, not the ABMG, that would set certification requirements for counselors and (currently under its offshoot, the Accreditation Council for Genetic Counseling) accreditation standards for genetic counseling programs (Gettig, 1992).

[4] Editors' note: While at the time of these events the organization was the ABMG, it is now the American Board of Medical Genetics and Genomics.

Ultimately, the vote in 1992 wasn't close: Nearly 1,000 ABMG members voted in favor of the split, and 200 in opposition (Spence, 1992). Many consider this divestiture from ABMG oversight to be the catalyst for the rapid expansion and growth of an independent genetic counseling profession, though at the time, some saw it as the beginning of the end.

Professional Advancement

One approach to promoting professional growth is the development of funding mechanisms that support research and activities that advance the profession. The NSGC Jane Engelberg Memorial Fund (JEMF) and Audrey Heimler Special Projects Award are both competitive financial awards that provide recipients dedicated time to complete a proposed project. Since 1993, when it was awarded to Katherine Schneider to write a book on cancer genetic counseling, the JEMF finances scholarly investigation to promote the practice of genetic counseling. That same year, Vivian Wang received a Special Projects Award to write a training handbook about cross-cultural counseling. It focuses on the direct provision of genetic services. That Special Projects Award has subsequently been renamed to acknowledge the vital role that Audrey Heimler has had in the profession. These NSGC funding mechanisms continue to provide opportunities for members to engage in scholarly activities that enhance genetic counseling knowledge, research, and practice.

Another mechanism used by the NSGC to grow the profession is the creation of awards or honors intended to recognize work that advances the profession. Dr. Beverly Rollnick and Beth Fine Kaplan, two early leaders of the organization, are memorialized during the annual conference. For the Dr. Beverly Rollnick lecture a speaker explores either the genetic counseling profession or the individuals and families counseled through a creative lens. Beth Fine Kaplan helped develop the Northwestern University Graduate Program in Genetic Counseling, and her dedication to educational excellence is recognized each year as a newly graduated student is honored with a Best Student Abstract Award in her name.

Licensure and Scope of Practice

From 1982 to 2000, the number of genetic counselors who demonstrated competency by successfully sitting for the certification exam grew. These certified genetic counselors were hired in academic settings, clinics, laboratories, and many other organizations, holding a wide range of responsibilities. However, as the field of genetics grew, many healthcare providers and self-proclaimed, untrained "counselors" were offering opinions regarding medical direction for patients. Some of those opinions were harmful. An incomplete understanding of Mendelian genetics, an inability to interpret a germline genetic test report (especially a variant of uncertain significance), and a paternalistic attitude or belief in how much a patient should be told have resulted in individuals making healthcare decisions they might not otherwise make if better informed. In the interest of public safety, genetic counselors started down the road to professional licensure (Bensend et al., 2014; Greendale & Pyeritz, 2001).

Though protection of the public was the first priority, a number of genetic counselors believed licensure would also foster the sustainability of the profession. It was recognized that genetic counselors needed to generate a revenue stream for healthcare organizations to invest in their employment. Part of this occurs when a profession is formally recognized by payors. Payors recognize credentialed healthcare professionals, and credentialing is most typically granted to licensed providers.

So began the effort to obtain licensure. In 2000, California was the first state to pass a licensure law (NSGC, 2023), followed by several years of developing the rules for the license application. The first genetic counselors were licensed in California in 2011. The Utah legislature passed a genetic counseling licensure law in spring of 2002, and because the rules committee had been proactive, the first genetic counselor licenses were issued that same year (NSGC, 2023). Early in that process, one of the key components was the right to exclusive use of the professional label "genetic counselor," another important step on the road to professionalism.

Another requirement of licensure is continuing education. As explained above, a cohort of genetic counselors were charter diplomates of the newly formed ABGC in 1993. When those genetic counselors first had become diplomates of the ABMG between 1982 and 1993, their certification did not come with formal continuing education requirements. The genetic counselors certified by the ABGC from 1996 forward were required to demonstrate proof of continuing education (or re-sit the exam), initially every 10 years, but since 2009, every 5 years.[5] One of the many ways in which licensure protects the public is that it requires genetic counselors to possess current knowledge in the field, so with licensure came documentation of continuing education for the charter genetic counselor ABGC diplomates.

With licensure laws comes codification of the clinical scope of practice for genetic counselors. While, as with many professions, genetic counselors are involved in administration, education, management, research, public health, and a variety of nonclinical roles, licensure focuses on clinical care (NSGC, 2020b). Specifically, it describes the range of responsibilities that a clinical professional is trained and competent to perform. While the profession can determine its scope of practice, state licensure laws also define the scope of practice for genetic counselors. Over half of the states in the United States have licensure laws in place, but their language varies considerably. It was not until 2007 that the NSGC offered model language for licensure (NSGC, 2020c). Still, legislators can modify the language to accommodate political and administrative requirements. One example of this was the inclusion of "conscientious objection" that was written directly into the genetic counseling regulations in several states. The concept of conscientious objection in healthcare is the ability of a provider to perform or educate based on moral or other personal beliefs. Recently, this conscientious objection clause has been invoked by providers who refuse to deliver (or refer patients to) services such as contraception or abortion. This language stands in tension with several of the NSGC position statements (NSGC, 2020a). However, since most laws regarding licensure of genetic counselors are part of the state legal code under an umbrella that includes all healthcare providers, and the conscientious objection language was originally written into that overarching law, it is now understood not to be an effort to legislate the comprehensive options that most genetic counselors offer in their clinical service.

[5] Details from correspondence between the authors and the ABGC.

Table 3.1 The National Society of Genetic Counselors' Model Legislative Provisions for Genetic Counselor Scope of Practice

The National Society of Genetic Counselors outlines the following for genetic counselor scope of practice:

a) obtain and evaluate individual, family, and medical histories to determine genetic risk for genetic/medical conditions and diseases in a patient, his/her offspring, and other family members;
b) discuss the features, natural history, means of diagnosis, genetic and environmental factors, and management of risk for genetic/medical conditions and diseases;
c) identify, order, and coordinate genetic laboratory tests and other diagnostic studies as appropriate for the genetic assessment;
d) integrate genetic laboratory test results and other diagnostic studies with personal and family medical history to assess and communicate risk factors for genetic/medical conditions and diseases;
e) explain the clinical implications of genetic laboratory tests and other diagnostic studies and their results;
f) evaluate the client's or family's responses to the condition or risk of recurrence and provide client-centered counseling and anticipatory guidance;
g) identify and utilize community resources that provide medical, educational, financial, and psychosocial support and advocacy; and
h) provide written documentation of medical, genetic, and counseling information for families and health care professionals.

Source: From NSGC (2020d).

Table 3.1 contains the elements that the NSGC suggests as model language for states considering licensing genetic counselors. Much of it is broad and relatively unchanged since the early days of genetic counseling, although the information has become more complex. However, one contentious point in the model language has to do with the ability to independently order genetic testing. While it has been common for genetic counselors to identify and coordinate genetic laboratory tests, and several studies have documented that physicians and other healthcare providers may not order and interpret genetic laboratory tests appropriately, the concern has to do with infringing on the scope of practice for other healthcare professionals (Baars et al., 2005; Hamilton et al., 2017; Wakefield et al., 2018).

Licensure is also essential to credentialing, which is the process of evaluating the qualifications and practice history of a medical provider. This assessment is usually conducted by a facility or agency and is often the final step before a genetic counselor can provide and bill for direct patient care.

Federal Recognition

Even with licensure, financial sustainability continues to be a challenge for the profession, as the CMS does not currently recognize genetic counselors as healthcare providers who can independently bill and receive reimbursement for services. The result is that genetic counselors are typically not reimbursed by the CMS for genetic counseling services, although that remains an option for physicians and nurse practitioners. On June 12, 2019, H.R. 3235, "Access to Genetic Counselor Services Act of 2019," was introduced to the U.S. House of Representatives by Rep. Dave Loebsack (D-IA) and Rep. Mike Kelly (R-PA). This bill would authorize the CMS to recognize certified genetic counselors as healthcare providers and therefore cover services furnished by genetic counselors under the Medicare program. This recognition would increase the opportunities to be recognized by other payors. The secretary of the Department of Health and Human Services will set criteria for regulations, which will be tied to licensure for the state in which genetic counselors are currently licensed. Until the other states enact licensure, ABGC certification will likely be used.

Conclusion

In a relatively short period of time, genetic counseling has established itself as a full-fledged health profession. Many steps along the way were taken by bold individuals who contributed to its growth. The profession of genetic counseling is inextricably connected with the explosive growth of human genetics in the second half of the 20th century and will likely continue to grow along with it. The range of clinical, research, commercial, laboratory, educational, and entrepreneurial choices that marked the first 40 years may well be matched by yet-unknown opportunities in the next 40 years.

References

Allain, D., & Ormond, K. (2005). The Genetic Counseling Foundation: A foundation of the national society of genetic counselors. *Perspectives in Genetic Counseling*, *27*(3), 1.

Baars, M. J., Henneman, L., & Ten Kate, L. P. (2005). Deficiency of knowledge of genetics and genetic tests among general practitioners, gynecologists, and pediatricians: A global problem. *Genetics in Medicine*, *7*(9), 605–610. https://doi.org/10.1097/01.gim.0000182895.28432.c7

Baty, B. J. (2018). Genetic counseling: Growth of the profession and the professional. *American Journal of Medical Genetics Part C: Seminars in Medical Genetics*, *178*(1), 54–62. https://doi.org/10.1002/ajmg.c.31601

Begleiter, M. L., Collins, D. L., & Greendale, K. (1981). NSGC Professional Status Survey. *Perspectives in Genetic Counseling*, *3*(4), 1.

Benkendorf, J. L., Callanan, N. P., Grobstein, R., Schmerler, S., & FitzGerald, K. T. (1992). An explication of the National Society of Genetic Counselors (NSGC) code of ethics. *Journal of Genetic Counseling*, *1*(1), 31–39. https://doi.org/10.1007/bf00960082

Bensend, T. A., Veach, P. M., & Niendorf, K. B. (2014). What's the harm? Genetic counselor perceptions of adverse effects of genetics service provision by non-genetics professionals. *Journal of Genetic Counseling*, *23*(1), 48–63. https://doi.org/10.1007/s10897-013-9605-3

Blumenthal, D., & Biesecker, B. (2005). Point-counterpoint: What's a better title? *Perspectives in Genetic Counseling*, *27*(1), 1.

Eunpu, D. L. (1992). Introductory statement. *Journal of Genetic Counseling*, *1*(1), 1–4. https://doi.org/10.1007/bf00960078

Forsyth, P. B., & Danisiewicz, T. J. (1985). Toward a theory of professionalization. *Work and Occupations, 12*(1), 59–76. https://doi.org/10.1177/0730888485012001004

Fraser, F. C. (1974). Genetic counseling. *American Journal of Human Genetics, 26*(5), 636–659.

Gettig, B. (1992). Restructuring of ABMG: NSGC to move toward healing; vision. *Perspectives in Genetic Counseling, 14*(4), 3.

Golbus, M. S., Loughman, W. D., Epstein, C. J., Halbasch, G., Stephens, J. D., & Hall, B. D. (1979). Prenatal genetic diagnosis in 3000 amniocenteses. *New England Journal of Medicine, 300*(4), 157–163. https://doi.org/10.1056/NEJM197901253000402

Greendale, K., & Pyeritz, R. E. (2001). Empowering primary care health professionals in medical genetics: How soon? How fast? How far? *American Journal of Medical Genetics, 106*(3), 223–232. https://doi.org/10.1002/ajmg.10010

Hamilton, J. G., Abdiwahab, E., Edwards, H. M., Fang, M., Jdayani, A., & Breslau, E. S. (2017). Primary care providers' cancer genetic testing-related knowledge, attitudes, and communication behaviors: A systematic review and research agenda. *Journal of General Internal Medicine, 32*(3), 315–324. https://doi.org/10.1007/s11606-016-3943-4

Heimler, A. (1979). From whence we've come: A message from the President. *Perspectives in Genetic Counseling, 1*(1), 1.

Heimler, A. (1997). An oral history of the National Society of Genetic Counselors. *Journal of Genetic Counseling, 6*(3), 315–336. https://doi.org/10.1023/a:1025680306348

Institute of Medicine. (2011). Institute of Medicine (US) Committee on standards for developing trustworthy clinical practice guidelines. In R. Graham, M. Mancher, D. Miller Wolman, S. Greenfield, & E. Steinberg (Eds.), *Clinical practice guidelines we can trust.* National Academies Press (US). https://doi.org/10.17226/13058

Kloza, E. M. (1989). EdNotes—Visions, viewpoints & valued opinions. *Perspectives in Genetic Counseling, 11*(4), 2.

Kloza, E. M. (1992). ABMS Report . . . Evaluating the counselors' status. *Perspectives in Genetic Counseling, 14*(1), 1.

Leopold, B. (1992). NSGC is not going to New Orleans. *Perspectives in Genetic Counseling, 14*(2), 1.

Means, C., Wojcik, A., Darnes, D., Rolf, B., & McGruder, C. (2023, October 17–21). Say my name, say my name: It's time to discuss the problem with the name "genetic counselor" [Plenary session]. *NSGC 42nd Annual Conference*, Chicago, IL, United States.

McInerney, J. D. (1979). Genetic education at the high school level: Some implications for counselors. *Perspectives in Genetic Counseling, 1*(4), 1.

National Center for Biotechnical Information. (2020, July 25). *NLM catalog.* https://www.ncbi.nlm.nih.gov/nlmcatalog/9206865

National Society of Genetic Counselors. (2014). *NSGC bylaws revised, October 2.* https://www.nsgc.org/Portals/0/Docs/About/NSGC%20Bylaws%20Revised%2010-2-2014.pdf?ver=4CeYP5phywOW-8M_ykqLfQ%3D%3D

National Society of Genetic Counselors. (2018). National Society of Genetic Counselors code of ethics. *Journal of Genetic Counseling, 27*(1), 6–8. https://doi.org/10.1007/s10897-017-0166-8

National Society of Genetic Counselors. (2020a). *National Society of Genetic Counselors (2020) position statement.* https://www.nsgc.org/POLICY/Position-Statements

National Society of Genetic Counselors. (2020b). *National Society of Genetic Counselors (2020) professional status survey.* https://www.nsgc.org/Research-and-Publications/Professional-Status-Survey/Past-Professional-Status-Surveys

National Society of Genetic Counselors. (2020c). *National Society of Genetic Counselors (2020) model legislative provisions.* https://www.nsgc.org/POLICY/State-Licensure-for-Genetic-Counselors/Model-Legislative-Provisions

National Society of Genetic Counselors. (2020d). *National Society of Genetic Counselors: Model legislative provisions.* https://www.nsgc.org/POLICY/State-Licensure-for-Genetic-Counselors/Model-Legislative-Provisions#scope

National Society of Genetic Counselors. (2022). *National Society of Genetic Counselors (2022). Dobbs v. Jackson Women's Health Organization, No. 19-1392, 597 U.S.* https://www.nsgc.org/Portals/0/Docs/Dobbs%20v%20Jackson%20Joint%20Statement%20ASHG%20ACMG%20NSGC%20Approved%206-24-22.pdf

National Society of Genetic Counselors. (2023). *National Society of Genetic Counselors (2023) states issuing licenses for genetic counselors.* https://www.nsgc.org/POLICY/State-Licensure-for-Genetic-Counselors/States-Issuing-Licenses

Palomaki, G. E. (1986). Collaborative study of Down syndrome screening using maternal serum alpha-fetoprotein and maternal age. *Lancet*, 2(8521-22), 1460. https://doi.org/10.1016/s0140-6736(86)92768-6

Reed, S. C. (1974). A short history of genetic counseling. *Social Biology*, *21*(4), 332–339. https://doi.org/10.1080/19485565.1974.9988131

Resta, R. G. (1993). Genetic library. *Journal of Genetic Counseling*, *2*(4), 295–298. https://doi.org/10.1007/bf00961577

Resta, R. G. (1997). Editorial introduction. *Journal of Genetic Counseling*, *6*(4), 373–374. https://doi.org/10.1023/A:1025640625004

Rollnick, B. R. (1981). The state of the society. *Perspectives in Genetic Counseling*, *3*(4), 4–5.

Schneider, K. A., & Resta, R. G. (1997). Editorial introduction. *Journal of Genetic Counseling*, *6*(2), 93–95. https://doi.org/10.1023/A:1025613315860

Senter, L., Bennet, R. L., Madeo, A. C., Noblin, S., Ormond, K. E., Schneider, K. W., Swan, K., Virani, A., & The National Society of Genetic Counselors Code of Ethics Review Task Force. (2018). National Society of Genetic Counselors code of ethics: Explication of 2017 revisions. *Journal of Genetic Counseling*, *27*(1), 9–15. https://doi.org/10.1007/s10897-017-0165-9

Spence, M. A. (1992). Letter to ABMG Diplomates. *Perspectives in Genetic Counseling*, *14*(4), 3.

Stoll, K. A., Mackison, A., Allyse, M. A., & Michie, M. (2017). Conflicts of interest in genetic counseling: Acknowledging and accepting. *Genetic Medicine*, *19*(8), 864–866. https://doi.org/10.1038/gim.2016.216

Venne, V. L., & Schneider, K. A. (2006). Editorial introduction: Genetic counseling challenges in cancer. *Journal of Genetic Counseling*, *15*(6), 407. https://doi.org/10.1007/s10897-006-9064-1

Wakefield, E., Keller, H., Mianzo, H., Nagaraj, C. B., Tawde, S., & Ulm, E. (2018). Reduction of health care costs and improved appropriateness of incoming test orders: The impact of genetic counselor review in an academic genetic testing laboratory. *Journal of Genetic Counseling*, *27*(5), 1067–1073. https://doi.org/10.1007/s10897-018-0226-8

Walker, A. (1979). Asilomar East. *Perspectives in Genetic Counseling*, *1*(3), 1.

Weiloch, S. (2005). NSGC introduces SmithBucklin as new executive director. *Perspectives in Genetic Counseling*, *27*(4), 1.

PART II

ENGAGING IN THE PRACTICE OF GENETIC COUNSELING

CHAPTER 4

A THEORY OF RESPONSIVE GENETIC COUNSELING PRACTICE

ROBIN E. GRUBS AND MARIA PIANTANIDA

INTRODUCTION

SINCE the inception of genetic counseling as a field of practice, conceptions of what constitutes "counseling" have been evolving. Early counseling models were predicated on the need to convey accurate scientific information (Kessler, 1997). More recently, however, models have expanded to address the psychosocial concerns associated with being at risk for a genetic condition; see Chapter 5—"The Reciprocal-Engagement Model of Genetic Counseling Practice," in this volume. The purpose of this chapter is to offer an overarching theoretical framework that encompasses both the information-giving and emotional support aspects of genetic counseling. The theory emerged from two interpretive grounded theory studies. One examined the experiences of women and couples who were at risk for a genetic condition due to advanced maternal age. The second focused on individuals with a family history of breast cancer and individuals who were at risk for having a child with a birth defect due to an abnormal maternal serum screening result.[1,2]

Emerging from these studies are four stances genetic counselors might enact in their work with clients:[3] information presenter, decision facilitator, information facilitator, and

[1] This second study was supported by the 2006 Jane Engelberg Memorial Fellowship. The Jane Engelberg Memorial Fellowship is an endowment from the Engelberg Foundation to the National Society of Genetic Counselors, Inc.

[2] See Appendix for additional details about the research process.

[3] We recognize that the terms "patient" and "client" are used interchangeably in the genetic counseling literature to describe the individual who is receiving genetic counseling services. As Biesecker (2018) notes, both descriptors are not equivalent as patients can be viewed as those who have a condition. For the purposes of this chapter, we chose to use the term "client" to provide a broader perspective of those who seek the services of a genetic counselor and to acknowledge our focus on the psychosocial dimensions of genetic counseling practice.

empathetic responder. Excerpts from the research interviews are used to illustrate variations in the needs and expectations clients bring to genetic counseling sessions.

The Need for a Theory of Practice

Sheldon Reed first introduced the phrase "genetic counseling" in 1947 and described three requirements of the practice: (a) "knowledge of human genetics"; (b) "a deep respect for the sensitivities, attitudes and reactions of the client"; and (c) "the desire to teach, and to teach the truth to the full extent that it is known" (Reed, 1955, pp. 11–12). As noted by Seymour Kessler, around the time of Reed's genetic counseling description, genetic counseling had its origins in biology, and as a result, genetic counseling practice was not grounded in psychology or psychiatry. This influenced the practice of the profession and is one reason why information transmission emerged as a major focus of the counseling session (Kessler, 1979). Kessler (1997) further argued that the strict adherence to a teaching approach for genetic counseling practice tends to ignore emotional concerns.

Today, the dual focus on education and emotional support is reflected in the definition of genetic counseling as developed by the National Society of Genetic Counselors:

> Genetic counseling is the process of helping people understand and adapt to the medical, psychological and familial implications of genetic contributions to disease. This process integrates the following: . . . Education about inheritance, testing, management, prevention, resources and research. Counseling to promote informed choices and adaptation to the risk or condition. (National Society of Genetic Counselors' Definition Task Force et al., 2006, p. 77)

The scope of genetic counselors' interactions with clients can be daunting, especially in an era when billing, reimbursement, and insurance coverage influence genetic counseling services and testing options available to clients. While scientific theories provide counselors with accurate information about the biological basis of genetic risk, they offer little guidance to counselors on how to balance the provision of information and support for clients' psycho-social-emotional concerns. For this, a theory of practice is needed.

Within the genetic counseling literature are calls for a theory of professional practice for genetic counselors (Eunpu, 1997; McAllister, 2001; Veach et al., 2002). Eunpu (1997) suggests that a theoretical basis of practice has the potential to enhance practitioners' counseling skills and, more practically, may help justify genetic counseling services to insurance providers. Historically, genetic counseling has drawn from other theoretical approaches in psychology, but as Veach et al. (2002) argue, genetic counseling is a "unique service" that merits its own theory (p. 188). In fact, Veach et al. (2007) developed the Reciprocal-Engagement Model, which outlines tenets, goals, strategies, and behaviors of genetic counseling practice; this model is described in Chapter 5—"The Reciprocal-Engagement Model of Genetic Counseling Practice," in this volume. In this chapter, we offer a theory of genetic counseling practice that encompasses both the information-giving and emotional support roles of genetic counseling. Different theoretical frameworks within a discipline provide educators, researchers, and students the opportunity to approach and examine practice from varied perspectives.

On the Nature of Theories of Practice

Within the scientific literature, the concept of theory typically connotes causal or correlational relationships among key variables. Describing the work of several scholars and philosophers, social scientist Bent Flyvbjerg points out that the aim is to generate knowledge claims that are "(1) explicit, (2) universal, and (3) abstract, . . . (4) discrete, . . . (5) systematic, . . . (6) complete and predictive" (Flyvbjerg, 2001, pp. 38–39). Mapping of the human genome is a stunning example of such scientific knowledge. On a less sweeping scale, the genetic counseling literature is replete with scientific research aimed at identifying associations and predictive relationships between specific client factors and particular decisions about genetic counseling and genetic testing (e.g., Allen et al., 2019; Biesecker et al., 2000; Kuppermann et al., 2006; Sweeny et al., 2014; Willis et al., 2017). As useful as these studies are, the knowledge they yield is not sufficient for expert practice. To guide practice, a different form of theory is needed, one grounded in assumptions that

- human actions (including decisions) are based on the meanings that individuals make of their experiences;
- meanings are made within the context of an individual's life—encompassing past, current, and imagined future experiences;
- it is neither possible nor particularly useful to try to predict a priori what meanings individuals will make of their experiences; and
- it is useful for practitioners to have a way of thinking about and responding to the variability of meanings that clients might ascribe to the prospect of genetic risk and genetic counseling.

Given that individuals can ascribe very different meanings to the same set of biologic facts, theories of practice offer not scientific certainty, but what Schwartz and Sharpe (2010) call "practical wisdom." Practical wisdom entails the ability to figure out "the right way to do the right thing in a particular circumstance, with a particular person, at a particular time" (Schwartz & Sharpe, 2010, pp. 5–6). In the profession of genetic counseling, practical wisdom is the capacity to discern each client's information needs, counseling expectations, and the meaning ascribed to being at risk. The proposed theory of practice places responsiveness to these variations of clients' needs at the center of genetic counseling.

A Theory of Responsive Genetic Counseling Practice

The matrix shown in Figure 4.1 illustrates four stances genetic counselors might enact in their practice. The horizontal axis contrasts two different ways of framing the experience of making a decision about genetic testing. The vertical axis contrasts two different ways in which counselors might frame their purpose when working with clients. The anchor points

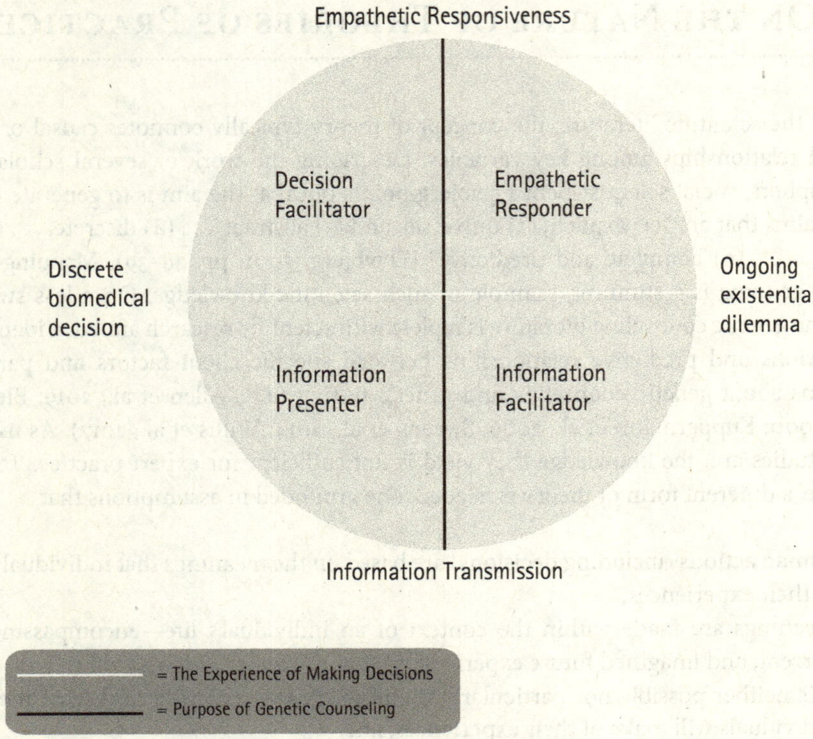

FIGURE 4.1 A theory of responsive genetic counseling practice.
(Adapted from Grubs, 2018, with permission from Learning Moments Press)

at the opposite ends of each axis are meant to illustrate points along a continuum, not absolute categories.

The experience of making decisions

The horizontal axis depicts a continuum regarding the experience of making decisions related to genetic counseling and testing.[4] On the left end of the continuum is a view grounded in a biomedical model that treats the decision as a one-time event with a discrete outcome—for example, either testing is accepted or testing is declined. Some early decision models, developed to predict and facilitate genetic decision making, exemplify this view. For example, Pauker and Pauker constructed (1977) and shared (1987) a decision analysis

[4] Not all genetic counseling sessions will involve a situation in which a client is facing a genetic testing decision. However, the research that generated this theory of practice focused on individuals who were offered prenatal genetic screening, prenatal genetic diagnostic testing, or *BRCA1/2* genetic testing. Therefore, decision making related to genetic testing is an element of the theory. We hope that over time, this theory can be expanded to address genetic counseling situations in which clients face other decisions (e.g., treatment or management decisions) or when decision making is not a focus of the session.

model with clients who were having difficulty deciding about amniocentesis. To reduce the amniocentesis decision to a series of "simpler decisions" for clients, Pauker and Pauker (1977) created a decision tree that examined the different outcomes related to the decision to pursue or decline amniocentesis—at each branch of the tree a particular outcome is examined, such as the possibility of miscarriage following an amniocentesis. They argued that the use of the decision tree reduces a "complex decision" into a sequence of "simpler ones," provides a manner to assess attitudes toward possible outcomes, and would allow a healthcare professional to suggest a "rational decision" to an individual/couple (Pauker & Pauker, 1977, p. 286). This decision-tree model tends to focus on the biological and medical aspects of genetic testing, and it is this focus that we associate with the left-hand side of the continuum.

Over time, decision aids have evolved and strive to enhance client education and facilitate decision making in a variety of settings (e.g., Green et al., 2004; Juan et al., 2008; Shickh et al., 2018; Wakefield et al., 2007, 2008; Wang et al., 2005). As Wakefield et al. (2007) point out, decision aids can occur in a number of formats and may incorporate clients' values into the decision-making process. One review of studies that examined the use of decision aids for cancer-related decision making identified a number of beneficial outcomes such as improved knowledge, risk perception accuracy, and decreased decisional conflict (McAlpine et al., 2018).

Beyond some early decision aids, when the decision to accept or refuse genetic testing is framed as a discrete biomedical decision, the ethical principle of "informed consent" underpins the client–counselor interaction. In *Making Health Care Decisions: A Report on the Ethical and Legal Implications of Informed Consent in the Patient-Practitioner Relationship* (United States President's Commission for the Study of Ethical Problems in Medicine Biomedical Behavioral Research, 1982), the authors argue, "The ethical foundation of informed consent can be traced to the promotion of two values: personal well-being and self-determination" (p. 2). We tend to associate the left hand of the continuum with the principle of self-determination. Manson and O'Neill (2007) argue that the principle of self-determination or client autonomy has traditionally been achieved through a "conduit model" (p. 50) of communication in which a professional transmits technical information to a client-recipient. While Manson and O'Neill offer a detailed critique of the conduit model of communication, a thorough review of their argument goes beyond the scope of this discussion. One limitation of the conduit model is its inadequate consideration of issues that may affect the client's emotional well-being or their right to make a decision that is in their best interests.

Although the principles of self-determination and well-being are interconnected, for the purposes of this discussion we focus on well-being to illuminate the right end of the continuum. Here, making a decision about genetic testing is seen as an existential dilemma, and possibly even a crisis. "Existential" is used to convey the idea that living with genetic risk can be a powerful and profound experience and that people recognize their responsibility in making genetic testing decisions. Moreover, facing a genetic-related decision is not a discrete event but part of an ongoing process in which people make meaning of the experience within the context of their lives.

Psychologist Rollo May (1977, 1983) suggests that the threat of "nonbeing" lies at the heart of an existential crisis. In genetic terms, "being at risk" carries a connotation that a human *being* is facing the possibility that their own life or that of an unborn child is in jeopardy.

May (1983) goes on to say that "Anxiety is the subjective state of the individual's becoming aware that his [*sic*] existence can become destroyed, that he can lose himself and his world, that he can become 'nothing'" (pp. 109–110). Although humans live with the knowledge of their own mortality, the prospect of "nonbeing" can often be relegated to some vaguely imagined, distant future. However, when the possibility of a genetic condition is raised along with a recommendation for testing, the prospect of nonbeing comes to the fore, which for some can engender a state of angst.

The concept of angst was used by European existentialists to describe an emotional state of profound anguish and dread. The English term "anxiety" is considered a weak translation of the German word "angst" (May, 1977). Regardless of what term is used, genetic counselors are working with clients who are likely to be in a state of heightened anxiety as they struggle with and make difficult choices. These choices are not common, everyday decisions but rather decisions that can be viewed as involving matters of life and death. For example, considering genetic testing might raise questions such as: Will I have to face the possible choice to abort a wanted pregnancy in the event I receive an abnormal test result? Should I have genetic testing for the breast cancer gene and risk learning that I might have passed it on to my children?

When the decision to accept or refuse genetic testing is framed as an existential dilemma, then focusing solely on the ethical principle of self-determination might offer too little guidance for the conscientious counselor. Although a client might fully understand the physiological or medical risks associated with the testing procedure per se, how the results of the tests reverberate through one's life can never be fully known in advance. However, when a counselor assumes a stance of responsiveness toward a client's concerns and is guided by the ethical principle of the client's well-being, the possibility of exploring emotional benefits and risks is enhanced.

Purpose of genetic counseling

The vertical axis depicts a continuum of purposes that genetic counselors might strive to achieve when working with clients who face the experience of making decisions about genetic testing. The purpose at the bottom of the continuum emphasizes the transmission of information, presumably to help clients become well enough informed to accept or refuse genetic testing. This approach is consistent with the "teaching model" outlined by Kessler (1997, p. 287). The goal of this model is to educate clients about medical and genetic facts, and a genetic counselor who adheres to the teaching model would "provide information and correct misinformation and misperceptions" (p. 288). Framing the purpose of genetic counseling as the transmission of information carries an ethical obligation to remain current with the best scientific information available to the field and values the educational aspect of a genetic counseling encounter, which is consistent with the Accreditation Council for Genetic Counseling (ACGC) practice-based competencies as shown in Box 4.1 (ACGC, 2023).

While mastery of relevant scientific knowledge is necessary for information transmission, it is not sufficient for responsive counseling. As Kessler (1997) contends, the teaching model has the tendency to ignore individual needs as the same information is often dispensed to

Box 4.1 Accreditation Council for Genetic Counseling Practice-Based Competencies

- Demonstrate knowledge of genetics and genomic principles and concepts.
- Apply knowledge of genetic conditions to the delivery of genetic services.
- Use a variety of approaches to communicate genetics and genomic information.

Box 4.2 Accreditation Council for Genetic Counseling Practice-Based Competencies

- Promote integration of psychosocial needs and client-centered decision making into genetic counseling interactions.
- Promote psychosocial adaptation.

all clients. Consequently, this model can hinder meaningful engagement with clients and fails to address their psychosocial concerns.

If the teaching model frames the purpose of genetic practice as information transmission, a counseling model frames the purpose as empathetic responsiveness, which is represented by the top of the vertical axis. Emphasis here is on understanding the meanings that clients ascribe to their being at risk. When the focus of the session is directed toward understanding clients' needs and concerns, the opportunity for developing an empathetic rapport is enhanced. The ACGC practice-based competencies address the importance of attending to the well-being of clients and responding empathetically to their concerns (see Box 4.2; ACGC, 2023).

When the two axes are juxtaposed, the resulting matrix depicts four different stances that genetic counselors might enact in their work with clients. By *stance* we mean a way of being with clients that encompasses a practitioner's beliefs, attitudes, and values about what it means to be a counselor and the nature of the counselor–client relationship.

Information presenter stance

The lower left quadrant exemplifies the stance of the genetic counselor as a presenter of scientifically factual information. The *information presenter* stance is predicated on the assumption that clients both want and need basic information about genetic conditions and/or genetic testing. Research eliciting the perspectives of genetic counselors and clients suggests that information provision is a desired goal of genetic counseling (Bernhardt et al., 2000; Davey et al., 2005; Lobb et al., 2001). Symbolic of this stance is the *Genetic Counseling Aids*, published by the Greenwood Genetic Center, which is a collection of pictures commonly shown during genetic counseling sessions and can be organized in a way that allows one to convey a great deal of complex genetic information in a short period of time. Maggie illustrates that some clients seek genetic counseling primarily for informational purposes:

> Maggie was 2 years old when her mother died of breast cancer at approximately 30 years of age. After learning about the availability of genetic testing, Maggie decided that she wanted to pursue testing. She said, "I realized it's kind of better to know, that way you can tackle it

> right from the beginning." When Maggie described her expectations of genetic counseling, she mentioned, "I kind of thought it was going to be more of a psychological mind play, trying to get into my feelings when really they just informed me of everything . . . so it really did help." She did not prefer a counselor "getting into her head" and instead desired receiving information about testing and her risk for carrying a pathogenic breast cancer gene variant. She was pleased with her genetic counseling session because ". . . it was informational and if I had any questions, the genetic counselors answered them." She stated, "I think they [genetic counselors] did a really great job is what I'm trying to say."

As Maggie's comments suggest, there are clients who desire medical and genetic information. In the early days of genetic counseling, it may have been reasonable to assume that this was the need of all or most individuals who sought the services of a genetic counselor. As the ACGC practice-based competencies indicate (see Box 4.1), information provision is still an important component of genetic counseling practice.

However, some clients may proactively seek information about their genetic risk and testing options from the internet, physicians, and trusted confidants. These clients are not necessarily representative of the socially and culturally diverse individuals who present for genetic counseling, but they do call attention to the limitation of framing counseling only as "information giving."

Mary, for example, illustrates the type of client who enters the genetic counseling session with a considerable store of factual information:

> Probably I'm a little bit more knowledgeable than your average, older patient because of my involvement at the medical center, but I knew straight away that yes, my age was a factor, but I think it's becoming less and less so. I mean there are more and more women my age having children but obviously as you get older the odds are that things will not progress as normally as one would hope and that the outcome might not be quite what one would hope. Certainly, the fact that there is testing available is attractive. It's just simply to be informed and prepared that seems like the logical thing to do. So, I fully expected to be offered testing and, indeed, if it had not been offered, I would have certainly inquired. . . .
>
> I was frankly just a little bit disappointed with my genetic counseling. I think I had all these expectations. I had it in my mind that there would be more discussion with me. But rather, what it seemed was just an imparting of information of how, where, why, what, and when. There were some little pretty pictures held up—this is how the CVS [chorionic villus sampling] will be done, this is where the catheter will go, the risks of, and things like that. But I had actually thought that there might be more interviewing about my background, what I knew of my parents, my husband's background, what he knew of his parents, and then probably more discussion about the "what ifs." But there was absolutely no discussion about the "what ifs."

Individuals like Mary already bring to the counseling session a considerable understanding of the risks they face. This understanding, however, does not exhaust the spoken or unspoken needs that they may have. Embedded within their stories may be emotional issues as well as dynamics between partners and their broader social circles that have the potential to create counseling challenges.

When the genetic counselor's stance is framed as *information presenter*, they may have little to offer clients who are as knowledgeable as Mary. Dissatisfaction with genetic counseling services might occur if the counselor spends the limited time in a session presenting information that the client already knows. The upper left quadrant represents a shift from conveying basic information to ascertaining where clients might be in the decision-making process.

Decision facilitator stance

Like the *information presenter* stance, the *decision facilitator* stance views the counseling session as an opportunity to help clients reach a decision about testing. However, rather than focusing on the presentation of standardized information, the counselor begins by exploring the client's concerns and questions. Information can then be shared in a way that helps clients work through potential struggles that are keeping them from reaching a decision. We place the *decision facilitator* stance in the upper left quadrant to suggest that this stance calls for establishing empathetic rapport with clients to elicit their questions and concerns about the facts of genetic risk and testing.

Dana and Sean might have benefited from meeting with a genetic counselor enacting a *decision facilitator* stance. Receiving pamphlets and having a brief discussion with their obstetrical provider left them feeling confused because they felt this limited information did not help them reach a decision. As Dana indicated:

> Well, I was very confused about testing at first. I mean not confused about the chances of something going wrong after 35, but I wasn't sure if I wanted to have prenatal testing done or not. I talked to a lot of people. I talked to my sister about it and my babysitter, and she has a sister-in-law who's a nurse and she said, "Well, I'll ask her what she thinks." Her sister-in-law really didn't say one way or the other either, but she just said the risks involved in it and everything and it depends on what you would do if you found out something was wrong. And I don't know if I would do anything and if I did go through with it and something was wrong, I don't know what I would have done.

Having experienced a late miscarriage in a previous pregnancy, Dana and Sean were worried about the risk associated with amniocentesis. Sean described his fear of possibly experiencing another pregnancy loss:

> One of our friends said, "Well, somebody had the test one time and it broke their water, and they lost the baby because of that." And I'm thinking, "Well, here we go again" because Dana had miscarried 3 years ago, and I don't know if I can deal with that emotional thing again. It ripped me up because it was a boy and it was like 5 months into it. I just wasn't ready for that emotional roller coaster again. Emotionally, I was ripped up, bawling my eyes out for a good couple days.

Dana and Sean thought that meeting with a genetic counselor would have been more helpful than "just getting pamphlets and reading on their own" when they were struggling to reach a decision about testing. A genetic counselor who enacted a stance of *decision facilitator* would strive to understand Dana and Sean's concerns to assist them in making a decision. Their obstetrician provided Dana and Sean with technical/medical information about genetic risks and testing options, but as their comments suggest, the provision of information was not completely useful. A *decision facilitator* who recognized Dana and Sean's fears regarding miscarriage could help them explore this fear in relation to the possible benefits of testing as well as what choices they might make had testing found a chromosome abnormality in their baby. By allowing Dana and Sean to consider the implications of different decisions within the context of their concerns, a *decision facilitator* could have possibly eased some of the difficulties Dana and Sean encountered when trying to make a testing decision.

Clients like Dana and Sean may not be able to assimilate information when they are preoccupied with concerns that a counselor is not recognizing or addressing. If, for example, a counselor starts by providing genetic information, a client may be unable to attend to what the counselor is saying when worried about the risk of a miscarriage. A *decision facilitator* tailors information to the questions and concerns of the client with the goal of helping clients reach a decision to either accept or reject testing. Although the *decision facilitator* stance represents a shift toward responsiveness to clients' concerns, the focus still remains on the conceptual or cognitive aspects of a client's decision.

Information facilitator stance

The stance of *information facilitator* places the need for a decision about testing within the broader context of a client's life. Like all competent genetic counselors, *information facilitators* draw from their store of scientific and technical knowledge to address information gaps or misconceptions that clients may bring to the counseling session. However, *information facilitators* customize the delivery of information in ways that acknowledge clients' evolving life experiences. Unlike the teaching model that may present information in a predetermined, uniform manner, *information facilitators* elicit information from clients to better understand the meaning of genetic risk within their life circumstances. Thus, the counseling session takes on a more conversational quality with greater give and take between counselor and client. Kathy and Mike exemplify clients who might be better served by the stance of *information facilitator* than *information presenter*:

> After undergoing infertility treatment for 4 years, Kathy and Mike became pregnant with their second child. During their pregnancy they elected for genetic counseling and amniocentesis. Prior to the counseling session, Mike had not really thought about the risk associated with Kathy's age. During the counseling session when he learned about the age-related risk and the risk associated with amniocentesis, Mike became concerned. Feeling overwhelmed with the information, Mike did not speak much during the session and shared, "I was definitely more quiet than Kathy. I hardly said a word as I recall. There were a lot of things running through my mind, it being the first time that I heard a lot of it."

Mike feared the possibility of miscarriage because he perceived the pregnancy as their "last chance" to complete their family. Had the pregnancy ended in a miscarriage, they planned on stopping the infertility treatment and trying to conceive. Mike shared that early in the pregnancy when he was on a hunting trip, he tried calling home but could not reach Kathy. He said:

> I called every 10 minutes because I had myself convinced that something was wrong, but it ended up that she was at her mother's house. I was very nervous throughout this entire pregnancy. I guess it was because we tried for so long, put so much effort into it, put so much emotion. If something bad would have happened, it would have been an emotional tragedy. We would have had a hard time dealing with it. I was on pins and needles throughout the pregnancy.

As Mike described, the prospect of facing a decision about a test that increases the risk for having a miscarriage "puts a moral dilemma on you."

Mike came to the genetic counseling session with little information about the risks associated with Kathy's age and with the testing procedures. The concerns generated by learning this information resulted in him becoming detached from the conversation during the counseling session. It is possible that clients like Mike whose emotions are heightened will encounter difficulty in comprehending information being conveyed during a counseling session. When sharing medical and genetic facts, an *information facilitator* tries to understand how clients interpret such facts within the context of their lives. This understanding would allow an *information facilitator* to recognize the angst that can be experienced when clients learn about their genetic risks and the potential complications associated with genetic testing.

An *information facilitator* tailors the delivery of information to the client's experience and needs, but the focus remains on information provision. This stance does not strive to be responsive to the profound emotions that can emerge when clients are living with genetic risk.

Empathetic responder stance

The upper right quadrant illustrates a stance predicated on the assumption that referral for genetic counseling and testing can be an event fraught with meaning within the context of a client's life experience. Thus, a counselor who embodies the stance of *empathetic responder* assumes that facing genetic risk can be a profound experience, touching on existential issues of life, disability, and death. Depending on the context within which counselors are practicing, it may or may not be possible to help clients come to grips with the emotions associated with such profound issues. Still, some acknowledgment of a client's angst may need to take precedence over the delivery of genetic and medical information. Although an informed decision may ultimately be necessary, automatically focusing on this discrete endpoint may not be sensitive to a client's immediate concerns.

Anne is a client who appears to have benefited from having a genetic counselor who was concerned with Anne's emotional well-being. Anne pursued *BRCA1/2* genetic testing after she was diagnosed with breast cancer. She has a family history of breast cancer and began to worry that her cancer was due to a genetic cause. When discussing her genetic counseling experience, she shared:

> My genetic counseling was very well done. I was tested; they drew blood the same day that I went for the counseling and the genetic counselor spent all of the time that I needed answering questions. A lot of the things that she normally explained I already knew from reading so we talked not so much about the science of the genetics but more of the emotional issues surrounding the testing. My sister was not at that appointment with me so there was no immediate pressure.

Anne discussed the challenges she faced with her testing process. One of her sisters pressured Anne to pursue testing earlier than she wanted. Anne had planned to discuss testing with her oncologist after completing chemotherapy treatment, but her sister pressured Anne to go for genetic counseling before that time. In addition, her husband, who had genetic testing for an autosomal dominant neurological condition, regretted his decision to have testing. Although he knew that Anne had testing, they never discussed her genetic counseling or testing results. She left the results on a table in the house so he would know the testing outcome. It seemed that Anne was lacking support from her family, and having an opportunity to discuss "emotional issues" with her genetic counselor left Anne feeling satisfied with the encounter.

Implications of the Proposed Theory for Genetic Counseling Practice

The positions along the horizontal and vertical continuum are not dichotomous, and by the same token, the stances are not discrete. Further, it is possible to develop highly sophisticated skills within any of the stances. A novice practitioner, for example, might initially focus heavily on the presentation of information in a more uniform manner. But with greater experience and comfort, they might develop a repertoire on explanations for translating technical information into client-friendly language. Similarly, advanced beginners might draw upon their experience to form more nuanced questions when enacting a *decision facilitator* stance. We contend, however, that counselors who are able to embrace the stance of *empathetic responder* have the broadest view of how they might attend to clients' needs. This affords them flexibility in shifting focus from the presentation of information to responsiveness to clients' emotional state of being. The broader the counselor's view of their purpose and role as well as the range of client needs, the greater the likelihood that they can respond intuitively to more complex situations such as those illustrated in the examples above.

It is worth noting that the practice of genetic counseling is often constrained by a number of contextual limitations. For example, because of cost, efficiency, and reimbursement concerns, counseling sessions may face considerable time limitations. This affords limited opportunity to respond substantively to clients' emotional needs. In some circumstances, counseling sessions are scheduled immediately before a genetic test is administered. This gives clients limited time to assimilate the information, consider their decision, and deal with the existential dimensions of being at risk. Issues related to the nature of services eligible for reimbursement can further constrain the amount of time available for counseling. We do not want to minimize the effect of these contextual factors on the opportunity to engage in client counseling. Dealing with such systemic issues may require action from the profession at large. That said, however, individual counselors have choices about how they want to approach and relate to clients. A stance of empathetic responsiveness may be conveyed through nonverbal aspects of communication such as posture, tone of voice, active listening, and gestures. Sometimes simply acknowledging the difficulty of a client's situation can convey a sense of caring and, in turn, engender a sense of comfort. Such manifestations of empathetic responsiveness take no more time than nonverbal communication that conveys a sense of detachment and lack of caring. Although counselors face time constraints, Kessler (1979) claims that responding to clients' psychological needs can save time because "one properly timed intervention, so to speak empathetically on the mark, may actually avoid needless explanations and diversions and may facilitate the transmission of factual material" (pp. 101–102).

When genetic counselors perceive that clients are in profound emotional distress that cannot be addressed within the constraints of their own practice, they should be prepared to offer the names of competent therapists with whom clients might work or other resources that can assist clients.

Conclusion

In concluding this chapter, we look at the implications of the proposed theory of responsive genetic counseling practice for the education of genetic counselors. Drawing on the work of Dreyfus and Dreyfus (1986), Flyvbjerg (2001) lays out five levels of learning associated with professional development:

(1) Novices act on the basis of context-independent elements and rules.
(2) Advanced beginners also use situational elements, which they have learned to identify and interpret on the basis of their own experience from similar situations.
(3) Competent performers are characterized by the involved choice of goals and plans as a basis for their actions. Goals and plans are used to structure and store masses of both context-dependent and context-independent information.
(4) Proficient performers identify problems, goals, and plans intuitively from their own experientially based perspective. Intuitive choice is checked by analytical evaluation prior to action.
(5) Finally, experts' behavior is intuitive, holistic, and synchronic, understood in the way that a given situation releases a picture of problem, goal, plan, decision, and action in one instant and with no division into phases. This is the level of true human expertise. Experts are characterized by a flowing, effortless performance, unhindered by analytic deliberations. (pp. 20–21)

Within this framework, those who rely primarily on conveying genetic information to clients may be operating at the novice level. The stance of *empathetic responder* is more congruent with the expert level of learning. When genetic counseling educators adopt a developmental view of student learning, they may help students to recognize where they might be in a trajectory of increasing competence. If novices think that they must immediately master learning at an expert level, then they may become overwhelmed and discouraged. When they understand this is a longer range goal, they can recognize the importance of ongoing professional development.

Within the developmental learning sequence outlined above, scientific knowledge lays a foundation for genetic counseling at the novice through competent levels of performance. Expert practice, however, is exemplified by responsiveness within the counselor–client relationship. Educational scholar Thomas Schwandt (2001) suggests that responsiveness

> is a unique kind of knowledge precisely because it avoids the extremes of an almost innocent immersion in experience (being awash in a sea of particulars), on one hand, and commitments to general principles, ends, theories, and the like, which are totally blind to fine-grained particularities of the immediate case, on the other. (p. 79)

A theory of practice such as that proposed in Figure 4.1 helps practitioners to avoid "being awash in a sea of particulars." It offers a framework for sorting through what form of response might be most helpful given the particulars of a client's experience and needs. Both the ACGC practice-based competencies (ACGC, 2023) and the National Society of Genetic Counselors scope of practice (National Society of Genetic Counselors, 2007) emphasize the importance of *responsiveness* to the concerns of clients. Thus, although the stances represented in the cells of the matrix are not mutually exclusive, we contend that empathetic responsiveness lies at the heart of a genetic counseling theory of practice.

Acknowledgments

The development of the theory described in this chapter was supported in part by the 2006 Jane Engelberg Memorial Fellowship, an endowment from the Engelberg Foundation to the National Society of Genetic Counselors, Inc. RE Grubs is grateful to Learning Moments Press for its permission to adapt Figure 4.1 from a previous chapter she wrote that recounted the process of her dissertation research and outlined a typology of existential angst that was generated from the research (Grubs, 2018).

APPENDIX

Research Process

The theory of responsive genetic counseling practice was constructed from two qualitative studies that explored the experiences of individuals who faced genetic risk. The first inquiry examined the experiences of women and couples who were offered genetic counseling and prenatal genetic testing because of advanced maternal age. The second study, funded by the Jane Engelberg Memorial Fellowship (JEMF),[5] focused on the experiences of being at risk for having a child with a birth defect due to an abnormal maternal serum screening result and being at risk for carrying a *BRCA1/2* pathogenic variant.

Conversational interviews were used in both studies to elicit accounts of being at risk and reaching a decision about genetic testing. In the first study, 24 individuals were interviewed (10 couples), and for the second study, 11 individuals were interviewed (three couples). These individuals and couples made different decisions regarding genetic testing; some pursued testing, while others did not. The studies were conducted using grounded theory, a qualitative method that was originally developed in the 1960s by two sociologists, Barney Glaser and Anselm Strauss (Glaser & Strauss, 1967). Since its inception, grounded theory has been adapted for use in a wide variety of disciplines including genetic counseling (Grubs & Piantanida, 2010; McAllister, 2001; Skirton, 2001). Grounded theory allows researchers to develop theoretical frameworks from lived experiences. Although other qualitative research methods also offer insight into human experience, grounded theory,

[5] The second study was supported by the 2006 Jane Engelberg Memorial Fellowship, an endowment from the Engelberg Foundation to the National Society of Genetic Counselors, Inc.

with its systematic process of coding and comparative analysis, offers a particularly powerful method for generating abstract concepts from the details of idiosyncratic experiences with the goal of constructing relationships among the concepts to develop a theory to portray the phenomenon under study.

References

Accreditation Council for Genetic Counseling. (2023). *Practice-based competencies for genetic counselors.* https://www.gceducation.org/wp-content/uploads/2023/12/ACGC_PracticeBasedCompetencies_2023.pdf

Allen, C. G., Roberts, M., & Guan, Y. (2019). Exploring predictors of genetic counseling and testing for hereditary breast and ovarian cancer: Findings from the 2015 U.S. National Health Interview Survey. *Journal of Personalized Medicine*, *9*(2), 26. https://doi.org/10.3390/jpm9020026

Bernhardt, B. A., Biesecker, B. B., & Mastromarino, C. L. (2000). Goals, benefits, and outcomes of genetic counseling: Client and genetic counselor assessment. *American Journal of Medical Genetics*, *94*(3), 189–197. https://doi.org/10.1002/1096-8628(20000918)94:3<189::aid-ajmg3>3.0.co;2-e

Biesecker, B. B. (2018). Genetic counselors as social and behavioral scientists in the era of precision medicine. *American Journal of Medical Genetics Part C: Seminars in Medical Genetics*, *178*(1), 10–14. https://doi.org/10.1002/ajmg.c.31609

Biesecker, B. B., Ishibe, N., Hadley, D. W., Giambarresi, T. R., Kase, R. G., Lerman, C., & Struewing, J. P. (2000). Psychosocial factors predicting BRCA1/BRCA2 testing decisions in members of hereditary breast and ovarian cancer families. *American Journal of Medical Genetics*, *93*(4), 257–263. https://doi.org/10.1002/1096-8628(20000814)93:4<257::aid-ajmg1>3.0.co;2-8

Davey, A., Rostant, K., Harrop, K., Goldblatt, J., & O'Leary, P. (2005). Evaluating genetic counseling: Client expectations, psychological adjustment and satisfaction with service. *Journal of Genetic Counseling*, *14*(3), 197–206. https://doi.org/10.1007/s10897-005-0519-6

Dreyfus, H., & Dreyfus, S. (1986). *Mind over machine: The power of human intuition and expertise in the era of the computer*. Free Press.

Eunpu, D. L. (1997). Systemically-based psychotherapeutic techniques in genetic counseling. *Journal of Genetic Counseling*, *6*(1), 1–20. https://doi.org/10.1023/A:1025630917735

Flyvbjerg, B. (2001). *Making social science matter: Why social inquiry fails and how it can succeed again* (S. Sampson, Trans.). Cambridge University Press.

Glaser, B. G., & Strauss, A. L. (1967). *The discovery of grounded theory: Strategies for qualitative research*. Aldine Publishing Company.

Green, M. J., Peterson, S. K., Baker, M. W., Harper, G. R., Friedman, L. C., Rubinstein, W. S., & Mauger, D. T. (2004). Effect of a computer-based decision aid on knowledge, perceptions, and intentions about genetic testing for breast cancer susceptibility: A randomized controlled trial. *JAMA*, *292*(4), 442–452. https://doi.org/10.1001/jama.292.4.442

Grubs, R. E. (2018). Reimagining grounded theory: Moving toward an interpretive stance. In N. B. Garman & M. Piantanida (Eds.), *The authority to imagine: The struggle toward representation in dissertation writing* (pp. 121–139). Learning Moments Press.

Grubs, R. E., & Piantanida, M. (2010). Grounded theory in genetic counseling research: An interpretive perspective. *Journal of Genetic Counseling*, *19*(2), 99–111. https://doi.org/10.1007/s10897-009-9270-8

Juan, A. S., Wakefield, C. E., Kasparian, N. A., Kirk, J., Tyler, J., & Tucker, K. (2008). Development and pilot testing of a decision aid for men considering genetic testing for breast and/or ovarian cancer-related mutations (BRCA1/2). *Genetic Testing*, *12*(4), 523–532. https://doi.org/10.1089/gte.2008.0035

Kessler, S. (1979). *Genetic counseling: Psychological dimensions*. Academic Press.

Kessler, S. (1997). Psychological aspects of genetic counseling. IX. Teaching and counseling. *Journal of Genetic Counseling*, *6*(3), 287–295. https://doi.org/10.1023/A:1025676205440

Kuppermann, M., Learman, L. A., Gates, E., Gregorich, S. E., Nease, R. F., Jr., Lewis, J., & Washington, A. E. (2006). Beyond race or ethnicity and socioeconomic status: Predictors of prenatal testing for Down syndrome. *Obstetrics and Gynecology*, *107*(5), 1087–1097. https://doi.org/10.1097/01.AOG.0000214953.90248.db

Lobb, E., Butow, P., Meiser, B., Tucker, K., & Barratt, A. (2001). How do geneticists and genetic counselors counsel women from high-risk breast cancer families? *Journal of Genetic Counseling*, *10*(2), 185–199. https://doi.org/10.1023/a:1009447932274

Manson, N. C., & O'Neill, O. (2007). *Rethinking informed consent in bioethics*. Cambridge University Press.

May, R. (1977). *The meaning of anxiety*. W.W. Norton & Co.

May, R. (1983). *The discovery of being: Writings in existential psychology*. W.W. Norton & Co.

McAllister, M. F. (2001). Grounded theory in genetic counseling research. *Journal of Genetic Counseling*, *10*(3), 233–250.

McAlpine, K., Lewis, K. B., Trevena, L. J., & Stacey, D. (2018). What is the effectiveness of patient decision aids for cancer-related decisions? A systematic review subanalysis. *JCO Clinical Cancer Informatics*, *2*, 1–13. https://doi.org/10.1200/CCI.17.00148

National Society of Genetic Counselors. (2007). *Genetic counselor scope of practice*. https://www.nsgc.org/p/cm/ld/fid=18#scope

National Society of Genetic Counselors' Definition Task Force, Resta, R., Biesecker, B. B., Bennett, R. L., Blum, S., Hahn, S. E., Strecker, M. N., & Williams, J. L. (2006). A new definition of Genetic Counseling: National Society of Genetic Counselors' Task Force report. *Journal of Genetic Counseling*, *15*(2), 77–83. https://doi.org/10.1007/s10897-005-9014-3

Pauker, S. P., & Pauker, S. G. (1977). Prenatal diagnosis: A directive approach to genetic counseling using decision analysis. *Yale Journal of Biological Medicine*, *50*(3), 275–289.

Pauker, S. P., & Pauker, S. G. (1987). The amniocentesis decision: Ten years of decision analytic experience. *Birth Defects Original Article Series*, *23*(2), 151–169.

Reed, S. C. (1955). *Counseling in medical genetics*. W.B. Saunders Company.

Schwandt, T. A. (2001). Responsiveness and everyday life. *New Directions for Evaluation*, *92*, 73–88. https://doi-org.pitt.idm.oclc.org/10.1002/ev.36

Schwartz, B., & Sharpe, K. (2010). *Practical wisdom: The right way to do the right thing*. Riverhead Books.

Shickh, S., Clausen, M., Mighton, C., Casalino, S., Joshi, E., Glogowski, E., Schrader, K. A., Scheer, A., Elser, C., Panchal, S., Eisen, A., Graham, T., Aronson, M., Semotiuk, K.M ., Winter-Paquette, L., Evans, M., Lerner-Ellis, J., Carroll, J. C., Hamilton, J. G., . . . Bombard, Y. (2018). Evaluation of a decision aid for incidental genomic results, the Genomics ADvISER: Protocol for a mixed methods randomised controlled trial. *BMJ Open*, *8*(4), e021876. https://doi.org/10.1136/bmjopen-2018-021876

Skirton, H. (2001). The client's perspective of genetic counseling—A grounded theory study. *Journal of Genetic Counseling*, *10*(4), 311–329.

Sweeny, K., Ghane, A., Legg, A. M., Huynh, H. P., & Andrews, S. E. (2014). Predictors of genetic testing decisions: A systematic review and critique of the literature. *Journal of Genetic Counseling, 23*(3), 263–288. https://doi.org/10.1007/s10897-014-9712-9

United States President's Commission for the Study of Ethical Problems in Medicine and Biomedical and Behavioral Research. (1982). *Making health care decisions: A report on the ethical and legal implications of informed consent in the patient-practitioner relationship.*

Veach, P. M., Bartels, D. M., & LeRoy, B. S. (2002). Commentary on genetic counseling—A profession in search of itself. *Journal of Genetic Counseling, 11*(3), 187–191. https://doi.org/10.1023/a:1015227106269

Veach, P. M., Bartels, D. M., & Leroy, B. S. (2007). Coming full circle: A reciprocal-engagement model of genetic counseling practice. *Journal of Genetic Counseling, 16*(6), 713–728. https://doi.org/10.1007/s10897-007-9113-4

Wakefield, C. E., Meiser, B., Homewood, J., Peate, M., Kirk, J., Warner, B., Lobb, E., Gaff, C., & Tucker, K. (2007). Development and pilot testing of two decision aids for individuals considering genetic testing for cancer risk. *Journal of Genetic Counseling, 16*(3), 325–339. https://doi.org/10.1007/s10897-006-9068-x

Wakefield, C. E., Meiser, B., Homewood, J., Ward, R., O'Donnell, S., Kirk, J., & Australian GENetic testing Decision Aid Collaborative Group (2008). Randomized trial of a decision aid for individuals considering genetic testing for hereditary nonpolyposis colorectal cancer risk. *Cancer, 113*(5), 956–965. https://doi.org/10.1002/cncr.23681

Wang, C., Gonzalez, R., Milliron, K. J., Strecher, V. J., & Merajver, S. D. (2005). Genetic counseling for BRCA1/2: A randomized controlled trial of two strategies to facilitate the education and counseling process. *American Journal of Medical Genetics Part A, 134A*(1), 66–73. https://doi.org/10.1002/ajmg.a.30577

Willis, A. M., Smith, S. K., Meiser, B., Ballinger, M. L., Thomas, D. M., & Young, M. A. (2017). Sociodemographic, psychosocial and clinical factors associated with uptake of genetic counselling for hereditary cancer: A systematic review. *Clinical Genetics, 92*(2), 121–133. https://doi.org/10.1111/cge.12868

CHAPTER 5

THE RECIPROCAL-ENGAGEMENT MODEL OF GENETIC COUNSELING PRACTICE

PATRICIA MCCARTHY VEACH AND
BONNIE S. LEROY

Introduction: The Importance of Practice Models

A model of practice defines and guides what genetic counselors do and why they do what they do in providing a clinical service. It is important to note that a model of *practice* is different from a model of *service delivery*. A service delivery model describes the means by which a service is provided, such as in-person genetic counseling, telephone genetic counseling, group genetic counseling, and telegenetics, which involves both video and audio access (Trepanier & Allain, 2020).

In contrast to a service delivery model, models of practice provide certain answers to critical questions such as:

> (a) What is the theoretical framework for the practice? (b) What are the goals of practice? (c) How do we know when we have met those goals? (d) How do we evaluate the service? (e) How do we improve services? and (f) How do we teach the practice? (McCarthy Veach et al., 2007, p. 714)

Specifically, a model of practice serves several important functions:

> A model of practice constitutes a systematic method of problem solving that is applied to clinical situations and is based on scientific process (Brazen 1992; Spielberger and Stenmark 1985). A model provides: (1) a tentative theoretical framework for organizing interrelated theory, research, and practice (Spielberger and Stenmark 1985); (2) a common frame of reference for the systematic assessment of patients and the development of interventions (Nix and Dillon 1986); (3) a common frame for all practitioners in the clinical setting, thereby facilitating

communication and agreement among staff regarding identified patient problems (Nix and Dillon 1986); and (4) consistency and continuity of care in the delivery of clinical services, thereby enhancing quality of care (Nix and Dillon 1986). (McCarthy Veach et al., 2007, p. 714)

The underlying objectives and values of genetic counseling have remained steady over the years, but the ways in which genetic counseling is practiced have changed dramatically since the field's inception. In 2005, when we undertook development of a model, rapid increases in the number and types of sophisticated genetic tests and technologies, intense media attention, and the expanded use of genetics in many areas of medicine were raising the demand for services and widening the scope of practice. Genetic counselors were addressing these ever-evolving needs, but the changes were not systematically incorporated into models that define and guide practice. At the time of its publication, the Reciprocal-Engagement Model (REM; McCarthy Veach et al., 2007) was the only empirically derived genetic counseling practice model.

In this chapter, we describe the development of the REM and how it encompasses the underlying values and goals of genetic counseling practice. We then review relevant literature that supports and extends the REM in clinical practice and describes its adaptation to supervision. Lastly, we discuss the REM's clinical utility and offer several research recommendations.

The Reciprocal-Engagement Model of Genetic Counseling Practice

Description

The REM (McCarthy Veach et al., 2007) is a distinct model of genetic counseling intended to guide clinical practice. The model "articulates a psychosocial basis to exploring genetic information and presumes that reciprocity is integral to the relationship that is genetic counseling" (McCarthy Veach et al., 2007, p. 726). The REM is grounded in the results of a 2005 consensus meeting of 23 program directors (or their representatives) of North American genetic counseling graduate programs. The meeting included experts in model development and multiculturalism and group discussions of stimulus questions aimed at determining the model(s) of genetic counseling practice. Participants were tasked with identifying components of the model of practice (i.e., what genetic counselors do in a session), which they taught to their students at that time. The resulting product consisted of initial tenets (fundamental assumptions) and goals (aims) describing clinical genetic counseling practice, as well as a few strategies (plans to achieve aims) and behaviors (actions/reactions) for addressing patient needs. We used these data to develop a preliminary model organized according to key components. Figure 5.1 illustrates the REM components, tenets, and genetic counseling outcomes.

As seen in Figure 5.1, there are three components: education, individual attributes, and relationship. There are five related tenets: (a) *genetic information is key*—the primary focus of genetic counseling is on imparting the genetic contributions to disease

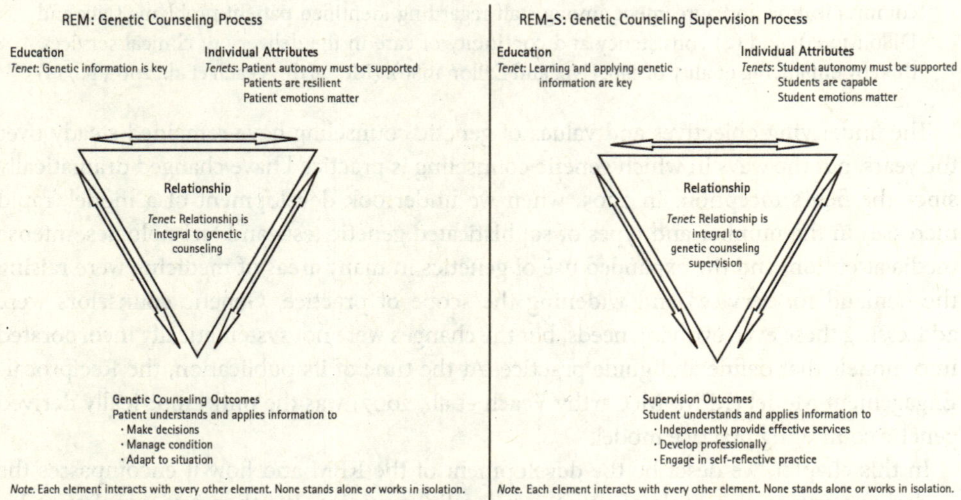

FIGURE 5.1 Comparison of the Reciprocal-Engagement Model of practice (REM) and the Reciprocal-Engagement Model of Supervision (REM-S).

(Reproduced with permission from McCarthy Veach et al. [2007] and Wherley et al. [2015])

and the value that being informed is better than being uninformed; (b) *relationship is integral to genetic counseling*—effective genetic counseling is characterized by good communication, and the counselor–patient(s) relationship is a positive and critical part of the process; (c) *patient autonomy must be supported*—this tenet articulates the belief that patients know their situations best and should be self-directed in their decisions, and their sociocultural and familial contexts should be respected and valued; (d) *patients are resilient*—they possess strength and the capacity to learn from the most difficult and painful situations; and (e) *patient emotions matter*—feelings are a relevant and important part of genetic counseling, and it is therefore essential to attend to the emotional impact of genetic information.

Seventeen goals correspond to the REM tenets (Table 5.1). These goals are intended to help patients understand and apply genetic information to achieve three broad outcomes (Figure 5.1): make decisions, manage their conditions, and adapt to their situations. As described by McCarthy Veach and colleagues, the REM tenets and goals signify that

> genetic counselors contextualize *scientific facts* within the intrapersonal, interpersonal, and cultural identities of a given patient and her or his family; and they take into consideration their patients' intrapersonal and interpersonal concerns as well as their own personal characteristics (values, biases, ethics, etc.) to accomplish desired outcomes in genetic counseling. (2007, p. 723)

The model is enacted through a reciprocal process in which each aspect mutually influences the other. The primary conduit for model enactment is the relationship between the genetic counselor and patient.

Table 5.1 Reciprocal-Engagement Model Factors and Associated Goals

Factor 1: Understanding and appreciation
Associated goals
- Counselor and patient reach an understanding of patient's family dynamics and their effects on the patient's situation
- Counselor promotes maintenance of or increase in patient self-esteem
- Counselor facilitates patient's feelings of empowerment
- Counselor integrates patient's familial and cultural context into the counseling relationship and decision making
- Counselor works with patient to recognize concerns that are triggering patient's emotions
- Counselor establishes a working contract with patient

Factor 2: Support and guidance
Associated goals
- Counselor recognizes patient strengths
- Counselor and patient establish a bond
- Counselor's characteristics positively influence the process of relationship building and communication between counselor and patient
- Counselor helps patient to gain new perspectives
- Counselor helps patient to adapt to the situation
- Counselor helps patient to feel in control

Factor 3: Facilitative decision making
Associated goals
- Counselor helps patient to feel informed
- Counselor knows what information to impart to each patient
- Counselor facilitates collaborative decisions with patient

Factor 4: Patient-centered education
Associated goals
- Counselor presents genetic information in a way that patient can understand
- Good counselor–patient communication occurs

Source: Factors found by Hartmann et al. (2015).

Extensions of the REM

We consider the REM, as described in our initial publication (McCarthy Veach et al., 2007), to be a working model. It's been our wish that further research and theorization would extend the model, particularly with respect to goals, strategies, and behaviors. Several subsequent studies have provided elaboration of the model.

Hartmann et al. (2015) surveyed 194 genetic counselors about how important they believed each of the 17 REM goals to be in their genetic counseling sessions. Average ratings indicated that participants viewed every goal as important. An exploratory factor analysis of their importance ratings for each goal yielded four factors. These factors and the REM goals associated with each factor are presented in Table 5.1. The four factors are as follows:

Factor 1: Understanding and appreciation. This factor contains six REM goals, which indicate the counselor and patient gain an understanding of the patient's individual, familial, and

> cultural characteristics. The counselor draws upon the patient's unique situation to set goals for the session and works with the patient in ways to allow the patient to feel involved and efficacious. (Hartmann et al., 2015, p. 230)
>
> *Factor 2: Support and guidance.* Six REM goals involve "the development of a supportive alliance comprised of rapport, trust, and recognition of patient strengths. Within this supportive relationship, the counselor guides patient perspective-taking, adaptation, and sense of control" (Hartmann et al., 2015, p. 230).
>
> *Factor 3: Facilitative decision making.* Three REM goals involve "counselor actions which promote informed, collaborative decision-making by patients" (Hartmann et al., 2015, p. 230).
>
> *Factor 4: Patient-centered education.* Two REM goals pertain to "effectively communicating information tailored to the patient's needs and characteristics. These goals comprise teaching objectives of genetic counseling" (Hartmann et al., 2015, p. 230).

Hartmann et al. (2015) also asked participants to rate the frequency with which they achieve each REM goal. Their frequency ratings were lower than for goal importance, suggesting that not all goals are easily attainable or relevant for every patient or every counseling situation.

Redlinger-Grosse et al. (2016) convened focus groups of practicing genetic counselors, program directors, and/or researchers. They tasked the groups with identifying a comprehensive set of genetic counseling session outcomes using the 17 REM goals as a frame to guide discussion. They obtained 194 possible outcomes reflecting one or more of the REM goals. Table 5.2 contains examples of outcomes that correspond to the REM factors and associated goals. Redlinger-Grosse et al. (2016) concluded that "Overall, the REM provides a comprehensive model of practice on which to base education, training, and clinical practice of genetic counselors" (p. 141).

Redlinger-Grosse et al. (2017) conducted an additional study to elaborate the REM by identifying strategies associated with REM goals. They conducted a secondary analysis of written descriptions of successful and unsuccessful genetic counseling sessions from a prior study (Hartmann et al., 2015) and transcripts of the focus group data concerning genetic counseling outcomes (Redlinger-Grosse et al., 2016). Using directed content analysis methods, they extracted 15 broad domains of strategies associated with the 17 REM goals. Some of the most prevalent domains are presented in Table 5.3. The researchers found that "A majority of the strategy domains . . . are also consistent with numerous practice-based competencies established by the Accreditation Council for Genetic Counseling" (Redlinger-Grosse et al., 2017, p. 1384). These findings further support the REM of genetic counseling practice.

Redlinger-Grosse et al. (2017) further found that the most prevalent strategies evident in successful sessions involved information giving and use of psychosocial skills and strategies. In unsuccessful sessions, the strategies that were often lacking were information giving and strategies to build a working alliance. The researchers concluded that the REM's emphasis on both patients' informational needs and psychosocial needs can promote successful genetic counseling processes and outcomes. They further concluded that the counselor–patient relationship is critical in genetic counseling sessions.

Ash (2017) describes motivational interviewing (MI) strategies and behaviors she believes are effective for accomplishing REM tenets and goals with some patients. Based on the work of Miller and Rollnick (2013), Ash (2017) defines MI as a

> collaborative, goal-oriented style of communication with particular attention to the language of change. It is designed to strengthen personal motivation for and commitment to a specific goal by eliciting and exploring the person's own reasons for change within an atmosphere of acceptance and compassion. (p. 300)

According to Ash (2017), MI has a strong focus on the relationship between counselor and patient, and this relationship is influenced by the counselor's attitude and communication style. A second major focus of MI is specific counseling strategies for giving and receiving information, prompting and reinforcing change talk by the patient, and encouraging patient motivation. Ash identifies open questions, affirmations, reflections, and summaries as behaviors related to these strategies; she asserts that their effective implementation promotes, among other effects, the counselor–patient relationship by building rapport and a working alliance. Using case excerpts, Ash illustrates MI strategies and behaviors and concludes that they can accomplish REM goals.

Schmidlen et al. (2018) conducted a study to develop a framework for providing genomic counseling services. Their framework includes operationalized descriptions of REM components and strategies that would "address secondary findings identified in broad-scale genomic testing, genomic screening (e.g., carrier testing, population screening), elective genomic testing in healthy individuals, and the combined effects of multiple genetic variants and environmental factors as effectors of disease risk" (Schmidlen et al., 2018, p. 1112).

Similar to the original REM, a core aspect of their counseling approach is patient centered. As Schmidlen and colleagues (2018) explain:

> The counseling agenda is patient-driven and action-oriented, with the end-goal being the activation of patients toward healthy behavior changes to reduce and manage their risk appropriately . . . through four components: (1) pre-test expectation setting and informed consent for genomic testing, (2) automated contracting and modality preference assessment, (3) tailoring of the session based on patient pre-session preferences, and (4) enhancing patient access and empowerment. (p. 1114)

The researchers concluded that their framework is a preliminary step in operationalization of the REM as a model for "(1) reducing risk for both common and rare diseases with genetic and genomic components in a proactive approach and (2) helping patients and families adapt to and cope with genetic health risks" (Schmidlen et al., 2018, p. 1125).

Shugar (2017) proposes an expansion of one of the broad REM outcomes—*patients understand and apply information to adapt to their situations*. Focusing on psychosocial adaptation, Shugar developed a genetic counseling adaptation continuum (GCAC) model and methodology to teach students counseling skills to assess and facilitate emotional, social, and psychological adaptation with respect to diagnosis, risk, and/or decision making in their patients. Shugar uses the term "purposeful psychosocial skills" to promote 13 outcomes identified by Redlinger-Grosse et al. (2016) that she considers particularly pertinent to psychosocial goals. The 13 outcomes are (Shugar, 2017, p. 217):

- A patient considers their family in decision-making;
- A change in a patient's resolution of crisis;
- A change in a patient's understanding of the long-term impact of their decision;

Table 5.2 Genetic Counseling Outcomes Identified in Multiple Reciprocal-Engagement Model (REM) Factors and Associated REM Goals

Genetic counseling outcome	Factor 1: Understanding and appreciation						Factor 2: Support and guidance						Factor 3: Facilitative decision making			Factor 4: Patient-centered education	
	1[a]	2[b]	3[c]	4[d]	5[e]	6[f]	7[g]	8[h]	9[i]	10[j]	11[k]	12[l]	13[m]	14[n]	15[o]	16[p]	17[q]
A change in communication regarding genetic information within patient's family			X										X				
A change in patient's ability to ask appropriate questions regarding their medical care												X	X				
A change in patient's ability to engage in the genetic counseling process				X	X			X	X	X			X		X		X
A change in patient's ability to gain a new perspective										X		X					
A change in patient's adaptation				X							X	X		X			
A change in patient's adherence to health behaviors											X						X
A change in patient's adjustment																X	X
A change in patient's anxiety										X						X	
A change in patient's autonomy					X										X		
A change in patient's comfort level with their decision			X											X	X		X
A change in patient's coping												X				X	
A change in patient's distress					X		X				X						
A change in patient's empowerment			X														X
A change in patient's feeling of stigma										X						X	X
A change in patient's genetic knowledge						X	X	X			X	X	X	X		X	
A change in patient's guilt										X				X			
A change in patient's locus of control		X					X										
A change in patient's medical follow-up							X										X
A change in patient's medical management			X			X	X				X	X		X		X	X
A change in patient's perceived power of control		X										X		X	X		
A change in patient's perception that they are supported															X		X
A change in patient's perception that they receive empathy						X					X						X
A change in patient's self- esteem		X				X											
A change in patient's understanding of implications of genetic information															X	X	

A change in patient's level of regret regarding their decision			X	X		X									X		
A change in the information exchanged between genetic counselor and patient																X	X
A collaborative conversation between patient and genetic counselor															X	X	
A patient is empowered		X		X		X							X				
A patient is satisfied with genetic counseling service				X		X	X				X			X			X
A patient perceives their decision to be consistent with their values										X				X			
A patient receives care that is congruent with their needs	X													X			
A patient receives competent care				X			X										
A patient receives relevant information				X										X			
A patient's decision making is autonomous				X										X	X		
A patient's emotional needs are addressed								X									X
A patient's informational needs are addressed								X									X
A patient's informational needs are met	X																X
A patient's informed decision making				X						X							
A patient's medical needs are addressed								X									X
A trust is formed between patient and genetic counselor								X									X
An alliance between patient and genetic counselor is formed				X	X	X	X	X								X	X

Note: REM goals: [a](1) Counselor and patient reach an understanding of patient's family dynamics and their effects on the patient's situation; [b](2) Counselor promotes maintenance of or increase in patient self-esteem; [c](3) Counselor facilitates patient's feelings of empowerment; [d](4) Counselor integrates patient's familial and cultural context into the counseling relationship and decision making; [e](5) Counselor works with patient to recognize concerns that are triggering patient's emotions; [f](6) Counselor establishes a working contract with patient; [g](7) Counselor recognizes patient strengths; [h](8) Counselor and patient establish a bond; [i](9) Counselor's characteristics positively influence the process of relationship building and communication between counselor and patient; [j](10) Counselor helps patient to gain new perspectives; [k](11) Counselor helps patient to adapt to their situation; [l](12) Counselor helps patient to feel in control; [m](13) Counselor helps patient to feel informed; [n](14) Counselor knows what information to impart to each patient; [o](15) Counselor facilitates collaborative decisions with patient; [p](16) Counselor presents genetic information in way that patient can understand; [q](17) Good counselor–patient communication occurs.
Reprinted with permission from the *Journal of Genetic Counseling.*
Source: Redlinger-Grosse et al. (2016, Table 8, pp. 252–253).

Table 5.3 Summary of Most Prevalent Strategy Domains Organized by Reciprocal-Engagement Model Tenets, Factors, and Individual Goals

Tenet: Genetic information is key	
Goal	Most prevalent strategy domain for each goal
Counselor helps the patient to gain new perspectives[b]	• Assessment • Use psychosocial counseling skills/strategies • Information giving
Counselor helps the patient to feel informed[c]	• Information giving • Use psychosocial counseling skills/strategies • Establish working alliance
Counselor knows what information to impart to each patient[c]	• Information giving • Use psychosocial counseling skills/strategies • Assessment
Counselor presents genetic information in a way that patient can understand[d]	• Information giving • Assessment • Use psychosocial counseling skills/strategies
Tenet: Relationship is integral to genetic counseling	
Goal	Most prevalent strategy domain for each goal
Counselor and patient establish a bond[b]	• Establish working alliance • Use psychosocial counseling skills/strategies • Information giving
Counselor's characteristics positively influence the process of relationship building and communication between counselor and patient[b]	• Use psychosocial counseling skills/strategies • Information giving • Establish working alliance • Practice self-awareness • Provide pre- and post-GC session care
Good counselor–patient communication occurs[d]	• Information giving • Use psychosocial counseling skills/strategies • Establish working alliance

Tenet: Patient autonomy must be supported	
Goal	**Most prevalent strategy domain for each goal**
Counselor integrates patient's familial and cultural context into the counseling relationship and decision making[a]	• Use psychosocial counseling skills/strategies • Information giving • Establish working alliance
Counselor establishes a working contract with patient[a]	• Establish GC goals and expectations • Information giving • Establish working alliance
Counselor helps patient to feel in control[b]	• Information giving • Use psychosocial counseling skills/strategies • Assessment
Counselor facilitates collaborative decisions with patient[c]	• Use psychosocial counseling skills/strategies • Assessment • Information giving

Tenet: Patients are resilient	
Goal	**Most prevalent strategy domain for each goal**
Counselor facilitates patient's feelings of empowerment[a]	• Information giving • Use psychosocial counseling skills/strategies • Provide care before and after GC sessions • Establish working alliance
Counselor recognizes patient strengths[a]	• Assessment • Use psychosocial counseling skills/strategies • Information giving
Counselor helps patient to adapt to their situation[b]	• Information giving • Assessment • Use psychosocial counseling skills/strategies

(continued)

Table 5.3 Continued

Tenet: Patient emotions make a difference

Goal	Most prevalent strategy domain for each goal[a]
Counselor and patient reach an understanding of patient's family dynamics and their effects on patient's situation[a]	• Use psychosocial counseling skills/strategies • Information giving • Assessment
Counselor promotes maintenance of or increase in patient self-esteem[a]	• Use psychosocial counseling skills/strategies • Provide resources • Empower patient
Counselor works with patient to recognize concerns that are triggering patient's emotions[a]	• Use psychosocial counseling skills/strategies • Information giving • Assessment

Note: GC = genetic counseling.
[a] Factor 1: Understanding and Appreciation.
[b] Factor 2: Support and Guidance.
[c] Factor 3: Facilitative Decision Making.
[d] Factor 4: Patient-Centered Education.
Source: Redlinger-Grosse et al. (2017, Table 1, pp. 1378–1379). Reprinted with permission from the *Journal of Genetic Counseling.*

- A change in a patient's self-esteem;
- A patient overcomes barriers to their care;
- A change in a patient's autonomy;
- A change in a patient's distress;
- A change in a patient's emotional stability;
- A change in a patient's feeling of stigma;
- A change in a patient's guilt;
- A change in a patient's ability to gain a new perspective;
- A change in a patient's comfort level with their decision; and
- A decision is made collaboratively between the genetic counselor and the patient.

Shugar also suggests specific strategies to help achieve each outcome. Her proposed strategies include, among others, contracting, active listening, looking for themes in a patient's narrative, primary empathy, asking clarifying questions, showing positive regard, immediacy, reframing, advanced empathy (formulating and sharing hunches), attending to a patient's verbal and nonverbal cues, and collaborating on a plan with the patient. These strategies overlap and are congruent with those identified in previous studies that support the REM as the model of genetic counseling practice.

Adaptations of the REM

Fox et al. (2007) noted at the time the REM was published that "the model should be evaluated with respect to ethno-cultural variations among individuals and client populations, and also in terms of genetic counseling as practiced in other parts of the world" (p. 730). We hoped researchers would determine whether variations in the model might be necessary due to genetic counseling specialty, patient condition, and/or patient cultural background. Some validation studies have occurred, and they generally provide support for the soundness of the model across specialties and patient and counselor characteristics.

Costa et al. (2018) used the REM to develop a 50-item scale assessing the quality of genetic counseling services in Portugal. Their measure has a strong focus on the patient–counselor relationship. They validated their scale on 81 genetic counseling sessions from various specialties and reported that the scale assesses five dimensions: education (provision of genetic information, patient understanding, and establishment of mutual agenda); patient characteristics that affect the genetic counseling process (patient's emotions and motivations, and decision-making support); the relationship between the counselor and the patient (therapeutic relationship, empathy, reflexive practice, and professionalism); potential effects of the genetic counseling process on the counselee (promotes empowerment); and provision of services (organization of services and preparation of counselee for the genetic counseling session). The first four dimensions align well with the REM elements of education, individual attributes, and relationship and with all five REM tenets (Figure 5.1; McCarthy Veach & LeRoy, 2018). Their fifth dimension pertains to "outside of session" activities, a dimension that is not part of the REM.

Parallel of the REM of practice with genetic counseling supervision

Wherley et al. (2015) propose a model of supervision to provide a comprehensive framework and direction for genetic counseling supervision of students and for supervisor training. Using the concept *form follows function*, they created a model of supervision that parallels the REM of genetic counseling practice. They named their model the Reciprocal-Engagement Model of Supervision (REM-S). The REM-S (illustrated in Figure 5.1) has parallel components (education, individual attributes, and relationship), tenets, goals, and outcomes. The five REM-S tenets are as follows: Learning and applying genetic information are key; relationship is integral to genetic counseling supervision; student autonomy must be supported; students are capable; and student emotions matter. As in the REM of genetic counseling practice, the relationship is central to achieving desired outcomes. There are 16 REM-S goals intended to achieve three outcomes that involve helping students understand and apply information to independently provide effective services, develop professionally, and engage in self-reflective practice. The following are examples of these goals: The supervisor knows what information to impart to the student; good supervisor–student communication occurs; supervisor characteristics positively influence the supervision process; the supervisor facilitates collaborative decisions; the supervisor recognizes the student's stage of development; and the supervisor addresses the student's feelings and responses to supervision and genetic counseling.

Wherley et al. (2015) suggest a few strategies they believe align with the REM-S but also call for researchers to "identify and evaluate the efficacy of strategies and behaviors congruent with REM-S tenets and goals" (p. 715). In response to this call, Suguitan et al. (2019) conducted focus group interviews with supervisors representing different practice specialties (prenatal, pediatric, cancer). To elaborate the REM-S, they asked participants to identify strategies they use when attempting to achieve each of the 16 REM-S goals. The authors extracted 14 different strategy domains from the interviews. The most prevalent strategy domains across the REM-S goals are to assess the student, practice self-reflection to increase supervisor self-awareness, and establish student goals and expectations.

Utility of the REM for Practice

A growing literature is drawing upon the REM and its implications for clinical practice. For instance, Burgess (2012), in a personal essay, describes a challenging genetic counseling session in which he had to explain a patient's positive *BRCA* results in a nonnative language. He writes:

> As genetic counsellors, we have training in the concepts of Person Centered therapy and are skilled at building rapport and engaging with our clients by using techniques such as active listening, non-judgmental approaches and empathy, but I wanted a model of practice. I did not think it is good enough to say I use an eclectic model of counselling. When I came across the Reciprocal-Engagement Model (2007), it really resonated with me. I agree that giving information and education is part of our role, but we do more than that. We are able to work

> with the individual attributes of our clients to achieve an appropriate genetic counselling outcome through the relationship that we build with our clients. (Burgess, 2012, p. 178)

Burgess asserts that building relationships with patients is key to promoting genetic counseling outcomes.

Hodgson and Gaff (2013) explore how genetic counseling discussions about the importance of family communication often pose ethical and professional challenges for counselors. They use the REM to describe these challenges and ways to resolve them. Consistent with the REM, they stress the importance of the counselor–patient relationship as a pivotal component for discussions about family communication. They note, "The counselor and patient are co-informants, with the counselor providing expertise in genetics and counseling and the patient contributing his or her life story. They work together to determine what is in the patient's best interests" (Hodgson & Gaff, 2013, p. 17).

Hodson and Gaff (2013) further assert that "genetic counseling around family communication—or rather, lack of family communication—brings the tenet of Genetic information is key (being informed is better than being uninformed) into conflict with that of Patient autonomy must be supported" (p. 17). The authors "explored these tensions by returning to the core principles or tenets of genetic counseling as described by the REM, and resolved them by drawing on the Rogerian principle of 'patient centred counseling' as it is applied to genetic counseling" (Hodson & Gaff, 2013, pp. 19–20).

Williams et al. (2017) use the REM tenet *relationship is integral to genetic counseling* as the theoretical basis of their qualitative study of the relationship between genetic counselors and prenatal patients who received a prenatal diagnosis that indicated a fetus with a life limiting condition. They interviewed both the counselors and patients. Of note, this is one of the first published studies to assess patients' perspective using the REM as a framework. Counselors and patients described three major categories of support provided by the genetic counselors: provision of information/education that is pertinent and understandable, displaying facilitative characteristics and attitudes (e.g., treating patients with respect and sensitivity, regarding patient as a priority, genuineness, compassion), and addressing patients' psychosocial needs (e.g., listening, normalization and validation of feelings, reinforcing patients' strengths).

The researchers conclude that their findings support all five REM tenets. In addition to the data supporting the pivotal role of the relationship (tenet 2), they note:

> The provision of information was one of the greatest sources of support during the time of crisis [tenet 1]. . . . The genetic counselor throughout the relationship acted as an advocate for the patient and supported patient autonomy [tenet 3]. . . . Many of the genetic counselors mentioned how impressed and inspired they were by the patient's resilience throughout the process [tenet 4] . . . [and] the genetic counselors empathized with the patient, proceeded at the patient's pace in terms of informational and psychosocial needs, and offered as much support as possible or necessary [tenet 5]. (Williams et al., 2017, p. 351)

Some researchers have used the REM to interpret the findings of their studies. For instance, Greve et al. (2020) studied proxy patient and genetic counselor perceptions of the skillfulness of various responses to a hypothetical prenatal patient's request for self-disclosure. They concluded that skillful responses generally were those that participants perceived as providing support and guidance to the patient. They recommended that, consistent with the REM, genetic counselors' responses should be based on the goals of providing support and guidance when prenatal patients request self-disclosure.

Miranda et al. (2016) interviewed 15 master's-level genetic counselor clinicians to identify their personal and professional characteristics. They found a number of prevalent characteristics, including curiosity, lifelong learners, self-reflection, authenticity, and desire to form collaborative and interactive relationships with patients. The researchers concluded that their findings "are consistent with the five tenets or underlying assumptions of the REM . . . [and] are also consistent with the REM view that counselor characteristics are a pivotal part of genetic counseling processes and outcomes" (Miranda et al., 2016, p. 780).

Future Research Recommendations

Ongoing efforts to validate and elaborate the REM will add support to its viability as a model of practice. Further studies should more fully characterize REM strategies and behaviors associated with the tenets and goals. The REM and most extant studies to date are based on genetic counseling practice in North America. The extent to which the REM will be a feasible model in other countries remains to be seen. Further validation of the model ideally will involve studies of actual or simulated genetic counseling sessions across practice specialties and with diverse patient populations in different settings. Most of the REM literature is from the perspective of practitioners. Studies assessing patients' reactions to the model will help to further establish its validity. Finally, we have been part of the research teams for many of the extant studies grounded in the REM. We look forward to additional investigations by other researchers to corroborate our findings.

Conclusion

Although the REM is a working model of genetic counseling practice, the components, tenets, and goals thus far appear to be withstanding the test of time. Empirical evidence is growing to support the REM, especially the tenets and goals. The three broad REM outcomes also generally appear to be applicable, but they are further enhanced by the articulation of more specific types of outcomes (e.g., Redlinger-Grosse et al., 2016; Shugar, 2017). While findings suggest that the counselor–patient relationship is central to all other aspects of the model, each component of the REM, alone, is necessary, but not sufficient for providing the highest quality of clinical genetic counseling services to patients. As we speculated in our initial publication of the model (McCarthy Veach et al., 2007), there may be greater individual, cultural, and contextual variation in the implementation of certain strategies and goals in genetic counseling sessions. Continued efforts to characterize the REM and its effects on genetic counseling processes and outcomes will not only contribute to "our understanding of how to prepare genetic counselors and the profession for the future" (Fox et al., 2007, p. 730) but also provide a framework for future genetic counseling research.

References

Ash, E. (2017). Motivational Interviewing in the Reciprocal Engagement Model of genetic counseling: A method overview and case illustration. *Journal of Genetic Counseling, 26*, 300–311.

Brazen, L. (1992). Project 2000: The difference between conceptual models, practice models. *AORN Journal, 56*, 840–844.

Burgess, M. (2012). Developing my preferred model of genetic counselling. *Journal of Genetic Counseling, 21*, 177–178.

Costa, C., Lemos, M. S., & Paneque, M. (2018). The contribution of the Reciprocal-Engagement Model as a theoretical framework of a Portuguese scale for quality assessment of genetic counseling. *Journal of Genetic Counseling, 27*, 1005–1007.

Fox, M., Weil, J., & Resta, R. (2007). Why we do what we do: Commentary on a reciprocal-engagement model of genetic counseling practice. *Journal of Genetic Counseling, 16*, 729–730.

Greve, V., McCarthy Veach, P., LeRoy, B. S., MacFarlane, I. M., & Redlinger-Grosse, K. (2020). Genetic counselor and proxy patient perceptions of genetic counselor responses to prenatal patient self-disclosure requests: Skillfulness is in the eye of the beholder. *Journal of Genetic Counseling, 29*(6), 894–909. https://doi.org/10.1002/jgc4.1190

Hartmann, J., McCarthy Veach, P., MacFarlane, I. M., & LeRoy, B. S. (2015). Genetic counselor perceptions of genetic counseling session goals: A validation study of the Reciprocal-Engagement Model. *Journal of Genetic Counseling, 24*, 225–237.

Hodgson, J., & Gaff, C. (2013). Enhancing family communication about genetics: Ethical and professional dilemmas. *Journal of Genetic Counseling, 22*, 16–21.

McCarthy Veach, P., & LeRoy, B. S. (2018). Response to Costa, Lemos, and Paneque Letter to the Editor. *Journal of Genetic Counseling, 27*, 1008.

McCarthy Veach, P., Bartels, D. M., & LeRoy, B. S. (2007). Coming full circle: A Reciprocal-Engagement Model of genetic counseling practice. *Journal of Genetic Counseling, 16*, 713–728. https://doi.org/10.1007/s10897-007-9113-4

Miller, W., & Rollnick, S. (2013). *Motivational interviewing: Helping people change* (3rd ed.). Guilford Press.

Miranda, C., McCarthy Veach, P., Martyr, M., & LeRoy, B. S. (2016). Portrait of the master genetic counselor: A qualitative investigation of expertise in genetic counseling. *Journal of Genetic Counseling, 25*, 767–785.

Nix, J., & Dillon, K. (1986). Short-term nursing therapy: A conceptual model for inpatient psychiatric care. *Hospital and Community Psychiatry, 37*, 493–496.

Redlinger-Grosse, K., McCarthy Veach, P., Cohen, S., LeRoy, B. S., MacFarlane, I. M., & Zierhut, H. (2016). Defining our clinical practice: The identification of genetic counselor outcomes utilizing the Reciprocal Engagement Model. *Journal of Genetic Counseling, 25*, 239–257.

Redlinger-Grosse, K., McCarthy Veach, P., LeRoy, B. S., & Zierhut, H. (2017). Elaboration of the Reciprocal-Engagement Model of genetic counseling practice: A qualitative investigation of goals and strategies. *Journal of Genetic Counseling, 26*, 1372–1387.

Schmidlen, T., Sturm, A. C., Hovick, S., Scheinfeldt, L., Scott Roberts, J., Morr, L., McElroy, J., Toland, A. E., Christman, M., O'Daniel, J. M., Gordon, E. S., Bernhardt, B. A., Ormond, K. E., & Sweet, K. (2018). Operationalizing the reciprocal engagement model of genetic counseling practice: A framework for the scalable delivery of genomic counseling and testing. *Journal of Genetic Counseling, 27*, 1111–1129.

Shugar, A. (2017). Teaching genetic counseling skills: Incorporating a genetic counseling adaptation continuum model to address psychosocial complexity. *Journal of Genetic Counseling, 26*, 215–223.

Spielberger, C. D., & Stenmark, D. E. (1985). Community psychology. In E. Altmeier & M. E. Meyer (Eds.), *Applied specialties in psychology* (pp. 75–97). Random House.

Suguitan, M. D., Redlinger-Grosse, K., McCarthy Veach, P., & LeRoy, B. S. (2019). Genetic counseling supervisor strategies: An elaboration of the Reciprocal-Engagement Model of supervision. *Journal of Genetic Counseling, 28*, 602–615.

Trepanier, A., & Allain, D. C. (2020). Adapting genetic counseling practice to different models of service delivery. In B. S. LeRoy, P. McCarthy Veach, & N. P. Callanan (Eds.), *Genetic counseling practice: Advanced concepts and skills* (2nd ed., pp. 317–339). John Wiley & Sons.

Wherley, C., McCarthy Veach, P., Martyr, M., & LeRoy, B. S. (2015). Form follows function: A model for clinical supervision practice in genetic counseling. *Journal of Genetic Counseling, 24*, 702–716. https://doi.org/10.1007/s10897-015-9837-5

Williams, S. R., Berrier, K. L., Redlinger-Grosse, K., & Edwards, J. G. (2017). Reciprocal relationships: The genetic counselor-patient relationship following a life-limiting prenatal diagnosis. *Journal of Genetic Counseling, 26*, 337–354.

CHAPTER 6

NEW PERSPECTIVES IN PSYCHOSOCIAL GENETIC COUNSELING

JON WEIL

Introduction

Psychosocial genetic counseling offers a perspective on all aspects of genetic counseling that go beyond the factual data or statistical/probability information that is provided. It is inclusive, with recognition of the multiple ways that individuals, families, and communities are affected by the risk of and occurrence of disorders with a genetic etiology or contribution and by the screening, testing, and treatment interventions that are involved. In a clinical situation it may be immediately applicable (e.g., the patient is devastated by the news they have just received), it may provide a useful means for understanding what is occurring (e.g., the patient is having difficulty understanding the information because of their anxiety), or it may have little or no relevance (e.g., at this time a clear, factual explanation of how the risk figure was determined is of paramount importance). In this chapter I will address a variety of topics from the psychosocial perspective. I will consider how it may be used to reframe long-standing issues, to identify connections and parallels among different issues, and to develop a more comprehensive understanding of the stresses and challenges that patients and genetic counselors confront in the present era. To this end I am intentionally speculative, pushing the boundaries of what is known and suggesting clinical approaches and research opportunities that, if judged to be valuable, will require further validation and development.

A Selective Review of the Historical Development of Risk Perception and Decision Making

Risk perception and decision making are central to genetic counseling. How they are understood and conceptualized has significant influence on clinical practice. A brief review of the historical development of these concepts will provide a framework for a number of the topics that will be discussed in this chapter. The review is limited and selective to serve this purpose.

From the early decades of the 20th century into the 1980s, as the rapidly developing science of genetics was applied to human disorders, the data presented as occurrence or recurrence risks were generally considered to be objective, which recipients could use to make rational decisions concerning the magnitude of the risk and the implications for their and their loved one's well-being (Palmer & Sainfort, 1993). During this period, genetic counseling was primarily the domain of White male geneticists and physicians working in heredity clinics and medical genetics departments (Fine, 1993; Stern, 2012). Their approach was often deeply embedded in eugenic thinking, although there was also often great compassion for the individuals and families who were being treated.[1] In addition, there was a diversity of opinion as well as ambiguity and change over time concerning the relative importance of the eugenic or "public health" role of genetic counseling as opposed to supporting the wishes and decisions of the individuals who were being counseled (Stern, 2012). The assumption of objective, actionable risk figures occurred within the context of increasing actuarial and risk studies after World War II, in which "the paramount assumption . . . was that individuals and societies behaved as rational decision makers, operating in accordance with utilitarian principles of self- or group maximization" (Stern, 2012, p. 37).

In 1979, four articles by Lippman-Hand and Fraser presented a radically deeper, nuanced view of patients' responses to receiving occurrence and recurrence risk information (Lippman-Hand & Fraser, 1979a, 1979b, 1979c, 1979d). Lippman-Hand and Fraser observed genetic counseling sessions in which patients received reproductive risk figures and then conducted in-depth interviews with the patients. Among their findings were the following: *Binarization*: In all 60 follow-up interviews, patients perceived the risk figure they were given as implying two alternatives, "either the child would be normal or affected" (Lippman-Hand & Fraser, 1979c, p. 57). This largely unconscious process converted the uncertainty of the risk figure into more tangible potential outcomes whose implications could be evaluated. *Scenarios*: This evaluation involved what Lippman-Hand and Fraser called a scenario—"the starting point for an imagined series of outcomes in which the dimensions most important to the woman were highlighted and her emotional responses to them surveyed" (Lippman-Hand & Fraser, 1979c, p. 63). *Existential burden of being at*

[1] Editors' note: For more in-depth discussion on early social eugenic programs in the United States, see Chapter 1 by Devon Stillwell in this volume.

risk: Being at risk and the need to make decisions in the face of uncertainty were experienced as burdens in and of themselves.

This research and the transformational articles it produced occurred during a period of profound changes in the knowledge and techniques of human/medical genetics and the attitudes and personnel of those involved in genetic counseling. In 1969 the genetic counseling master's degree program at Sarah Lawrence College accepted its first students, and by 1981 graduates from six master's degree programs were establishing the new profession of master's-level genetic counselors. Concurrently, in 1971 an ad hoc committee of the American Society of Human Genetics concluded that genetic counseling should only be provided by physicians with training in genetics, a position that was explicitly reversed in 1974 (Stern, 2012). These changes, in turn, occurred within the context of vast social–political changes including the civil rights, feminist rights, counterculture, and anti–Vietnam War movements and protests (Stern, 2009).

The articles by Lippman-Hand and Fraser initiated an era in which many aspects of patient experiences were examined and conceptualized. Wertz et al. (1986) found that patients who had received a similar risk figure (e.g., 25%) varied widely in the verbal descriptor they applied to it (from 3% who called it "very low" through 37% indicating "moderate" to 14% using "very high"). Conversely, Burke and Kolker (1994) asked 36 genetic counselors to assess the one-in-200 risk of spontaneous abortion following prenatal diagnosis, with the majority describing it as "low" or "very low." When asked about the same risk for a genetic disorder, it was most commonly described as "moderate." These and other studies demonstrated the inadequacy of considering risk figures as facts and led to the conceptualization and further investigation of *risk perception*.

In 1993, Palmer and Sainfort addressed the complex nature of risk and uncertainty and proposed a new formulation in which the central concept was *uncertainty*—the need to make decisions in the face of unknown potential outcomes (Palmer & Sainfort, 1993). Because genetic counseling involves Mendelian inheritance patterns and empiric risk figures, uncertainty is operationalized as *probabilities*. Whereas probabilities are neutral, *risk* implies that one or more potential outcomes will have adverse effects. Palmer and Sainfort proposed that risk and the process of risk assessment involve both the probability of an event and the assessment of the adversity involved should it occur. "The *presence* of both uncertainty and adversity is the relevant and necessary aspect of our view of risk, not the *amount*. Risk perception serves as the individual-specific measure of the amount of risk present in a decision situation" (Palmer & Sainfort, 1993, p. 288, italics in original). Building on Lippman-Hand and Fraser's concept of scenarios, they said:

> The judgment of the level of adversity associated with having a child with an abnormality is really the judgment of the adversity of a myriad of consequences, or potential events which make up that abnormality. Each consequence may have a different influence on the overall judgment of adversity. Therefore, it is important to organize the consequences associated with an outcome as a hierarchy of events. (Palmer & Sainfort, 1993, p. 289)

In an elaboration of the concept of scenarios, they called this process an *event structure*. As an example, they presented an event structure for achondroplasia. Eleven components were identified. These included employment, relationships with school peers, ear infections, and (lumbar spinal) stenosis, illustrating the great variety of factors that might influence a reproductive decision based on the physical, emotional, and financial resources and the beliefs and values of those making the decision.

In subsequent years, a large body of research has developed concerning the manner in which patients understand, evaluate, and act upon the information they receive. Sivell et al. (2008) reviewed 59 studies that investigated risk perception, construction, interpretation, and effects on decision making. They found multiple, complex factors affecting each of these components. The majority of the studies involved cancer genetics, most often breast/ovarian, and predominantly serving White patients. Within these limitations they stated:

> This review highlights a tension between studies that address understanding of risk as a numerical entity to be recalled and/or modified . . . and those that demonstrate that understanding of risk is a process of making meaning and responding to the potential threat that risk represents. When risk communication is described as a two-way exchange of information and opinion about risk . . . , genetic counseling can be seen to assimilate these different perspectives, providing "objective" information while also giving the individual an opportunity to explore the understanding they hold of their situation and the meaning they make of any new information. The factors influencing the process [include] environmental factors, occupation, diet, stress and worry, physical resemblance to an affected relative, as well as genetic or family history. (Sivell et al., 2008, pp. 59–60)

In 2010 Skirton and Bylund addressed the clinical implications of patients' need to deal with uncertainty (Skirton & Bylund, 2010). Drawing on work from other disciplines, they introduced the principles of uncertainty management theory (UMT) in the context of communication and risk assessment in genetic counseling. Three concepts are central: (a) Attempts to reduce or eliminate uncertainty may create greater uncertainty (e.g., when a genetic test identifies a pathogenic variant whose penetrance and expressivity are variable); (b) patients may choose to maintain or increase uncertainty (e.g., when a decision is made not to pursue genetic testing); and (c) there are situations in which uncertainty cannot be reduced (e.g., a genetic condition for which a definitive test is not available).

Subsequent work has advanced this line of research and its clinical applications. Fisher et al. (2017) used UMT as the basis for investigating how genetic practitioners helped women receiving *BRCA1/2* counseling manage multiple aspects of uncertainty about themselves and their daughters. Among many valuable results they identified five uncertainty management strategies: addressing myths, misunderstandings, or misconceptions; using science-based uncertainty (e.g., future scientific/technological developments; the ambiguity of *BRCA* testing) to introduce hope; encouraging information seeking and sharing of family medical history; reaffirming and validating previous behavior and decisions; and minimizing the probability of personal or family members' risk. Barlow Stewart (2018) provides a concise summary of UMT theory, research, and clinical applications in genetic counseling.

This review provides the background for several topics that will be discussed later. It also illustrates two broad concepts: First, major developments such as those of Lippman-Hand and Fraser (1979a, 1979b, 1979c, 1979d) and Skirton and Bylund (2010) build upon advances in knowledge and techniques in clinical/medical genetics as well as other medical/scientific disciplines. In addition, although it is beyond the scope of this review, they reflect broader technological developments as well as changes in societal values and concerns (Stern, 2009). Second, although less frequently commented upon, the historical changes described involve profound changes in the implicit view of the patient—in brief, from a rational evaluator of risk data, to an individual who assesses the personal meaning of such data, to a person undertaking complex conscious and unconscious psychological processes, to a person whose life is embedded in multiple forms of uncertainty regarding both information and the future. The latter includes, as Fisher et al. (2017) state regarding *BRCA1/2*, "families . . . learning how to manage a complex web of uncertainty that can challenge them for a lifetime" (p. 456). The implications of these broader concepts will also be addressed later in the chapter, including in the final section.

New Perspectives on Enduring Issues

Scenarios: A broadly applicable concept

As discussed in the preceding section, the concept of scenarios, in which women receiving prenatal genetic counseling evaluated the implications of the possible outcomes they faced, was one among several findings by Lippman-Hand and Fraser (1979c) that qualitatively changed consideration of how patients respond to genetic counseling. Palmer and Sainfort (1993) expanded this concept, using the term "event structure," to examine the great diversity of issues that could in principle be involved—ranging, for achondroplasia, from childhood ear infections to future employment opportunities. Other scholars have considered similar constructs and their impact on decision making (Shiloh, 2006; Sivell et al., 2008). These and most other studies have addressed the issue from a research perspective: How are scenarios constructed and how do they influence decision making? However, the concept is also relevant from the perspective of clinical practice: How can genetic counselors help patients develop scenarios that best serve them in assessing potential outcomes and making decisions that are consistent with their circumstances, values, and wishes?

Over many years of teaching and consulting, drawing primarily on Lippman-Hand and Fraser's conceptualization, I have discussed three elements of the latter question: How accurate is the scenario in terms of the information and perceptions involved? How representative is it—that is, is it based on a sufficiently broad set of examples or circumstances, with a reasonably correct understanding of the relative frequency of different possible outcomes? And how rich in detail is it? Helping patients explore, correct, refine, and enrich these components of their scenario or scenarios can improve the value of the decisions to which they contribute. However, Palmer and Sainfort's (1993) analysis makes clear that an immense variety of issues may be relevant to a given patient, and research concerning uncertainty indicates that the various forms of uncertainty associated with testing, clinical services, and the condition or disorder that is involved are also relevant (Fisher et al., 2017; Skirton & Bylund, 2010).

Attention to and guidance in the formation of the patient's scenario(s) are broadly applicable. This may begin during the contracting stage of a session, when the genetic counselor initiates the process of trying to understand and respond to the patient's concerns and hopes for the session. For some patients the most important concerns may involve the immediate or near future, whereas for others they may be more long term. For some the most pressing issue may be "How can I get through this undesired mandatory counseling session as quickly as possible?" With such patients it is useful to consider the relevant scenario to be that involving the session itself. Discussing the accuracy, representativeness, and richness of detail of the patient's perceptions concerning the session, uncertainty about what will occur, and more long-term concerns (e.g., Am I starting a process that I will regret?) provides one means for addressing their resistance.

Continuing with this example, to the extent that the patient becomes engaged, the next scenario will involve the issues for which the session has been requested or the patient has been referred. This may initially focus on the medical implications of the disorder, as described by a referring physician. When these have been addressed, the discussion may turn to the resources available to the patient, which they may describe in terms of financial resources. The genetic counselor can broaden and enrich this scenario by asking about family and social support and then about personal resources based on faith, hope, previous experience, and other factors.

Although the essentially unbounded set of possible scenarios makes it difficult to think about applying this approach to clinical encounters, it is also an asset: It has sufficient breadth to serve as a unifying concept across a number of issues that the patient, and thus the genetic counselor, may confront. Genetic counselors have the mandate to provide increasingly complex information, with major components of uncertainty, while attempting to address psychosocial issues the patient or patients confront (Skirton, 2018). Conceptualizing the genetic counseling interaction in terms of refining the patient's evolving scenario or scenarios provides an additional way to undertake this process. It may also be helpful when planning a session as well as when reviewing a session with respect to potential follow-up and more broadly in terms of what can be learned from the session.

The interventions I have discussed above are well-established components of psychosocial genetic counseling. I suggest that conceptualizing them in terms of scenarios is a useful way to understand the strengths and limitations of the patient's knowledge and ability to evaluate the meaning of the information provided, and thus to effectively address them.

Reframing Patient Resistance as Communication

In his seminal article, "Bearing Bad News: Dealing with the Mimics of Denial," Lubinsky (1994) says of disbelief, a type of resistance in which the patient understands the information but does not accept or believe it, "Our explanations are heard, but not understood. People are left trying to comprehend something outside of normal experience, something that goes against their common sense and everything their hearts want to believe" (p. 7). How might genetic counselors reframe our understanding of patient resistance to more fully approach Lubinsky's level of empathy and compassion?

Patient resistance, which I have previously defined as "attitudes, behaviors, emotions and ways of thinking by which a patient limits full engagement with the process of genetic counseling," occurs frequently and is to be expected (Weil, 2010a, p. 155). It may be expressed in multiple ways whose effects range from a minor impediment or discontinuity to a major disruption of the session. Examples include providing incomplete or inaccurate information; failing to recognize the severity or significance of a situation; avoiding meaningful discussion or informed decision making; expressing anger, hostility, and withdrawal verbally and/or through behavior; and questioning the competence of the genetic counselor or the value of genetic counseling.

Resistance can be understood as an attempt to protect self and/or family and loved ones. In its most limited forms this may involve momentary discomfort, anxiety, or confusion. In more protracted or intense forms, it is an attempt to provide protection against devastating news, loss of hopes and dreams, emotional and financial difficulties, insufficient empathy from the genetic counselor, and other actual, perceived, or feared threats to well-being and self-esteem.

From the perspective of its self-protective role, and drawing on the work of others, I proposed three principles that are central to addressing patient resistance: *empathy* based on an understanding of the reasons for and protective role of resistance, *acceptance of the normality* of resistance, and *attention to the* very substantial *countertransference* that resistance can invoke (Weil, 2010a). This represents a well-established practice- and theory-driven approach to addressing patient resistance (McCarthy Veach et al., 2018). I now propose a more explicitly client-oriented approach, beginning with the following revised definition:

> Resistance is a normal and essential mechanism by which patients communicate their confusion, fear, anger, pain, and other responses to the genetic counseling process and the situations they face.

In the moment when a patient expresses resistance, it embodies their experience or concern. It may be limited and quickly over; it may affect the process of the session in a way that is fairly readily managed; or, when it involves anger or rejection, it may be highly disruptive or bring the session to an end. Thus, depending on the circumstances and the genetic counselor's judgment, it may be the most important aspect of the interaction to address. When responding to resistance, I propose that the genetic counselor can more effectively understand and attend to the patient's experience or concern by accepting the resistance as communication rather than perceiving it as an impediment. Indeed, when resistance is expressed through behavior (e.g., distractedness, failure to answer questions) or in angry or indirect speech combined with behavior (e.g., rejection of the genetic counselor's knowledge), the fact that the communication is verbally inarticulate may help the genetic counselor understand the level of concern or despair that the patient is experiencing.

I suggest that this approach will have the following effects: It may increase empathy because the genetic counselor's response is shifted from perceiving the resistance as an impediment toward trying to understand it as an attempt, perhaps anguished or desperate, to communicate. It may shift countertransference away from anger, defensiveness, and self-doubt concerning professional competence toward concern for trying to understand the patient's unmet informational or psychological needs. It will not necessarily reduce the intensity of the countertransference; there may still be a strong negative response, and the depth of the patient's anger or pain may be more keenly experienced if it is perceived as an attempt to communicate. Most importantly, it may make the genetic counselor's responses or interventions more effective because they address the basis for the resistance more directly and can be adjusted as necessary from this perspective.

The Challenge of Diversity

With continuing expansion of the types of genetic counseling services provided (e.g., oncology, neurogenetics) and populations served including individuals and groups that have experienced migration and displacement, issues of diversity and inclusivity have become critically important. There are many resources and methods available to assist genetic counselors, individually and collectively, in investigating and advancing with respect to these issues (e.g., see Chapter 29—"Cultural Responsiveness and Linguistic Competence in Genetic Counseling: Taking Responsibility" in this volume; Genetic Counseling Toolkit, n.d.; Kfir et al., 2020). What follows draws on many resources. However, it is also an attempt to find an individual path toward greater awareness and understanding, which I undertake for three reasons. First, I hope it will have value in and of itself. Second, it exemplifies my belief that any such effort must draw on multiple resources to find its own direction based on the populations served, the nature of that service, and the circumstances and background of the genetic counselor or genetic counselors who are involved. Third, I hope it will receive thorough, critical review. Elaboration of the material I present would be useful. However, alternative viewpoints, including those that involve opposing perspectives, are potentially more valuable because they represent the essence of addressing issues of diversity.

Diversity is highly multidimensional and has many interrelated forms. Although not a complete list of possible characteristics that could be used to define diversity, the following is a brief compilation:

- Ethnocultural
- Religious/spiritual
- Socioeconomic
- Gender identity
- Sexual orientation
- Abled–disabled
- Age
- Stable versus unstable circumstances

Each of these is in turn multidimensional and may change over time (Zayts-Spence et al., 2021). For example, many individuals and families are of mixed, often complex ethnicity and culture with respect to genetic lineage and self-identity (Fennel, 2021). Stable versus unstable circumstances include homelessness and immigrant, refugee, or displaced status (Fennel, 2021). Abled–disabled includes a broad array of situations that genetic counselors are accustomed to considering (Crowe et al., 2018; Finucane, 2012). Diversity is also fluid, changing with time while retaining elements from the past (Fennel, 2021; Weil, 2000). For example, the patient or genetic counselor may have overcome substantial adversity to achieve the current level of socioeconomic stability and security but continues to have substantial anxiety about the permanence of their situation.

From this perspective a genetic counseling session may be thought of as comprising many aspects of diversity of varying degrees and importance. One benefit of this approach is to help the genetic counselor explore the specific circumstances and needs of a given patient or family. For example, in a given case the most salient initial issue might be ethnocultural.

However, as the session proceeds the opinion of a family member affected by a different disorder (abled–disabled) may be highly significant, and financial concerns and limited healthcare (socioeconomic) may constrain both medical and psychosocial options. Applied more broadly, this conceptualization supports the genetic counselor in avoiding stereotypes and preconceptions.

In a genetic counseling session or comparable interaction such as a telephone conversation, the patient and their circumstances make up one focus of the encounter. The other involves the genetic counselor with their circumstances that include personal, social, and cultural components as well as the medical/genetic counseling context within which they work. I find it helpful to think in geometric terms, so I visualize the interaction as involving two points in a highly multidimensional hyperspace. Thus, the genetic counselor and patient may be distant in some dimensions, be relatively close in others, and occupy almost identical positions in yet others.

Many sources agree on the importance of being aware of and sensitive to one's own beliefs, emotions, self-identity, and circumstances vis-à-vis the multiple components of diversity just discussed (e.g., see Chapter 29—"Cultural Responsiveness and Linguistic Competence in Genetic Counseling: Taking Responsibility" in this volume; Genetic Counseling Toolkit, n.d.; Sharif et al., 2020; Weil, 2000; Wilson, 2014).

From the wealth of approaches and resources for undertaking self-examination individually and collectively, I propose the following approach to self-exploration:

Many interactions in the genetic counselor's life involve a degree of diversity that provides an opportunity to explore relevant issues. For encounters that are relatively straightforward and unproblematic, one may ask questions such as:

- What are the nature and extent of differences between my values, beliefs, perceptions, actions, and worldview and those of the other person?
- What are the nature and extent of similarities between my values, beliefs, perceptions, actions, and worldview and those of the other person?
- Would my evaluations change if I reversed the order of the previous two questions?
- What are the origins of my values, beliefs, perceptions, actions, and worldview in my personal history, my family's history, and my cultural background and experiences?
- How accurate is my knowledge of the other person's personal history, family history, cultural background, and experiences? What questions does that raise about how accurately I understand my own?

For interactions that are more difficult, confrontive, and/or thrust upon someone, later review may involve questions about one's core beliefs and values, including questions such as:

- How much flexibility do I have for accommodating the other person's position where there is divergence and for increasing agreement and understanding where there is overlap?
- To what extent is my flexibility or inflexibility a matter of unexamined beliefs or values and to what extent does it seem firmly grounded in well-thought-out beliefs and values?
- Which values and behaviors are or were essential to preserve the physical and emotional well-being of myself, my family, my forbears, and/or my culture in the face

of current and historical discrimination, persecution, and other destructive or existential threats? Of these, which are potentially inclusive of the other person (e.g., strength through caring for others) and which are potentially exclusive?

A related opportunity for increased self-awareness occurs when one's stereotypes, prejudices, or other forms of unrecognized bias are unexpectedly revealed. In 1978, while studying clinical genetics and genetic counseling after 15 years conducting basic research with bacteriophage, I read a paper on reconstructive surgery for individuals with profound facial dysmorphology. As I looked at the figures, I realized with shock that I was assuming intellectual disability when looking at photographs taken before surgery but not when looking at those illustrating successful surgical outcomes. I have had a number of such experiences since then within and outside genetic counseling, involving both interpersonal interactions and resources such as journal articles. Each has contributed to my awareness of an important bias, stereotype, or presupposition that had been unconscious. Collectively they have made me aware of the value of being open to such self-observation.

Self-exploration, whether alone, with assistance, or collectively, may reveal or increase one's awareness of issues that range from uncomfortable to deeply distressing. The beliefs, biases, and stereotypes may themselves be upsetting. However, underlying them there can be a loss of self-esteem and sense of personal or professional identity as well as an awareness of significant internal conflicts or contradictions. To address these issues as effectively as possible, it is important insofar as possible to accept them as normal human responses rather than reacting to them with avoidance or denial.

Research into unconscious bias described by Eberhardt (2019) provides one approach to acceptance and normalization. She and associates investigated the previously well-documented finding "that people are much better at recognizing faces of their own race than faces of other races" (Eberhardt, 2019, p. 13). This differential response, which begins as early as 3 months of age and increases during adolescence, is influenced by the ethnicity of others in the individual's social environment, not by the individual's ethnicity. Using functional magnetic resonance imaging with White and Black volunteers responding to pictures of the faces of White and Black individuals, they investigated neural activity in the fusiform face area (FFA), an area of the brain associated with facial recognition. "We found that the FFA was responding more vigorously to faces that were the same race as the study participant" (Eberhardt, 2019, p. 18). These and other data demonstrate that the differential recognition is in large part socially determined and neurologically based. Interpreting this research, undertaken to address critical issues involving police–community interactions, Eberhardt states:

> Categorization—grouping like things together—is not some abhorrent feature of the human brain, a process that some people engage in and others do not. Rather, it is a universal function of the brain that allows us to organize and manage the overload of stimuli that constantly bombard us. It's a system that brings coherence to a chaotic world; it helps our brains make judgments more quickly and efficiently by instinctively relying on patterns that seem predictable. (Eberhardt, 2019, pp. 23–24)

Schaa et al. (2015) investigated the relationship between genetic counselors' implicit racial attitudes and their interactions with simulated clients portrayed by Black, non-Hispanic White, or Hispanic professional actors. Racial attitudes were assessed with a web-based survey. Simulated cases involved a woman seeking preamniocentesis counseling based on advanced maternal age or information about *BRCA1/2* testing with a family history of breast/ovarian cancer. Participants chose which case they preferred, with some cases portraying the woman alone and the remainder including a partner. Coding of the videotaped sessions included a particular focus on patient-centered communication styles such as verbal dominance, socioemotional and psychosocial communication, and biomedical information giving.

Among the results were the following: Genetic counselors who indicated stronger pro-White bias displayed less rapport building and positive affect in sessions with minority simulated clients and were significantly less verbally dominant than other genetic counselors in sessions with White simulated clients. They received higher ratings on overall communication from White simulated clients, and their degree of pro-White bias was positively correlated with ratings of their nonverbal communication. No relationship was established between degree of pro-White bias and self-ratings of communication, which may result from the largely unconscious aspects of implicit bias.

The research conducted by Eberhardt (2019) and Schaa et al. (2015) was undertaken to support and advance the value of self-awareness and other demonstrated methods for addressing unconscious attitudes and bias. Based on their work and that of others (e.g., National Society of Genetic Counselors/JEDI Online Course; Wilson, 2014), I propose the following: Personal and professional development regarding diversity is aided and in part dependent upon recognizing that the psychological processes involved are normal and, under appropriate circumstances, adaptive. However, as I have previously argued with respect to countertransference (Weil, 2010b), I also believe they are very valuable sources of information and learning. Recognizing the origins of one's biases can help reduce them in one's personal development and socially through understanding their depth and power communally and historically. This in turn can heighten one's awareness and understanding of the depth of analogous personal and historical experiences in those with whom one interacts. Using these approaches and the many others that are available, an aspirational goal would be to have at least as detailed and in-depth an understanding of one's own relationship to the components of diversity presented at the beginning of this section as one does for another individual or group.[2]

A Contextual Proposal for Genetic Counseling

Many rapidly evolving, interrelated issues confront genetic counseling. A given test (e.g., chromosomal microarray [CMA], exome sequencing) can produce multiple findings that vary in reliability, interpretability, and clinical utility. The identification and interpretation of such results rest on a vast, expanding network of interrelated databases including population sampling, sequencing data, patient medical and demographic data, and clinical trials of pharmaceutical and other interventions (Lappalainen & MacArthur, 2021; Visscher et al.,

[2] See Chapters 29, 31, and 32 in this volume for further analyses and discussion of other components of diversity that complement this chapter.

2021). The clinical utility of a given result may depend medically on the specific disorder involved or psychosocially on the patient's circumstances and concerns and may change over time. Much of the data collection, combining of diverse data sets, and curation occur before results are reported to the clinic or other ordering entity. It is the reported results, with their multiple complexities, that affect the work of the clinical genetic counselor, both with respect to their understanding and interpretation and in determining how to provide adequate pretest counseling and which results and in what manner to inform patients postcounseling (Lattimore et al., 2015; Resta et al., 2019; Schmidt et al., 2019). Another layer of complexity arises from the marketing of genomic tests and information by for-profit companies (Dwarte et al., 2019; Schmidt et al., 2019). The result is a thick web of information, services, and sources of information into which the genetic counselor may enter at many different points under a wide variety of circumstances.

The research literature documents the potential impact of this situation for patients. For example, Bernhardt and colleagues interviewed 26 women in a research protocol who had an invasive procedure for karyotype analysis and were then offered CMA with pretest counseling. Among the findings, women whose fetus had a normal karyotype but who then received an abnormal CMA felt "blindsided"; were initially "shocked, anxious, confused, and overwhelmed"; and were "often left with lingering uncertainties" due in some cases to contradictory information from counselors, physicians, and the internet. Many wished they had not received the information, which was characterized as "toxic knowledge" (Bernhardt et al., 2013, all quotations pp. 141–142).

Kaphingst et al. (2015) conducted semi-structured interviews with 60 women diagnosed with breast cancer at age 40 or younger to determine their interest in six types of incidental findings from hypothetical genome sequencing. All respondents stated that "it was important to be able to choose the results to receive" (Kaphingst et al., 2015, p. 10). For some this involved control or ownership over the information; for others it was to limit results to only those that were actionable. Although the greatest interest involved actionable results, actionable "meant a range of potential actions . . . including lifestyle changes, disease surveillance, medications, environmental changes, and discussions with doctors or treatment response" (Kaphingst et al., 2015, p. 8). Furthermore, variants of unknown significance were only of interest to women with no or moderate family history of breast cancer and no identified *BRCA1/2* pathogenic variant because of the possibility that future research would provide information that made them actionable.

A comparable literature documents the impact on genetic counselors. In 10 telephone interviews and a much larger survey, Bernhardt et al. (2014) investigated genetic counselors' experiences with CMA testing. Among the findings, the lack of information concerning many copy number variants led to frustration over the inability to provide patients with a definite risk figure or accurate information about the potential nature and severity of a disability. This, in turn, contributed to a strongly felt need to try to obtain further information, to uncertainty about how to help patients make decisions and cope with their frustration and anxiety, and to countertransference such as relief when a physician provided additional information. One respondent spoke movingly of the issue of toxic knowledge:

> But then when [the patient] said things like "I wish I didn't know this information" and "what am I supposed to do with this information?", then I felt more like . . . I guess I didn't really know what to say because I probably wouldn't know what to do either. (Bernhardt et al., 2014, p. 941)

In a wide-ranging consideration of the issues facing genetic counselors and genetic counseling training programs, Hooker et al. (2014) discussed the need for genetic counselors to have a practical and theoretical understanding of variant classification and interpretation, including complexities such as splice variants. They addressed the complexities of serving patients who obtain results from sequencing for other indications or from direct-to-consumer services. They further stated:

> The informed consent process has expanded to include agreeing to a vague notion of uncertainty about the type of results to be returned, when they will be returned, and how they will be returned. Individuals undergoing testing will be increasingly faced with variants predicting increased risk for conditions not predicted by their personal or family history, and therefore the informed consent process will be inherently different from the "traditional" genetic testing consent process. (Hooker et al., 2014, p. 448)

Based on the preceding discussion and a large body of additional literature, it is clear that the focus of genetic counseling has shifted from one involving decision making based on the evaluation of a relatively definable, if at times large, set of data to one in which evaluating, interpreting, and giving prior consideration to the parameters for accessing massive amounts of complex data characterize both the scientific and the counseling domains. While this transformation is described in much of the recent literature, I believe it is now time to identify and develop a more broadly based interpretation of the implications for psychosocial genetic counseling.

The issues confronting patients in pretest counseling (e.g., understanding and making decisions regarding the potential types of results that may be returned) and posttest counseling (e.g., responding to a variant of unknown significance, confronting toxic information) are ubiquitous in and representative of contemporary life. To begin with a specific example: An email in a full inbox may raise the same questions and concerns as a variant of unknown significance or an unanticipated result from exome sequencing: What is its level of importance? Will it require an immediate response? If so, is there sufficient information to do so? Will it require further investigation? Will it facilitate or impede a desired action? What is the probability that it contains toxic information or malware? More broadly, an online search for an apartment; online dating; and filtering, evaluating, and responding to the deluge of information, misinformation, and disinformation that confronted millions of people during the COVID-19 pandemic of 2019–2021 involve the same sorts of questions and quandaries.

These individual and collective events are a vast, largely untapped source of patient knowledge and experience. Thus, in pretest counseling a genetic counselor might ask, "Have you had a similar experience with a large amount of information of varying reliability? If so, what ways helped you evaluate what was potentially useful, recognize ways to use the most relevant, and discard the rest?" When relevant, posttest counseling could include, "Have you had other situations in which you inadvertently received information that you regretted receiving about a person or a family or work situation? If so, did you find ways to limit the impact of that information, avoid thinking about it excessively, but make long-range plans as needed? Were there family, friends, individuals in a similar situation, or online resources that helped you do so?" Interventions such as these might initiate helpful exploration of the patient's broader experience relevant to addressing the genomic issues.

Genetic counselors have ongoing responsibilities to understand and evaluate large amounts of data in case preparation and counseling, formal and informal professional development, and, for some, activities that are a specified component of their employment in genomic research and services (Patch & Middleton, 2018). They too can draw on personal experience and knowledge to think more broadly about how to address the relevant issues. However, they also have shared experience with relevant issues in the workplace such as evaluating, discussing, and acting on laboratory data and clinical procedures of many sorts. Furthermore, there are opportunities for collective discussion of this approach among the members of a clinic or other work unit, at professional meetings, in online forums, and at the level of national and international contacts, collaborations, meetings, and publications.

Using illustrative cases chosen for in-depth analysis by a consortium of genetic counselors, Brett et al. (2018) addressed the concern that genetic counseling will lead to a new form of information overload in which the attempt to explain the complex issues will further reduce the time spent addressing the patient's basic concerns. The authors identified key psychosocial issues in each case, illustrated how they might be effectively addressed, and identified the relevant core genetic counseling competencies. Incorporating broader aspects of the patient's experience, as I propose, provides a complementary approach. It helps transform the process from one in which the genetic counselor must explain complex information requiring difficult decisions into a more dynamic discussion in which the genetic counselor helps guide the patient to understanding and possible responses. It thus supports, rather than competes with, the psychosocial component of genetic counseling because it addresses the patient's concerns, values, and circumstances in the process of providing the requisite information.

This proposal has particular relevance to situations in which genetic counselors work with patients who have had prior genetic services within the healthcare system or from for-profit companies as well as those who have obtained information from the internet or other sources. As has been well documented, this can result in uncertainty and confusion for patients and genetic counselors as well as concerns regarding the role of genetic counseling as a profession (Patch & Middleton, 2018). My proposal would facilitate genetic counselors framing the issue as one of evaluating and acting on diverse sources of sometimes conflicting information and providing guidance in using the patients' prior experience to do so. In addition to helping the patient, this approach provides a broader perspective with which to address the complexities of such counseling situations. Equally important, I believe conceptualizing the role of genetic counseling in this way creates a stronger argument for the role of genetic counseling in the contemporary environment of genomic medicine and services.

In 2010 Skirton and Bylund introduced the concept of uncertainty management theory, although, as they stated, "its applicability to family communication [about genetics] has not yet been fully explored" (Skirton & Bylund, 2010, p. 136). As discussed in the first section of this chapter, a broad expansion of research and knowledge concerning uncertainty in genetic counseling occurred in the decade that followed. In a similar manner, my proposal encourages an exploration of the sources of theory and practice that are available regarding the complex issues of evaluating and acting upon large amounts of interrelated data. To the extent that this is successful, it will more fully integrate genetic counseling into the lived experience of patients and into the intellectual and technological environment in which it provides services.

Conclusion

There is a central theme guiding the issues discussed in this chapter: In a world saturated with information, data, and theories, including in the scientific and psychosocial domains of genetic counseling, are there ways to understand the experiences of patients and genetic counselors that will advance our ability to address patients' psychosocial concerns?

The first section discusses the profound changes that genetic counseling has undergone since its origins in the first part of the 20th century and its professional initiation in the 1970s. There has been a continuous elaboration of theory and practice, punctuated by seminal papers that have opened new opportunities for research and clinical practice. I believe it is equally important to recognize historical changes in the implicit view of the patient, which is to say, in the attitudes and perceptions of the genetic counselor, which will continue to evolve in the future.

The second section reframes two concepts that have received extensive research and clinical development in a way that promotes more direct involvement with the patient. Using scenarios as a way to understand and guide the beliefs and assumptions with which a patient makes decisions helps the genetic counselor better understand that individual's circumstances and worldview. Accepting patient resistance as communication is a new perspective that informs understanding of the patient's primary concern in the moment.

In writing about diversity, I have explored the experience of interacting with another individual in terms of one's own beliefs, values, stereotypes, and conscious and unconscious biases; the similarities and differences between two individuals, including the degree of flexibility and openness to change of each; and the immense multidimensionality of diversity among and between individuals. In addition, I find that conceptualizing diversity as involving two (or more) individuals is helpful within the context of genetic counseling interactions. Instead of focusing on oneself or the other person, it directs attention to the cognitive and emotional issues in the interaction.

The final section returns to the historical themes of the first section and proposes another expansion of theory and practice including a reconceptualization of the patient and their place in modern life.

Acknowledgments

I thank Margie Goldstein, Jan Hodgson, and Kelly Ormond for long friendships and shared professional interests that have been an invaluable source of support and have greatly influenced my thinking about issues in genetic counseling.

References

Barlow Stewart, K. (2018). The certainty of uncertainty in genomic medicine: Managing the challenge. *Journal of Healthcare Communications*, 3(3:37), 1–4. https://doi.org/10.4172/2472-1654.100147

Bernhardt, B. A., Kellom, K., Barbarese, A., Faucett, W. A., & Wapner, R. J. (2014). An exploration of genetic counselors' needs and experiences with prenatal chromosomal microarray testing. *Journal of Genetic Counseling, 23*, 938–947. https://doi.org/10.1007/s10897-014-9702-y

Bernhardt, B. A., Soucier, D., Hanson, K., Savage, M. S., Jackson, L., & Wapner, R. J. (2013). Women's experiences receiving abnormal prenatal chromosomal microarray testing results. *Genetics in Medicine, 15*, 139–145. https://doi.org/10.1038/gim.2012.113

Brett, G. R., Wilkins, E. J., Creed, E. T., West, K., Jarmolowicz, A., Valente, G. M., Prawer, Y., Lynch, E., & Macciocca, I. (2018). Genetic counseling in the era of genomics: What's all the fuss about? *Journal of Genetic Counseling, 27*, 1010–1021. https://doi.org/10.1007/s10897-018-0216-x

Burke, B. M., & Kolker, A. (1994). Variation in content in prenatal genetic counseling interviews. *Journal of Genetic Counseling, 3*, 23–38.

Crowe, L., Graham, R. H., Robson, S. C., & Rankin, J. (2018). Negotiating acceptable termination of pregnancy for non-lethal fetal anomaly: A qualitative study of professional perspectives. *BMJ Open, 8*, e020815. https://doi.org/10.1136/bmjopen-2017-020815

Dwarte, T., Barlow-Stewart, K., O'Shea, R., Dinger, M. E., & Terrill, B. (2019). Role and practice evolution for genetic counseling in the genomic era: The experience of Australian and UK genetics practitioners. *Journal of Genetic Counseling, 28*, 378–387. https://doi.org/10.1002/jgc4.1053

Eberhardt, J. L. (2019). *Biased: Uncovering the hidden prejudice that shapes what we see, think, and do*. Viking.

Fennell, S. J. (Ed.). (2021). *Wild tongues can't be tamed: 15 voices from the Latinx diaspora*. Flatiron Books.

Fine, B. A. (1993). The evolution of nondirectiveness in genetic counseling and implications of the human genome project. In D. M. Bartels, B. S. LeRoy, & A. L. Caplan (Eds.), *Genetic counseling: Ethical challenges and consequences* (pp. 101–117). Routledge. https://doi.org/10.4324/9780203790953

Finucane, B. (2012). Introduction to the Special Issue on Developmental Disabilities. *Journal of Genetic Counseling, 21*, 749–751.

Fisher, C. L., Roccotagliata, T., Rising, C. J., Kissane, D. W., Glogowski, E. A., Bylund, C. L., & Carma, L. (2017). "I don't want to be an ostrich": Managing mothers' uncertainty during BRCA1/2 genetic counseling. *Journal of Genetic Counseling, 26*, 455–468. https://doi.org/10.1007/s10897-016-9998-x

Genetic Counseling Toolkit. (n.d.). https://www.geneticcounselingtoolkit.com

Hooker, G. W., Ormond, K. E., Sweet, K., & Biesecker, B. B. (2014). Teaching genomic counseling: Preparing the genetic counseling workforce for the genomic era. *Journal of Genetic Counseling, 23*, 445–451. https://doi.org/10.1007/s10897-014-9689-4

Kaphingst, K., Ivanovich, J., Biesecker, B., Dresser, R., Seo, J., Dressler, L., Goodfellow, P., & Goodman, M. (2015). Preferences for return of incidental findings from genome sequencing among women diagnosed with breast cancer at a young age. *Clinical Genetics, 89*, 378–384. https://doi.org/10.1111/cge.12597.

Kfir, N. C., Rudolf, M., Bentwich, M. E., Dickman, N., & Fali-Zaccai, T. C. (2020). "LEADERS": A culturally tailored approach to genetic counseling for minority populations. *Journal of Genetic Counseling, 30*, 70–74. https://doi.org/10.1002/jgc4.1369

Lappalainen, T., & MacArthur, D. G. (2021). From variant to function in human disease. *Science, 373*(6562), 1464–1468.

Lattimore, V., Currie, M., Lintott, C., Sullivan, J., Robinson, B. A., & Walker, L. C. (2015). Meeting the challenges of interpreting variants of unknown clinical significance in BRCA testing. *New Zealand Medical Journal, 128*, 56–61.

Lippman-Hand, A., & Fraser, F. C. (1979a). Genetic counseling: Parents' responses to uncertainty. *Birth Defects, 15*(5C), 325–339.

Lippman-Hand, A., & Fraser, F. C. (1979b). Genetic counseling: Provision and reception of information. *American Journal of Medical Genetics*, 3, 113–127.

Lippman-Hand, A., & Fraser, F. C. (1979c). Genetic counseling—The postcounseling period I. Parent's perceptions of uncertainty. *American Journal of Medical Genetics*, 4, 51–71.

Lippman-Hand, A., & Fraser, F. C. (1979d). Genetic counseling—The postcounseling period II. Making reproductive choices. *American Journal of Medical Genetics*, 4, 73–87.

Lubinsky, M. S. (1994). Bearing bad news: Dealing with the mimics of denial. *Journal of Genetic Counseling*, 3, 5–12.

McCarthy Veach, P., LeRoy, B. S., & Callanan, N. P. (2018). *Facilitating the genetic counseling process: Practice-based skills* (2nd ed.). Springer.

Palmer, C. G. S., & Sainfort, F. (1993). Toward a new conceptualization and operationalization of risk perception within the genetic counseling domain. *Journal of Genetic Counseling*, 2, 275–294.

Patch, C., & Middleton, A. (2018). Genetic counselling in the era of genomic medicine. *British Medical Bulletin, 126*, 27–36. https://doi.org/doi:10.1093/bmb/ldy008

Resta, R. G., Sullivan, J., & McConkie-Rosell, A. (2019). Introduction to exploring the exome special issue. *Journal of Genetic Counseling, 28*, 181. https://doi.org/10.1002/jgc4.1113

Schaa, K. L., Roter, D. L., Biesecker, B. B., Cooper, L. A., & Erby, L. H. (2015). Genetic counselors' implicit racial attitudes and their relationship to communication. *Health Psychology, 34*, 111–119. https://doi.org/10.1037/hea0000155

Schmidt, J. L., Maas, R., & Altmeyer, S. R. (2019). Genetic counseling for consumer-driven whole exome and whole genome sequencing: A commentary on early experiences. *Journal of Genetic Counseling, 28*, 449–455. https://doi.org/10.1002/jgc4.1109

Sharif, S. M., Blyth, M., Ahmed, M., Sheridan, E., Saltus, R., Yu, J., Tonkin, E., & Kirk, M. (2020). Enhancing inclusion of diverse populations in genomics: A competence framework. *Journal of Genetic Counseling, 29*, 282–292. https://doi.org/10.1002/jgc4.1263

Shiloh, S. (2006). Illness representations, self-regulation, and genetic counseling: A theoretical review. *Journal of Genetic Counseling, 15*, 325–337. https://doi.org/10.1007/s10897-006-9044-5

Sivell, S., Elwyn, G., Gaff, C. L., Clarke, A. J., Iredale, R., Shaw, C., Dundon, J., Thornton, H., & Edwards, A. (2008). How risk is perceived, constructed and interpreted by clients in clinical genetics, and the effects on decision making: Systematic review. *Journal of Genetic Counseling, 17*, 30–63. https://doi.org/10.1007/s10897-007-9132-1

Skirton, H. (2018). More than an information service: Are counselling skills needed by genetics professionals in the genomic era? *European Journal of Human Genetics, 26*, 1239–1240. https://doi.org/10.1038/s41431-018-0133-3

Skirton, H., & Bylund, C. L. (2010). Management of uncertainty. In C. L. Gaff & C. L. Bylund (Eds.), *Family communication about genetics: Theory and practice* (pp. 136–151). Oxford University Press.

Stern, A. M. (2009). A quiet revolution: The birth of the genetic counselor at Sarah Lawrence College, 1969. *Journal of Genetic Counseling, 18*, 1–11. https://doi.org/10.1007/s10897-008-9186-8

Stern, A. M. (2012). *Telling genes: The story of genetic counseling in America*. Johns Hopkins University Press.

Visscher, P. M., Yengo, L., Cox, N. J., & Wray, N. R. (2021). Discovery and implications of polygenicity of common diseases. *Science*, *373*(6562), 1468–1473.

Weil, J. (2000). *Psychosocial genetic counseling*. Oxford University Press.

Weil, J. (2010a). Resistance and adherence: Understanding the patient's perspective. In B. S. LeRoy, P. McCarthy Veach, & D. M. Bartels (Eds.), *Genetic counseling practice: Advanced concepts and skills* (pp. 155–174). Wiley-Blackwell.

Weil, J. (2010b). Countertransference: Making the unconscious conscious. In B. S. LeRoy, P. McCarthy Veach, & D. M. Bartels (Eds.), *Genetic counseling practice: Advanced concepts and skills* (pp. 175–197). Wiley-Blackwell.

Wertz, D. C., Sorenson, J. R., & Heeren, T. C. (1986). Clients' interpretation of risks provided in genetic counseling. *American Journal of Medical Genetics*, *39*, 253–264.

Wilson, A. (2014). Addressing uncomfortable issues: Reflexivity as a tool for culturally safe practice in Aboriginal and Torres Strait Islander health. *Australian Journal of Indigenous Education*, *43*(2), 218–230. https://doi.org/10.1017/jie.2014.24

Zayts-Spence, O., Fung, J. L. F., & Chung, B. H. Y. (2021). "Do language and culture really matter?": A trans-disciplinary investigation of cultural diversity in genetic counseling in Hong Kong. *Journal of Genetic Counseling*, *30*, 75–84. https://doi.org/10.1002/jgc4.1385

PART III

CONTEXTS OF GENETIC COUNSELING PRACTICE

CHAPTER 7

PRENATAL GENETIC COUNSELING

SANDRA A. DARILEK AND JENNIFER HOSKOVEC

Introduction

APPROXIMATELY 3% of all children born in the Unites States have a major birth defect, 20% of which have an underlying genetic etiology (Martin et al., 2017). In an effort to allow for earlier diagnosis and management of affected pregnancies, prenatal testing was developed using screening modalities and diagnostic tests to provide risk assessments and diagnostic information about an unborn fetus.

Over the past 70 years, the tools and techniques used in prenatal diagnostics have evolved rapidly and will likely continue to do so. Effective clinical integration of these new technologies often requires genetic counseling as part of the workflow. Clinically available tests such as genetic carrier screening, aneuploidy screening, ultrasound examination, and molecular testing have unique benefits, limitations, and clinical and personal utility that should be considered before use. Testing decisions made during the prenatal period are often also complicated by psychosocial and timing aspects, some of which are unique to testing in the antenatal period. Pretest and posttest counseling for families considering such testing is integral in appropriate clinical integration and informed decision making.

Genetic counselors are uniquely positioned to provide support to both patients and providers in the prenatal setting. While discussion of these available genetic screening and testing options is a component of prenatal genetic counseling, it is not the only goal. Given the optional nature of most genetic tests, balanced and accurate information is key for patients to make informed choices that are in line with their personal values, needs, and desires for them and their families.

Prenatal Testing and Screening

Carrier screening

Carrier screening has been an evolving and multifaceted testing option in the prenatal arena. Carrier screening is generally defined as genetic testing performed on asymptomatic individuals with the aim of determining whether they carry a genetic variant associated with a particular inherited condition that would result in a current or future pregnancy being at increased risk for a specific genetic condition. Determination of carrier status provides individuals and couples the ability to use prenatal or preimplantation genetic testing to identify an affected fetus or embryo and allows for more informed reproductive decision making both prior to and during pregnancy. Information about this option should be given to every individual during pregnancy but should ideally be performed prior to pregnancy to allow for the greatest access to available reproductive testing options (American College of Obstetricians and Gynecologists, 2017b).

Approaches and technology

Carrier screening typically focuses on identifying carriers of select autosomal recessive and X-linked conditions. The conditions for which an individual is screened depend on the screening approach selected. In general, it is recommended that conditions included in carrier screening panels meet several of the following criteria: a carrier frequency of one in 100 to 200 or greater; a well-defined phenotype; onset in infancy/childhood; cause cognitive, physical, or quality-of-life impairment; or require medical or surgical intervention (American College of Obstetricians and Gynecologists, 2017a; Gregg et al., 2021).

Acceptable strategies for carrier screening have included ethnicity-based, panethnic, and expanded carrier screening (American College of Obstetricians and Gynecologists, 2017a). Ethnicity-based carrier screening uses the ethnic background of an individual to limit the conditions to those with an increased frequency in the ethnic population of the individual who is undergoing screening. A limitation of this strategy is that some individuals have mixed ancestry or have inaccurate or limited knowledge of their ethnic background. Conversely, panethnic and expanded carrier screening do not rely on knowledge of ethnic background. These testing panels vary in size and can include up to several hundred conditions. It should be kept in mind that, in addition to size, the makeup of panethnic or expanded carrier screening panels can also vary widely between testing labs. More recent recommendations have moved from focusing on ethnic background to a more ethnicity-neutral approach (Gregg et al., 2021). Of note, when there is a known family history of an autosomal recessive or X-linked condition, the at-risk individual should be offered targeted carrier testing for the familial pathogenic variant, if known, or offered sequencing for the associated disease gene. This type of familial carrier testing does not replace, but instead complements, the other carrier screening approaches. Additionally, consanguineous couples benefit from consideration of larger carrier screening panels due to the increased chance of both members of the couple being found to be carriers of the same condition(s).

The methods generally used for carrier screening are genotyping and sequence analysis. Genotyping only assesses well-described disease-causing variants for the conditions screened, while most newer screening assays use next-generation sequencing of most or the entire coding regions of included genes to report pathogenic or likely pathogenic variants detected. A limitation of the genotyping method is that while it works well for specific conditions in select ethnic populations, it generally has a lower carrier detection rate compared to the sequencing method. Alternatively, while the sequencing approach allows for reporting of all variants classified as pathogenic or likely pathogenic, over time it is possible that some pathogenic variants may be reclassified to be variants of uncertain significance or benign or vice versa. For some conditions, both approaches may use other additional assays for carrier detection, including copy number analysis of exon 7 of the *SMN1* gene for spinal muscular atrophy, polymerase chain reaction and/or Southern blotting to determine CGG repeat size in the *FMR1* gene, AGG interruption analysis of the *FMR1* gene for premutation carriers, hexosaminidase A enzyme activity for Tay-Sachs disease, and a complete blood count with red blood cell indices and hemoglobin electrophoresis for hemoglobinopathies.

In addition to panel selection and technology method, another aspect of carrier screening to be considered is the approach to testing a couple. Carrier screening can be offered in a sequential or simultaneous (concurrent) manner. For sequential carrier screening, one member of a couple undergoes carrier screening, and the partner then undergoes testing only if the tested individual has positive results. With simultaneous carrier screening, both members of a couple undergo screening at the same time. Sequential carrier screening may be a cost-saving approach, but when there are time constraints for reproductive decision making, concurrent screening is suggested (American College of Obstetricians and Gynecologists, 2017b). Additionally, when carrier screening is performed using sequencing analysis, concurrent testing through the same laboratory may prove beneficial in situations where variant reclassification occurs and is reported by the laboratory, leading to newly determined carrier status in one partner. In these cases, if both parents have been screened concurrently with the same carrier screening panel, the provider will already have information regarding the other partner's carrier status for the condition affected by the reclassification, saving valuable time in determining risk to the pregnancy. Variant reclassification occurs more frequently with larger carrier screening panels. Laboratories have varying policies and processes in place regarding reporting of reclassifications on carrier screening panels.

Additional considerations

While available recommendations state that ethnicity-based, panethnic, and expanded carrier screening are all valid approaches to screening, providers are encouraged to be consistent in the approach they offer (American College of Obstetricians and Gynecologists, 2017a). It is important that individuals undergoing carrier screening receive pretest counseling that includes information about the testing panel(s) being offered, the benefits of obtaining this information, the reproductive and testing options available to them should they be determined to be a carrier of a genetic condition, and the general limitations of carrier screening and the specific panel offered. Limitations of carrier screening include that no carrier screening panel screens for all inherited conditions, that carrier screening does not provide information about genetic conditions that are typically not inherited such as chromosome abnormalities, and that while negative carrier screening results significantly reduce carrier risk, they do not eliminate carrier risk for the screened conditions. Additionally, individuals should be counseled that while carrier status for most conditions included on screening panels has no health implications for the carrier individual, there are select conditions for which carrier status is associated with health risks, such as increased risk for cancer, Parkinson's disease, or anesthesia-related complications, and that our knowledge of risks associated with carrier status for additional conditions may change over time.

There are additional considerations that should be taken into account when utilizing expanded carrier screening through a large panel and/or using sequencing technology. When sequencing technology is utilized, it is important to consider the possibility that an individual may need to be recontacted with updated carrier screening results should lab review and reclassification of variants lead to a change in carrier status. For example, most carrier screening labs do not report variants of uncertain significance (VUSs) detected on screening. More and more carrier screening labs are performing variant review, and if review of the variant later leads to reclassification of the variant to a likely pathogenic or pathogenic variant, an updated report may be provided that changes the patient's carrier status. This information then needs to be communicated to the patient by the provider. An additional consideration for partner testing is panel selection. When coordinating carrier screening for an individual whose partner has already had a carrier screen performed, it is important to keep in mind that both size and composition of carrier screening panels can differ between labs. In this instance it is usually best to perform carrier screening for the partner using the same panel. If a partner is screened with a different panel and determined to be a carrier of a condition not included on their partner's initial screening panel, this could lead to retesting, which can be inefficient and costly.

If paternity is inaccurate or the reproductive partner of an individual is not available for testing, then carrier screening may be of limited benefit. Additional special circumstances to consider include individuals who are adopted and have no information about their biological relatives and consanguineous couples. For these, expanded carrier screening is often a preferred option.

Noninvasive screening

An increasing number of noninvasive screening options are available during pregnancy as a means to adjust risk for select genetic conditions in a fetus. These range from traditional serum screening options that provide risk estimates for trisomy 21, trisomy 18, and open neural tube defects (ONTDs) to cell-free DNA (cfDNA) screening that standardly assesses risk for trisomy 13, 18, and 21 but also has the ability to screen for sex chromosome aneuploidy and select microdeletion disorders and an increasing potential to screen for both select de novo and inherited conditions. To determine the most appropriate screening option for a particular pregnancy, a priori risk along with clinical circumstances should be considered. It is paramount to keep in mind that noninvasive screening options are not considered diagnostic testing and any individual with positive screening results should be offered diagnostic testing to confirm the screening results.

Biochemical screening

Biochemical screening includes first-trimester screening (FTS), second-trimester screening, and combinations of both first- and second-trimester screening that incorporate select maternal serum protein and hormone levels with or without a nuchal translucency measurement to assess risk for trisomy 21, trisomy 18 (or in some cases trisomy 18 and trisomy 13), and/or ONTDs. See Table 7.1 for a comparison of Down syndrome detection rates for the various options.

FTS is performed between 11 and 14 weeks gestation. It incorporates gestational age, maternal age-related risk, and ultrasound measurement of fetal nuchal translucency (NT) along with maternal serum human chorionic gonadotrophin (hCG) or free β-hCG, plasma-associated protein of pregnancy A (PAPP-A), and, in some algorithms, alpha-fetoprotein (AFP) to provide a risk estimate for trisomy 21 and trisomy 18 (or combined risk estimate for trisomy 18 and trisomy 13). When the calculated risk estimate exceeds a predetermined cut-off, the screen is classified as positive or increased risk.

Second-trimester screening is performed through triple, quadruple, or penta screening. It is performed between 15 and 22 weeks gestation. The algorithm for the triple screen incorporates gestational age, maternal age-related risk, and maternal weight and ethnicity, along with measurement of maternal serum levels of hCG, unconjugated estriol (uE3), and AFP, while the quadruple screen adds measurement of dimeric inhibin A (DIA) and the penta screen adds DIA along with hyperglycosylated hCG (h hCG). These screens provide a risk for trisomy 21, trisomy 18, and ONTDs. As with FTS, a positive result indicates that the risk for one or more of these conditions exceeds a predetermined threshold. Of note, only the maternal serum AFP (MSAFP) measurement is used to assess risk for ONTDs and can

Table 7.1 Down Syndrome Detection Rates for Biochemical Screening Options

Trimester	Screening test	Detection rate[a]
First trimester		
	First-trimester screen	82%–87%
Second trimester		
	Triple screen	69%
	Quadruple screen	81%
Combined first and second trimester		
	Integrated screen	96%
	Serum integrated screen	88%
	Stepwise sequential screen	95%
	Contingent sequential screen	88%–94%

[a] Detection rate at a 5% screen-positive rate.

Source: Adapted from Table 2 in American College of Obstetricians and Gynecologists. (2016). Practice Bulletin Number 163: Screening for fetal aneuploidy. *Obstetrics and Gynecology, 127*(5), 979–981.

be used as a standalone screening for ONTDs in the second trimester for individuals who have already had other screening for aneuploidy performed in the pregnancy. Additionally, other anomalies such as abdominal wall defects and fetal renal disease can also lead to elevated MSAFP levels. In cases where elevated MSAFP levels are unexplained by these causes, there may be an increased risk for pregnancy complications or in rare cases a risk for maternal disease, such as a liver tumor.

Combinations of first- and second-trimester screening were developed to increase the detection rate for Down syndrome provided by maternal serum screening. While these options have the benefit of an increased detection rate, they also have the limitation of requiring both a first- and second-trimester blood draw and with some approaches a delay of the screening result until the second trimester. Integrated and serum integrated use first- and second-trimester analytes either alone (serum integrated) or in combination with the NT measurement (integrated) to provide a single risk assessment that is provided in the second trimester. Conversely, sequential screens, which are performed in either a stepwise or contingent manner, provide patients a first-trimester screening result so that the option of early diagnostic testing through chorionic villus sampling (CVS) is still an option available to them should the first-trimester portion provide a positive result. In stepwise sequential screening a positive first-trimester result is followed by an offer of diagnostic testing and a negative result is followed by the second-trimester screening portion, with the risk assessment incorporating both the first- and second-trimester results. In contrast, in contingent sequential screening a positive first-trimester result is followed by an offer of diagnostic testing, a negative result leads to no further testing, and an intermediate result leads to the second-trimester screening portion, again providing a risk assessment using both the first- and second-trimester results.

Cell-free DNA screening

In an ongoing effort to improve prenatal screening detection rates and with the aim to decrease the need for, or even replace, diagnostic testing procedures, cfDNA testing methodologies have been developed for use in screening for aneuploidy during pregnancy and have the potential to also allow for screening, and possibly even diagnosis, of single gene disorders.

cfDNA screening for aneuploidy, also referred to as noninvasive prenatal testing (NIPT), evaluates the risk for aneuploidy in a pregnancy through analysis of short segments of placental-derived DNA fragments present in the maternal bloodstream. These fragments, referred to as the fetal fraction, account for approximately 3% to 13% of all circulating cfDNA in maternal plasma (American College of Obstetricians and Gynecologists, 2016b). This screening can be performed as early as 8 weeks gestation. Labs performing this testing typically utilize one of two methodologies: single nucleotide polymorphism (SNP)-based analysis or massively parallel sequencing. The SNP-based analysis approach examines relative allele frequencies of SNPs by using targeted polymerase chain reaction (PCR) amplification and sequencing of SNPs on select chromosomes (Ryan et al., 2016). Alternatively, the massively parallel sequencing approach is based on sequencing large numbers of DNA fragments and then allocating them to their chromosome of origin, counting them, and identifying abnormal amounts of DNA from the chromosome(s) of interest relative to reference chromosomes (Palomaki et al., 2012). The positive predictive value (PPV) of cfDNA screening depends on the particular screened condition's a priori risk as well as the sensitivity and specificity reported for that condition by the performing lab. The PPV of cfDNA screening is superior to that of multiple marker screening. cfDNA screening for Down syndrome is reported to have a detection rate of 99% with a screen-positive rate of 0.5% (American College of Obstetricians and Gynecologists, 2016b).

The standard approach of this screening focuses on evaluation for aneuploidy of chromosomes 13, 18, and 21, with the ability to also assess for fetal sex and sex chromosome aneuploidy. However, most laboratories performing this screening also allow for opt-in screening for other rarer trisomies, such as trisomy 16 and trisomy 22, and specific microdeletion conditions, such as the chromosome 22q11.2 deletion syndrome. At least one laboratory offers a genome-wide approach that allows for assessment of all chromosomes and is reported to have the ability to detect deletions and duplications of chromosome material larger than 7 Mb (Lefkowitz et al., 2016). More recently, focus has been moving to the development of noninvasive prenatal diagnosis (NIPD) approaches. Interest in this area began with the development of a noninvasive approach to determining fetal RhD status. Focus then shifted to trying to identify inherited paternal variants or de novo pathogenic variants. With the advent of next-generation sequencing, this area of noninvasive testing has now expanded to include more complex genetic analysis to try to allow for the diagnosis of recessive and X-linked conditions as well as dominant conditions inherited from the mother (Hayward & Chitty, 2018). While NIPD is not widely utilized as of the writing of this chapter, these screening options show much promise and could revolutionize prenatal diagnosis.

Additional considerations

Before undergoing prenatal screening, an individual should be informed that the screening test is voluntary and is not diagnostic and that it is recommended that all positive screening (increased risk) results be confirmed by diagnostic testing. While negative results, particularly negative cfDNA screening results, are reassuring, negative results do not eliminate the risk for any of the screened conditions. All of the screening options perform better in singleton pregnancies than in pregnancies with multiples and may not be able to be performed in all multiple-gestation pregnancies. Additionally, an increased risk for aneuploidy in a twin pregnancy is not able to provide information about whether one or both twins are at risk/affected with the condition of concern.

Additionally with respect to cfDNA screening, since the cfDNA fragments assessed originate from the placenta, abnormal screening results could be suggestive of confined placental mosaicism and not actually representative of the fetus. As a result, amniocentesis is typically considered to be the most appropriate follow-up diagnostic test, though other clinical factors such as timing, ultrasound findings, and patient preference need to be taken into account when selecting the most appropriate follow-up test. Another consideration with cfDNA screening is the possibility of a nonreportable result. Fetal fraction measurement is a key component to cfDNA screening, and as such, low fetal fraction, typically considered to be less than 2% to 4%, may lead to a nonreportable result. It has been reported that low fetal fraction is associated with an increased risk for fetal aneuploidy but also with maternal obesity, maternal hypertension, early gestational age, and maternal anticoagulation therapy (Burns et al., 2017). In rare cases, cfDNA screening may provide unexpected results related to the presence of a maternal condition such as fibroids (benign uterine tumors), cancer, or a maternal chromosome abnormality, such as low-level mosaicism for monosomy X or the presence of a previously unidentified maternal microdeletion. Lastly, with respect to cfDNA testing for single gene disorders, there is a potential to unmask misattributed paternity. Pretest counseling is important to provide individuals with thorough information about the benefits, limitations, and potential for unexpected information that may be provided by cfDNA screening results.

Fetal ultrasound and imaging

As many chromosomal and single gene disorders are associated with structural anomalies, ultrasound remains a valuable tool in trying to identify fetuses at increased risk for genetic disease. For several decades second-trimester ultrasound has been used to assess for major structural anomalies. It is well established that the presence of a major structural anomaly increases the risk for fetal aneuploidy, and it has been shown that certain constellations of ultrasound findings can be suggestive of certain single gene disorders (American College of Obstetricians and Gynecologists, 2007). Additionally, it has been shown that soft markers, nonspecific physical characteristics that can be noted on ultrasound (e.g., thickened nuchal fold, renal pelvis dilation, echogenic bowel), may also confer a somewhat increased risk for aneuploidy (American College of Obstetricians and Gynecologists, 2016b). However, these soft markers are also common in unaffected pregnancies. With increasing improvement in ultrasound imaging, first-trimester ultrasounds are also proving to be helpful in early detection of findings that may be suggestive of the presence of a genetic condition. This is probably best demonstrated by the detection of increased nuchal translucency at 11 to 14 weeks gestation and the association of this finding with an increased risk for fetal aneuploidy, cardiac disease, and a number of single gene disorders. Fetal echocardiogram and fetal magnetic resonance imaging are additional imaging modalities that are commonly and increasingly being used to provide additional detailed information about certain fetal structural anomalies (e.g., cardiac anomalies, neural tube defects, brain anomalies, lung anomalies) to help inform prenatal management and testing decisions.

All fetal imaging has limitations, particularly compared to postnatal imaging. Prenatal imaging can be limited by the gestational age of the fetus, fetal positioning, maternal habitus, and multiple gestation. Additionally, some structural anomalies can be challenging to diagnose prenatally (e.g., cleft palate) or can evolve over the course of a pregnancy (e.g., ventriculomegaly, findings suggestive of a skeletal dysplasia). Thus, postnatal imaging may still be needed to better characterize a prenatally diagnosed structural anomaly to inform management.

Diagnostic testing

Prenatal diagnostic genetic testing can identify inherited or de novo genetic conditions, including chromosomal aneuploidy, copy number variants, or pathogenic variants associated with single gene conditions. Currently, prenatal diagnosis is available only via an invasive procedure such as CVS or amniocentesis, though as noted previously this may be changing with the evolution of cfDNA testing. These procedures provide either fetal or placental DNA, allowing for an array of different genetic testing to be performed. Prenatal diagnosis provides individuals/couples with information to aid reproductive decision making and management of an ongoing pregnancy.

Procedures

CVS involves obtaining a sample of placental cells from the chorionic villi via either transabdominal needle aspiration or transcervical catheter aspiration dependent on placental location. This procedure is typically performed at 10 to 14 weeks gestation. Amniocentesis is performed by transabdominal needle aspiration of amniotic fluid containing fetal cells and can be performed after 15 weeks gestation. The procedure-related loss rate with amniocentesis has been reported to be one in 300 to 500, with even lower loss rates reported in experienced centers. While the overall pregnancy loss rate after CVS is greater than the loss rate after amniocentesis, because of the increased background rate of spontaneous pregnancy loss at 9 to 16 weeks gestation, it has been shown that the loss rate for CVS appears to approach and may be the same as the rate for amniocentesis (American College of Obstetricians and Gynecologists, 2007). It should be noted that because the sample obtained through CVS is placental in origin, individuals undergoing CVS should be counseled about the 1% to 2% occurrence of confined placental mosaicism and the potential need in those cases for a follow-up amniocentesis to clarify the fetus's genetic status.

Testing methodologies

Cytogenetic analysis

The mainstay of prenatal diagnosis for chromosomal abnormalities has been karyotyping. Karyotyping allows for detection of full chromosome aneuploidy as well as large structural chromosome rearrangements (e.g., translocations, inversions, marker chromosomes) of greater than 10 Mb in size. Karyotyping requires cell culture, and results typically take 2 weeks but can take longer depending on the culture growth and quality. As a means of obtaining faster results, typically within 48 to 72 hours, rapid analysis can be performed through fluorescence in situ hybridization (FISH) or quantitative fluorescence PCR for the common aneuploidies.

Molecular analysis

To allow for a more robust assessment of fetal chromosomal status, karyotyping is often being supplemented or replaced by chromosomal microarray analysis (CMA). CMA detects gains (duplications) and losses (deletions), referred to as copy number variants (CNVs), throughout the genome. In addition to identifying the large aneuploidies detectable by karyotyping, it has the ability to also detect submicroscopic CNVs that are too small to be detected by traditional testing (American College of Obstetricians and Gynecologists, 2016a). Results are typically available within 10 to 14 days when direct analysis is performed but can take 3 to 4 weeks if cell culture is required. It has been shown that 6% of pregnancies with a structural abnormality and 1.7% of pregnancies without a structural abnormality are found to have a clinically significant CNV on CMA following a normal karyotype, demonstrating the clinical utility of CMA in prenatal diagnosis (Wapner et al., 2012). It should be noted that in 1.5% to 1.6% of cases a VUS may be identified on prenatal CMA (Brady et al., 2014; Wapner et al., 2012). It is important that individuals considering this testing be counseled about the benefits and limitations of CMA along with a discussion of the potential types of test results that may be obtained, including the identification of a disease-causing CNV, a negative result, and a finding of a VUS, in order to allow for fully informed decision making. Additionally, though not common, it is possible that identification of a CNV in a fetus may provide information about an adult-onset condition or disease risk for the fetus. If follow-up testing indicates the CNV was inherited, results may be suggestive of a risk for or diagnosis of an adult-onset condition or disease in one of the parents. Finally, it is possible that subsequent parental testing after abnormal fetal CMA results could unmask misattributed paternity.

In the case of a known inherited genetic risk, prenatal molecular genetic testing is best performed by known familial variant testing. To facilitate this type of prenatal testing, the disease-causing variant(s) first need(s) to be identified in an affected family member or carrier parents to allow for targeted analysis in the fetus. When prenatal ultrasound findings are suggestive of a potential single gene condition, single gene testing or panel testing for a group of genetic conditions through sequence analysis may be warranted. This may be considered when previous chromosomal-based testing proved nondiagnostic or when there is high suspicion for a particular condition or type of condition (e.g., skeletal dysplasia, ciliopathy). When prenatal single gene or panel testing is performed, individuals need to be counseled that results may take more time than chromosomal-based testing. While test results for a known familial variant can take as little as 2 weeks, results for panel testing can take 4 to 6 weeks or more depending on the culture requirements and genes included in the testing. With single gene and panel sequencing tests, individuals again need to be counseled about the benefits and limitations of the testing, including the fact that negative results will not rule out all genetic conditions, and the possible test results, including the potential for a VUS.

More recently increasing attention is being given to the potential use of exome or genome sequencing (ES or GS) for prenatal diagnosis, particularly due to its successful use in pediatric and adult populations to diagnose Mendelian disorders. As a prenatal testing approach, ES/GS uses sequencing of DNA from the exome or genome as a means to try to identify the underlying etiology of anomalies noted in a fetus. While not a standard prenatal test at the time of the writing of this chapter, this testing is available on both a research and clinical basis for certain indications, and while data is limited, early studies suggest that a genetic abnormality may be detected in up to 20% to 30% of fetuses with multiple anomalies for which other prenatal genetic testing has proven nondiagnostic (Drury et al., 2015). ES/GS provides the advantage of producing the broadest set of genetic data to assist in diagnosis of fetal disease. However, there are a number of considerations that need to be taken into account, some of which are specific to the prenatal setting. As with all molecular genetic sequencing–based testing, the potential for the identification of VUSs is also present with ES/GS, and is even greater when ES/GS is used for prenatal diagnosis. While the resolution or clarification of a finding of a VUS in the pediatric or adult setting can be difficult, this can be even more challenging in the prenatal setting where clinicians are limited by the data that ultrasound can provide. To an even greater extent than with prenatal CMA, there is the potential to identify pathogenic variants in genes not associated with the prenatal phenotype (incidental findings) or associated with other disease risk (secondary or medically actionable findings). These types of findings can be difficult for families to deal with, particularly when options such as whether to continue a pregnancy may be being considered. Likewise, the potential to learn information about parental disease risk is again an important consideration with prenatal ES/GS. The American College of Medical Genetics and Genomics (ACMG) provides guidance about the reporting of these types of results and specific considerations to be taken into account in the prenatal testing realm. Additionally, labs performing ES/GS typically have policies specific to their reporting of these results in prenatal cases (Monaghan et al., 2020).

Preimplantation Genetic Testing

For couples who are interested in reducing the risk for a genetic disease in a pregnancy, preimplantation genetic testing (PGT) is available. PGT was first performed in 1990 in an effort to reduce the risk for an X-linked disorder by determining the sex of the embryos (Handyside et al., 1990). Since that time PGT has evolved to allow for testing for chromosomal aneuploidies and a large number of inherited genetic conditions. PGT requires a couple to undergo in vitro fertilization (IVF), which includes ovarian stimulation, egg retrieval, and fertilization typically by intracytoplasmic injection followed by embryo culture. For PGT to be performed, five to 10 cells are biopsied from the trophectoderm after 5 days of embryo culture. The embryos are then cryopreserved to allow for testing to be performed prior to transfer. Following testing, embryos expected to be unaffected based on test results are then selected, thawed, and transferred in hopes of producing a pregnancy. PGT has been divided into three types depending on the type of condition being tested for: PGT-A for general aneuploidy screening, PGT-SR for testing for structural chromosome rearrangements, and PGT-M for testing for monogenic conditions.

PGT-A for aneuploidy and PGT-SR for structural rearrangements

PGT-A is used to identify embryos with chromosomal aneuploidy in an effort to improve pregnancy rate and reduce miscarriage rate. It is typically performed for individuals of advanced reproductive age or for individuals with a history of recurrent pregnancy loss or previously failed IVF cycles. PGT-SR is used to identify embryos with an unbalanced structural rearrangement when one parent is known to carry a balanced chromosomal translocation or inversion. Until recently, PGT-A and PGT-SR were performed by FISH or microarray analysis, but currently both PGT-A and PGT-SR are performed by next-generation sequencing (NGS), which allows for detection of whole chromosomal trisomy or monosomy and large chromosomal deletions and duplications (segmental aneuploidies). NGS also allows for the detection of mosaicism in biopsy samples.

PGT-M for monogenic disorders

PGT-M is utilized when a pregnancy is at increased risk for an autosomal dominant, autosomal recessive, or X-linked condition. PGT-M is most commonly performed by targeted haplotyping of polymorphic markers that are closely linked to the gene of interest. While targeted mutation analysis can also be performed, if used, it is typically performed in conjunction with haplotyping to provide higher detection rates and lower false-positive or false-negative results. For PGT-M to be offered, a familial pathogenic variant(s) must be identified. Prior to PGT-M being performed, the testing laboratory will request DNA samples from relevant family members to set up an assay to detect the linked haplotype or familial variant(s) specific to the family.

Practical considerations and limitations

Any patient or couple undergoing a form of PGT should have pretest counseling that includes a discussion about the benefits, risks, and limitations of PGT. The discussion should describe the risk for false-positive or false-negative results due to possible allele dropout (when one or both alleles at a genetic locus fail to be amplified and provide a result in genetic testing) for single gene conditions, due to mosaicism for chromosomal disorders, and due to contamination. PGT-A has lower resolution than prenatal or postnatal chromosomal-based testing and as a result cannot detect most chromosomal microdeletions or microduplications. Due to the potential for embryo mosaicism, abnormal PGT-A results may not be fully representative of the chromosomal makeup of an embryo since the trophectoderm may not be representative of the inner cell mass, which becomes the fetus. Conversely, while normal PGT-A results reduce the risk for chromosomal aneuploidy, they do not eliminate this risk. For all of these reasons, a follow-up diagnostic test (CVS or amniocentesis) is offered if pregnancy is achieved.

While PGT-SR has the ability to detect unbalanced forms of a chromosomal translocation or inversion, it typically cannot differentiate between embryos carrying a balanced chromosomal rearrangement and those with no chromosomal rearrangement. Additionally, the size of the chromosomal translocation and inversion affects how or if PGT-SR can be performed. Since PGT-M typically requires a haplotype approach, test setup may be difficult if samples are not available from other family members carrying the familial variant, such as cases of de novo autosomal dominant conditions. When PGT-M is performed for autosomal recessive or X-linked disorders, the carrier parent(s) must have their carrier status confirmed molecularly. Sometimes carrier testing of additional family members is required for PGT-M assay development. For diseases caused by a triplet repeat expansion (such as fragile X syndrome), certain gene inversions (as in hemophilia A), or a large gene deletion, most testing labs only perform analysis by haplotyping as the mutation itself is often difficult to detect through direct mutation analysis. When an affected family member has been found to have a VUS, the ability to perform PGT-M will be at the discretion of the testing laboratory and consideration of PGT test setup may require documentation explaining why the variant is believed to be potentially pathogenic. Additionally, further counseling documenting the couple's understanding of the limitations of PGT-M in the context of a VUS may be required. PGT is not offered for certain disorders, such as conditions caused by mutations in mitochondrial DNA. Finally, every couple undergoing PGT should be made aware that after testing is performed there may be no unaffected embryos available for transfer and should be asked to consider what they will do with any unaffected embryos that may remain after they have completed their family.

Counseling

Risk assessment

Risk assessment is an essential component of most genetic counseling sessions. While the type of risk assessment is dependent on the patient's indication, effective execution of other components of the genetic counseling session, including but not limited to test interpretation, test selection, and personalized counseling, rely on proper risk assessment. Risk assessment may include specifics of the patient's medical, family, pregnancy, exposure, and travel history as well as ethnicity, age, and previous test results specific to the current pregnancy. This information allows proper determination of a patient's a priori risk for certain conditions such as aneuploidy, as well as specific risks that may be unique to them based on history. These initial risk assessments may then be refined based on additional medical information such as test results for the patient and/or their partner, ultrasound imaging, and/or other prenatal screening results.

Family history

The focus on family history in a prenatal genetic counseling session varies depending on indication. At times, the family history is the focus of the session and the primary component of the risk assessment. This is true, for example, for a patient referred for a family history of intellectual disabilities, birth defects, or a known genetic condition. In other circumstances, the family history assessment is uniquely broad and independent of referral indication. In this case, the family history evaluation is aimed at identifying patients with increased risks for genetic conditions, birth defects, hereditary cancer, and other conditions with a possible genetic predisposition, particularly when this could impact pregnancy management or testing options available to the patient. In cases where the family history is not the focus of the session based on indication, it remains an important component of comprehensive genetic counseling. Studies have shown that 6% to 27% of the time a genetic risk factor that was not identified as part of the patient's referral indication was documented during the family history evaluation of a prenatal genetic counseling session (McClatchey et al., 2018; Pompilii et al., 2014).

Pretest counseling

Pretest counseling is an essential component of the genetic testing process, allowing for thorough consideration of and informed consent for testing. Provided that prenatal genetic tests are optional in nature, a nondirective approach with sensitivity toward the patient's culture, education level, language, and values is important. The extent of the pretest counseling will vary based on the particular test being offered; however, the conversation should include information about the purpose of the testing; how the test is performed; test performance data; the benefits, risks, and limitations of the test; possible results and potential implications of those results; and any incidental information that may be uncovered by the test technology (see Box 7.1).

A variety of counseling aids are available to supplement pretest counseling and can be effective and increase efficiency, particularly with regard to the medical and scientific details of the tests. However, prior to utilization of such aids, careful attention should be paid to ensure they are appropriately developed for the education level of the patient as well as unbiased with regard to test specifics and utility. In addition, discussion of the benefits and limitations of testing should be approached with regard to each individual patient's

Box 7.1 Pretest Counseling Components

- Purpose of the test
- Sample requirements
  - Blood sample
  - Saliva sample
  - Invasive procedure
- Test performance data
  - Sensitivity
  - Specificity
- Risks of testing
  - Procedure-related complications
  - Uncertain results
  - Incidental findings
  - Increased anxiety or stress to patient
- Benefits of testing
  - Refined risk assessment
  - Diagnosis of condition
  - Information for management
  - Treatment or prevention available
  - Reduced anxiety or stress to patient
- Possible results
  - Positive or high risk
  - Negative or low risk
  - Uncertain
  - No results
- Turnaround time for results
- Plan for communication of results
- Possible implications of test results for partner or other family members
- Insurance coverage of the test
- Optional nature of the test and alternative testing options available

desire for information. A patient's threshold for uncertainty, risk, and various options for management of the pregnancy are all considerations that may impact how the benefits and limitations of testing options are perceived and weighed in the decision-making process. Anticipatory guidance regarding the possible test results and their associated meaning, impact, follow-up, and management options will help set the stage for effective results disclosure and posttest counseling.

Posttest counseling

Prenatal genetic tests are reported in a variety of ways, and for many, a normal test result comes with a residual risk for the condition(s) of interest. All genetic tests will have a residual risk in the presence of a negative or normal result. This risk may be presented in a variety of ways, such as a posttest risk number or a negative predictive value, which is the chance the condition is not present given a negative result. Regardless of the specifics of the residual risk or the way it is reported by the laboratory, clear communication of this residual risk to patients is an important component of posttest counseling. Additionally, not all genetic tests are comprehensive, and the normal test results should be reviewed in the context of the limitations of the testing technology.

With regard to abnormal or positive test results, disclosure should be in line with the patient's knowledge level and done in a culturally and emotionally sensitive manner. If the posttest counseling is performed by the same person who performed pretest counseling, then anticipatory guidance and discussion from the pretest session will help set the tone for a productive conversation with a common agenda. If this is not the case, then it is important to determine the patient's baseline understanding of the potential results and the extent to which they have considered a possible abnormal result early in the conversation. Components of posttest counseling may include discussion of the condition characteristics and etiology, degree of risk versus a diagnostic result, data specific to the result such as positive predictive value (the chance the condition is present given a positive result), follow-up testing options, available treatment and therapies for the condition, pregnancy management options (when applicable), and available support resources (if appropriate). Depending on the trajectory of the conversation and the likelihood of follow-up counseling sessions, information such as recurrence risks and potential impact for other family members may be appropriate to discuss in the posttest counseling session.

Documentation

It is important to document all aspects of the genetic counseling session, including referral indication, risk assessment (with all applicable components), decision making, and plans for follow-up. While the specifics of documentation are variable from provider to provider, it is important that the information is clear and comprehensive and updated frequently to ensure the most up-to-date information is available for the patient's medical management.

Special considerations

Fetal intervention

With improvements in both prenatal imaging modalities and techniques to try to correct or improve fetal congenital anomalies, the number of fetal interventions available has grown and continues to expand. Interventions currently available include in utero repair of spina bifida; balloon atrial septostomy and balloon dilation of the aortic valve for hypoplastic left heart syndrome; endoscopic tracheal occlusion for congenital diaphragmatic hernia; open fetal surgery for sacrococcygeal teratoma, vascular tumors, and lung masses; amniotic band resection; fetal shunt placement for lower urinary tract obstructions; selective fetoscopic laser photocoagulation for twin-to-twin transfusion syndrome; ex utero intrapartum treatment for conditions expected to cause severe breathing difficulties at delivery; and intrauterine transfusion for severe fetal anemia. The logistics of fetal interventions can be challenging, and the benefits and risks to both the fetus or fetuses and the pregnant parent have to be weighed. Fetal intervention is typically performed in tertiary care centers where multidisciplinary teams work together to evaluate a pregnancy, formulate a treatment or management plan, and counsel the patient or couple about the benefits, risks, and alternatives to fetal intervention. In many cases, prenatal genetic testing is part of the evaluation process to help determine whether a fetus is a good candidate for intervention and whether an underlying genetic condition may complicate an intervention under consideration. Prenatal genetic counselors often are members of this team to provide insight into possible genetic etiologies for conditions being treated, input and coordination for appropriate genetic testing, and counseling and psychosocial support, particularly when a genetic diagnosis is confirmed or suspected.

Termination of pregnancy

Elective termination of pregnancy as a pregnancy management option should be explored with all patients considering prenatal genetic testing. It is important for providers to understand that legal and institutional policies vary greatly across the United States and they must stay up to date on the policies and laws governing this option in the location in which they practice. Availability of procedures, gestational age restrictions, insurance coverage, and other policies, such as a mandatory waiting period or review of specific informational materials, are just some of the aspects regarding termination of pregnancy options that providers should be aware of when discussing this option with patients. Additionally, every patient and family will have their own unique perspective of the various pregnancy management options, and exploration of these options in an unbiased and supportive environment is essential to ensuring all patients have access to termination of pregnancy as a management option. These conversations can be aided by an understanding of differing cultural and religious views of termination that may be relevant to a patient.

Perinatal autopsy

Knowing the underlying cause of fetal anomalies or a fetal demise or neonatal death is vital to being able to provide families with accurate recurrence risk estimates and future reproductive testing options. Perinatal autopsy is an often underutilized tool to aid in these circumstances, often due to a lack of awareness of its availability, the difficulty some health-care providers have in bringing up this topic with families, and misperceptions families have about the autopsy process. Prenatal imaging can be limited by factors including, but not limited to, maternal habitus, fetal lie, and gestational age at the time of imaging, which can lead to having a limited phenotype on which to base genetic test choice or results interpretation. As a result, being able to obtain additional information about fetal phenotype through fetal autopsy can be invaluable, particularly in cases of termination of pregnancy or fetal demise. Perinatal autopsy has the potential to provide additional details about fetal anatomy that may help guide additional testing or clarify a diagnosis. Even pathological evaluation of products of conception tissue or additional postmortem imaging can provide additional vital details that may aid in narrowing down a diagnosis. Genetic counselors can be instrumental in making families aware of this option, discussing the type of information autopsy might provide, and helping them make an informed decision while being sensitive to the loss they have suffered.

Resource identification

With the overwhelming amount of readily available information, it is important for genetic counselors to provide guidance to patients and families regarding useful, accurate, and supportive resources, particularly in an environment where unvetted, nonexpert, and biased resources abound. Quality patient resources can be used to supplement care and enhance the patient's experience and ability to continue to learn about and adapt to new information.

Support resources for patients are vast and will not be one size fits all. Written information about genetic conditions can be in the form of brochures, books, and most often websites. Given the rapid changes in the field of genetics, one must ensure that the information provided to the patient is up to date and medically accurate. Interactive resources for patients are often helpful, and it is important to recognize that, for some patients, the desire for interaction with others in a similar situation may not be immediate. For some patients, an online forum is preferred, while others may be looking for an in-person experience. For some genetic conditions, there are robust support groups that focus specifically on one condition, while other genetic conditions are so rare that families may find only a more general support group available to them. Genetic counselors are often uniquely positioned to be aware of or find these types of resources for the families they serve.

Perinatal hospice is one form of ongoing support and management during the pregnancy for patients with a lethal or life-limiting diagnosis. Perinatal hospice and palliative care programs exist across the country and are a model of care that begins at diagnosis and supports families and their babies throughout the pregnancy, birth, and death experience. These programs support patients through birth planning, preliminary medical decision making, and emotional and spiritual support and typically use a multidisciplinary team approach. The perinatal hospice and palliative care website is one resource where providers and patients can learn more about this option and available programs across the country (http://www.perinatalhospice.org).

Psychosocial counseling challenges particular to prenatal genetic counseling

Providing genetic counseling during pregnancy has inherent challenges that may not be encountered in other subspecialties of genetic counseling, particularly the aspects of time constraints for making testing and management decisions, the dual patient scenario of the pregnant individual and fetus, and, at times, complicated family or pregnancy dynamics. Time constraints for decisions making are the norm in prenatal genetic counseling. This is due to certain testing options only being available during select windows of time during pregnancy and test turnaround times that are often 2 weeks or longer being superimposed on legal limitations for the timing of decisions such as termination of pregnancy. Additionally, the fact that fetal imaging often provides more detailed information in the late second trimester and that fetal intervention availability may also be limited by gestational age makes time of the essence in prenatal genetics. The urgency that is often felt in prenatal genetic counseling can make decision making more challenging for families during this time period, particularly when irreversible decisions are being considered. An additional complexity of prenatal genetic counseling is the duality of the patient, with both the well-being of the pregnant patient and the fetus or fetuses being considered in most management and testing decisions. At times, families have to consider possible consequences of management decisions for both the pregnant patient and the fetus or for one fetus versus another and in some circumstances may be forced to place the well-being of one above the other. Lastly, all of these decision-making processes are superimposed on family dynamics, which can at times be complicated and made more challenging by aspects particular to pregnancy. For example, while both parents' opinions should be taken into account in decisions about a pregnancy, often the pregnant individual's choice has more weight because they are carrying the pregnancy. Decision making in pregnancies of teenagers may be challenging due to the teenager's parents wanting to have control over pregnancy management decisions or the teenage patient deferring to their parents' decisions. In pregnancies that involve third-party reproduction, such as a gestational carrier, there is an additional party beyond the biological parents who has to agree to any testing, intervention, and management decisions that are made. Genetic counselors have the skills to help families negotiate these delicate conversations, see all sides of the decision at hand, and hopefully facilitate a decision that is best for all involved.

Conclusion

Genetic counseling has been and continues to be an integral aspect of reproductive healthcare. The expertise of genetic counselors assists both patients and providers in navigating the ever-evolving landscape of screening, testing, and management options. Genetic counselors are uniquely positioned to stay abreast of developments within reproductive medicine, which allows them to guide patients through the array of options available to them to assess and manage their reproductive genetic risk. Additionally, genetic counselors arm patients with the tools needed to effectively utilize the information they learn along the way, support patients in making personalized healthcare decisions, and advocate for access to the care needed and desired.

References

American College of Obstetricians and Gynecologists. (2007). ACOG Practice Bulletin No. 88, December 2007: Invasive prenatal testing for aneuploidy. *Obstetrics and Gynecology, 110*(6), 1459–1467.

American College of Obstetricians and Gynecologists. (2016a). Committee on Genetics and the Society for Maternal-Fetal Medicine. Committee Opinion No. 682: Microarrays and next-generation sequencing technology: The use of advanced genetic diagnostic tools in Obstetrics and Gynecology. *Obstetrics and Gynecology, 128*(6), e262–e268.

American College of Obstetricians and Gynecologists. (2016b). Practice Bulletin No. 163: Screening for fetal aneuploidy. *Obstetrics and Gynecology, 127*(5), 979–981.

American College of Obstetricians and Gynecologists. (2017a). Committee Opinion No. 690: Carrier screening in the age of genomic medicine. *Obstetrics and Gynecology, 129*(3), e35–e40.

American College of Obstetricians and Gynecologists. (2017b). Committee Opinion No. 691: Carrier screening for genetic conditions. *Obstetrics and Gynecology, 129*(3), e41–e55.

Brady, P. D., Chiaie, B. D., Christenhusz, G., Dierickx, K., Van Den Bogaert, K., Menten, B., Janssens, S., Defoort, P., Roets, E., Sleurs, E., Keymolen, K., De Catte, L., Deprest, J., de Ravel, T., Van Esch, H., Fryns, J. P., Devriendt, K., & Vermeesch, J. R. (2014). A prospective study of the clinical utility of prenatal chromosomal microarray analysis in fetuses with ultrasound abnormalities and an exploration of a framework for reporting unclassified variants and risk factors. *Genetics in Medicine, 16*(6), 469–476.

Burns, W., Koelper, N., Barberio, A., Deagostino-Kelly, M., Mennuti, M., Sammel, M. D., & Dugoff, L. (2017). The association between anticoagulation therapy, maternal characteristics, and a failed cfDNA test due to a low fetal fraction. *Prenatal Diagnosis, 37*(11), 1125–1129.

Drury, S., Williams, H., Trump, N., Boustred, C., GOSGene, Lench, N., Scott, R. H., & Chitty, L. S. (2015). Exome sequencing for prenatal diagnosis of fetuses with sonographic abnormalities. *Prenatal Diagnosis, 35*(10), 1010–1017.

Gregg, A. R., Arabi, M., Klugman, S., Leah, N. T., Bashford, M., Goldwaser, T., Chen, E., Sparks, T. N., Reddi, H. V., Rajkovic, A., Dungan, J. S., ACMG Professional Practice and Guidelines Committee. (2021). Screening for autosomal recessive and X-linked conditions during pregnancy and preconception: A practice resource of the American College of Medical Genetics and Genomics (ACMG). *Genetics in Medicine, 23*, 1793–1806.

Handyside, A. H., Kontogianni, E. H., Hardy, K., & Winston, R. M. (1990). Pregnancies from biopsied human preimplantation embryos sexed by Y-specific DNA amplification. *Nature, 19*(344), 768–770.

Hayward, J., & Chitty, L. S. (2018). Beyond screening for chromosomal abnormalities: Advances in non-invasive diagnosis of single gene disorders and fetal exome sequencing. *Seminars in Fetal & Neonatal Medicine, 23*(2), 94–101.

Lefkowitz, R. B., Tynan, J. A., Liu, T., Wu, Y., Mazloom, A. R., Almasri, E., Hogg, G., Angkachatchai, V., Zhao, C., Grosu, D. S., McLennan, G., & Ehrich, M. (2016). Clinical validation of a noninvasive prenatal test for genomewide detection of fetal copy number variants. *American Journal of Obstetrics and Gynecology, 215*(2), 227.e1–227.e16.

Martin, J. A., Hamilton, B. E., Osterman, M. J., Driscoll, A. K., & Mathews, T. J. (2017). Births: Final data for 2015. *National Vital Statistics Reports, 66*(1), 1.

McClatchey, T., Lay, E., Strassberg, M., & Van den Veyver, I. B. (2018). Missed opportunities: Unidentified genetic risk factors in prenatal care. *Prenatal Diagnosis, 38*(1), 75–79.

Monaghan, K. G., Leach, N. T., Pekarek, D., Prasad, P., Rose, N. C., & ACMG Professional Practice and Guidelines Committee. (2020). The use of fetal exome sequencing in prenatal diagnosis: A points to consider document of the American College of Medical Genetics and Genomics (ACMG). *Genetics in Medicine*, *22*(4), 675–680.

Palomaki, G. E., Deciu, C., Kloza, E. M., Labert-Messerlian, G. M., Haddow, J. E., Neveux, L. M., Ehrich, M., van den Boom, D., Bombard, A. T., Brody, W. W., Nelson, S. F., & Canick, J. A. (2012). DNA sequencing of maternal plasma reliable identifies trisomy 18 and trisomy 13 as well as Down syndrome: An international collaborative study. *Genetics in Medicine*, *14*(3), 296–305.

Pompilii, E., Astolfi, G., Calabrese, O., Calzolari, E., Ferlini, A., Lucci, M., Parmeggiani, G., Seri, M., & Baroncini, A. (2014). Prenatal genetic counseling referrals for advanced maternal age: Still room for improvement. *Prenatal Diagnosis*, *34*(1), 71–74.

Ryan, A., Hunkapiller, N., Banjevic, M., Vankayalapati, N., Fong, N., Jinnett, K. N., Demko, Z., Zimmermann, B., Sigurjonsson, S., Gross, S. J., & Hill, M. (2016). Validation of an enhanced version of a single-nucleotide polymorphism-based noninvasive prenatal test for detection of fetal aneuploidies. *Fetal Diagnosis and Therapy*, *40*(3), 219–223.

Wapner, R. J., Martin, C. L., Levy, B., Ballif, B. C., Eng, C. M., Zachary, J. M., Savage, M., Platt, L. D., Saltzman, D., Grobman, W. A., Klugman, S., Scholl, T., Simpson, J. L., McCall, K., Aggarwal, V. S., Bunke, B., Nahum, O., Patel, A., Lamb, A. N., Thom, E. A. (2012). Chromosomal microarray versus karyotyping for prenatal diagnosis. *New England Journal of Medicine*, *367*(23), 2175–2184.

CHAPTER 8

PEDIATRIC GENETIC COUNSELING

CAROL S. WALTON

Introduction

Pediatrics is a long-established area of practice for genetic counselors. Genetic counseling focusing on the provision of genetic recurrence risk information to parents of children diagnosed with genetic conditions was promoted as a specific role of pediatricians and sometimes also nonphysician human geneticists during the 1950s and 1960s as the underlying basis of some conditions was identified. The sensitive nature of these discussions and the value of having an established relationship with families, including awareness of socioeconomic and psychologic factors impacting a family's receipt of genetic information, were noted (Fraser, 1958; Thompson, 1967). As the first graduates of master's-level genetic counseling programs sought positions during the 1970s, they most often worked with clinical geneticists in pediatric or prenatal genetics clinics (Baty, 2018; Walker, 2009). Navigating a landscape where clinical geneticists were accustomed to being the sole provider of genetic counseling services and establishing a professional scope that appropriately recognized and utilized the genetic counselors' training and expertise were early challenges for these pioneers (Heimler, 1997). Pediatrics is now one of the most diverse and rapidly evolving practice areas. According to the 2020 Professional Status Survey of the National Society of Genetic Counselors (NSGC), 25% of all genetic counselors and 31% of genetic counselors providing direct patient care report practicing in pediatrics (NSGC, 2020a). Next-generation sequencing (NGS) and other genetic testing advances have vastly expanded the ability to diagnose genetic conditions in infants, children, and adolescents. The provision of client-centered genetic counseling to these young patients and their families is a critical component of quality, comprehensive care in diverse pediatric settings.

Individually, many of the conditions affecting pediatric patients are rare, but collectively they are common. Birth defects, which are any abnormalities affecting body structure or function that are present from birth, affect one in every 33 newborns in the United States annually and account for one in every five infant deaths, representing the leading cause of infant deaths (Centers for Disease Control and Prevention, 2008; Christianson et al., 2006;

Mai et al., 2012; Matthews et al., 2015). Globally, at least 6% of total births have a serious birth defect of genetic or partially genetic origin (Christianson et al., 2006). An estimated 25 to 50 million Americans and 30 million Europeans have a rare disease, often initially recognized at birth or during infancy but sometimes not apparent until much later depending on the order and intensity of presenting symptoms (Fernandez-Marmiesse et al., 2018). The recent emergence of NGS technology and its applications to clinical genetic testing such as multigene panels and broad exome or genome sequencing have enabled relatively fast and inexpensive identification of genetic etiologies underlying many of these conditions and increased the diagnostic yield severalfold over older genetic testing approaches. While a specific genetic cause still cannot be determined in many of the patients presenting for genetic evaluation, ongoing gene discovery and increased understanding of the roles of copy number variants (CNVs), somatic mosaicism, polygenic inheritance, epigenetic effects on gene function and regulation, and other novel mechanisms as the basis for birth defects and rare diseases will continue to decrease the proportion of patients who remain undiagnosed (Fernandez-Marmiesse et al., 2018; Thiffault et al., 2019).

Newborns and young infants may be seen for genetic evaluation as hospital inpatients or in outpatient clinic settings depending on the acuity of their medical issues. Infants and toddlers are often referred for genetics evaluations due to delays in achieving expected developmental milestones or delayed identification of congenital anomalies. Differences in behavior or learning may not become apparent until the child starts preschool or elementary school. Among the reasons for referral in later childhood or adolescence are new onset or worsening of symptoms, atypical progression of puberty, or identification of new concerns in the family history that may increase the pediatric patient's risk for an inherited condition. Table 8.1 outlines common referral indications for genetic evaluation of pediatric patients.

Models, Settings, and Genetic Counselor Roles in Pediatrics

Traditionally, genetic counselors in pediatrics partnered on genetics teams with physician clinical geneticists. This continues to be a common model, especially for general pediatric genetics clinics focusing on diagnostic evaluation and management of children with known or suspected genetic conditions (Stein et al., 2018). Genetic counselors and clinical geneticists may interact with patients in a synchronous fashion, each taking the lead for elements of a patient's visit as determined by the reason for referral and their respective scopes of practice but conducting the visit and subsequent case management activities jointly. To accommodate expanding demand for genetics services, increase efficiency, and promote top-of-scope practice by all providers on the team, some clinics have adopted asynchronous approaches. For instance, a genetic counselor may conduct the patient's initial triage and risk assessment and coordinate guideline-driven first-tier genetic testing for common referral indications, such as autism spectrum disorder. A clinical geneticist then sees the patient when test results are available to conduct a thorough review of systems and physical examination, determine genotype–phenotype correlation, discuss the test results and any associated diagnostic information, and make recommendations for

Table 8.1 Common Referral Indications for Genetic Evaluation in Pediatrics

Referral indication	Examples
Single or multiple congenital anomalies	Dysmorphic features, cleft palate, microtia, aniridia, myelomeningocele, congenital heart defect, craniosynostosis, brain malformation, polydactyly, renal dysplasia, ectodermal dysplasia, ambiguous genitalia
Neurological or neuromuscular symptoms	Microcephaly, macrocephaly, hydrocephalus, seizures, ataxia, hypotonia, weakness, neuropathy, myotonia, joint contractures, fasciculations, regression, neurodegeneration
Growth or feeding concerns	Small or large for gestational age, prenatal- or postnatal-onset short stature, failure to thrive, generalized overgrowth, obesity, hyperphagia, asymmetric growth
Sensory disorders	Congenital or postnatal-onset hearing loss, congenital or postnatal-onset vision impairment, anosmia, pain insensitivity
Abnormal newborn genetic screening	Inborn errors of metabolism, hemoglobinopathies, cystic fibrosis, spinal muscular atrophy, others
Hematological disorders	Hemoglobinopathies, hemophilia, von Willebrand disease, hereditary thrombophilia, Fanconi pancytopenia syndrome
Atypical pubertal development	Turner syndrome, Klinefelter syndrome, Kallmann syndrome, McCune-Albright syndrome
Hereditary cancer predisposition	Retinoblastoma, familial polyposis conditions, PTEN hamartoma tumor syndrome, Li-Fraumeni syndrome, DICER1, multiple endocrine neoplasia syndromes, hereditary neuroblastoma, Von Hippel-Lindau syndrome, RASopathies, Bloom syndrome
Developmental delay, intellectual disability, autism spectrum disorder, other learning or behavioral disorders	Chromosomal anomalies, Mendelian disorders (e.g., fragile X syndrome, PTEN hamartoma tumor syndrome, neurofibromatosis type 1, tuberous sclerosis, Rett syndrome), inborn errors of metabolism, teratogen exposures
Postnatal evaluation of prenatally identified concerns	Fetal ultrasound anomalies, karyotype abnormality on CVS or amniocentesis, positive cell-free fetal DNA testing (NIPT)
Family history of genetic disorder or genetic predisposition	Sibling, parent, or other family member(s) with known or suspected chromosome abnormality, Mendelian disorder, multifactorial condition or other genetic diagnosis. Prior stillbirth, unexplained neonatal/infant death and/or multiple miscarriages, especially when within the child's sibship, may also prompt referral to genetics.

Note: CVS = chorionic villus sampling; NIPT = noninvasive prenatal testing.

additional testing or specific medical management. Conversely, a clinical geneticist may conduct the initial patient evaluation and initiate the genetic testing process. The genetic counselor subsequently meets with the patient and family upon completion of the testing to discuss the test results and their implications. Recognizing that not all pediatric patients require a physical examination or other specific services from a physician geneticist, some centers have established genetic counseling clinics staffed solely by genetic counselors, with clinical geneticists functioning in a medical advisory role should a medically complex patient be identified. Examples of genetic counseling clinic referrals include family history of a genetic condition, counseling about carrier status, and discussion of outside test results with clear-cut implications or prompting the need for coordination of cascade testing of other relatives (Hannig et al., 2014). Other variations of these approaches exist and are influenced by staffing, clinic- and institutional-level policies, state licensure and other relevant regulations, the credentialing practices of hospitals and third-party payers, and billing and reimbursement considerations.

Inherited metabolic disease clinics for patients with inborn errors of metabolism (IEMs) have long incorporated genetic counselors on teams with clinical biochemical geneticists, registered dieticians, nurses, and other professionals. A genetic counselor may be the initial point of contact with a state newborn screening laboratory that has identified a positive test result on a baby that requires expeditious follow-up to confirm or exclude the presence of an IEM. The genetic counselor's expertise in communicating with the laboratory, family, hospital, and primary care provider is critical to ensure clear understanding of the need for additional testing, referral to the IEM clinic, and initiation of interim medical care as determined by the suspected diagnosis and its implications for potential acute morbidity or mortality. Genetic counselors in the IEM setting play critical roles in providing longitudinal, age-appropriate education; reproductive planning and recurrence risk discussions; and support for children and their parents coping with these chronic conditions (Hartley et al., 2011). New treatment options such as enzyme replacement therapies for lysosomal storage disorders are revolutionizing management of IEMs (Regier et al., 2017), and genetic counselors may work with patients undergoing treatment or enrolled in clinical trials for these emerging therapeutics. Finally, genetic counselors provide expertise and advocacy on behalf of patients with IEMs to public health and other government officials who determine policy and funding for newborn screening programs, IEM clinics, and related initiatives (McWalter et al., 2015).

Increasingly, genetic counselors have become integral members of pediatric multidisciplinary teams practicing alongside nongenetics physicians in neurology, cardiology, developmental pediatrics, hematology, oncology, otolaryngology, pulmonology, and many other specialties that have widely adopted genetic testing in the diagnosis and management of their patients (Stein et al., 2018). Genetic counselors in these settings ensure that genetic testing is conducted appropriately in terms of test and laboratory selection, patient education, informed consent and decision making, test results disclosure, coordination of follow-up referrals, and provision of psychosocial support and resources as indicated by the test results. Through collection and assessment of patient histories and pedigrees, genetic counselors may triage patients with more complex findings that suggest an underlying syndrome to be evaluated by a clinical geneticist, if one is not a member of the multidisciplinary team. Multidisciplinary clinics may also serve as the referral centers for babies identified through state newborn screening programs with cystic fibrosis, hemoglobinopathies, and other nonmetabolic genetic conditions. Timely coordination of confirmatory diagnostic and genetic testing and provision of expert genetic counseling are increasingly important in facilitating early therapeutic treatment of newborns identified through these programs. The recent addition of spinal muscular atrophy to some newborn screening programs to facilitate early identification and entry of affected newborns into therapeutic trials is one such example (Glascock et al., 2018).

Genetic counselors also play critical roles in newborn and pediatric intensive care units and other inpatient hospital settings. Families are often in crisis dealing with a child's unexpected, serious illness or congenital anomalies or with acute exacerbation of a chronic genetic condition. The genetic counselor may be the first person to sit down with a family to sensitively explain a new genetic diagnosis and introduce the family to resources and a roadmap to move forward. Rapid exome or genome sequencing are also increasingly being used in the diagnosis of critically ill pediatric patients. These approaches have demonstrated high clinical utility for providing actionable information that parents and healthcare teams can use for making real-time decisions about medical and surgical management, therapeutics, palliative care, and other critical matters (Dimmock et al., 2020; Petrikin et al., 2018). Genetic counselors help to ensure that complex pretest parental education and informed consent discussions are conducted in an understandable, client-centered manner that mitigates potential harms and illuminates all available options and other sometimes nuanced issues such as genetic discrimination and the future autonomy of the child. Genetic counselors provide parents with needed support for optimal decision making under what are often emotionally overwhelming and time-sensitive circumstances. Likewise, genetic counselor participation in results disclosure can help promote clear communication about diagnostic results or other identified variants and aid parents in their processing of this information as they navigate difficult decision making about next steps for their child's care and process how these results may impact other family members (Ayres et al., 2019; Cakici et al., 2020; Clowes Candadai et al., 2019; Lantos, 2019; Petrikin et al., 2015; Smith et al., 2019; Szego et al., 2019). When the child's prognosis is poor, the genetic counselor may engage in supportive and culturally sensitive discussions with parents about resources such as palliative care services (Wool & Dudek, 2013). If the child dies, with or without establishment of a diagnosis prior to death, a genetic counselor can be a source of immediate support to the parents as well as a future resource should they seek information about reproductive planning, reproductive recurrence risks, and testing options.

Roles for genetic counselors in pediatrics have expanded beyond the physical walls of the clinic or hospital. Telegenetics services staffed by genetic counselors are an effective means to expand access to patients located in rural areas or who otherwise would have to travel significant distances to be seen in a traditional hospital-based genetics clinic (Hilgart et al., 2012). If the nature of a child's medical concerns or other special needs makes in-person clinic attendance logistically difficult, then meeting with a genetic counselor for discussion via telegenetics can be a welcome alternative. Additionally, commercial laboratories offering genetic tests that are often ordered by pediatricians for patients with autism spectrum disorder and other specific clinical indications employ genetic counselors via telegenetics platforms to help ensure that pre- and posttest activities such as correct test selection, informed consent, accurate results interpretation, and referrals to clinical specialists based on the results can be facilitated (Cohen et al., 2016).

The Genetic Counseling Appointment in Pediatrics

Genetic counselors work with pediatric patients and their families in many different contexts, often until the child reaches young adulthood. When a child is referred for an initial diagnostic genetic evaluation, the genetic counselor may serve as the patient's primary point of contact with the genetics service. This may extend from the information-gathering phase during an initial clinic visit through the genetic testing process, sharing of results, and provision of patient education. It includes supporting families coping with a new genetic diagnosis and families receiving no diagnosis and processing how best to move forward (Stein et al., 2018). Genetic counselors often have continuity of involvement with children with established genetic diagnoses who return periodically for follow-up management of their condition, enabling the genetic counselor to assess and address the family's changing needs and questions over time. Often, the focus at the time of the child's initial diagnosis is on understanding its immediate implications for medical and developmental prognosis and management, while helping to facilitate the family's adjustment to this "new normal." Parents considering expanding their families may have questions about the chance of recurrence of the condition in future children and options available to them or extended family members for carrier, preimplantation, prenatal, or postnatal genetic testing. With age, the child with the genetic condition may begin asking questions about the diagnosis and the genetic counselor may model age-appropriate and developmentally appropriate responses. Families may also seek help talking to their other children, extended family members, or other professionals such as the child's teachers about the diagnosis and how best to support the child's needs outside of the home environment. Finally, as children enter puberty and the teen years, they may have their own questions about inheritance of the condition and future family planning that can be addressed with a genetic counselor.

Preparing for the appointment

There are some practical steps that can help pediatric patients and their families feel more comfortable and prepared for a genetics visit. Providing general information about the clinic, its services, and the team members and their roles can help families better understand why their child is being seen and what to expect during an appointment. Informing families that genetics appointments can be lengthy allows them to bring necessities like formula and diapers for infants and favorite, quiet toys or activities to occupy older patients and any siblings in attendance. Bringing along another adult who can watch the child(ren) outside of the clinic room or utilizing the hospital's childcare center can ensure that parents can engage in important, uninterrupted discussions with providers. Older pediatric patients should be actively encouraged to participate in the genetic counseling session and discussion about their diagnosis, any misconceptions they may have, difficulties they are experiencing, and needs for support. The genetic counselor may help them vocalize experiences and feelings about their genetic condition, such as challenges that they are having in school or social settings that they are otherwise hesitant to share. The extent of the pediatric patient's direct engagement in the session will depend on their age, maturity, interest, and cognitive level. It can be helpful to explore this with parents as part of preappointment communications, especially when there are concerns about the patient's ability to understand or cope with discussions about topics that are sensitive or potentially scary for them. Where available, professional child life specialists can be included in appointments to help the child who experiences anxiety in clinical settings cope better and to provide therapeutic respite during extended appointments or difficult discussions. Inclusion of other professionals in the appointment, such as a social worker or child psychologist, may be indicated in some situations.

Preclinic case preparation by the genetic counselor and other team members helps to ensure that the genetic counseling visit goes smoothly and meets the family's needs. Access to relevant medical records and patient history questionnaires prior to the visit can direct the genetic counselor's review of relevant published genetics literature, genetic testing directories, variant databases, and resources for support. The genetic counselor can subsequently focus on gaps and clarification of unclear information and better target lines of inquiry during the intake and pedigree to aid in risk assessment. If the patient is scheduled to see multiple providers in addition to the genetic counselor, preclinic meetings or other coordinated communications among the team members can establish a cohesive plan for the visit. If the clinic model includes same-day or on-call scheduling of patients to see a genetic counselor, advance case preparation may not be possible. The initial visit with the genetic counselor may focus on history and pedigree collection to enable the genetic counselor to conduct preliminary education and risk assessment, address the patient's and family's immediate needs, and formulate a plan of next steps and future contact.

Setting the agenda

At the outset of a genetic counseling session in pediatrics, the genetic counselor will typically engage in a process of contracting by exploring the family's understanding of and reasons for seeking genetics services and establishing goals for the visit (McCarthy Veach et al., 2018). In addition to supporting mutual understanding, effective contracting helps to build trust and clarify the roles of the genetic counselor and any other team members participating in the visit. Contracting can provide insight about what the family has already been told and understands so far about the patient's condition. It may also inform and prioritize the genetic counselor's next steps, such as addressing possible misunderstandings about why the patient was referred or what genetics can offer. As the session progresses, information is exchanged, and interpersonal dynamics evolve, the genetic counselor may engage in continuous contracting so that the appointment remains client centered and meets intended goals.

Genetic counseling in pediatric settings is usually directed to the parents or guardians of the child who is the patient. Children have diverse and sometimes quite fluid family structures. Biological parents, adoptive parents, stepparents, foster parents, grandparents, and other guardians may be involved in genetic counseling appointments (Pew Research Center, 2015). It is important for the genetic counselor to ascertain who is involved in the ongoing care and medical decision making about the patient. For instance, if the child's parents are divorced but share custody, the genetic counselor will need to explore whether their concerns and understanding of the patient's needs are well aligned. Do they have different perspectives about undertaking diagnostic genetic testing for the child or, if the child's diagnosis is known, the effective management of the child's condition? Likewise, if the genetic counselor ascertains that the child lives in a multigenerational household and has several regular care providers, then it is important to explore the extent to which everyone involved in the child's care understands the child's diagnosis and consistently provides and reinforces recommended management, be it a specialized diet or therapeutic behavioral reinforcements. One-quarter of children in the United States live in a single-parent household (Pew Research Center, 2015), which may place additional demands on the parent, especially when the patient has multiple special needs related to the genetic condition. Genetic counselors can provide an outlet for parents to express feelings such as stress and needs for referrals around self-care, respite services, or other resources. When multiple extended family members attend a child's clinic visits, their love and support for the child are usually evident, but competing agendas sometimes emerge. In these instances, skillful management of the session dynamics is necessary so that those in attendance feel heard and valued while prioritizing the needs and best interests of the patient.

Pediatric intake histories

Depending on the composition of the clinic team seeing a patient, the genetic counselor may collect all or only some of the elements of the intake history. In pediatrics, these typically include the patient's prenatal history, birth and neonatal history, medical history, developmental and school history, and relevant social history and a minimum three-generation family history or pedigree. Some elements may be emphasized more than others based on the patient's reason for referral. Table 8.2 outlines key elements of the medical and developmental intake history for pediatric genetic evaluation.

Obtaining the pedigree

Genetic counselors are skilled at obtaining family histories and typically document these in the form of a pedigree constructed using standardized nomenclature (Bennett et al., 1995, 2008, 2022). A minimum of three generations is typically obtained, though targeted expansion of the pedigree may be indicated depending on the clinical indication, phenotypic variability, and other factors. The pedigree aids in conducting genetic risk assessment based on the phenotypes and potential patterns of inheritance identified in the family. It guides counseling about reproductive recurrence risks, offering cascade genetic testing to extended family members or identifying other individuals at risk for a genetic condition identified in the patient. Knowledge of the patient's ethnicity and ancestors' countries of origin, if known, may guide test ordering, aid variant interpretation, identify consanguinity, and support the genetic counselor in employing a culturally sensitive approach (Bennett, 2019). See Chapter 19—"Family History in Contemporary Genetics" in this volume for further details on pedigree collection and use in genetic counseling.

Pedigree collection should be targeted to the child's referral indication(s). The pedigree collected for a positive family history indication will focus primarily on symptoms of that

Table 8.2 Elements of the Medical and Developmental Intake History for Pediatric Genetic Evaluation

Element	Examples
Pregnancy history	
Obstetric history	Number of term births, preterm births, abortions (including spontaneous abortions and termination of pregnancy), living children, stillbirths; relevant complications in prior pregnancies; infertility (underlying etiology, treatment/interventions used)
Parental ages	Maternal age-related risks for nondisjunction events, paternal age-related risks for new pathogenic variants
Exposures	Medications, recreational substances, occupational, household, TORCH infections, chronic maternal disease, diagnostic radiation
Genetic screening or diagnostic testing results	Preimplantation genetic testing, cell-free fetal DNA (NIPT), maternal serum screening (first trimester, second trimester, combined), chorionic villus sampling, amniocentesis, percutaneous umbilical blood sampling
Fetal imaging results	Ultrasound, fetal echocardiogram, fetal MRI
Complications	Late prenatal care, multiple gestation, bleeding, placental insufficiency, limited fetal activity, size-dates discrepancy, gestational diabetes, preeclampsia, preterm labor, HELLP syndrome, fetal distress
Birth and neonatal history	
Gestational age at delivery by LMP	Extremely preterm (<28 weeks), preterm (28–36 $^6/_7$ weeks), term (37–41$^6/_7$ weeks), postterm (42 weeks and over)
Delivery mode	Spontaneous vaginal, assisted vaginal (forceps, vacuum), cesarean
Location of birth	Hospital, home, home with subsequent transport to hospital (and any associated newborn complications)
Birth parameters	Birth weight, length, and head circumference (OFC); appropriate for gestational age, small for gestational age, large for gestational age
Apgar scores	Score from 1 to 10 at 1 minute, 5 minutes, and 10 minutes or longer, if indicated
Complications and treatments provided	Cyanosis, apnea, congenital heart defect, oxygen requirement, meconium aspiration, jaundice/hyperbilirubinemia, sepsis, hypoglycemia, feeding difficulties and method(s), intracranial hemorrhage, seizures, neonatal abstinence syndrome, others
Specialists/consults	Neonatology, genetics/metabolism, cardiology, neurology, ENT, ophthalmology, gastroenterology, surgery, others
Newborn screening results	Newborn metabolic/genetic screening, newborn hearing screening, critical congenital heart defects screening
Length of stay in hospital and status	Days/weeks in routine-level nursery or NICU if indicated, age at discharge to home, supports needed at discharge (e.g., supplemental oxygen, special feeding devices or nutritional support, others)

(continued)

Table 8.2 Continued

Element	Examples
Medical history	
General health	Healthy with primarily developmental/behavioral concerns vs. chronic/complex medical concerns
Major medical concerns	Age of onset, natural history over time, and current status of each
Growth and feeding	Growth charts for height, weight, and OFC; prenatal vs. postnatal onset of undergrowth or overgrowth; feeding or nutrition concerns
Specialist evaluations and recommendations	Cardiology, neurology, developmental pediatrics, endocrinology, gastroenterology, rehabilitation medicine, ENT, ophthalmology, others
Genetic and biochemical testing and results	Chromosomal microarray, fragile X testing, next-generation sequencing panels (targeted to symptoms and differential), exome or genome sequencing, serum amino acids, urine organic acids, acylcarnitine and carnitine profile, urine mucopolysaccharide screen, lysosomal enzymes, very long chain fatty acids, lactate, pyruvate, others
Other labs and results	Thyroid profile, creatine kinase, complete blood count with differential, electrolytes, blood gases, comprehensive metabolic panel, liver function studies, ammonia, glucose, urinalysis, ketones, others
Imaging and results	X-ray, skeletal survey, bone age, ultrasound (e.g., cranial, renal, abdominal), computed tomography, MRI, echocardiogram, others
Developmental history	
Age of attainment of milestones	Gross motor, fine motor, communication, social/emotional, cognitive; comparison to expected norms for age
Regression	Specific examples of any previously attained skills that were lost and any associated events
Behavior	Atypical/unusual behaviors for age such as poor eye contact, diminished social interaction, routines or repetitive behaviors, echolalia, self-injury, aggression toward others, emotional outbursts, others
Cognitive and adaptive abilities	Academic challenges, learning disability, intellectual disability, difficulty making friends, limited self-care skills for age
Developmental screening and testing results	Screenings done by pediatrician or early childhood program, psychology or neuropsychology evaluations, autism assessment, others
Interventions and services	Individual Education Plan or 504 Plan, physical therapy, occupational therapy, speech therapy, applied behavior analysis therapy, individual or family therapy, respite care, others

Note: The specific elements obtained and in what detail they are explored should be individualized according to the patient's referral indication(s) and the differential diagnosis being considered. Review of available medical and developmental records, history questionnaires completed by the family and/or direct interviews may be used to collect the information necessary for genetic evaluation and counseling.

ENT = ears, nose, and throat; HELLP = hemolysis, elevated liver enzymes, low platelets; LMP = last menstrual period; MRI = magnetic resonance imaging; NICU = neonatal intensive care unit; NIPT = noninvasive prenatal testing; OFC = occipital frontal circumference; TORCH = toxoplasmosis, other, rubella, cytomegalovirus, herpes simplex virus.

condition. Conversely, if the child is referred due to a constellation of medical and developmental symptoms that could manifest across a wide phenotypic spectrum or be genetically heterogenous, then the pedigree content may be relatively broad, encompassing physical, developmental, learning, and reproductive outcome histories of family members. A pedigree collected for a pediatric indication often identifies conditions in other family members that are not directly related to the child's reason for referral but may indicate a different concern, such as a possible hereditary predisposition to cancer. These important but secondary issues may be addressed briefly, with subsequent referral of the family to a hereditary cancer clinic or other resource that can provide comprehensive assessment while maintaining current focus on the child's primary referral indications.

Exploring the social history

Each child's medical and developmental concerns exist against a background of psychosocial factors in the household, school, and community. Exploring the child's and family's social history allows the genetic counselor to consider how these factors contribute to the overall risk assessment and determine what needs for supports or other resources the family may have. Exploring these issues is often most effectively accomplished through active listening and responding in the moment to statements made by the family as well as verbal and nonverbal cues noted by the genetic counselor. For instance, exploring how a child's extended hospitalization following surgery for a congenital anomaly may have impacted emerging developmental milestones or contributed to the development of a new behavior informs the team's understanding of possible multifactorial contributors to the observed developmental phenotype. If a child with a genetic condition spends time in multiple households, probing further into how effectively the different caregivers implement medical or behavioral interventions may identify inconsistencies in understanding about the child's condition and prompt the need for additional education and reinforcement of important management recommendations.

Establishing a plan

Just as a genetic counseling session utilizes contracting at the beginning to establish a clear, mutual agenda, the later part of the session should clearly delineate a plan for what will take place next and how this will be accomplished. When genetic testing has been offered and the family decides to move forward with this after proper informed consent, the logistics of test ordering, sample collection, authorization for payment coverage by insurance or other means, and the timeline and process for reporting of results should be discussed. Should the child's genetic testing necessitate collection of samples from parents or other family members, either at the time that the child's sample is sent or in a reflex fashion based on the child's results, the purposes of doing so should be clearly explained. The scope of the testing being performed on other family members should also be explained clearly, as it may be of a more limited or targeted nature than the child's test. With the increasing use of exome and genome sequencing methodologies that are often performed on a trio basis with patient and parental samples, genetic counseling discussions must comprehensively address the primary testing as well as any opt-in or opt-out testing and disclosure options for secondary findings (Green et al., 2013; Kalia et al., 2017). This ensures that individual autonomy is supported and informed consent is obtained from all parties involved. Flexibility to consider patient-only or duo testing is needed when one or both parents do not consent to participate in a trio approach due to concerns about their own genetic privacy or for other reasons.

Providing an expected timeline for completion of testing and reporting of results allows the family and other providers to manage their expectations and plan accordingly. This is especially important when decisions about medical management for the child or reproductive planning by the parents are dependent upon the genetic test results. Genetic testing is often completed in multiple tiers, so revising the plan and timeline as new tiers are pursued may be necessary. Results disclosure may take place in person or by phone, as most appropriate to the situation, and should be arranged in a timely manner. If other recommendations were also made by the genetics team, then the genetic counselor or other team members responsible for coordinating these should inform the family how this will be done.

Effective communication with families

An important component of most genetic counseling sessions is discussion of genetic concepts relevant to the child's diagnosis or any recommended genetic testing. Recognizing the spectrum of medical and scientific literacy among one's clients is critical to tailoring explanations that enable them to effectively integrate genetic information into their understanding and decision making. Asking a parent, "What is your understanding of the cause of your child's condition?" or "What does the term 'genetics' mean to you?" can provide insight into how accurate or sophisticated their understanding may be, enabling the genetic counselor to properly tailor the subsequent conversation. Simplifying technical terminology to more familiar words and simple analogies can make difficult concepts clearer. When the pediatric patient is an active participant in the discussion, exploring what they already know about how the human body and genetics work from science or health classes at school can be helpful. Having the patient share their understanding of their condition can set the stage for age-appropriate discussion. Incorporating visual aids can support the verbal discussion of genetic diagnoses, genetic testing, test results, and inheritance patterns. Employing published genetics visual aids, developing visual aids specific to the patient's test results or diagnosis, or even hand-drawing pictures or simple diagrams while explaining key concepts can be effective. Using child-friendly visuals or written materials may support more active engagement in the session and understanding of genetics concepts by pediatric patients (Newcomb et al., 2014).

Genetic counselors in the pediatric setting often work with families with limited English proficiency. Children who are bilingual are frequently more fluent in the language spoken by the genetic counselor than are their parents, and it may be the norm for their family to rely on them to assist with communication in healthcare and community settings. However, pediatric patients or other accompanying minors should not be used as interpreters during genetic counseling sessions. Professional medical interpreters employ their knowledge of language, cultural aspects of clinical communication, and linguistic tools such as contextualization to streamline complex genomic information, facilitate culturally sensitive discussion of difficult topics, and bridge sociocultural gaps between language-discordant family members and genetic counselors (Gutierrez et al., 2019). Ensuring that appropriate interpretation services are available to meet the communication needs of all clients participating in genetic counseling is critical. This may include in-person or remote telephone or video language interpreters, as well as use of technologies such as text telephone relay during phone calls and inclusion of subtitles during video telegenetics appointments with children or their family members with deafness.

Clinical documentation and additional resources

Documenting the genetic counseling provided to pediatric patients and their families helps to ensure continuity of the patient's medical care. It provides written affirmation of the information that was discussed during the visit for later reference by the family and the rest of the child's care team. Documentation may be in the form of a separate genetic counseling note or a focused genetic counseling entry as part of a larger team-generated note when multiple providers are involved in a clinic visit. In some settings, one set of documentation written in medical language and directed primarily at the child's primary care and referring medical providers is generated to share impressions and recommendations from the appointment, while a separate genetic counseling letter is written at a lay level for the family. In other settings, one correspondence is generated that is meant to strike a reasonable balance between medical and lay content (Baker et al., 2002; Lochner Doyle, 2009; VandenBoom et al., 2018). Given the complexity of genetics and testing, some review of foundational concepts may be beneficial for all audiences. The referring provider and other specialists working with the patient may receive questions about the genetics visit from the family, and this can help them accurately review and reinforce the genetic counseling information that was provided.

Many excellent resources exist for patient-friendly information about genetic conditions, genetic testing, and other topics commonly discussed during genetic counseling visits. This includes government-sponsored online consumer health sites dedicated to genetic information such as the U.S. Library of Medicine's MedlinePlus Genetics (https://medlineplus.gov/genetics/), online searchable directories such as Disease InfoSearch (https://www.diseaseinfosearch.org/), and hundreds of genetic disease advocacy and support organizations that have developed condition-specific educational resources. Materials may be printed out for families, or URL links to online sites vetted by the genetic counselor for relevance and currency of information may be provided to families when the genetic counselor has first confirmed the family's ability to readily access the internet. These lay materials may supplement or, when appropriate, replace a separate lay family letter.

Genetic Testing in Pediatrics

Genetic testing of pediatric patients is determined by multiple factors including, but not limited to, their reasons for referral, available testing options, recommendations of the healthcare team, insurance coverage, and the desires of the family. Where available, clinical guidelines addressing appropriate inclusion of genetic testing in pediatric care should be considered (Alford et al., 2014; Miller et al., 2014; Waggoner et al., 2018). However, as genetic testing technologies continue to evolve at a pace outstripping existing guidelines, it is incumbent upon genetic counselors to consult the published genetics literature, available databases, and their colleagues in clinical and laboratory settings to optimize the genetic testing approach for each patient.

Genetic counselors in both clinical and laboratory settings participate in utilization management or stewardship of genetic testing by ensuring that the right genetic test is performed at the right time and for the right reasons for each patient. Responsible genetic test selection endeavors to answer the clinical question(s) being asked in the context of the child's history, direct the sample to a laboratory qualified to perform and interpret the test, and consider factors including efficiency and cost savings (Dickerson et al., 2014; Miller et al., 2014; Wakefield et al., 2018). Examples of practical considerations in test selection in pediatrics include the availability of multiple sample type options, such as the ability to use a buccal DNA collection when a child with behavioral concerns is averse to phlebotomy, or the efficiencies of a laboratory's approach to sample collection and billing when parental samples are requested to help resolve the clinical interpretation of a variant of uncertain significance (VUS).

Genetic testing can be expensive, coverage by third-party payers is variable, and not all patients have insurance or adequate insurance, potentially leading to substantial out-of-pocket costs to families when genetic testing is recommended for a child or their family members. While public healthcare programs or financial subsidies provided by some hospitals may enable specific patient groups to undergo medically necessary genetic testing at no cost, many patients do not qualify. Discussion of the financial aspects of genetic testing and how this influences families' ability and decisions to pursue genetic testing is integral to genetic counseling practice in pediatrics (Brown et al., 2018; Stein et al., 2018). Genetic counselors often must advocate on behalf of the patient when coverage of recommended genetic testing is denied by a payer. Understanding the reasons for the denial, citing any existing genetic testing guidelines for the child's clinical presentation, and clearly explaining the medical necessity of the testing and potential adverse ramifications of not completing the testing are all strategies that a genetic counselor may employ to craft a letter of medical necessity or engage in direct peer-to-peer conversation with the third-party payer to effect reversal of an initial adverse coverage decision (Uhlmann et al., 2017). If the child's genetic testing is not covered, then the genetic counselor may work to identify testing options with discounted self-pay rates or other payment options that are acceptable to the family. Tiering genetic testing in an order that addresses the most likely diagnostic possibilities or the most pressing concerns first and then offering subsequent tiers of testing when first-tier results are uninformative can sometimes allow a family to have more control over out-of-pocket costs. Genetic counselors may also help families consider subsidized testing options offered by commercial laboratories, which offer substantially discounted testing options often with the mandate of sharing genetic data generated by sequencing.

Unfortunately, genetic testing may remain financially or logistically out of reach for some families who desire it. In this case, it is important to discuss what options exist for medical management, surveillance, and provision of therapies to the child in the absence of information potentially afforded by genetic testing. A child's parents may have questions about their own family planning and recurrence risks that a genetic counselor should try to address as accurately and realistically as possible in the absence of genetic testing results. The parents' timeline for making family planning decisions can also be considered. For instance, parents who are not planning another pregnancy immediately may be reassured that genetic testing options can be pursued at any time in the future should their insurance coverage or other financial resources change.

The reasons for and goals of genetic testing of a child vary among families. Often, genetic testing is pursued to establish or clarify a diagnosis suspected clinically based on the child's phenotype. Sometimes, genetic testing of a child is pursued based on a family history of a genetic condition in a family member and concern that the child may have inherited the condition and be at risk for medical or developmental impacts of the condition. Future reproductive planning of an affected child's parents, other family members, or the patient as they reach teenage years may also drive testing. In any case, the provision of informed consent is essential. Considerations for doing so are covered elsewhere in this volume[1] and addressed in several position statements by professional organizations (ACMG Board of Directors, 2015; Botkin et al., 2015; Kalia et al., 2017; NSGC, 2018a, 2018b, 2020b).

Parents seeking genetic testing for a child often expect it to provide a conclusive diagnosis, offer clear-cut answers to guide future medical or other management, or possibly even lead to a cure (Hayeems et al., 2016; Krabbenborg et al., 2016). While sometimes this is the case, the results of genetic testing are often more nuanced. Providing accurate information and helping to establish realistic expectations for each genetic test offered are important. Discussion may include the likelihood of finding a positive result given the child's clinical presentation and what subsequent actions might be informed by a positive versus a negative test result. Understandably, many parents hope that genetic testing will clarify uncertainty about their child's future. It is important that they are informed of the inherent limitations of even a positive, diagnostic test result. For instance, a test result might show that an infant with multiple congenital anomalies and developmental delay has a known pathogenic variant in a gene that correlates with the clinical presentation and confirms that the child has a specific genetic syndrome. However, identification of this variant most likely will not predict how severe the child's medical course will be over time or exactly what the patient's cognitive function will be in adolescence or adulthood. Confirming a genetic diagnosis may guide recommendations for screening or evaluation of the child for known potential clinical complications and help ensure that appropriate anticipatory guidance is provided. However, the extent and depth of knowledge about specific genetic conditions varies widely. As broad-based genetic testing methodologies such as chromosomal microarray, exome sequencing, and genome sequencing increasingly make possible the diagnosis of novel genetic conditions, it is critical that genetic counselors adequately prepare families for the possibility that their child's genetic testing may identify a rare genetic diagnosis about which very little is currently known (Bowdin et al., 2016; Kiedrowski et al., 2016; Krabbenborg et al., 2016; Reiff et al., 2012; Wynn et al., 2018).

Depending on the type of testing being performed, it may be appropriate to inform families of the possibility that it will identify a VUS. Identification of a VUS result may

[1] Editors' note: For more on informed consent and genetic testing of minors, see Chapter 15 by Kelly E. Ormond and Chapter 26 by Dena S. Davis in this volume.

leave a child's family in a state of uncertainty (Hayeems et al., 2016; Kiedrowski et al., 2016). When a child undergoes multiple genetic tests, it is possible that VUS results may arise on more than one test. Through the course of trying to properly classify a VUS identified in a child, parental testing may also identify the VUS in a parent. In some situations, this may provide some degree of reassurance that the VUS likely does not explain the child's findings. In other cases, identifying the same VUS in both the child and a parent may raise more uncertainty, such as when the variant has been seen in both symptomatic and asymptomatic individuals, and may potentially impact parental self-concept or cause feelings of guilt or blame (Kiedrowski et al., 2016; Reiff et al., 2012). While genetic counseling may help parents understand the scientific limitations of VUS results and the possibility that a VUS may be reclassified as either benign or pathogenic based on new information in the future, parental reactions to a VUS or other nondiagnostic results may vary significantly. It is important that the genetic counselor explore the family's feelings about the lack of a diagnostic test result. Some will express relief, viewing each nondiagnostic result as a reprieve from receiving news of an irreparable genetic anomaly that might impose limitations on expectations for their child or dampen hope (Reiff et al., 2012; Wilkins et al., 2016). Other families may experience disappointment because they sought confirmation of a specific genetic diagnosis that would provide actionable guidance for their child's care, a clearer prognosis, access to more services or support resources, or better clarity for their own reproductive planning (Kiedrowski et al., 2016). Parents who have been pursuing genetic testing for their child over an extended period with few answers may express ambivalence about yet another nondiagnostic test result or take a generally pragmatic view of how the information relates to their understanding of their child. They may be able to balance their desire for additional information about their child's concerns with a recognition that genetic testing is not a panacea and flexibly incorporate uncertain results into their family's experience and approach to life (Wilkins et al., 2016).

Genetic counselors working in pediatrics recognize the importance of including the possibilities of identifying consanguinity or misattributed parentage in the pretest discussion of any genetic test that may readily inform on biological relationships. For example, single nucleotide polymorphism–based chromosomal microarray can identify regions of long-contiguous stretches of homozygosity (LCSH), which, if present on two or more chromosomes, is assumed to indicate that the regions are identical by descent, implying consanguinity and enabling an estimate of the degree of parental relationship. LCSH of 6% in a child suggests that the parents are first cousins, while LCSH of 12.5% arouses suspicion of incest (Gardner & Amor, 2018). A child's parents may know or suspect that they are consanguineous, either because it is a common practice in their culture to marry within the family or because they know that their ancestors lived in the same geographic area. However, other families may be surprised by this information when revealed unexpectedly by their child's testing. Genetic testing that involves comparing parental DNA samples to the child's sample, such as parental chromosomal microarray studies or trio NGS panel or exome testing, may reveal that biological relationships are not consistent with the reported social relationships in the family. Informing both presumed parents during the pretest consent process of the test's ability to inform on biological relationships prior to providing their samples is critical (Botkin et al., 2015; Prero et al., 2019). This affords an opportunity for a parent to elect not to provide a sample or to request a private discussion of any concerns with the genetic counselor. Offering the option for parents to submit their samples at some time after the child's clinic visit, rather than requiring that they proceed directly to the laboratory for sample collection, is one approach of creating some time for all those involved to determine how to best navigate any concerns prompted by the pretest discussion.

Genetic counselors working in pediatrics are often met with genetic testing requests from families or other healthcare providers that necessitate careful consideration of not only the clinical utility of the testing but also relevant ethical, legal, and social factors. Weighing the potentially competing interests of the parties involved and recognizing that there may be complex cultural, social, or interpersonal dynamics influencing requests for genetic testing of children are critical to formulating an appropriate, individualized response. For instance, under what circumstances is it appropriate to perform genetic testing of a child for a typically adult-onset condition? If testing identifies a pathogenic variant in a gene that confirms a diagnosis in a symptomatic child, then what should be the genetic counselor's response to the child's parents should they request testing for the variant in the child's clinically unaffected siblings? What considerations should guide a response to parental requests for reproductive carrier testing of healthy siblings of a child affected with a Mendelian disorder or for a familial translocation? Genetic counselors may also receive requests from families or social services case managers for genetic testing of children who are being considered for adoptive placement. Understanding and articulating the clinical facts of each situation, the motivations driving such requests, and the potential benefits versus harms of testing are paramount in these situations. It is beyond the scope of this chapter to provide in-depth analyses of these issues. Fortunately, several thoughtful points to consider have been illuminated and recommendations have been made by professional genetics and pediatrics organizations to assist clinicians who may receive these requests (Botkin et al., 2015; Committee on Bioethics, Committee on Genetics, and American College of Medical Genetics and Genomics Social, Ethical, & Legal Issues Committee, 2013; Green et al., 2013; NSGC, 2018a, 2018b; Ross et al., 2013). Formal consultations with ethics committees through an employing institution or national professional organizations can also provide valuable guidance for particularly challenging situations.[2]

Families may seek genetic testing of children based on information they find on the internet or through other popular sources (Barton et al., 2019). These self-referrals sometimes represent a parent's astute observation that a child's features mirror those of a recognized genetic syndrome that can then be confirmed by the genetics team. In other cases, genetic testing requests are based on information and claims that are widely promoted but not scientifically substantiated or clinically indicated. In these circumstances, it can be helpful to explore the family's motivation for seeking such testing and acknowledge what is often a very genuine desire to use the testing to benefit the child's care. Respectfully explaining why such testing is not endorsed by the genetics community while partnering with the family to try to identify other credible options to assist their child may be an effective strategy.

While in-home or direct-to-consumer (DTC) genetic testing initially emerged as a means for adults to seek personal insights into their ancestry or participate in recreational identification of genetic characteristics, it has more recently expanded to include genetic testing of children for clinical indications such as autism spectrum disorder. Use of DTC testing in children has been discouraged by professional organizations, citing

[2] Editors' note: For more on the ethical and social issues related to the genetic testing of minors, see Chapter 26 by Dena S. Davis in this volume.

concerns about inaccurate results and interpretation, harmful interventions, altered family dynamics, and privacy, among others (Ross et al., 2013). As with other consumer-driven medical products, such testing will likely continue to expand, barring increased regulation limiting access. Supporting the expanded genetic literacy of pediatricians and other healthcare professionals caring for children in this landscape is critical so that they may have informed discussions with parents. In turn, encouraging families to share the results of in-home genetic testing with their child's healthcare providers will help to ensure that these results are interpreted correctly, that the potential benefits and limitations of the testing are clear, and that children who should receive formal evaluation by a genetics team are appropriately referred (Clayton, 2020).

The diagnostic odyssey

Genetic counselors often work with parents who have searched for answers and embarked on an extended diagnostic odyssey with their child with a suspected genetic condition lasting months or years. This journey may have begun even before their child was born if fetal anomalies were noted during the pregnancy. Multiple consultations with the pediatric genetics team and many rounds of genetic and other testing may have occurred over time. For parents seeking a genetic diagnosis to explain their child's symptoms, each nondiagnostic test result prolongs the search for answers as to what the future may hold and may contribute to an ongoing emotional odyssey that can adversely impact their physical and mental health, finances, and family dynamics (Macnamara et al., 2019; McConkie-Rosell et al., 2018; Rosenthal et al., 2001; Spillmann et al., 2017). Parental feelings of depression and anxiety may coexist with positive coping self-efficacy, active engagement in their child's healthcare, and apparent tolerance for the uncertainty associated with an undiagnosed condition, sometimes making it difficult for genetic counselors and other professionals to recognize parental needs for support unless this is actively assessed (McConkie-Rosell et al., 2018). The parents may be advised to continue to follow up with genetics periodically to see if the child's features evolve or "grow into" a recognizable syndrome or if anticipated advances in genetics may offer further options for diagnostic testing in the future. To the extent possible, acknowledging and normalizing parents' feelings of uncertainty and frustration around the lack of a diagnosis while providing clear next steps and optimizing symptomatic management of the child's medical and developmental concerns by the child's primary care provider and specialists may help alleviate parental worries that important needs are being missed. Exploring avenues of support for parents based not on a specific genetic diagnosis but rather on the shared experience of being on a diagnostic odyssey with their children may reduce feelings of isolation and promote feelings of engagement and empowerment with research efforts and other activities (Macnamara et al., 2019). Additionally, some parents of undiagnosed children may find participation in support groups centered around a predominant medical or developmental concern of their child, or in groups with a more general focus that connect families based on a shared language or culture, to be valuable.

Eventually finding a genetic diagnosis for a child's symptoms may affirm or change medical or other management, provide access to additional resources, relieve concerns that they did or did not do something that caused the child's health concerns, or allow the parents to move forward with greater clarity in their reproductive planning based on more information about inheritance, recurrence risks, and options for prenatal testing. The degree to which this is true for an individual child and family may depend on the child's age, how common and well understood the new diagnosis is, and how much knowledge and experience with available treatment or management approaches exist. Families receiving a rare diagnosis based on broad-based genetic testing such as exome sequencing may find that very little beyond the causal pathogenic variant(s) is currently understood. They may transition from a diagnostic odyssey to a therapeutic odyssey—another extended "waiting game" as they continue to support their child's needs symptomatically while hoping that additional, detailed reports of others with the same condition are published and that research advances in ways that produce concrete benefits for their child (Ayres et al., 2019; Brosco, 2018; Krabbenborg et al., 2016). Even when ending the diagnostic odyssey provides meaningful insights about their child's condition, complex emotions that evolved over the months or years of searching for answers may persist for parents. Grieving missed opportunities, receiving confirmation of a life-limiting diagnosis or a less hopeful prognosis than desired, mourning the loss of whom they perceived their child to be, experiencing ongoing feelings of isolation due to the rarity of the condition or loss of previous peer support from parents whose children remain undiagnosed, and feeling disappointed that the newly confirmed diagnosis does not positively impact the child's care as much as anticipated have all been reported by parents (Ayres et al., 2019; Krabbenborg et al., 2016; Macnamara, 2019).

Test results disclosure

When sharing a new diagnosis for a child, genetic counselors can help parents reduce feelings of uncertainty and create meaning as well as feel supported, more in control, and empowered (Helm, 2015; Lipinski et al., 2006). The genetic counselor is tasked with discussing the diagnosis in an informative, balanced, and sensitive manner while simultaneously attending to parents' affective responses that may reflect the adequacy of their understanding and how they are receiving and coping with the information (McGlynn & Langfelder-Schwind, 2020). Results disclosure discussions should clearly address what can be said with certainty based on the test results, such as confirmation of the underlying genetic mechanism, versus what remains less certain, such as the long-term prognosis for the child's cognitive abilities. Discussion of the implications of a new diagnosis should be based whenever possible on current and accurate published, peer-reviewed literature, as well as additional resources such as materials developed by reputable family support organizations. Helping parents understand what gaps currently exist in the understanding of their child's condition and potential future avenues to help address these gaps is also important. Honesty and transparency in the team's approach to results disclosure are important in promoting credibility and a sense of partnership with the family. Parents naturally want to find and maintain hope for their child's future. Balancing parental hope with encouraging realistic expectations can be challenging. However, many genetic conditions do present along a clinical spectrum that leaves the door open for each child to chart and define an individual, optimal course for the future. It can be useful to remind parents that a child's new genetic diagnosis exists within the context of other aspects of the child's genetic background as well as social, cultural, and environmental factors that all contribute to the child's outcomes.

Life-limiting conditions

Genetic counselors in pediatrics likely will work with families whose infant or older child has been diagnosed with a congenital, progressive, or otherwise life-limiting genetic condition. Some conditions that were once presented to families as incompatible with life and not amenable to intervention, such as trisomy 13 or trisomy 18, are now increasingly approached in a more individualized manner that recognizes the full clinical spectrum of the condition and that surgical or other technological advances in care may be available as options to extend survival or promote improved quality of life. These discussions are complex and often involve a multidisciplinary team, each member of which contributes their respective clinical expertise and recommendations about what options are clinically appropriate to offer for the patient. Even when options are limited, it is important that the genetic counselor and other team members maintain a collaborative, open-minded approach to such discussions so that they genuinely hear and appreciate the parents' values, perspectives, and wishes for their child during whatever time they do have together as a family (Andrews et al., 2016; Kaulfus et al., 2019). Genetic counselors may be able to assist families who wish to speak with parents of children with the same condition who have faced similar complex decisions. Genetic counselors may also facilitate referrals to pediatric palliative care services to help the child and family achieve the best quality of life when it is determined that the child's condition will ultimately lead to a shortened life.

Conclusion

Genetic counselors in pediatric settings help to ensure that families receive timely, relevant, accessible, client-centered care and support to meet their informational, decision-making, emotional, and resource needs when facing a known or suspected genetic diagnosis in their child. They employ expertise in the clinical and genetic aspects of pediatric syndromes and in the appropriate uses, selection, and interpretation of genetic testing to help families navigate the diagnostic process and understand its outcomes and implications for their child's care, now and in the future. For families who are still actively building their families at the time of a child's diagnosis with a genetic condition, genetic counselors help parents understand recurrence risks, available testing options, and alternatives such as adoption, as desired. Importantly, genetic counselors in pediatrics recognize the diagnostic and therapeutic odyssey many families experience and the importance of presenting difficult news, balanced whenever possible with hope, when talking to parents of a child who is expected to have chronic, lifelong medical or cognitive effects and needs for services and supports due to a genetic diagnosis.

This is an exciting time for pediatric genetic counseling practice. Genotype-first approaches that leverage broad genetic testing methods and robust bioinformatics capabilities to process vast amounts of medical records and phenotypic data about patients will allow genetic diagnoses to be confirmed sooner and more often. This will substantially shorten or bypass altogether the diagnostic odyssey for many families. As translational research continues to advance the understanding of rare genetic disorders and devise novel treatments and interventions, the therapeutic odyssey may also be shortened or eliminated, brightening the prognosis and outlook for many children. Parents will continue to seek answers, guidance, and resources that will empower them to optimize the health, quality of life, and expanding opportunities for their children as they grow. As children mature into adolescents, helping them understand the long-term medical, reproductive, and other implications of their genetic condition and effectively transition into adulthood become priorities; these issues are addressed in Chapter 14—"Genetic Counseling Approaches for Adolescents and Young Adults" in this volume. As the field of genetics continues to expand, pediatric genetic counselors are well poised to play an integral role, partnering with clinicians and families as genetics and genomics are increasingly incorporated into clinical care.

References

ACMG Board of Directors. (2015). ACMG policy statement: Updated recommendations regarding analysis and reporting of secondary findings in clinical genome-scale sequencing. *Genetics in Medicine, 17*(1), 68–69. https://doi.org/10.1038/gim.2014.151

Alford, R. L., Arnos, K. S., Fox, M., Lin, J. W., Palmer, C. G., Pandya, A., Rehm, H. L., Robin, N. H., Scott, D. A., Yoshinaga-Itano, C., ACMG Working Group on Update of Genetics Evaluation Guidelines for the Etiologic Diagnosis of Congenital Hearing Loss, & Professional Practice and Guidelines Committee. (2014). American College of Medical Genetics and Genomics guideline for the clinical evaluation and etiologic diagnosis of hearing loss. *Genetics in Medicine, 16*(4), 347–355. https://doi.org/10.1038/gim.2014.2

Andrews, S. E., Downey, A. G., Showalter, D. S., Fitzgerald, H., Showalter, V. P., Carey, J. C., & Hulac, P. (2016). Shared decision making and the pathways approach in the prenatal and postnatal management of the trisomy 13 and trisomy 18 syndromes. *American Journal of Medical Genetics Part C: Seminars in Medical Genetics, 172*(3), 257–263. https://doi.org/10.1002/ajmg.c.31524

Ayres, S., Gallacher, L., Stark, Z., & Brett, G. R. (2019). Genetic counseling in pediatric acute care: Reflections on ultra-rapid genomic diagnoses in neonates. *Journal of Genetic Counseling, 28*(2), 273–282. https://doi.org/10.1002/jgc4.1086

Baker, D. L., Eash, T., Schuette, J. L., & Uhlmann, W. R. (2002). Guidelines for writing letters to patients. *Journal of Genetic Counseling, 11*(5), 399–418. https://doi.org/10.1023/A:1016841731426

Barton, K. S., Wingerson, A., Barzilay, J. R., & Tabor, H. K. (2019). "Before Facebook and before social media . . . we did not know anybody else that had this": Parent perspectives on internet and social media use during the pediatric clinical genetic testing process. *Journal of Community Genetics, 10*(3), 375–383. https://doi.org/10.1007/s12687-018-0400-6

Baty, B. J. (2018). Genetic counseling: Growth of the profession and the professional. *American Journal of Medical Genetics Part C: Seminars in Medical Genetics, 178*(1), 54–62. https://doi.org/10.1002/ajmg.c.31601

Bennett, R. L. (2019). Family health history: The first genetic test in precision medicine. *Medical Clinics of North America, 103*(6), 957–966. https://doi.org/10.1016/j.mcna.2019.06.002

Bennett, R. L., French, K. S., Resta, R. G., & Austin, J. (2022). Practice resource-focused revision: Standardized pedigree nomenclature update centered on sex and gender inclusivity: A practice resource of the National Society of Genetic Counselors. *Journal of Genetic Counseling, 31*(6), 1238–1248. https://doi.org/10.1002/jgc4.1621

Bennett, R. L., French, K. S., Resta, R. G., & Doyle, D. L. (2008). Standardized human pedigree nomenclature: Update and assessment of the recommendations of the National Society of Genetic Counselors. *Journal of Genetic Counseling, 17*(5), 424–433. https://doi.org/10.1007/s10897-008-9169-9

Bennett, R. L., Steinhaus, K. A., Uhrich, S. B., O'Sullivan, C. K., Resta, R. G., Lochner-Doyle, D., Markel, D. S., Vincent, V., & Hamanishi, J. (1995). Recommendations for standardized human pedigree nomenclature. Pedigree Standardization Task Force of the National Society of Genetic Counselors. *American Journal of Human Genetics, 56*(3), 745–752.

Botkin, J. R., Belmont, J. W., Berg, J. S., Berkman, B. E., Bombard, Y., Holm, I. A., Levy, H. P., Ormond, K. E., Saal, H. M., Spinner, N. B., Wilfond, B. S., & McInerney, J. D. (2015). Points to consider: Ethical, legal, and psychosocial implications of genetic testing in children and adolescents. *American Journal of Human Genetics, 97*(1), 6–21. https://doi.org/10.1016/j.ajhg.2015.05.022

Bowdin, S. C., Hayeems, R. Z., Monfared, N., Cohn, R. D., & Meyn, M. S. (2016). The SickKids Genome Clinic: Developing and evaluating a pediatric model for individualized genomic medicine. *Clinical Genetics, 89*(1), 10–19. https://doi.org/10.1111/cge.12579

Brosco, J. P. (2018). Whose odyssey is it? Family-centered care in the genomic era. *Hastings Center Report, 48*(Suppl. 2), S20–S22. https://doi.org/10.1002/hast.879

Brown, S., Puumala, S., Leonhard, J., Bell, M., Flanagan, J., Dean, L. W., & Stein, Q. (2018). Genesurance counseling: Genetic counselors' roles and responsibilities in regards to genetic insurance and financial topics. *Journal of Genetic Counseling, 27*(4), 800–813. https://doi.org/10.1007/s10897-017-0180-x

Cakici, J. A., Dimmock, D. P., Caylor, S. A., Gaughran, M., Clarke, C., Triplett, C., Clark, M. M., Kingsmore, S. F., & Bloss, C. S. (2020). A prospective study of parental perceptions of rapid whole-genome and -exome sequencing among seriously ill infants. *American Journal of Human Genetics, 107*(5), 953–962. https://doi.org/10.1016/j.ajhg.2020.10.004

Centers for Disease Control and Prevention (CDC). (2008). Update on overall prevalence of major birth defects—Atlanta, Georgia, 1978–2005. *MMWR Morbidity and Mortality Weekly Report, 57*(1), 1–5.

Christianson, A., Howson, C. P., & Modell, B. (2006). *March of Dimes global report on birth defects: The hidden toll of dying and disabled children*. March of Dimes Birth Defects Foundation.

Clayton, E. W. (2020). Be ready to talk with parents about direct-to-consumer genetic testing. *JAMA Pediatrics, 174*(2), 117–118. https://doi.org/10.1001/jamapediatrics.2019.5006

Clowes Candadai, S. V., Sikes, M. C., Thies, J. M., Freed, A. S., & Bennett, J. T. (2019). Rapid clinical exome sequencing in a pediatric ICU: Genetic counselor impacts and challenges. *Journal of Genetic Counseling, 28*(2), 283–291. https://doi.org/10.1002/jgc4.1116

Cohen, S. A., Huziak, R. C., Gustafson, S., & Grubs, R. E. (2016). Analysis of advantages, limitations, and barriers of genetic counseling service delivery models. *Journal of Genetic Counseling, 25*(5), 1010–1018. https://doi.org/10.1007/s10897-016-9932-2

Committee on Bioethics, Committee on Genetics, and American College of Medical Genetics and Genomics Social, Ethical, & Legal Issues Committee. (2013). Ethical and policy issues in genetic testing and screening of children. *Pediatrics, 131*(3), 620–622. https://doi.org/10.1542/peds.2012-3680

Dickerson, J. A., Cole, B., Conta, J. H., Wellner, M., Wallace, S. E., Jack, R. M., Rutledge, J., & Astion, M. L. (2014). Improving the value of costly genetic reference laboratory testing with active utilization management. *Archives of Pathology & Laboratory Medicine, 138*(1), 110–113. https://doi.org/10.5858/arpa.2012-0726-OA

Dimmock, D. P., Clark, M. M., Gaughran, M., Cakici, J. A., Caylor, S. A., Clarke, C., Feddock, M., Chowdhury, S., Salz, L., Cheung, C., Bird, L. M., Hobbs, C., Wigby, K., Farnaes, L., Bloss, C. S., Kingsmore, S. F., & RCIGM Investigators. (2020). An RCT of rapid genomic sequencing among seriously ill infants results in high clinical utility, changes in management, and low perceived harm. *American Journal of Human Genetics, 107*(5), 942–952. https://doi.org/10.1016/j.ajhg.2020.10.003

Fernandez-Marmiesse, A., Gouveia, S., & Couce, M. L. (2018). NGS technologies as a turning point in rare disease research, diagnosis and treatment. *Current Medicinal Chemistry, 25*(3), 404–432. https://doi.org/10.2174/0929867324666170718101946

Fraser, F. C. (1958). Genetic counselling in some common paediatric diseases. *Pediatric Clinics of North America, 5*(2), 475–491. https://doi.org/10.1016/s0031-3955(16)30662-9

Gardner, M., & Amor, D. (2018). *Gardner and Sutherland's chromosome abnormalities and genetic counseling* (5th ed.). Oxford University Press.

Glascock, J., Sampson, J., Haidet-Phillips, A., Connolly, A., Darras, B., Day, J., Finkel, R., Howell, R. R., Klinger, K., Kuntz, N., Prior, T., Shieh, P. B., Crawford, T. O., Kerr, D., & Jarecki, J. (2018). Treatment algorithm for infants diagnosed with spinal muscular atrophy through newborn screening. *Journal of Neuromuscular Diseases, 5*(2), 145–158. https://doi.org/10.3233/JND-180304

Green, R. C., Berg, J. S., Grody, W. W., Kalia, S. S., Korf, B. R., Martin, C. L., McGuire, A. L., Nussbaum, R. L., O'Daniel, J. M., Ormond, K. E., Rehm, H. L., Watson, M. S., Williams, M. S., Biesecker, L. G., & American College of Medical Genetics and Genomics. (2013). ACMG recommendations for reporting of incidental findings in clinical exome and genome sequencing. *Genetics in Medicine, 15*(7), 565–574. https://doi.org/10.1038/gim.2013.73

Gutierrez, A. M., Statham, E. E., Robinson, J. O., Slashinski, M. J., Scollon, S., Bergstrom, K. L., Street, R. L., Jr, Parsons, D. W., Plon, S. E., & McGuire, A. L. (2019). Agents of empathy: How medical interpreters bridge sociocultural gaps in genomic sequencing disclosures with Spanish-speaking families. *Patient Education and Counseling, 102*(5), 895–901. https://doi.org/10.1016/j.pec.2018.12.012

Hannig, V. L., Cohen, M. P., Pfotenhauer, J. P., Williams, M. D., Morgan, T. M., & Phillips, J. A., 3rd. (2014). Expansion of genetic services utilizing a general genetic counseling clinic. *Journal of Genetic Counseling, 23*(1), 64–71. https://doi.org/10.1007/s10897-013-9608-0

Hartley, J. N., Greenberg, C. R., & Mhanni, A. A. (2011). Genetic counseling in a busy pediatric metabolic practice. *Journal of Genetic Counseling, 20*(1), 20–22. https://doi.org/10.1007/s10897-010-9324-y

Hayeems, R. Z., Babul-Hirji, R., Hoang, N., Weksberg, R., & Shuman, C. (2016). Parents' experience with pediatric microarray: Transferrable lessons in the era of genomic counseling. *Journal of Genetic Counseling, 25*(2), 298–304. https://doi.org/10.1007/s10897-015-9871-3

Heimler, A. (1997). An oral history of the National Society of Genetic Counselors. *Journal of Genetic Counseling, 6*(3), 315–336. https://doi.org/10.1023/A:1025680306348

Helm, B. M. (2015). Exploring the genetic counselor's role in facilitating meaning-making: Rare disease diagnoses. *Journal of Genetic Counseling, 24*(2), 205–212. https://doi.org/10.1007/s10897-014-9812-6

Hilgart, J. S., Hayward, J. A., Coles, B., & Iredale, R. (2012). Telegenetics: A systematic review of telemedicine in genetics services. *Genetics in Medicine, 14*(9), 765–776.

Kalia, S. S., Adelman, K., Bale, S. J., Chung, W. K., Eng, C., Evans, J. P., Herman, G. E., Hufnagel, S. B., Klein, T. E., Korf, B. R., McKelvey, K. D., Ormond, K. E., Richards, C. S., Vlangos, C. N., Watson, M., Martin, C. L., & Miller, D. T. (2017). Recommendations for reporting of secondary findings in clinical exome and genome sequencing, 2016 update (ACMG SF v2.0): A policy statement of the American College of Medical Genetics and Genomics. *Genetics in Medicine, 19*(2), 249–255. https://doi.org/10.1038/gim.2016.190

Kaulfus, M. E., Gardiner, H., Hashmi, S. S., Mendez-Figueroa, H., Miller, V. J., Stevens, B., & Carter, R. (2019). Attitudes of clinicians toward cardiac surgery and trisomy 18. *Journal of Genetic Counseling, 28*(3), 654–663. https://doi.org/10.1002/jgc4.1089

Kiedrowski, L. A., Owens, K. M., Yashar, B. M., & Schuette, J. L. (2016). Parents' perspectives on variants of uncertain significance from chromosome microarray analysis. *Journal of Genetic Counseling, 25*(1), 101–111. https://doi.org/10.1007/s10897-015-9847-3

Krabbenborg, L., Vissers, L. E., Schieving, J., Kleefstra, T., Kamsteeg, E. J., Veltman, J. A., Willemsen, M. A., & Van der Burg, S. (2016). Understanding the psychosocial effects of WES test results on parents of children with rare diseases. *Journal of Genetic Counseling, 25*(6), 1207–1214. https://doi.org/10.1007/s10897-016-9958-5

Lantos, J. D. (2019). Ethical and psychosocial issues in whole genome sequencing (WGS) for newborns. *Pediatrics, 143*(Suppl. 1), S1–S5. https://doi.org/10.1542/peds.2018-1099B

Lipinski, S. E., Lipinski, M. J., Biesecker, L. G., & Biesecker, B. B. (2006). Uncertainty and perceived personal control among parents of children with rare chromosome conditions: The role of genetic counseling. *American Journal of Medical Genetics Part C: Seminars in Medical Genetics, 142C*(4), 232–240. https://doi.org/10.1002/ajmg.c.30107

Lochner Doyle, D. (2009). Medical documentation. In W. R. Uhlmann, J. L. Schuette, & B. M. Yashar (Eds.), *A guide to genetic counseling* (2nd ed., pp. 313–329). Wiley-Blackwell.

Macnamara, E. F., Schoch, K., Kelley, E. G., Fieg, E., Brokamp, E., Undiagnosed Diseases Network, Signer, R., LeBlanc, K., McConkie-Rosell, A., & Palmer, C. G. S. (2019). Cases from the Undiagnosed Diseases Network: The continued value of counseling skills in a new genomic era. *Journal of Genetic Counseling, 28*(2), 194–201. https://doi.org/10.1002/jgc4.1091

Mai, C. T., Petersen, E. E., & Miller, A. (2012). Public perception of birth defects terminology. *Birth Defects Research Part A: Clinical and Molecular Teratology, 94*(12), 984–989. https://doi.org/10.1002/bdra.23080

Matthews, T. J., MacDorman, M. F., & Thoma, M. E. (2015). Infant mortality statistics from the 2013 period linked birth/infant death data set. *National Vital Statistics Reports, 64*(9), 1–30.

McCarthy Veach, P., LeRoy, B. S., & Callanan, N. P. (2018). Structuring genetic counseling sessions: Initiating, contracting, ending, and referral. In *Facilitating the genetic counseling process: Practice-based skills* (2nd ed., pp. 139–172). Springer. https://doi.org/10.1007/978-3-319-74799-6_6

McConkie-Rosell, A., Hooper, S. R., Pena, L. D. M., Schoch, K., Spillmann, R. C., Jiang, Y. H., Cope, H., Undiagnosed Diseases Network, Palmer, C., & Shashi, V. (2018). Psychosocial profiles of parents of children with undiagnosed diseases: Managing well or just managing? *Journal of Genetic Counseling, 27*(4), 935–946. https://doi.org/10.1007/s10897-017-0193-5

McGlynn, J. A., & Langfelder-Schwind, E. (2020). Bridging the gap between scientific advancement and real-world application: Pediatric genetic counseling for common syndromes and single-gene disorders. *Cold Spring Harbor Perspectives in Medicine, 10*(10), a036640. https://doi.org/10.1101/cshperspect.a036640

McWalter, K. M., Sdano, M. R., Dave, G., Powell, K. P., & Callanan, N. (2015). Public health genetic counselors: Activities, skills, and sources of learning. *Journal of Genetic Counseling, 24*(3), 438–451. https://doi.org/10.1007/s10897-014-9795-3

Miller, C. E., Krautscheid, P., Baldwin, E. E., Tvrdik, T., Openshaw, A. S., Hart, K., & Lagrave, D. (2014). Genetic counselor review of genetic test orders in a reference laboratory reduces unnecessary testing. *American Journal of Medical Genetics Part A, 164A*(5), 1094–1101. https://doi.org/10.1002/ajmg.a.36453

National Society of Genetic Counselors. (2018a, April 12). *Position statement: Genetic testing of minors for adult-onset conditions*. https://www.nsgc.org/p/bl/et/blogaid=860

National Society of Genetic Counselors. (2018b, October 9). *Position statement: Genetic testing of children in the adoption process*. https://www.nsgc.org/p/bl/et/blogid=47&blogaid=1065

National Society of Genetic Counselors. (2020a, May 4). *Professional status survey 2020: Work environment*. https://www.nsgc.org/Policy-Research-and-Publications/Professional-Status-Survey

National Society of Genetic Counselors. (2020b, March 23). *Position statement: Secondary and incidental findings in genetic testing*. https://www.nsgc.org/p/bl/et/blogaid=30

Newcomb, P., Hudlow, R., Heilskov, J., Martinez, C. D., & Le, H. (2014). Conversations with children about DNA and genes using an original children's book. *Journal of Pediatric Health Care*, *28*(6), 497–506. https://doi.org/10.1016/j.pedhc.2014.02.006

Petrikin, J. E., Cakici, J. A., Clark, M. M., Willig, L. K., Sweeney, N. M., Farrow, E. G., Saunders, C. J., Thiffault, I., Miller, N. A., Zellmer, L., Herd, S. M., Holmes, A. M., Batalov, S., Veeraraghavan, N., Smith, L. D., Dimmock, D. P., Leeder, J. S., & Kingsmore, S. F. (2018). The NSIGHT1-randomized controlled trial: Rapid whole-genome sequencing for accelerated etiologic diagnosis in critically ill infants. *NPJ Genomic Medicine*, *3*, 6. https://doi.org/10.1038/s41525-018-0045-8

Petrikin, J. E., Willig, L. K., Smith, L. D., & Kingsmore, S. F. (2015). Rapid whole genome sequencing and precision neonatology. *Seminars in Perinatology*, *39*(8), 623–631. https://doi.org/10.1053/j.semperi.2015.09.009

Pew Research Center. (2015, December 17). *Parenting in America: Outlook, worries, aspirations are strongly linked to financial situation*. https://www.pewresearch.org/wp-content/uploads/sites/3/2015/12/2015-12-17_parenting-in-america_FINAL.pdf

Prero, M. Y., Strenk, M., Garrett, J., Kessler, A., Fanaroff, J. M., & Lantos, J. D. (2019). Disclosure of misattributed paternity. *Pediatrics*, *143*(6), e20183899. https://doi.org/10.1542/peds.2018-3899

Regier, D. S., Ferreira, C. R., Hart, S., Hadley, D. W., & Muenke, M. (2017). Medical genetics and genomic medicine in the United States. Part 2: Reproductive genetics, newborn screening, genetic counseling, training, and registries. *Molecular Genetics & Genomic Medicine*, *5*(6), 621–630. https://doi.org/10.1002/mgg3.343

Reiff, M., Bernhardt, B. A., Mulchandani, S., Soucier, D., Cornell, D., Pyeritz, R. E., & Spinner, N. B. (2012). "What does it mean?": Uncertainties in understanding results of chromosomal microarray testing. *Genetics in Medicine*, *14*(2), 250–258. https://doi.org/10.1038/gim.2011.52

Rosenthal, E. T., Biesecker, L. G., & Biesecker, B. B. (2001). Parental attitudes toward a diagnosis in children with unidentified multiple congenital anomaly syndromes. *American Journal of Medical Genetics*, *103*(2), 106–114. https://doi.org/10.1002/ajmg.1527

Ross, L. F., Saal, H. M., David, K. L., Anderson, R. R., American Academy of Pediatrics, & American College of Medical Genetics and Genomics. (2013). Technical report: Ethical and policy issues in genetic testing and screening of children. *Genetics in Medicine*, *15*(3), 234–245. https://doi.org/10.1038/gim.2012.176

Smith, E. E., du Souich, C., Dragojlovic, N., CAUSES Study, RAPIDOMICS Study, & Elliott, A. M. (2019). Genetic counseling considerations with rapid genome-wide sequencing in a neonatal intensive care unit. *Journal of Genetic Counseling*, *28*(2), 263–272. https://doi.org/10.1002/jgc4.1074

Spillmann, R. C., McConkie-Rosell, A., Pena, L., Jiang, Y. H., Undiagnosed Diseases Network, Schoch, K., Walley, N., Sanders, C., Sullivan, J., Hooper, S. R., & Shashi, V. (2017). A window into living with an undiagnosed disease: Illness narratives from the Undiagnosed

Diseases Network. *Orphanet Journal of Rare Diseases, 12*(1), 71. https://doi.org/10.1186/s13023-017-0623-3

Stein, Q., Loman, R., & Zuck, T. (2018). Genetic counseling in pediatrics. *Pediatrics in Review, 39*(7), 323–331. https://doi.org/10.1542/pir.2017-0194

Szego, M. J., Meyn, M. S., Shuman, C., Zlotnik Shaul, R., Anderson, J. A., Bowdin, S., Monfared, N., & Hayeems, R. Z. (2019). Views from the clinic: Healthcare provider perspectives on whole genome sequencing in paediatrics. *European Journal of Medical Genetics, 62*(5), 350–356. https://doi.org/10.1016/j.ejmg.2018.11.029

Thiffault, I., Farrow, E., Zellmer, L., Berrios, C., Miller, N., Gibson, M., Caylor, R., Jenkins, J., Faller, D., Soden, S., & Saunders, C. (2019). Clinical genome sequencing in an unbiased pediatric cohort. *Genetics in Medicine, 21*(2), 303–310. https://doi.org/10.1038/s41436-018-0075-8

Thompson, M. W. (1967). Genetic counseling in clinical pediatrics. What to do with inquiries about heritable disorders. *Clinical Pediatrics, 6*(4), 199–209. https://doi.org/10.1177/000992286700600405

Uhlmann, W. R., Schwalm, K., & Raymond, V. M. (2017). Development of a streamlined work flow for handling patients' genetic testing insurance authorizations. *Journal of Genetic Counseling, 26*(4), 657–668. https://doi.org/10.1007/s10897-017-0098-3

VandenBoom, E., Trepanier, A. M., & Carmany, E. P. (2018). Assessment of current genetic counselor practices in post-visit written communications to patients. *Journal of Genetic Counseling, 27*(3), 681–688. https://doi.org/10.1007/s10897-017-0163-y

Waggoner, D., Wain, K. E., Dubuc, A. M., Conlin, L., Hickey, S. E., Lamb, A. N., Martin, C. L., Morton, C. C., Rasmussen, K., Schuette, J. L., Schwartz, S., Miller, D. T., & ACMG Professional Practice and Guidelines Committee. (2018). Yield of additional genetic testing after chromosomal microarray for diagnosis of neurodevelopmental disability and congenital anomalies: A clinical practice resource of the American College of Medical Genetics and Genomics (ACMG). *Genetics in Medicine, 20*(10), 1105–1113. https://doi.org/10.1038/s41436-018-0040-6

Wakefield, E., Keller, H., Mianzo, H., Nagaraj, C. B., Tawde, S., & Ulm, E. (2018). Reduction of health care costs and improved appropriateness of incoming test orders: The impact of genetic counselor review in an academic genetic testing laboratory. *Journal of Genetic Counseling, 27*(5), 1067–1073. https://doi.org/10.1007/s10897-018-0226-8

Walker, A. P. (2009). The practice of genetic counseling. In W. R. Uhlmann, J. L. Schuette, & B. M. Yashar (Eds.), *A guide to genetic counseling* (pp. 1–35). Wiley-Blackwell.

Wilkins, E. J., Archibald, A. D., Sahhar, M. A., & White, S. M. (2016). "It wasn't a disaster or anything": Parents' experiences of their child's uncertain chromosomal microarray result. *American Journal of Medical Genetics Part A, 170*(11), 2895–2904. https://doi.org/10.1002/ajmg.a.37838

Wool, C., & Dudek, M. (2013). Exploring the perceptions and the role of genetic counselors in the emerging field of perinatal palliative care. *Journal of Genetic Counseling, 22*(4), 533–543. https://doi.org/10.1007/s10897-013-9581-7

Wynn, J., Ottman, R., Duong, J., Wilson, A. L., Ahimaz, P., Martinez, J., Rabin, R., Rosen, E., Webster, R., Au, C., Cho, M. T., Egan, C., Guzman, E., Primiano, M., Shaw, J. E., Sisson, R., Klitzman, R. L., Appelbaum, P. S., Lichter-Konecki, U., Anyane-Yeboa, K., & Chung, W. K. (2018). Diagnostic exome sequencing in children: A survey of parental understanding, experience and psychological impact. *Clinical Genetics, 93*(5), 1039–1048. https://doi.org/10.1111/cge.13200

CHAPTER 9

CANCER GENETIC COUNSELING

STEPHANIE A. COHEN

Introduction

The first descriptions of hereditary cancer syndromes appeared in the late 1800s and included familial adenomatous polyposis (Cripps, 1882; Dukes, 1952), retinoblastoma (Griffith & Sorsby, 1944), and hereditary colon cancer (Warthin, 1913). However, for most of the next century, many believed that families with common cancers such as colon and breast cancer were exposed to similar environments, which largely explained the common cancer history, in spite of exhaustive documentation of autosomal dominant inheritance (Lynch & Krush, 1971). The 1960s brought about many new descriptions of syndromic hereditary cancer families, such as Gorlin syndrome (Gorlin & Goltz, 1960), hereditary nonpolyposis colorectal cancer syndrome by Henry Lynch in 1966 (Lynch et al., 1966), Muir-Torre (now known to be caused by the same genes that cause Lynch syndrome; Muir et al., 1967; Torre, 1968), multiple endocrine neoplasia (MEN; Schimke et al., 1968), and Li-Fraumeni syndrome (Li & Fraumeni, 1969). The discovery of the first causative genes in the 1980s to explain hereditary cancer families finally brought credence to the idea that cancer can be hereditary. Today, it is widely accepted that 5% to 10% of most cancers are due to hereditary causes (Mandelker et al., 2017). A timeline of gene discovery is provided in Table 9.1 and offers a glimpse into the discovery of genes and their availability in clinical testing.

Over time, genetic testing has become more widely available, less expensive, and better covered by insurance. The passage of the Genetic Information Nondiscrimination Act (GINA) in 2008 offered unaffected individuals protection from health insurance discrimination, allowing more individuals to consider predictive genetic testing. Advances in technology have improved detection rates over the years as well. A good example is testing for the *BRCA1/* genes. Initially, *BRCA1/2* testing was done by single gene sequencing. Large gene rearrangement analysis of five common sites in the *BRCA1* gene was added in 2003 and expanded to include both *BRCA1* and *BRCA2* and any large rearrangement in 2006 (Table 9.1). However, it wasn't until 2013 that comprehensive

Table 9.1 Timeline of Hereditary Cancer Gene Discovery and Test Availability

Gene discovered	Year	Gene testing available at one or more commercial labs[a]
RB1	1987	
TP53, NF1	1990	
APC	1991	
MSH2, RET, NF2, VHL	1993	
BRCA1, MLH1, PMS2, CDKN2A	1994	
BRCA2, ATM	1995	*BRCA1/2* (Myriad) *RET* (Quest)
PTCH	1996	
MEN1, PTEN, MSH6, STK11	1997	
	1999	*RB1* (Impact Genetics) *TP53* (City of Hope) *APC* sequencing and deletion/duplication (Baylor) *NF1*[b] (protein truncation testing)
SDHC, SDHD	2000	*MLH1/MSH2* (Myriad) *PTEN, RET, STK11, PTCH, CDKN2A* (GeneDx)
CHEK2, FH, SDHB, MUTYH	2001	
FLCN, MUTYH	2002	*APC* sequencing (Myriad) *MEN1* (GeneDx)
	2003	*BRCA1/2* five-site rearrangement analysis added (Myriad) *ATM* (City of Hope)
	2004	*FH* and *VHL* (GeneDx) *MLH1/MSH2* del/dup (Myriad) *APC* del/dup (Myriad) *MUTYH* founder mutations (Myriad)
BRIP1	2005	*MLH1/MSH2/MSH6, MUTYH* (Baylor) *MSH6* sequencing (Myriad) *MUTYH* sequencing (Myriad)
	2006	Large gene rearrangement analysis of *BRCA1/2* available on request (Myriad) *FLCN* (GeneDx) *CHEK2* (City of Hope)
PALB2	2007	
	2008	*SDHx* (GeneDx) *PTEN* (Baylor)
DICER1, EPCAM	2009	*TP53* (Baylor)
RAD51C	2010	
RAD51D, BAP1	2011	*BMPR1A/SMAD4* (GeneDx) *MSH6* del/dup (Myriad) *PMS2* sequencing and del/dup (Myriad) *EPCAM* sequencing and del/dup (Myriad)
	2012	Next-generation sequencing panels (Ambry) *MUTYH* del/dup (Myriad)

Table 9.1 Continued

Gene discovered	Year	Gene testing available at one or more commercial labs[a]
POLE, POLD1	**2013**	Comprehensive *BRCA1/2* gene rearrangement analysis routinely included *BRCA1/2* added to next-generation sequencing cancer panels (multiple labs)
	2014	*CHEK2, ATM* (Baylor)
	2017	SNP-based testing (Myriad)

Note: Myriad data from their website, accessed March 7, 2020, and from Eric Rosenthal, August 3, 2020, personal communication. GeneDx data from Jessica Mester, April 7, 2020, personal communication. Quest data from Kate Wilson, April 9, 2020, personal communication. Baylor data from Eric Schmitt, August 1, 2020, personal communication. Impact Genetics data inferred from website, accessed February 20, 2021. City of Hope data from Bita Nehoray/Barbara Choi, February 22, 2021, personal communication.

[a] This table does not include tests that may have been available from all laboratories or on a research basis. Information on first testing available is not complete given limited ability to retrieve this historic information from each laboratory or rarity of testing prior to next-generation sequencing panels.

[b] Mention in publication of commercial testing (Rasmussen & Friedman, 2000).

Sources: Rahman (2014), Schmidt (2013), and Al-Tassan et al. (2002).

deletion/duplication testing was routinely performed as part of *BRCA1/2* genetic testing. The Supreme Court's decision to overturn Myriad Genetics' patent on the sequence of *BRCA1/2* opened up the market for other testing companies to offer *BRCA1/2* as part of a next-generation sequencing panel, thus beginning the era of multigene panel testing (Kesselheim et al., 2013).

Another example of test evolution is the *APC* gene, where testing was initially done with protein truncation analysis at a detection rate of about 80% (Ballhausen, 2000). Sequencing and large gene rearrangement analysis of the *APC* gene have improved the diagnostic rate for classic familial adenomatous polyposis (FAP) to better than 98% (Yen et al., 1998).

The timeline of availability of genetic testing is more than just interesting—it is practically important. Individuals who previously had negative genetic testing may need additional genetic testing, as the detection rate for some tests (such as *APC* or *BRCA1/2*) has improved. It is important to note the actual methodology of testing; some genes initially were evaluated only for a few common point variants (such as *MUTYH*, where initially just two founder variants were evaluated) or for a few exons (as in the case for *PMS2*, where initially some exons were excluded from analysis due to the challenges posed by the presence of pseudogenes), and some testing did not initially include promoter regions (e.g., the *PTEN* and *APC* genes). Finally, updated genetic testing that includes newer genes related to hereditary causes for cancer may allow for explanation of the family history of cancer, identification of at-risk relatives, and changes in clinical management (Crawford et al., 2017).

Causes of Cancer

The majority of cancer is sporadic and occurs as a result of an accumulation of genetic damage over time. Although sporadic cancers are thought of as related to age or environmental factors, such as smoking, the etiology of most common cancers remains unknown. Certain exposures, such as asbestos and sunburn, have clear cause and effect. Obesity, alcohol exposure, and smoking contribute to the development of many types of cancers (Whiteman & Wilson, 2016). However, not everyone who smokes develops lung cancer, suggesting there may be genetic influences even within these defined exposures. As much as 20% of all cancers are considered "familial," occurring within clusters in a family without an identifiable hereditary cause. Up to 10% of all cancers are hereditary, considered to be due to a constitutional pathogenic variant that contributes to the development of cancer. However, even among individuals who inherit a pathogenic variant in a high-risk gene predisposing to cancer, there is considerable variation in the likelihood to actually develop cancer. Figure 9.1 depicts the etiology of cancers as we know it today.

Hereditary Cancer Syndromes

Families with a hereditary cause for cancer tend to have multiple individuals affected with the same type of cancer or a combination of certain types of cancers over multiple generations. Ages of onset among hereditary cancers tend to be younger than the average age of onset for the cancer type in the general population, and rare cancers may be present (Figure 9.2). Certain cancer types warrant investigation for a hereditary cause, due to the association with a pathogenic gene variant. Sometimes identifying a pathogenic variant allows for consideration of different management, such as additional surveillance, prophylactic surgery, and different cancer treatment regimens. The discovery of the mechanism for how genes protect cells from the development of cancer has allowed for the development of new targeted therapies, whether the pathogenic variant was sporadically acquired or inherited. Specifically, poly(ADP-ribose) polymerase (PARP) inhibitors (PARPi) to treat ovarian, prostate, and pancreatic cancers with homologous repair defects (specifically *BRCA1/2* and possibly some other genes) may improve outcomes (Tung et al., 2020). The use of immunotherapy for cancer with mismatch repair deficiency (such as in Lynch syndrome) has resulted in improved outcomes, and even full remission in some cases (Lemery et al., 2017; Marabelle et al., 2020).

Highly penetrant genes

Hereditary cancer genes tend to be highly penetrant, with a defined phenotype and guidelines for surveillance (Table 9.2). The National Comprehensive Cancer Network (NCCN) is an organization that monitors evidence-based literature and agrees upon and

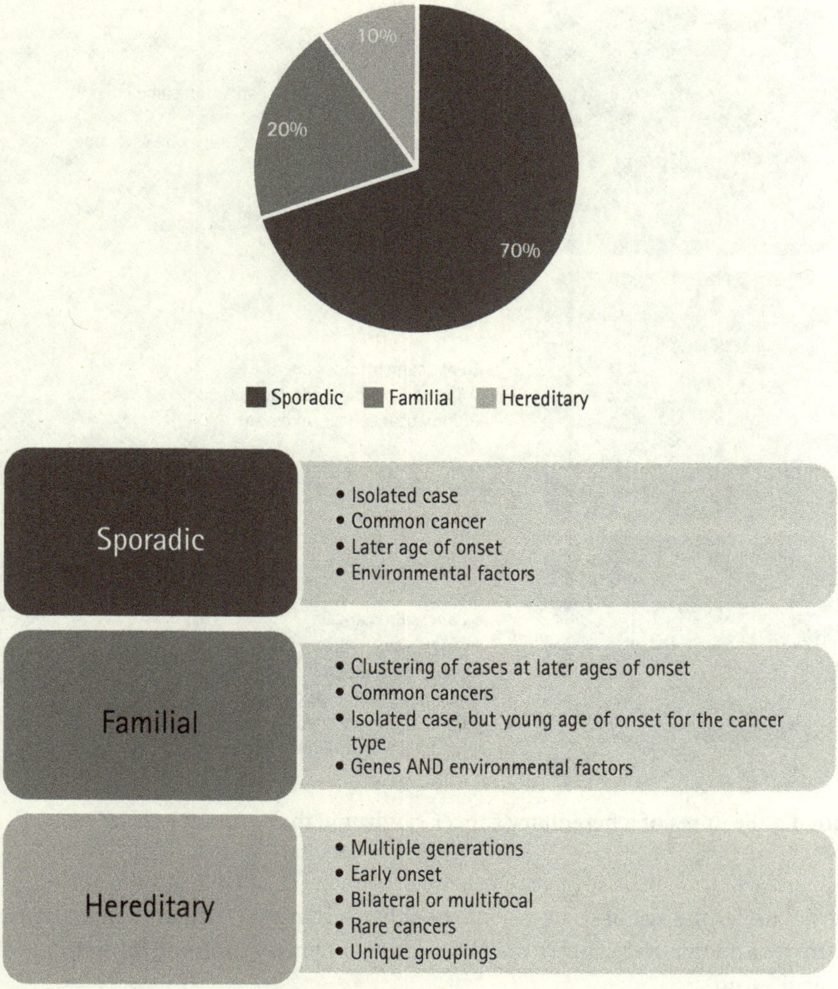

FIGURE 9.1 Hereditary contribution to cancer.

publishes surveillance guidelines based on this emerging evidence. These are updated at least annually and should be reviewed frequently for changes (https://www.nccn.org).

Several studies have now demonstrated that among individuals with breast cancer and features of a hereditary cancer syndrome, approximately 8% have a pathogenic variant (Kurian et al., 2019). Although the most common hereditary cause is an inherited pathogenic variant in the *BRCA1* or *BRCA2* gene, there are many other genes that can cause an increased risk for breast cancer (Couch et al., 2017; Domchek, 2015; Kurian et al., 2019). Up to 20% of ovarian cancer has been demonstrated to be due to hereditary causes, frequently by pathogenic variants in *BRCA1/2* (10% to 15% of all ovarian cancers and 90% of hereditary ovarian cancers), although other genes have been implicated (Norquist et al., 2016). As much as 3% of all colon cancers, regardless of age at onset or family history, are due to Lynch syndrome (Hampel et al., 2005), and as much as 10% of all colon cancers

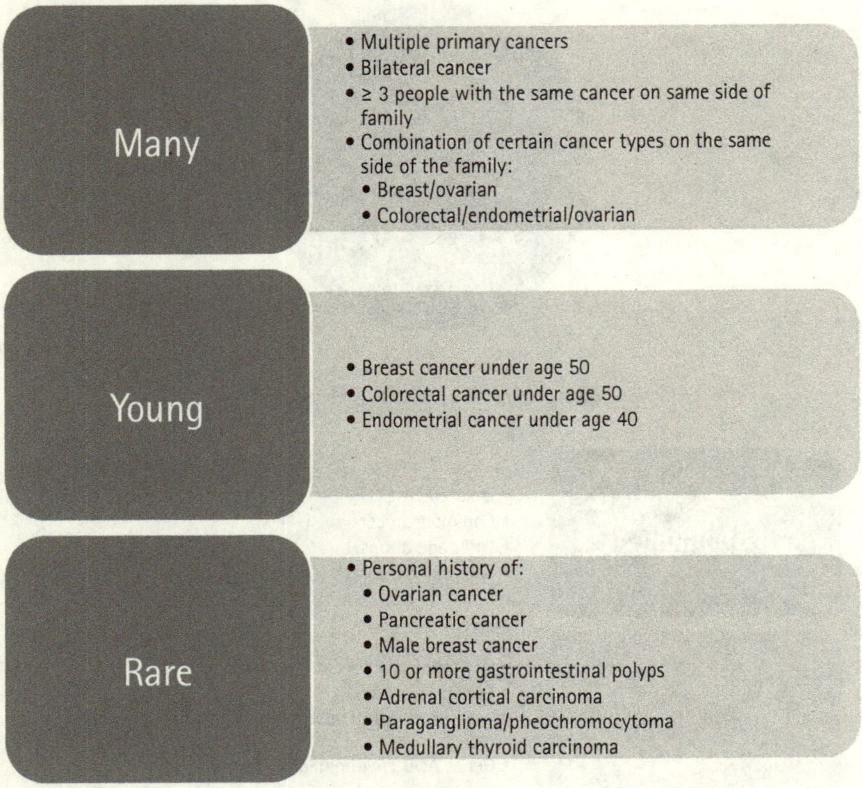

FIGURE 9.2 Features of a hereditary cancer syndrome that warrant evaluation.

diagnosed under the age of 50 have some hereditary cause (Pearlman et al., 2017; Yurgelun et al., 2017). Endometrial cancers may be related to Lynch syndrome in up to 3% of cases (Ryan et al., 2019).

While hereditary breast and ovarian cancer and Lynch syndrome remain the most commonly recognized hereditary causes for cancer, there are many other genes that have been described as highly penetrant with well-recognized presentations (Table 9.2).

Moderately penetrant genes

Many of the genes that are considered to have moderate penetrance rely on family history to provide guidance for surveillance recommendations, rather than a certain set of agreed-upon standards. When compared to high-risk genes, moderately penetrant genes may not have as high of a risk for cancer and cancer may be diagnosed at a later age of onset (Table 9.3). Some of the genes in this category have guidelines for management, but data are emerging and likely to change. Therefore, the management guideline is often presented for consideration, rather than a recommendation, leaving ambiguity in many cases. This poses challenges for clinicians and patients as they attempt to decide the best course of action. Family history can play a vital role in evaluating how the gene has behaved in other

Table 9.2 Examples of Highly Penetrant Genes with Published Guidelines

	Lifetime cancer risks							
Gene(s) (syndrome)	Breast	Ovarian	Endometrial	Colon	Pancreatic	Prostate	Kidney/ urinary tract	Other features
BRCA1/2 **(Hereditary breast and ovarian cancer syndrome)** (Chen et al., 2020; Kuchenbaecker et al., 2017)	40%–60%	20%–40%	Unknown/ unclear	Unknown/ unclear	5%	20%–30%	N/A	Melanoma
BMPR1A, SMAD4 **(Juvenile polyposis syndrome)** (Brosens et al., 2011)	N/A	N/A	N/A	40%	N/A	N/A	N/A	Hamartomas, gastric cancer, HHT (*SMAD4*)
CDH1 **(Hereditary diffuse gastric cancer)** (Xicola et al., 2019)	40% (lobular breast cancer)	N/A	N/A	N/A	N/A	N/A	N/A	Gastric cancer
MLH1/MSH2/MSH6/PMS2/EPCAM **(Lynch syndrome)** (Dominguez-Valentin et al., 2019; Moller et al., 2017)	10%–15%	10%	20%–60%	20%–60%	5%	Unknown/ unclear	5%–10%	Sebaceous adenoma/ carcinoma
PALB2 (Antoniou et al., 2015; Yang, Leslie, et al., 2020)	40%	5%	N/A	Unknown/ unclear	3%–5%	N/A	N/A	N/A
PTEN **(Cowden syndrome)** (Ngeow et al., 2017; Pilarski, 2019)	25%–50%	N/A	15%–20%	10%	N/A	N/A	5%	Thyroid cancer, hamartomas, macrocephaly
STK11 **(Peutz–Jeghers syndrome)** (Daniell et al., 2018; Syngal et al., 2015)	40%	20% (ovarian sex cord tumors with annular tubules)	10%	40%	25%	N/A	N/A	Gastric, small bowel, lung, and testicular cancer
TP53 **(Li–Fraumeni syndrome)** (Mai et al., 2016; Shin et al., 2020)	50%–60%	Unknown/unclear	N/A	Unknown/ unclear	Unknown/ unclear	N/A	N/A	ACC, brain, leukemia, osteosarcoma
VHL **(von Hippel Lindau syndrome)** (Maher & Sandford, 2019; Rednam et al., 2017)	N/A	N/A	N/A	N/A	N/A	N/A	25-50%	Hemangioblastoma, pheochromocytoma

Note: ACC = adrenocortical carcinoma; HHT = hereditary hemorrhagic telangiectasia.

Table 9.3 Examples of Moderately Penetrant Genes

Gene	Lifetime cancer risk				
	Breast	Ovarian	Endometrial	Colon	Other
CHEK2 (Näslund-Koch et al., 2016; Schmidt et al., 2016)	20%–40%	Unknown/ unclear	Unknown/ unclear	8%–10%	Thyroid, kidney, prostate
ATM (Marabelli et al., 2016)	20%–40%	Unknown/ unclear	N/A	Unknown/ unclear	Pancreatic cancer
BRIP1 (Easton et al., 2016; Rafnar et al., 2011)	Unknown/ unclear	10%	N/A	N/A	N/A
RAD51C, *RAD51D* (Yang, Song, et al., 2020)	20%	11%–13%	N/A	N/A	N/A

family members and may provide insight on the age to begin surveillance. It is likely that the range of risk is modified by other as-of-yet-undiscovered genes and/or environmental factors.[1]

Genes with limited or unknown clinical significance

There have been genes identified that may have a modestly increased risk, but studies accounting for bias and sample size have brought their significance into question. Some genes that fall into this category include genes that have been identified but not yet studied well enough to determine if there is any meaningful impact on risk. These should probably be considered to fall into the "familial" piece of the pie (Figure 9.1), where their significance may be amplified or muted by other genes or other environmental factors.

Single nucleotide polymorphisms

Single nucleotide polymorphisms (SNPs) largely represent population variation, although some of this variation may have a relationship to cancer risk, at a very modest level. Efforts are ongoing to use SNPs to attempt to modify the interpretation of a pathogenic variant in a high-risk gene, such as *BRCA1/2*. At this moment in time, the clinical relevance of SNPs remains limited since management recommendations for gene carriers are unlikely to change based on SNP data (Gordon et al., 2020; Mavaddat et al., 2019). However, it may become possible to incorporate SNP data into personalized risk assessment as these models are further developed, and some commercial labs have begun to incorporate polygenic risk scores into patient genetic testing.

[1] Editors' note: For further discussion on family history, see Chapter 19 by Debra L. Collins and Devin M. Cox in this volume.

Autosomal recessive hereditary cancer syndromes

Most of the high-risk, well-described hereditary cancer syndromes are inherited in an autosomal dominant manner. However, there are a few adult-onset hereditary cancer syndromes that are recessive, including multiple adenomatous polyposis (MAP) syndrome, caused by biallelic pathogenic variants in the *MUTYH* gene (Sutcliffe et al., 2019), and NTHL1-associated polyposis, caused by biallelic pathogenic variants in the *NTHL1* gene (Groves et al., 2019).

Pediatric Cancer Syndromes

Several pediatric cancer syndromes were recognized initially due to the association of dysmorphic features, such as in nevoid basal cell carcinoma syndrome (formerly known as Gorlin syndrome) or neurofibromatosis type 1 (NF1). These syndromes can be recognized clinically and may not require genetic testing, although it can be useful to rule out the condition in unaffected family members who do not have obvious clinical features as part of cascade testing. There are several autosomal recessive hereditary syndromes diagnosed in childhood that cause an increased risk for cancer, including ataxia telangiectasia, Fanconi anemia, Bloom syndrome, Nijmegen breakage syndrome, and xeroderma pigmentosum (Scollon et al., 2017). A more newly described syndrome, constitutional mismatch repair deficiency (CCMRD) syndrome, is caused by biallelic inheritance of pathogenic variants in mismatch repair genes that cause Lynch syndrome. CCMRD is characterized by café-au-lait macules similar to those seen in NF1. CCMRD is associated with colon polyposis and risks for childhood-onset brain tumors, leukemia, lymphoma, and colon cancer (Durno et al., 2015). Finally, other pediatric syndromes that can be associated with an increased risk for cancer include Down syndrome, Turner syndrome, and Beckwith-Wiedemann syndrome (Scollon et al., 2017). Table 9.4 lists some of the more commonly recognized pediatric hereditary cancer syndromes.

Some hereditary cancer syndromes have known risks in childhood, such as Li-Fraumeni syndrome and FAP, although the major risks exist in adulthood. Predictive testing for a hereditary cancer syndrome in children should be limited to genes that have actionable recommendations at their current age. For example, it is reasonable to test a child for the *RET* gene in a family with MEN type 2 at birth as thyroidectomy may be indicated within the first year of life to avoid the risk for medullary thyroid cancer. Other syndromes, such as FAP, may have indications to test in childhood, because colonoscopy surveillance is recommended to begin by age 10. Testing children for *BRCA1/2*, Lynch syndrome, and other adult-onset syndromes is not recommended, since surveillance does not typically begin until adulthood and an individual would be old enough to participate in the decision-making process for genetic testing. It should be noted that these genes are included on the American College of Medical Genetics list of genes to consider as secondary findings. When exome or genome sequencing is performed to evaluate children for a hereditary syndrome, there should be discussion about what kind of results parents want to receive (see Chapter 21—"Risk Assessment of Secondary Findings" in this

Table 9.4 Hereditary Pediatric Cancer Syndromes

Name	Gene	Primary risks in childhood	Age of onset of surveillance	Adult-onset cancers	Other (noncancerous) features
Constitutional mismatch repair deficiency (CCMRD) syndrome (Durno et al., 2015; Vasen et al., 2014; Wimmer et al., 2014)	Biallelic *MLH1*, *MSH2*, *MSH6*, or *PMS2*	Brain tumors, colon cancer, leukemia, lymphoma	6–12 months	Lynch-associated cancers	Polyposis, café-au-lait macules
DICER1 syndrome (Khan et al., 2018; Stewart et al., 2019)	*DICER1*	Pleuropulmonary blastoma, cystic nephroma, Wilms tumor, ovarian sex cord-stromal tumors, thyroid cancer, nasal chondromesenchymal hamartoma, ciliary body medulloepithelioma, embryonal rhabdomyosarcoma, brain tumors	0–12 months	Ovarian sex cord-stromal tumors	Thyroid nodules, macrocephaly, structural anomalies in renal collecting system, retinal abnormalities
Familial adenomatous polyposis (Dinarvand et al., 2019; Galiatsatos & Foulkes, 2006; Yen, 1998)	*APC*	Hepatoblastoma polyposis	6 months 10 years	Colon cancer, gastric cancer, thyroid cancer, desmoid tumors	Supernumerary teeth, CHRPE
Li-Fraumeni syndrome (Amadou et al., 2018; Bojadzieva et al., 2018; Shin et al., 2020)	*TP53*	Osteosarcoma, soft tissue sarcoma, leukemia, adrenocortical cancer, brain tumors	Birth	Breast, pancreatic, brain tumors, leukemia, lymphoma, colorectal cancer	N/A
Multiple endocrine neoplasia type 2 (MEN2, MEN2A, and FMTC) (Raue & Frank-Raue, 2010; Wells et al., 2015)	*RET*	Medullary thyroid cancer	Birth	Pheochromocytoma, medullary thyroid cancer	Parathyroid adenoma MEN2B: mucosal neuromas, marfanoid habitus, ganglioneuromas of GI tract

Nevoid basal cell (Gorlin) syndrome (Evans & Farndon, 1993; Foulkes et al., 2017; Huq et al., 2018)	*PTCH1* and *SUFU*	Medulloblastoma	Birth	Basal cell neoplasms	Macrocephaly, skeletal anomalies, cardiac and ovarian fibromas, jaw cysts, palmar pits, cleft lip/palate
Retinoblastoma (Imbert-Bouteille et al., 2019; Kamihara et al., 2017; Marees et al., 2008)	*RB1*	Retinoblastoma	Birth	Osteosarcoma, soft tissue sarcoma, second primary malignancies	N/A
Rhabdoid tumor predisposition (Foulkes et al., 2017)	*SMARCB1*, *SMARCA4*	Atypical teratoid/rhabdoid tumor, extracranial malignant rhabdoid tumor	Birth	Small cell carcinoma of ovary	Schwannomas
Tuberous sclerosis (Annear et al., 2019)	*TSC1*, *TSC2*	Subependymal giant cell astrocytomas, cardiac rhabdomyoma	Birth	Renal cell carcinoma, lymphangioleiomyomatosis, neuroendocrine tumors	Seizures, intellectual disability, skin lesions (shagreen patches, angiofibromas), renal disease and lesions

Note: CHRPE = congenital hypertrophy of the retinal pigmented epithelium; FMTC = familial medullary thyroid cancer; GI = gastrointestinal.

Source: Scollon et al. (2017).

volume). Additionally, consideration for protection from genetic discrimination should be given. The GINA does prevent health insurance companies and employers from discriminating based on gene status but does not include provisions to prevent life and long-term insurance companies from doing so. Finally, possible psychosocial concerns may arise in children and adolescents when testing for a known adult-onset hereditary condition and the potential for harm is likely greater than any theoretical benefits (Bradbury et al., 2010; Tercyak et al., 2019).

Identification of Hereditary Cancer Syndromes

Hereditary cancer syndromes may be recognized by their likelihood to present at young ages, occur many times within a family over multiple generations, and present with unusual or rare tumors and certain combinations of tumors, such as breast and ovarian cancer or colon and endometrial cancer (Figure 9.2). Guidelines for when genetic counseling should be offered have been created by multiple organizations, which can be complicated and challenging for clinicians to recognize (Daly et al., 2020; Gupta et al., 2019; Heald et al., 2020; Nelson et al., 2019; Robson et al., 2015; Singer et al., 2018). Some cancer types have recommendations for testing all patients, due to the strong association with a hereditary cause for that cancer type and/or the type of cancer being very rarely seen in the general population, simplifying this process (Table 9.5; Banks et al., 2013). More cancers are being added to this list with the availability of treatments, such as PARPi to treat *BRCA*-related cancers and immunotherapy to treat tumors with mismatch repair deficiency. This is changing the paradigm of cancer genetics services, as testing is now needed quickly, often at the point of care. Newer models that embed genetic counselors into cancer clinics (Kentwell et al., 2017; Pederson et al., 2018; Senter et al., 2017), use genetic counselor extenders (Cohen & Nixon, 2016), or refer for posttest genetic counseling only (Schmidlen et al., 2018) are being studied to determine the best way to deliver high-quality care in a timely fashion (Rayes et al., 2019).

Risk models can be used to predict the likelihood that a person has a pathogenic variant and typically depend on the family history (type and ages of onset of cancers). A particular threshold may be arbitrarily used to identify those who should be offered genetic testing, although there is no evidence-based guidance on what this threshold should be. Common risk models to identify those at risk for hereditary breast and ovarian cancer include the BRCAPro, Tyrer-Cuzick, and BOADICEA models, all of which estimate both the risk for a *BRCA1/2* pathogenic variant and the likelihood to develop cancer based on this risk (Amir et al., 2010; Gail, 2015). Some of these models have been incorporated into mammogram screening software (Bellcross et al., 2009, 2019) or an electronic health platform (Crump et al., 2018; Del Fiol et al., 2020; Goshen et al., 2018) to automate the process of patient identification. Follow-through to genetic counseling and/or testing has been somewhat limited with these automated efforts (Kne et al., 2017), driving the need for more research to educate patients and their healthcare providers about the benefits of hereditary cancer risk

Table 9.5 Cancer Types Where There Is Evidence to Test All Patients

Cancer type	Likelihood of a gene mutation	Genes associated
Ovarian (Konstantinopoulos et al., 2020; Norquist et al., 2016)	20%	*BRCA1/2, MLH1/MSH2/MSH6/PMS2, BRIP1, ATM, PALB2*
Pancreatic (Rainone et al., 2020; Young et al., 2018)	10%	*BRCA1/2, ATM, PALB2, MLH1/MSH2/MSH6/PMS2, CDKN2A, TP53, STK11*
Adrenocortical (Else et al., 2014)	50%–80% in children 5%–7% in adults	*TP53, MEN1, FAP, MLH1/MSH2/MSH6/PMS2*
Medullary thyroid cancer (Wells et al., 2015)	25%–30%	*RET*
Pheochromocytoma and paraganglioma (Muth et al., 2019)	20%	*SDHx, FH, NF1, RET, VHL, MEN1, TMEM127, MAX*

assessment and motivating patients to apply this knowledge to improved health behaviors (Albada et al., 2015; Morman et al., 2017; Paskett et al., 2020).

Identification of individuals at increased risk for a hereditary cause of their cancer can be done by screening tumors at the time of diagnosis, as in the case of Lynch syndrome. Microsatellite instability testing or immunohistochemical staining for the presence or absence of the MLH1/MSH2/MSH6/PMS2 proteins on colon and endometrial cancers identifies those who need genetic counseling and consideration of genetic testing (Latham et al., 2019; Yurgelun & Hampel, 2018). Universal screening of endometrial and colon tumors has been demonstrated to be cost effective, particularly when considering cascade testing of relatives who are then identified as at risk and can begin appropriate surveillance (Hampel, 2016; Mvundura et al., 2010).

Challenges of multigene panels: Overlapping phenotypes and coinheritance

Next-generation sequencing panels have revealed significant gaps in our knowledge of hereditary cancer syndromes. First, there is significant clinical overlap among syndromes once believed to have very clear clinical presentations (Rosenthal et al., 2017). For example, there is overlap in the presentation of Lynch syndrome and MAP syndrome (Castillejo et al., 2014). Additionally, there is genetic heterogeneity for some cancers, such as ovarian cancer, where a number of different genes may confer an increased risk (Angeli et al., 2020; Norquist et al., 2016).

Second, some pathogenic variants do not present as expected or present with very little family history (Idos et al., 2019; LaDuca et al., 2019). There is wide variability in the phenotype of hereditary cancer syndromes, and the clinical criteria described early on in the identification of hereditary cancer syndromes have evolved to include a more broad presentation. As panels uncover unexpected pathogenic variants, the understanding of associated phenotypes and risks continues to evolve. For example, Lynch syndrome, a hereditary colon and endometrial cancer syndrome, may confer a modestly increased risk for breast cancer. As breast cancer is a relatively common cancer, affecting as many as one in eight women (12% lifetime risk), it has been difficult to determine whether breast cancer present within a Lynch syndrome kindred is due to general population risk or whether there is a true increase in the risk for breast cancer due to a pathogenic mismatch repair gene (Kohlmann, 2020; Nguyen-Dumont et al., 2020; Stoll et al., 2020). Molecular studies have confirmed the presence of mismatch repair deficiencies in some breast tumors among women with Lynch syndrome, documenting that at least a few of these breast cancers are a result of defective mismatch repair (Win et al., 2013). However, so far, there is not enough evidence that these tumors arise at an age or at a level warranting additional surveillance (Stoll et al., 2020).

Another challenge is the coinheritance of multiple pathogenic variants. Panel testing simultaneously evaluates multiple genes, including many that occur with a relatively high frequency, such as *MUTYH* (one in 50 to one in 100) or *CHEK2* (one in 100). Panels may now be considered when there is a family history of a known pathogenic variant, due to emerging evidence that as many as 5% of individuals will have a second pathogenic variant detected (Tsaousis et al., 2019). This highlights the likely underrecognized frequency of pathogenic variants in the general population (Gordon et al., 2020; Grzymski et al., 2020). There is little information about cancer risks when an individual inherits a pathogenic variant in two cancer predisposition genes, although there are a few publications about those with a *BRCA1* and *BRCA2* mutation (Lavie et al., 2011; Rebbeck et al., 2016), suggesting that the risk is not significantly increased from those with a single *BRCA1* or a *BRCA2* pathogenic variant. However, biallelic carriers of pathogenic variants in the *CHEK2* gene may face a higher lifetime risk for breast cancer than those with a single pathogenic variant in *CHEK2* (Rainville et al., 2020). Even less is known about carriers of a pathogenic variant in two different cancer predisposing genes, with only scattered case reports (Andrés et al., 2019; Cohen et al., 2016; Gong et al., 2012; Sokolenko et al., 2014; Thiffault et al., 2004). As more genetic testing is performed, cases become published more often, and data from registries such as the Inherited Cancer Registry (https://www.inheritedcancer.net) are collated, our understanding of the impact of having pathogenic variants in two cancer predisposing genes will improve.

Finally, it has been recognized that autosomal recessive conditions like Fanconi anemia can be caused by biallelic inheritance of pathogenic variants in *BRCA2*, *PALB2*, *BRIP1*, or the *FANC* genes (Barroso et al., 2009) and ataxia telangiectasia is caused by biallelic inheritance of pathogenic variants in the *ATM* gene (van Os et al., 2016). CCMRD syndrome is a result of biallelic inheritance of two mismatch repair genes, such as *PMS2* (Durno et al., 2015). Therefore, when one of these gene variants is identified, besides the increased risk for cancer in the individual and the risks to other family members to inherit the familial variant, the risk for autosomal recessive syndromes needs to be addressed as part of genetic counseling. For individuals of childbearing age, preimplantation and prenatal diagnosis options should be mentioned in these scenarios.

Essential Elements of a Cancer Genetic Counseling Session

The essential elements of a genetic counseling session are extensively described elsewhere (Riley et al., 2012), and some organizations have endorsed a certain list of topics that should be included in quality genetic counseling for hereditary cancer (Heald et al., 2020; Newman, 2019; Sarantou et al., 2017). A consolidated list of these elements can be found in Figure 9.3. Some organizations' recommendations also address who should be covering these elements of genetic counseling, traditionally provided by board-certified genetic counselors. There are ongoing efforts to improve efficiency in providing hereditary cancer risk assessment, genetic counseling and testing, as well as addressing workforce issues, such as the use of electronic tools to collect family history (Li et al., 2019; Stefansdottir et al., 2019; Welch et al., 2018), the introduction of videos or chatbots to review educational and/or informed consent components (Hurtado-de-Mendoza et al., 2019; Schmidlen et al., 2019; Watson et al., 2016), and the use of other healthcare providers in straightforward cases or to cover some elements of genetic counseling with appropriate educational supports (Cohen & Nixon, 2016).

When a pathogenic variant associated with an increased risk for hereditary cancer is identified, prenatal and preconception genetic testing may be appropriate to discuss with individuals of childbearing age, not only due to the 50% chance of passing on a pathogenic

Pretest genetic counseling

- Collect 3-generation pedigree
  - Assess risk for cancer
  - Assess likelihood of a pathogenic variant
- Conduct psychosocial assessment
- Educate
  - Include review of test options
- Obtain informed consent
  - Purpose of test
  - Possible test results
  - Accuracy
  - Possibility for inconclusive/uncertain result
  - Describe how results may impact care
  - Review laws that protect from genetic discrimintation
  - Discuss alternatives to testing
- Agree on plan to share results
- Document the encounter

Posttest genetic counseling

- Interpret/explain the result
- Assess cancer risk based on family history and genetic test result
- Review surveillance guidelines
- Review risks to family members based on family history and genetic test result
- Address psychosocial and family issues
- Develop a plan for long-term follow-up
  - Research
  - Updates to interpretation/surveillance guidelines/changes in testing options
- Document the encounter

FIGURE 9.3 Essential elements of genetic counseling for hereditary cancer.

variant associated with cancer risk, but also in some cases because an autosomal recessive condition may result, as in the case of biallelic pathogenic variants in *BRCA2* causing Fanconi anemia, or biallelic inheritance of a mismatch repair gene causing CCMRD. Although these recessive conditions are fairly rare, the incidence of carriers for pathogenic variants in genes such as *BRCA2* or those causing Lynch syndrome may be as high as 1 in 200 to 1 in 300 in the general population (Grzymski et al., 2020; Manickam et al., 2018).

Cascade testing to identify at-risk relatives is an important component of genetic counseling, which may be overlooked by healthcare providers focused solely on the care of their patient. Genetic counselors have long recognized that they not only support the patient in front of them but also have a responsibility to discuss the impact of genetic testing on the entire family (Young et al., 2020). Identification of at-risk relatives can allow for meaningful changes in surveillance, allowing for earlier identification or prevention of some cancers, as in the case of prophylactic surgery or polypectomy. There remain significant barriers to acceptance of cascade testing, including logistical, financial, and accessibility to experts (Kurian & Katz, 2020). Efforts such as telephone or online outreach to at-risk relatives may improve accessibility and uptake, but more research is needed to optimize communication among family members and acceptance of cascade testing (Caswell-Jin et al., 2019; Frey et al., 2020; Schwiter et al., 2018).

Another important element to the genetic counseling process is the consideration of long-term follow-up. Although many genetic counseling sessions are one or two encounters in a pre- and/or posttest setting, there should be a mechanism for updating the patient and the patient's physician when new guidelines are published and/or when new tests become available (Carrieri et al., 2019). Patients with a pathogenic variant linked to hereditary cancer should be offered participation in a registry or research study specific to their hereditary cause when available. This not only allows for advancement in the understanding of their gene variant among the broader medical community but also may allow the patient a mechanism to increase their knowledge about their own hereditary risks and stay updated.

It should also be recognized that family histories are not stagnant. Rather, they are evolving entities, which require updating over time. The majority of individuals who consider or undergo genetic testing will not actually be documented to have a pathogenic variant in a known hereditary cancer risk gene. However, there may still be an increased risk for cancer, and there may be some as-of-yet-unidentified hereditary contribution to the cancer history. Patients and their healthcare providers should be encouraged to contact the genetics clinic with changes in personal and/or family history, as the opportunity for updated risk assessment and/or genetic testing may emerge over time.

Likewise, cancer genetics clinics should have a policy to update patients as the interpretation of variants of uncertain significance changes over time. Some genetic testing laboratories will notify the ordering healthcare provider when a variant of uncertain significance has been reclassified. This is an opportune time to update family history information and consider re-evaluation. Clinicians can also request reanalysis, which should be considered when there are changes to a personal or family history. Obtaining a release of information at the time of genetic testing can facilitate the process for communicating with a patient's relative if that patient has died in the interval between when the testing was completed and when the variant was reclassified.

Finally, a formal registry or an informal, internal database may be helpful for tracking clinic activities (e.g., that a test was ordered/completed, that a patient was notified, etc.), test results, updates to variants, and other appointment metrics (e.g., time spent with a patient; length of time from referral to appointment; how the genetic counseling was delivered—telephone, televideo, in person, etc.). A database can be useful for reporting and documenting that certain criteria are met for accreditation by organizations such as the Commission on Cancer, and it may be valuable to implement and document quality improvement.

Precision Medicine in Oncology

Tumor testing is becoming more widespread as the understanding of cancer genomics improves and new therapies are developed that target driver mutations. The use of immunotherapy to treat tumors with mismatch repair deficiency and the use of PARPi to treat tumors with homologous repair deficiency arose directly as a result of studies on individuals with Lynch syndrome and those with pathogenic variants in *BRCA1/2* (Biller et al., 2019; Le et al., 2017; Tung et al., 2020). Although the number of treatments continues to increase, the majority of tumor testing does not result in a change of management or therapy options (Marquart et al., 2018; Singh et al., 2020).

With the increased use of somatic tumor genomic sequencing for treatment purposes, hereditary cancer syndromes will be inadvertently identified (Clark et al., 2019). Individuals with a pathogenic variant in a gene associated with a hereditary cancer syndrome should be referred for genetic counseling and consideration of germline genetic testing (Forman & Sotelo, 2020). It is important to recognize that pathogenic variants in somatic samples do not always correlate with germline findings (Moody et al., 2019), and some pathogenic variants are commonly found in certain cancer types (Jain et al., 2016). Another issue is the way in which somatic testing is performed. Some laboratories pair somatic and germline testing, subtracting out pathogenic variants that are present in both samples, to assist with the variant interpretation. In doing so, however, this can lead to the failure to detect a pathogenic germline variant that may have both treatment and familial implications (Thavaneswaran et al., 2019). Molecular tumor boards must include genetics professionals to ensure that there is adequate identification of individuals who should consider genetic counseling and testing (AlDubayan, 2019; Clark et al., 2019; Fishler et al., 2019).

Conclusion

The field of cancer genetics has been one of the first areas of genetics where identification of the underlying hereditary cause allowed for changes in management, treatment, and prevention. Much work still needs to be done to improve identification of individuals with a hereditary predisposition to take advantage of this opportunity to improve outcomes, particularly with cascade testing. The practice of cancer genetic counseling continues to evolve rapidly, and it is critical for genetic counselors to stay current. Genetic counselors will need to educate front-line healthcare providers who may be ordering genetic testing, and collaboration will be key to ensuring that patients receive high-quality genetic services (K. Stoll et al., 2018).

References

Albada, A., Dulmen, S., Dijkstra, H., Wieffer, I., Witkamp, A., & Ausems, M. G. E. M. (2015). Counselees' expressed level of understanding of the risk estimate and surveillance recommendation are not associated with breast cancer surveillance adherence. *Journal of Genetic Counseling*, *25*(2), 279–289. https://doi.org/10.1007/s10897-015-9869-x

AlDubayan, S. H. (2019). Leveraging clinical tumor-profiling programs to achieve comprehensive germline-inclusive precision cancer medicine. *JCO Precision Oncology*, *3*, 1–3. https://doi.org/10.1200/po.19.00108

Al-Tassan, N., Chmiel, N. H., Maynard, J., Fleming, N., Livingston, A. L., Williams, G. T., Hodges, A. K., Davies, D. R., David, S. S., Sampson, J. R., & Cheadle, J. P. (2002). Inherited variants of MYH associated with somatic G:C-->T:A mutations in colorectal tumors. *Nature Genetics*, *30*(2), 227–232. https://doi.org/10.1038/ng828

Amadou, A., Achatz, M. I. W., & Hainaut, P. (2018). Revisiting tumor patterns and penetrance in germline TP53 mutation carriers: Temporal phases of Li-Fraumeni syndrome. *Current Opinions in Oncology*, *30*(1), 23–29. https://doi.org/10.1097/cco.0000000000000423

Amir, E., Freedman, O. C., Seruga, B., & Evans, D. G. (2010). Assessing women at high risk of breast cancer: A review of risk assessment models. *Journal of the National Cancer Institute*, *102*(10), 680–691. https://doi.org/10.1093/jnci/djq088

Andrés, R., Menao, S., Arruebo, M., Quílez, E., & Cardiel, M. J. (2019). Double heterozygous mutation in the BRCA1 and ATM genes involved in development of primary metachronous tumours: A case report. *Breast Cancer Research and Treatment*, *177*(3), 767–770. https://doi.org/10.1007/s10549-019-05343-4

Angeli, D., Salvi, S., & Tedaldi, G. (2020). Genetic predisposition to breast and ovarian cancers: How many and which genes to test? *International Journal of Molecular Sciences*, *21*(3), 1128. https://doi.org/10.3390/ijms21031128

Annear, N. M. P., Appleton, R. E., Bassi, Z., Bhatt, R., Bolton, P. F., Crawford, P., Crowe, A., Tossi, M., Elmslie, F., Finlay, E., Gale, D. P., Henderson, A., Jones, E. A., Johnson, S. R., Joss, S., Kerecuk, L., Lipkin, G., Morrison, P. J., O'Callaghan, F. J., . . . Kingswood, J. C. (2019). Tuberous sclerosis complex (TSC): Expert recommendations for provision of coordinated care. *Frontiers in Neurology*, *10*, 1116. https://doi.org/10.3389/fneur.2019.01116

Antoniou, A. C., Foulkes, W. D., & Tischkowitz, M. (2015). Breast cancer risk in women with PALB2 mutations in different populations. *Lancet Oncology*, *16*(8), e375–e376. https://doi.org/10.1016/S1470-2045(15)00002-9

Ballhausen, W. G. (2000). Genetic testing for familial adenomatous polyposis. *Annals of the New York Academy of Sciences*, *910*, 36–47; discussion 47–39. https://doi.org/10.1111/j.1749-6632.2000.tb06699.x

Banks, K., Moline, J., Marvin, M., Newlin, A., & Vogel, K. (2013). 10 rare tumors that warrant a genetics referral. *Familial Cancer*, *12*(1), 1–18. https://doi.org/10.1007/s10689-012-9584-9

Barroso, E., Pita, G., Arias, J. I., Menendez, P., Zamora, P., Blanco, M., Benitez, J., & Ribas, G. (2009). The Fanconi anemia family of genes and its correlation with breast cancer susceptibility and breast cancer features. *Breast Cancer Research and Treatment*, *118*(3), 655–660. https://doi.org/10.1007/s10549-009-0439-5

Bellcross, C. A., Hermstad, A., Tallo, C., & Stanislaw, C. (2019). Validation of Version 3.0 of the Breast Cancer Genetics Referral Screening Tool (B-RST). *Genetics in Medicine*, *21*(1), 181–184. https://doi.org/10.1038/s41436-018-0020-x

Bellcross, C. A., Lemke, A. A., Pape, L. S., Tess, A. L., & Meisner, L. T. (2009). Evaluation of a breast/ovarian cancer genetics referral screening tool in a mammography population. *Genetics in Medicine*, *11*(11), 783–789. https://doi.org/10.1097/GIM.0b013e3181b9b04a

Biller, L. H., Syngal, S., & Yurgelun, M. B. (2019). Recent advances in Lynch syndrome. *Familial Cancer*, *18*(2), 211–219. https://doi.org/10.1007/s10689-018-00117-1

Bojadzieva, J., Amini, B., Day, S. F., Jackson, T. L., Thomas, P. S., Willis, B. J., Throckmorton, W. R., Daw, N. C., Bevers, T. B., & Strong, L. C. (2018). Whole body magnetic resonance imaging (WB-MRI) and brain MRI baseline surveillance in TP53 germline mutation carriers: Experience from the Li-Fraumeni Syndrome Education and Early Detection (LEAD) clinic. *Familial Cancer*, *17*(2), 287–294. https://doi.org/10.1007/s10689-017-0034-6

Bradbury, A. R., Patrick-Miller, L., Egleston, B., Sands, C. B., Li, T., Schmidheiser, H., Feigon, M., Ibe, C. N., Hlubocky, F. J., Hope, K., Jackson, S., Corbman, M., Olopade, O. I., Daly, M., & Daugherty, C. K. (2010). Parent opinions regarding the genetic testing of minors for BRCA1/2. *Journal of Clinical Oncology*, *28*(21), 3498–3505. https://doi.org/10.1200/jco.2009.27.2971

Brosens, L. A., Langeveld, D., van Hattem, W. A., Giardiello, F. M., & Offerhaus, G. J. A. (2011). Juvenile polyposis syndrome. *World Journal of Gastroenterology*, *17*(44), 4839–4844. https://doi.org/10.3748/wjg.v17.i44.4839

Carrieri, D., Howard, H. C., Benjamin, C., Clarke, A. J., Dheensa, S., Doheny, S., Hawkins, N., Halbersma-Konings, T. F., Jackson, L., Kayserili, H., Kelly, S. E., Lucassen, A. M., Mendes, A., Rial-Sebbag, E., Stefansdottir, V., Turnpenny, P. D., van El, C. G., van Langen, I. M., Cornel, M. C., . . . European Society of Human Genetics. (2019). Recontacting patients in clinical genetics services: Recommendations of the European Society of Human Genetics. *European Journal of Human Genetics*, *27*(2), 169–182. https://doi.org/10.1038/s41431-018-0285-1

Castillejo, A., Vargas, G., Castillejo, M. I., Navarro, M., Barberá, V. M., González, S., Hernandez-Illan, E., Brunet, J., Ramon y Cajal, T., Balmana, J., Oltra, S., Iglesias, S., Velasco, A., Solanes, A., Campos, O., Sanchez Heras, A. B., Gallego, J., Carrasco, E., Gonzalez Juan, D., . . . Soto, J. L. (2014). Prevalence of germline MUTYH mutations among Lynch-like syndrome patients. *European Journal of Cancer*, *50*(13), 2241–2250. https://doi.org/10.1016/j.ejca.2014.05.022

Caswell-Jin, J. L., Zimmer, A. D., Stedden, W., Kingham, K. E., Zhou, A. Y., & Kurian, A. W. (2019). Cascade genetic testing of relatives for hereditary cancer risk: Results of an online initiative. *Journal of the National Cancer Institute*, *111*(1), 95–98. https://doi.org/10.1093/jnci/djy147

Chen, J., Bae, E., Zhang, L., Hughes, K., Parmigiani, G., Braun, D., & Rebbeck, T. R. (2020). Penetrance of breast and ovarian cancer in women who carry a BRCA1/2 mutation and do not use risk-reducing salpingo-oophorectomy: An updated meta-analysis. *JNCI Cancer Spectrum*, *4*(4), pkaa029. https://doi.org/10.1093/jncics/pkaa029

Clark, D. F., Maxwell, K. N., Powers, J., Lieberman, D. B., Ebrahimzadeh, J., Long, J. M., McKenna, D., Shah, P., Bradbury, A., Morrissette, J. J. D., Nathanson, K. L., & Domchek, S. M. (2019). Identification and confirmation of potentially actionable germline mutations in tumor-only genomic sequencing. *JCO Precision Oncology*, *3*, 1–11. https://doi.org/10.1200/po.19.00076

Cohen, S. A., & Nixon, D. M. (2016). A collaborative approach to cancer risk assessment services using genetic counselor extenders in a multi-system community hospital. *Breast Cancer Research and Treatment*, *159*(3), 527–534. https://doi.org/10.1007/s10549-016-3964-z

Cohen, S. A., Tan, C. A., & Bisson, R. (2016). An individual with both MUTYH-associated polyposis and Lynch syndrome identified by multi-gene hereditary cancer panel testing: A case report. *Frontiers in Genetics*, *7*(36), 36. https://doi.org/10.3389/fgene.2016.00036

Couch, F. J., Shimelis, H., Hu, C., Hart, S. N., Polley, E. C., Na, J., Hallberg, E., Moore, R., Thomas, A., Lilyquist, J., Feng, B., McFarland, R., Pesaran, T., Huether, R., LaDuca, H., Chao, E. C., Goldgar, D. E., & Dolinsky, J. S. (2017). Associations between cancer predisposition testing panel genes and breast cancer. *JAMA Oncology*, *3*(9), 1190–1196. https://doi.org/10.1001/jamaoncol.2017.0424

Crawford, B., Adams, S. B., Sittler, T., van den Akker, J., Chan, S., Leitner, O., Ryan, L., Gil, E., & van't Veer, L. (2017). Multi-gene panel testing for hereditary cancer predisposition in unsolved high-risk breast and ovarian cancer patients. *Breast Cancer Research and Treatment*, *163*(2), 383–390. https://doi.org/10.1007/s10549-017-4181-0

Cripps, H. (1882). Two cases of disseminated polypus of the colon. *Transactions of the Pathological Society of London*, *33*, 165–168.

Crump, J. K., Del Fiol, G., Williams, M. S., & Freimuth, R. R. (2018). Prototype of a standards-based EHR and genetic test reporting tool coupled with HL7-compliant infobuttons. *AMIA Joint Summits on Translational Science Proceedings*, *2017*, 330–339.

Daly, M. B., Pilarski, R., Yurgelun, M. B., Berry, M. P., Buys, S. S., Dickson, P., Domchek, S. M., Elkhanany, A., Friedman, S., Garber, J. E., Goggins, M., Hutton, M. L., Khan, S., Klein, C., Kohlmann, W., Kurian, A. W., Laronga, C., Litton, J. K., Mak, J. S., . . . Darlow, S. D. (2020). NCCN guidelines insights: Genetic/familial high-risk assessment: Breast, ovarian, and pancreatic, version 1.2020. *Journal of the National Comprehensive Cancer Network*, *18*(4), 380–391. https://doi.org/10.6004/jnccn.2020.0017

Daniell, J., Plazzer, J.-P., Perera, A., & Macrae, F. (2018). An exploration of genotype-phenotype link between Peutz-Jeghers syndrome and STK11: A review. *Familial Cancer*, *17*(3), 421–427. https://doi.org/10.1007/s10689-017-0037-3

Del Fiol, G., Kohlmann, W., Bradshaw, R. L., Weir, C. R., Flynn, M., Hess, R., Schiffman, J. D., Nanjo, C., & Kawamoto, K. (2020). Standards-based clinical decision support platform to manage patients who meet guideline-based criteria for genetic evaluation of familial cancer. *JCO Clinical Cancer Informatics*, *4*, 1–9. https://doi.org/10.1200/cci.19.00120

Dinarvand, P., Davaro, E. P., Doan, J. V., Ising, M. E., Evans, N. R., Phillips, N. J., Lai, J., & Guzman, M. A. (2019). Familial adenomatous polyposis syndrome: An update and review of extraintestinal manifestations. *Archives of Pathology and Laboratory Medicine*, *143*(11), 1382–1398. https://doi.org/10.5858/arpa.2018-0570-RA

Domchek, S. M. (2015). Evolution of genetic testing for inherited susceptibility to breast cancer. *Journal of Clinical Oncology*, *33*(4), 295–296. https://doi.org/10.1200/jco.2014.59.3178

Dominguez-Valentin, M., Sampson, J. R., Seppälä, T. T., ten Broeke, S. W., Plazzer, J.-P., Nakken, S., Engel, C., Aretz, S., Jenkins, M. A., Sunde, L., Bernstein, I., Capella, G., Balaguer, F., Thomas, H., Evans, D. G., Burn, J., Greenblatt, M., Hovig, E., de Vos Tot Nederveen

Cappel, W. H., . . . Møller, P. (2019). Cancer risks by gene, age, and gender in 6350 carriers of pathogenic mismatch repair variants: Findings from the Prospective Lynch Syndrome Database. *Genetics in Medicine, 22*(1), 15–25. https://doi.org/10.1038/s41436-019-0596-9

Dukes, C. E. (1952). Familial intestinal polyposis. *Annals of Eugenics, 17*(Part 1), 1–29. https://doi.org/10.1111/j.1469-1809.1953.tb02531.x

Durno, C. A., Sherman, P. M., Aronson, M., Malkin, D., Hawkins, C., Bakry, D., Bouffet, E., Gallinger, S., Pollett, A., Campbell, B., Tabori, U., & International Biallelic Mismatch Repair Deficiency Consortium. (2015). Phenotypic and genotypic characterisation of biallelic mismatch repair deficiency (BMMR-D) syndrome. *European Journal of Cancer, 51*(8), 977–983. https://doi.org/10.1016/j.ejca.2015.02.008

Easton, D. F., Lesueur, F., Decker, B., Michailidou, K., Li, J., Allen, J., Luccarini, C., Pooley, K. A., Shah, M., Bolla, M. K., Wang, Q., Dennis, J., Ahmad, J., Thompson, E. R., Damiola, F., Pertesi, M., Voegele, C., Mebirouk, N., Robinot, N., . . . Chenevix-Trench, G. (2016). No evidence that protein truncating variants in BRIP1 are associated with breast cancer risk: Implications for gene panel testing. *Journal of Medical Genetics, 53*(5), 298–309.

Else, T., Kim, A. C., Sabolch, A., Raymond, V. M., Kandathil, A., Caoili, E. M., Jolly, S., Miller, B. S., Giordano, T. J., & Hammer, G. D. (2014). Adrenocortical carcinoma. *Endocrine Reviews, 35*(2), 282–326. https://doi.org/10.1210/er.2013-1029.

Evans, D. G., & Farndon, P. A. (1993). Nevoid basal cell carcinoma syndrome. In M. P. Adam, H. H. Ardinger, R. A. Pagon, S. E. Wallace, L. J. H. Bean, K. Stephens, & A. Amemiya (Eds.), *GeneReviews®*. University of Washington, Seattle.

Fishler, K. P., Breese, E. H., Walters-Sen, L., & McGowan, M. L. (2019). Experiences of a multidisciplinary genomic tumor board interpreting risk for underlying germline variants in tumor-only sequencing results. *JCO Precision Oncology, 3*, 1–8. https://doi.org/10.1200/po.18.00216

Forman, A., & Sotelo, J. (2020). Tumor-based genetic testing and familial cancer risk. *Cold Spring Harbor Perspectives in Medicine, 10*(8), a036590. https://doi.org/10.1101/cshperspect.a036590

Foulkes, W. D., Kamihara, J., Evans, D. G. R., Brugières, L., Bourdeaut, F., Molenaar, J. J., Walsh, M. F., Brodeur, G. M., & Diller, L. (2017). Cancer surveillance in Gorlin syndrome and rhabdoid tumor predisposition syndrome. *Clinical Cancer Research, 23*(12), e62–e67. https://doi.org/10.1158/1078-0432.ccr-17-0595

Frey, M. K., Kahn, R. M., Chapman-Davis, E., Tubito, F., Pires, M., Christos, P., Anderson, S., Mukherjee, S., Jordan, B., Blank, S. V., Caputo, T. A., Sharaf, R. N., Offit, K., Holcomb, K., & Lipkin, S. (2020). Prospective feasibility trial of a novel strategy of facilitated cascade genetic testing using telephone counseling. *Journal of Clinical Oncology, 38*(13), 1389–1397. https://doi.org/10.1200/jco.19.02005

Gail, M. H. (2015). Twenty-five years of breast cancer risk models and their applications. *Journal of the National Cancer Institute, 107*(5), djv042. https://doi.org/10.1093/jnci/djv042

Galiatsatos, P., & Foulkes, W. D. (2006). Familial adenomatous polyposis. *American Journal of Gastroenterology, 101*(2), 385–398.

Gong, P., Charles, S., Rosenblum, N., Wang, Z., & Witkiewicz, A. K. (2012). A case of endometrial cancer in the context of a BRCA2 mutation and double heterozygosity for Lynch syndrome. *Gynecologic Oncology Case Reports, 2*(3), 69–72. https://doi.org/10.1016/j.gynor.2012.03.001

Gordon, A. S., Zouk, H., Venner, E., Eng, C. M., Funke, B. H., Amendola, L. M., Carrell, D. S., Chisholm, R. L., Chung, W. K., Denny, J. C., Fedotov, A., Hakonarson, H., Kullo,

I. J., Larson, E. B., Leduc, M. S., Leppig, K. A., Lennon, N. J., Linder, J. E., Muzny, D. M., . . . Jarvik, G. P. (2020). Frequency of genomic secondary findings among 21,915 eMERGE network participants. *Genetics in Medicine*, *22*(9), 1470–1477. https://doi.org/10.1038/s41436-020-0810-9

Gorlin, R. J., & Goltz, R. W. (1960). Multiple nevoid basal-cell epithelioma, jaw cysts and bifid rib. A syndrome. *New England Journal of Medicine*, *262*, 908–912. https://doi.org/10.1056/nejm196005052621803

Goshen, R., Choman, E., Ran, A., Muller, E., Kariv, R., Chodick, G., Ash, N., Narod, S., & Shalev, V. (2018). Computer-assisted flagging of individuals at high risk of colorectal cancer in a large health maintenance organization using the ColonFlag Test. *JCO Clinical Cancer Informatics*, 2, 1–8. https://doi.org/10.1200/cci.17.00130

Griffith, A. D., & Sorsby, A. (1944). The genetics of retinoblastoma. *British Journal of Ophthalmology*, *28*(6), 279–293. https://doi.org/10.1136/bjo.28.6.279

Groves, A., Gleeson, M., & Spigelman, A. D. (2019). NTHL1-associate polyposis: First Australian case report. *Familial Cancer*, *18*(2), 179–182. https://doi.org/10.1007/s10689-018-0107-1

Grzymski, J. J., Elhanan, G., Morales Rosado, J. A., Smith, E., Schlauch, K. A., Read, R., Rowan, C., Slotnick, N., Dabe, S., Metcalf, W. J., Lipp, B., Reed, H., Sharma, L., Levin, E., Kao, J., Rashkin, M., Bowes, J., Dunaway, K., Slonim, A., . . . Lu, J. T. (2020). Population genetic screening efficiently identifies carriers of autosomal dominant diseases. *Nature Medicine*, *26*(8), 1235–1239. https://doi.org/10.1038/s41591-020-0982-5

Gupta, S., Provenzale, D., Llor, X., Halverson, A. L., Grady, W., Chung, D. C., Haraldsdottir, S., Markowitz, A. J., Slavin, T. P., Jr., Hampel, H., Ness, R. M., Weiss, J. M., Ahnen, D. J., Chen, L. M., Cooper, G., Early, D. S., Giardiello, F. M., Hall, M. J., Hamilton, S. R., . . . Ogba, N. (2019). NCCN guidelines insights: Genetic/familial high-risk assessment: Colorectal, version 2.2019. *Journal of National Comprehensive Cancer Network*, *17*(9), 1032–1041. https://doi.org/10.6004/jnccn.2019.0044

Hampel, H. (2016). Genetic counseling and cascade genetic testing in Lynch syndrome. *Familial Cancer*, *15*(3), 423–427. https://doi.org/10.1007/s10689-016-9893-5

Hampel, H., Frankel, W. L., Martin, E., Arnold, M., Khanduja, K., Kuebler, P., Nakagawa, H., Sotamaa, K., Prior, T. W., Westman, J., Panescu, J., Fix, D., Lockman, J., Comeras, I., & de la Chapelle, A. (2005). Screening for the Lynch syndrome (hereditary nonpolyposis colorectal cancer). *New England Journal of Medicine*, *352*(18), 1851–1860. https://doi.org/10.1056/NEJMoa043146

Heald, B., Hampel, H., Church, J., Dudley, B., Hall, M. J., Mork, M. E., Singh, A., Stoffel, E., Stoll, J., You, Y. N., Yurgelun, M. B., Kupfer, S. S., & The Collaborative Group of the Americas on Inherited Gastrointestinal Cancer. (2020). Collaborative Group of the Americas on Inherited Gastrointestinal Cancer Position statement on multigene panel testing for patients with colorectal cancer and/or polyposis. *Familial Cancer*, *19*(3), 223–239. https://doi.org/10.1007/s10689-020-00170-9

Huq, A. J., Walsh, M., Rajagopalan, B., Finlay, M., Trainer, A. H., Bonnet, F., Sevenet, N., & Winship, I. M. (2018). Mutations in SUFU and PTCH1 genes may cause different cutaneous cancer predisposition syndromes: Similar, but not the same. *Familial Cancer*, *17*(4), 601–606. https://doi.org/10.1007/s10689-018-0073-7

Hurtado-de-Mendoza, A., Graves, K. D., Gómez-Trillos, S., Song, M., Anderson, L., Campos, C., Carrera, P., Ostrove, N., Peshkin, B. N., Schwartz, M. D., Ficca, N., Cupertino, A. P., Gonzalez, N., Otero, A., Huerta, E., & Sheppard, V. B. (2019). Developing a culturally targeted video to enhance the use of genetic counseling in Latina women at increased risk for hereditary breast and ovarian cancer. *Journal of Community Genetics*, *11*(1), 85–89. https://doi.org/10.1007/s12687-019-00423-w

Idos, G. E., Kurian, A. W., Ricker, C., Sturgeon, D., Culver, J. O., Kingham, K. E., Koff, R., Chun, N. M., Rowe-Teeter, C., Lebensohn, A. P., Levonian, P., Lowstuter, K., Partynski, K., Hong, C., Mills, M. A., Petrovchich, I., Ma, C. S., Hartman, A. R., Allen, B., . . . Gruber, S. B. (2019). Multicenter prospective cohort study of the diagnostic yield and patient experience of multiplex gene panel testing for hereditary cancer risk. *JCO Precision Oncology*, *3*, 1–12. https://doi.org/10.1200/po.18.00217

Imbert-Bouteille, M., Gauthier-Villars, M., Leroux, D., Meunier, I., Aerts, I., Lumbroso-Le Rouic, L., Lejeune, S., Delnatte, C., Abadie, C., Pujol, P., Houdayer, C., & Corsini, C. (2019). Osteosarcoma without prior retinoblastoma related to RB1 low-penetrance germline pathogenic variants: A novel type of RB1-related hereditary predisposition syndrome? *Molecular Genetics and Genomic Medicine*, *7*(12), e913. https://doi.org/10.1002/mgg3.913

Jain, R., Savage, M. J., Forman, A. D., Mukherji, R., & Hall, M. J. (2016). The relevance of hereditary cancer risks to precision oncology: What should providers consider when conducting tumor genomic profiling? *Journal of the National Comprehensive Cancer Network*, *14*(6), 795–806.

Kamihara, J., Bourdeaut, F., Foulkes, W. D., Molenaar, J. J., Mossé, Y. P., Nakagawara, A., Parareda, A., Scollon, S. R., Schneider, K. W., Skalet, A. H., States, L. J., Walsh, M. F., Diller, L. R., & Brodeur, G. M. (2017). Retinoblastoma and neuroblastoma predisposition and surveillance. *Clinical Cancer Research*, *23*(13), e98–e106. https://doi.org/10.1158/1078-0432.Ccr-17-0652

Kentwell, M., Dow, E., Antill, Y., Wrede, C. D., McNally, O., Higgs, E., Hamilton, A., Ananda, S., Lindeman, G. J., & Scott, C. L. (2017). Mainstreaming cancer genetics: A model integrating germline BRCA testing into routine ovarian cancer clinics. *Gynecologic Oncology*, *145*(1), 130–136. https://doi.org/10.1016/j.ygyno.2017.01.030

Kesselheim, A. S., Cook-Deegan, R. M., Winickoff, D. E., & Mello, M. M. (2013). Gene patenting—The Supreme Court finally speaks. *New England Journal of Medicine*, *369*(9), 869–875. https://doi.org/10.1056/NEJMhle1308199

Khan, N. E., Ling, A., Raske, M. E., Harney, L. A., Carr, A. G., Field, A., Harris, A. K., Williams, G. M., Dehner, L. P., Messinger, Y. H., Hill, D. A., Schultz, K. A. P., & Stewart, D. R. (2018). Structural renal abnormalities in the DICER1 syndrome: A family-based cohort study. *Pediatric Nephrology (Berlin, Germany)*, *33*(12), 2281–2288. https://doi.org/10.1007/s00467-018-4040-1

Kne, A., Zierhut, H., Baldinger, S., Swenson, K. K., Mink, P., Veach, P. M., & Tsai, M. L. (2017). Why is cancer genetic counseling underutilized by women identified as at risk for hereditary breast cancer? Patient perceptions of barriers following a referral letter. *Journal of Genetic Counseling*, *26*(4), 697–715. https://doi.org/10.1007/s10897-016-0040-0

Kohlmann, W. (2020). Lynch syndrome and breast cancer risk: Weighing the data. *JCO Precision Oncology*, *4*, 128–130. https://doi.org/10.1200/po.19.00376

Konstantinopoulos, P. A., Norquist, B., Lacchetti, C., Armstrong, D., Grisham, R. N., Goodfellow, P. J., Kohn, E. C., Levine, D. A., Liu, J. F., Lu, K. H., Sparacio, D., & Annunziata, C. M. (2020). Germline and somatic tumor testing in epithelial ovarian cancer: ASCO guideline. *Journal of Clinical Oncology*, *38*(11), 1222–1245. https://doi.org/10.1200/jco.19.02960.

Kuchenbaecker, K. B., Hopper, J. L., Barnes, D. R., Phillips, K. A., Mooij, T. M., Roos-Blom, M. J., Jervis, S., van Leeuwen, F. E., Milne, R. L., Andrieu, N., Goldgar, D. E., Terry, M. B., Rookus, M. A., Easton, D. F., Antoniou, A. C., BRCA1 and BRCA2 Cohort Consortium,

McGuffog, L., Evans, D. G., Barrowdale, D., . . .Olsson, H. (2017). Risks of breast, ovarian, and contralateral breast cancer for BRCA1 and BRCA2 mutation carriers. *Journal of the American Medical Association*, *317*(23), 2402–2416. https://doi.org/10.1001/jama.2017.7112

Kurian, A. W., & Katz, S. J. (2020). Emerging opportunity of cascade genetic testing for population-wide cancer prevention and control. *Journal of Clinical Oncology*, *38*(13), 1371–1374. https://doi.org/10.1200/jco.20.00140

Kurian, A. W., Ward, K. C., Howlader, N., Deapen, D., Hamilton, A. S., Mariotto, A., Miller, D., Penberthy, L. S., & Katz, S. J. (2019). Genetic testing and results in a population-based cohort of breast cancer patients and ovarian cancer patients. *Journal of Clinical Oncology*, *37*(15), 1305–1315. https://doi.org/10.1200/jco.18.01854

LaDuca, H., Polley, E. C., Yussuf, A., Hoang, L., Gutierrez, S., Hart, S. N., Yadav, S., Hu, C., Na, J., Goldgar, D. E., Fulk, K., Smith, L. P., Horton, C., Profato, J., Pesaran, T., Gau, C. L., Pronold, M., Davis, B. T., Chao, E. C., . . . Dolinsky, J. S. (2019). A clinical guide to hereditary cancer panel testing: Evaluation of gene-specific cancer associations and sensitivity of genetic testing criteria in a cohort of 165,000 high-risk patients. *Genetics in Medicine*, *22*(2), 407–415. https://doi.org/10.1038/s41436-019-0633-8

Latham, A., Srinivasan, P., Kemel, Y., Shia, J., Bandlamudi, C., Mandelker, D., Middha, S., Hechtman, J., Zehir, A., Dubard-Gault, M., Tran, C., Stewart, C., Sheehan, M., Penson, A., DeLair, D., Yaeger, R., Vijai, J., Mukherjee, S., Galle, J., . . . Stadler, Z. K. (2019). Microsatellite instability is associated with the presence of Lynch syndrome pan-cancer. *Journal of Clinical Oncology*, *37*(4), 286–295. https://doi.org/10.1200/jco.18.00283

Lavie, O., Narod, S., Lejbkowicz, F., Dishon, S., Goldberg, Y., Gemer, O., & Rennert, G. (2011). Double heterozygosity in the BRCA1 and BRCA2 genes in the Jewish population. *Annals of Oncology*, *22*(4), 964–966. https://doi.org/10.1093/annonc/mdq460

Le, D. T., Durham, J. N., Smith, K. N., Wang, H., Bartlett, B. R., Aulakh, L. K., Lu, S., Kemberling, H., Wilt, C., Luber, B. S., Wong, F., Azad, N. S., Rucki, A. A., Laheru, D., Donehower, R., Zaheer, A., Fisher, G. A., Crocenzi, T. S., Lee, J. J., . . . Diaz, L. A. (2017). Mismatch-repair deficiency predicts response of solid tumors to PD-1 blockade. *Science*, *357*(6349), 409–413. https://doi.org/10.1126/science.aan6733

Lemery, S., Keegan, P., & Pazdur, R. (2017). First FDA approval agnostic of cancer site—When a biomarker defines the indication. *New England Journal of Medicine*, *377*(15), 1409–1412. https://doi.org/10.1056/NEJMp1709968

Li, F. P., & Fraumeni, J. F., Jr. (1969). Soft-tissue sarcomas, breast cancer, and other neoplasms. A familial syndrome? *Annals of Internal Medicine*, *71*(4), 747–752. https://doi.org/10.7326/0003-4819-71-4-747

Li, W., Murray, M. F., & Giovanni, M. A. (2019). Obtaining a genetic family history using computer-based tools. *Current Protocols in Human Genetics*, *100*(1), e72. https://doi.org/10.1002/cphg.72

Lynch, H. T., & Krush, A. J. (1971). Cancer family "G" revisited: 1895–1970. *Cancer*, *27*(6), 1505–1511.

Lynch, H. T., Shaw, M. W., Magnuson, C. W., Larsen, A. L., & Krush, A. J. (1966). Hereditary factors in cancer. Study of two large midwestern kindreds. *Archives of Internal Medicine*, *117*(2), 206–212.

Maher, E. R., & Sandford, R. N. (2019). von Hippel-Lindau disease: An update. *Current Genetic Medicine Reports*, *7*(4), 227–235. https://doi.org/10.1007/s40142-019-00180-9

Mai, P. L., Best, A. F., Peters, J. A., DeCastro, R. M., Khincha, P. P., Loud, J. T., Bremer, R. C., Rosenberg, P. S., & Savage, S. A. (2016). Risks of first and subsequent cancers among TP53 mutation carriers in the National Cancer Institute Li-Fraumeni syndrome cohort. *Cancer, 122*(23), 3673–3681. https://doi.org/10.1002/cncr.30248

Mandelker, D., Zhang, L., Kemel, Y., Stadler, Z. K., Joseph, V., Zehir, A., Pradhan, N., Arnold, A., Walsh, M. F., Li, Y., Balakrishnan, A. R., Syed, A., Prasad, M., Nafa, K., Carlo, M. I., Cadoo, K. A., Sheehan, M., Fleischut, M. H., Salo-Mullen, E., . . . Offit, K. (2017). Mutation detection in patients with advanced cancer by universal sequencing of cancer-related genes in tumor and normal DNA vs guideline-based germline testing. *JAMA, 318*(9), 825–835. https://doi.org/10.1001/jama.2017.11137

Manickam, K., Buchanan, A. H., Schwartz, M. L. B., Hallquist, M. L. G., Williams, J. L., Rahm, A. K., Rocha, H., Savatt, J. M., Evans, A. E., Butry, L. M., Lazzeri, A. L., Lindbuchler, D. M., Flansburg, C. N., Leeming, R., Vogel, V. G., Lebo, M. S., Mason-Suares, H. M., Hoskinson, D. C., Abul-Husn, N. S., . . . Murray, M. F. (2018). Exome sequencing-based screening for BRCA1/2 expected pathogenic variants among adult biobank participants. *JAMA Network Open, 1*(5), e182140. https://doi.org/10.1001/jamanetworkopen.2018.2140

Marabelle, A., Le, D. T., Ascierto, P. A., Di Giacomo, A. M, Jesus-Acosta, A. D., Delord, J. P., Geva, R., Gottfried, M., Penel, N., Hansen, A. R., Piha-Paul, S. A., Doi, T., Gao, B., Chung, H. C., Lopez-Martin, J., Bang, Y. J., Frommer, R. S., Shah, M., Ghori, R., . . . Diaz, L. A. (2020). Efficacy of pembrolizumab in patients with noncolorectal high microsatellite instability/mismatch repair–deficient cancer: Results from the phase II KEYNOTE-158 study. *Journal of Clinical Oncology, 38*(1), 1–10. https://doi.org/10.1200/jco.19.02105

Marabelli, M., Cheng, S. C., & Parmigiani, G. (2016). Penetrance of ATM gene mutations in breast cancer: A meta-analysis of different measures of risk. *Genetic Epidemiology, 40*(5), 425–431. https://doi.org/10.1002/gepi.21971

Marees, T., Moll, A. C., Imhof, S. M., de Boer, M. R., Ringens, P. J., & van Leeuwen, F. E. (2008). Risk of second malignancies in survivors of retinoblastoma: More than 40 years of follow-up. *Journal of the National Cancer Institute, 100*(24), 1771–1779. https://doi.org/10.1093/jnci/djn394

Marquart, J., Chen, E. Y., & Prasad, V. (2018). Estimation of the percentage of US patients with cancer who benefit from genome-driven oncology. *JAMA Oncology, 4*(8), 1093–1098. https://doi.org/10.1001/jamaoncol.2018.1660

Mavaddat, N., Michailidou, K., Dennis, J., Lush, M., Fachal, L., Lee, A., Tyrer, J. P., Chen, T. H., Wang, Q., Bolla, M. K., Yang, X., Adank, M. A., Ahearn, T., Aittomaki, K., Allen, J., Andrulis, I. L., Anton-Culver, H., Antonenkova, N. N., Arndt, V., . . . Easton, D. F. (2019). Polygenic risk scores for prediction of breast cancer and breast cancer subtypes. *American Journal of Human Genetics, 104*(1), 21–34. https://doi.org/10.1016/j.ajhg.2018.11.002

Moller, P., Seppala, T. T., Bernstein, I., Holinski-Feder, E., Sala, P., Gareth Evans, D., Lindblom, A., Macrae, F., Blanco, I., Sijmons, R. H., Jeffries, J., Vasen, H. F. A., Burn, J., Nakken, S., Hovig, E., Rodland, E. A., Tharmaratnam, K., de Vos Tot Nederveen Cappel, W. H., Hill, J., . . . Capella, G. (2017). Cancer risk and survival in path_MMR carriers by gene and gender up to 75 years of age: A report from the Prospective Lynch Syndrome Database. *Gut, 67*(7), 1306–1316. https://doi.org/10.1136/gutjnl-2017-314057

Moody, E. W., Vagher, J., Espinel, W., Goldgar, D., Hagerty, K. J., & Gammon, A. (2019). Comparison of somatic and germline variant interpretation in hereditary cancer genes. *JCO Precision Oncology, 3*, 1–8. https://doi.org/10.1200/po.19.00144

Morman, N. A., Byrne, L., Collins, C., Reynolds, K., & Bell, J. G. (2017). Breast cancer risk assessment at the time of screening mammography: Perceptions and clinical management outcomes for women at high risk. *Journal of Genetic Counseling*, *26*(4), 776–784. https://doi.org/10.1007/s10897-016-0050-y

Muir, E. G., Bell, A. J., & Barlow, K. A. (1967). Multiple primary carcinomata of the colon, duodenum, and larynx associated with kerato-acanthomata of the face. *British Journal of Surgery*, *54*(3), 191–195.

Muth, A., Crona, J., Gimm, O., Elmgren, A., Filipsson, K., Stenmark Askmalm, M., Sandstedt, J., Tengvar, M., & Tham, E. (2019). Genetic testing and surveillance guidelines in hereditary pheochromocytoma and paraganglioma. *Journal of Internal Medicine*, *285*(2), 187–204. https://doi.org/10.1111/joim.12869.

Mvundura, M., Grosse, S. D., Hampel, H., & Palomaki, G. E. (2010). The cost-effectiveness of genetic testing strategies for Lynch syndrome among newly diagnosed patients with colorectal cancer. *Genetics in Medicine*, *12*(2), 93–104. https://doi.org/10.1097/GIM.0b013e3181cd666c

Näslund-Koch, C., Nordestgaard, B. G., & Bojesen, S. E. (2016). Increased risk for other cancers in addition to breast cancer for CHEK2*1100delC heterozygotes estimated from the Copenhagen General Population Study. *Journal of Clinical Oncology*, *34*(11), 1208–1216. https://doi.org/10.1200/jco.2015.63.3594

Nelson, H. D., Pappas, M., Cantor, A., Haney, E., & Holmes, R. (2019). Risk assessment, genetic counseling, and genetic testing for BRCA-related cancer in women: Updated evidence report and systematic review for the US Preventive Services Task Force. *JAMA*, *322*(7), 666–685. https://doi.org/10.1001/jama.2019.8430

Newman, L. (2019). US Preventive Services Task Force breast cancer recommendation statement on risk assessment, genetic counseling, and genetic testing for BRCA-related cancer. *JAMA Surgery*, *154*(10), 895–896. https://doi.org/10.1001/jamasurg.2019.3184

Ngeow, J., Sesock, K., & Eng, C. (2017). Breast cancer risk and clinical implications for germline PTEN mutation carriers. *Breast Cancer Research and Treatment*, *165*(1), 1–8. https://doi.org/10.1007/s10549-015-3665-z

Nguyen-Dumont, T., Steen, J. A., Winship, I., Park, D. J., Pope, B. J., Hammet, F., Mahmoodi, M., Tsimiklis, H., Theys, D., Clendenning, M., Giles, G. G., Hopper, J. L., & Southey, M. C. (2020). Mismatch repair gene pathogenic germline variants in a population-based cohort of breast cancer. *Familial Cancer*, *19*(3), 197–202. https://doi.org/10.1007/s10689-020-00164-7

Norquist, B. M., Harrell, M. I., Brady, M. F., Walsh, T., Lee, M. K., Gulsuner, S., Bernards, S. S., Casadei, S., Yi, Q., Burger, R. A., Chan, J. K., Davidson, S. A., Mannel, R. S., DiSilvestro, P. A., Lankes, H. A., Ramirez, N. C., King, M. C., Swisher, E. M., & Birrer, M. J. (2016). Inherited mutations in women with ovarian carcinoma. *JAMA Oncology*, *2*(4), 482–490. https://doi.org/10.1001/jamaoncol.2015.5495

Paskett, E. D., Bernardo, B. M., Young, G. S., Katz, M. L., Reiter, P. L., Tatum, C. M., Oliveri, J. M., DeGraffinreid, C. R., Gray, D. M., Pearlman, R., & Hampel, H. (2020). Comparative effectiveness of two interventions to increase colorectal cancer screening for those at increased risk based on family history: Results of a randomized trial. *Cancer Epidemiology Biomarkers & Prevention*, *29*(1), 3–9. https://doi.org/10.1158/1055-9965.Epi-19-0797

Pearlman, R., Frankel, W. L., Swanson, B., Zhao, W., Yilmaz, A., Miller, K., Bacher, J., Bigley, C., Nelsen, L., Goodfellow, P. J., Goldberg, R. M., Paskett, E., Shields, P. G., Freudenheim, J. L., Stanich, P. P., Lattimer, I., Arnold, M., Liyanarachchi, S., Kalady, M., . . . Ohio Colorectal Cancer Prevention Initiative Study Group. (2017). Prevalence and spectrum of germline cancer susceptibility gene mutations among patients with early-onset colorectal cancer. *JAMA Oncology*, *3*(4), 464–471. https://doi.org/10.1001/jamaoncol.2016.5194

Pederson, H. J., Hussain, N., Noss, R., Yanda, C., O'Rourke, C., Eng, C., & Grobmyer, S. R. (2018). Impact of an embedded genetic counselor on breast cancer treatment. *Breast Cancer Research and Treatment*, *169*(1), 43–46. https://doi.org/10.1007/s10549-017-4643-4

Pilarski, R. (2019). PTEN hamartoma tumor syndrome: A clinical overview. *Cancers (Basel)*, *11*(6), 844. https://doi.org/10.3390/cancers11060844

Rafnar, T., Gudbjartsson, D. F., Sulem, P., Jonasdottir, A., Sigurdsson, A., Jonasdottir, A., Besenbacher, S., Lundin, P., Stacey, S. N., Gudmundsson, J., Magnusson, O. T., le Roux, L., Orlygsdottir, G., Helgadottir, H. T., Johannsdottir, H., Gylfason, A., Tryggvadottir, L., Jonasson, J. G., de Juan, A., . . . Stefansson, K. (2011). Mutations in BRIP1 confer high risk of ovarian cancer. *Nature Genetics*, *43*(11), 1104–1107. http://www.nature.com/ng/journal/v43/n11/abs/ng.955.html#supplementary-information

Rahman, N. (2014). Realizing the promise of cancer predisposition genes. *Nature*, *505*(7483), 302–308. https://doi.org/10.1038/nature12981.

Rainone, M., Singh, I., Salo-Mullen, E. E., Stadler, Z. K., & O'Reilly, E. M. (2020). An emerging paradigm for germline testing in pancreatic ductal adenocarcinoma and immediate implications for clinical practice: A review. *JAMA Oncology*, *6*(5), 764–771. https://doi.org/10.1001/jamaoncol.2019.5963.

Rainville, I., Hatcher, S., Rosenthal, E., Larson, K., Bernhisel, R., Meek, S., Gorringe, H., Mundt, E., & Manley, S. (2020). High risk of breast cancer in women with biallelic pathogenic variants in CHEK2. *Breast Cancer Research and Treatment*, *180*(2), 503–509. https://doi.org/10.1007/s10549-020-05543-3

Rasmussen, S. A., & Friedman, J. M. (2000). NF1 gene and neurofibromatosis 1. *American Journal of Epidemiology*, *151*(1), 33–40. https://doi.org/10.1093/oxfordjournals.aje.a010118

Raue, F., & Frank-Raue, K. (2010). Update multiple endocrine neoplasia type 2. *Familial Cancer*, *9*(3), 449–457. https://doi.org/10.1007/s10689-010-9320-2

Rayes, N., Bowen, D. J., Coffin, T., Nebgen, D., Peterson, C., Munsell, M. F., Gavin, K., Lechner, R., Crase, J., Polinsky, D., Romero, I., Blank, S. V., Levine, D. A., Norquist, B. M., Swisher, E. M., & Lu, K. H. (2019). MAGENTA (Making Genetic testing accessible): A prospective randomized controlled trial comparing online genetic education and telephone genetic counseling for hereditary cancer genetic testing. *BMC Cancer*, *19*(1), 648. https://doi.org/10.1186/s12885-019-5868-x

Rebbeck, T. R., Friebel, T. M., Mitra, N., Wan, F., Chen, S., Andrulis, I. L., Apostolou, P., Arnold, N., Arun, B. K., Barrowdale, D., Benitez, J., Berger, R., Berthet, P., Borg, A., Buys, S. S., Caldes, T., Carter, J., Chiquette, J., Claes, K. B., . . . Ramus, S. J. (2016). Inheritance of deleterious mutations at both BRCA1 and BRCA2 in an international sample of 32,295 women. *Breast Cancer Research*, *18*(1), 112. https://doi.org/10.1186/s13058-016-0768-3

Rednam, S. P., Erez, A., Druker, H., Janeway, K. A., Kamihara, J., Kohlmann, W. K., Nathanson, K. L., States, L. J., Tomlinson, G. E., Villani, A., Voss, S. D., Schiffman, J. D., & Wasserman, J. D. (2017). Von Hippel–Lindau and hereditary pheochromocytoma/paraganglioma syndromes: Clinical features, genetics, and surveillance recommendations in childhood. *Clinical Cancer Research*, *23*(12), e68–e75. https://doi.org/10.1158/1078-0432.Ccr-17-0547

Riley, B., Culver, J., Skrzynia, C., Senter, L., Peters, J., Costalas, J., Callif-Daley, F., Grumet, S. C., Hunt, K. S., Nagy, R. S., McKinnon, W. C., Petrucelli, N. M., Bennett, R. L., & Trepanier, A. (2012). Essential elements of genetic cancer risk assessment, counseling, and testing: Updated Recommendations of the National Society of Genetic Counselors. *Journal of Genetic Counseling*, *21*(2), 151–161. https://doi.org/10.1007/s10897-011-9462-x

Robson, M. E., Bradbury, A. R., Arun, B., Domchek, S. M., Ford, J. M., Hampel, H. L., Lipkin, S. M., Syngal, S., Wollins, D. S., & Lindor, N. M. (2015). American Society of Clinical Oncology policy statement update: Genetic and genomic testing for cancer susceptibility. *Journal of Clinical Oncology, 33*(31), 3660–3667. https://doi.org/10.1200/jco.2015.63.0996

Rosenthal, E. T., Bernhisel, R., Brown, K., Kidd, J., & Manley, S. (2017). Clinical testing with a panel of 25 genes associated with increased cancer risk results in a significant increase in clinically significant findings across a broad range of cancer histories. *Cancer Genetics, 218–219*(Suppl. C), 58–68. https://doi.org/10.1016/j.cancergen.2017.09.003

Ryan, N. A. J., Glaire, M. A., Blake, D., Cabrera-Dandy, M., Evans, D. G., & Crosbie, E. J. (2019). The proportion of endometrial cancers associated with Lynch syndrome: A systematic review of the literature and meta-analysis. *Genetics in Medicine, 21*(10), 2167–2180. https://doi.org/10.1038/s41436-019-0536-8

Sarantou, T., Rabinowitz, B., Baron, P., Boudreaux, C., Chagpar, A., Connolly, J., Dietz, J., Everett, J. N., Fischer-Cartlidge, E., Heckel, T., Kurtzman, S., Laidley, A., Lee, C., O'Regan, R., Rosenberg, R., Smetherman, D., Weissman, S., & Winchester, D. J. (2017). *National accreditation program for Breast Centers Standards Manual 2018 edition*. American College of Surgeons.

Schimke, R. N., Hartmann, W. H., Prout, T. E., & Rimoin, D. L. (1968). Syndrome of bilateral pheochromocytoma, medullary thyroid carcinoma and multiple neuromas. *New England Journal of Medicine, 279*(1), 1–7. https://doi.org/10.1056/nejm196807042790101

Schmidlen, T., Schwartz, M., DiLoreto, K., Kirchner, H. L., & Sturm, A. C. (2019). Patient assessment of chatbots for the scalable delivery of genetic counseling. *Journal of Genetic Counseling, 28*(6), 1166–1177. https://doi.org/10.1002/jgc4.1169

Schmidlen, T., Sturm, A. C., Hovick, S., Scheinfeldt, L., Scott Roberts, J., Morr, L., McElroy, J., Toland, A. E., Christman, M., O'Daniel, J. M., Gordon, E. S., Bernhardt, B. A., Ormond, K. E., & Sweet, K. (2018). Operationalizing the reciprocal engagement model of genetic counseling practice: A framework for the scalable delivery of genomic counseling and testing. *Journal of Genetic Counseling, 27*(5), 1111–1129. https://doi.org/10.1007/s10897-018-0230-z

Schmidt, L. S. (2013). Birt-Hogg-Dubé syndrome: From gene discovery to molecularly targeted therapies. *Familial Cancer, 12*(3), 357–364. https://doi.org/10.1007/s10689-012-9574-y

Schmidt, M. K., Hogervorst, F., van Hien, R., Cornelissen, S., Broeks, A., Adank, M. A., Meijers, H., Waisfisz, Q., Hollestelle, A., Schutte, M., van den Ouweland, A., Hooning, M., Andrulis, I. L., Anton-Culver, H., Antonenkova, N. N., Antoniou, A. C., Arndt, V., Bermisheva, M., Bogdanova, N. V., . . . Easton, D. F. (2016). Age- and tumor subtype–specific breast cancer risk estimates for CHEK2*1100delC carriers. *Journal of Clinical Oncology, 34*(23), 2750–2760. https://doi.org/10.1200/jco.2016.66.5844

Schwiter, R., Rahm, A. K., Williams, J. L., & Sturm, A. C. (2018). How can we reach at-risk relatives? Efforts to enhance communication and cascade testing uptake: A mini-review. *Current Genetic Medicine Reports, 6*(2), 21–27. https://doi.org/10.1007/s40142-018-0134-0

Scollon, S., Anglin, A. K., Thomas, M., Turner, J. T., & Wolfe Schneider, K. (2017). A comprehensive review of pediatric tumors and associated cancer predisposition syndromes. *Journal of Genetic Counseling, 26*(3), 387–434. https://doi.org/10.1007/s10897-017-0077-8

Senter, L., O'Malley, D. M., Backes, F. J., Copeland, L. J., Fowler, J. M., Salani, R., & Cohn, D. E. (2017). Genetic consultation embedded in a gynecologic oncology clinic improves compliance with guideline-based care. *Gynecologic Oncology, 147*(1), 110–114. https://doi.org/10.1016/j.ygyno.2017.07.141

Shin, S. J., Dodd-Eaton, E. B., Peng, G., Bojadzieva, J., Chen, J., Amos, C. I., Frone, M. N., Khincha, P. P., Mai, P. L., Savage, S. A., Ballinger, M. L., Thomas, D. M., Yuan, Y., Strong, L. C., & Wang, W. (2020). Penetrance of different cancer types in families with Li-Fraumeni syndrome: A validation study using multicenter cohorts. *Cancer Research*, *80*(2), 354–360. https://doi.org/10.1158/0008-5472.Can-19-0728

Singer, C. F., Balmana, J., Burki, N., Delaloge, S., Filieri, M. E., Gerdes, A. M., Grindedal, E. M., Han, S., Johansson, O., Kaufman, B., Krajc, M., Loman, N., Olah, E., Paluch-Shimon, S., Plavetic, N. D., Pohlodek, K., Rhiem, K., Teixeira, M., & Evans, D. G. (2018). Genetic counselling and testing of susceptibility genes for therapeutic decision-making in breast cancer—An European consensus statement and expert recommendations. *European Journal of Cancer*, *106*, 54–60. https://doi.org/10.1016/j.ejca.2018.10.007

Singh, A. P., Shum, E., Rajdev, L., Cheng, H., Goel, S., Perez-Soler, R., & Halmos, B. (2020). Impact and diagnostic gaps of comprehensive genomic profiling in real-world clinical practice. *Cancers (Basel)*, *12*(5), 1156. https://doi.org/10.3390/cancers12051156

Sokolenko, A. P., Bogdanova, N., Kluzniak, W., Preobrazhenskaya, E. V., Kuligina, E. S., Iyevleva, A. G., Aleksakhina, S. N., Mitiushkina, N. V., Gorodnova, T. V., Bessonov, A. A., Togo, A. V., Lubinski, J., Cybulski, C., Jakubowska, A., Dork, T., & Imyanitov, E. N. (2014). Double heterozygotes among breast cancer patients analyzed for BRCA1, CHEK2, ATM, NBN/NBS1, and BLM germ-line mutations. *Breast Cancer Research and Treatment*, *145*(2), 553–562. https://doi.org/10.1007/s10549-014-2971-1

Stefansdottir, V., Skirton, H., Johannsson, O. T., Olafsdottir, H., Olafsdottir, G. H., Tryggvadottir, L., & Jonsson, J. J. (2019). Electronically ascertained extended pedigrees in breast cancer genetic counseling. *Familial Cancer*, *18*(2), 153–160. https://doi.org/10.1007/s10689-018-0105-3

Stewart, D. R., Best, A. F., Williams, G. M., Harney, L. A., Carr, A. G., Harris, A. K., Kratz, C. P., Dehner, L. P., Messinger, Y. H., Rosenberg, P. S., Hill, D. A., & Schultz, K. A. P. (2019). Neoplasm risk among individuals with a pathogenic germline variant in DICER1. *Journal of Clinical Oncology*, *37*(8), 668–676. https://doi.org/10.1200/jco.2018.78.4678

Stoll, J., Rosenthal, E., Cummings, S., Willmott, J., Bernhisel, R., & Kupfer, S. S. (2020). No evidence of increased risk of breast cancer in women with Lynch syndrome identified by multigene panel testing. *JCO Precision Oncology*, *4*, 51–60. https://doi.org/10.1200/po.19.00271

Stoll, K., Kubendran, S., & Cohen, S. A. (2018). The past, present and future of service delivery in genetic counseling: Keeping up in the era of precision medicine. *American Journal of Medical Genetics. Part C Seminars in Medical Genetics*, *178*(1), 24–37. https://doi.org/10.1002/ajmg.c.31602

Sutcliffe, E. G., Bartenbaker Thompson, A., Stettner, A. R., Marshall, M. L., Roberts, M. E., Susswein, L. R., Wang, Y., Klein, R. T., Hruska, K. S., & Solomon, B. D. (2019). Multi-gene panel testing confirms phenotypic variability in MUTYH-Associated Polyposis. *Familial Cancer*, *18*(2), 203–209. https://doi.org/10.1007/s10689-018-00116-2

Syngal, S., Brand, R. E., Church, J. M., Giardiello, F. M., Hampel, H. L., & Burt, R. W. (2015). ACG clinical guideline: Genetic testing and management of hereditary gastrointestinal cancer syndromes. *American Journal of Gastroenterology*, *110*(2), 223–262. https://doi.org/10.1038/ajg.2014.435

Tercyak, K. P., Bronheim, S. M., Kahn, N., Robertson, H. A., Anthony, B. J., Mays, D., O'Neill, S. C., Peterson, S. K., Miesfeldt, S., Peshkin, B. N., & DeMarco, T. A. (2019). Cancer genetic health communication in families tested for hereditary breast/ovarian cancer risk: A qualitative investigation of impact on children's genetic health literacy and psychosocial adjustment. *Translational Behavioral Medicine*, *9*(3), 493–503. https://doi.org/10.1093/tbm/ibz012

Thavaneswaran, S., Rath, E., Tucker, K., Joshua, A. M., Hess, D., Pinese, M., Ballinger, M. L., & Thomas, D. M. (2019). Therapeutic implications of germline genetic findings in cancer. *Nature Reviews Clinical Oncology*, *16*(6), 386–396. https://doi.org/10.1038/s41571-019-0179-3

Thiffault, I., Hamel, N., Pal, T., McVety, S., Marcus, V. A., Farber, D., Cowie, S., Deschênes, J., Meschino, W., Odefrey, F., Goldgar, D., Graham, T., Narod, S., Watters, A. K., MacNamara, E., Du Sart, D., Chong, G., & Foulkes, W. D. (2004). Germline truncating mutations in both MSH2 and BRCA2 in a single kindred. *British Journal of Cancer*, *90*(2), 483–491. https://doi.org/10.1038/sj.bjc.6601424

Torre, D. (1968). Multiple sebaceous tumors. *Archives of Dermatology*, *98*(5), 549–551.

Tsaousis, G. N., Papadopoulou, E., Apessos, A., Agiannitopoulos, K., Pepe, G., Kampouri, S., Diamantopoulos, N., Floros, T., Iosifidou, R., Katopodi, O., Koumarianou, A., Markopoulos, C., Papazisis, K., Venizelos, V., Xanthakis, I., Xepapadakis, G., Banu, E., Eniu, D. T., Negru, S., . . . Nasioulas, G. (2019). Analysis of hereditary cancer syndromes by using a panel of genes: Novel and multiple pathogenic mutations. *BMC Cancer*, *19*(1), 535. https://doi.org/10.1186/s12885-019-5756-4

Tung, N. M., Boughey, J. C., Pierce, L. J., Robson, M. E., Bedrosian, I., Dietz, J. R., Dragun, A., Gelpi, J. B., Hofstatter, E. W., Isaacs, C. J., Jatoi, I., Kennedy, E., Litton, J. K., Mayr, N. A., Qamar, R. D., Trombetta, M. G., Harvey, B. E., Somerfield, M. R., & Zakalik, D. (2020). Management of hereditary breast cancer: American Society of Clinical Oncology, American Society for Radiation Oncology, and Society of Surgical Oncology guideline. *Journal of Clinical Oncology*, *38*(18), 2080–2106. https://doi.org/10.1200/jco.20.00299

van Os, N. J., Roeleveld, N., Weemaes, C. M., Jongmans, M. C., Janssens, G. O., Taylor, A. M., Hoogerbrugge, N., & Willemsen, M. A. (2016). Health risks for ataxia-telangiectasia mutated heterozygotes: A systematic review, meta-analysis and evidence-based guideline. *Clinical Genetics*, *90*(2), 105–117. https://doi.org/10.1111/cge.12710

Vasen, H. F., Ghorbanoghli, Z., Bourdeaut, F., Cabaret, O., Caron, O., Duval, A., Entz-Werle, N., Goldberg, Y., Ilencikova, D., Kratz, C. P., Lavoine, N., Loeffen, J., Menko, F. H., Muleris, M., Sebille, G., Colas, C., Burkhardt, B., Brugieres, L., Wimmer, K., & EU-Consortium Care for CMMR-D (C4CMMR-D). (2014). Guidelines for surveillance of individuals with constitutional mismatch repair-deficiency proposed by the European Consortium "Care for CMMR-D" (C4CMMR-D). *Journal of Medical Genetics*, *51*(5), 283–293. https://doi.org/10.1136/jmedgenet-2013-102238

Warthin, A. S. (1913). Heredity with reference to carcinoma: As shown by the study of the cases examined in the pathological laboratory of the University of Michigan, 1895–1913. *Archives of Internal Medicine*, *12*(5), 546–555.

Watson, C. H., Ulm, M., Blackburn, P., Smiley, L., Reed, M., Covington, R., Bokovitz, L., & Tillmanns, T. (2016). Video-assisted genetic counseling in patients with ovarian, fallopian and peritoneal carcinoma. *Gynecologic Oncology*, *143*(1), 109–112. https://doi.org/10.1016/j.ygyno.2016.07.094

Welch, B. M., Wiley, K., Pflieger, L., Achiangia, R., Baker, K., Hughes-Halbert, C., Morrison, H., Schiffman, J., & Doerr, M. (2018). Review and comparison of electronic patient-facing family health history tools. *Journal of Genetic Counseling*, *27*(2), 381–391. https://doi.org/10.1007/s10897-018-0235-7

Wells, S. A., Jr., Asa, S. L., Dralle, H., Elisei, R., Evans, D. B., Gagel, R. F., Lee, N., Machens, A., Moley, J. F., Pacini, F., Raue, F., Frank-Raue, K., Robinson, B., Rosenthal, M. S., Santoro, M., Schlumberger, M., Shah, M., Waguespack, S. G., & American Thyroid Association Guidelines Task Force on Medullary Thyroid Carcinoma. (2015). Revised American Thyroid Association guidelines for the management of medullary thyroid carcinoma. *Thyroid*, *25*(6), 567–610. https://doi.org/10.1089/thy.2014.0335

Whiteman, D. C., & Wilson, L. F. (2016). The fractions of cancer attributable to modifiable factors: A global review. *Cancer Epidemiology*, *44*, 203–221. https://doi.org/10.1016/j.canep.2016.06.013

Wimmer, K., Kratz, C. P., Vasen, H. F., Caron, O., Colas, C., Entz-Werle, N., Gerdes, A. M., Goldberg, Y., Ilencikova, D., Muleris, M., Duval, A., Lavoine, N., Ruiz-Ponte, C., Slavc, I., Burkhardt, B., Brugieres, L., & EU Corsorium Care for CMMRD. (2014). Diagnostic criteria for constitutional mismatch repair deficiency syndrome: Suggestions of the European consortium 'care for CMMRD' (C4CMMRD). *Journal of Medical Genetics*, *51*(6), 355–365. https://doi.org/10.1136/jmedgenet-2014-102284

Win, A., Lindor, N., & Jenkins, M. (2013). Risk of breast cancer in Lynch syndrome: A systematic review. *Breast Cancer Research*, *15*(2), R27.

Xicola, R. M., Li, S., Rodriguez, N., Reinecke, P., Karam, R., Speare, V., Lopez-Giraldez, F., Choi, J., Emmadi, R., Alagiozian-Angelova, V., Kupfer, S. S., Ellis, N. A., & Llor, X. (2019). Clinical features and cancer risk in families with pathogenic CDH1 variants irrespective of clinical criteria. *Journal of Medical Genetics*, *56*(12), 838–843. https://doi.org/10.1136/jmedgenet-2019-105991

Yang, X., Leslie, G., Doroszuk, A., Schneider, S., Allen, J., Decker, B., Dunning, A. M., Redman, J., Scarth, J., Plaskocinska, I., Luccarini, C., Shah, M., Pooley, K., Dorling, L., Lee, A., Adank, M. A., Adlard, J., Aittomaki, K., Andrulis, I. L., . . . Tischkowitz, M. (2020). Cancer risks associated with germline PALB2 pathogenic variants: An international study of 524 families. *Journal of Clinical Oncology*, *38*(7), 674–685. https://doi.org/10.1200/jco.19.01907

Yang, X., Song, H., Leslie, G., Engel, C., Hahnen, E., Auber, B., Horvath, J., Kast, K., Niederacher, D., Turnbull, C., Houlston, R., Hanson, H., Loveday, C., Dolinsky, J. S., LaDuca, H., Ramus, S. J., Menon, U., Rosenthal, A. N., Jacobs, I., . . . Antoniou, A. C. (2020). Ovarian and breast cancer risks associated with pathogenic variants in RAD51C and RAD51D. *Journal of the National Cancer Institute*, *112*(12), 1242–1250. https://doi.org/10.1093/jnci/djaa030

Yen, T., Stanich, P. P., Axell, L., & Patel, S. G. (1998). APC-Associated Polyposis Conditions. In M. P. Adam, H. H. Ardinger, R. A. Pagon, S. E. Wallace, L. J. H. Bean, K. Stephens, & A. Amemiya (Eds.), *GeneReviews®* [Internet]. University of Washington, Seattle. https://www.ncbi.nlm.nih.gov/books/NBK1345/

Young, A. L., Butow, P. N., Tucker, K. M., Wakefield, C. E., Healey, E., & Williams, R. (2020). When to break the news and whose responsibility is it? A cross-sectional qualitative study of health professionals' views regarding disclosure of BRCA genetic cancer risk. *BMJ Open*, *10*(2), e033127–e033127. https://doi.org/10.1136/bmjopen-2019-033127

Young, E. L., Thompson, B. A., Neklason, D. W., Firpo, M. A., Werner, T., Bell, R., Berger, J., Fraser, A., Gammon, A., Koptiuch, C., Kohlmann, W. K., Neumayer, L., Goldgar, D. E., Mulvihill, S. J., Cannon-Albright, L. A., & Tavtigian, S. V. (2018). Pancreatic cancer as a sentinel for hereditary cancer predisposition. *BMC Cancer*, *18*(1), 697. https://doi.org/10.1186/s12885-018-4573-5.

Yurgelun, M. B., & Hampel, H. (2018). Recent advances in Lynch syndrome: Diagnosis, treatment, and cancer prevention. *American Society of Clinical Oncology Educational Book*, *38*, 101–109. https://doi.org/10.1200/edbk_208341

Yurgelun, M. B., Kulke, M. H., Fuchs, C. S., Allen, B. A., Uno, H., Hornick, J. L., Ukaegbu, C. I., Brais, L. K., McNamara, P. G., Mayer, R. J., Schrag, D., Meyerhardt, J. A., Ng, K., Kidd, J., Singh, N., Hartman, A. R., Wenstrup, R. J., & Syngal, S. (2017). Cancer susceptibility gene mutations in individuals with colorectal cancer. *Journal of Clinical Oncology*, 35(10), 1086–1095. https://doi.org/10.1200/jco.2016.71.0012

CHAPTER 10

SPECIALIZATION AND SUBSPECIALIZATION IN GENETIC COUNSELING

Trends and Drivers

CATHERINE A. WICKLUND AND
ANGELA M. TREPANIER

Introduction

Genetic counselors increasingly work in a variety of settings and in a range of roles. While most genetic counselors were employed in prenatal, pediatric, and general genetics settings in primarily clinical roles when the profession was first established, they now work in a wide array of direct and nondirect patient care subspecialties. In contrast to physicians, who must complete a fellowship and/or residency to practice in a specific area of medicine, genetic counselors are trained as generalists and can currently practice in any specialty. As a result, there is not a clear distinction between specialization and subspecialization for genetic counselors. For the purposes of this chapter, we are using the terms interchangeably to describe the various specialty areas within which genetic counselors work. In addition, this chapter is mainly written through a North American lens. It is important to recognize that specialization trends may vary from country to country. There are several drivers that propelled genetic counselors into new roles and settings, including a highly transferrable skill set, the rapid evolution of genomic technologies, institutional needs, personal motivations, and sometimes just serendipity (Davis et al., 2020).

Evolution of Subspecialization

The first genetic counseling training program was established in 1969 by Melissa Richter at Sarah Lawrence College in Bronxville, New York. The impetus for training genetic associates, as they were originally called, was to help geneticists meet the growing demand for genetics services (Marks & Richter, 1976). In the early days of the profession, genetic counselors largely trained and worked in the pediatric genetics setting (Baty, 2018). Genetic counselors worked closely with medical geneticists and played a key role in educating and supporting families who had a child with a suspected genetic condition. For those families in which a diagnosis was made, the focus of these sessions was often on an assessment of the pedigree and recurrence risks based on Mendelian probabilities. In the absence of a diagnosis, pedigree assessment to provide a recurrence risk estimate was standard (Corson & Bernhardt, 2021; Stern, 2009).

During the late 1960s and early 1970s, prenatal testing procedures such as amniocentesis became available and diagnostic testing through karyotype analysis and genetic or biochemical tests expanded. These developments created an opportunity for genetic counselors to work in reproductive genetics. The number of amniocenteses performed from 1967 to 1971 in the United States was extremely limited due to the lack of information regarding the safety of the procedure. However, once further research demonstrated the relative safety of amniocentesis and accuracy of genetic testing, the number of procedures performed in the United States increased significantly (Stern, 2009). Concurrently, the number of genetic counselors working in prenatal settings increased as well. Whereas genetic counselors primarily worked with medical geneticists in pediatric genetics clinics, they began to work closely with obstetricians and maternal fetal medicine specialists in prenatal settings (Cohen, 2020; National Society of Genetic Counselors [NSGC] Professional Status Survey [PSS], 1980–2002).

Subspecialization gained traction in pediatric settings as genetic counselors branched out to work in specialty clinics and/or on multidisciplinary teams in addition to their work in general genetics clinics. Subspecialties included but were not limited to connective tissue disorders, bone dysplasias, craniofacial disorders, and neurocutaneous syndromes. The subspecialty clinics were staffed by either medical geneticists and genetic counselors or genetic counselors working closely with nongenetics specialists such as cardiologists and dermatologists. In some respects, these early experiences were reflective of what was to come—genetic counselors not only working with medical geneticists but also working independently with other specialized healthcare providers (NSGC PSS, 1980–2002; NSGC PSS, 2022).

In the early 1990s a new specialty joined the mix of prenatal and pediatric genetic counseling services—cancer genetics. Cancer genetic counseling gained momentum around the time the *BRCA1* gene was identified as a cause of hereditary breast and ovarian cancer (Futreal et al., 1994; Miki et al., 1994). A 1994 survey of NSGC members who indicated an interest in cancer genetic counseling showed that a majority had been providing the service for less than 2 years (Schneider & Marnane, 1997). Further, most had not received adequate training in cancer genetic counseling in their graduate programs given the limited information available. As such, genetic counselors gained cancer genetics knowledge through reading the medical literature and attending continuing education sessions at their professional conferences (Schneider & Marnane, 1997).

The development of cancer genetic counseling as a specialty provides an excellent example of how genetic counselors and the professional organizations that support them adapt and thrive in the changing landscape of genetic and genomic technology. Whereas early cancer genetic counselors largely had to educate themselves, didactic education and internships in cancer genetics are now required components of genetic counseling student training (Accreditation Council for Genetic Counseling [ACGC], 2023b), at least in some parts of the world. Content on cancer genetics is included on board certification exams such as the American Board of Genetic Counseling exam. Genetic counselor professional organizations provide extensive cancer genetics education at their annual conferences. Through special interest groups, cancer genetic counselors keep each other up to date on best practices. Genetic counselors have written books about cancer genetic counseling (Schneider, 2012), developed genetic counselor practice guidelines and practice resources (Berliner & Fay, 2007; Berliner et al., 2012; Riley et al., 2011; Trepanier et al., 2004), and participated in multidisciplinary groups developing guidelines for the use of cancer genetics services (Hampel et al., 2015). In other words, genetic counselors went from novices in cancer genetics to experts in a relatively short period of time.

When asked to designate all their areas of practice, cancer genetic counseling was the most common among genetic counselors in the United States and Canada, with 42% of respondents to the 2022 NSGC PSS selecting cancer genetics (adults; NSGC PSS, 2022). It is important to note, however, that the availability of cancer genetic counseling services varies by country. Factors such as having a limited number of genetic counselors and needing to provide other, more high-priority genetics services impact the extent to which these services are available worldwide (Laurino et al., 2018).

While pediatric, prenatal, and cancer genetics remain the three largest areas of practice in the United States and Canada, genetic counselors have branched out into numerous other specialty areas in both direct and nondirect patient care settings. Even during the very early years of the profession, genetic counselors began taking on roles outside of clinical settings. In 1985, an ad hoc committee was appointed to explore how genetic counselors were applying their skills in ways that were not originally anticipated when the field was established (Heimler, 1997). The role of the laboratory genetic counselor is one example. Due to increasing numbers of genetic testing options, many laboratories recognized the value of employing a genetic counselor to serve as a liaison between the laboratory and the ordering healthcare provider. The NSGC PSS included diagnostic laboratory as a work setting as early as 2000. Since that time, the PSS has added additional details and changed terminology regarding laboratory work settings, reflecting the evolving landscape of laboratory-related positions. These changes have made it difficult to track growth in laboratory positions longitudinally; however, looking broadly at this category, the number of genetic counselors who reported working in a diagnostic laboratory has grown from 5% in 2000 to 20% in 2022 (NSGC PSS, 1980–2002; NSGC PSS, 2022).

The trend toward specialization and subspecialization continues as the profession evolves. In the 2000 NSGC PSS, the most common specialties/subspecialties were prenatal (60%), pediatric (39%), cancer (34%), adult (26%), multiple marker screening (22%), teratogens (20%), and specialty disease (17%). Other practice areas included molecular, biochemical, and cytogenetic testing (12%); neurogenetics (7%); public health/newborn screening (6%); infertility/in vitro fertilization/assisted reproductive technology (6%); and psychiatric genetic counseling (1%). Emerging roles in genetic counseling over the last two decades include cardiology, precision oncology, pediatric arrhythmias, and pediatric oncology (Desrosiers et al., 2019; Everett et al., 2014, Helm et al., 2018, Ingles et al., 2011;

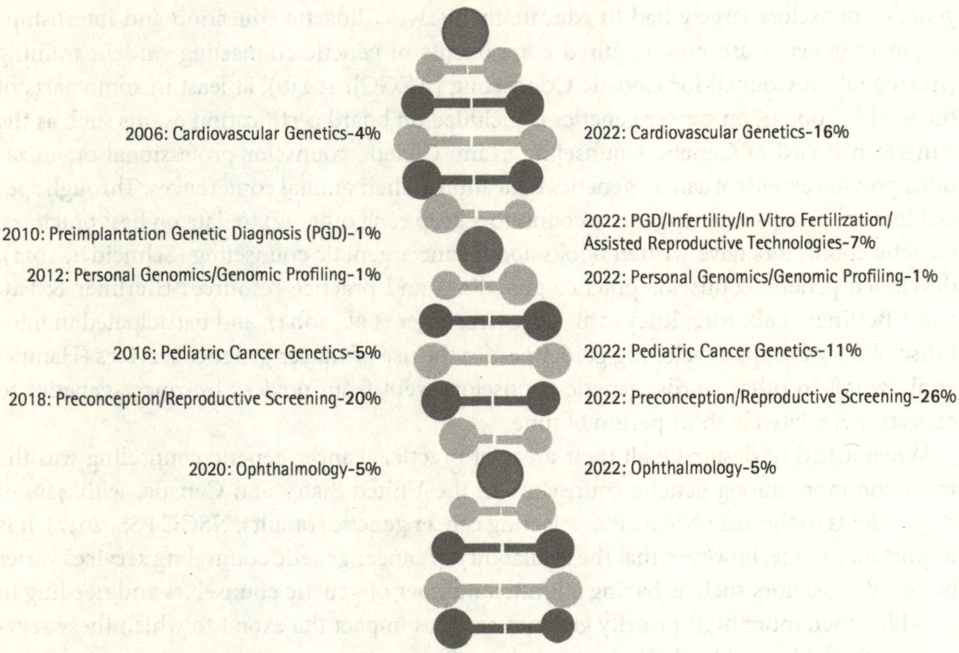

FIGURE 10.1 Emergence and growth of select subspecialties per the NSGC Professional Status Surveys. Percentages reflect the proportion of respondents who indicated they practice in the subspecialty when asked to denote all areas of practice (versus primary area of practice).

Powell et al., 2010). These changes and others are reflected in the NSGC PSSs, as described briefly below and in Figure 10.1 (NSGC PSS, 1980–2002; NSGC PSS 2006, 2008; NSGC PSS, 2010, 2012, 2014, 2016; NSGC PSS, 2018, 2019, 2020, 2021, 2022).

There have been changes in laboratory positions over time, but it is hard to quantify these in terms of practice areas since some of the designations have changed. For instance, molecular/cytogenetics/biochemical testing was redesignated as laboratory science/variant interpretation in 2022. An area called laboratory was added in 2010 and then changed to laboratory operations in 2018. Many other new areas have been added and at times removed from the NSGC PSSs. Examples include genomic medicine, population-based/biobanking, pharmacogenomics, research, administration, public policy, and education (public or professional).

As of 2022, most PSS respondents reported their primary area of practice as either adult cancer, prenatal, or pediatric genetics at 32%, 18%, and 13%, respectively; 37% of respondents indicated that their primary area of practice is outside of these common practice areas (NSGC PSS, 2022). Other subspecialties not designated in the PSSs but reported in a study by Haverbusch et al. (2019) include pulmonology/cystic fibrosis, autism, craniofacial genetics, gastroenterology, exome sequencing, disorders of sex development, neurofibromatosis, and skeletal dysplasias. Participants of this study also reported that they worked within a broader specialty such as pediatrics, cancer, and prenatal. This implies that while some genetic counselors spend all their time in one subspecialty, others work in a broader specialty and spend some of their clinical time in a subspecialized setting (Haverbusch et al., 2019). While the NSGC PSS is a good resource for tracking and documenting the evolution of specialties and subspecialties, it has limitations, and clear timelines for the emergence of each subspecialty do not exist. Furthermore, the NSGC PSSs primarily capture responses from genetic counselors in the United States and Canada and as such do not provide a global perspective of the practice of genetic counseling. Nonetheless, the PSSs and the literature give a broad view of how genetic counseling practice areas have expanded over time.

Drivers of Subspecialization

What has led to the tremendous growth of subspecialization in genetic counseling? Below are some key factors that have fueled this trend.

Training and core skills

Genetic counselors are trained to develop core competencies in seven areas: genetics and genomics expertise, risk assessment, counseling, communication, research, healthcare systems, and professional identity, as described by the ACGC Practice-Based Competencies for Genetic Counselors (ACGC, 2023a) and reflected in other genetic counselor training standard documents including the Canadian Association of Genetic Counsellors (2012) Practice-Based Competencies for Canadian Genetic Counsellors; the European Board of Medical Genetics (2010) Professional and Educational Standards for Genetic Counsellors in Europe; and the Human Genetics Society of Australasia (2022) Competency Standards for Genetic Counsellors. Through coursework and experiential learning, genetic counselor trainees gain expertise in recognizing a broad range of genetic and genomic conditions; collecting robust, targeted family and personal medical histories; assessing genetic risk; identifying and ordering appropriate genetic/genomic tests; providing case management; and critically evaluating the rapidly changing medical genomics literature. Genetic counselors are one of only a few professions (e.g., genetic nurses, physician geneticists, lab geneticists) with such extensive knowledge of medical genetics. Programs have had to adapt their training over time to integrate and reprioritize content to accommodate these growing practice areas. It is no longer feasible to provide trainees with didactic and experiential learning about all conditions, settings, and roles. However, the core knowledge, skills, and attitudes are transferable, preparing trainees to be generalists, capable of working in all areas of practice.

Training in education skills helps genetic counselors explain complex genetic information in ways that optimize patient understanding and promote patient use of the information to make decisions. Training includes instruction in topics such as health literacy, effective risk communication, and providing balanced information. In addition, genetic counselors are trained to communicate clinical and scientific material in a manner that makes the information accessible to individuals from a wide variety of educational backgrounds, ranging from lay audiences to medical professionals. Training in how to develop written educational materials such as brochures and website content, how to document clinical encounters for both patient and professional audiences, and how to give educational presentations to a broad range of audiences are typical and often required components of any ACGC-accredited genetic counseling program curriculum (ACGC, 2023b).

Training in interpersonal communication and psychosocial counseling skills provides genetic counselors the opportunity to assess and acknowledge the psychosocial impact of genetic information; identify patients' beliefs, values, and cultural traditions; facilitate informed and value-based decision making; and promote adaptation to genetic risk. Such skills are used to help patients identify and manage their thoughts and feelings related to genetic information, recognize and adhere to clinical management recommendations, identify and use support mechanisms, and share genetic risk information with their relatives and pertinent healthcare providers. The goal is to promote patient empowerment and adaptation and to maximize quality of life. The extent to which genetic counselors incorporate psychotherapeutic approaches versus a more education-oriented approach into practice varies from country to country (Ormond et al., 2018) and among genetic counselors themselves. However, mounting evidence suggests that utilizing psychotherapeutic techniques improves patient outcomes (Austin et al., 2014) and as such the value of genetic counseling. One important caveat to recognize when discussing patient empowerment is that this is a predominantly Western concept and may not be the goal in all cultural groups, such as those with a collectivist worldview.

The professional development and practice domain of genetic counseling training encompasses several different competencies. These include demonstrating ethical and legal conduct and recognizing potential conflicts of interest, conducting research and being able to identify research opportunities for patients, utilizing multiple service delivery models, identifying and providing support resources for patients and families, and serving as an advocate on a larger scale for issues that impact those with genetic conditions or risk. Genetic counselors are also trained to utilize evidence-based practice, to understand how healthcare systems operate, to recognize their role in the bigger healthcare team and work effectively with other providers, to help other providers integrate genetics into practice, and to promote the responsible use of genetics technologies (ACGC, 2023a; Canadian Association of Genetic Counselors, 2012; Human Genetics Society of Australasia, 2022).

It is this unique combination of knowledge and skills in genetics expertise, education, communication, psychosocial assessment and counseling, ethical–legal aspects of clinical genetics, evidence-based practice, healthcare systems, advocacy, service delivery models, research, and interprofessional collaboration that has paved the way for genetic counselor subspecialization. For instance, Davis et al. (2020) conducted a study of genetic counselors who had sought advanced training, either informally or formally, to advance their careers. The results showed that individuals' past experiences in genetic counseling training, clinical work, and volunteering, combined with their personal attributes (reflective practice, desire for change/novelty) and contextual factors such as trends in medicine and new job opportunities, facilitated their overall career development. Some sought advanced degrees, but many were able to change the focus of their careers (e.g., practice area, work environment) based on the attributes mentioned above and informal training such as continuing education (Davis et al., 2020).

The fact that genetic counselors are trained as generalists helps them be able to change specialties/subspecialties. Training involves didactic content and experiential learning in a broad array of genetics specialties including but not limited to reproductive, cancer, cardiovascular, pediatric, and adult genetics as well as neurogenetics, public health genomics, and genetics laboratories. Upon graduation, genetic counselors can practice in any of these settings and can readily transition between specialties without additional formal training or certification. In fact, most genetic counselors work in more than one practice area. In 2022, only 40% of genetic counselors (all position types) reported working in one practice area in their current position (NSGC PSS, 2022). About one-quarter (26%) reported working in two practice areas; 15% and 19% reported working in three and four or more practice areas, respectively (NSGC PSS, 2022). This ability to work in multiple practice areas and theoretically move from specialty to specialty over the course of a career is likely one of the factors that has allowed broad and rapid subspecialization in genetic counseling. However, it is possible that genetic counselors may be able to move with greater ease from one specialty to another based on work experience and the other aforementioned personal attributes (Davis et al., 2020).

Technological advances

With the completion of the Human Genome Project in 2003, a genetic blueprint for human beings became available to provide insight into the structure, organization, and function of genes. This publicly available tool was widely disseminated to scientists and physicians to utilize in their research to advance testing, diagnoses, and, importantly, prevention and treatment. Scientists are now able to sequence genes directly to look for variations that may cause disease, while in the past they relied heavily on linkage analysis as a means for locating and identifying a gene that may play a role in the condition in question. This, coupled with the development of massively parallel sequencing developed by Lynx Therapeutics in 2000, accelerated the discovery of disease-causing genes, and in 2004 several companies launched second- and third-generation sequencing platforms (Durmaz et al., 2015). As a result of this technology, gene discovery accelerated at a rapid pace, with almost 80,000 genetic tests available in 2023 compared to just 25,000 in 2014 (National Library of Medicine, n.d.).

Subspecialization in genetic counseling, as in medicine (Oren et al., 2020), is driven in large part by advances in scientific knowledge, technology, and subsequent clinical applications. For instance, as mentioned previously, cancer genetic counseling emerged as a genetic counseling specialty in the early 1990s, around the time the *BRCA1* gene was identified as a cause of hereditary breast and ovarian cancer (Futreal et al., 1994; Miki et al., 1994). Similarly, the emergence of cardiovascular genetic counseling, which was included as a subspecialty for the first time in the 2006 NSGC PSS, coincided with the availability of genetic testing for inherited cardiovascular diseases (Moscarello & Caleshu, 2019; NSGC PSS, 2006). As the number of cardiovascular genetic tests increased, so did the proportion of genetic counselors who provide services in this subspecialty (Moscarello & Caleshu, 2019). Other clinical subspecialties that emerged as a result of advances in genomics include genomic medicine (2008), pharmacogenetics (2008), preimplantation genetic diagnosis (2010), and personal genomics/genomic profiling (2012; NSGC PSS, 2008; NSGC PSS, 2010, 2012; Figure 10.1).

Technological advances may impact the emergence and practice of a subspecialty but do not always result in its growth, as is the case with neurogenetics. Neurogenetics has been denoted as a genetic counseling subspecialty since the first PSSs were administered in the

1980s and 1990s (NSGC PSS, 1980–2002). However, according to the 2021 NSGC PSS, only 2% of genetic counselors reported neurogenetics as their primary area of practice, and 11% reported that their practice involved some neurogenetics, demonstrating a stable trend over the last three decades (NSGC PSS, 2021). Genetic testing has expanded tremendously in neurology from single gene tests and karyotyping to chromosomal microarrays, multigene panels, and exome and genome sequencing. Indications have expanded from testing for well-delineated single gene or chromosomal disorders to identifying the etiology of a wide array of movement, seizure, autism spectrum, and polyneuropathy disorders as well as conditions associated with dementia.

Why has the proportion of genetic counselors working in neurogenetics not grown in response? It may be that genetic testing can be and has been successfully implemented in general neurology clinics such that genetic counselors are only consulted when a patient has a complicated result (e.g., variant of uncertain significance) or a positive result warranting consideration of familial testing (Bardakjian et al., 2018). Given the limited number of genetic counselors, this type of model has the potential to improve patient access to genetic testing and to genetic counselors when needed. Or it may be that requests for neurogenetic counseling and testing are still seen through general pediatric or adult genetics services rather than separate neurogenetics specialty clinics. Such a possibility is consistent with findings that genetic counselors are about five times more likely to indicate that they work with neurogenetics patients than to designate neurogenetics as their primary specialty (NSGC PSS, 2021).

Policy change

Policy change has also led to the growth of certain genetic counselor subspecialties. For example, in 2012, the Commission on Cancer (CoC) of the American College of Surgeons established a new cancer genetics risk assessment and genetic counseling standard for CoC-accredited sites. The standard required that patients have access to genetic counseling services onsite or by referral and that they be provided by a qualified genetics professional such as a genetic counselor (Vogel & Weissman, 2012). According to the NSGC PSSs, the proportion of clinical genetic counselors who spent at least 50% of their time providing cancer genetics services increased from 26% in 2012 to 48% in 2016 (NSGC PSS, 2012, 2016).

Consumerism

Consumers are increasingly more aware of how genetics impacts their health and therefore also expect their providers to be knowledgeable about genetic testing. In parallel with the increased number of genetic tests, a new genetic service delivery model, called direct-to-consumer (DTC) testing, emerged in the mid-2000s (Allyse et al., 2018). DTC testing allows consumers to have direct access to genetic tests, bypassing the healthcare system and ordering providers. Initially these companies faced widespread criticism from the genetics community and subsequently drew attention from regulatory bodies in the United States, such as the Food and Drug Administration, the Federal Trade Commission, and the

Government Accountability Office. Since that time, DTC testing has evolved into a more hybrid model, with many companies having physicians who work either for them or at an outside physician network who can order the test and offer access to genetic counselors. In 2015, mainstream molecular diagnostic companies also began to enter this space and have subsequently coined the term "consumer-driven genomic testing" (CD-GT) to describe this type of testing.[1]

With both the increased number of available genetic tests and the development of DTC and CD-GT, there is even more pressure on nongenetics providers to become familiar with genetics and genomics. Physicians should be competent in ordering genetic tests and subsequently interpreting the results. This requires a deeper knowledge base of genetics and genomics to understand the analytical validity, clinical validity, and utility of the test. In addition, they must be confident in and comfortable with communicating information about testing and the implications of the test results with their patients. Unfortunately, it has been repeatedly reported that physicians are not confident in or comfortable with ordering and interpreting genetic tests (Ong et al., 2022). This has been exacerbated by the increasing number and complexity of genetic tests. Providers are also expected to make decisions regarding ordering a single gene, multigene panel, or exome/genome test. The degree to which medical genetics and genomics have been incorporated into medical education has varied over the years and remains highly dependent on the educational institution. While genetics education has been incorporated into most medical school curricula, the content, depth, and emphasis are not consistent (Haspel et al., 2021; Rubanovich et al., 2018). In addition, for those physicians who trained several decades ago, medical genetics may not have been incorporated at all. In some cases, this lack of confidence and knowledge in providers has led to more reliance on genetic counselors.

While one purpose of DTC testing and CD-GT is to bypass the healthcare system, they do offer multiple new opportunities for genetic counselors. Several genetic counselors were employed by these early DTC companies to help develop consumer-facing platforms, create education materials, and determine testing options. In addition, some companies offer the option of posttest counseling, which became more desirable as an optional service as DTC companies faced increased regulatory oversight. The landscape of DTC/CD-GT has evolved and further subspecialization has emerged, such as ancestry genetic counseling, providing additional opportunities for genetic counselors in this sector (Kirkpatrick & Rashkin, 2017).

Therapeutics and precision medicine

Historically, treatment for genetic disorders was generally lacking. However, there has been expanded use of genetic testing in multiple areas including precision therapeutics and pharmacology. While precision therapeutics has primarily been led by providers in pertinent specialties, genetic counselors became integrated in these areas when it became apparent

[1] Editors' note: For further discussion on DTC genetic testing and CD-GT, see Chapter 11 by Anne E. Greb in this volume.

that a deep knowledge of genetics/genomics was necessary to properly interpret and apply results. For example, genetic counselors became involved in tumor profiling for therapeutic purposes when it was realized that tumor sequencing results could identify potential risk for germline pathogenic variants as well.

Precision therapeutics is a relatively new specialty for genetic counselors. Early in the profession there were very few opportunities to provide treatment to individuals diagnosed with genetic conditions, except for metabolic disorders. While genetic counselors work with patients who have metabolic disorders, treatment decisions are primarily made by physician geneticists and nurses. With more and more opportunities for treatment based on genomic test results, training programs have integrated this new area of practice into their curriculum (Loudon et al., 2021). It has also put a new focus on genetic counselors' scope of practice and the line between interpreting genetic test results and decisions regarding treatment. Precision therapeutics has highlighted the continued importance of genetic counselor–physician collaborations and has re-emphasized the importance of informed consent when testing for somatic variants. It is still unknown how many genetic counselors will be integrated into this area of practice. Most likely, integration will depend on the individual genetic counselor's readiness and acceptance of this new role and institutional and individual provider needs.

Using genomic information to determine the right drug at the right dose for the right individual has been an area of growth for the past several years. The Clinical Pharmacogenomics Implementation Consortium was established to help providers understand how to optimize drug therapy. Currently there are multiple published guidelines (available at https://cpicpgx.org/). It has been noted that utilizing the skills of genetic counselors would be beneficial for the implementation of pharmacogenomics. However, very few genetic counselors work primarily in pharmacogenomics (NSGC PSS, 2022). Implementation of pharmacogenomics can happen in several ways, including physicians independently electing to order genetic testing to guide drug management and/or institutional precision medicine programs, which may also integrate other genetic testing such as variants in genes associated with hereditary conditions recommended by the American College of Medical Genetics and Genomics (Kalia et al., 2017). Depending on the setting, genetic counselors have been integral to the implementation of these large-scale initiatives and work directly with physicians, patients, and other providers who are potentially impacted by these results (Blout Zawatsky et al., 2022).

Other factors

Haverbusch et al. (2019) investigated factors that led to the development of new clinical subspecialties in genetic counseling. Specifically, clinical genetic counselors working in subspecialties were asked how the need for their subspecialty was identified and how positions were developed. Survey respondents worked in a broad array of subspecialties. About half provided cardiovascular genetics and neurogenetics services. Other specialties represented included assisted reproductive technologies, autism, craniofacial genetics, cystic fibrosis/pulmonology, disorders of sex development (DSDs), gastroenterology, hematology/hemoglobinopathies, metabolic genetics, neurofibromatosis, ophthalmologic genetics, pediatric oncology, skeletal dysplasias, and exome sequencing. Of note, according to the 2022 NSGC PSS Work Environment report, 3% and 2%, respectively, of genetic counselors working in direct patient care positions reported cardiovascular genetics and neurogenetics as their primary area of practice. In contrast, 1% or less denoted any of the other subspecialties as their primary area of practice. Some subspecialties (craniofacial genetics, cystic fibrosis/pulmonology, DSDs, gastroenterology, neurofibromatosis, and skeletal dysplasias) are not currently listed as subspecialties in the 2022 NSGC PSS (NSGC PSS, 2022).

Factors that led to the development of subspecialty positions included the availability of genetic tests (e.g., technological advances), physician interest, research funding, and/or institution-identified need for a genetic counselor. Additional factors included increased patient volumes, development of a new clinic, and genetic counselor–driven change (Haverbusch et al., 2019). Reasons that genetic counselors chose to move into subspecialty positions included having a particular interest or some experience in a specialty area, having a desire to be an expert in an area of practice, and/or wanting to have more autonomy (Haverbusch et al., 2019).

The above examples are most relevant in countries where the genetic counseling profession is well established. In some countries, the profession is in its infancy. As such, the emphasis necessarily must first be on developing a workforce to provide services rather than focusing on subspecialization (Cutiongco-de la Paz et al., 2019).

Challenges of Subspecialization

There are both pros and cons of specialization and subspecialization. Examples from physician practice show that the increased training and knowledge associated with subspecialization can lead to improved patient outcomes. However, there can be detrimental impacts associated with having a narrow focus of practice, especially when managing patients with a wide range of comorbidities (Oren et al., 2020). Overspecialization, defined as redundant or overlapping specialty areas, can lead to longer appointment wait times and reduced patient access to care (Oren et al., 2020). In addition, there can be a point where subspecialization leads to costlier patient care (Oren et al., 2020).

Penom-Portmann et al. (2020) investigated the genetics workforce in California and access to genetics services. They identified that workforce shortages and geographic barriers negatively impacted access to care. Furthermore, subspecialization may be compounding access issues in the state given that 27% of genetics providers are not practicing in clinical settings (Penom-Portmann et al., 2020).

It is particularly important to examine trends in subspecialization moving forward in the context of genome and exome sequencing. While technology has been a driver in subspecialization, genome and exome sequencing could impact the practice of genetic counseling in an alternate way. If sequencing is implemented on a population level, then the needs of individuals will be different from those who had testing for a specific indication (e.g., cardiac, cancer, or neurological risk). Results will most likely be given over a person's lifetime, necessitating access to pediatric, reproductive, and adult genetics care. The timing of services will depend on what is medically relevant at that point in a person's life. The expectation that an individual will need to see multiple different specialized genetic counselors depending on their test results may cause barriers to access and care. This could especially be a concern for individuals who live in rural areas (Penom-Portmann et al., 2020).

It is conceivable that genetic counselors may need to evolve (back) into generalists to be able to meet the needs of those who are receiving results that are not specific to symptoms and are receiving more than one result at a given time. This will also depend on geographical location, with those in urban areas having access to specialized genetic counselors and those in rural areas most likely not. The increasing acceptance of telehealth genetic counseling as an equally viable option to in-person genetic counseling may also impact how genome-based genetic counseling practice evolves. It is reasonable to anticipate that generalization and continued specialization will evolve in parallel, dependent on access, population demographics, and geographical location. Given this, it will be important to preserve genetic counselors' ability to practice as generalists and switch specialties, without burdensome requirements such as specialty credentialing and additional state regulatory oversight. While there is no evidence to suggest changing specialties causes patient harm, it will be important to monitor this as the field evolves.

Conclusion

Although early genetic counselors primarily worked in a handful of specialty areas, in the four decades that have ensued they have branched out into a multitude of specialties/subspecialties. Genetic counselors are trained as generalists with a highly transferrable skill set, which has enabled them to take on various new roles and expand their practice in multiple settings. As such, genetic counselors are uniquely positioned to practice in new specialties as genomic knowledge and its impact on health increase.

This chapter explored potential drivers of specialization such as advancing genomic technology with subsequent availability of genetic testing and treatment, institutional needs, and the personal motivations of the genetic counselor. As individual genetic counselors, whether we move toward subspecialization or generalization likely depends on the needs of a specific community. Factors like geographic access to services, the specific culture of the community being served, the comfort level of nongenetics providers in assessing genetic risk and ordering and interpreting genetic/genomic testing, and genetic counselor accessibility will all have an impact. As such, even as genetic counselors become more specialized, it is important that we maintain our generalist abilities to best meet the needs of the communities we serve and promote equitable access to the full scope of genomic medicine advances.

References

Accreditation Council for Genetic Counseling. (2023a). *Practice-based competencies for genetic counselors*. https://www.gceducation.org/wp-content/uploads/2023/12/ACGC_PracticeBasedCompetencies_2023.pdf

Accreditation Council for Genetic Counseling. (2023b). *Standards of accreditation for graduate programs in genetic counseling.* https://www.gceducation.org/wp-content/uploads/2023/11/ACGC_StandardsOfAccreditation_2023.pdf

Allyse, M. A., Robinson, D. H., Ferber, M. J., & Sharp, R. R. (2018). Direct-to-consumer testing 2.0: Emerging models of direct-to-consumer genetic testing. *Mayo Clinic Proceedings, 93*(1), 113–120. https://doi.org/10.1016/j.mayocp.2017.11.001

Austin, J. E., Semaka, A., & Hadjipavlou, G. (2014). Conceptualizing genetic counseling as psychotherapy in genomic medicine. *Journal of Genetic Counseling, 23*(6), 903–909. https://doi.org/10.1007/s10897-014-9728-1

Bardakjian, T. M., Helbig, I., Quinn, C., Elman, L. B., McCluskey, L. F., Scherer, S. S., & Gonzalez-Alegre, P. (2018). Genetic test utilization and diagnostic yield in adult patients with neurological disorders. *Neurogenetics, 19,* 105–110. https://doi.org/10.1007/s10048-018-0544-x

Baty, B. J. (2018). Genetic counseling: Growth of the profession and professional. *American Journal of Medical Genetics, 178C,* 54–62. https://doi.org/10.1002/ajmg.c.31601

Berliner, J. L., & Fay, A. M. (2007). Risk assessment and genetic counseling for hereditary breast and ovarian cancer: Recommendations of the National Society of Genetic Counselors. *Journal of Genetic Counseling, 16*(3), 241–260. https://doi.org/10.1007/s10897-007-9090-7

Berliner, J. L., Fay, A. M., Cummings, S. A., Burnett, B., & Tillmans, T. (2012). NSGC Practice Guideline: Risk assessment and genetic counseling for hereditary breast and ovarian cancer. *Journal of Genetic Counseling, 22*(2), 155–163. https://doi.org/10.1007/s10897-012-9547-1

Blout Zawatsky, C. L., Leonhard, J. R., Bell, M., Moore, M. M., Petry, N. J., Platt, D. M., Green, R. C., Hajek, C., & Christensen, K. D. (2022). Workforce considerations when building a precision medicine program. *Journal of Personalized Medicine, 12,* 1929. https://doi.org/10.3390/jpm12111929

Canadian Association of Genetic Counsellors. (2012). *Practice-based competencies for Canadian genetic counsellors.* https://www.cagc-accg.ca/doc/cagc%20practice%20based%20competencies.pdf

Cohen, L. (2020). The decoders: A historical perspective of the genetic counseling profession. *Birth Defects Research, 112,* 307–315. https://doi.org/10.1002/bdr2.1629

Corson, V. L., & Bernhardt, B. A. (2021). The evolution of genetic counseling at Johns Hopkins Hospital and beyond. *American Journal of Medical Genetics, 185A,* 3230–3235. https://doi.org/10.1002/ajmg.a.62374

Cutiongco-de la Paz, E. M., Chung, B. H., Faradz, S. M. H., Thong, M. K., David-Padilla, C., Lai, P. S., Lin, S. P., Chen, Y. H., Sura, T., & Laurino, M. (2019). Training in clinical genetics and genetic counseling in Asia. *American Journal of Medical Genetics. Part C, Seminars in Medical Genetics, 181*(2), 177–186. https://doi.org/10.1002/ajmg.c.31703

Davis, C., Baty, B. J., Hippman, C., Trepanier, A., & Erby, L. (2020). Genetic counselors with advanced skills: II. A new career trajectory framework. *Journal of Genetic Counseling, 29,* 771–785. https://doi.org/10.1002/jgc4.1204

Desrosiers, L. R., Quinn, E., Cramer, S. & Dobek, W. (2019). Integrating genetic counseling and testing in the pediatric oncology setting: Parental attitudes and influencing factors. *Pediatric Blood & Cancer, 66,* e27907. https://doi.org/10.1002/pbc.27907

Durmaz, A. A., Karaca, E., Demkow, U., Toruner, G., Schoumans, J., & Cogulu, O. (2015). Evolution of genetic techniques: Past, present, and beyond. *BioMed Research International,* 2015, 461524. https://doi.org/10.1155/2015/461524

European Board of Medical Genetics. (2010). *Professional and educational standards for genetic counsellors in Europe*. https://www.ebmg.eu/fileadmin/GCGN_Downloads/EBMGProfessionalAndEducationalStandardsForGeneticCounsellors-July2010.pdf

Everett, J. N., Gustafson, S. L., & Raymond, V. M. (2014). Traditional roles in a non-traditional setting: Genetic counseling in precision oncology. *Journal of Genetic Counseling*, *23*(4), 655660. https://doi.org/10.1007/s10897-014-9698-3

Futreal, P. A., Liu, Q., Shattuck-Eidens, D., Cochran, C., Harshman, K., Tavtigian, S., Bennett, L. M., Haugen-Strano, A., Swensen, J., Miki, Y., Eddington, K., McClure, M., Frye, C., Weaver-Feldhaus, J., Ding, W., Gholami, Z., Söderkvist, P., Terry, L., Jhanwar, S., . . . Wiseman, R. (1994). BRCA1 mutations in primary breast and ovarian carcinomas. *Science*, *266*(5182), 120–122. https://doi.org/10.1126/science.7939630

Hampel, H., Bennett, R. B., Buchanan, A., Pearlman, R., & Wiesner, G. L. (2015). A practice guideline from the American College of Medical Genetics and Genomics and the National Society of Genetic Counselors: Referral indications for cancer predisposition assessment. *Genetics in Medicine*, *17*, 70–87. https://doi.org/10.1038/gim.2014.147

Haspel, R. L., Genzen, J. R., Wagner, J., Fong, K., & the Undergraduate Training in Genomics (UTRIG) Working Group. (2021). Call for improvement in medical school training in genetics: Results of a national survey. *Genetics in Medicine*, *23*(6), 1151–1157. https://doi.org/10.1038/s41436-021-01100-5

Haverbusch, V. C. E., Heise, E. M., Foreman, A. K. M., & Callanan, N. P. (2019). An examination of factors contributing to the expansion of subspecialty genetic counseling. *Journal of Genetic Counseling*, *28*, 616–625.

Heimler, A. (1997). An oral history of the National Society of Genetic Counselors. *Journal of Genetic Counseling*, *6*, 315–336. https://doi.org/10.1023/A:1025680306348

Helm, B. M. Freeze, S. L., Spoonamore, K. G., Ware, S. M. Ayers, M. D., & Kean, A. C. (2018). The genetic counselor in the pediatric arrhythmia clinic: Review and assessment services. *Journal of Genetic Counseling*, *27*, 588–564. https://doi.org/10.1007/s10897-017-0169-5

Human Genetics Society of Australasia. (2022). *Competency standards for genetic counsellors*. https://www.hgsa.org.au/common/Uploaded%20files/pdfs/policies,%20position%20statements%20and%20guidelines/genetic%20counselling/Competency%20Standards%20for%20GCs.pdf

Ingles, J., Zodgekar, P. R., Yeates, L., Macciocca, I., Semsarian, C., Fatkin, D., & CSANZ Cardiac Genetic Diseases Council Writing Group. (2011). Guidelines for genetic testing of inherited cardiac disorders. *Heart, Lung, and Circulation*, *20*(11), 681–687. https://doi.org/10.1016/j.hlc.2011.07.013

Kalia, S. S., Adelman, K., Bale, S. J., Chung, W. K., Eng, C., Evans, J. P., Herman, G. E., Hufnagel, S. B., Klein, T. E., Korf, B. R., McKelvey, K. D., Ormond, K. E., Richards, C. S., Vlangos, C. N., Watson, M., Martin, C. L., & Miller, D. T. (2017). Recommendations for reporting of secondary findings in clinical exome and genome sequencing, 2016 update (ACMG SF v2.0): A policy statement of the American College of Medical Genetics and Genomics. *Genetics in Medicine*, *19*(2), 249–255. https://doi.org/10.1038/gim.2016.190

Kirkpatrick, B. E., & Rashkin, M. D. (2017). Ancestry testing and the practice of genetic counseling. *Journal of Genetic Counseling*, *26*(1), 6–20. https://doi.org/10.1007/s10897-016-0014-2.

Laurino, M. Y., Leppig, K. A., Abad, P. J., Cham, B., Chu, Y. W. Y., Kejriwal, S., Lee, J. M. H., Sternen, D. L., Thompson, J. K., Burgess, M. J., Chien, S., Elackatt, N., Lim, J. Y., Sura, T., Faradz, S., Padilla, C., Paz, E. C. D., Nauphar, D., Nguyen, K. N., . . . Thong, M. K. (2018). A report on ten Asian Pacific countries on current status and future directions of the genetic counseling profession: The establishment of the Professional Society of Genetic Counselors in Asia. *Journal of Genetic Counseling, 27*, 21–32. https://doi.org/10.1007/s10897-017-0115-6

Loudon, E., Scott, S. A., Rigobello, R., Scott, E. R., Zinberg, R., & Naik, H. (2021). Pharmacogenomic education among genetic counseling training programs in North America. *Journal of Genetic Counseling, 30*, 1500–1508. https://doi.org/10.1002/jgc4.1417

Marks, J. H., & Richter, M. L. (1976). The genetic associate: A new health professional. *American Journal of Public Health, 66*(4), 388–390.

Miki, Y., Swensen, J., Shattuck-Eidens, D., Futreal, P. A., Harshman, K., Tavtigian, S., Liu, Q., Cochran, C., Bennett, L. M., & Ding, W. (1994). A strong candidate for the breast and ovarian cancer susceptibility gene BRCA1. *Science, 266*(5182), 66–71. https://doi.org/10.1126/science.7545954

Moscarello, T., & Caleshu, C. (2019). A review of the emergence of and expansion of cardiovascular genetic counseling. *Current Cardiovascular Reports, 13*, 36–45. https://doi.org/10.1007/s12170-019-0631-z

National Library of Medicine. (n.d.). *Genetic testing registry*. https://www.ncbi.nlm.nih.gov/gtr/

National Society of Genetic Counselors. (1980–2002). *Professional status surveys, 1980–2002 PSS trends report, (archived)*. https://www.nsgc.org/Research-and-Publications/Professional-Status-Survey/Archived-Professional-Status-Survey. Members only section.

National Society of Genetic Counselors. (2000). *Professional status survey, (archived)*. https://www.nsgc.org/Policy-Research-and-Publications/Professional-Status-Survey/Archived-Professional-Status-Survey?folderId=152&view=gridview&pageSize=10. Members only section.

National Society of Genetic Counselors. (2002). *Professional status survey, 2002 (archived)*. https://www.nsgc.org/Policy-Research-and-Publications/Professional-Status-Survey/Archived-Professional-Status-Survey?folderId=152&view=gridview&pageSize=10. Members only section.

National Society of Genetic Counselors. (2004). *Professional status survey, 2004 (archived)*. https://www.nsgc.org/Research-and-Publications/Professional-Status-Survey/Archived-Professional-Status-Survey. Members only section.

National Society of Genetic Counselors. (2006). *Professional status survey, 2006 (archived)*. https://www.nsgc.org/Research-and-Publications/Professional-Status-Survey/Archived-Professional-Status-Survey. Members only section.

National Society of Genetic Counselors. (2008). *Professional status survey, 2008 (archived)*. https://www.nsgc.org/Research-and-Publications/Professional-Status-Survey/Archived-Professional-Status-Survey. Members only section.

National Society of Genetic Counselors. (2010). *Professional status survey, 2010 (archived)*. https://www.nsgc.org/Research-and-Publications/Professional-Status-Survey/Archived-Professional-Status-Survey. Members only section.

National Society of Genetic Counselors. (2012). *Professional status survey, 2012 (archived)*. https://www.nsgc.org/Research-and-Publications/Professional-Status-Survey/Archived-Professional-Status-Survey. Members only section.

National Society of Genetic Counselors. (2014). *Professional status survey, 2014 (archived)*. https://www.nsgc.org/Research-and-Publications/Professional-Status-Survey/Archived-Professional-Status-Survey. Members only section.

National Society of Genetic Counselors. (2016). *Professional status survey, 2016 (archived)*. https://www.nsgc.org/Research-and-Publications/Professional-Status-Survey/Archived-Professional-Status-Survey. Members only section.

National Society of Genetic Counselors. (2018). *Professional status survey, work environment reports, 2018 (archived).*https://www.nsgc.org/Research-and-Publications/Professional-Status-Survey/Archived-Professional-Status-Survey. Members only section.

National Society of Genetic Counselors. (2019). *Professional status survey, work environment reports, 2019 (archived).* https://www.nsgc.org/Research-and-Publications/Professional-Status-Survey/Archived-Professional-Status-Survey. Members only section.

National Society of Genetic Counselors. (2020). *Professional status survey, work environment reports, 2020 (archived).*https://www.nsgc.org/Research-and-Publications/Professional-Status-Survey/Archived-Professional-Status-Survey. Members only section.

National Society of Genetic Counselors. (2021). *Professional status survey, work environment reports, 2021 (archived).*https://www.nsgc.org/Research-and-Publications/Professional-Status-Survey/Archived-Professional-Status-Survey. Members only section.

National Society of Genetic Counselors. (2022). *Professional status survey, work environment reports, 2022 (archived).*https://www.nsgc.org/Research-and-Publications/Professional-Status-Survey/Archived-Professional-Status-Survey. Members only section.

Ong, C. S. B., Fok, R. W., Tan, R. C. A., Fung, S. M., Sun, S., & Ngeow, J. Y. Y. (2022). General practitioners' (GPs) experience, attitudes and needs on clinical genetic services: A systematic review. *Family Medicine Community Health, 10*(4), e001515. https://doi.org/10.1136/fmch-2021-001515

Oren, O., Gersh, B. J., & Bhatt, D. L. (2020). On the pearls and perils of sub-subspecialization. *The American Journal of Medicine, 133*(2), 158–159. https://doi.org/10.1016/j.amjmed.2019.06.052

Ormond, K. E., Laurino, M. Y., Barlow-Steward, K., Wessels, T-M., Macaulay, S., Austin J., & Middleton, A. (2018). Genetic counseling globally: Where are we now? *American Journal of Medical Genetics, 178C*, 98–107. https://doi.org/10.1002/ajmg.c.31607

Penon-Portmann, M., Chang, J., Cheng, M., & Shieh, J. T. (2020). Genetics workforce: Distribution of genetics services and challenges to health care in California. *Genetics in Medicine, 22*(1), 227–231. https://doi.org/10.1038/s41436-019-0628-5

Powell, K. P., Hasegawa, L., & McWalter, K. (2010). Expanding roles: A survey of public health genetic counselors. *Journal of Genetic Counseling, 19*(6), 593–605. https://doi.org/10.1007/s10897-010-9313-1

Riley, B. D., Culver, J. O., Skrzynia, C., Senter, L. A., Peters, J. A., Costalas, J. W., Callif-Daley, F., Grumet, S. C., Hunt, K. S., Nagy, R., McKinnon, W. C., Petrucelli, N. M., Bennett, R. L., & Trepanier, A. M. (2011). Essential elements of genetic cancer risk assessment, counseling, and testing: Updated recommendations of the National Society of Genetic Counselors. *Journal of Genetic Counseling, 21*(2), 151–161. https://doi.org/10.1007/s10897-011-9462-x

Rubanovich, C. K., Cheung, C., Mandel, J., & Bloss, C. S. (2018). Physician preparedness for big genomic data: A review of genomic medicine education initiatives in the United States. *Human Molecular Genetics, 27*(R2), R250–R258. https://doi.org/10.1093/hmg/ddy170

Schneider, K. A. (2012). *Counseling about cancer: Strategies for genetic counselors* (3rd ed.). John Wiley & Sons.

Schneider, K. A., & Marnane, D. (1997). Cancer risk counseling: How is it different? *Journal of Genetic Counseling, 6*(2), 97–109.

Stern, A. M. (2009). A quiet revolution: The birth of the genetic counselor at Sarah Lawrence College, 1969. *Journal of Genetic Counseling, 18*, 1–11.

Trepanier, A., Ahrens, M., McKinnon, W., Peters, J., Stopfer, J., Grumet, S. C., Manley, S., Culver, J. O., Acton, R., Larsen-Haidle, J., Correia, L. A., Bennett, R., Pettersen, B., Ferlita, T. D., Costalas, J. W., Hunt, K., Donlon, S., Skrzynia, C., Farrell, C., . . . National Society of Genetic

Counselors. (2004). Genetic cancer risk assessment and counseling: Recommendations of the National Society of Genetic Counselors. *Journal of Genetic Counseling*, *13*, 83–114. https://doi.org/10.1023/B:JOGC.0000018821.48330.77

Vogel, K. J., & Weissman, S. M. (2012). The Commission on Cancer genetics standard: Risk assessment and genetic counseling. *Oncology Practice Management*, 2(5), 1–6.

CHAPTER 11

THE GENETIC COUNSELOR'S ROLE IN DIRECT-TO-CONSUMER GENETIC TESTING

ANNE E. GREB

Introduction

Direct-to-consumer (DTC) genetic testing as a method to access personal genetic information has been available since the early 2000s, resulting in tens of millions of consumers accessing genetic testing outside of the traditional healthcare setting (Gollust et al., 2003; Regalado, 2019). The popularity of ancestry tests is one driver in the DTC testing market, but many consumers also seek genetic health information. In fact, early adopters of DTC genetic testing were motivated by the promised health benefits of human genome discoveries (Gollust et al., 2011; McGowan et al., 2010).

Tests today include a broad range of services. Most start around $100, and in addition to ancestry, people can learn about genetic health risks (GHRs) or carrier status for specific recessive diseases. Some tests provide pharmacogenetics information and polygenic risk scores for common complex conditions and diseases. Consumers can get information on how genetics plays a role in a variety of phenotypic traits and wellness characteristics. There are tests that claim to provide information about nutrition, weight loss, athletic ability, sleep, and even wine preferences.

Consumers can access and download uninterpreted raw genetic data files to further explore their genetic information. DTC genetic testing provides opportunities for consumers to participate in research. Genetic genealogists use DTC tests to find biological relatives and deduce relationships between individuals. Sharing and comparing the information with family and friends, an entertainment or fun factor, is often part of the experience. The term "recreational genomics" is sometimes used to describe the fun or entertainment value some seek in DTC genetic testing (Felzman, 2015).

By definition, *a DTC genetic test is a type of genetic test that is marketed directly to consumers without the involvement of a healthcare provider* (Food and Drug Administration

[FDA], 2019b). The consumer never has to leave their home or meet with a provider. They do not need a doctor's order or prescription for the test. Consumers directly obtain a test kit from the company and then send back a saliva sample or buccal swab for analysis. Results are later available on a secure website or mobile app for the consumer to privately access.

Despite its popularity, DTC genetic testing remains controversial (Evans & Green, 2009; Hogarth et al., 2008; Khoury, 2017; Su, 2013). Proponents argue for patient autonomy and that access to personal genetic information is an individual right. Some see DTC testing as a safer option for protection against genetic discrimination than having their information in a medical record system (Critchley et al., 2015; Haeusermann et al., 2018). Others point out that DTC testing has raised public awareness and enthusiasm about genetics and has the potential to improve genetic literacy and empower individuals to take a more active role in their healthcare (Crow, 2019). Also, given the large consumer genetics databases and the willingness of consumers to participate in research, DTC testing can accelerate research and creates a unique opportunity to engage underrepresented populations and diversify databases (National Academies of Sciences, Engineering, and Medicine [NAS], 2020).

Critics of DTC genetic testing express concerns about the quality and accuracy of tests and lack of scientific evidence supporting claims made by some companies (McCabe & McCabe, 2004). There are worries consumers do not understand test results and their limitations and may make health decisions based on inaccurate or misleading information (Gill et al., 2018). Opponents raise concerns about the privacy of consumers' genetic data including its storage, sharing, and use by companies (Laestadius et al., 2017). There are uncertainties about the impact on the healthcare system and whether providers can answer patient questions and interpret DTC test results (Goldsmith et al., 2012; McGrath et al., 2019; Powell et al., 2012).

Many genetic counselors have limited experience and express discomfort discussing DTC testing with patients (Brett et al., 2012; Hock et al., 2011). In a 2018 survey of 482 genetic counselors, only one-third of respondents indicated they were comfortable providing genetic counseling about DTC testing, and 56.4% were negative or very negative toward DTC genetic testing (Hsieh et al., 2020). The uptake of genetic counseling services following DTC is relatively small, although consumers do express interest in genetic counseling if it is accessible (Darst et al., 2013; Koeller et al., 2017). While genetic societies recommend genetics professionals be involved in helping consumers understand DTC test results (American College of Medical Genetics and Genomics, 2016; Hudson et al., 2007; National Society of Genetic Counselors, 2019), the attitudes of genetic counselors toward DTC genetic testing have remained relatively negative and they are divided on their role (Hsieh et al., 2020). Some feel their expertise is needed, while others feel DTC genetic testing is outside their scope of practice (Harris et al., 2013; Hawkins & Ho, 2012; Hock et al., 2011).

There is much to learn about DTC genetic testing and its impact on healthcare, on society, and on individuals and their families who take these tests. DTC testing has implications for clinical care, research, and education. Genetic counselors have an opportunity to address these questions and function as thought leaders and influencers as genetic testing moves outside the traditional clinical setting. The purpose of this chapter is to provide a foundational framework for informed discussions and debates within the genetic counseling profession about DTC genetic testing.

Expanding Service Delivery Model

DTC genetic testing as a new service delivery model providing increased access to genetic testing is expanding and evolving in real time (Allyse et al., 2018; NAS, 2020; Weissman et al., 2019). There is a spectrum of health and nonhealth services offered and molecular methods used in testing. Services differ in regulatory oversight, whether a healthcare provider is involved in the process, and how services are marketed and delivered to consumers. It is important to understand these distinctions among different services offered since they are core to much of the confusion and debate surrounding DTC genetic testing.

A broader category of testing referred to as *consumer driven* includes DTC tests as well as tests that require the involvement of a physician (K. A. Phillips et al., 2019; Precision Medicine Advisors, 2019; Stoll, 2020). These tests, considered a hybrid model, are initiated by a consumer, but a physician must sign off on the request before the test can be processed and results returned to the consumer. Companies usually provide consumers access to an ordering physician through a third-party network, although the order can be written within the context of a traditional physician–patient relationship. This type of consumer-driven genetic testing is referred to as *consumer initiated, physician mediated* and is different from DTC testing, which allows the consumer to initiate testing and access their genetic information with no required involvement of a physician or other healthcare provider. The current genetic testing service delivery models are depicted in Figure 11.1.

The molecular techniques used and tests performed in consumer-driven testing depend on the nature of the genetic information provided and services offered by a company. Generally, the techniques include DNA sequencing in genomic areas of interest and genotyping using single nucleotide polymorphism (SNP) microarrays to look for known disease-associated and other variants of interest. Consumer-driven testing tends to be broad, covering a range of conditions, whereas clinical genetic testing tends to be targeted

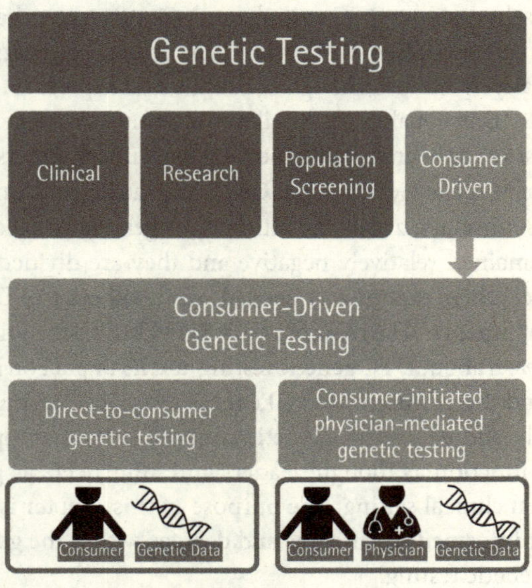

FIGURE 11.1 Genetic testing service delivery models.

to the clinical indication for testing. Not all clinical genetic tests are comprehensive, and not all consumer-driven tests have limited coverage. For example, some consumer-driven tests include comprehensive gene panels, and clinical testing can include single-site family variant testing.

Typically, DTC genetic tests are not intended to answer a specific clinical or diagnostic question about an individual or their family. In these circumstances, genetic testing is performed in a clinical setting where testing depends on the assessment of a healthcare provider who has an established relationship with the patient and is familiar with their personal and family history. Since consumer-driven genetic testing is not tailored to a clinical indication, conceptually it is more similar to a population screening test. Population genetic screening is broadly offered to healthy populations not known to be at increased risk. Screening identifies people who have or are at risk for a medical condition in themselves or that they could pass on to future offspring. Clinical genetics professionals are typically not involved in initiating testing in population genetic screening programs but are available to provide follow-up clinical genetic services for those identified as at increased risk. Screening genetic tests tend to be less expensive than clinical diagnostic tests, which makes them more accessible to larger groups of people (Godard et al., 2003).

Consumer-driven testing for health information is often most informative for healthy people not otherwise known to be at increased risk. Tests may be marketed directly to consumers using print, broadcast, and social media. Some tests are delivered through employee health insurance plans or in collaboration with healthcare systems. When GHRs and other health information are discovered, consumers should be encouraged to talk to a healthcare provider about follow-up evaluation and care. There is variability in the range of pretest evaluation and posttest follow-up services offered to consumers. Some companies offer genetic counseling services or information and links about how to access these services. Most companies provide educational information and resources, although the quality of these resources may vary.

Government Oversight

To appreciate the nuances and complexities of government regulation of DTC genetic tests, it is helpful to be familiar with the oversight of genetic tests in general. Regulatory oversight of genetic testing includes inspection of the laboratories that perform the tests and review of the tests themselves (National Human Genome Research Institute [NHGRI], 2020b). The term "genetic test" is defined by the Secretary's Advisory Committee on Genetics, Health, and Society (SACGHS), a former government policy committee, as "the analysis of human chromosomes, DNA, RNA, genes and/or gene products, and are predominately used to detect heritable or somatic mutation, genotypes, or phenotypes related to disease and health" (Ferreira-Gonzalez et al., 2008, p. 3). The Centers for Medicare and Medicaid Services (CMS) under the Clinical Laboratory Improvement Amendments (CLIA) has primary authority for regulating the procedural aspects of testing laboratories. CLIA regulations are designed to ensure the analytical validity of tests by overseeing the quality of laboratory procedures and qualifications of technicians (CMS, 2020). Laboratories may also undergo voluntary accreditation by the College of American Pathologists (CAP) by meeting standards typically more rigorous than CLIA requirements.

The FDA is responsible for the regulatory oversight of specific genetic tests, which are considered medical devices. A medical device is "intended for use in the diagnosis of a disease or other conditions, or in the cure, mitigation, treatment, or prevention of disease" (FDA, 2018f, Overview section). Some medical devices are considered in vitro diagnostics (IVD) since their intended use is to collect, prepare, and examine specimens taken from the human body (FDA, 2019a). Some consumer-driven genetic tests, such as specific DTC health tests, are considered IVD medical devices. Others, such as ancestry tests, are not considered medical devices (FDA, 2019b).

The FDA regulates medical devices based on how they come to market and their intended uses. Test kits are sample collection kits that are manufactured and sold for use in multiple laboratories as a unit. Laboratory-developed tests (LDTs) are tests designed, manufactured, and used within a single laboratory (FDA, 2018g). The FDA regulates genetic tests considered test kits but generally exercises enforcement discretion over most other types, meaning it has the authority to regulate them but chooses not to enforce those regulations in most cases. Historically, the FDA has used enforcement discretion on genetic tests that are LDTs and tests ordered by physicians (FDA, 2018g). An overview of the regulatory framework used to evaluate genetic tests is shown in Figure 11.2 (McDonough & Armstrong, 2017).

Regulatory oversight of all types of genetic tests is evolving as testing expands and has more relevance to health. The FDA recognizes the increasing high complexity of LDTs for genetic

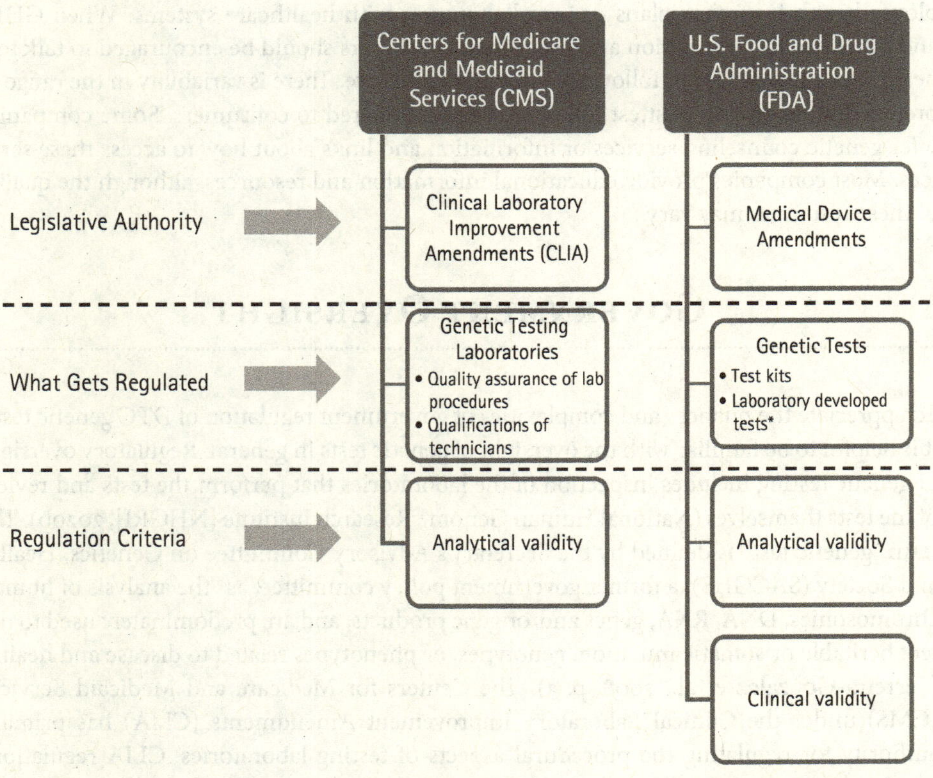

FIGURE 11.2 Genetic testing regulatory framework.

(Adapted from McDonough & Armstrong 2017)

testing, such as next-generation sequencing (NGS) for exome and genome testing, and has drafted guidelines on how it intends to regulate NGS tests (FDA, 2018d). Pharmacogenetics is another testing area for which the FDA has considered oversight guidelines even though most pharmacogenetics tests are LDTs (FDA, 2018e). In October 2018, the FDA issued a safety communication public alert about pharmacogenetics tests with unapproved claims (FDA, 2018h). When it comes to DTC genetic tests, the FDA enforces premarket review and labeling requirements for categories of health tests felt to have a higher impact on medical care. As of this writing, these categories are GHR, carrier screening, cancer predisposition, and pharmacogenetics (FDA, 2019b).

The FDA assesses the safety and effectiveness of DTC health categories based on analytical validity, clinical validity, and user comprehension studies (FDA, 2018c, 2019b). Analytical validity refers to test accuracy and knowing if a specific variant is present or not. Tests must meet standards for accuracy and reproducibility. Clinical validity refers to knowing what having or not having that genetic variant means for an individual's health. The genetic variants included in a test must have published evidence indicating that they are related to the presence (or risk of) or absence of a specific disease. User comprehension studies must demonstrate a high level (90% or greater) of understanding of key concepts in the reports explaining test results.

The FDA has worked to streamline its regulation of DTC genetic tests and has expressed an openness to working with companies to develop reasonable and efficient pathways for new types of DTC genetic tests (FDA, 2018a, 2018b). For example, carrier screening tests are considered moderate-risk devices that are exempt from FDA premarket review provided the manufacturer conforms to special controls, which are regulatory requirements established to ensure safety and effectiveness. Companies can offer additional GHR tests without premarket review once they receive initial FDA clearance on their first test and continue to conform to special controls. The FDA more closely regulates cancer susceptibility GHR tests requiring all tests to go through premarket review and clearance. Updated information about FDA oversight of DTC genetic tests can be found on the FDA's website (https://www.fda.gov) under "direct-to-consumer genetic tests."

Since the FDA generally does not enforce premarket reviews of LDTs, most genetic tests enter the healthcare and nonhealthcare market without FDA evaluation for safety, effectiveness, or accuracy. Although tests may be performed in a CLIA-certified laboratory, CLIA does not address clinical validity or utility or review laboratory marketing practices. Despite molecular genetic tests being classified as moderate to high complexity, CLIA does not have specific category and proficiency standards for genetic testing as it does for other high-complexity tests (NHGRI, 2020c). Genetic tests performed in CLIA-certified laboratories that also have CAP accreditation may be held to higher standards similar to other high-complexity laboratory tests.

Regulatory History of DTC Genetic Tests

The first U.S. government public statement about DTC genetic testing was in 2006 when the Government Accountability Office (GAO) voiced concerns after a review of nutrigenomic testing concluded that information from DTC companies was misleading, was ambiguous, and did not provide meaningful information to consumers (GAO, 2006). In 2008, the SACGHS issued a report identifying major gaps in the overall regulation of genetic testing, including DTC genetic tests, and recommended increased FDA regulatory oversight (Ferreira-Gonzalez et al., 2008). As it turned out, it was the states and not the federal government who acted first. In 2008, California and New York sent cease-and-desist letters to a number of consumer genetics companies warning them that they were operating without necessary state licenses (Magnus et al., 2009). Companies were forced to change their practices in these states, and some stopped selling directly to consumers. During this time period, the genetic testing regulatory landscape continued to remain uncertain at the federal level despite the SACGHS report. Meanwhile, public awareness and interest in DTC continued to grow and "The Retail DNA Test" was named the *TIME* invention of the year in 2008 (Lombardi, 2008).

A congressional hearing held in 2010 on "Direct-to-Consumer Genetic Testing and the Consequences to Public Health" included a discussion of a new GAO report on an undercover investigation of 15 consumer genetics companies (GAO, 2010). The investigation involved sending "donor" samples to various companies and making undercover calls to companies seeking health advice. The report detailed how 10 companies had engaged in "deceptive marketing, misinformation, and questionable practices" (GAO, 2010, p. 15). The scientific basis for risk predictions was questionable because of discordant results across companies and results that were inconsistent with donors' clinical histories. The GAO report concluded that a lack of government oversight made it difficult for consumers to determine whether a DTC genetic test provides meaningful scientifically based information.

In early 2010, Pathway Genomics announced a partnership with Walgreens to sell its genetic testing service in its stores (Pollack, 2010). This prompted the FDA to act by publicly voicing its concerns about the arrangement, which ultimately resulted in Walgreens severing the relationship (Vorhaus, 2010a). The FDA then sent letters to five DTC companies (23andMe, Navigenics, deCODE Genetics, Knome, and Ilumina) informing them they could find no record of the necessary FDA clearance or approval for their tests, which the FDA deemed to be medical devices. One month later, the FDA sent letters to 14 additional companies. DTC companies were surprised by this move as the FDA had not told companies such approval was necessary and it remained unclear the steps needed to comply with the FDA (Vorhaus, 2010b). The FDA letters led some companies to drop out of the DTC market and others to discontinue their health-related tests. In November 2013, the FDA sent a warning letter to 23andMe, which had continued to offer its health testing despite the 2010 FDA letter (Pollack, 2013). Consequently, 23andMe stopped offering health testing in 2013, although it did continue its ancestry service.

There was opposition to the FDA's move to regulate DTC genetic tests. Opponents pointed out that concerns about harm from DTC genetic testing were never based on actual evidence and that overcautious regulation violates consumers' rights to obtain personal genetic information, therefore preventing individuals from taking actions that could improve their health (Green & Farahany, 2014; TechFreedom, 2013). Others felt the FDA's involvement should instead focus on facilitating consumer discussions about test results with healthcare providers. In a 2014 Hastings Center Report essay, the authors maintained that the risk of harm from DTC genetic testing resulting from consumer misunderstanding is only "exceptionally high" within a clinical setting, where most reasonable healthcare professionals would mitigate this risk. For example, they argued that most physicians would not perform a mastectomy based solely on DTC test results (Edwards & Huang, 2014).

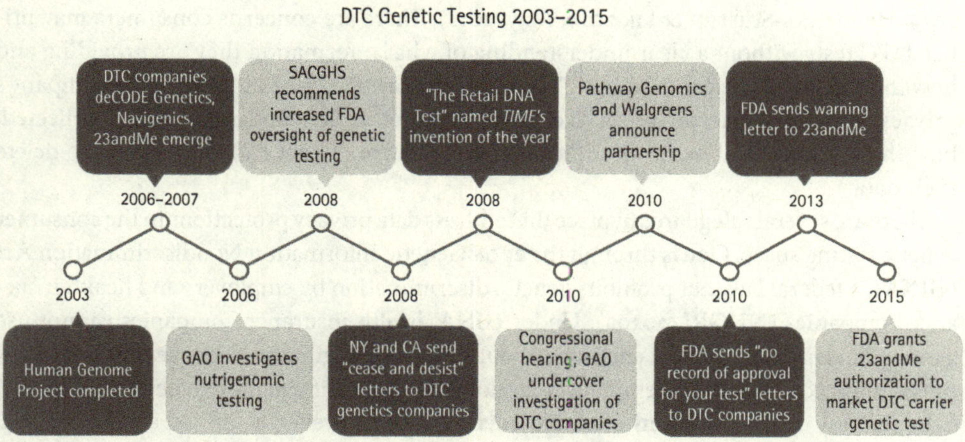

FIGURE 11.3 Selected milestones in the regulatory history of DTC genetic tests 2003–2015. DTC = direct-to-consumer; GAO = Government Accountability Office; SACGHS = Secretary's Advisory Committee on Genetics, Health, and Society; FDA = Food and Drug Administration.

The FDA's intervention in 2010 in the marketing of DTC genetic tests was the first time it imposed regulatory oversight of any genetic test. Of the 19 DTC companies who received letters from the FDA, 23andMe was the only company to go back to the FDA and submit a premarket application for its health test under the de novo submission pathway. In 2015, the FDA granted 23andMe authorization to market a carrier test for Bloom syndrome, providing a regulatory framework for future submissions of DTC genetic tests. Figure 11.3 shows a timeline of the key events in the regulatory history of DTC genetic testing from 2003 to 2015.

In the years since the FDA's crackdown on the marketing of DTC genetic tests, relatively few consumer genetics companies have sought FDA clearance or authorization to market their health tests. Many companies instead require a physician's authorization before a consumer can proceed with testing, creating the consumer initiated, physician mediated model. Consumer driven companies tend to make the requirement of a physician ordered test as seamless as possible by offering to solicit the physician's order for the consumer. The level of involvement of the ordering physician varies. In some instances, physicians and/or genetic counselors are involved to assess if the genetic test requested by a consumer is appropriate. Some companies provide their customers with access to a genetic counselor to discuss test results. For other companies, the involvement of the physician is limited to ordering the test (STAT, 2018; Stoll, 2020).

Privacy Protections and Consumer Choice

The importance of having safeguards to minimize potential harm and protect personal genetic information obtained through consumer driven testing is well recognized, just as it was for genetic information obtained for medical and research reasons (Clayton et al.,

2019; Hendricks-Sturrup & Lu, 2019; May, 2018). There are concerns consumers may utilize DTC tests without a clear understanding of what information they are providing and how their data may be used. Although consumers are encouraged to review the company's privacy policies and terms of service, some may not understand what data is collected, how their data is used, with whom it may be shared, and what rights they have to delete their data.

There are several safeguards in place that address data privacy protections in the consumer genetic testing space. One is through the 2008 Genetic Information Nondiscrimination Act (GINA), a federal law that prohibits genetic discrimination by employers and health insurance companies (NHGRI, 2020a). Under GINA, health insurance companies cannot use genetic information to make decisions about insurance eligibility, coverage, underwriting, or premium costs. Similarly, employers cannot use genetic information to determine hiring, firing, or any other conditions of employment. GINA, however, is limited and has several gaps in protections, namely in not extending its protections to limit providers in using genetic information for life, disability, or long-term care insurance decisions. GINA also does not apply to employers with fewer than 15 employees, the U.S. military, the Veterans Health Administration, or Indian Health Service. Another safeguard is the Health Insurance Portability and Accountability Act (HIPAA), which protects against unauthorized disclosure of health information by covered entities such as healthcare systems. Although consumer genetics companies are not covered entities, consumer health information shared with a healthcare provider is protected under HIPAA within the healthcare system.

Many states have approached privacy by enacting their own genetic privacy laws to provide safeguards against the misuse of genetic information that go beyond GINA. State consumer privacy laws such as the 2018 California Consumer Privacy Act and the California Privacy Rights Act of 2020 create additional protections around the use of consumer information, including genetic information (State of California, 2018).

Without a comprehensive federal genetic privacy law, a number of consumer genetics companies have chosen to self-regulate and hold themselves accountable to their users. Industry self-regulation includes establishing best practices, monitoring for compliance, and enforcing regulations. In an effort to establish self-regulation in the consumer genetics industry, industry leaders, academics, and policymakers collaborated on defining industry best practices for the collection, use, and storage of consumer genetic data. In 2018, the Future of Privacy Forum, a nonprofit group, published the *Privacy Best Practices for Consumer Genetic Testing Services*, a code of conduct outlining these standards (Future of Privacy Forum, 2018). These best practices focus on transparency in terms of providing straightforward information in language consumers can understand, providing consumers with a choice as far as how their genetic information is used and shared, offering enhanced privacy protections to include not sharing data with employers and insurance companies, and requiring a valid legal process for any disclosure of genetic data to law enforcement.

Although there are benefits to self-regulation such as efficiency, flexibility, and creating an internal commitment to corporate ethics and responsibility, there are also limitations. Inherent conflicts of interest and lack of transparency may exist due to overriding company business interests. Since agreements to comply with regulations are voluntary in nature and involve self-policing, there can be irregularities in monitoring and enforcing sanctions (Castro, 2011). Companies that agree to follow industry best practices can be motivated by the desire for a favorable public image or by fear of a negative image. For example, the Future of Privacy Forum made public the names of eight consumer genetics companies that supported its best practices and then publicly called out and removed one company when that company made an agreement with the FBI, which conflicted with the industry best practices. Consumer protection laws, which are in place to prevent unfair and deceptive business practices, can also help enforce best practices among consumer genetics companies (Federal Trade Commission, 2013).

Many consumer genetics companies provide opt-in options and consent-based features to promote consumer choice. For example, some companies give customers the choice of which genetic results they want to view and require an additional opt-in to connect with DNA matches in their database. Companies should ensure their research programs have Institutional Review Board oversight and pursue acquiring a Certificate of Confidentiality issued by the Department of Health and Human Services. Certificates of confidentiality protect the privacy of research participants in research that involves the collection of sensitive data by prohibiting disclosure of identifiable, sensitive research information to anyone not connected to the research. Data protection, however, also depends on the privacy policies and practices of academic, nonprofit, pharmaceutical, and other industry organizations if companies share consumer data.

There are policy guidelines that address genetic testing in minors in the clinical context. If a minor is suspected of having a genetic condition, then genetic testing is viewed as appropriate for diagnostic and treatment purposes. However, predictive or presymptomatic testing in childhood or adolescence is generally discouraged unless early preventative actions are indicated. The rationale is that individuals should be able to make informed decisions about genetic testing as competent adults (Committee on Bioethics, Committee on Genetics, and The American College of Medical Genetics and Genomics Social, Ethical, and Legal Issues Committee, 2013; Botkin et al., 2015; National Society of Genetic Counselors, n.d.-b). Guidelines now address DTC genetic testing in children, which is universally discouraged (National Society of Genetic Counselors, n.d.-a). There is acknowledgment, however, of situations when parents may pursue testing in their children. For example, ancestry testing in children who are adopted or donor conceived can identify ethnicity and provide a sense of cultural identity or connection to biological relatives (Weissman et al., 2019). In these cases, it is recommended that testing be considered in collaboration with clinical genetics experts to ensure understanding of the potential benefits, limitations, and risks of testing.

When considering a DTC genetic test, consumers have a role to play in protecting their privacy, which includes being knowledgeable of a company's policies and aware of the choices they have as customers. Consumers should be aware of a company's policies when it comes to sharing or selling consumer genetic data before agreeing to participate in research. If consumers choose to upload their uninterpreted raw genetic data to third-party services, then they should read the terms of service and privacy policies of these services and consumer options before they share their data files.

Services Provided

The popularity of DTC genetic testing is best understood by looking at consumer motivations and the nature of genetic information consumers obtain through testing. Factors that affect consumer participation in DTC testing have shifted since the 2000s (Hendricks-Sturrup & Lu, 2020; A. M. Phillips, 2016). Social factors influence the uptake of DTC genetic testing; experiences of family and friends, receiving a test kit as a gift, social media, and marketing likely impact whether or not someone decides to take a DTC genetic test. Some consumers are enticed by the entertainment or fun in learning more about themselves and sharing and comparing trait and ancestry information or amount of Neanderthal DNA with friends and family members (Ruhl et al., 2019; Turrini & Prainsack, 2016).

Today health-related results obtained from DTC genetic testing can include information about disease predisposition and risk, drug processing, and carrier status. Polygenic scores are being advanced in the DTC space and have the potential to identify individuals at increased likelihood for complex, adult-onset conditions. Some tests also provide information about lifestyle and wellness attributes, although the validity of the information from these tests varies considerably. Similar to other genetic databases, consumer databases currently lack diversity, making their tests most relevant for European ancestry populations and raising ethical and scientific challenges related to equitable access to genetic information (Martin et al., 2019).

When reviewing test results, it is important to check if the results are from the same company the patient sent their sample to or from a third-party interpretive service. The uninterpreted genetic data used by third-party services has not been validated, so results may be inaccurate or misinterpreted. DTC genetic tests are not meant to be a substitute for traditional healthcare, and medically relevant results should be confirmed in a clinical setting (FDA, 2019b). Additionally, the patient's personal and family history, ethnicity, and reasons for testing should be considered when reviewing results.

Health tests

GHR tests provide information about genetic variants known to be associated with an increased risk for specific diseases or conditions, ranging from neurodegenerative to cancer predispositions. The information provided by GHR tests is meant to help individuals make better lifestyle decisions and to inform discussions with healthcare providers. Since environment, lifestyle, and other genetic factors also contribute to the occurrence of most genetic conditions, GHR tests are not able to provide an overall risk of developing a genetically related condition. The FDA enforces premarket review and labeling requirements for GHR tests.

Examples of GHR tests available through DTC genetic testing include Centers for Disease Control and Prevention (CDC) Tier 1 conditions such as familial hypercholesterolemia and hereditary breast and ovarian cancer. Tier 1 genetic tests have enough scientific evidence to support their clinical value and implementation in everyday clinical practice (CDC, 2014). Consumers identified as having disease-associated variants for familial hypercholesterolemia or hereditary breast and ovarian cancer need follow-up genetic counseling and specialized medical care. DTC genetic test results should be confirmed in a clinical setting. Since these conditions are inherited, other family members should consider testing.

GHR tests can also include conditions such as hereditary thrombophilia. Consumers identified as having the common factor V Leiden variant in the *F5* gene are at increased risk for developing venous thromboembolism. Since factors such as age, pregnancy, obesity, and immobility also contribute to risk, clinical management will depend on a patient's clinical and family history. Alpha-1-antitrypsin deficiency is another GHR test available through DTC testing. Consumers found to have the PI*Z variant in each *SERPINA1* gene are at increased risk of developing lung and liver disease. Patients with the PI*ZZ genotype may be candidates for enzyme replacement therapy.

Other possible GHR tests may include neurological conditions such as Alzheimer's and Parkinson's disease. Consumers who learn they have one or more e4 variants in their *APOE* gene are at an increased risk of developing late-onset Alzheimer's disease (Farrer et al., 1997). Despite a lack of prevention or cure, some consumers seek this information to help with life planning and other decisions. Results like this, with limited clinical benefit, can still have high personal value (Roberts et al., 2017).

Similar to other screening tests, GHR test results will likely be negative or indicate variant not detected for most conditions for most consumers. When interpreting a GHR test result, it is important to know the test's sensitivity or variant coverage, which varies depending on the testing technology used, the number of known genes and variants associated with the condition, and relevant ethnicities. It is important that consumers understand the meaning of a negative DTC or any other genetic test result so they are not falsely reassured.

GHR tests offer an opportunity to identify individuals with specific disease-associated variants who are not identified through traditional medical practices such as regular collection and analysis of family health information or ethnicity-based testing (Tennen et al., 2020). GHR tests are not intended for individuals with a known family history of inherited disease. In these situations, genetic testing should be offered and interpreted within the context of a clinical relationship with a genetic counselor or other healthcare provider.

Carrier screening tests provide information about variants known to be associated with recessive diseases such as cystic fibrosis, sickle cell anemia, and Tay-Sachs disease. Tests are intended to provide individuals and couples with carrier status information that could indicate an autosomal recessive disease in future offspring. Like GHR tests, the sensitivity, or variant coverage, of carrier screening tests varies depending on the testing technology used, number of known genes and variants associated with a specific autosomal recessive condition, nature and number of autosomal recessive diseases included in the test, and relevant ethnicities. DTC carrier screening tests provide an opportunity for widespread preconceptual population carrier screening. DTC carrier screening tests may not meet standards established by organizations such as the American College of Medical Genetics and Genomics and the American College of Obstetrics and Gynecology (ACOG), and therefore additional testing in a clinical setting should be offered for those who are pregnant or contemplating pregnancy (ACOG, 2017; Grody et al., 2013).

Pharmacogenetics tests include information about how genetics may play a role in an individual's response to drugs and include variants associated with medication processing. A common example is the *CYP2C19* gene and the drug clopidogrel. Consumers with a *2 variant in each of their *CYP2C19* genes are considered poor metabolizers and often cannot activate clopidogrel, so other platelet inhibitors may be better options for them. The FDA enforces premarket review and labeling requirements for pharmacogenetics tests. Initially, FDA authorization of pharmacogenetics test labeling did not include interpretive drug information. In 2020, the FDA granted 23andMe a 510(k) clearance for a pharmacogenetics report on two medications, clopidogrel and citalopram, allowing 23andMe to provide interpretive drug information and remove their requirement for confirmatory testing.

Genetic counselors' training in genetics, risk communication, and counseling well positions them as leaders in the delivery of comprehensive pharmacogenetics services for both patients and clinicians. DTC genetic testing will likely raise awareness about pharmacogenetics given the prevalence of clinically relevant variants in genes such as *CYP2C19* in the general population (Ionova et al., 2020). Increased awareness provides educational opportunities for genetic counselors to help patients and other healthcare providers understand the value and limitations of pharmacogenetics tests (Lu et al., 2017).

Wellness tests

Wellness is a broad category and can include information such as how well someone digests lactose or breaks down alcohol. Other types of wellness testing include food sensitivities, muscle composition, sleep movement, and genetic weight. A general wellness test is considered a low-risk device by the FDA if its intended use is related to maintaining or encouraging a healthy lifestyle or if its intended use is to reduce the risk or impact of a chronic disease where healthy lifestyle choices are known to play an important role in prevention and medical management. Based on this definition, the FDA currently uses enforcement discretion for the oversight of most general wellness tests (FDA, 2019b).

Wellness test results can be based on the analysis of one or more variants with a known association. For example, consumers can learn if they have a variant near their *LCT* gene, which is associated with lactose intolerance, or a variant in their *ALDH2* gene, and are more likely to flush red in the face after consuming alcohol. Other tests are based on data from genome-wide association studies (GWASs), which analyze hundreds to thousands of variants using statistical models that provide polygenic scores and risk or likelihood estimates. For example, information about the likelihood of dog and cat allergies based on GWASs is available in the DTC genetics marketplace. Other results include information about risks for common adult-onset complex diseases such as type 2 diabetes, coronary artery disease, and high blood pressure. The rationale is that polygenic scores, which identify those at increased risk for complex conditions, may provide motivation for healthy lifestyle behavior.

The DTC wellness industry is rapidly growing. Critical evaluation of wellness tests is important since not all tests on the market have scientific evidence to support the claims made to consumers (Drabsch & Holzapfel, 2019; Floris et al., 2020). Some companies sell supplements, skincare, and other products to their customers based on genetic test results. Despite these limitations, consumers see value in using genetic information in their health and wellness efforts.

Trait tests

Traits refer to nonmedical characteristics of an individual such as physical features, taste preferences, ability to detect certain smells, and even personality insights. The curiosity factor among consumers in learning about traits is one of the reasons consumers pursue testing and is sometimes referred to as "edutainment" (NAS, 2020). Just like medical conditions and diseases, traits can be determined by genes, the environment, or the interaction of both. Like wellness tests, some trait information is based on the analysis of variants in or near a single gene, such as the *OR2M7* gene and asparagus urine odor detection and the *MC1R* gene and red hair color. Other results depend on the analysis of variants in several genes, such as variants in the *SLC45A2* and *SLC24A5* genes associated with skin color in individuals of European and African ancestry. Since many traits are complex in their inheritance, traits reports are often based on GWAS studies and provide a statistical likelihood of having a specific trait. Often companies power their own research databases to run GWAS to provide a wide range of trait information to their customers. Like other categories of DTC genetic information, trait information is most applicable for European populations.

Leveraging consumer interest in wellness and trait information is an opportunity for genetic counselors to talk about genetics in creative ways, providing teachable moments to explain genetic mechanisms and etiologies and to demonstrate that genetics is not always deterministic. It is a chance to talk about the potential of genetics, its current limitations, and how environment and lifestyle factors play an equally significant role.

Uninterpreted genetic data files

Consumer genetics companies provide reports on only a subset of the genetic information generated from their testing assay. As a result, a vast amount of uninterpreted genetic information still remains. Companies typically allow customers to access and download their uninterpreted or raw genetic data. Uninterpreted data generated through SNP genotyping technology includes all identified single nucleotide variants (SNVs or SNPs) and small insertions and deletions (INDELs) included in the company's assay. The information is digitized and available to consumers in some type of text format, such as the variant call format (VCF). The VCF includes the marker or SNP name (either the reference SNP [rs] ID or an internal ID number), the genomic location, possible variants associated with that marker, and the customer's genotype. The NCBI human reference genome build (e.g., human genome assembly GRCh37) used by the company and whether the data is referring to the positive (+) or negative (−) DNA strand are needed if the customer plans to transfer their data file to a third-party service. Nomenclature for deletions and no data should also be clarified. An example of a raw genetic data text file is shown in Figure 11.4.

Raw data has typically not been validated for accuracy and is meant for research or educational purposes, not for medical or diagnostic use. A variety of third-party interpretive services are available to consumers since most are not able to process their genetic data on their own (Badalato et al., 2017; Takano, 2020). Most are free, whereas some charge a fee for their services. Some services offer a range of information, while others focus on specific areas of interest such as research, genealogy, relative matching, and health and wellness. Individuals who share and explore their uninterpreted data using third-party services do so for many reasons such as seeking further health information, trying to find more relatives, looking for additional ancestry insights, or wanting to participate in research (Nelson et al., 2019).

```
# This data file generated on Mon Nov 02 13:04:35 2020

# This file contains raw genotype data, including data that is not used in our
# reports. This data has undergone a general quality review however only a subset
# of markers have been individually validated for accuracy. As such, this data
# is suitable only for research, educational, and informational use and not for
# medical or other use.
#
# Below is a text version of your data. Fields are TAB-separated
# Each line corresponds to a single SNP. For each SNP, we provide its identifier
# (an rsid or an internal id), its location on the reference human genome, and
# the genotype call oriented with respect to the plus strand on the human
# reference sequence. We are using reference human assembly build 37 (also known
# as Annotation Release 104). Note that it is possible that data downloaded at
# different times may be differnet due to ongoing improvements in our ability to
# call genotypes.
#
# More information on reference human assembly builds:
# https://www.ncbi.nlm.nih.gov/assembly/GCF_000001405.13/

rsid          chromosome position    genotype
rs548049170       1      69869          TT
rs9283150         1      565508         AA
rs116587930       1      727841         GG
rs3131972         1      752721         GG
rs12184325        1      754105         CC
rs12567639        1      756268         AA
rs114525117       1      759036         GG
rs12124819        1      776546         AA
rs12127425        1      794332         GG
rs79373928        1      801536         TT
rs7538305         1      824398         AC
rs28444699        1      830181         AA
rs116452738       1      834830         GG
rs72631887        1      835092         TT
rs28678693        1      838665         TT
rs4970382         1      840753         CC
rs4475691         1      846808         CT
rs72631889        1      851390         GG
rs7537756         1      854250         AG
rs13302982        1      861808         GG
rs376747791       1      863130         AA
rs2880024         1      866893         TT
(Report continues with listing of 600,000-700,000 SNPs)
```

FIGURE 11.4 Example of text file containing raw uninterpreted genetic data for single nucleotide polymorphism (SNP) genotyping platform.

Some are seeking health information because of a personal or family history, while others may be searching for a diagnosis of an unknown illness in themselves or a family member. Consumers can learn about additional genetic health information, which, if confirmed through clinical genetic testing, may lead to a diagnosis, changes in medical management, or lifestyle modifications. Promethease is one example of a third-party service that consumers use to obtain personal DNA health-related reports based on information in the SNPedia database (Promethease, n.d.). Additional genealogy information and connecting with biological relatives have the potential to expand family health information. GEDmatch is an online service commonly used by genetic genealogists and others when searching for biological relatives that compares autosomal DNA data files from different testing companies (GEDmatch, n.d.). Contributing to research by sharing genotypic and phenotypic data on crowdsourcing platforms such as Open Humans further promotes research and provides those consumers with a sense of goodwill (Open Humans, n.d.).

Consumers can gain additional genetic information as a result of their DTC testing experience; however, there are risks associated with interpreting raw data and transferring it from the original company to a third party. Unlike the data companies use to provide test reports to their customers, the remaining data has not been validated for accuracy and meaning (Tandy-Connor et al., 2018; Wu et al., 2019). The results provided by third-party interpretative services, which are largely unregulated, may not be accurate or clearly communicated to consumers (Guerrini et al., 2020). These limitations can result in false-positive and false-negative results. False-positive information can lead to unnecessary worry, emotional distress, follow-up tests and procedures, and financial hardship (Horton et al., 2019). Additionally, once a consumer downloads their uninterpreted data file, it is no longer protected by the original company's privacy and security measures (May, 2018; Moscarello et al., 2019). Consumers should read the privacy and security policies of any third-party service they are considering using.

There are additional concerns about public genealogy and other relative matching services. One involves law enforcement agencies' use of genealogy DNA databases to solve crimes, which raises privacy and ethical issues about the unauthorized or unintended uses of this information. GEDmatch was used in 2018 by law enforcement to solve the Golden State Killer case in California (Chamary, 2020). Site users were not aware that their DNA was being used for this purpose. Another concern is that people with malicious intent who are not actual relatives could upload fake genetic profiles to deduce information about a consumer based on matching sections of DNA. Lastly, the more databases a consumer utilizes, the greater the likelihood of unexpected findings such as the discovery of previously unknown close relatives.

Despite the limitations and risks involved in transferring and interpreting raw genetic data files, there is a growing consensus that consumers, research participants, and patients have a right to access their genetic data (May et al., 2020; Schickhardt et al, 2020). Some argue that genetic data access is an individual right based on GINA and HIPAA (Dreyfus & Sobel, 2018). HIPAA specifically provides individuals a legal right to obtain their laboratory test results, including genomic data (Evans, 2018).

Ancestry tests

Ancestry tests are used for various reasons and cross over into the health space (Smart et al., 2017). One reason for their use is to learn more about genetic ancestry or ethnicity, or one's biogeographical origins. A second reason is to search for and contact genetic relatives; DNA relative matching features typically involve an additional opt-in process. A third reason is to access uninterpreted raw genetic data files. Using their uninterpreted data, consumers can access online tools independently of the company to further explore their genetic information, including health-related SNPs, as discussed previously (B. E. Kirkpatrick & Rashkin, 2017; Yin et al., 2020).

FamilyTreeDNA, founded in 2000, was the first company established for genealogy purposes (FamilyTreeDNA, n.d.). Early ancestry tests included Y chromosome and mitochondrial DNA analysis. Ancestry testing today also includes autosomal and X chromosome DNA testing (Wallace & Bean, 2019). Y chromosome DNA tests comprise short tandem repeat (STR) and SNP analysis. SNP testing identifies paternal haplogroups that align with a direct line of male ancestors. Because of the stability of the Y chromosome, testing provides information about ancient migration routes taken by paternal ancestors going back tens of thousands of years. A comparison of STR markers looks for male matches that have a common recent ancestor. Y chromosome testing combined with surname databases helps in searches for male relatives along a paternal lineage. Women who want to know their paternal lineage need to obtain haplotype information from a paternally related male relative (International Society of Genetic Genealogy [ISOGG] Wiki, 2015; Royal et al., 2010).

Mitochondrial DNA testing for purposes of ancestry testing can include SNP testing, sequencing of hypervariable regions 1 and 2, and sequencing of the full mitochondrial genome. Mitochondrial DNA tests identify maternal haplogroups, providing information about the origins and migrations patterns of a person's ancient maternal lineage. Mitochondrial DNA results can be helpful when researching potential maternal biological relatives. Both males and females can be assigned a maternal haplogroup. Autosomal and X chromosome DNA tests involve primarily SNP testing but can include STR analysis. Autosomal DNA tests allow for more comprehensive searching, including using chromosome browser tools, and are not restricted to parental lineage (ISOGG Wiki, 2015; Royal et al., 2010).

Genetic ancestry

Estimating genetic ancestry or ethnicity is primarily done using markers or variants called ancestry-informative markers that are associated with populations of specific geographical areas from around the world (Via et al., 2009). As with other genetic association studies, testing looks for similarities in DNA among those with common self-identified ancestries. Based on reference populations, testing reveals the admixture of ancestral origins or ethnicity estimations of an individual (Royal et al., 2010). Companies use algorithms to assign segments of DNA to different populations and at varying levels of specificity depending on currently available reference group data. Ancestry information typically includes percentile breakdowns of various ethnicities. Typically, through a company's secure online portal, consumers can see a pie chart and geographical map of their ethnic background. An example of an ancestry test result is shown in Figure 11.5. DNA testing for genetic ancestry usually provides information about more recent populations; however, some ancestry results go further back.

Genetic ancestry results do not always coincide with what consumers expect based on family knowledge of ancestry (Resnick, 2019; Rubanovich et al., 2020). There are some technical reasons that this can happen:

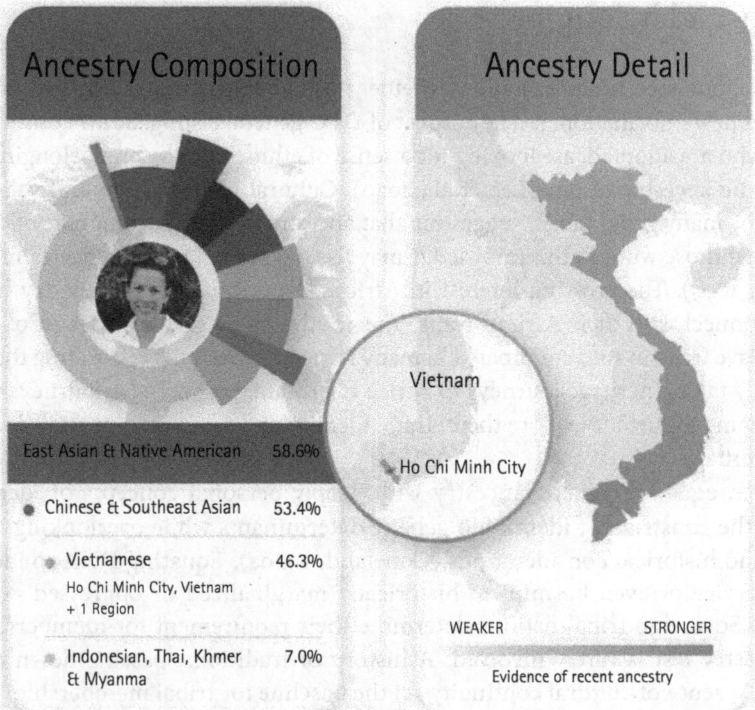

FIGURE 11.5 Display of a consumer's genetic ancestry results showing broad and detailed ancestry estimations for one continental area.

(Reproduced with permission from 23andMe)

1. Certain populations are difficult to tell apart since they share a common history (e.g., British and Irish; French and German).
2. Genetic ancestry is defined by genetically similar groups of people and not necessarily the political borders of countries.
3. Recent migration of certain groups may not be reflective of the reference populations used to assign genetic ancestry.
4. There may not be a robust reference population or enough specificity for some groups.
5. The knowledge of a specific ethnicity in a distant ancestor does not mean all descendants inherited DNA from that ancestor.

There can also be discrepancies in the information received from different companies, and genetic ancestry information from one company can change over time. This is because different companies may use different reference groups or different algorithms to assign ancestry. Results are often updated as the company's database grows and algorithms improve. Because of these limitations and confusion surrounding concepts such as ancestry and race, some argue that caution should be taken in how genetic ancestry information is used in healthcare (Blell & Hunter, 2019).

Identity and belonging

Curiosity about ancestry information, whether it is to confirm information already known or to learn new information, is a key aspect of DTC genetic testing. Some consumers, such as those who are adopted, are looking for a sense of ethnic identity and belonging through their genetic ancestry results (Lee et al., 2020). Cultural identification and values can be retained for many generations, suggesting that ancestry is an important part of one's identity and that those without this knowledge may feel a sense of loss and uncertainty (Bhugra & Becker, 2005). The growing interest in African American genetic ancestry has helped many reconnect with their African roots. The 400th anniversary of the start of the trans-Atlantic slave trade in 1619 culminated in many African Americans celebrating their genetic ancestry by taking heritage journeys to Africa (Germani, 2019). These journeys reflect the need for some to further explore their ethnic identity and celebrate a previously unknown cultural heritage.

However, equating genetic ancestry with deeply personal concepts of identity risks reducing the construct of identity to genetic determinants while overlooking important cultural and historical considerations (Copeland, 2020a). Equating DNA to identity can be a disservice or even harmful to historically marginalized or oppressed groups. For example, "Sovereign tribal nations determine their requirement for membership. A genetic ancestry test is rarely involved. A history of traditions, passing down crafts and skills, and a sense of cultural continuity set the baseline for tribal membership" (NHGRI, 2019, What it really means to be Native American section). The use of genetic ancestry testing to claim tribal heritage for purposes of personal gains, such as access to minority scholarships, raises concerns about misappropriated uses of a claimed identity (Walajahi et al., 2019).

Genetic counselors recognize how the variables that make up one's identity are integral in decision making about genetic testing and coping with a genetic condition. How consumers incorporate (or not) their genetic ancestry results into their sense of identity will vary (Shim et al., 2018). Engaging with patients about their motivations for DTC testing and what they learned about their genetic ancestry and its meaning to them presents opportunities for enriching discussions with patients and culturally competent care.

Relative matching and searching

Autosomal DNA tests are used to identify individuals within a database who have shared segments of DNA and are related by sharing one or more common ancestors (ISOGG Wiki, 2015). Companies provide estimates of relatedness between a matching pair by comparing sequences of markers including total length (based on centimorgans) and number of shared segments (Bettinger, 2017). The relatedness of a matching pair is estimated as first-degree relatives (full sibling, parent, child), second-degree relatives (half-sibling, aunt/uncle, niece/nephew, grandparent/grandchild), and third-degree and more distant cousin relatives. Companies often use demographic information, such as self-reported birth dates, to better specify relationships within a relatedness group. Nuances that can complicate relationship estimations include an atypical generational timespan or the unique genetic histories of different ethnic groups impacted by events such as endogamy or population bottlenecks (Southard, 2019).

Consumers who opt in to relative-matching features see their matches when they log in to their online portal, which can include close and more distant relatives. Matches may opt in to communicate with each other via email or an internal customer messaging system. Consumers can typically edit estimated relationships if they identify errors as well as clarify and expand their family tree by sharing genealogy information with their matches. Some services include tools and sorting features to help consumers explore how their matches might fit into their family tree.

Relative search strategies include genetic testing and genetic genealogy methods combined with traditional genealogy or adoption search methods (B. Kirkpatrick & Combs-Bennett, 2019). The approach typically involves testing at one or more of the major DTC genetic testing companies with large databases (ISOGG Wiki, 2015). Matches that are second cousins or closer are the most helpful for finding close relatives. If the search with the first company is unsuccessful, then individuals may consider testing with another major company, and so on.

Consumers often utilize third-party tools and services to extend and further refine their relative searches. This involves the transfer of a consumer's raw data file from the original source to the third-party service. GEDmatch is one third-party service used by genealogists and others searching for biological relatives (ISOGG Wiki, 2015). Consumers should read the terms and privacy policies of these services and consumer options before they share their data files. Genetic genealogy specialists and support communities are available to provide guidance to those undertaking a search. The ISOGG is a resource for information and strategies for finding biological relatives (ISOGG Wiki, 2015).

DTC genetic testing not only is an important tool for genealogists but also has transformed the process of searching for biological families for adoptees, those who are donor conceived, and others with unknown parentage (B. Kirkpatrick & Combs-Bennett, 2019; Lee et al., 2020). Some are searching for a birth parent hoping to connect with extended biological family members. Some want to be more certain about their current relationships, including who to date and marry, and pursue testing to rule out a biological relationship. Some use DTC testing because they are interested in genetic ancestry or want health-related information.

The decision to search for a biological family member is a major undertaking in terms of time and financial resources and can create emotional challenges. Some find birth parents and other family members and are able to happily welcome them into their lives. For others their search is unsuccessful, they are rebuffed by those they reach out to, or they are disappointed in the nature of their new relationships or distressed by some other discovery (B. Kirkpatrick & Combs-Bennett, 2019).

Adoptees interested in genetic health information can consider genetic testing beyond DTC health tests. Additional testing options include expanded carrier screening, pharmacogenomics panels, and exome or genome screening. Uninterpreted data files can be used to gain additional health information; however, as was previously discussed, there are risks and limitations with interpreting raw genetic data.

The ability to connect with biological relatives and learn genetic ancestry information through DTC genetic testing provides useful information for genetic counseling practice.

Consumers' genealogy and searching efforts can clarify and expand information about biological relationships, family health information, and ethnicity. Genetic counselors are an important resource for those searching for a biological family as they navigate genetic testing, use complex genetic strategies and principles in their searches, sort through a sense of identity and belonging, and experience a wide range of emotions inherent in looking for biological relatives. In fact, helping consumers navigate family searches and its consequences has become a unique area of specialization in genetic counseling practice (Watershed DNA, n.d.).

Unexpected Findings

The interest in discovering and contacting biological relatives is contributing to increased openness to publicly sharing genetic information and some unintended consequences. Emerging data reveal that a significant proportion of consumers discover unexpected information as a result of their DTC testing experience (Copeland, 2020b; Grab et al., 2019; Yin et al., 2020). People discover among their DNA matches previously unknown relatives, such as half-siblings, or that they are not matching with assumed biological relatives who also tested with the same company. Explanations can include technical or reporting issues, but often it is the beginning of the uncovering of a family secret. Besides discovering half-siblings, others learn that they were conceived using donor gametes, or their understanding of existing relationships is altered as in the cases of misattributed paternity. Third-party services offering tools that evaluate for regions of homozygosity can reveal consanguinity or incest (GEDmatch, n.d.).

The term "nonpaternity event" (NPE) was originally used to explain that a person's attributed father is not their biological father. Today the term is used more broadly to include misattributed parentage, so the acronym can also mean "not parent expected." NPEs result from adoptions, donor conceptions, infidelity, nonconsensual sex, medical errors, and even cases of kidnapping (NPE Friends Fellowship, n.d.). Individuals who donated sperm or eggs or placed a child up for adoption are no longer guaranteed the anonymity once promised (Dominus, 2019). Undisclosed relationships may be revealed regardless of whether or not all the parties involved have taken a DTC test (Khan & Mittelman, 2018).

DTC genetic testing has led to a surprising number of individuals discovering an NPE within their own families (Copeland, 2020a). There can be surprising but happy unions or major upheavals to existing relationships. Although some may feel empowered by the truth, for others it is devastating and results in a complex set of reactions and emotions (B. E. Kirkpatrick & Rashkin, 2017). The frequency of NPEs has led to the formation of online support and other groups (NPE Friends Fellowship, n.d.; Watershed DNA, n.d.).

Genetic counselors have dealt with the issue of misattributed paternity since the early days of genetic testing, helping families cope with the complex ethical and psychosocial ramifications (Hercher & Jamal, 2016). The possibility of the disclosure of misattributed paternity and other NPEs is regularly discussed during a genetic counseling session as part of the informed consent process prior to genetic testing. This risk associated with testing can then be factored into patient decision making and genetic counselors can offer support and anticipatory guidance if needed. Despite the challenges of helping patients cope with unrealized risks such as an NPE after genetic testing, genetic counselors have the skills and experience to provide support and guidance as NPEs and other "DNA surprises" become more commonplace as a result of DTC genetic testing. This includes educating other healthcare providers about how to help their patients navigate this unexpected consequence of DTC and other genetic tests.

Clinical and Personal Utility

Genetic tests, like other types of diagnostic tests, can be evaluated based on their clinical utility (Burke, 2014). Clinical utility refers to whether a test can provide information about the diagnosis, treatment, management, or prevention of disease. Since genetic testing is relatively new, evidence is being accumulated and reviewed about various genetic tests and their use in healthcare and screening programs. The CDC's Public Health Genomics and Precision Health Knowledge Base evaluates how well genetic and genomic discoveries are translated, or applied, to healthcare and disease prevention (CDC, 2014). Assessing the clinical utility of DTC genetic tests is important since test results can have clinical implications requiring follow-up care in a healthcare setting. Like clinical genetic tests, it will take time to gather enough evidence to determine whether or not DTC genetic tests have clinical value. A confounding variable is that physicians and other healthcare providers are not confident in interpreting DTC results or answering patient questions about DTC testing (Brothers & Knapp, 2018; Haga et al., 2019; Powell et al., 2012).

Studies are also looking at the psychological and behavioral effects of DTC genetic testing. Information, however, is limited since most of the published data are from three cohort studies: the Impacts of Personal Genomics (PGen) study (Gollust et al., 2017; Roberts et al., 2017), the Scripps Genomic Health Initiative (Bloss et al., 2011; Darst et al., 2013), and the National Institutes of Health Multiplex Initiative (Kaphingst et al., 2012). Participants from these studies were recruited over a decade ago and likely represent early adopters and not current DTC genetic testing consumers. Most participants were Caucasians of high socioeconomic status.

A 2018 meta-analysis of 11 studies looked at health-related behavior change, psychological responses, undesired consequences of testing, and sharing behaviors as a consequence of DTC genetic testing (Stewart et al., 2018). The analysis concluded that behavior changes were measurable but modest (one-quarter reported health behavior change). There was little evidence of serious adverse psychological responses among consumers, although there were a few potentially concerning reports of consumers changing prescriptions and over-the-counter medications based on test results. The analysis showed that consumers share information with family, and over one-third share results with healthcare providers. This early data suggests that DTC genetic testing only modestly improves health outcomes and is not detrimental to its users.

Other reasons consumers pursue testing have to do with personal and social factors. Personal utility refers to the nonmedical motivations and information that has personal value. Some consumers are seeking health information regardless of whether or not it influences their medical care (Turrini & Prainsack, 2016). For example, a sought-after DTC health test is for late-onset Alzheimer's disease despite a lack of prevention or cure

(Ostergren et al., 2015). The pursuit of DTC testing to learn about genetic ancestry, to look for biological relatives, to participate in research, and even just out of curiosity has personal value. This information for many consumers has a significant and far-reaching impact despite its lack of clinical utility.

Research Opportunities

Consumers have surprisingly embraced the opportunity to participate in research as part of their DTC genetic testing experience (Haeusermann et al., 2017; Ruhl et al., 2020). People use their genetic information to do good by contributing to research, which has value for society or social utility (Haeusermann et al., 2017). More recently, customers typically must opt in to participate in research and may have the option to opt out of continued participation. It is important for consumer genetics companies to be transparent and provide straightforward explanations on genetic data collection, how it is used, and how it is retained. Companies should provide clear choices and ask consumers to give express and separate consent for biological sample storage and use of their genetic data in research studies (Future of Privacy Forum, 2018; Niemiec & Howard, 2016).

Genetic data are usually deidentified and then used to look for genotype–phenotype associations at the population level. Large DTC genetic databases with high consumer participation in research and willingness to answer survey questions offer a unique platform for large-scale genomic studies. Consumer genetics companies share aggregated results of analyses with external researchers, furthering opportunities for genetic research (Ryan et al., 2020). In some instances, consumers are offered genotyping to participate in disease-specific research communities based on their personal and family history (23andMe, n.d.-b). Some who are frustrated with the slow progress in finding effective treatments and cures for familial diseases realize that DTC genetic testing provides a mechanism for them to personally contribute to genetic research.

Individuals from underrepresented groups can be recruited and offered genotyping to participate to help diversify genetic databases (23andMe, 2016a, 2016b). Some argue that the accessibility of DTC genetic tests, along with growing interest among Hispanic and non-Hispanic Black populations, may offer an opportunity to engage underrepresented groups in genetic testing and research (Carroll et al., 2019; NAS, 2020; Roberts et al., 2017). Research opportunities for consumers also exist through third-party services such as Open Humans (n.d.). Consumers should read the terms of service and privacy policies of these services before they download and transfer their raw data files.

Genetic Counseling and Education

As the DTC genetic testing market continues to grow, genetic counselors can help consumers and patients understand the value and limitations of DTC tests. Patients may seek genetic counseling to discuss their DTC test results, or DTC testing may come up incidentally in genetic counseling sessions. Consumers often seek genetic counseling services following

DTC testing because of health concerns, including seeking a diagnosis and uncertainty about results (Koeller et al., 2017).

Goal setting with patients who want to discuss DTC test results requires a realignment since some of the traditional genetic counseling goals do not apply. For example, the decision to have genetic testing has already been made. Patients' reasons for DTC testing and concerns about their results should be explored. Genetic counseling practice is based on the ability to recognize what motivates patients to pursue or not pursue genetic testing, which can be extended to understanding why patients decide to take DTC genetic tests. Additionally, patients' expectations of DTC testing may be unrealistic. Genetic counselors should realign these expectations without undermining patients' desire for information or belief in genetics. Patients need clear explanations about any potentially clinically relevant results and why confirmatory testing and other follow-up actions may be necessary (Marzulla et al., 2020).

Patient motivations for elective exome or genome sequencing are also applicable to DTC genetic testing. Three "patient types" have been described: (a) the "healthy and curious" who are not anticipating significant health results but want reassurance, (b) those who are looking for something specific based on a personal or family history, and (c) the "undiagnosed and searching" who have unexplained symptoms and are seeking validation that they are ill (Schmidt et al., 2019). This last group, who may be frustrated with doctors and the healthcare system, could particularly benefit from genetic counseling. In one small study of 15 participants, a third of patients seeking genetic counseling to discuss DTC test results self-reported a diagnosis of Ehlers-Danlos syndrome type III, which is underdiagnosed (Marzulla et al., 2020).

Genetic counselors can be a resource for primary care providers who are on the frontlines answering patients' questions about DTC genetic testing. Despite the growing appreciation for the potential of genomic medicine, many healthcare providers still do not feel adequately prepared to use genetic and genomic information in the care of their patients (Powell et al., 2012). Primary care and other healthcare providers need to recognize when results contain important health information requiring confirmation and follow-up care. There are opportunities in primary care to take advantage of patient discussions about DTC testing. These include the chance to update and discuss family health information, including any new biological relatives. Primary care providers who often have long-standing relationships with patients may be best positioned to offer support when patients discover unexpected findings as a result of DTC testing. Healthcare providers can inquire about genetic ancestry results, which may have relevance for health. Discussions about a patient's reasons for DTC testing offer opportunities to leverage patient engagement and motivation to discuss prevention and other health and wellness goals. A checklist to help primary care providers address DTC genetic testing in patient encounters is shown in Figure 11.6.

Conclusion

The Human Genome Project started in 1990 with the goal of determining the DNA sequence of the entire human genome. Today for a couple hundred dollars consumers can access their personal genetic information without the involvement of a healthcare provider.

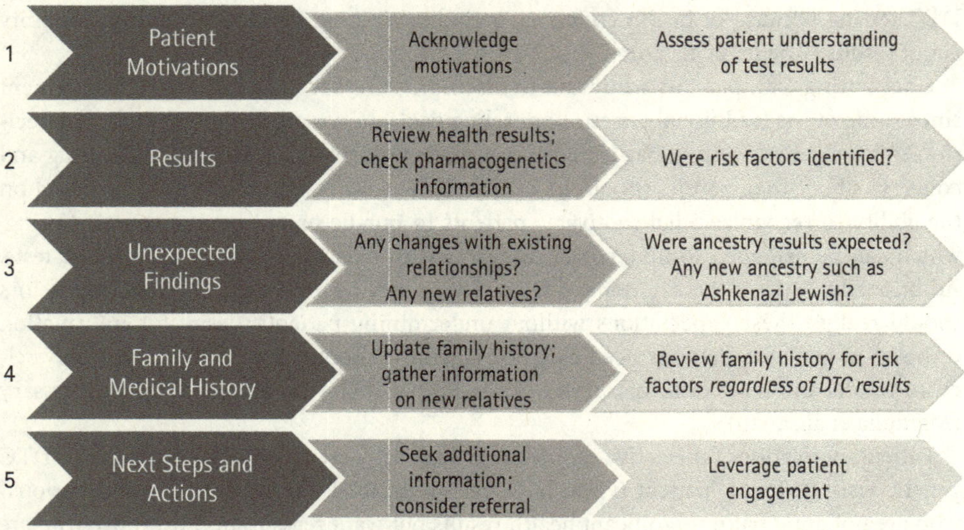

FIGURE 11.6 Primary care provider checklist for DTC genetic testing patient encounters. DTC = direct-to-consumer.

The accessibility and popularity of DTC genetic testing have helped to generate greater awareness and education about the role of genetics in health and identity. Uptake of DTC genetic testing is likely to continue to grow, with increasing numbers of consumers sharing their information with healthcare providers. There are aspects of DTC genetic testing that are unique from other types of genetic tests and important for genetic counselors to know. These are summarized in Box 11.1.

Genetic counselors have been integral in helping to adapt human genome discoveries and emerging technologies into clinical care by advocating that genetic information and technologies be used appropriately, that patients know the benefits and limitations of testing, and that patients make decisions based on their own values and beliefs. The emergence of DTC genetic testing occurred outside of the traditional clinical setting and has mostly evolved without significant input from genetic counselors. The ability of people to obtain genetic information outside of the context of genetic counseling has disrupted core genetic counseling values. The majority of genetic counselors are not comfortable counseling a patient about their DTC test results, while others refuse to even discuss health-related DTC testing in the first place. Despite the debates and controversies within the genetic counseling profession, genetic counselors' expertise and input are needed in the consumer genetics space.

Genetic counselors have an opportunity to lead and guide the responsible and ethical mainstreaming of genetics and health outside of the traditional healthcare model and within the context of consumer engagement and curiosity. They can advocate for regulatory standards and privacy protections for consumer genetic data. Genetic counselors can help consumers better understand what they are consenting to when they agree to participate in research and how their data might be used when it is uploaded to third-party services. Genetic counselors can participate in ongoing debates about consumer access to uninterpreted genetic data and help develop standards for evaluation of third-party services.

Box 11.1 Important Facts About DTC Genetic Testing

1. Models for consumer-driven genetic testing are evolving; only those with no required involvement of a health care provider are "true" DTC tests.
2. Consumers are interested in genealogy, ancestry, and health information and often want access to their raw genetic data files. A curiosity or fun factor may be part of the testing experience.
3. FDA evaluation of DTC tests involves assessing analytical and clinical validity as well as user comprehension studies.
4. Limitations include concerns about lack of scientific evidence, particularly in the wellness category; consumer misunderstanding of test results; breach of privacy of consumer data; and limited health care resources to provide follow-up.
5. Privacy protections for consumer genetic data are addressed by GINA, HIPAA, state genetic and consumer privacy laws, and consumer genetics industry standards for the collection, use, and storage of consumer genetic data.
6. Consumers may be engaged with research participation, creating unique opportunities to leverage large consumer databases for genetics research.
7. Consumers may upload their raw genetic data files to third-party interpretive services to gain more health information and find more DNA relatives. There are concerns about the validity of raw data, quality of third-party services, and privacy of genetic data once it is downloaded from the original company.
8. Health information related to ancestry tests includes genetic ancestry (ethnicity), clarification of biological relationships, and expanded knowledge of DNA relatives.
9. Discrepancies can occur with genetic ancestry results. Whether or not consumers integrate ancestry information into their concept of identity varies.
10. Unexpected findings, such as "not parents expected" or NPE, occur as a consequence of testing and have psychosocial and medical ramifications for consumers.
11. Evidence so far suggests DTC testing modestly improves health outcomes and is not detrimental to its users. One-third of consumers share test results with their health care providers.

DTC = direct-to-consumer; FDA = Food and Drug Administration; GINA = Genetic Information Nondiscrimination Act; HIPAA = Health Insurance Portability and Accountability Act.

They can develop educational resources to help people navigate the consumer genomics market and make informed decisions about tests that are based on scientific evidence.

Genetic counselors can participate in policy discussions involving the use of genetic ancestry information in healthcare, including educating other healthcare professionals about its significance, limitations, and potential for misuse. Genetic counselors are well versed in the ethical, legal, and social issues related to genetic testing in minors and should raise these issues within the context of DTC genetic testing. Genetic counselors can focus on strategies and innovations within the medical community that take advantage of consumer interest in genetics. Consumer genetics presents a teachable moment to educate and support other healthcare providers about genetic principles and issues, which will also help address the coming needs of precision medicine. DTC genetic testing is here to stay. Instead of viewing consumer genetics as an adversary, genetic counselors should leverage consumer engagement and awareness around it as human genome discoveries and technologies continue to advance both within and outside of healthcare.

Acknowledgments

I would like to thank Stacey Detweiler, MS, LCGC; Brianne Kirkpatrick, MS, LCGC; and Samantha Ancona Esselmann, PhD, for providing helpful feedback and insight on the contents of this chapter.

References

23andMe. (n.d.-a). *23andMe Research Innovation Collaborations Program*. https://research.23andme.com/research-innovation-collaborations/

23andMe. (n.d.-b). *Parkinson's disease research*. https://www.23andme.com/pd/

23andMe. (2016a, April 5). *23andMe scientists improving diversity in genetic research*. 23andMe Blog. https://blog.23andme.com/news/announcements/23andme-scientists-improving-diversity-in-genetic-research/

23andMe. (2016b, October 12). *The African Genetics Project*. 23andMe Blog. https://blog.23andme.com/23andme-research/the-african-genetics-project/

Allyse, M. A., Robinson, D. H., Ferber, M. J., & Sharp, R. R. (2018). Direct-to-consumer testing 2.0: Emerging models of direct-to-consumer genetic testing. *Mayo Clinic Proceedings*, *93*(1), 113–120. https://doi.org/10.1016/j.mayocp.2017.11.001

American College of Medical Genetics and Genomics. (2016). Direct-to-consumer genetic testing: A revised position statement of the American College of Medical Genetics and Genomics. *Genetics in Medicine*, *18*(2), 207–208. https://doi.org/10.1038/gim.2015.190

American College of Obstetricians and Gynecologists. (2017, March). *Carrier screening for genetic conditions*. https://www.acog.org/en/Clinical/Clinical Guidance/Committee Opinion/Articles/2017/03/Carrier Screening for Genetic Conditions

Badalato, L., Kalokairinou, L., & Borry, P. (2017). Third party interpretation of raw genetic data: An ethical exploration. *European Journal of Human Genetics*, *25*(11), 1189–1194. https://doi.org/10.1038/ejhg.2017.126

Bettinger, B. (2017, August 26). *August 2017 update to the Shared cM Project—The Genetic Genealogist*. https://thegeneticgenealogist.com/2017/08/26/august-2017-update-to-the-shared-cm-project/

Bhugra, D., & Becker, M. (2005). Migration, cultural bereavement and cultural identity. *World Psychiatry*, *4*(1), 18–24.

Blell, M., & Hunter, M. A. (2019). Direct-to-consumer genetic testing's red herring: "Genetic ancestry" and personalized medicine. *Frontiers in Medicine*, *6*, 48. https://doi.org/10.3389/fmed.2019.00048

Bloss, C. S., Schork, N. J., & Topol, E. J. (2011). Effect of direct-to-consumer genomewide profiling to assess disease risk. *New England Journal of Medicine*, *364*(6), 524–534. https://doi.org/10.1056/NEJMoa1011893

Botkin, J. R., Belmont, J. W., Berg, J. S., Berkman, B. E., Bombard, Y., Holm, I. A., Levy, H. P., Ormond, K. E., Saal, H. M., Spinner, N. B., Wilfond, B. S., & McInerney, J. D. (2015). Points to consider: Ethical, legal, and psychosocial implications of genetic testing in children and adolescents. *American Journal of Human Genetics*, *97*(1), 6–21. https://doi.org/10.1016/j.ajhg.2015.05.022

Brett, G. R., Metcalfe, S. A., Amor, D. J., & Halliday, J. L. (2012). An exploration of genetic health professionals' experience with direct-to-consumer genetic testing in their clinical practice. *European Journal of Human Genetics, 20*(8), 825–830. https://doi.org/10.1038/ejhg.2012.13

Brothers, K. B., & Knapp, E. E. (2018). How should primary care physicians respond to direct-to-consumer genetic test results? *AMA Journal of Ethics, 20*(9), 812–818. https://doi.org/10.1001/amajethics.2018.812.

Burke, W. (2014). Genetic tests: Clinical validity and clinical utility. *Current Protocols in Human Genetics, 81*, 9.15.1–8. https://doi.org/10.1002/0471142905.hg0915s81

Carroll, N. M., Blum-Barnett, E., Madrid, S. D., Jonas, C., Janes, K., Alvarado, M., Bedoy, R., Paolino, V., Aziz, N., McGlynn, E. A., & Burnett-Hartman, A. N. (2020). Demographic differences in the utilization of clinical and direct-to-consumer genetic testing. *Journal of Genetic Counseling, 29*(4), 634–643. https://doi.org/10.1002/jgc4.1193

Castro, D. (2011, December 13). *Benefits and limitations of industry self-regulation for online behavioral advertising.* https://itif.org/publications/2011/12/13/benefits-and-limitations-industry-self-regulation-online-behavioral/

Centers for Disease Control and Prevention. (2014, March 6). *Tier 1 genomics applications and their importance to public health.* https://www.cdc.gov/genomics/implementation/toolkit/tier1.htm

Centers for Medicare and Medicaid Services. (2020, October 1). *Clinical Laboratory Improvement Amendments (CLIA).* https://www.cms.gov/Regulations-and-Guidance/Legislation/CLIA

Chamary, J. (2020, June 30). *How genetic genealogy helped catch the Golden State Killer.* https://www.forbes.com/sites/jvchamary/2020/06/30/genetic-genealogy-golden-state-killer/#66b072205a6d

Clayton, E. W., Evans, B. J., Hazel, J. W., & Rothstein, M. A. (2019). The law of genetic privacy: Applications, implications, and limitations. *Journal of Law and the Biosciences, 6*(1), 1–36. https://doi.org/10.1093/jlb/lsz007

Committee on Bioethics, Committee on Genetics, and The American College of Medical Genetics and Genomics Social, Ethical, and Legal Issues Committee (2013). Ethical and policy issues in genetic testing and screening of children. *Pediatrics, 131*(3), 620–622. https://doi.org/10.1542/peds.2012-3680

Copeland, L. (2020a). *The lost family: How DNA testing is upending who we are* (Illustrated ed.). Abrams Press.

Copeland, L. (2020b, May 15). DNA testing is radically reshaping the definition of family. *Washington Post.* https://www.washingtonpost.com/outlook/dna-testing-is-radically-reshaping-the-definition-of-family/2020/05/14/2d7a746e-5e6c-11ea-b29b-9db42f7803a7_story.html

Critchley, C., Nicol, D., Otlowski, M., & Chalmers, D. (2015). Public reaction to direct-to-consumer online genetic tests: Comparing attitudes, trust and intentions across commercial and conventional providers. *Public Understanding of Science (Bristol, England), 24*(6), 731–750. https://doi.org/10.1177/0963662513519937

Crow, D. (2019). A new wave of genomics for all. *Cell, 177*(1), 5–7. https://doi.org/10.1016/j.cell.2019.02.041

Darst, B. F., Madlensky, L., Schork, N. J., Topol, E. J., & Bloss, C. S. (2013). Perceptions of genetic counseling services in direct-to-consumer personal genomic testing. *Clinical Genetics, 84*(4), 335–339. https://doi.org/10.1111/cge.12166

Dominus, S. (2019, June 26). Sperm donors can't stay secret anymore. Here's what that means. *New York Times.* https://www.nytimes.com/2019/06/26/magazine/sperm-donor-questions.html

Drabsch, T., & Holzapfel, C. (2019). A scientific perspective of personalised gene-based dietary recommendations for weight management. *Nutrients, 11*(3), 617. https://doi.org/10.3390/nu11030617

Dreyfus, J. C., & Sobel, M. E. (2018). Concern about justifying the release of genomic data as a civil right. *American Journal of Human Genetics, 103*(1), 163–165. https://doi.org/10.1016/j.ajhg.2018.06.003

Edwards, K. T., & Huang, C. J. (2014). Bridging the consumer-medical divide: How to regulate direct-to-consumer genetic testing. *Hastings Center Report, 44*(3), 17–19. https://doi.org/10.1002/hast.310

Evans, B. J. (2018). HIPAA's individual right of access to genomic data: Reconciling safety and civil rights. *American Journal of Human Genetics, 102*(1), 5–10. https://doi.org/10.1016/j.ajhg.2017.12.004

Evans, J. P., & Green, R. C. (2009). Direct to consumer genetic testing: Avoiding a culture war. *Genetics in Medicine, 11*(8), 568–569. https://doi.org/10.1097/GIM.0b013e3181b2e96e

FamilyTreeDNA. (n.d.). *DNA testing for ancestry & genealogy*. https://www.familytreedna.com/

Farrer, L. A., Cupples, L. A., Haines, J. L., Hyman, B., Kukull, W. A., Mayeux, R., Myers, R. H., Pericak-Vance, M. A., Risch, N., & van Duijn, C. M. (1997). Effects of age, sex, and ethnicity on the association between apolipoprotein E genotype and Alzheimer disease. A meta-analysis. APOE and Alzheimer Disease Meta Analysis Consortium. *JAMA, 278*(16), 1349–1356.

Federal Trade Commission. (2013, March 12). *Bureau of Consumer Protection*. https://www.ftc.gov/about-ftc/bureaus-offices/bureau-consumer-protection

Felzmann, H. (2015). 'Just a bit of fun': How recreational is direct-to-customer genetic testing? *New Bioethics, 21*(1), 20–32. https://doi.org/10.1179/2050287715Z.00000000062

Ferreira-Gonzalez, A., Teutsch, S., Williams, M. S., Au, S. M., FitzGerald, K. T., Miller, P. S., & Fomous, C. (2008). US system of oversight for genetic testing: A report from the Secretary's Advisory Committee on Genetics, Health and Society. *Personalized Medicine, 5*(5), 521–528. https://doi.org/10.2217/17410541.5.5.521

Floris, M., Cano, A., Porru, L., Addis, R., Cambedda, A., Idda, M. L., Steri, M., Ventura, C., & Maioli, M. (2020). Direct-to-consumer nutrigenetics testing: An overview. *Nutrients, 12*(2), 566. https://doi.org/10.3390/nu12020566

Food and Drug Administration. (2018a, February 22). *Statement from FDA Commissioner Scott Gottlieb, M.D., on implementation of agency's streamlined development and review pathway for consumer tests that evaluate genetic health risks*. https://www.fda.gov/news-events/press-announcements/statement-fda-commissioner-scott-gottlieb-md-implementation-agencys-streamlined-development-and

Food and Drug Administration. (2018b, March 7). *FDA authorizes, with special controls, direct-to-consumer test that reports three mutations in the BRCA breast cancer genes*. https://www.fda.gov/news-events/press-announcements/fda-authorizes-special-controls-direct-consumer-test-reports-three-mutations-brca-breast-cancer

Food and Drug Administration. (2018c, March 28). *FDA allows marketing of first direct-to-consumer tests that provide genetic risk information for certain conditions*. https://www.fda.gov/news-events/press-announcements/fda-allows-marketing-first-direct-consumer-tests-provide-genetic-risk-information-certain-conditions

Food and Drug Administration. (2018d, April 12). *FDA finalizes guidances to accelerate the development of reliable, beneficial next generation sequencing-based tests*. https://www.fda.gov/

news-events/press-announcements/fda-finalizes-guidances-accelerate-development-reliable-beneficial-next-generation-sequencing-based

Food and Drug Administration. (2018e, June 15). *Pharmacogenetic tests and genetic tests for heritable markers*. https://www.fda.gov/regulatory-information/search-fda-guidance-documents/pharmacogenetic-tests-and-genetic-tests-heritable-markers

Food and Drug Administration. (2018f). *Medical device overview*. https://www.fda.gov/industry/regulated-products/medical-device-overview

Food and Drug Administration. (2018g, September 27). *Laboratory developed tests*. https://www.fda.gov/medical-devices/vitro-diagnostics/laboratory-developed-tests

Food and Drug Administration. (2018h). *The FDA warns against the use of many genetic tests with unapproved claims to predict patient response to specific medications: FDA safety communication*. https://www.fda.gov/medical-devices/safety-communications/fda-warns-against-use-many-genetic-tests-unapproved-claims-predict-patient-response-specific

Food and Drug Administration. (2019a, October 25). *In vitro diagnostics*. https://www.fda.gov/medical-devices/products-and-medical-procedures/vitro-diagnostics

Food and Drug Administration. (2019b). *Direct-to-consumer tests*. https://www.fda.gov/medical-devices/vitro-diagnostics/direct-consumer-tests

Future of Privacy Forum. (2018, July). *Privacy best practices for consumer genetic testing services*. https://fpf.org/wp-content/uploads/2018/07/Privacy-Best-Practices-for-Consumer-Genetic-Testing-Services-FINAL.pdf

GEDmatch. (n.d.). *GEDmatch login*. https://www.gedmatch.com/login1.php

Germani, C. (2019, August 26). On US slavery's 400th anniversary, how ancestry quests help heal. *Christian Science Monitor*. https://www.csmonitor.com/USA/Society/2019/0826/On-US-slavery-s-400th-anniversary-how-ancestry-quests-help-heal

Gill, J., Obley, A. J., & Prasad, V. (2018). Direct-to-consumer genetic testing: The implications of the US FDA's first marketing authorization for BRCA mutation testing. *JAMA*, *319*(23), 2377–2378. https://doi.org/10.1001/jama.2018.5330

Godard, B., ten Kate, L., Evers-Kiebooms, G., & Aymé, S. (2003). Population genetic screening programmes: Principles, techniques, practices, and policies. *European Journal of Human Genetics*, *11*(2), S49–S87. https://doi.org/10.1038/sj.ejhg.5201113

Goldsmith, L., Jackson, L., O'Connor, A., & Skirton, H. (2012). Direct-to-consumer genomic testing: Systematic review of the literature on user perspectives. *European Journal of Human Genetics*, *20*(8), 811–816. https://doi.org/10.1038/ejhg.2012.18

Gollust, S. E., Gordon, E. S., Zayac, C., Griffin, G., Christman, M. F., Pyeritz, R. E., Wawak, L., & Bernhardt, B. A. (2011). Motivations and perceptions of early adopters of personalized genomics: Perspectives from research participants. *Public Health Genomics*, *15*(1), 22–30. https://doi.org/10.1159/000327296

Gollust, S. E., Gray, S. W., Carere, D. A., Koenig, B. A., Lehmann, L. S., McGuire, A. L., Sharp, R. R., Spector-Bagdady, K., Wang, N. A., Green, R. C., Roberts, J. S., & PGen Study Group. (2017). Consumer perspectives on access to direct-to-consumer genetic testing: Role of demographic factors and the testing experience. *Milbank Quarterly*, *95*(2), 291–318. https://doi.org/10.1111/1468-0009.12262

Gollust, S. E., Wilfond, B. S., & Hull, S. C. (2003). Direct-to-consumer sales of genetic services on the Internet. *Genetics in Medicine*, *5*(4), 332–337. https://doi.org/10.1097/01.GIM.0000076972.83711.48

Government Accountability Office. (2006). *Nutrigenetic testing: Tests purchased from four web sites mislead consumers. GAO-06-977T*. https://www.gao.gov/products/GAO-06-977T

Government Accountability Office. (2010). *Direct-to-consumer genetic tests: Misleading test results are further complicated by deceptive marketing and other questionable practices. GAO-10-847T*. https://www.gao.gov/assets/gao-10-847t.pdf

Grab, N. (2019, August 6). *Mail-in DNA test results bring surprises about family history for many users*. Pew Research Center. https://www.pewresearch.org/fact-tank/2019/08/06/mail-in-dna-test-results-bring-surprises-about-family-history-for-many-users/

Green, R. C., & Farahany, N. A. (2014). Regulation: The FDA is overcautious on consumer genomics. *Nature News*, *505*(7483), 286. https://doi.org/10.1038/505286a

Grody, W. W., Thompson, B. H., Gregg, A. R., Bean, L. H., Monaghan, K. G., Schneider, A., & Lebo, R. V. (2013). ACMG position statement on prenatal/preconception expanded carrier screening. *Obstetrical & Gynecological Survey*, *68*(12), 785–787.

Guerrini, C. J., Wagner, J. K., Nelson, S. C., Javitt, G. H., & McGuire, A. L. (2020). Who's on third? Regulation of third-party genetic interpretation services. *Genetics in Medicine*, *22*(1), 4–11. https://doi.org/10.1038/s41436-019-0627-6

Haeusermann, T., Fadda, M., Blasimme, A., Tzovaras, B. G., & Vayena, E. (2018). Genes wide open: Data sharing and the social gradient of genomic privacy. *AJOB Empirical Bioethics*, *9*(4), 207–221. https://doi.org/10.1080/23294515.2018.1550123

Haeusermann, T., Greshake, B., Blasimme, A., Irdam, D., Richards, M., & Vayena, E. (2017). Open sharing of genomic data: Who does it and why? *PloS One*, *12*(5), e0177158. https://doi.org/10.1371/journal.pone.0177158

Haga, S. B., Kim, E., Myers, R. A., & Ginsburg, G. S. (2019). Primary care physicians' knowledge, attitudes, and experience with personal genetic testing. *Journal of Personalized Medicine*, *9*(2), 29. https://doi.org/10.3390/jpm9020029

Harris, A., Kelly, S. E., & Wyatt, S. (2013). Counseling customers: Emerging roles for genetic counselors in the direct-to-consumer genetic testing market. *Journal of Genetic Counseling*, *22*(2), 277–288. https://doi.org/10.1007/s10897-012-9548-0

Hawkins, A. K., & Ho, A. (2012). Genetic counseling and the ethical issues around direct to consumer genetic testing. *Journal of Genetic Counseling*, *21*(3), 367–373. https://doi.org/10.1007/s10897-012-9488-8

Hendricks-Sturrup, R. M., & Lu, C. Y. (2019). Direct-to-consumer genetic testing data privacy: Key concerns and recommendations based on consumer perspectives. *Journal of Personalized Medicine*, *9*(2). https://doi.org/10.3390/jpm9020025

Hendricks-Sturrup, R. M., & Lu, C. Y. (2020). What motivates the sharing of consumer-generated genomic information? *SAGE Open Medicine*, *8*, 2050312120915400. https://doi.org/10.1177/2050312120915400

Hercher, L., & Jamal, L. (2016). An old problem in a new age: Revisiting the clinical dilemma of misattributed paternity. *Applied & Translational Genomics*, *8*, 36–39. https://doi.org/10.1016/j.atg.2016.01.004

Hock, K. T., Christensen, K. D., Yashar, B. M., Roberts, J. S., Gollust, S. E., & Uhlmann, W. R. (2011). Direct-to-consumer genetic testing: An assessment of genetic counselors' knowledge and beliefs. *Genetics in Medicine*, *13*(4), 325–332. https://doi.org/10.1097/GIM.0b013e3182011636

Hogarth, S., Javitt, G., & Melzer, D. (2008). The current landscape for direct-to-consumer genetic testing: Legal, ethical, and policy issues. *Annual Review of Genomics and Human Genetics*, *9*, 161–182. https://doi.org/10.1146/annurev.genom.9.081307.164319

Horton, R., Crawford, G., Freeman, L., Fenwick, A., & Lucassen, A. (2019). Direct-to-consumer genetic testing with third party interpretation: Beware of spurious results. *Emerging Topics in Life Sciences*, *3*(6), 669–674. https://doi.org/10.1042/ETLS20190059

Hsieh, V., Braid, T., Gordon, E., & Hercher, L. (2020). Direct-to-consumer genetic testing companies tell their customers to "see a genetic counselor." How do genetic counselors feel about direct-to-consumer genetic testing? *Journal of Genetic Counseling*, *30*, 191–197. https://doi.org/10.1002/jgc4.1310

Hudson, K., Javitt, G., Burke, W., & Byers, P. (2007). ASHG statement* on direct-to-consumer genetic testing in the United States. *American Journal of Human Genetics*, *81*(3), 635–637. https://doi.org/10.1086/521634

Ionova, Y., Ashenhurst, J., Zhan, J., Nhan, H., Kosinski, C., Tamraz, B., & Chubb, A. (2020). CYP2C19 allele frequencies in over 2.2 million direct-to-consumer genetics research participants and the potential implication for prescriptions in a large health system. *Clinical and Translational Science*, *13*, 1298–1306. https://doi.org/10.1111/cts.12830

ISOGG Wiki. (2015, October). *ISOGG Wiki*. https://isogg.org/wiki/Wiki_Welcome_Page

Kaphingst, K. A., McBride, C. M., Wade, C., Alford, S. H., Reid, R., Larson, E., Baxevanis, A. D., & Brody, L. C. (2012). Patients' understanding of and responses to multiplex genetic susceptibility test results. *Genetics in Medicine*, *14*(7), 681–687. https://doi.org/10.1038/gim.2012.22

Khan, R., & Mittelman, D. (2018). Consumer genomics will change your life, whether you get tested or not. *Genome Biology*, *19*(1), 120. https://doi.org/10.1186/s13059-018-1506-1

Khoury, M. (2017, April 18). *Direct to consumer genetic testing: Think before you spit, 2017 edition!* https://blogs.cdc.gov/genomics/2017/04/18/direct-to-consumer-2/

Kirkpatrick, B., & Combs-Bennett, S. (2019). *The DNA guide for adoptees: How to use genealogy and genetics to uncover your roots, connect with your biological family, and better understand your medical history*. Brianne Kirkpatrick and Shannon Combs-Bennett.

Kirkpatrick, B. E., & Rashkin, M. D. (2017). Ancestry testing and the practice of genetic counseling. *Journal of Genetic Counseling*, *26*(1), 6–20. https://doi.org/10.1007/s10897-016-0014-2

Koeller, D. R., Uhlmann, W. R., Carere, D. A., Green, R. C., Roberts, J. S., & PGen Study Group. (2017). Utilization of genetic counseling after direct-to-consumer genetic testing: Findings from the Impact of Personal Genomics (PGen) study. *Journal of Genetic Counseling*, *26*(6), 1270–1279. https://doi.org/10.1007/s10897-017-0106-7

Laestadius, L. I., Rich, J. R., & Auer, P. L. (2017). All your data (effectively) belong to us: Data practices among direct-to-consumer genetic testing firms. *Genetics in Medicine*, *19*(5), 513–520. https://doi.org/10.1038/gim.2016.136

Lee, H., Vogel, R. I., LeRoy, B., & Zierhut, H. A. (2020). Adult adoptees and their use of direct-to-consumer genetic testing: Searching for family, searching for health. *Journal of Genetic Counseling*, *30*, 144–157. https://doi.org/10.1002/jgc4.1304

Lombardi, C. (2008, October 30). *23andMe named best 2008 invention*. CNET. https://www.cnet.com/news/23andme-named-best-2008-invention/

Lu, M., Lewis, C. M., & Traylor, M. (2017). Pharmacogenetic testing through the direct-to-consumer genetic testing company 23andMe. *BMC Medical Genomics*, *10*(1), 47. https://doi.org/10.1186/s12920-017-0283-0

LunaDNA. (n.d.). *Upload raw DNA data & your health info to advance medicine*. https://www.lunadna.com/

Magnus, D., Cho, M. K., & Cook-Deegan, R. (2009). Direct-to-consumer genetic tests: Beyond medical regulation? *Genome Medicine*, *1*(2), 17. https://doi.org/10.1186/gm17

Martin, A. R., Kanai, M., Kamatani, Y., Okada, Y., Neale, B. M., & Daly, M. J. (2019). Clinical use of current polygenic risk scores may exacerbate health disparities. *Nature Genetics*, *51*(4), 584–591. https://doi.org/10.1038/s41588-019-0379-x

Marzulla, T., Roberts, J. S., DeVries, R., Koeller, D. R., Green, R. C., & Uhlmann, W. R. (2020). Genetic counseling following direct-to consumer genetic testing: Consumer perspectives. *Journal of Genetic Counseling*, *30*, 329–334. https://doi.org/10.1002/jgc4.1309

May, T. (2018). Sociogenetic risks—Ancestry DNA testing, third-party identity, and protection of privacy. *New England Journal of Medicine*, *379*(5), 410–412. https://doi.org/10.1056/NEJMp1805870

May, T., Nakano-Okuno, M., Kelley, W. V., East, K., Moss, I. P., Sodeke, S., Korf, B., & Barsh, G. (2020). Return of raw data in genomic testing and research: Ownership, partnership, and risk-benefit. *Genetics in Medicine*, *22*(1), 12–14. https://doi.org/10.1038/s41436-019-0607-x

McCabe, L. L., & McCabe, E. R. B. (2004). Direct-to-consumer genetic testing: Access and marketing. *Genetics in Medicine*, *6*(1), 58–59. https://doi.org/10.1097/01.gim.0000105753.01536.be

McDonough, R., & Armstrong, J. (2017). Technology assessment and the road to reimbursement of genomic based diagnostics. In G. S. Ginsburg & H. F. Willard (Eds.), *Genomic and precision medicine* (3rd ed., pp. 343–355). Academic Press. https://doi.org/10.1016/B978-0-12-800681-8.00023-2

McGowan, M. L., Fishman, J. R., & Lambrix, M. A. (2010). Personal genomics and individual identities: Motivations and moral imperatives of early users. *New Genetics and Society*, *29*(3), 261–290. https://doi.org/10.1080/14636778.2010.507485

McGrath, S. P., Walton, N., Williams, M. S., Kim, K. K., & Bastola, K. (2019). Are providers prepared for genomic medicine: Interpretation of direct-to-consumer genetic testing (DTC-GT) results and genetic self-efficacy by medical professionals. *BMC Health Services Research*, *19*(1), 844. https://doi.org/10.1186/s12913-019-4679-8

Moscarello, T., Murray, B., Reuter, C. M., & Demo, E. (2019). Direct-to-consumer raw genetic data and third-party interpretation services: More burden than bargain? *Genetics in Medicine*, *21*(3), 539–541. https://doi.org/10.1038/s41436-018-0097-2

National Academies of Sciences, Engineering, and Medicine. (2020). *Exploring the current landscape of consumer genomics: Proceedings of a workshop* (S. H. Beachy, J. Alper, S. Addie, & M. Hackmann, Eds.). National Academies Press. http://www.ncbi.nlm.nih.gov/books/NBK559862/

National Society of Genetic Counselors. (n.d.-a). *At-home genetic testing position statement*. https://www.nsgc.org/Policy-Research-and-Publications/Position-Statements/Position-Statements/Post/at-home-genetic-testing-position-statement

National Society of Genetic Counselors. (n.d.-b). *Genetic testing of minors for adult-onset conditions*. https://www.nsgc.org/Policy-Research-and-Publications/Position-Statements/Position-Statements/Post/genetic-testing-of-minors-for-adult-onset-conditions

National Human Genome Research Institute. (2019, May 19). *DNA tests stand on shaky ground to define Native American identity*. https://www.genome.gov/news/news-release/DNA-tests-stand-on-shaky-ground-to-define-Native-American-identity

National Human Genome Research Institute. (2020a, May 5). *Genetic Information Nondiscrimination Act of 2008*. Genome.Gov. https://www.genome.gov/about-genomics/policy-issues/Genetic-Discrimination

National Human Genome Research Institute. (2020b, September 25). *Regulation of genetic tests*. https://www.genome.gov/about-genomics/policy-issues/Regulation-of-Genetic-Tests

National Human Genome Research Institute. (2020c, September 25). *Regulation of genetic tests, CMS regulation, CLIA factsheet*. https://www.genome.gov/about-genomics/policy-issues/Regulation-of-Genetic-Tests

National Society of Genetic Counselors. (2019, June). *At-home genetic testing position statement*. https://www.nsgc.org/p/bl/ar/blogaid=1119

Nelson, S. C., Bowen, D. J., & Fullerton, S. M. (2019). Third-party genetic interpretation tools: A mixed-methods study of consumer motivation and behavior. *American Journal of Human Genetics, 105*(1), 122–131. https://doi.org/10.1016/j.ajhg.2019.05.014

Niemiec, E., & Howard, H. C. (2016). Ethical issues in consumer genome sequencing: Use of consumers' samples and data. *Applied & Translational Genomics, 8*, 23–30. https://doi.org/10.1016/j.atg.2016.01.001

NPE Friends Fellowship. (n.d.). *Awareness · community · education*. https://npefellowship.org/

Open Humans. (n.d.). *Home—Open Humans*. https://www.openhumans.org/

Ostergren, J. E., Gornick, M. C., Carere, D. A., Kalia, S. S., Uhlmann, W. R., Ruffin, M. T., Mountain, J. L., Green, R. C., Roberts, J. S., & PGen Study Group. (2015). How well do customers of direct-to-consumer personal genomic testing services comprehend genetic test results? Findings from the Impact of Personal Genomics Study. *Public Health Genomics, 18*(4), 216–224. https://doi.org/10.1159/000431250

Phillips, A. M. (2016). Only a click away—DTC genetics for ancestry, health, love . . . and more: A view of the business and regulatory landscape. *Applied & Translational Genomics, 8*, 16–22. https://doi.org/10.1016/j.atg.2016.01.001

Phillips, K. A., Trosman, J. R., & Douglas, M. P. (2019). Emergence of hybrid models of genetic testing beyond direct-to-consumer or traditional labs. *JAMA, 321*(24), 2403–2404. https://doi.org/10.1001/jama.2019.5670

Pollack, A. (2010, May 11). Start-up may sell genetic tests through Walgreens. *New York Times*. https://www.nytimes.com/2010/05/11/health/11gene.html

Pollack, A. (2013, November 25). F.D.A. orders genetic testing firm to stop selling DNA analysis service. *New York Times*. https://www.nytimes.com/2013/11/26/business/fda-demands-a-halt-to-a-dna-test-kits-marketing.html

Powell, K. P., Cogswell, W. A., Christianson, C. A., Dave, G., Verma, A., Eubanks, S., & Henrich, V. C. (2012). Primary care physicians' awareness, experience and opinions of direct-to-consumer genetic testing. *Journal of Genetic Counseling, 21*(1), 113–126. https://doi.org/10.1007/s10897-011-9390-9

Precision Medicine Advisors. (2019, November 21). *The expanding landscape of consumer genetic health testing*. https://www.precisionmedicineadvisors.com/precisionmedicine-blog/2019/11/21/the-expanding-landscape-of-consumer-genetic-health-testing

Promethease. (n.d.). *Promethease*. https://promethease.com/ondemandagreed

Regalado, A. (2019, February 11). More than 26 million people have taken an at-home ancestry test. *MIT Technology Review*. https://www.technologyreview.com/2019/02/11/103446/more-than-26-million-people-have-taken-an-at-home-ancestry-test/

Resnick, B. (2019, May 23). *The limits of ancestry DNA tests, explained*. Vox. https://www.vox.com/science-and-health/2019/1/28/18194560/ancestry-dna-23-me-myheritage-science-explainer

Roberts, J. S., Gornick, M. C., Carere, D. A., Uhlmann, W. R., Ruffin, M. T., & Green, R. C. (2017). Direct-to-consumer genetic testing: User motivations, decision making, and perceived utility of results. *Public Health Genomics, 20*(1), 36–45. https://doi.org/10.1159/000455006

Royal, C. D., Novembre, J., Fullerton, S. M., Goldstein, D. B., Long, J. C., Bamshad, M. J., & Clark, A. G. (2010). Inferring genetic ancestry: Opportunities, challenges, and implications. *American Journal of Human Genetics, 86*(5), 661–673. https://doi.org/10.1016/j.ajhg.2010.03.011

Rubanovich, C. K., Taitingfong, R., Triplett, C., Libiger, O., Schork, N. J., Wagner, J. K., & Bloss, C. S. (2020). Impacts of personal DNA ancestry testing. *Journal of Community Genetics*, *12*, 37–52. https://doi.org/10.1007/s12687-020-00481-5

Ruhl, G. L., Hazel, J. W., Clayton, E. W., & Malin, B. A. (2020). Public attitudes toward direct to consumer genetic testing. *AMIA Annual Symposium Proceedings*, *2019*, 774–783.

Ryan, K. A., Krenz, C. D., & Trinidad, M. G. (2020). What motivates the sharing of consumer-generated genomic information? *SAGE Open Medicine*, *8*. https://doi.org/10.1177/2050312120915400

Schickhardt, C., Fleischer, H., & Winkler, E. C. (2020). Do patients and research subjects have a right to receive their genomic raw data? An ethical and legal analysis. *BMC Medical Ethics*, *21*(1), 7. https://doi.org/10.1186/s12910-020-0446-y

Schmidt, J. L., Maas, R., & Altmeyer, S. R. (2019). Genetic counseling for consumer-driven whole exome and whole genome sequencing: A commentary on early experiences. *Journal of Genetic Counseling*, *28*(2), 449–455. https://doi.org/10.1002/jgc4.1109

Shim, J. K., Alam, S. R., & Aouizerat, B. E. (2018). Knowing something versus feeling different: The effects and non-effects of genetic ancestry on racial identity. *New Genetics and Society*, *37*(1), 44–66. https://doi.org/10.1080/14636778.2018.1430560

Smart, A., Bolnick, D. A., & Tutton, R. (2017). Health and genetic ancestry testing: Time to bridge the gap. *BMC Medical Genomics*, *10*, 1–9. https://doi.org/10.1186/s12920-016-0240-3

Southard, D. (2019, February 23). *DNA testing and endogamy*. Your DNA Guide. https://www.yourdnaguide.com/ydgblog/2019/2/23/endogamy

STAT. (2018, March 16). *Genetic tests ordered by doctors race to market, while DTC tests seek FDA approval*. https://www.statnews.com/2018/03/16/genetic-tests-fda-regulation/

State of California. (2018, October 15). *California Consumer Privacy Act (CCPA)*. State of California, Department of Justice, Office of the Attorney General. https://oag.ca.gov/privacy/ccpa

Stewart, K. F. J., Wesselius, A., Schreurs, M. A. C., Schols, A. M. W. J., & Zeegers, M. P. (2018). Behavioural changes, sharing behaviour and psychological responses after receiving direct-to-consumer genetic test results: A systematic review and meta-analysis. *Journal of Community Genetics*, *9*(1), 1–18. https://doi.org/10.1007/s12687-017-0310-z

Stoll, K. (2020, January 16). *Is there a doctor in the house? Physician-mediated DTC genetic testing*. The DNA Exchange. https://thednaexchange.com/2020/01/16/is-there-a-doctor-in-the-house-physician-mediated-dtc-genetic-testing/

Su, P. (2013). Direct-to-consumer genetic testing: A comprehensive view. *The Yale Journal of Biology and Medicine*, *86*(3), 359–365.

Takano, T. (2020, October 24). *Best free DNA upload sites to upload raw DNA data*. https://blog.genomelink.io/posts/best-raw-dna-data-upload-sites

Tandy-Connor, S., Guiltinan, J., Krempely, K., LaDuca, H., Reineke, P., Gutierrez, S., Gray, P., & Davis, B. T. (2018). False-positive results released by direct-to-consumer genetic tests highlight the importance of clinical confirmation testing for appropriate patient care. *Genetics in Medicine*, *20*(12), 1515. https://doi.org/10.1038/gim.2018.38

TechFreedom. (2013, December 17). *FDA oversteps on genetic testing: Berin Szoka in USA Today*. https://techfreedom.org/fda-oversteps-on-genetic-testing-berin-szoka-in/

Tennen, R. I., Laskey, S. B., Koelsch, B. L., McIntyre, M. H., & Tung, J. Y. (2020). Identifying Ashkenazi Jewish BRCA1/2 founder variants in individuals who do not self-report Jewish ancestry. *Scientific Reports*, *10*(1), 7669. https://doi.org/10.1038/s41598-020-63466-x

Turrini, M., & Prainsack, B. (2016). Beyond clinical utility: The multiple values of DTC genetics. *Applied & Translational Genomics, 8*, 4–8. https://doi.org/10.1016/j.atg.2016.01.008

Via, M., Ziv, E., & Burchard, E. G. (2009). Recent advances of genetic ancestry testing in biomedical research and direct to consumer testing. *Clinical Genetics, 76*(3), 225–235. https://doi.org/10.1111/j.1399-0004.2009.01263.x

Vorhaus, D. (2010a, May 11). *Where to next for personal genomics?* WIRED. https://www.wired.com/2010/05/where-to-next-for-personal-genomics/

Vorhaus, D. (2010b, August 5). *The past, present and future of DTC genetic testing regulation*. The Privacy Report. https://theprivacyreport.com/2010/08/05/the-past-present-and-future-of-dtc-genetic-testing-regulation/

Walajahi, H., Wilson, D. R., & Hull, S. C. (2019). Constructing identities: The implications of DTC ancestry testing for tribal communities. *Genetics in Medicine, 21*(8), 1744–1750. https://doi.org/10.1038/s41436-018-0429-2

Wallace, S. E., & Bean, L. J. (2019). *Resources for genetics professionals—Direct-to-consumer genetic testing*. University of Washington, Seattle. https://www.ncbi.nlm.nih.gov/books/NBK542335/

Watershed DNA. (n.d.). *Watershed DNA*. https://www.watersheddna.com

Weissman, S. M., Kirkpatrick, B., & Ramos, E. (2019). At-home genetic testing in pediatrics. *Current Opinion in Pediatrics, 31*(6), 723–731. https://doi.org/10.1097/MOP.0000000000000824

Wu, S., Pollard, J., Chowdry, A., Scheller, R., & Gentleman, R. (2019). Addressing the accuracy of direct-to-consumer genetic testing. *Genetics in Medicine, 21*(3), 758. https://doi.org/10.1038/s41436-018-0094-5

Yin, Z., Song, L., Clayton, E. W., & Malin, B. A. (2020). Health and kinship matter: Learning about direct-to-consumer genetic testing user experiences via online discussions. *PLOS ONE, 15*(9), e0238644. https://doi.org/10.1371/journal.pone.0238644

CHAPTER 12

GENETIC COUNSELORS AS RESEARCHERS

JULIA WYNN AND TARA SCHMIDLEN

Introduction

Genetic counselors have been engaged in research as long as the profession has been in existence. In this chapter, we highlight some of the seminal moments for genetic counseling research, current roles for genetic counselors in research, and types of research genetic counselors are conducting to continue to advance the field. This chapter is an examination of the role of genetic counselors in research and is not intended to provide instruction on how to conduct genetic counseling research. As the field continues to build a body of evidence to illustrate the value of genetic counseling, it will be important to examine how the roles of genetic counselors in research continue to evolve.

Genetic Counselors and Research

The critical importance of genetic counselor involvement in research is woven into genetic counseling training program accreditation standards and practice-based competencies. Genetic counselors need to have the ability to critically review, understand, and translate evidence from the primary literature into practice. They must be able to apply relevant research to patient care and be able to communicate it to patients and fellow healthcare providers. The provision of counseling to promote informed choices and adaptation to genetic risk or disease requires familiarity with research methods and the ability to distill outcomes reported in scientific literature into meaningful guidance for patients and their families.

The Accreditation Council for Genetic Counseling (ACGC) requires genetic counseling students to perform research and "other scholarly activities" (ACGC, 2023b, p. 23). For students to have the requisite skills for this work, the ACGC standards also require accredited master's programs to have curriculum content that covers quantitative and qualitative research methodologies, development of research questions, data collection and data analysis approaches, protection of human subjects, and the role of the Institutional Review Board (IRB).

The ACGC maintains the Practice-Based Competencies for Genetic Counselors that provides guidance for genetic counseling training as well as assessment of competency for practicing genetic counselors. Research is one of the competencies and is defined as the ability to "synthesize the evidence base relevant to genetic counseling," and within this competency are the following three subcompetencies: "Critically interpret data and literature. Apply data and literature considering its strengths, weaknesses, and limitations. Demonstrate knowledge of how genetic counselors engage and contribute to the research process" (ACGC, 2023a, p. 4).

Completion of a formal thesis, capstone, or other independent research project is a key component of a genetic counselor's training. A number of training programs require the dissemination of student research findings via both oral defense and written report. Submission of abstracts to national conferences and development of manuscripts for submission to peer-reviewed journals for publication are highly encouraged.

Beyond the application of research to genetic counseling clinical practice, research on genetic counseling service delivery, outcomes, and policies, among other areas, will be critical to continue to move the field forward. Genetic counselors have the appropriate expertise and perspective to lead these efforts. Genetic counselors are well positioned to identify pertinent knowledge gaps in genetic counseling practice and have the training needed to craft well-designed studies to address these gaps.

Seminal Events in Genetic Counseling Research

The field of genetic counseling is founded on and continues to be guided by research. Research established a need for genetic counselors, informed the development of the field, and evolves genetic counseling practice. Numerous people have contributed to the field of genetic counseling research, and a review of seminal works is helpful to see how these efforts have shaped the profession. In her book *Telling Genes: The Story of Genetic Counseling in America*, Alexandra Minna Stern offers a comprehensive summary of the early work that established the field of genetic counseling and genetic counseling research (Stern, 2012). In 2019, Robert Resta published a review of research related to genetic counseling outcomes (Resta, 2019). The following section summarizes the history that has been thoroughly reviewed by Stern and Resta and offers some additional observations of key developments in genetic counseling research.

Shaping the profession through research

Nongenetic counselors conducted some of the early research on genetic counseling as the profession was still being established. These works contributed to the formal development of the profession and eventually paved the way for genetic counseling research. Early work focused on exploring the experiences, impact, and effectiveness of genetic counseling. In 1979, Evers-Kiebooms and Van den Berghe published a review of studies assessing the impact of genetic counseling (Evers-Kiebooms & Van Den Berghe, 1979). Many of the studies examined patients' comprehension of recurrence risk and the factors that impact their comprehension including their genetic knowledge as well as socioeconomic and cultural background (Evers-Kiebooms & Van Den Berghe, 1979). These issues continue to challenge the field.

Evers-Kiebooms and Van den Berghe examined these studies for evidence that successful genetic counseling resulted in a reduction in the incidence of disease. This premise was based on what we now know to be a too simplistic assumption that all individuals are motivated to reduce disease burden in their family and population. Most of these studies were qualitative, though some collected more quantitative data via pre- and postcounseling patient surveys. Evers-Kiebooms and Van den Berghe concluded that these studies were limited by their design and recommended an arguably unethical design of randomized controlled trials where one group does not receive genetic counseling (Evers-Kiebooms & Van Den Berghe, 1979). The field continues to struggle with how to measure the impact of genetic counseling, which we now recognize to be multidimensional.

Around the same time as Evers-Kiebooms and Van den Berghe's work, geneticist F. Clark Fraser and epidemiologist Abby Lippman-Hand first documented that genetic counselors and parents do not always share the same views and understanding of genetic risk (Lippman-Hand & Fraser, 1979). Their study reviewed audio recordings of pediatric genetic counseling sessions and interviewed people who had received genetic counseling. They described the importance of distinguishing between patient perception and factual information. In particular, they noted a tendency of patients to conceptualize risk as binary—it will happen or it will not happen—regardless of the magnitude of risk (Lippman-Hand & Fraser, 1979).

In this same vein, James Sorenson led a landmark large-scale, multi-institutional longitudinal survey study of genetic counseling recipients (Sorenson et al., 1981). This study helped to highlight the importance of studying patient-reported outcome measures and that the reported outcomes should not focus solely on the provider's goals of the session but also on the patient's needs and goals. He proposed that outcome studies should not just focus on whether or not the provider's goals are met but also assess the needs of the patient and how well they are addressed.

Finally, it is important to recognize the significant impact of psychologist Seymour Kessler's work on the genetic counseling profession. Kessler is often credited with the movement of genetic counseling to a more psychologically based approach. His work focused on understanding the psychosocial aspects of a patient's choices and actions and emphasized the frequent discordance between the genetic counselor's and patient's session goals. He published seminal papers on the psychological aspects of genetic counseling that helped the field make the transition to studying psychological impact as an outcome of genetic counseling (Kessler, 1992).

These individuals and others conducted work that enhanced genetic counseling practice and advanced understanding of how to study the practice. Qualitative and quantitative studies examining patient interviews, recorded genetic counseling sessions, and patient-reported outcome measures are critical areas of research and remain integral topics of interest for genetic counseling researchers.

Refining the Research of Genetic Counseling

Genetic counselors are leading efforts to set research priorities for the field as well as continue to elevate the quality and rigor of the evidence generated. Genetic counseling outcomes studies are critical in establishing the value of our practice as well as understanding the effectiveness of interventions or novel approaches to genetic counseling practice. In particular, as genomic medicine becomes more widespread and as medicine is increasingly using technology to provide accessible and scalable care, there has been a movement to assess and promote evidence-based clinical applications of genetic counseling. To address this, the National Society of Genetic Counselors (NSGC) convened a task force of experts in genetic counseling practice who developed standards for reporting genetic counseling interventions and in 2017 published the Genetic Counseling Intervention Reporting Standards (Hooker et al., 2017). The final standards include 23 items across eight domains to provide guidelines across a range of different study designs. The standards specify that the following domains should be reported in all outcomes research: (a) indication for genetic counseling; (b) interventions that occurred, if any, at the time of genetic counseling such as offering genetic testing; (c) how the intervention was delivered (in person, telephone); (d) who provided the intervention (genetic counselor, other healthcare provider); (e) risk/educational content included in session; (f) psychotherapeutic content included in session; (g) the length of the intervention; and (h) the number of interventions. The goal of these standards is to improve the assessment, reporting, and evaluation of genetic counseling interventions, which is critical to achieve desirable patient outcomes as the field moves toward a more evidence-based practice.

Genetic counseling research has also been important in developing models of genetic counseling practice and frameworks to conceptualize genetic counseling theories. In 2007, work by psychologist Patricia McCarthy Veach, nursing and family social science expert Dianne Bartels, and genetic counselor Bonnie LeRoy led to the development of the Reciprocal-Engagement Model (Veach et al., 2007). This model is based on input from over 20 genetic counseling program directors. It established five tenets of genetic counseling that focused on genetic education, the patient–provider relationship, patient autonomy, patient resiliency, and patient emotions. See Chapter 5—"The Reciprocal-Engagement Model of Genetic Counseling Practice" in this volume for further details on the Reciprocal-Engagement Model.

Heather Zierhut and Deborah Cragun developed a framework to conceptualize communication strategies in practice. They completed a comprehensive review and thematic analysis of genetic counseling outcome literature to develop the "Framework for Outcomes of Clinical commUnication Services" (FOCUS), which contains the domains of communication strategy; communication process measures; patient care experience, patient changes, and patient health; and family changes (https://www.focusoutcomes.com). They developed an accompanying website to provide a step-by-step guide (Cragun & Zierhut, 2018).

Effective analysis of the practice of genetic counseling is important to facilitate evidence-based practice that integrates the best evidence from studies and patient care data with clinician expertise and patient preferences and value. Understanding the impact of genetic counseling on patient and healthcare outcomes can inform practice guidelines and demonstrate the value of genetic counselors for payers and institutions. The development, validation, and implementation of patient-reported outcome measures can generate this evidence. One utilized outcome measure is the Genetic Counseling Outcome Scale (GCOS) and the short-form scale, the Genetics Outcomes Scale (GOS; Grant et al., 2019; McAllister et al., 2011). The GCOS has been used across genetic counseling disciplines and multiple languages and demonstrates reliability and validity (Burns et al., 2018; Gerrard et al., 2020; Muñoz-Cabello et al., 2018; Voorwinden et al., 2019). Other genetic counseling–specific patient outcome measures have also been developed including the Genetic Counseling Satisfaction Scale, which was validated in women receiving hereditary cancer genetic counseling (DeMarco et al., 2004). Given the diversity of genetic counseling practice settings, it is particularly challenging to create a single scale that captures all genetic counseling outcomes across all areas of practice. In response, additional scales have been developed to measure desired outcomes of genetic counseling. An example of this is the Multidimensional Measure of Informed Choice, which aims to assess whether a patient has made an informed decision by measuring knowledge, attitudes, and uptake of a test. This scale has been used to measure informed choice for prenatal Down syndrome screening (Dormandy et al., 2002). Another scale was developed to measure patient empowerment following genetic counseling and testing (McConkie-Rosell et al., 2019). Scales have also been developed to measure the value of genetic counseling. Press Ganey, a private organization that measures patient satisfaction in healthcare and is frequently used by payers to guide value-based payment structures, has a medical practice survey specifically for genetic counseling services (Presson et al., 2017). A full examination of outcome and value measures is beyond the scope of this chapter. This is a very active area of genetic counseling research. A publication by Higgs and colleagues (Higgs et al., 2022) on the landscape and future directions of this field and the Genetic Counseling Literature Repository (GCLR) are both excellent resources to stay abreast of these topics. The GCLR is a searchable, PMID-linked database within the NSGC's website, designed to identify articles that (a) document the value and quality of genetic counseling services and (b) describe clinical and research outcomes relevant to genetic counseling patients. It includes indexing to identify studies utilizing outcome and value measures (NSGC, n.d.).

Genetic Counselors Leading Research

Genetic counselors contribute enormously to research within the genetics community. Because of their unique placement at the intersection of clinical care and research, the research is often translational, addressing how new technologies and discoveries are integrated into clinical care. In the 2010s, genetic counselor Barbara Bernhardt led the qualitative work exploring patients' experiences of prenatal chromosome microarray testing, at the time a new diagnostic technology (Bernhardt et al., 2013). This work continues to inform genetic counseling for genomic analysis and studies exploring prenatal genomic sequencing. Genetic counselors have contributed to the establishment of new domains of genetic counseling as well as expanding existing domains. The work of Jehannine Austin, a genetic counselor and neuropsychiatric genetics expert, laid the foundation establishing the specialty of psychiatric genetic counseling and continues to inform this practice area

(Austin & Honer, 2007; Peay et al., 2008). Genetic counselor Jodie Ingles is a leader in cardiogenetics exploring issues such as the challenges of interpreting genetic variants but also the psychosocial impacts of having an inherited cardiac condition (Ingles et al., 2011). Christina Palmer has been integral in guiding culturally competent genetic counseling for the Deaf community. Her work helped to define the role and impact of genetic testing in this community and guide the training of genetic counselors (Alford et al., 2014; Nagakura et al., 2015). Marion McAllister, genetic counselor and social scientist, is a leader in the field of patient-reported outcomes in genetic counseling. See Chapter 30—"Genetic Counseling Outcomes, Patient Empowerment, and the Genetic Counseling Outcome Scale" in this volume for further details on the value of measuring patient outcomes from genetic counseling. She developed the GCOS discussed previously and continues to work on identifying and measuring genetic counseling outcomes and establishing an evidence base for genetic counseling (Thomas & McAllister, 2019). These are just a few of the examples of how hundreds of research genetic counselors from study coordinators to principal investigators across all genetic research disciplines are impacting the profession and practice.

One interesting and unique aspect of genetic counseling research is the diversity of practice settings to which individual researchers can contribute. Many prominent research genetic counselors are not specialized to a specific area but rather, related to their academic positions, clinical roles, and training program involvement, have contributed across several research disciplines. For example, Barbara Biesecker has led or contributed to developing genetic counseling outcome scales, assessing novel platforms for the delivery of genetic counseling services, and exploring patient experiences of receiving secondary findings from genomic sequencing (Biesecker et al., 2017; Hart et al., 2018; Lewis et al., 2018). Another example is Amy Curry Sturm, whose body of work is focused on cardiovascular genetics (VanDyke et al., 2021) but also includes exploring issues in cancer genetics (Campbell-Salome et al., 2021), pharmacogenetics (Schmidlen et al., 2020), and precision medicine (Buchanan et al., 2020). Diverse research across topics and study designs is a unique opportunity among scientific researchers where often very specialized expertise is required. Having a high-level expertise in any one domain is frequently a criterion for funding, and therefore, a diverse research portfolio may create challenges when applying for funding.

Roles in Research

Genetic counselors serve in a variety of roles with respect to the conduct of research. Many begin their research careers in the role of the research coordinator. Research coordinators work under the supervision of the study principal investigator and carry out many study essential duties. These tasks can include drafting and assembling the study protocol and IRB submission, writing the informed consent document, recruiting subjects, collecting and documenting subject informed consent, drafting questionnaires or interview guides, providing genetic counseling to study participants, documenting and reporting any adverse events, preparing continuing review updates to the IRB, drafting abstracts and manuscripts reporting study data, participating in the administrative tasks of closing out a study, and myriad other research tasks necessary to maintain study operations.

Genetic counselors are also increasingly occupying leadership roles in research, such as serving as the study principal investigator (PI). In research, the PI is responsible for the design, conduct, and reporting of the project as well as coordination and management of any external collaborative partners. Principal investigators are also responsible for the oversight of research compliance, study budget, and all study personnel. To achieve this, they coordinate with their university, department, and administrative personnel to ensure that their research is conducted according to federal regulations and the policies and procedures required by their institution and/or sponsoring agency. Many institutions may require that individuals serving in the PI role have doctoral-level training, faculty status, or both. Some institutions will only grant faculty status to those with doctoral-level training, which may limit available avenues to master's-level genetic counselors wishing to obtain grant funding.

Another avenue for genetic counselor leadership in research is the co–principal investigator (co-PI) or coinvestigator (co-I) role. The Co-PI/co-I have responsibilities very similar to that of the PI on research projects. While the study PI maintains the ultimate responsibility for research conduct and oversight, the co-PI/co-I is also obligated to ensure that the study is conducted in a manner compliant with applicable laws, research regulations, and institutional policies. Often co-Is/co-PIs will take responsibility for a specific aim of a research project related to their subject matter expertise. Alternatively, they may serve as the leader of all of the research aims for a satellite location of a multisite research project. Institutions and funding agencies vary with regard to criteria on who is eligible to serve as PI or co-I. Doctoral degree, faculty status, and/or support of an academic department or academic administrator such as a dean may be required.

Outside of academia, genetic counselors can provide expertise to industry or other stakeholders by serving as a research consultant. Research consultants collect and analyze data on various topics and present their findings to stakeholders. Duties of a research consultant may vary widely but typically include designing and implementing a research strategy and estimating time for completion, conducting literature reviews and summarizing existing data, collecting additional new data, analyzing and interpreting data, and summarizing research outcomes into written reports and presentations.

Genetic counselors working within industry may also fill roles that require research expertise. Increasingly, genetic testing laboratories are employing genetic counselors with research experience to serve as "medical affairs" or "clinical science" liaisons between the laboratory, academic, biopharmaceutical, biotechnology and other research partners. Counselors in these roles often provide project management support and may also be charged with identifying and vetting research collaboration requests.

The core competencies of a master's-level genetic counselor provide a firm foundation for further on-the-job research skill development. Upon graduation from an accredited program, genetic counselors must demonstrate understanding of the research process described in the aforementioned practice-based competencies.

Opportunities for genetic counselors to gain research training are also increasing. Some research genetic counselors come to the profession with doctorate-level training or pursue a doctoral degree after obtaining a master's degree in genetic counseling. A doctoral degree is historically a requirement to hold research faculty positions at academic institutions. Doctorate-level genetic counselors have represented less than 2% of the genetic counseling community since these data were initially collected by the Professional Status Survey (PSS; NSGC, 2000; NSGC, 2022). Many research genetic counselors, including those working solely in research, develop or enhance their research skills through on-the-job training often with dedicated mentoring and peer support. Increasingly, institutions are recognizing the capacity of master's-level genetic counselors to conduct research. In 2020 the National Institutes of Health (NIH) released a call for the first-ever genetic counseling training grant: "Notice of Special Interest (NOSI): Availability of Administrative Supplements for Providing Research Experiences in Genomic Research for Genetic Counselors." As genetic counselors are increasingly recognized as integral partners in research, it is likely that these types of opportunities will grow for both master's-level and doctorate-level genetic counselors. Importantly, as these opportunities are presented, it is imperative that genetic counselors step in to lead this research in collaboration with other integral disciplines including bioethicists, psychologists, and health economists, among others.

Types of Research

The types of research genetic counselors are conducting are as diverse as the roles that they serve in research. In the era of precision medicine, genetic counselors are well positioned to lead efforts that will answer the social and behavioral research questions that arise as genomic medicine becomes further integrated into clinical care. Genetic counselors are engaged in research investigating key areas of genomic medicine including identifying the best ways to educate and empower a diverse array of clients to utilize genomic information to make health decisions and finding the most effective strategies to help individuals adapt to unexpected or uncertain information (e.g., secondary findings, variants of uncertain significance, etc.). In addition to research aimed at improving the patient experience, there is a pressing need for research to examine alternative genetic counseling service delivery models that leverage emerging technologies such as online interactive web portals, video education modules, and chatbots. Noninferior alternatives to the traditional face-to-face genetic counseling model are needed to expand access to genetic counseling services in a manner that allows all patients who need genetics services to receive them while preserving the limited pool of genetic counselors for in-person sessions that involve more complex health issues and more significant psychosocial burdens.

In addition to facilitating the integration of genomics into clinical care, genetic counselors are contributing their unique skills to a wide variety of other research activities including natural history studies, clinical trials, research consortiums, and the assimilation of research outcomes into evidence-based practice guidelines to guide the practice of genetic counselors.

Genomics is becoming increasingly important in the execution of clinical trials as researchers work to develop more effective targeted therapies. In the clinical trial setting, genetic counselors can assist with genetic testing for patient identification and enrollment of eligible patients as they are uniquely poised to explain expectations and implications of genetic tests to potential trial participants. Genetic counseling can also improve participant satisfaction, which may help improve engagement and retention during clinical trials in addition to creating a more positive experience with trial participation (Zierhut & Austin, 2011).

Genetic counselors have been an integral part of several large research consortia in genomics tackling gene and variant curation (ClinGen), integrating genome sequencing into the clinical care of diverse and medically underserved individuals (CSER), combining the power of biorepositories with electronic medical record systems for genomic discovery and genomic medicine implementation research (eMERGE), and incorporating genomic information into the electronic medical record with appropriate clinical decision support (IGNITE), to highlight just a few of the many genomics consortiums in existence. Genetic counselors are involved in these consortia at all levels, from clinical research coordinators to investigators. Involvement in these types of consortia enables genetic counselors to grow in their careers by engaging in new research opportunities and providing mentorship desired by colleagues who wish to gain research skills.

Genetic counselors are playing a critical role in helping research participants understand genomic test results returned by the largest longitudinal study in the history of the United States, the All of Us Research Program. The All of Us Research Program plans to build a diverse cohort of at least 1 million volunteer participants in the United States with the goals of accelerating biomedical research and improving health. All of Us currently recruits participants 18 years of age or older from more than 300 recruitment sites. All of Us volunteers will contribute biospecimens and their health data via questionnaires, electronic health records, and digital health technology to a centralized national database. This database will serve as a platform for research capable of identifying individual differences in disease etiology and natural history by examining variability in genes, environment, and lifestyle. In August 2019, the National Institutes of Health awarded $4.6 million to Color, a privately held health technology company based in California, to establish a nationwide genetic counseling resource to support the All of Us Research Program, using software and digital tools to address traditional barriers to genetic counseling. Genetic counselors with Color and the All of Us Research Program are working with participants to return results, provide genetic counseling, and connect participants to local healthcare providers to address their specific health risks.

Leading the assimilation and dissemination of key research outcomes into evidence-based clinical practice guidelines is another important role for genetic counselors in the research setting. Clinical practice guidelines are statements that include recommendations intended to optimize patient care. They are informed by a systematic review of evidence and an assessment of the benefits and harms of alternative care options. The NSGC established the Practice Guidelines Committee (PGC) in 2012 to oversee the development of the NSGC's evidence-based practice guidelines and to review endorsement requests for practice guidelines sponsored by external organizations. The NSGC's genetic counseling practice guidelines help demonstrate that genetic counseling is an integral part of healthcare delivery and quality care. These documents contain recommendations for using certain genetic information in healthcare, which include but are not limited to referral practices, disease screening, predictive testing, disease diagnosis, and treatment. Recommendations may also address accessing, evaluating, and/or delivering genetic counseling services.

Milestones in Genetic Counselor Research

The NSGC PSS is an annual survey of NSGC membership that examines various aspects of the genetic counseling profession, including work environments and faculty status. The PSS has collected information about genetic counselors' research involvement since 2000, and the data indicate a consistent proportion of genetic counselors' participation in research at varying levels. Initially, the survey collected information about the proportion of genetic counselors who reported research to be a component of their job, and nearly a third (27% to 32%) of genetic counselors from 2000 to 2006 reported it was (NSGC, 2000, 2002, 2004, 2006). After 2006, the PSS began collecting information about the number of respondents who report researcher, research scientist, or study coordination as their primary role, and this number has ranged from 1.5% to 4.5% through 2021 (NSGC, 2008; NSGC, 2010, 2012, 2014, 2016, 2018, 2019, 2020, 2021b). During these years, the PSS also gathered information about research-related activities. For example, the 2023 NSGC PSS found that 15% of genetic counselor respondents wrote or developed protocols that were approved by an IRB, 17% worked on peer-reviewed publications, and approximately 7% contributed to funded grant applications (NSGC, 2023). Overall, data from the PSS indicate that research has been and continues to be important in the profession of genetic counseling.

The growing involvement of genetic counselors in research is reflected in the growth of opportunities for genetic counselors engaged in research. In 1996 the NSGC launched special interest groups (SIGs), which are now under the umbrella of NSGC communities (NSGC, 2021a). The SIGs bring together genetic counselors working in similar areas of practice or who are focused on specific issues to create a peer group. They also serve as a place for genetic counselors to identify specific expertise. The NSGC Research SIG was founded in 2000 (NSGC, 2021a) and continues to be an active community of the full spectrum of genetic counselors involved in research at every career stage. The Research SIG maintains a listserv and research-related resources and consistently contributes to the NSGC annual conference through the development of educational breakout sessions and pre- and postconference symposia.

In March of 1992, the first edition of the *Journal of Genetic Counseling* (JoGC) was published. At that time, Editor-in-Chief Deborah L. Eunpu outlined the journal's goals: (a) increase the number of papers that address the interface of advancing technologies and the needs of the genetic patient/client and (b) "improve the quality and richness of material published" about the field of genetic counseling (Eunpu, 1992, p. 1). The inaugural issue included a spectrum of content for which the journal has become known. In his seminal piece, psychologist Seymour Kessler interrogates the concepts of both nondirective and directive genetic counseling, comparing and contrasting both (Kessler, 1992). Another article addressed how Asian ethnocultural perspectives on autonomy (collective versus individual), informed consent, and nondirective counseling conducted from a Western perspective may contribute to misinterpretations of the normative decision-making process and misconceptions about normalcy and result in less effective care (Wang & Marsh, 1992). The NSGC Code of Ethics was also published in full (NSGC, 1992). In addition, the first edition included the abstracts from the most recent NSGC Annual Education Conference (1990), which it continued to publish until 2018. Nearly 30 years, five editors, and over 2,000 articles later, the JoGC is the leader in publications related to the field of genetic counseling. The journal has risen in visibility and scope, and articles extend beyond genetic counseling theory and practice. The journal now includes articles on genetics and genetic counseling as they relate to public health, public policy, and access and delivery service issues; ethical, legal, and social issues; and education, workforce, and risk assessment. The editorial board considers a variety of different article types for publication, from original research, case series, and reviews to invited commentary and book reviews. The journal also publishes the NSGC practice guidelines and resources. Regularly, new guest editors are invited to compile special editions as topical issues arise; some special editions include Minorities and Health Disparities in Genetic Counseling and Genomic Medicine (2020), Exploring the Exome: New Genetic Counseling Insights (2019), Technology in Practice (2018), Working With Psychological and Social Complexity (2017), and Genetic Counselor Professional Development (2016). Further indicative of the rising profile of genetic counseling research, the JoGC is now indexed in PubMed with a steadily increasing impact factor.

The first funding opportunity from the NSGC began in 1989 with the Audrey Heimler Special Project Award (AHSPA). The AHSPA was established to honor genetic counselor Audrey Heimler, who graduated in the first class of the Sarah Lawrence College Genetic Counseling Program in 1971 and was a founding member and first president of the NSGC in 1979. The AHSPA is a competitive grant application awarded annually to fund projects focused on informing the future of the profession and/or the provision of genetic services.

Just 2 years later, informed by the success of the AHSPA, the Jane Engelberg Memorial Fellowship (JEMF) was established. The JEMF commemorates genetic counselor Jane Engelberg, who passed away from Hodgkin's disease after 15 years as a genetic counselor. Engelberg graduated from the Sarah Lawrence College Genetic Counseling Program in 1973 and specialized in prenatal and hematology counseling. The Engelberg Foundation funded and now endows the JEMF. The JEMF is a competitive grant application awarded to fund 2 years of research relevant to the field of genetic counseling. The call for funds is purposely broad to allow research projects to address timely topics in the field. Student JEMFs are awarded to genetic counseling students to fund their scholarly projects completed as part of their Master in Genetic Counseling training.

In 2020, the research funding opportunity focused on the genetic counseling process by the NIH was released (RFA-HG-20-048). This unique funding initiative allowed for nondoctoral- and doctoral-level applicants and supported investigator-initiated research on genetic counseling processes and practices in genomic medicine. It called for applications to address research to optimize the genetic counseling process in the context of limited resources. Additionally, several funding opportunities, for which genetic counseling training programs were well positioned to be successful applicants, designed to add to the profession of genetic counselor researchers were launched in 2021. The first was 1 to 2 years of mentored research training experiences for master's-level genetic counselors (PAR-21-074), and another provided funding to develop undergraduate training programs for students interested in careers in genetic research (RFA-HG-21-033). Finally, in 2021, genetic counselors working in research became eligible to apply for the NIH Loan Repayment Program (LRP). The NIH LRP pays up to $50,000 annually of a researcher's "qualified educational debt" when they agree to participate in "NIH mission-relevant research" (NIH, 2021). The emergent recognition of the NIH to train and support genetic counselor researchers is a critical step forward for our profession.

Genetic counselors are uniquely positioned at the intersection of research and clinical care, and these funding opportunities have enabled them to conduct high-quality, timely research to inform the profession and other areas of genetics. Despite these opportunities, there remains a need for additional funding opportunities for genetic counselors. Some of this need is being met with small funding opportunities awarded by several NSGC SIGs and some of the NSGC committees for research on topics related to their interests. While these funds are generally modest, they can be used to fund pilot studies to test proof of concept and collect data for larger grant applications.

The growing recognition of genetic counseling–focused research by the NSGC continues to benefit the field. In the 2019–2021 Strategic Plan, the NSGC set out to develop an infrastructure to accelerate research to evaluate genetic counseling processes and outcomes. In service of this goal, a formal Research, Quality, and Outcomes (RQO) Committee was established in 2018 and charged with developing a research agenda detailing the high-level questions to identify and evaluate best practices and outcomes in the delivery of genetic counseling. Among its many activities, this committee conducted a full review of the current environment of NSGC research-related activities and developed a research agenda for the NSGC. Additionally, the committee has several collaborations underway to validate patient-reported outcome measures and is working to develop an infrastructure to support additional funding of genetic counseling–led research. We expect the RQO Committee will continue to have a key role in the development of the necessary tools and creation of pathways for genetic counselors to design and implement high-quality research that generates evidence to elevate the profession.

We anticipate that the areas highlighted in this section represent only the tip of the iceberg of seminal times for genetic counselors in research. We expect that the type and number of opportunities for genetic counselors to participate in, conduct, and lead research will continue to expand.

Conclusion

We are in an era of growth in genetic counseling research. There has never before been a time where there have been so many opportunities for genetic counselor–led research and research on the practice of genetic counseling. There are also increasing opportunities for genetic counselors to broaden their research skill set beyond their graduate program training. There are unanswered research questions within the field of genetic counseling that genetic counselors have the expertise to answer. The genomic era of medicine has resulted in an unprecedented need for genetic counseling services and with it comes a growing list of research questions such as how to scale our services to meet the expanding needs, how to leverage technology and artificial intelligence, and how to ensure equity in the benefits of genomic medicine. The very nature of our profession is to evolve as technology changes, and genetic counseling research is imperative to informing this evolution.

As a profession we need to take advantage of available research resources and continue to seek out more so we can lead the direction of our profession. While genetic counseling research conducted by individuals outside the field has advanced the profession, research conducted by genetic counselors will be critical to direct the advancement of the field in a manner consistent with our unique goals, values, and expertise.

We need to continue to train our community in how to conduct this research. Historically, much of this training has happened through formal and informal mentorships with established genetic counselor and nongenetic counselor researchers. We feel that there is still a place for this type of training. The interplay between clinical experience and research design often results in the most insightful research questions.

Resources

We would like to direct readers to resources that provide more in-depth discussions in specific areas. In particular, the book *Genetic Counseling Research: A Practical Guide* is a comprehensive, accessible guide to genetic counseling research. Robert Resta's article "What Have We Been Trying to Do and Have We Been Any Good at It? A History of Measuring the Success of Genetic Counseling" is an insightful review of genetic counseling research with a focus on outcomes research (Resta, 2019). *Telling Genes: The Story of Genetic Counseling in America* by Alexandra Minna Stern provides a discussion of the history of genetic counseling in America and the research that informed it. For guidance on study design, we recommend *Research Design: Qualitative, Quantitative, and Mixed Methods Approaches* by John W. Creswell and J. David Creswell. For quantitative studies, we recommend *Quantitative Research Methods: From Theory to Publication* by Nicholas Harkiolakis and the classic biostatistics textbook *Principles of Biostatistics* by Marcello Pagano and Kimberlee Gauvreau. For qualitative research, we recommend *Qualitative Research & Evaluation Methods: Integrating Theory and Practice* by Michael Quinn Patton, and for guidance on coding we recommend *The Coding Manual for Qualitative Researchers* by Johnny Saldaña.

References

Accreditation Council for Genetic Counseling. (2023a). *Practice-based competencies for genetic counselors.* https://www.gceducation.org/wp-content/uploads/2023/12/ACGC_PracticeBasedCompetencies_2023.pdf

Accreditation Council for Genetic Counseling. (2023b). *Standards of accreditation for graduate programs in genetic counseling.* https://www.gceducation.org/wp-content/uploads/2023/11/ACGC_StandardsOfAccreditation_2023.pdf

Alford, R. L., Arnos, K. S., Fox, M., Lin, J. W., Palmer, C. G., Pandya, A., Rehm, H. L., Robin, N. H., Scott, D. A., & Yoshinaga-Itano, C. (2014). American College of Medical Genetics and Genomics guideline for the clinical evaluation and etiologic diagnosis of hearing loss. *Genetics in Medicine, 16*(4), 347–355. https://doi.org/10.1038/GIM.2014.2

Austin, J. C., & Honer, W. G. (2007). The genomic era and serious mental illness: A potential application for psychiatric genetic counseling. *Psychiatric Services (Washington, D.C.)*, *58*(2), 254–261. https://doi.org/10.1176/PS.2007.58.2.254

Bernhardt, B. A., Soucier, D., Hanson, K., Savage, M. S., Jackson, L., & Wapner, R. J. (2013). Women's experiences receiving abnormal prenatal chromosomal microarray testing results. *Genetics in Medicine*, *15*(2), 139–145. https://doi.org/10.1038/gim.2012.113

Biesecker, B. B., Woolford, S. W., Klein, W. M. P. P., Brothers, K. B., Umstead, K. L., Lewis, K. L., Biesecker, L. G., & Han, P. K. J. J. (2017). PUGS: A novel scale to assess perceptions of uncertainties in genome sequencing. *Clinical Genetics*, *92*(2), 172–179. https://doi.org/10.1111/cge.12949

Buchanan, A. H., Lester Kirchner, H., Schwartz, M. L. B., Kelly, M. A., Schmidlen, T., Jones, L. K., Hallquist, M. L. G., Rocha, H., Betts, M., Schwiter, R., Butry, L., Lazzeri, A. L., Frisbie, L. R., Rahm, A. K., Hao, J., Willard, H. F., Martin, C. L., Ledbetter, D. H., Williams, M. S., & Sturm, A. C. (2020). Clinical outcomes of a genomic screening program for actionable genetic conditions. *Genetics in Medicine*, *22*(11), 1874–1882. https://doi.org/10.1038/S41436-020-0876-4

Burns, C., James, C. A., & Ingles, J. (2018). Communication of genetic information to families with inherited rhythm disorders. *Heart Rhythm*, *15*(5), 780–786. https://doi.org/10.1016/J.HRTHM.2017.11.024

Campbell-Salome, G., Buchanan, A. H., Hallquist, M. L. G., Rahm, A. K., Rocha, H., & Sturm, A. C. (2021). Uncertainty management for individuals with Lynch Syndrome: Identifying and responding to healthcare barriers. *Patient Education and Counseling*, *104*(2), 403–412. https://doi.org/10.1016/J.PEC.2020.07.017

Cragun, D., & Zierhut, H. (2018). Development of FOCUS-GC: Framework for Outcomes of Clinical Communication Services in Genetic Counseling. *Journal of Genetic Counseling*, *27*(1), 33–58. https://doi.org/10.1007/S10897-017-0145-0

Creswell, J. W., & Creswell, J. D. (2017). *Research design: Qualitative, quantitative, and mixed methods approaches*. Sage Publications.

DeMarco, T. A., Peshkin, B. N., Mars, B. D., & Tercyak, K. P. (2004). Patient satisfaction with cancer genetic counseling: A psychometric analysis of the Genetic Counseling Satisfaction Scale. *Journal of Genetic Counseling*, *13*(4), 293–304.

Dormandy, E., Hooper, R., Michie, S., & Marteau, T. M. (2002). Informed choice to undergo prenatal screening: A comparison of two hospitals conducting testing either as part of a routine visit or requiring a separate visit. *Journal of Medical Screening*, *9*(3), 109–114. https://doi.org/10.1136/JMS.9.3.109

Eunpu, D. L. (1992). Introductory statement. *Journal of Genetic Counseling*, *1*(1), 1–4. https://doi.org/10.1007/BF00960078

Evers-Kiebooms, G., & Van Den Berghe, H. (1979). Impact of genetic counseling: A review of published follow-up studies. *Clinical Genetics*, *15*(6), 465–474. https://doi.org/10.1111/J.1399-0004.1979.TB00827.X

Gerrard, S., Inglis, A., Morris, E., & Austin, J. (2020). Relationships between patient- and session-related variables and outcomes of psychiatric genetic counseling. *European Journal of Human Genetic*, *28*(7), 907–914. https://doi.org/10.1038/s41431-020-0592-1

Grant, P. E., Pampaka, M., Payne, K., Clarke, A., & McAllister, M. (2019). Developing a short-form of the Genetic Counselling Outcome Scale: The Genomics Outcome Scale. *European Journal of Medical Genetics*, *62*(5), 324–334. https://doi.org/10.1016/j.ejmg.2018.11.015

Harkiolakis, N. (2017). *Quantitative research methods: From theory to publication*. CreateSpace Independent Publishing Platform.

Hart, M. R., Biesecker, B. B., Blout, C. L., Christensen, K. D., Amendola, L. M., Bergstrom, K. L., Biswas, S., Bowling, K. M., Brothers, K. B., Conlin, L. K., Cooper, G. M., Dulik, M. C., East, K. M., Everett, J. N., Finnila, C. R., Ghazani, A. A., Gilmore, M. J., Goddard, K. A. B., Jarvik, G. P., . . . Hindorff, L. A. (2018). Secondary findings from clinical genomic sequencing: Prevalence, patient perspectives, family history assessment, and health-care costs from a multisite study. *Genetics in Medicine*, *21*(5), 1261–1262. https://doi.org/10.1038/s41436-018-0308-x

Higgs, E., Wain, K. E., Wynn, J., Cho, M. T., Higgins, S., Blaisdell, D., Dugan, D., Valek, S., & Cohen, S. (2022). Measuring quality and value in genetic counseling: The current landscape and future directions. *Journal of Genetic Counseling*, *32*(2), 315–324. https://doi.org/10.1002/JGC4.1657

Hooker, G. W., Babu, D., Myers, M., Zierhut, H., & McAllister, M. (2017). Standards for the Reporting of Genetic Counseling Interventions in Research and Other Studies (GCIRS): An NSGC Task Force Report. *Journal of Genetic Counseling*, *26*(3), 355–360. https://doi.org/10.1007/S10897-017-0076-9

Ingles, J., Zodgekar, P. R., Yeates, L., Macciocca, I., Semsarian, C., & Fatkin, D. (2011). Guidelines for genetic testing of inherited cardiac disorders. *Heart, Lung, and Circulation*, *20*(11), 681–687. https://doi.org/10.1016/j.hlc.2011.07.013

Kessler, S. (1992). Psychological aspects of genetic counseling. VII. Thoughts on directiveness. *Journal of Genetic Counseling*, *1*(1), 9–17. https://doi.org/10.1007/BF00960080

Lewis, K. L., Umstead, K. L., Johnston, J. J., Miller, I. M., Thompson, L. J., Fishler, K. P., Biesecker, L. G., & Biesecker, B. B. (2018). Outcomes of counseling after education about carrier results: A randomized controlled trial. *American Journal of Human Genetics*, *102*(4), 540–546. https://doi.org/10.1016/J.AJHG.2018.02.009

Lippman-Hand, A., & Fraser, F. C. (1979). Genetic counseling: Provision and reception of information. *American Journal of Medical Genetics*, *3*(2), 113–127. https://doi.org/10.1002/ajmg.1320030202

MacFarlane, I. M., Veach, P. M., & LeRoy, B. S. (2014). *Genetic counseling research: A practical guide*. Oxford Academic. https://doi.org/10.1093/med/9780199359097.001.0001

McAllister, M., Wood, A., Dunn, G., Shiloh, S., & Todd, C. (2011). The Genetic Counseling Outcome Scale: A new patient-reported outcome measure for clinical genetics services. *Clinical Genetics*, *79*(5), 413–424. https://doi.org/10.1111/J.1399-0004.2011.01636.X

McConkie-Rosell, A., Schoch, K., Sullivan, J., Cope, H., Spillmann, R., Palmer, C. G. S., Pena, L., Jiang, Y. H., Daniels, N., Walley, N., Tan, K. G., Hooper, S. R., & Shashi, V. (2019). The genome empowerment scale: An assessment of parental empowerment in families with undiagnosed disease. *Clinical Genetics*, *96*(6), 521–531. https://doi.org/10.1111/CGE.13635

Muñoz-Cabello, P., García-Miñaúr, S., Espinel-Vallejo, M. E., Fernández-Franco, L., Stephens, A., Santos-Simarro, F., Lapunzina-Badía, P., & McAllister, M. (2018). Translation and cross-cultural adaptation with preliminary validation of GCOS-24 for use in Spain. *Journal of Genetic Counseling*, *27*(3), 732–743. https://doi.org/10.1007/S10897-017-0154-Z

Nagakura, H., Schneider, G., Morris, J., Lafferty, K. A., & Palmer, C. G. S. (2015). Assessing deaf awareness training: Knowledge and attitudes of recent genetic counseling graduates. *Journal of Genetic Counseling*, *24*(1), 104–116. https://doi.org/10.1007/S10897-014-9742-3

National Institutes of Health. (2021, December 28). *Division of loan repayment*. https://www.lrp.nih.gov/

National Society of Genetic Counselors. (n.d.). *Genetic counseling literature repository*. https://www.nsgc.org/Research-and-Publications/Genetic-Counseling-Literature-Repository
National Society of Genetic Counselors. (1992). Code of ethics. *Journal of Genetic Counseling*, *1*(1), 41–43. https://doi.org/10.1007/BF00960083
National Society of Genetic Counselors. (2000). *Professional status surveys, 2000 (archived)*. https://www.nsgc.org/Policy-Research-and-Publications/Professional-Status-Survey/Archived-Professional-Status-Survey?folderId=152&view=gridview&pageSize=10. Members only section.
National Society of Genetic Counselors. (2002). *Professional status surveys, 2002 (archived)*. https://www.nsgc.org/Policy-Research-and-Publications/Professional-Status-Survey/Archived-Professional-Status-Survey?folderId=152&view=gridview&pageSize=10. Members only section.
National Society of Genetic Counselors. (2004). *Professional status surveys, 2004 (archived)*. https://www.nsgc.org/Policy-Research-and-Publications/Professional-Status-Survey/Archived-Professional-Status-Survey?folderId=152&view=gridview&pageSize=10. Members only section.
National Society of Genetic Counselors. (2006). *Professional status surveys, 2006 (archived)*. https://www.nsgc.org/Policy-Research-and-Publications/Professional-Status-Survey/Archived-Professional-Status-Survey?folderId=152&view=gridview&pageSize=10. Members only section.
National Society of Genetic Counselors. (2008). *Professional status surveys, 2008 (archived)*. https://www.nsgc.org/Policy-Research-and-Publications/Professional-Status-Survey/Archived-Professional-Status-Survey?folderId=152&view=gridview&pageSize=10. Members only section.
National Society of Genetic Counselors. (2010). *Professional status surveys work environment reports, 2010 (archived)*. https://www.nsgc.org/Policy-Research-and-Publications/Professional-Status-Survey/Archived-Professional-Status-Survey?folderId=152&view=gridview&pageSize=10. Members only section.
National Society of Genetic Counselors. (2012). *Professional status surveys work environment reports, 2012 (archived)*. https://www.nsgc.org/Policy-Research-and-Publications/Professional-Status-Survey/Archived-Professional-Status-Survey?folderId=152&view=gridview&pageSize=10. Members only section.
National Society of Genetic Counselors. (2014). *Professional status surveys work environment reports, 2014 (archived)*. https://www.nsgc.org/Policy-Research-and-Publications/Professional-Status-Survey/Archived-Professional-Status-Survey?folderId=152&view=gridview&pageSize=10. Members only section.
National Society of Genetic Counselors. (2016). *Professional status surveys work environment reports, 2016 (archived)*. https://www.nsgc.org/Policy-Research-and-Publications/Professional-Status-Survey/Archived-Professional-Status-Survey?folderId=152&view=gridview&pageSize=10. Members only section.
National Society of Genetic Counselors. (2018). *Professional status surveys, work environment reports, 2018*. https://www.nsgc.org/Research-and-Publications/Professional-Status-Survey/Past-Professional-Status-Surveys. Members only section.
National Society of Genetic Counselors. (2019). *Professional status surveys, work environment reports, 2019*. https://www.nsgc.org/Research-and-Publications/Professional-Status-Survey/Past-Professional-Status-Surveys. Members only section.

National Society of Genetic Counselors. (2020). *Professional status surveys, work environment reports, 2020*. https://www.nsgc.org/Research-and-Publications/Professional-Status-Survey/Past-Professional-Status-Surveys. Members only section.

National Society of Genetic Counselors. (2021a, January 28). *NSGC timeline*. https://www.nsgc.org/About/About-NSGC/Timeline

National Society of Genetic Counselors. (2021b). *Professional status surveys, work environment reports, 2021*. https://www.nsgc.org/Research-and-Publications/Professional-Status-Survey/Past-Professional-Status-Surveys. Members only section.

National Society of Genetic Counselors. (2022). *Professional status survey, demographics & methodology report*. https://www.nsgc.org/Research-and-Publications/Professional-Status-Survey/Past-Professional-Status-Surveys. Members only section.

National Society of Genetic Counselors. (2023). *Professional status survey*. https://www.nsgc.org/Research-and-Publications/Professional-Status-Survey. Members only section.

Pagano, M., Gauvreau, K., & Mattie, H. (2022). *Principles of biostatistics*. Chapman and Hall/CRC.

Patton, M. Q. (2014). *Qualitative research & evaluation methods: Integrating theory and practice*. Sage Publications.

Peay, H. L., Veach, P. M. C., Palmer, C. G. S., Rosen-Sheidley, B., Gettig, E., & Austin, J. C. (2008). Psychiatric disorders in clinical genetics I: Addressing family histories of psychiatric illness. *Journal of Genetic Counseling*, *17*(1), 6–17. https://doi.org/10.1007/S10897-007-9120-5

Presson, A. P., Zhang, C., Abtahi, A. M., Kean, J., Hung, M., & Tyser, A. R. (2017). Psychometric properties of the Press Ganey® Outpatient Medical Practice Survey. *Health and Quality of Life Outcomes*, *15*(1). https://doi.org/10.1186/S12955-017-0610-3

Resta, R. G. (2019). What have we been trying to do and have we been any good at it? A history of measuring the success of genetic counseling. *European Journal of Medical Genetics*, 62(5), 300–307. https://doi.org/10.1016/j.ejmg.2018.11.003

Saldaña, J. (2021). *The coding manual for qualitative researchers*. Sage Publications.

Schmidlen, T., Sturm, A. C., & Scheinfeldt, L. B. (2020). Pharmacogenomic (PGx) counseling: Exploring participant questions about PGx test results. *Journal of Personalized Medicine*, *10*(2). https://doi.org/10.3390/JPM10020029

Sorenson, J., Swazey, J., Scotch, N., Kavanagh, C., & Matthews, D. (1981). Reproductive pasts, reproductive futures. Genetic counseling and its effectiveness—PubMed. *Birth Defects Original Article Series*, *17*(4), 191–192.

Stern, A. M. (2012). *Telling genes: The story of genetic counseling in America*. Johns Hopkins University Press.

Thomas, C., & McAllister, M. (2019). Establishing the minimum clinically important difference for the Genetic Counseling Outcome Scale (GCOS-24). *Journal of Genetic Counseling*, *28*(5), 1003–1010. https://doi.org/10.1002/JGC4.1152

VanDyke, R. E., Hashimoto, S., Morales, A., Pyatt, R. E., & Sturm, A. C. (2021). Impact of variant reclassification in the clinical setting of cardiovascular genetics. *Journal of Genetic Counseling*, *30*(2), 503–512. https://doi.org/10.1002/JGC4.1336

Veach, P. M. C., Bartels, D. M., & LeRoy, B. S. (2007). Coming full circle: A reciprocal-engagement model of genetic counseling practice. *Journal of Genetic Counseling*, *16*(6), 713–728. https://doi.org/10.1007/S10897-007-9113-4

Voorwinden, J. S., Plantinga, M., Krijnen, W., Ausems, M., Knoers, N., Velthuizen, M., Birnie, E., Lucassen, A. M., van Langen, I. M., & Ranchor, A. V. (2019). A validated PROM in genetic counselling: The psychometric properties of the Dutch version of the Genetic

Counselling Outcome Scale. *European Journal of Human Genetics*, *27*(5), 681–690. https://doi.org/10.1038/S41431-018-0318-9

Wang, V., & Marsh, F. H. (1992). Ethical principles and cultural integrity in health care delivery: Asian ethnocultural perspectives in genetic services. *Journal of Genetic Counseling*, *1*(1), 81–92. https://doi.org/10.1007/BF00960087

Zierhut, H., & Austin, J. (2011). How inclusion of genetic counselors on the research team can benefit translational science. *Science Translational Medicine*, *3*(74), 74cm7. https://doi.org/10.1126/SCITRANSLMED.3001898

CHAPTER 13

GENETIC COUNSELORS IN MARKETING AND INDUSTRY

ELISSA LEVIN AND EDGAR MACBEAN

The Value of Genetic Counselors in Industry

The genetic counseling profession was created, in part, to meet a critical need to enhance the communication of complex genetic information—genetic translators for patients and providers who are unfamiliar with the technologies, utility, and implications of genetic testing. With the growth of genomics, the need for genetic counselors has expanded beyond the clinic. As a result, genetic counselors have increasingly entered the commercial sector over the past few decades. To capture this growth, the National Society of Genetic Counselors' (NSGC) Professional Status Survey (PSS) began including additional designations to assess what percentage of the workforce works in nondirect patient care either full time or part time. As of 2021, the NSGC PSS found that 25% of members identify as having a nondirect patient care role and 22% as having a mixed patient care role, indicating that a significant portion of the membership is working in industry or other nonclinical settings (NSGC, 2021b). While the field has been rapidly growing, many have been closely following the movement of genetic counselors out of the clinic (Cohen & Tucker, 2018). An unpublished survey of industry genetic counselors from five of the largest commercial diagnostic laboratories in 2017 found that 73.2% reported moving to industry from a clinical position (Bergner & Babu, 2017).

One potential explanation for the growth in opportunity for and success of genetic counselors in industry is the effective application of genetic counselors' core skill set in a variety of roles and settings. During the 2012 NSGC president-elect address, Brenda Finucane discussed the findings of the Core Skills Task Force that identified the following: a deep and broad knowledge of genetics; the ability to tailor, translate, and communicate complex information in a simple, relevant way for diverse audiences; strong interpersonal skills; emotional intelligence and self-awareness; the ability to dissect and analyze a complex problem; research skills; and an in-depth knowledge of healthcare delivery (Finucane, 2011). This distillation perfectly encompasses why genetic counselors have and continue to see such expansion of roles and opportunities in the commercial sector.

Another driving factor for the growth in opportunities for genetic counselors is the technological advances in genomics. It is a relatively straightforward formula—the more technology delves into the genome, the more data becomes available, and the greater the need for skilled professionals who fundamentally understand the science as well as the nuances, challenges, and opportunities for enabling access to this information. The advent of next-generation sequencing, for example, has made testing more ubiquitous, affordable, and efficient and has expanded the amount of information covered by any one test (such as multigene panels, exome sequencing, genome sequencing). The speed of innovation was further accelerated when the U.S. Supreme Court determined that naturally occurring genes cannot be patented (*Association for Molecular Pathology vs. Myriad*, 2013). The use of these technologies in areas such as noninvasive prenatal testing, liquid biopsies, and the microbiome also creates novel opportunities for individuals who understand both the technology and its applications for individual and population health.

Why do some genetic counselors choose to work in industry? The decision may be driven by a desire to innovate, the potential to have a broader impact outside of an in-person clinical setting, the speed of change, feeling valued, and, in some cases, career development, including leadership and management opportunities as well as the potential for better compensation (Cohen & Tucker, 2018; Rabideau et al., 2016).

Regardless of how and why, the fact remains that genetic counselors continue to successfully expand their roles, take on new responsibilities, and create new opportunities outside of the clinic. They now fill a broad spectrum of roles including marketing, sales, test development, test interpretation and analysis, telehealth, complex case management, client services, bioinformatics, information technology, product development, education, management, and leadership. With the continued growth of startup companies across the science, health, and technology sectors, opportunities for genetic counselors continue to expand in breadth and scope (Rabideau et al., 2016).

The NSGC PSS identified that genetic counselors in nondirect patient care positions were significantly more satisfied with their current positions than those in direct patient care roles (NSGC, 2021a). An earlier study of laboratory-based genetic counselors found that 96.7% of respondents reported job satisfaction as either "very satisfied" or "satisfied" (Waltman et al., 2016). Several also mentioned that autonomy and the variety of roles and opportunities their position provided positively affected their overall satisfaction. Research has also highlighted that genetic counselors in industry tend to have high levels of job satisfaction with salary, benefits, recognition, and opportunities for advancement (Cohen et al., 2017; Field et al., 2016; Waltman et al., 2016).

It is important to note that choosing to work in industry comes with an element of risk and uncertainty that typically is not encountered in more traditional clinical care settings. Startup companies as well as seemingly well-established businesses can face financial challenges. Some may simply go out of business. Some may be merged with another organization. Other companies may acquire additional businesses to meet their strategic and financial objectives. These shifting business models and organizational structures often impact the size, scope, or requisite subject matter expertise of their employees. As a result, long-term job security may not be as sound as those within larger health systems. Underscoring this reality, some of the companies mentioned in this chapter are no longer in business or have been acquired by or merged with other companies.

A Brief History: The Growth of the Genetics Industry and Emerging Roles for Genetic Counselors

Through the 1980s, relatively few genetic counselors worked in industry. Beginning in the mid- to late 1980s, Genzyme, a pharmaceutical company, began hiring genetic counselors to staff clinics. While some nonclinical business roles were emerging, most genetic counselors employed by the company were providing direct, in-person prenatal genetic counseling services. During this time, some genetic counselors in academic and hospital settings began working with internal testing labs, providing a range of functions including writing consent forms, creating lab reports, developing educational materials, and supporting the providers who ordered testing.

In the early 1990s, there were significantly fewer commercial labs in existence, as much of the diagnostic and research testing was still performed in academic medical centers and hospital labs. The large reference labs began hiring genetic counselors as they recognized the value of core genetic counseling skills, including the ability to translate and communicate complex information to both patients and providers (T. Brown, personal communication, June 2020). The early lab-based genetic counselors were described as "clinical genetics educators who provide physicians with genetics expertise that they would not otherwise be able to access" (Amos & Gold, 1998, p. 294). Genetic counselors also played key roles in test development, communicating test methodologies, managing complex cases, and facilitating result reporting. An important goal was to make complicated information consumable.

More professional opportunities for genetic counselors became available in the mid- to late 1990s as internal industry leadership began to further recognize that the core skills genetic counselors embodied were valuable in a variety of ways (S. Keiles, personal communication, June 2020). More genetic counselors were hired into roles to provide subject matter expertise, translation, communication, and coordination for central lab services. Major labs such as the Nichols Institute and Smith Klein (both later acquired by Quest) placed genetic counselors in the lab to develop diagnostic coordination and support. LabCorp leveraged genetic counseling leadership to commercialize new technologies as their existing frameworks for commercialization were not sufficient for the emerging molecular diagnostics business (T. Brown, personal communication, June 2020). As testing demand grew, so did the genetic counselor workforce—in the lab and in the field. By the early 2000s the role of the medical science liaison (MSL) emerged, initially driven by Myriad. MSLs functioned as the clinical genomics expert on the commercial sales team to educate providers about new types of tests and became established clinical partners in delivering complex new tests into the market. Gradually, the scope of responsibility broadened to include management, business development, education, research, and variant interpretation (Cho & Guy, 2020).

The NSGC Industry Special Interest Group (SIG) was formed in the 1990s and continues to exist today. At its inception, it was composed of a small group of genetic counselors employed by a handful of commercial testing labs. Throughout the 1990s and 2000s, the number of testing labs and number of genetic tests on the market continued to grow. Many of these emerging labs hired one or two genetic counselors. For some labs, there was an understanding that they "needed a genetic counselor" as key opinion leaders advised a genetic counselor would be a valuable addition to the organization. Despite acting on such advice, a number were uncertain about how to leverage genetic counseling expertise. This path paved the way for many genetic counselors to demonstrate their value and create their own career trajectory within the organization.

From the public's perspective, before the 2000s, awareness about genetic testing was limited, as it largely occurred in clinics and focused on rare disease. Starting in 2002, Myriad Genetics (which at the time held the patent for the *BRCA1* and *BRCA2* genes) launched the first marketing campaign for a genetic test. It ran a 5-month test campaign in two cities—Denver and Atlanta—to drive consumer awareness of its BRCAnalysis. The advertisement provided information about hereditary breast and ovarian cancer risk and availability of testing and encouraged individuals to speak with their doctor, who would be required to order the test. While the company stated that the advertisement successfully drove a significant increase in inquiries and testing, the genetic counseling community strongly pushed back on the campaign, fearing the overutilization of unnecessary testing, the potential for false reassurance based on negative tests, and a lack of healthcare provider knowledge about the test combined with an insufficient number of genetic counselors to address the volume of testing. Myriad paused and spent the next 5 years focusing, in part, on provider education and relaunched the campaign in 2007. There was growing concern among genetic professionals about direct-to-consumer advertising and eventually investigations by regulators occurred (Pollock, 2007).

Starting in the early 2000s, pharmaceutical and life science companies began shifting focus to the orphan drug market as a number of trends converged including "patents expiring, academia's growing interest in rare disorder research, regulatory incentives, and the advocacy work of patient organizations" (Hirschler, 2013). From 2001 to 2010, the orphan drug market saw 25.8% growth. Companies like Biomarin, Ultragenyx, and Biogen began developing genome-guided therapies and sought genetic counselors with specialized clinical expertise to contribute to both the strategic development and execution of clinical market development plans. Critical components of drug development are engaging key stakeholders, understanding the needs of the community, and translating genomic information to a wide variety of clinical and nonclinical audiences. This has created clear opportunities for genetic counselors (Field et al., 2016). In recent years, large pharmaceutical companies as well as a growing number of more specialized companies have focused efforts on rare diseases or companion molecular diagnostics, providing additional opportunities for genetic counselors.

At this point in time, the internet created new channels for education and awareness, and genetic counselors began to work as content experts. They worked alongside software developers to innovate consumer access for those seeking information and answers. Additionally, consumer genomics companies started to enter the scene where the few genetic counselors employed by direct-to-consumer companies played roles, from directly supporting consumers to strategic development, as well as building and marketing products (e.g., DNA Direct, Pathway Genomics, Navigenics). During this era, we also witnessed the first genetic counselors hired into manufacturing companies not only to support commercial market growth but also to lead efforts in advocacy, public policy, and government affairs (e.g., Affymetrix).

The consumer genetics industry sparked new debate within the genetic counseling community. Where the Myriad marketing campaign had been an example of direct-to-consumer advertising, the consumer genetics companies further pushed boundaries by offering consumers direct access to genetic testing. Companies used a variety of physician authorization approaches, most of which were compliant with existing regulatory requirements, to allow individuals to order testing on their own. Some of these companies employed genetic counselors and offered support services—both before and after testing—while others chose not to provide genetic counseling services or engage genetic counselors in their product development efforts. As criticism continued to mount, the Government Accountability Office (GAO) investigated the consumer genetics industry as "experts remain concerned that the test results mislead consumers" (GAO, 2010, p. 2). The report prompted a congressional hearing that called several leaders of the companies to the witness stand. The hearing had long-lasting impact on the consumer genetics industry, shifting greater focus to analytic and clinical validity and regulatory oversight. One outcome was that some companies that had previously refrained from hiring genetic counselors began to do so.

In part driven by the consumer genetics industry, some employers began to offer genetic screening as one of their wellness benefits to employees. This trend, combined with a growing belief that pharmacogenomic testing could positively impact patient health, compliance, and healthcare costs, motivated pharmaceutical benefit management (PBM) companies such as Medco to start hiring genetic counselors into operational and strategic business roles, including developing commercial wellness programs. Quickly, a new type of health management company emerged, focused on genetic benefit management (GBM). One such company, Generation Health, was formed in 2008 to help employers and healthcare plans manage medical costs and improve health outcomes by optimizing utilization of genetic testing. A few genetic counselors played critical roles in the early evolution of these businesses. As of 2022, Color Genomics and other companies continue to offer genetic screening to employers as part of employee benefits programs, including genetic counseling, though broad adoption has not become standard.

Technological advances around the 2010s enabled companies like Counsyl to enter the market with expanded carrier screening. Counsyl hired many genetic counselors early on in the company's development, allowing for significant influence as the company built foundations for its clinical, marketing, and product development strategies. The advent of noninvasive prenatal testing further drove the emergence of new companies such as Natera, Verinata, Ariosa, and Sequenom, all of which benefited from hiring genetic counselors into a broad range of roles. Two leading manufacturers in the genomics space also began hiring genetic counselors during this time. Life Technologies, which was eventually subsumed into Thermo Fisher, hired its first genetic counselors. One of the innovative programs that resulted is the IMPACT program, the first genetic benefits program established by an employer to enable its employees to access cutting-edge clinical molecular technologies (S. Kieran, personal communication, July 2020). Illumina established the Understand Your Genome program to drive market awareness and interest in genome sequencing.

Since the turn of the century, the dramatic growth in both the genomics and technology sectors has offered a rich array of professional opportunities, further expanding the roles available to genetic counselors. While the number of genetic counselors has essentially doubled since 2006, overall, there is a decrease in the proportion providing direct patient counseling (Hoskovec et al., 2018). In conjunction with the scope of genomic tests that continue to enter the market, the growing sector of telehealth and other clinical implementation technology solutions remains an area ripe for genetic counseling leadership and innovation.

The Perception of Genetic Counselors in Industry

Genetic counseling roots are in the clinic, most strongly in academic medical centers. The gradual shift of counselors into industry has, at times, created tension. Such tensions are not new and certainly exist in other areas of medicine. An often-cited sentiment is the idea that physicians who choose to work in biopharma have "gone to the dark side" (Strohmeyer et al., 2023). Similar sentiments have seemed to pervade the genetic counseling community over the past several decades, creating challenges for both those in industry and those outside industry.

Underlying this perception are topics such as perceived conflict of interest, misconceptions of motivations and intentions, a lack of comfort with the speed of growth and commercialization of tests, and greater access to information that may not yet be deemed standard of care. In addition, over the years, the NSGC PSS has demonstrated that generally genetic counselors in industry have higher compensation and additional benefits, including more financial support for continuing education, travel, and attending professional conferences. In some cases, this has further fueled feelings among clinical genetic counselors of being undervalued (Cohen & Tucker, 2018). The outward projection of these sentiments has been internalized by some genetic counselors in industry. As one study found, some genetic counselors in laboratory settings were concerned about their professional image, citing negative perceptions of laboratory genetic counselors by nonlaboratory genetic counselors (Groepper et al., 2015).

Further, many genetic counselors in industry have struggled with a sense of discordance in their own professional identity—both as an individual and as a member of the community. As one genetic counselor in industry explained:

> I think many of us who've been in industry for a long time or who have left clinical jobs to go to industry . . . you've gone to the dark side. There's this feeling . . . you're not doing what you're trained to be doing. . . . And I think that's a natural feeling, but for NSGC to be inclusive of all genetic counselors regardless of their role . . . would go a long way to people like me and others who have forged new paths and still identify as a genetic counselor. (Davis et al., 2020, p. 773)

Challenges with professional identity have influenced career path decision making and overall career trajectories. It underscores some of the tensions that arise from how one defines themselves as a genetic counselor and how the broader professional community may perceive roles outside of direct patient care (Davis et al., 2020).

The emergence of consumer-initiated genetic testing, starting around 2005, also elicited strong sentiments from the genetic counseling community (Hawkins & Ho, 2012). Many critics of the consumer genetics industry called for both pretest and posttest genetic counseling to be provided to all consumers. The scope of genetic counseling services offered has ranged from no services, to fee-for-service genetic counseling, to in-house genetic counseling offered at no additional charge, with all versions of support being offered through some form of telehealth. Regardless of the model, the reality is that consumer-initiated testing has impacted genetic counselors in the clinic. A survey of genetic counselors found that 40% of respondents reported that they have consulted patients in clinic about consumer-initiated test results. Most (56.4%) felt negative or very negative about direct-to-consumer genetic testing, while only 6.9% felt positive or very positive. The vast majority (90.9%) believed that the involvement of genetic counselors would improve consumer genetic testing, but the majority (68.8%) were not comfortable providing this service (Hsieh et al., 2021). From this study, it is evident that the field continues to struggle with the existence of the consumer genetic testing industry.[1]

While these issues remain important points of discussion and continue to be studied more closely in the literature, generally there has been growing acceptance of genetic counselors in industry, with an acknowledgment of the growth and impact of opportunities afforded by commercial roles. Another study noted that "As of 2018, the landscape of genetic counseling has shifted. Genetic counselors who work in industry settings are no longer considered as having 'moved to the dark side'" (McWalter et al., 2018, p. 46).

Expanding the Definition of Patient Care

Many genetic counselors working in commercial roles contribute to the development of products and services that support patient needs in ways other than direct, in-person patient contact. Technology has allowed the field to develop tools and solutions that can potentially impact large populations despite not "seeing" individual patients. A thorough examination of this topic is beyond the scope of this chapter, but the concept of providing patient care continues to broaden. For example, genetic counselors are participating in the design of digital tools, such as risk assessment algorithms and family health history tools, that may eventually be presented to many people learning about their clinical risk for cancer. Similarly, a genetic counselor writing the scripts for a chatbot to engage individuals with questions about the appropriateness of a genetic test or what should be considered in making an informed decision is bringing their knowledge and expertise into the design of these tools to emulate the best practices used in clinical settings. How the field thinks about supporting patients and providers from the perspective of technology solutions—such as patients directly engaging with their personal health information and providers utilizing point-of-care support tools—will continue to evolve, and genetic counselors are and will continue to be core stakeholders in the development and delivery process.

[1] Editors' note: For more on consumer-initiated genetic testing, see Chapter 11 by Anne E. Greb in this volume.

Applying the Genetic Counseling Skillset to Industry Roles

Industry offers many opportunities for genetic counselors to build on their training and apply their core skills in a wide range of areas. Some companies are looking for genetic counselors to work in roles that are closely aligned with the responsibilities of a genetic counselor seeing patients in clinic. Others look to leverage genetic counselors' expertise in genomics and precision health to support a broad range of functional needs within their organization. The highly cross-functional nature of many roles provides access to various departments and professionals with skills, work styles, and motivations.

Often there is a period of adaptation for genetic counselors transitioning from more clinical or academic settings to industry as they acclimate to the differences in a corporate environment. The ability of genetic counselors to listen, educate, and problem-solve, as well as effectively translate and communicate complex information, provides a foundation for success in these environments.

Broadly, we identified five main areas where genetic counselors have thrived in industry: marketing, commercial, product development, education, and policy.

Marketing

Marketing is a general term that includes many subdisciplines, but there are roles for genetic counselors in all of them. One central aspect of marketing is helping to set the corporate strategy and how a company can differentiate itself in the marketplace. In this role, the value of a genetic counselor will vary based on the type of company. For example, genetic counselors can contribute to developing competitive landscape analyses for companies that offer molecular testing products. This may include detailing technical differences of tests available on the market and how ancillary services (such as genetic counseling) distinguish different companies' commercial offerings.

Another marketing function is in generating content to support the company's products or services. This includes visual and textual messaging that reflect a company's values, products, and services. Especially for companies that serve clinical customers, the experience and perspective of a genetic counselor as a clinician are extremely valuable in getting that messaging right. Genetic counselors can also help marketing teams figure out the best ways to get those messages out and in front of clinical decision makers.

In many companies, marketing is also responsible for sales training. Once again, the genetic counselor is highly regarded as a trusted resource to help train the sales team on both the technical details of a product and how to engage with and communicate effectively with potential clients.

Commercial

Working within commercialization or business teams in industry is another opportunity for genetic counselors. There is a surprising parallel between the core skills of genetic counselors and those who are successful at business development and sales. Educating, contracting, understanding needs and motivations, and facilitating informed decision making are critical skills applied in business development and sales. The nondirective approach that genetic counselors are trained in is valuable in helping successfully operate within commercial entities. Yet it is also important to recognize that the sales side of the company will have explicit goals and will apply directive approaches to meet those goals. Understanding fellow colleagues and their motivations and goals is no different than understanding the needs of a patient. It is simply the context that is different.

For companies selling to clinical customers, the experience of having been a clinician brings a critical degree of trust and respect that is highly valued. This has created opportunities to serve as a medical/scientific liaison, helping to "speak the language" of clinicians as well as ensure that their concerns are being addressed in a way that can be difficult for nonclinicians. This function can be structured in a number of commercial roles, such as technical sales, where the genetic counselor will be called upon to address the scientific and technical questions about a company's products. It is also common for genetic counselors to take on more general sales roles where that clinical experience and the associated level of trust will help close deals and bring on partners. Sales offers a different experience from an in-person clinical genetic counseling role, sometimes including extensive travel and meeting with many individuals at all levels of an organization.

Product development

Sales teams need products to sell, and this has created another opportunity for genetic counselors in industry. A product team will be focused on the user experience and will strive to develop an interface with their products that is intuitive and that the customer will embrace and use. To achieve that, they will often seek the insights of the end-user, listen to and observe what needs to be solved, and test and iterate the development of the product. Genetic counselors are uniquely positioned to work with designers and developers and often seamlessly integrate into interaction design teams to ensure a user experience that embodies a patient-centered approach, addresses the nuanced psychosocial realities of genetic testing, and directly handles challenges in existing clinical implementation workflows. Genetic counselors are trained to communicate complex genetic concepts into language that diverse audiences can understand, and this expertise can be useful in writing the content and designing the flow of information that is critical to the success of a product. The role of genetic translator also applies to the internal team, as they need to communicate the requirements to design and engineering teams, who need to understand the core concepts at hand and the nuances that can impact the product being developed.

Education

Genetic counselors are trained to convey complex genomic information in understandable ways and play an important role in educating commercial and product teams. However, limited genomic literacy remains a significant concern (Boerwinkel et al., 2017; Chapman et al., 2019), and even in a company that is focused on providing genomic services, there are employees who do not have a genetics background and are eager to learn from an experienced expert. This may include executive leadership who want the clinical perspective as they set the strategy for the company. There are also employees who work in support functions such as human resources, engineering, or accounting who want to better understand the company's products, services, and mission. Genetics is an interesting and dynamic field, and people are often curious to hear the experience and perspective of genetic counselors.

Education is also extremely important when implementing a new service, especially within a clinical environment. Researchers, clinicians, and administrators will have questions about how to support a new service and how it will affect their jobs. From clinicians, topics include understanding a report, knowing its limitations and what clinical steps can be taken based on that information, and being prepared for questions they might anticipate from their patients. Administrators will seek guidance to help them evaluate important policy questions for their organization, including issues related to privacy, ethics, and appropriate clinical care. These are not always easy questions, and it is important for administrators to understand the potential concerns and best practices to avoid unintended consequences as they develop their own programs.

Policy

Genetic counselors are trained to understand the complex ethical, legal, and societal questions that are raised by the ability to read and interpret an individual's DNA. Genomic technologies are impacting law enforcement, raising questions of privacy, data sharing, data access, and artificial intelligence (AI) and introducing new opportunities for managing public health in different ways. Once again, there is a key role for genetic counselors to play in helping policymakers and advisory groups to understand the current issues, trends, and possible solutions to help them make informed decisions and set effective policy. Many companies have hired genetic counselors to advise or to directly influence (lobby) on the company's behalf.

Many of these roles did not exist a few years ago, and as genomics continues to expand, there will likely be more new and exciting policy-related roles for genetic counselors in industry.

The Current Industry Landscape

The commercial market offers expansive job opportunities for genetic counselors across various industry settings. The NSGC PSSs have continued to expand the survey structure to accommodate the growing scope of practice and employment settings as genetic counselors have continued to venture outside of clinical practice into industry (and other) settings. The 2021 NSGC PSS Work Environment Report includes an overview of employer settings reported by genetic counselors. Table 13.1, which is from the 2021 NSGC PSS, highlights

Table 13.1 Genetic Counselor Employer Settings—2021 National Society of Genetic Counselors Work Environment Report

Employer work setting	Direct patient care		Nondirect patient care		Mixed position		All positions	
	N	%	*N*	%	*N*	%	*N*	%
Diagnostic laboratory—noncommercial, academic	1	<1%	29	4%	10	2%	40	1%
Diagnostic laboratory—commercial, academic	5	<1%	51	7%	10	2%	66	2%
Diagnostic laboratory—commercial, nonacademic	46	3%	346	48%	91	14%	483	17%
Government organization or agency	14	1%	8	1%	21	3%	43	1%
Health advocacy organization	0	0%	1	<1%	3	1%	4	<1%
Hospital/medical facility—academic medical center	621	40%	41	6%	279	44%	941	32%
Hospital/medical facility—private (nonprofit or for profit)	456	30%	24	3%	89	14%	569	20%
Hospital/medical facility—public	229	15%	8	1%	34	5%	271	9%
Insurance company/benefit management company	0	0%	26	4%	0	0%	26	1%
Not-for-profit organization—other	13	1%	15	2%	12	2%	40	1%
Pharmaceutical company	1	<1%	28	4%	2	<1%	31	1%
Physician's private practice	45	3%	0	0%	8	1%	53	2%
Private company—biotechnology/research development	1	<1%	18	2%	5	1%	24	1%
Private company—digital health/software	1	<1%	12	2%	0	0%	13	<1%
Private company—genetic consulting	11	1%	4	1%	8	1%	23	1%
Private company—telegenetics	53	3%	9	1%	16	3%	78	3%
Private company—utilization management	0	0%	33	5%	0	0%	33	1%
Private company—other	3	<1%	10	1%	5	1%	18	1%
Professional organization	1	<1%	2	0%	0	0%	3	<1%
Self-employed/private practice	4	<1%	0	0%	5	1%	9	<1%
University	22	1%	53	7%	40	6%	115	4%
Other work setting	8	1%	5	1%	2	1%	15	1%
Total	**1,535**	**100%**	**723**	**100%**	**640**	**100%**	**2,898**	**100%**

both industry and nonindustry employers as well as the type of patient care offered (direct, nondirect, or mixed).

While each of these sectors represents new areas for genetic counselors to apply their expertise in novel ways, it should be noted that with this innovation there can be significant volatility. Most of the companies listed below are successful businesses, but some are no longer in business, and there are others that never established a viable place in the market. Even those that have succeeded to date experience periods of volatility, and that can translate into the loss of jobs for many individuals, including genetic counselors. This is not limited to small startups, and even large and well-established companies have laid off genetic counselors as part of strategic shifts, cost-cutting efforts, or company reorganization. In 2022, Sema4/GeneDx announced the layoff of 700 individuals and Invitae laid off more than 1,000 as part of a year-long restructuring. Similarly, Illumina announced that it would be reducing its global workforce by 5%, or more than 9,000 employees globally. It is unknown how many of those cuts are affecting genetic counselors, and none of this should be interpreted as affecting the appeal of genetic counselors in industry. However, unlike more traditional clinical care, industry is more prone to periods of substantial growth followed by periods of retraction, and it would be reasonable to expect a higher degree of volatility and a greater likelihood of working for different companies over a career.

Laboratories

The number of labs has been growing over the past couple of decades, as has the wide range of test offerings. In 2021, it was estimated that there were about 160,000 genetic tests on the market, up from approximately 10,000 in 2012, with an average of 30 new tests being added daily (Concert Genetics, 2021). Large national labs, such as Quest and Labcorp, offer a range of molecular and nonmolecular tests, germline and somatic. Hundreds of smaller, independent labs have emerged. Examples of some of the largest labs today include Ambry Genetics, Exact Sciences, Foundation Medicine, GeneDx, Helix, Invitae, Myriad, Natera, and Tempus (listed alphabetically). As new technologies are developed, it is unlikely that the trend of new labs entering the market will change in the near future. However, there is a simultaneous trend in consolidation in recent years, with acquisition of smaller labs by larger ones. These acquisitions have served to diversify the product portfolio of larger labs while enabling the smaller labs to continue to offer their product(s) in a competitive market, which may otherwise not have been possible (Scheuner et al., 2021).

The percentage of genetic counselors citing diagnostic laboratories as their primary work setting increased from 6% in the 2002 NSGC PSS (it is important to note that at that time the PSS did not differentiate commercial from hospital settings) to 20% in the 2021 PSS, with 17% working for commercial labs (NSGC, 2002, 2021b). The expanding number of genetic counselors who work in a laboratory setting is a result of increased laboratory services and genetic testing menus, as well as growing job opportunities (Zetzsche et al., 2013).

In the lab setting, genetic counselors provide information in the preanalytic, analytic, and postanalytic stages of testing. A study of the roles and responsibilities of lab-based genetic counselors found that almost all performed customer liaison/case coordination (95%) and interpretation and result reporting (88%). The researcher noted:

> The most frequently performed tasks within these categories involved addressing questions from clients, making phone calls with genetic testing results, obtaining clinical or family history information for results interpretation, and composing case-specific interpretations for

> unique results and/or obtaining literature references to support interpretations. (Waltman et al., 2016, p. 786)

The study further documented expanding roles in variant interpretation and management responsibilities (Waltman et al., 2016).

As mentioned previously, sales and marketing are critical functions in which genetic counselors excel. The survey by Waltman et al. (2016) found that about 10% of genetic counselors were performing marketing and sales functions, of whom 52% never or rarely contacted or met with clients or clinicians, and 63% reported no direct outreach to promote testing. However, the role of the MSL is focused on direct outreach to clients and clinicians. Some of the additional responsibilities include creating, editing, and/or reviewing marketing materials as well as other external commercial activities such as staffing booths at conferences and events.

Telegenetics Services

A growing number of companies are creating telehealth platforms. The global COVID-19 pandemic further fueled the need for telehealth services (Demeke et al., 2021), including specialized genetic counseling services (Mills et al., 2021). One report estimated that telehealth use increased 38-fold from the pre-COVID-19 baseline (Bestsennyy et al., 2021). Many companies are leveraging telehealth technology to offer genetic counseling services directly to individuals. Examples of leading providers in this space are GeneMatters (subsequently acquired), Genome Medical, InformedDNA, and PWN Health (subsequently acquired), though there are many others. These businesses emerged to address the need to scale genetic counseling services to meet the growing patient demand using telehealth. They are focused on driving efficiencies with technology solutions, increasing access across geographies, and complementing in-person genetic counseling services with flexible telehealth visits. Their services may be driven directly by consumers who have questions about a test they have ordered online or through direct integration with physician workflows to provide access to general and specialized genetic counseling services not otherwise available. The genetic counseling provided by these companies is typically similar to what might be offered in a clinical setting and can offer genetic counselors the ability to provide counseling on a broader range of tests and to a wider patient demographic than in a single health system or clinic.

One study of this expanding workforce found that 91% of genetics counselors who had provided telegenetics services were satisfied or very satisfied with their position, citing an innovative approach to healthcare delivery and flexibility of work environment as reasons. Interestingly, of those genetic counselors who had not engaged in telegenetics services, 92% expressed some interest, highlighting an openness and curiosity about this evolving service delivery model (Zeirhut et al., 2018).

Beyond the support services, genetic counselors employed by telehealth or telegenetics companies serve in a number of other roles, including business development, product development, sales and marketing, and implementation or operations. These and other expanding commercial support services have provided genetic counselors with the opportunity to expand their roles to include recruiting, hiring, and adapting training and operational protocols (McWalter et al., 2016).

Interpretation Tools and Services

There are also companies that service genomic research and interpretation businesses. While these generally do not provide wet lab or direct patient services, many employ genetic counselors who can define the clinical requirements the product or service must develop to support its clients' needs. These genetic counselors serve as subject matter experts and often engage in product design, testing, and go-to-market planning. One subcategory is composed of companies that offer tools for interpretation of genomic data in either a research or clinical environment. Some provide general tools, while others provide more specialized tools. There are too many of these to list within the scope of this chapter, but some examples include Fabric Genomics, GoldenHelix, and YouScript as well as multinational companies like Decode (part of Amgen), Illumina, Sophia Genetics, and Genuity Science (previously WuxiNextCode).

Digital Health Solutions

The clinical setting continues to adopt technology solutions to address both provider and patient demands. For healthcare professionals, these solutions address the need to increase scale, improve efficiency, and decrease costs. For patients, these solutions can address barriers to increase access and engagement. Some of this is occurring directly within the electronic health record (EHR), while other solutions are evolving in parallel, with some integration points into the EHR and others as standalone products. When considering the end-to-end experience an individual may have during their genetic testing journey, each aspect of the journey lends the opportunity to develop technology solutions to improve the user experience and, ideally, to effectively and efficiently aggregate clinically relevant data to impact healthcare decisions and outcomes. Some examples include family health history tools that enable individuals to enter their information in a guided digital interface prior to a clinic visit, risk assessment tools that leverage guidelines to stratify patient risk, dynamic education interfaces to assist with informed consent and the delivery of results, and tools that facilitate cascade testing for at-risk relatives.

Genetic counselors contribute to these solutions by providing the subject matter expertise to inform product design, guide development, and ensure quality and accuracy. This has proven to be a small but growing sector where the products are highly attractive acquisition targets for large testing labs. For example, Clear Genetics, which developed chatbots to increase the productivity of genetic counselors; GenomeSmart, which leveraged AI to help identify and recommend appropriate testing for individuals; and Medneon, which developed a clinical decision support tool, were recently acquired by well-known diagnostic labs.

Payers and Utilization Management

As the breadth of genomic testing has significantly expanded in recent years, so has the scope of genetic counseling roles within healthcare delivery companies. Insurance providers are struggling to keep up with the pace of technological development and need to evaluate an endless supply of new molecular tests, technologies, and applications in making policy and coverage decisions. While there are genetic counselors employed in test utilization roles in both academia and industry, genetic counselors have continued to play major roles with insurers as subject matter experts, not only working to vet the vast number of tests on the market but also driving health economic outcomes research and becoming experts in interpreting Current Procedural Terminology (CPT) and International Classification of Diseases (ICD) coding systems that often obscure the coverage and reimbursement decision process. One early study identified the benefits of genetic counselor review of complex molecular test orders, in which 26% of test requests were changed or deemed unnecessary, resulting in $1.2 million in savings over a 21-month period (Miller et al., 2014). Genetic counselors have been instrumental in helping move payers toward more innovative policies and approaches to personalized medicine. In addition to those working within the payer system, opportunities have emerged for those working in data analytics, aggregating data from key stakeholders like insurance companies, labs, and health systems, to identify trends, barriers, and opportunities for cost-effective innovation (e.g., Concert Genomics).

Understanding the Business Side

Historically, the majority of genetic counselors in industry have not had formal business training (NSGC, 2022), although a growing number are choosing to secure additional degrees in areas such as organizational management, finance, marketing, and operations. The skills obtained during genetic counseling training, as mentioned above, serve as a valuable foundation that has allowed many genetic counselors to learn the business side experientially and be successful. However, those who have pursued more formal education may be better equipped, at least initially, to cater to the commercial demands of industry.

For any genetic counselor considering a move to industry, it is important to be cognizant of a few key concepts and expectations to enable success as well as professional satisfaction: the value of a business case, negotiating your value, and the importance of titles.

What is a business case?

One challenge encountered by many genetic counselors entering industry is embracing the need to develop a business case. This skill also proves highly valuable in noncommercial settings, including advocating for workforce expansion in a clinic, salary negotiations, or integration of tools and resources to enable greater efficiency in a clinical setting.

A business case is the rationale for proceeding with an idea or a project. Preparing a business case enables one to take a disciplined approach to critically examine the opportunity, the alternatives, the project stages, and the financial investment in order to make a recommendation for the best course of action to create the business value. It outlines the value of the project, the reason for initiating the project, the potential impact of the project, the benefits and risks, the alternatives, and the financial justification for the project, including short- and/or long-term impact. For example, in the genomics industry, parameters such as market size, market share, addressable market, and reimbursement can be critical components to a business case.

Genetic counseling training provides the intuitive foundation to identify what should be done, but in a business context, one needs to be prepared to articulate the why, how, and how much. It may sound daunting, but it is a cornerstone to success in industry.

Negotiating your value

There continues to be an increase in awareness about the term "genetic counselor" and a general grasp of the value of the skills that the profession brings. However, one should not assume that those outside the field fundamentally understand how genetic counseling expertise translates to different roles and responsibilities. Consider a scenario where it is necessary to explain the value of a genetic test in the context of a patient's medical history. Similarly for professional development, genetic counselors need to be able to represent the value they bring with tangible examples in the context of any new role they may seek.

These same principles of demonstrating value and investment can be applied to other aspects of business, including one's value as an employee. The benchmarks for advancement can be quite different in corporate as compared to clinical settings. There is a fundamental difference in promotion versus merit. Performance is not only based on merit, meeting and exceeding expectations, but also vision, overperforming, and creating opportunity. A genetic counselor navigating the commercial world must be aware of and prepared for appropriate expectation setting and purposeful career development goals. Growth and promotion within a company aren't just about performance, tenure, or meeting expectations. Advancement needs to be deliberate.

When negotiating compensation, it is important to recognize that salary and benefits are not the only levers. Compensation packages can vary significantly in terms of stock, options, and long-term equity depending on the size, stage, and financing of the company. In addition, personal risk tolerance is an important consideration in selecting the best personal fit for a role in industry. Some prefer more well-founded, established, and successful companies with a well-structured organization. Others may gravitate toward smaller, more agile, and faster-paced companies with less structure and more flexibility. The scope of compensation will depend on the context.

Titles matter

Whether as a new employee or during the trajectory of professional growth, it is important to not underestimate the value of a job title. In more clinical settings, the title of "genetic counselor" is broadly accepted. In industry, the designation can bring respect and authority, but for those who are not involved in directly servicing patients or providers, it may have less significance. As described above, companies have different departments or verticals, each often having its own career track or career ladders. The development of career ladders is an important mechanism to document and pursue career advancement opportunities for genetic counselors (Nagy et al., 2014). Selecting where one can grow and build relevant skills within a company is an important first step and, depending on the size and focus of the company, can often yield additional professional opportunities in other areas. While the core skill set embodied by genetic counselors can set someone up for success across a range of functions, growth comes from defining what successes have been achieved within a commercial business.

Emerging Trends, Future Opportunities

Awareness about the field of genetic counseling has continued to grow, as evidenced by genetic counseling being one of the leading job opportunities, with the Bureau of Labor Statistics projecting a 21.5% growth in employment between 2019 and 2029 (U.S. News and World Report, 2019). As a result, the public is becoming more familiar with what genetic counselors do and the value of their skills. More genetic counselors are founding companies and serving in executive leadership positions. Yet, there is more work to be done to expand awareness about the broad scope of roles that genetic counselors can fulfill.

The promise and potential for genomics to positively impact all lives is no longer a vision—it is rapidly becoming a reality. Genetic counselors have the opportunity to influence how genomics integrates into healthcare and empower individuals with both traditional and innovative solutions. Genetic counselors will continue to directly and indirectly translate the complexities and nuances of genomic data to meet the current and future needs of all stakeholders.

As aptly summarized by Bamshad and colleagues:

> To maximize [the] potential [of widespread precision health], approaches to genetic counseling and the role of genetic counselors will need to adapt to fit changing clinical and commercial needs worldwide. This will require overcoming multiple challenges including an inadequate workforce; development and implementation of alternate models of service delivery; integration of new technologies to improve, extend, and expand services; and support for equitable education and counseling among all populations. Genetic counselors are aptly poised to take on these challenges. (Bamshad et al., 2018, p. 6)

We believe several trends are here to stay:

- The cost of sequencing will continue to decrease due to technical enhancements and a competitive marketplace, while the ability to miniaturize and scale sequencing will increase. All of these market realities are leading to the commoditization of generating genomic data—for both research and clinical use.

- The technical ability to read genomic and other "omic" data has and will continue to generate vast amounts of information that requires rigorous study, clinical validation, and translation, leveraging both technical and human channels. AI and machine learning require skilled professionals to navigate inputs, create vetted clinical content, and develop the user experience to enable accurate and impactful insights.
- Telehealth and digital medicine, along with consumer-initiated health and wellness trends, will continue to empower individuals to seek information and services both within and outside the traditional healthcare system.
- The concept that one can have their DNA sequenced once, stored, and accessed for clinically relevant, on-demand interpretation throughout the lifecycle is a growing reality. Realizing the promise of the genome is limited not by patient or physician interest and demand but by information technology (EHRs), implementation (access points), policy (population-wide evidence), diversity (representative research driving equitable translational insights), and economics (who pays for what and when).
- The growth in other types of informational tests ("omics") that tell us about our genome will also bring new needs for "translators" in biochemical genetics, methylation/epigenetics, transcriptome, microbiome, and related disciplines.
- The demand for genetic counselors in industry will continue to expand—from small startups to the largest technology manufacturers and healthcare companies.

The growth in population health genomics over the past several years is likely the tip of the iceberg. Many health systems have invested in a research-first approach to enabling access to actionable genomic insights for their patients by consenting patients to large-scale research programs that may provide information on clinically actionable results (e.g., Geisinger's MyCode, Renown's Healthy Nevada Project). Some are taking a clinical-first approach, where patients consent to receive actionable clinical genomic results (e.g., Northshore Hospital's DNA 10k Program, Sanford Health's Imagenetics Program). As more hospitals and other healthcare delivery stakeholders institute these programs, more people will have access to information about what their DNA can tell them. While these programs are occurring within traditional healthcare delivery channels, behind the scenes industry players are driving much of the implementation, execution, and research partnerships (Helix, Color Genomics, Regeneron, and Genome Medical, to name a few). It remains to be seen exactly who will ultimately drive the funding and integration of genomics longitudinally, but it will likely include health systems, payers, and biopharma research. Genetic counselors can be critical players in helping these organizations with the strategy, implementation, and execution of these programs.

The global COVID-19 pandemic, arguably one of the most devastating catastrophes of our lifetime, also served to trigger awareness. As we have seen historically, such vast devastation often yields change and innovation. We have already seen the acceleration of adoption of and reimbursement for telehealth services. There is a national discussion about taking action to address gaps in underserved communities. We are beginning to see investment across healthcare technology to address some of the challenges faced by existing healthcare systems. And we will hopefully see a greater focus on bolstering public health programs in the future, including the integration of genomic data into risk stratification and clinical decision making.

Conclusion

Industry presents a growing spectrum of career opportunities for genetic counselors, expanding upon skills core to the profession. As technology continues to advance, the reality is that patients, providers, and other stakeholders will increasingly have access to genomic information. The ensuing gaps in translating that information to responsible clinical applications will drive evolving roles and opportunities for genetic counselors. There is no doubt that genetic counselors will play significant roles in the strategy, development, and implementation of solutions to meet the needs of the moment. It is up to the field, and its individual contributors, to ensure that genetic counselors remain key players who are able to positively impact the power of genomics and precision medicine, at the level of the individual and the broader population.

References

Amos, J., & Gold, B. (1998). Testing environment for single-gene disorders in U.S. reference laboratories. *Human Mutation*, *12*(5), 293–300.

Association for Molecular Pathology (AMP) et al. v. Myriad Genetics, Inc. et al., 569 U.S. (2013). http://www.supremecourt.gov/opinions/12pdf/12-398_1b7d.pdf

Bamshad, M. J., Magoulas, P. L., & Dent, K. M. (2018). Genetic counselors on the frontline of precision health. *Journal of Genetic Counseling*, *178*(1), 5–9.

Bergner, A. L., & Babu, D. (2017, March 21–25). *Characteristics of genetic counselors in industry-based roles: Considerations for ongoing workforce discussions* [Conference abstract]. ACMG Annual Meeting, Phoenix, AZ.

Bestsennyy, O., Gilbert, G., Harris, A., & Rost, J. (2021). *Telehealth: A quarter-trillion-dollar post-COVID-19 reality?* McKinsey & Company Report. https://www.mckinsey.com/industries/healthcare-systems-and-services/our-insights/telehealth-a-quarter-trillion-dollar-post-covid-19-reality

Boerwinkel, D. J., Yarden, A., & Waarlo, A. J. (2017). Reaching a consensus on the definition of genetic literacy that is required from a twenty-first-century citizen. *Science & Education*, *26*, 1087–1114.

Chapman, R., Likhanov, M., Selita, F., Zakharon, I., Smith-Woolley, E., & Kovas, Y. (2019). New literacy challenge for the twenty-first century: Genetic knowledge is poor even among well educated. *Journal of Community Genetics*, *10*, 73–84.

Cho, M. T., & Guy, C. (2020). Evolving roles of genetic counselors in the clinical laboratory. *Cold Spring Harbor Perspectives in Medicine*, *10*(10), a036574.

Cohen, S. A., & Tucker, M. E. (2018). Movement of genetic counselors from clinical to non-clinical positions: Identifying driving forces. *Journal of Genetic Counseling*, *27*(4), 792–799.

Cohen, S. A., Tucker, M. E., & Delk, P. (2017). Genetic counselor workforce issues: A survey of genetic counselors licensed in the state of Indiana. *Journal of Genetic Counseling*, *26*(3), 567–575.

Concert Genetics. (2021). *The Genetic Testing Unit (GTU)*. [White paper]. https://www.concertgenetics.com/resources/concert-genetic-testing-unit-gtu/

Davis, C., Baty, B. J., Hippman, C., Trepanier, A., & Erby, L. (2020). Genetic counselors with advanced skills: II. A new career trajectory framework. *Journal of Genetic Counseling*, *29*(5), 771–785.

Demeke, H. B., Merali, S., Marks, S., Pao, L. Z., Romero, L., Sandhu, P., Clark, H., Clara, A., McDow, K. B., Tindall, E., Campbell, S., Bolton, J., Le, X., Skapik, J. L., Nwaise, I., Rose, M. A., Strona, F. V., Nelson, C., & Siza, C. (2021). Trends in use of telehealth among health centers during the COVID-19 pandemic—United States, June 26–November 6, 2020. *MMWR Morbidity and Mortality Weekly Report*, *70*(7), 240–244.

Field, T., Brewster, S. J., Towne, M., & Campion, M. A. (2016). Emerging genetic counselor roles within the biotechnology and pharmaceutical industries: As industry interest grows in rare genetic disorders, how are genetic counselors joining the discussion? *Journal of Genetic Counseling*, *25*, 708–719.

Finucane, B. (2011). National Society of Genetic Counselors presidential address: Maintaining our professional identity in an ever-expanding genetics universe. *Journal of Genetic Counseling*, *21*(1), 3–6.

Government Accountability Office. (2010). *Direct-to-consumer genetic tests: Misleading test results are further complicated by deceptive marketing and other questionable practices.* https://www.gao.gov/products/gao-10-847t

Groepper, D., McCarthy, V. P., LeRoy, B. S., & Bower, M. (2015). Ethical and professional challenges encountered by Laboratory Genetic Counselors. *Journal of Genetic Counseling*, *24*, 580–596.

Hawkins, A. K., & Ho, A. (2012). Genetic counseling and the ethical issues around direct to consumer genetic testing. *Journal of Genetic Counseling*, *21*(3), 367–373.

Hirschler, B. (2013, January 3). *Analysis: Entering the age of the $1 million medicine.* Reuters. https://www.reuters.com/article/2013/01/03/us-rarediseases-idUSBRE9020C120130103

Hoskovec, J. M., Bennett, R. L., Carey, M. E., DaVanzo, J. E., Dougherty, M., Hahn, S. E., LeRoy, B. S., O'Neal, S., Richardson, J. G., & Wicklund, C. A. (2018). Projecting the supply and demand for certified genetic counselors: A workforce study. *Journal of Genetic Counseling*, *27*(1), 16–20.

Hsieh, V., Braid, T., Gordon, E., & Hercher, L. (2021). Direct-to-consumer genetic testing companies tell their customers to "see a genetic counselor." How do genetic counselors feel about direct-to-consumer genetic testing? *Journal of Genetic Counseling*, *30*(1), 191–197.

McWalter, K., Cho, M. T., Hart, T., Nusbaum, R., Sebold, C., Knapke, S., Klein, R., Friedman, B., Willaert, R., Singleton, A., Williams, L., Butler, E., & Juusola, J. (2018). Genetic counseling in industry settings: Opportunities in the era of precision health. *Journal of Genetic Counseling*, *178*(1), 46–53.

Miller, C. E., Krautscheid, P., Baldwin, E. E., Tvrdik, T., Openshaw, A. S., Hart, K., & Lagrave, D. (2014). Genetic counselor review of genetic test orders in a reference laboratory reduces unnecessary testing. *American Journal of Medical Genetics*, *164A*(5), 1094–1101.

Mills, R., MacFarlane, I. M., Caleshu, C., Ringler, M. A., & Zeirhut, H. A. (2021). Genetic counselor experiences with telehealth before and after COVID-19. *Journal of Genetic Counseling*, *30*(4), 999–1009.

Nagy, R., Peay, H., Hicks, M., Kloos, J., Westman, R., & Conway, L. (2014). Genetic counselors' and genetic counseling students' attitudes around the clinical doctorate and other advanced educational options for genetic counselors: A report from the genetic counseling advanced degree task force. *Journal of Genetic Counseling*, *24*(4), 626–634.

National Society of Genetic Counselors. (2002). *NSGC 2002 professional status survey*. https://www.nsgc.org/LinkClick.aspx?fileticket=hPybqdUhYSc%3d&portalid=0&timestamp=1695215104533.

National Society of Genetic Counselors. (2021a). *NSGC 2021 professional status survey special report professional diversity, inclusion and satisfaction*. https://www.nsgc.org/Research-and-Publications/Professional-Status-Survey/Past-Professional-Status-Surveys

National Society of Genetic Counselors. (2021b). *NSGC 2021 professional status survey work environment report*. https://www.nsgc.org/Research-and-Publications/Professional-Status-Survey/Past-Professional-Status-Surveys

National Society of Genetic Counselors. (2022). *NSGC 2022 professional status survey salary and benefits report*. https://www.nsgc.org/Research-and-Publications/Professional-Status-Survey/Past-Professional-Status-Surveys

Pollock, A. (2007, September 11). A genetic test that very few need, marketed to the masses. *New York Times*. https://www.nytimes.com/2007/09/11/business/media/11genetics.html

Rabideau, M. M., Wong, K., Gordon, E. S., & Ryan, L. (2016). Genetic counselors in startup companies: Redefining the genetic counselor role. *Journal of Genetic Counseling*, 25, 649–657.

Scheuner, M. T., Douglas, M. P., Sales, P., Ackerman, S. L., & Phillips, K. A. (2021). Laboratory business models and practices: Implications for availability and access to germline genetic testing. *Genetics in Medicine*, 23, 1681–1688.

Strohmeyer, J., Arjunan, A., Ryan, L., Pan, V., Wicklund, C., & Witherington, S. (2023) No longer "non-traditional": Genetic counselors' perceptions towards laboratory and industry roles. *Journal of Genetic Counseling*, 32, 646–655.

U.S. News and World Report. (2019). *Best jobs report*. https://money.usnews.com/careers/best-jobs/genetic-counselor

Waltman, L., Runke, C., Balcom, J., Riley, J. D., Lilley, M., Christian, S., Zetzsche, L., & Goodenberger, M. L. (2016). Further defining the role of the laboratory genetic counselor. *Journal of Genetic Counseling*, 25(4), 786–798.

Zeirhut, H. A., MacFarlane, I. M., Ahmed, Z., & Davies, J. (2018). Genetic counselors' experiences and interest in telegenetics and remote counseling. *Journal of Genetic Counseling*, 27(2), 329–338.

Zetzsche, L. H., Kotzer, K. E., & Wain, K. E. (2013). Looking back and moving forward: An historical perspective from laboratory genetic counselors. *Journal of Genetic Counseling*, 23, 363–370.

CHAPTER 14

GENETIC COUNSELING APPROACHES FOR ADOLESCENTS AND YOUNG ADULTS

MELANIE F. MYERS AND WENDY R. UHLMANN

Introduction

Most genetic counselors in clinical practice will encounter adolescents and young adults (AYAs) in clinic. AYAs may be seen by a genetics provider for a variety of reasons, such as management of a lifelong condition, workup of a suspected genetic condition, or risk assessment and management based on family history or a positive genetic test result. Medical factors that may influence how genetic counseling is approached include whether (a) the condition is known or unknown, (b) the AYA is symptomatic or asymptomatic, (c) the condition is congenital or has onset in childhood or onset in adulthood, (d) the condition is medically actionable in childhood, and (e) the family history is positive or negative. Additional patient and family factors that may impact the genetic counseling approach include the patient's cognitive abilities, maturity, psychological status, and frame of mind; family communication about the genetic condition or risk; and family dynamics. As with any patient, socioeconomic factors, cultural issues, language differences, health literacy, and views and perceptions of healthcare providers and medical care can also impact the clinic visit.

AYAs may also seek genetic services as a result of primary or secondary findings identified through genomic sequencing, through research studies where results were returned, through participation in a carrier screening program (e.g., sickle cell anemia, Tay-Sachs disease), or for follow-up after undergoing direct-to-consumer genetic testing.

Providing genetic counseling and facilitating healthcare decisions for AYAs presents some unique considerations and must balance AYAs' needs with parental involvement. While neurotypically developing individuals over the age of 18 years legally have full decision-making autonomy over their healthcare, parents have legal decision-making autonomy for individuals under 18 years of age and are expected to make decisions in the best interest of the child (Clayton, 2015; Ross, 2013). However, there is no consensus on how to weigh the child's present versus future interests, the parent's interests and that of other family members, and the child's current and future autonomy when considering the child's best interest (Ross, 2013). While recognition of adolescents' growing autonomy and the importance of engaging them in healthcare decisions is increasing (Sabatello & Appelbaum, 2016), there are few resources or best practice models for providing genetic counseling to AYA patients (Duncan & Young, 2013; Wainstein et al., 2022; Young et al., 2020). This chapter will explore AYA development and decision making, considerations in providing genetic counseling, and the healthcare decisions faced by young adults.

Adolescent Development and Decision Making

Adolescent development

Adolescence is the period of growth from puberty until adulthood, marked by completion of frontal lobe development. The frontal lobe contains the prefrontal cortex, which is responsible for executive functioning, including cognition, abstract thinking, planning, and impulse control (Halpern-Feshler, 2009; Steinberg, 2005). The age span that encompasses "adolescence" varies by culture and has changed over time as patterns of biological growth and social role transitions have evolved (Sawyer et al., 2018). Adolescence is a time of biological, social, emotional, and cognitive development and can be divided into three general stages: early adolescence from onset of puberty to 13 years, middle adolescence from 14 to 17 years, and late adolescence (or young/emerging adulthood) from 18 through the early to mid-20s (Allen & Waterman, 2019; Sawyer et al., 2018).

In early adolescence, puberty brings about body changes, which can bring on emotional lability, curiosity, anxiety, and questions about gender identity. Adolescents in this stage may have more concrete thinking and are often self-conscious. They often begin to push boundaries and feel an increased need for privacy (Allen & Waterman, 2019). In middle adolescence, physical changes continue. Teens tend to affiliate with similar-aged peers and become interested in romantic relationships. Their actions may be influenced by feelings and social/peer influences (Allen & Waterman, 2019; Halpern-Feshler, 2009; Steinberg, 2005). Adolescents in this stage may reach a stage of cognitive development that allows abstract thinking (Katz et al., 2016) but may not have the impulse control to apply it in the moment or in emotionally charged situations (Diekema, 2020). Risk taking and exploratory behaviors are more common, as are arguments with parents (Allen & Waterman, 2019). Brain maturation continues into late adolescence, with the prefrontal cortex being the last to mature (Diekema, 2020). Adolescents in this stage often experience a strong need for individual autonomy and privacy that must be balanced with the need for parental support (Pichini et al., 2016; Tse et al., 2013).

Overall, adolescents want to "fit in" and not be seen as different. Feeling different from one's peers can lead to low self-esteem and difficulty with peer and family relationships.

There can also be feelings of stigmatization (Pichini et al., 2016). AYAs with differing appearance and/or physical abilities may feel self-conscious and may hold back from participating in social activities. Peers may be reluctant to interact with AYAs who are differently abled. If the genetic condition impacts mobility, AYAs may find it difficult to be less mobile, remaining dependent at a time when peers are becoming more independent, including driving and moving toward living independently.

Adolescent decision making

Abstract reasoning and adolescent decision-making abilities develop over time as cognitive, social, and emotional abilities advance (Hein et al., 2012). Decision making relies on two systems in the brain: a socioemotional system composed of limbic and paralimbic structures and a cognitive-control system composed of prefrontal and parietal cortical structures (Katz et al., 2016; Diekema, 2020). The former matures in early to mid-adolescence, whereas the latter matures in the mid- to late 20s (Diekema, 2020). Studies suggest that most minors demonstrate a level of cognitive competency equivalent to that of adults around age 14 (Weithorn & Campbell, 1982) and are capable of rational decision making (Reyna & Farley, 2006). However, as noted, development of executive functioning and reasoning continues into the mid-20s (Diekema, 2020). Males and females also mature at different rates and may differ in their perceptions about health-related risks. Cultural and ethnic variations as well as life experiences can also impact understanding, as well as the ability to consider risks and benefits (Halpern-Feshler, 2009; Hein et al., 2015).

There is an ethical and legal obligation to obtain permission for clinical or research tests involving minors from the minor's parent or legal guardian (hereafter "parent" refers to either parent or legal guardian). However, parent–child collaboration is an important aspect in decision making, particularly as children mature developmentally and cognitively (Lipstein et al., 2015; V. A. Miller et al., 2008). Adolescents should be involved in health-related decisions about themselves, and assent ought to be solicited from adolescents in a developmentally appropriate manner, gradually increasing as they mature. Assent involves soliciting the minor's willingness to accept a medical intervention or to participate in a research study. The required elements of assent may vary in clinical and research settings, as well as by institution and the minor's age (Committee on Bioethics et al., 2013; Katz et al., 2016; V. A. Miller & Nelson, 2006).

In the guidance provided by the American Academy of Pediatrics (AAP), assent should be sought whenever appropriate and potentially can be obtained from children as young as age 7. Age 7 is typically when the concrete operations stage of development starts, "allowing for limited logical thought processes and the ability to develop a reasoned decision" (Katz et al., p. 2).

The AAP has issued both a policy statement and a technical report on informed consent in decision-making in pediatric practice that provide relevant information on the process of informed consent in decision-making in pediatric practice. Issues unique to pediatrics are addressed, including the content of the informed consent/assent discussion, surrogate decision-making for children and adolescents, engaging children and adolescents as medical decision-makers, and legal considerations based on varying scenarios (Katz et al., 2016).

Since joint decision-making precedes full decision-making independence (McCabe, 1996; V. A. Miller & Nelson, 2006), taking a developmental approach that respects shared decision making (SDM) between parents and children is optimal (Joffe, 2003) and fits well with the tenets of genetic counseling practice. SDM takes into account evidence-based information, provider knowledge and experience, and the patient's values and preferences (Agency for Healthcare Research and Quality, 2014). The provider and patient work together to make a healthcare decision that is best for the patient based on the patient's values and preferences. SDM can be more challenging in a pediatric setting since the preferences and values of both the child and the parent must be considered (Boland et al., 2019) and because there is a power differential between parents and their children. However, SDM can foster congruence when decisional preferences are discordant (Pervola et al., 2019). In a genetics setting, studies suggest that facilitation of collaborative decision making by a provider may increase the likelihood of keeping both parents and adolescents engaged and involved in decisions about genomic results rather than relying on parental decisional preferences alone (V. A. Miller et al., 2017).

Decisional autonomy

Research with adolescents indicates that they want to be involved in decision making about genetic testing and return of incidental findings from genomic sequencing (Geller et al., 2003; Hufnagel et al., 2016; Levenseller et al., 2014; McGowan et al., 2018). Parents and adolescents have suggested that involvement in the decision-making process about genomic research may vary based on the adolescent's age, maturity level, and personality (Geller et al., 2003; Hufnagel et al., 2016; Levenseller et al., 2014; Miner et al., 2022). In a clinical setting, adolescents' personal experiences with treatment or other medical choices due to the course of their condition should also be considered (Bush et al., 2018). Cultural influences may also significantly impact the decision-making process.

Parents and adolescents may have varying perceptions as to the amount of decisional autonomy they would like the other to have (Levenseller et al., 2014; V. A. Miller et al., 2008; Miner et al., 2022; Pervola et al., 2019). Although minors may recognize that their parent must be involved in genetic testing decisions (McGowan et al., 2018), when given choices and the option to learn genetic information about themselves, adolescents will not always make the same genetic testing decisions for themselves that parents make for them (Myers et al., 2020).

Although parental permission is required for genetic testing of minors, there are some situations when a minor can make their own healthcare decisions—for example, based on specific health conditions or categories, or if a state law designates a minor as emancipated or grants adolescents "mature minor" status (Katz et al., 2016). Most states grant adolescents the authority to make their own healthcare decisions for the diagnosis and treatment of sexually transmitted infections, contraceptive services, substance abuse and mental health treatment, and pregnancy-related care (Katz et al., 2016; Clayton, 2015; Diekema, 2020). In a genetic counseling setting, pregnant teens should be offered the same screening that would be offered to any pregnant patient. However, some pregnant adolescents may struggle with adolescent developmental tasks and pregnancy simultaneously (Peters-Brown

& Fry-Mehltretter, 1996). States generally recognize adolescents as emancipated when they are married, living separately from their parents and self-supporting, or serving active duty with the armed forces (Diekema, 2020). States may legally grant minors "mature minor" status based on considerations of the minor's age, maturity, cognitive abilities, and social and medical situation (Katz et al., 2016). However, adolescents' consent to services does not always protect their confidentiality.

Privacy

Legally, minors have few, if any, rights to stop genetic testing for which parents have given permission. In some cases, clinicians will not test a minor who does not want genetic testing based on ethical guidelines. In other cases, a clinician can refuse testing if they feel it is inappropriate. Regardless, parents can seek a different provider who will proceed with the testing (Clayton, 2015) or even pursue genetic testing online (i.e., consumer-initiated and direct-to-consumer testing).

When testing is performed, adolescents have little control over parental access to and sharing of their genetic test results (Clayton, 2015), even if the adolescent prefers such information not be shared. There is also the potential that parents and/or adolescents may share genomic information on social media platforms, which could lead to misuse of adolescents' genetic information by school officials, future employers, insurers, and others (Sabatello & Appelbaum, 2016). It has been proposed that shared or joint decision making could help safeguard adolescents' genomic privacy and help avert disclosure of medical information without regard for their preferences (Sabatello & Appelbaum, 2015).

Adolescents can make certain healthcare decisions before 18 (most often related to mental health, reproductive health, and substance abuse). However, age 18 is when the young adult is considered independent for healthcare management/decisions in the United States, unless the parent has legal guardianship due to cognitive impairment/disabilities associated with the genetic condition or guardianship for other reasons (e.g., significant impairment due to psychiatric disorder). When a parent states they have legal guardianship but it is not documented in the medical record, it is appropriate to ask to see this documentation to confirm. While parent(s) may still financially cover the cost of clinic visits and/or pay for healthcare insurance for young adults, the young adults' medical issues will no longer be known by the parent(s) unless shared by the young adult or if the parent has guardianship.

Counseling Adolescents and Young Adults

General approaches to providing genetic counseling for AYAs

Although adolescents should be engaged in the counseling session and decision-making processes, it can be challenging to know how to best encourage and support their participation (Werner-Lin et al., 2016). There is emerging literature that highlights strategies for and challenges of working with AYAs (Callard et al., 2012; Godino et al., 2016; Pichini et al.,

2016; Tse et al., 2013) and models for working with AYAs (Young et al., 2020) in a genetic counseling setting. Some of the strategies include:

- Explain the role of the genetic counselor and how genetic counseling may benefit the AYA before the session. This can be in the form of directing them to informational websites, emailing them, an information sheet accompanying the appointment letter, or a phone discussion.
- *Assess* but do not *assume* the AYA's educational, social, and developmental states and how they may impact understanding and decision making.
- Allow adolescents to choose who they prefer to be present for the session. Ideally, the adolescent should have the opportunity to choose *before* the session. Explain that having time alone with the adolescent is routine practice. Be aware of cultural or family influences on the adolescent's decision. The same principles hold for young adults, although young adults may prefer to attend sessions without a parent.
- Ascertain the AYA's prior knowledge of their condition or the reason for their visit. Confirm or clarify this information and provide age-appropriate resources for them to improve their knowledge. When clarifying information, avoid doing so in an authoritative manner as this may make the AYA hesitant to share their understanding of topics in the session.
- Engage directly with the AYA whenever possible throughout the scheduling process, the session itself, and follow-up. Encourage them to ask and answer questions. Do not answer questions for the AYA. Try to use open-ended questions.
- Use visual aids, particularly videos or animations, to aid understanding. Do not assume the AYA's literacy level or that they understand the subtleties of healthcare. Conduct psychosocial assessments and counseling as appropriate for age, ascertaining and asking about the AYA's unique lived experiences. Normalize the AYA's genetic condition and explore their personal identity and how they see themselves compared to their peers.
- Ask about sources of support. Offer support groups where available to assist with support and normalization of having a genetic condition.
- In cases where AYAs are struggling with worry about the outcome of their decision (e.g., approval from peers), asking how their peers might feel or act in a similar situation may be helpful. Alternatively, presenting a possible outcome of a decision and asking how the AYA would feel about it may assist them in seeing long-term implications of the decision, particularly around testing decisions.
- Ask questions about their school, work, or social environments and if they have experienced bullying or abuse.
- When sending visit summary letters, discuss how and to whom such letters are sent to ensure the AYA has access. Electronic communication may be preferable for AYAs.
- Provide resources and strategies to the AYA for self-management of their care. Offer to call or see them again for another visit in the future if they develop new concerns or questions.
- If counseling multiple members of a family, make sure to schedule extended visits. If possible, assign the AYA their own clinician rather than one clinician for all family members at the same time to enhance trust.

- Change in behavior, speech, or mannerisms to "get on their level" may be viewed as "fake" and untrustworthy by the AYA. However, some change in language may be needed to promote understanding of the information given. Continually assess understanding throughout the session.
- Ask about future reproductive plans and discuss recurrence risks and prenatal testing as appropriate to the individual.
- Explain consent, privacy, and confidentiality regarding testing, research, and so forth.
- The clinic space should be age appropriate. Consider blocks of appointment times dedicated to AYAs. Try to avoid scheduling that causes an AYA to be in a waiting room with all young children or older adults as this can hamper normalization.
- Continuously seek out educational opportunities related to caring for AYAs.

When exploring values and opinions, asking adolescents their thoughts first, followed by the parent's, can lead to a more in-depth discussion that ensures the adolescent perspective is heard. Additionally, eliciting the AYA's perspective before the parent's perspective, if applicable, can facilitate a collaborative decision-making process that maximizes the AYA's input (Myers et al., 2020; Pervola et al., 2019) and minimizes parental coercion.

If the AYA has intellectual disabilities, it remains important to greet the AYA and make sure to involve them in the visit to the extent possible. Maintaining eye contact with the AYA so that the AYA feels included and presenting information slowly and in simpler terms, especially if the AYA has the intellectual capacity to participate in decision making, can be helpful. Addressing developmental characteristics of individuals with intellectual disability (e.g., concreteness, irreversibility), genetic counseling approaches that are more conversational than teaching, shifting the focus from facts to feelings, and legal and ethical considerations are beyond the scope of this chapter (Finucane, 2010).

LGBTQIA+

Providing genetic counseling to AYAs who are LGBTQIA+ (lesbian, gay, bisexual, transgender, queer or questioning, intersex, asexual or ally, plus others who identify with a sexual orientation or gender identity not included in the acronym) requires sensitivity. Adolescence is a time of emerging sexual and gender identity. Adolescents may or may not feel comfortable sharing their sexual or gender identity due to feelings of self-consciousness or fear of stigmatization and lack of acceptance by peers, family, healthcare providers, or society. Genetic counseling research specific to adolescents who are LGBTQIA+ is lacking. However, interviews with adult members of the transgender and nonbinary community suggest that regardless of the patient's age, genetic counseling should create a safe environment and provide clarity about the clinical importance of both sex assigned at birth and gender identity for trans patients (Barnes et al., 2020). Two specific strategies suggested by Barnes et al. (2020) include (a) validating gender identity by asking preferred pronouns, preferred name, sex assigned at birth, and gender identity and (b) using inclusive and well-defined pedigree symbols that denote both sex assigned at birth and gender identity. While there is a growing need for best practices and resources for training genetic counselors to work with LGBTQIA+ youth (Sacca et al., 2019), the National Society of Genetic Counselors practice resource on standardized pedigree nomenclature provides guidance on terminology and pedigree symbols centered on sex and gender inclusivity (Bennett et al., 2022).

Parent–child dynamics and having time alone with the AYA

Parent–child dynamics and communication can affect the transition to the AYA taking a more active role in their care. During a clinic visit, tensions between the parent and child may be apparent. For example, the parent may take over the conversation or answer questions from the healthcare provider without allowing the AYA to first respond.

Balancing the needs of the adolescent and parent (or young adult whose parent is present) while being sensitive to the family context can be challenging (Gaff et al., 2006). The provider may need to proactively state that the AYA should answer the questions first with the parent assisting as needed and may need to interject, remind, and redirect when appropriate. In addition to asking the AYA questions directly, encouraging active participation from the AYA by ascertaining their views, giving them time to respond, and acknowledging and reflecting back information shared can lead to feelings of empowerment and increased autonomy.

It may be possible to give older adolescents the choice to have their parents in the session or present for the physical exam. Indeed, the AAP recommends that adolescents be given some time alone with providers (Rasch, 2012). Allowing such opportunities may increase feelings of respect and give adolescents a sense of control over their own health. Having time with the adolescent alone may also facilitate the sharing of information that might not be disclosed with the parent present (Pichini et al., 2016; Tse et al., 2013). The physical exam can be a time to ask the adolescent or young adult some sensitive questions (e.g., alcohol use, smoking, drug use, sexual activity/sexuality) that may not be readily shared if the parent is present. There also can be reluctance for AYAs to ask questions in front of their parents that could reveal poor adherence to treatment or involvement in risky behaviors (Maslyanskaya & Alderman, 2019). Being nonjudgmental, providing reassurance about confidentiality, and deciding with the adolescent or young adult what information to share with the parent are critical when sensitive information is disclosed (Callard et al., 2012; Duncan & Young, 2013).

Elements of the Genetic Counseling Session

Contracting and establishing rapport

As with any patient, the genetic counselor should maintain a nonjudgmental demeanor and provide unconditional positive regard (Pichini et al., 2016). Depending on the age of the patient, cognitive abilities, maturity, and other psychosocial and family factors, the AYA may or may not be an active participant in the clinic visit. If affected, the AYA may resent having a genetic condition and having to go to clinic appointments and may therefore not engage in the visit. Other AYAs may be accepting of their condition, approach it as "all that they have ever known," and be more comfortable engaging with healthcare providers. In fact, adolescents may welcome the visit for the opportunity to learn about the genetics of their condition and receive anticipatory guidance about the future (Pichini et al., 2016).

Asking the AYA what they expect from the genetic counseling session and following up by clarifying what will happen are recommended to facilitate engagement. Unfamiliarity with the genetic counseling process and how it differs from other medical visits can result in the AYA having unclear expectations and few questions or goals for the clinic visit (Pichini et al., 2016). It can be helpful to acknowledge that it can be hard to deal with health issues at their young age and that it's okay to be nervous or not sure what questions to ask.

When in person and possible, try to be seated near the AYA or in their direct line of sight. Taking the time to contract and establish rapport at the beginning of the appointment can make it clear that their involvement is valued and lead to better communication. It can also empower the AYA to actively participate in their own healthcare. The healthcare provider should direct questions to the AYA unless there is significant cognitive impairment and/or the AYA is not responding.

Asking the AYA questions about themselves can make them feel "seen" and sends the message that they are encouraged to be actively involved in the visit. Pichini et al. (2016) noted that making the adolescent the focus of the clinic visit and providing choices when possible are important for their feeling respected and having a sense of ownership and control of their health. For AYAs who may be used to parents taking care of visits, making sure they are engaged and not "tuning out" is important since ultimately this is about their bodies/health.

Possible considerations to develop rapport with the AYA include asking about their hobbies, work, school/college (favorite subjects/major), and any activities they might be engaged in and even commenting on a shirt logo or color of clothing. Cell phones make it easy to show artwork, a pet, or a photo taken. Asking adolescents if they have learned about genetics in a biology class may help make connections but has not consistently been shown to lead to more engagement (Werner-Lin et al., 2016). Since the quality of genetics education in grades 9 through 12 is not consistent, it is best to not make assumptions about knowledge (Dougherty et al., 2011; Sabatello et al., 2018). Initially asking some close-ended questions that can be readily answered may pave the way for responding to open-ended questions as the clinic visit progresses (Peters-Brown & Fry-Mehltretter, 1996; Weil, 2000).

Genetic counselors should pay attention to what is said/not said and be attuned to body language. The AYA may seem "shut down," reticent to respond, or not engaged out of anxiety from not knowing what is going to happen. The AYA may completely defer to their parent or give "I don't know. Whatever. Just ask my mother" responses. Given the emotional roller coaster of adolescence, a young patient's emotional state may be completely unrelated to the clinic visit (e.g., issue with friends). However, it is also important to assess (through direct questioning or administration of validated instruments) whether the AYA is dealing with depression and/or anxiety and consider referral to a therapist as indicated.

For patients with a lifelong condition, transition to adult care comes from "aging out" of pediatric care, generally resulting in transfer to new healthcare providers. During this transition, some AYAs may experience a sense of loss, particularly if they have an established, long-term relationship with their pediatric healthcare providers. Others may feel uncertainty and anxiety about establishing a new relationship with an adult provider and whether the physician will have the expertise to handle their medical issues. Time may be needed for new healthcare providers to learn about the AYA and their genetic condition. In addition, transition to adult care may represent a transition of the young adult taking on ownership of their healthcare. Acknowledging these issues associated with transitions in healthcare can help with setting realistic expectations.

Below are some open-ended general questions to directly ask and explore with AYAs, many of which are similar to questions often asked of adult patients being seen in a genetics clinic:

- What is your understanding of why you are here today?
- What questions or concerns do you have that you would like to discuss?
- What is hardest/most challenging for you day to day (if symptomatic)?
- What is your understanding of the condition?
- What is your understanding of your risk for the condition (if asymptomatic)?
- Have you talked about genetics in any of your classes?
- Have you searched the internet for information about the genetic condition? Have you found helpful information? Do you remember some of the sites?
- Are you part of a Facebook/online group or chat online?
- Have you talked about the condition/risk with your friends?
- What are your sources of support?
- What would be helpful to you?

Obtaining a family history and what can be learned

Taking a family history is important for risk assessment, rapport building, and determining how the AYA fits into the context of their family. Take the time to introduce the family history, explain why it is being taken and the symbols used, and show the final pedigree. Unless there are significant cognitive issues, try to engage the AYA when taking the family history, asking them ages of their siblings, parents, and potentially other family members. Relevant information may be provided in partnership with a parent or deferred to the parent, but at least the AYA will have been given the opportunity to participate.

Taking the family history can yield relevant information about how the genetic condition is inherited, who is affected or at risk, and what symptoms have been experienced by family members.[1] Keep in mind that during the family history the AYA may be hearing about family members' health conditions and/or being affected with a genetic condition for the first time. Furthermore, with some genetic conditions (e.g., hereditary cancers), the genetic condition is not visible and therefore may be a surprise for the AYA to learn.

Education about the condition and inheritance counseling

How informed the AYA is about a genetic condition will depend partly on what has been shared by parents and healthcare providers and what was understood. Information may have been intentionally or nonintentionally shared. Even when conveyed by the parent,

[1] Editors' note: For further discussion on family history, see Chapter 19 by Debra L. Collins and Devin M. Cox in this volume.

information may not have seemed salient or might not have been fully or accurately understood. What the AYA knows about the genetic condition will also depend on whether the AYA is the only family member with the genetic condition, if other family members are symptomatic, and the extent of contact with affected family members (none, limited, regular).

Providing education about the condition, including natural history, etiology, inheritance, and future personal and reproductive risks, can provide needed information and facilitate feeling increased personal control and conceptualizing the condition as part of their identity (Pichini et al., 2016). It may be helpful to tie in etiology and inheritance discussions with what the AYA has learned in school. Information can then be better tailored to the AYA (Tse et al., 2013). However, AYAs may not have liked their science courses, and they should be reassured that there will be no judgment regarding what they remember from class. Additionally, when appropriate, they should be informed that after the visit, a summary of the session and additional resources will be provided.

As with any patient, it is best to provide the AYA with information in understandable terms. A "less is more" approach may work well with adolescents. Acknowledging that the information may be complicated could help promote asking questions. Using diagrams and counseling aids during the visit can help focus attention, break down complex information into manageable segments, and facilitate education and engagement. "Chunking information" and stopping to ask about understanding and remaining questions are important for any patient and especially for AYAs. Using a computer or tablet to show video clips and animations of inheritance or biological processes may be helpful (Lewis et al., 2020; Pichini et al., 2016; Sabatello et al., 2018).

AYAs tend to be very comfortable with digital media (Sabatello et al., 2018). It is reasonable to ask what information they have already accessed on the internet and acknowledge the benefits and limitations of posted information. In this era where anything can be "googled," withholding information or asking the AYA to avoid searching for information on the internet is not practical.

Genetic counselors should proactively think about what questions, concerns, and fears an AYA may have and be prepared to provide this information, even when not directly asked. Presenting information and sharing questions as "other patients your age with this condition have wondered/asked/shared this concern . . ." can help normalize these questions and concerns. Lifespan, medical, psychosocial, and reproductive issues should all be addressed, including if there is no impact. Should surveillance be indicated, communicating what, how, and who will be involved can help provide anticipatory guidance and set realistic expectations for ongoing management. Being transparent and sharing what is known about medical and lifespan issues in a developmentally appropriate manner can build trust and understanding.

Answering the questions below and the extent to which some of these questions are addressed may be influenced by the AYA's age, condition, maturity, cognitive functioning, and psychosocial status:

- Will my condition worsen over time (if symptomatic)?
- If/when will I develop symptoms (if asymptomatic)?
- Will I be able to drive?
- Will I be able to have sex?

- Will I be able to have children?
- What is the risk to my children to have the same genetic condition?
- Will I be able to live independently?
- Will I be able to work?
- What can I expect? Is there anything I can do?
- Will I die at a younger age?

Providing genetic condition resources and national organization information

Linking affected individuals to the national organization for the genetic condition is one way to help connect them to individuals who are facing similar challenges. In the absence of a family history of the genetic condition, helping the AYA connect with other affected individuals may help to address feelings of isolation ("no one else like me in the family") and provide a community of individuals who may be facing similar issues (Pichini et al., 2016).

Organizations for the genetic condition can be found by internet search for the specific condition and through national organizations including the Genetic and Rare Diseases Information Center (GARD), Genetic Alliance, and National Organization for Rare Disorders, and internationally, Orphanet. MedlinePlus and GARD have developed patient-friendly information with web links on genetic conditions. Many genetics support groups have specifically developed resources geared toward AYAs, and academic institutions may have AYA support groups as well. It takes just a few minutes to show patients relevant content on a website to facilitate their accessing this information. There may also be social media groups and other online opportunities to connect, conferences, camps, local support group meetings, fundraising walks, and other activities. Some national organizations specifically have resources for talking with children about a genetic condition.

In general, the AYA should be provided with the resources since the appointment is for them. Even though the AYA may pass the resources over to a parent, at least it is clear that the resources were specifically intended for them and may be reviewed later. If providing paper copies, it can be helpful to have two copies—one for the patient and one for the parent(s). Consider providing the adolescent a copy of your card, in addition to the parent(s), to facilitate their contacting you with questions. If a summary letter of the clinic visit is generally provided to patients, then letting them know this can help take the pressure off trying to remember all the information. When possible, address the letter from the clinic visit to the adolescent and the parent and encourage that it be read by both. If the patient is 18 years of age or older, the letter should be addressed directly to the patient.

Having a visible genetic condition can be difficult especially since adolescence and young adulthood can be a time when "looks matter" and there is considerable focus on appearance. In addition to sharing information/resources from local/state and national organizations for the genetic condition, making young patients aware of Positive Exposure might be helpful. Founded by fashion photographer Rick Guidotti, Positive Exposure's mission is to promote "a more equitable, compassionate world for individuals and communities at risk of stigma and exclusion through photography, film, community storytelling, education, and advocacy" (Positive Exposure, 2023). In addition to photographs on the website, many featuring genetic conditions, there is a blog section (PEARLS Project) where AYAs share their stories.

Genetic Testing

Genetic testing may be considered for the AYA to establish, confirm, or rule out a diagnosis or to determine risk for a condition with childhood or adult onset. When a child is symptomatic or at risk for a childhood-onset condition, genetic testing is generally clinically indicated. However, genetic testing of minors for carrier status and adult-onset conditions, even if based on family history, is more controversial.

Predictive genetic testing and carrier testing

Professional guidelines recommend deferring both carrier testing and predictive genetic testing for conditions for which there is no intervention in childhood until the individual reaches the age of majority (18 years of age in the United States). Reasons to defer such testing include to facilitate autonomous decision making and to protect adolescents' right to an open future and minimize psychosocial harms (Botkin et al., 2015; Committee on Bioethics et al., 2013; Davis, 1997; National Society of Genetic Counselors, 2017). However, predictive genetic testing may be requested by the parent or the AYA because of lived experience with an affected parent or sibling (Fenwick et al., 2017; Mand et al., 2013). AYAs who have grown up either seeing family members with a genetic condition or having it openly discussed will have context for considering their own risk for the genetic condition and decisions about genetic testing. For AYAs where there was limited to no contact with affected relatives and/or the genetic condition was not openly discussed, there may be no context for considering their risks and decisions.

Testing decisions may be based on the anxiety of finding out about a family history of a genetic condition and wanting to be relieved from the anxiety of not knowing their status (ACMG Board of Directors, 2013). However, decisions made based on wanting relief from anxiety may not be carefully weighed or consider the different options and the long-term implications. AYAs may focus on immediate issues, and thus discussing long-term implications of testing decisions is critical.

There are multiple routes—clinical, nonclinical, and research—where parents and AYAs may learn their carrier status and/or risk for adult-onset conditions. If diagnostic genomic sequencing is ordered clinically, then parents may have the option to learn secondary findings about the minor child that could reveal risk for adult-onset conditions and possibly carrier status for some recessive conditions (Kalia et al., 2017; D. T. Miller et al., 2022). There are also increasing opportunities for pediatric populations to learn carrier status and risk for some adult-onset conditions through direct-to-consumer (DTC) genetic testing (although the AAP recommends against DTC genetic testing for children) and genomic research studies that offer return of results.

Professional guidelines also provide some guidance about disclosure with adolescents (Table 14.1). Although limited, evidence does not suggest that receiving genetic test results

Table 14.1 Professional Statements Regarding Predictive Genetic Testing of Minors

Organization	Statement	Assent of minor?	Adolescents mentioned?	Disclosure
AAP and ACMG (Committee on Bioethics et al., 2013)	Decisions driven by best interest of child. Parents[a] can authorize but recommend deferring unless intervention in childhood or to lessen diagnostic uncertainty	Yes	Parents should be involved even if minor is mature	Parents encouraged to inform child at appropriate age and to honor request of mature adolescent
ACMG (Bush et al., 2018)	Specific to sequencing (not predictive genetic testing)—encourage a robust engagement process with mature older child and adolescent to facilitate meaningful conversation to aid in decision making and return of results	Yes, child should be actively engaged and have opportunity to express feelings and opinions	Encourage engagement process with children over age 8 that includes the following information: 1. Sequencing may not provide diagnosis 2. Some test results may be more important to learn as an adult 3. New information may be learned over time 4. Test might uncover unexpected information and may lead to more tests	Some information may be reported to parent only and disclosed to child in the future (e.g., adult-onset condition with no childhood intervention). Continued discussion over time is optimal as relevancy of genomic information may change with life stage and as new data emerge
ASHG (Botkin et al., 2015)	Can be justified in certain situations (e.g., to alleviate substantial psychosocial distress or facilitate life-planning decisions). However, if no clinical intervention in childhood, parents should be encouraged to defer until adulthood or the child is an older adolescent who can participate in decision making in mature manner	Yes, for research, carrier, direct-to-consumer, and secondary findings. Children should be included in the informed assent or consent process to the extent that they are capable	Adolescents should be encouraged to defer until adulthood because of potential impact of the information at formative life stages	In context of secondary findings, clinicians should offer to disclose secondary findings for a child to the child's parents if the information has clear clinical utility for the child and/or family members
NSGC (NSGC, 2017)	Defer until minor has capacity to weigh risks/benefits/limitations if results won't impact child's management	Yes	No	If not disclosed to child, discuss strategy to share by age of majority

Note: AAP = American Academy of Pediatrics; ACMG = American College of Medical Genetics and Genomics; ASHG = American Society of Human Genetics; NSGC = National Society of Genetic Counselors.

[a] "Parent" is used to refer to parent or legal guardian.

leads to significant psychosocial harms to children (Lillie et al., 2022; Mand et al., 2013; Michie et al., 2001; Wade et al., 2010). However, more research is needed on disclosure practices (Miner et al., 2022), as well as to understand the impact of learning nonactionable genetic information in adolescence.

Possible questions to explore when an AYA wants to pursue genetic testing for an adult-onset condition include the following:

- What is their understanding of the genetic condition, age of onset, and what can be done if found to have the gene change for the condition?
- Why are they considering genetic testing at this time?
- What have they read/based their testing decision on?
- Are they feeling pressured to be tested by parent(s), other family members, or other individuals?
- What would they do if results were positive? Negative? Uncertain?
- What result are they expecting?
- What insurance coverage do they have?

Insurance coverage and implications

As parents are responsible for covering healthcare prior to age 18, 18-year-olds are new to thinking about health insurance coverage, let alone thinking about other types of insurance that could be impacted by genetic test results. In making decisions about genetic testing, young adults likely will not have an understanding of the potential long-term insurance implications. This is particularly an issue when considering predictive genetic testing for hereditary neurological conditions for which there currently is no cure (e.g., Huntington's disease, early-onset Alzheimer's disease, amyotrophic lateral sclerosis). Generally, genetic counselors should discuss having desired insurance coverage—health, life, long-term disability, and long-term care insurance—prior to undergoing predictive genetic testing.

Generally, in the United States, youth are covered by their parents' insurance while they are minors and through the Affordable Care Act up to age 26. College students may have health insurance through their school while they remain students. The young adult may not recognize the time limitations of insurance coverage through school or the Affordable Care Act and the fact that it only applies to health insurance. Those who work may have health insurance through their employer. Although those working may have the option of health and other types of insurance through their employer, they may not have considered purchasing it or may not have the funds to cover copayments or other costs. Young adults covered by Medicaid insurance may not recognize that this only applies for healthcare and in fact, depending on the plan, may not even cover genetic testing. Some young adults may have no health insurance.

How positive predictive genetic test results could impact young adults' ability to obtain needed insurance coverage is an important discussion topic. This particularly applies to life, long-term disability, and long-term care insurance. AYAs may not even be aware of these types of insurance, what they cover, why they are potentially needed, and the costs involved. The Genetic Information Nondiscrimination Act only applies to health insurance and employment (Genetic Alliance et al., 2024); AYAs may not be aware of this legislation or, if aware, may not be aware of these limitations.

Anxiety about blood draw

Patients of any age can have anxieties about having a blood sample drawn, even more so if the AYA is afraid of needles or has never had their blood drawn. Anxiety about a blood draw can make it hard to focus on the genetic counseling session. If collection of a saliva or cheek swab sample is not an option, then it may help to address concerns about a blood draw directly by letting the patient know that they have some control and can decide (a) left arm or right arm, (b) blood draw sitting or lying down, and (c) parent near or just in the room or not. Listening to music or suggesting that they look at videos and photos on their cell phone can provide a distraction. Giving phlebotomy "a heads up" if it is the patient's first time having a blood sample drawn and/or that the patient is anxious can be helpful. The institution or phlebotomy station may also have protocols or trained staff for drawing blood from young or anxious patients. Should time permit, consider being present with the AYA for the blood draw as this may help lessen their anxiety. Fortunately, many labs now offer the options of having a saliva or cheek swab sample provided in place of a blood sample for genetic testing.

Conclusion

Most genetic counselors in clinical practice will encounter AYAs. Providing genetic services to AYAs requires a different approach than working with adults and presents unique challenges specific to their developmental stage, health literacy, verbal expressive ability, family situations, experience with the healthcare system, and other factors described in the chapter. Resources for best practices when working with adolescents and theoretical models are emerging that can be integrated into genetics training and practice.

Depending on the AYA's genetic condition and cognitive abilities, there is a tightrope to walk in managing autonomy, privacy, and confidentiality while balancing the needs of the patient and their parent(s). From the initial contracting to providing genetic counseling and discussing genetic testing, it is important to take the time and make intentional efforts to engage the AYA to promote understanding of their genetic condition and to empower the AYA to become a partner in their own healthcare.

Acknowledgments

Melanie F. Myers and Wendy R. Uhlmann contributed equally to the writing of this chapter.

References

ACMG Board of Directors. (2013). Points to consider for informed consent for genome/exome sequencing. *Genetics in Medicine*, *15*(9), 748–749. https://doi.org/10.1038/gim.2013.94

Agency for Healthcare Research and Quality. (2014, October 2020). *The SHARE approach*. https://www.ahrq.gov/health-literacy/professional-training/shared-decision/index.html

Allen, B., & Waterman, H. (2019). *Stages of adolescence*. https://www.healthychildren.org/English/ages-stages/teen/Pages/Stages-of-Adolescence.aspx

Barnes, H., Morris, E., & Austin, J. (2020). Trans-inclusive genetic counseling services: Recommendations from members of the transgender and non-binary community. *Journal of Genetic Counseling*, *29*(3), 423–434. https://doi.org/10.1002/jgc4.1187

Bennett, R. L., French, K. S., Resta, R. G., & Austin, J. (2022). Practice resource-focused revision: Standardized pedigree nomenclature update centered on sex and gender inclusivity: A practice resource of the National Society of Genetic Counselors. *Journal of Genetic Counseling*, *31*(6), 1238–1248. https://doi.org/10.1002/jgc4.1621

Boland, L., Graham, I. D., Legare, F., Lewis, K., Jull, J., Shephard, A., Lawson, M. L., Davis, A., Yameogo, A., & Stacey, D. (2019). Barriers and facilitators of pediatric shared decision-making: A systematic review. *Implementation Science*, *14*(1), 7. https://doi.org/10.1186/s13012-018-0851-5

Botkin, J. R., Belmont, J. W., Berg, J. S., Berkman, B. E., Bombard, Y., Holm, I. A., Levy, H. P., Ormond, K. E., Saal, H. M., Spinner, N. B., Wilfond, B. S., & McInerney, J. D. (2015). Points to consider: Ethical, legal, and psychosocial implications of genetic testing in children and adolescents. *American Journal of Human Genetics*, *97*(1), 6–21. https://doi.org/10.1016/j.ajhg.2015.05.022

Bush, L. W., Bartoshesky, L. E., David, K. L., Wilfond, B., Williams, J. L., & Holm, I. A. (2018). Pediatric clinical exome/genome sequencing and the engagement process: Encouraging active conversation with the older child and adolescent: Points to consider—A statement of the American College of Medical Genetics and Genomics (ACMG). *Genetics in Medicine*, *20*(7), 692–694. https://doi.org/10.1038/gim.2018.36

Callard, A., Williams, J., & Skirton, H. (2012). Counseling adolescents and the challenges for genetic counselors. *Journal of Genetic Counseling*, *21*(4), 505–509. https://doi.org/10.1007/s10897-011-9460-z

Clayton, E. W. (2015). How much control do children and adolescents have over genomic testing, parental access to their results, and parental communication of those results to others? *Journal of Law Medicine & Ethics*, *43*(3), 538–544. https://doi.org/10.1111/jlme.12296

Committee on Bioethics, Committee on Genetics, American College of Medical Genetics, & Genomics Social Ethical Legal Issues Committee. (2013). Ethical and policy issues in genetic testing and screening of children. *Pediatrics*, *131*(3), 620–622. https://doi.org/10.1542/peds.2012-3680

Davis, D. S. (1997). Genetic dilemmas and the child's right to an open future. *Hastings Center Report*, *27*(2), 7–15. https://www.ncbi.nlm.nih.gov/pubmed/9131346

Diekema, D. S. (2020). Adolescent brain development and medical decision-making. *Pediatrics*, *146*(Suppl. 1), S18–S24. https://doi.org/10.1542/peds.2020-0818F

Dougherty, M. J., Pleasants, C., Solow, L., Wong, A., & Zhang, H. (2011). A comprehensive analysis of high school genetics standards: Are states keeping pace with modern genetics? *CBE Life Sciences Education*, *10*(3), 318–327. https://doi.org/10.1187/cbe.10-09-0122

Duncan, R. E., & Young, M. A. (2013). Tricky teens: Are they really tricky or do genetic health professionals simply require more training in adolescent health? *Personalized Medicine*, *10*(6), 589–600. https://doi.org/10.2217/pme.13.49

Fenwick, A., Plantinga, M., Dheensa, S., & Lucassen, A. (2017). Predictive genetic testing of children for adult-onset conditions: Negotiating requests with parents. *Journal of Genetic Counseling*, *26*(2), 244–250. https://doi.org/10.1007/s10897-016-0018-y

Finucane, B. (2010). Genetic counseling for women with intellectual disabilities. In B. S. LeRoy, P. M. Veach, & D. M. Bartels (Eds.), *Genetic counseling practice: Advanced concepts and skills* (pp. 281–303). Wiley-Blackwell.

Gaff, C. L., Lynch, E., & Spencer, L. (2006). Predictive testing of eighteen year olds: Counseling challenges. *Journal of Genetic Counseling, 15*(4), 245–251. https://doi.org/10.1007/s10897-006-9028-5

Geller, G., Tambor, E. S., Bernhardt, B. A., Fraser, G., & Wissow, L. S. (2003). Informed consent for enrolling minors in genetic susceptibility research: A qualitative study of at-risk children's and parents' views about children's role in decision-making. *Journal of Adolescent Health, 32*(4), 260–271. https://doi.org/10.1016/s1054-139x(02)00459-7

Genetic Alliance, Genetics and Public Policy Center, & National Coalition for Health Professional Education in Genetics. (2024). *GINA: Genetic Information Nondiscrimination Act*. https://www.ginahelp.org

Godino, L., Turchetti, D., Jackson, L., Hennessy, C., & Skirton, H. (2016). Impact of presymptomatic genetic testing on young adults: A systematic review. *European Journal of Human Genetics, 24*(4), 496–503. https://doi.org/10.1038/ejhg.2015.153

Halpern-Feshler, B. (2009). Adolescent decision making: An overview. *Prevention Researcher, 16*(2), 3–7.

Hein, I. M., Troost, P. W., Broersma, A., de Vries, M. C., Daams, J. G., & Lindauer, R. J. (2015). Why is it hard to make progress in assessing children's decision-making competence? *BMC Medical Ethics, 16*, 1. https://doi.org/10.1186/1472-6939-16-1

Hein, I. M., Troost, P. W., Lindeboom, R., de Vries, M. C., Zwaan, C. M., & Lindauer, R. J. L. (2012). Assessing children's competence to consent in research by a standardized tool: A validity study. *BMC Pediatrics, 12*, 156. https://doi.org/10.1186/1471-2431-12-156

Hufnagel, S. B., Martin, L. J., Cassedy, A., Hopkin, R. J., & Antommaria, A. H. (2016). Adolescents' preferences regarding disclosure of incidental findings in genomic sequencing that are not medically actionable in childhood. *American Journal of Medical Genetics Part A, 170*(8), 2083–2088. https://doi.org/10.1002/ajmg.a.37730

Joffe, S. (2003). Rethink "affirmative agreement," but abandon "assent." *American Journal of Bioethics, 3*(4), 9–11. https://doi.org/10.1162/152651603607067 23

Kalia, S. S., Adelman, K., Bale, S. J., Chung, W. K., Eng, C., Evans, J. P., Herman, G. E., Hufnagel, S. B., Klein, T. E., Korf, B. R., McKelvey, K. D., Ormond, K. E., Richards, C. S., Vlangos, C. N., Watson, M., Martin, C. L., & Miller, D. T. (2017). Recommendations for reporting of secondary findings in clinical exome and genome sequencing, 2016 update (ACMG SF v2.0): A policy statement of the American College of Medical Genetics and Genomics. *Genetics in Medicine, 19*(2), 249–255. https://doi.org/10.1038/gim.2016.190

Katz, A. L., Webb, S. A., & Committee on Bioethics. (2016). Informed consent in decision-making in pediatric practice. *Pediatrics, 138*(2), e20161485. https://doi.org/10.1542/peds.2016-1485

Levenseller, B. L., Soucier, D. J., Miller, V. A., Harris, D., Conway, L., & Bernhardt, B. A. (2014). Stakeholders' opinions on the implementation of pediatric whole exome sequencing: implications for informed consent. *Journal of Genetic Counseling, 23*(4), 552–565. https://doi.org/10.1007/s10897-013-9626-y

Lewis, C., Sanderson, S. C., Hammond, J., Hill, M., Searle, B., Hunter, A., Patch, C., & Chitty, L. S. (2020). Development and mixed-methods evaluation of an online animation for young people about genome sequencing. *European Journal of Human Genetics, 28*(7), 896–906. https://doi.org/10.1038/s41431-019-0564-5

Lillie, N., Prows, C. A., McGowan, M. L., Blumling, A. A., & Myers, M. F. (2022). Experiences of adolescents and their parents after receiving adolescents' genomic screening results. *Journal of Genetic Counseling, 31*(3), 608–619. https://doi.org/10.1002/jgc4.1528

Lipstein, E. A., Brinkman, W. B., Fiks, A. G., Hendrix, K. S., Kryworuchko, J., Miller, V. A., Prosser, L. A., Ungar, W. J., & Fox, D. (2015). An emerging field of research: Challenges in pediatric decision making. *Medical Decision Making, 35*(3), 403–408. https://doi.org/10.1177/0272989X14546901

Mand, C., Gillam, L., Duncan, R. E., & Delatycki, M. B. (2013). "It was the missing piece": Adolescent experiences of predictive genetic testing for adult-onset conditions. *Genetics in Medicine, 15*(8), 643–649. https://doi.org/10.1038/gim.2013.15

Maslyanskaya, S., & Alderman, E. M. (2019). Confidentiality and consent in the care of the adolescent patient. *Pediatrics in Review, 40*(10), 508–516. https://doi.org/10.1542/pir.2018-0040

McCabe, M. A. (1996). Involving children and adolescents in medical decision making: Developmental and clinical considerations. *Journal of Pediatric Psychology, 21*(4), 505–516.

McGowan, M. L., Prows, C. A., DeJonckheere, M., Brinkman, W. B., Vaughn, L., & Myers, M. F. (2018). Adolescent and parental attitudes about return of genomic research results: Focus group findings regarding decisional preferences. *Journal of Empirical Research on Human Research Ethics, 13*(4), 371–382. https://doi.org/10.1177/1556264618776613

Michie, S., Bobrow, M., & Marteau, T. M. (2001). Predictive genetic testing in children and adults: A study of emotional impact. *Journal of Medical Genetics, 38*(8), 519–526. https://doi.org/10.1136/jmg.38.8.519

Miller, D. T., Lee, K., Abul-Husn, N. S., Amendola, L. M., Brothers, K., Chung, W. K., Gollob, M. H., Gordon, A. S., Harrison, S. M., Hershberger, R. E., Klein, T. E., Richards, C. S., Stewart, D. R., Martin, C. L., & ACMG Secondary Findings Working Group. (2022). ACMG SF v3.1 list for reporting of secondary findings in clinical exome and genome sequencing: A policy statement of the American College of Medical Genetics and Genomics (ACMG). *Genetics in Medicine, 24*(7), 1407–1414. https://doi.org/10.1016/j.gim.2022.04.006

Miller, V. A., & Nelson, R. M. (2006). A developmental approach to child assent for nontherapeutic research. *Journal of Pediatrics, 149*(1 Suppl.), S25–S30. https://doi.org/10.1016/j.jpeds.2006.04.047

Miller, V. A., Reynolds, W. W., & Nelson, R. M. (2008). Parent-child roles in decision making about medical research. *Ethics & Behavior, 18*(2–3), 161–181.

Miller, V. A., Werner-Lin, A., Walser, S. A., Biswas, S., & Bernhardt, B. A. (2017). An observational study of children's involvement in informed consent for exome sequencing research. *Journal of Empirical Research on Human Research Ethics, 12*(1), 6–13. https://doi.org/10.1177/1556264616674096

Miner, S. A., Similuk, M., Jamal, L., Sapp, J., & Berkman, B. E. (2022). Genomic tools for health: Secondary findings as findings to be shared. *Genetics in Medicine*, 24(11), 2220–2227. https://doi.org/10.1016/j.gim.2022.07.015

Myers, M. F., Martin, L. J., & Prows, C. A. (2020). Adolescents' and parents' genomic testing decisions: Associations with age, race, and sex. *Journal of Adolescent Health, 66*(3), 288–295. https://doi.org/10.1016/j.jadohealth.2019.08.028

National Society of Genetic Counselors. (2017). *Genetic testing of minors for adult-onset conditions.* https://www.nsgc.org/Policy-Research-and-Publications/Position-Statements/Position-Statements/Post/genetic-testing-of-minors-for-adult-onset-conditions

Pervola, J., Myers, M. F., McGowan, M. L., & Prows, C. A. (2019). Giving adolescents a voice: The types of genetic information adolescents choose to learn and why. *Genetics in Medicine, 21*(4), 965–971. https://doi.org/10.1038/s41436-018-0320-1

Peters-Brown, T., & Fry-Mehltretter, L. (1996). Genetic counseling for pregnant adolescents. *Journal of Genetic Counseling, 5*(4), 155–168. https://doi.org/10.1007/BF01408370

Pichini, A., Shuman, C., Sappleton, K., Kaufman, M., Chitayat, D., & Babul-Hirji, R. (2016). Experience with genetic counseling: The adolescent perspective. *Journal of Genetic Counseling*, *25*(3), 583–595. https://doi.org/10.1007/s10897-015-9912-y

Positive Exposure. (2023). *Who we are*. https://positiveexposure.org/who-we-are/

Rasch, H. (2012). Adolescents need some private time with their doctor. *AAP News*, *33*(5), 24.

Reyna, V. F., & Farley, F. (2006). Risk and rationality in adolescent decision making: Implications for theory, practice, and public policy. *Psychological Science in the Public Interest*, *7*(1), 1–44. https://doi.org/10.1111/j.1529-1006.2006.00026.x

Ross, L. F. (2013). Predictive genetic testing of children and the role of the best interest standard. *Journal of Law, Medicine, and Ethics*, *41*(4), 899–906, Table of Contents. https://doi.org/10.1111/jlme.12099

Sabatello, M., & Appelbaum, P. S. (2015). Honey, I sequenced the kids: Preventive genomics and the complexities of adolescence. *American Journal of Bioethics*, *15*(7), 19–21. https://doi.org/10.1080/15265161.2015.1039722

Sabatello, M., & Appelbaum, P. S. (2016). Raising genomic citizens: Adolescents and the return of secondary genomic findings. *Journal of Law, Medicine, and Ethics*, *44*(2), 292–308. https://doi.org/10.1177/1073110516654123

Sabatello, M., Chen, Y., Sanderson, S. C., Chung, W. K., & Appelbaum, P. S. (2018). Increasing genomic literacy among adolescents. *Genetics in Medicine*, *21*(4), 994–1000. https://doi.org/10.1038/s41436-018-0275-2

Sacca, R. E., Koeller, D. R., Rana, H. Q., Garber, J. E., & Morganstern, D. E. (2019). Trans-counseling: A case series of transgender individuals at high risk for BRCA1 pathogenic variants. *Journal of Genetic Counseling*, *28*(3), 708–716. https://doi.org/10.1002/jgc4.1046

Sawyer, S. M., Azzopardi, P. S., Wickremarathne, D., & Patton, G. C. (2018). The age of adolescence. *Lancet Child and Adolescent Health*, 2(3), 223–228. https://doi.org/10.1016/S2352-4642(18)30022-1

Steinberg, L. (2005). Cognitive and affective development in adolescence. *Trends in Cognitive Science*, *9*(2), 69–74. https://doi.org/10.1016/j.tics.2004.12.005

Tse, C., Sahhar, M., Wallace, J., & Duncan, R. E. (2013). "There's a whole different way of working with adolescents": Interviews with Australian Genetic Counselors about their experiences with adolescent clients. *Journal of Genetic Counseling*, *22*(5), 674–684. https://doi.org/10.1007/s10897-013-9601-7

Wade, C. H., Wilfond, B. S., & McBride, C. M. (2010). Effects of genetic risk information on children's psychosocial wellbeing: A systematic review of the literature. *Genetics in Medicine*, *12*(6), 317–326. https://doi.org/10.1097/GIM.0b013e3181de695c

Wainstein, T., Marshall, S. K., Ross, C. J. D., Virani, A. K., Austin, J. C., Elliott, A. M., & Gen, C. S. (2022). Experiences with genetic counseling, testing, and diagnosis among adolescents with a genetic condition: A scoping review. *JAMA Pediatrics*, *176*(2), 185–195. https://doi.org/10.1001/jamapediatrics.2021.4290

Weil, J. (2000). *Psychosocial genetic counseling*. Oxford University Press.

Weithorn, L. A., & Campbell, S. B. (1982). The competency of children and adolescents to make informed treatment decisions. *Child Development*, *53*(6), 1589–1598.

Werner-Lin, A., Tomlinson, A., Miller, V., & Bernhardt, B. A. (2016). Adolescent engagement during assent for exome sequencing. *AJOB Empirical Bioethics*, *7*(4), 275–284. https://doi.org/10.1080/23294515.2016.1197983

Young, M. A., Thompson, K., Lewin, J., & Holland, L. (2020). A framework for youth-friendly genetic counseling. *Journal of Community Genetics*, *11*(2), 161–170. https://doi.org/10.1007/s12687-019-00439-2

PART IV

NAVIGATING CONTEMPORARY ISSUES IN GENETIC TESTING AND GENETIC COUNSELING PRACTICE

CHAPTER 15

CONSIDERATIONS BEFORE TESTING

Patient Education, Decision Making, and Informed Consent

KELLY E. ORMOND

Introduction

THERE is a significant body of literature (Bernhardt et al., 2000; National Society of Genetic Counselors' Definition Task Force et al., 2006; Wang et al., 2004) that suggests that after performing a risk assessment and identifying relevant genetic testing options for clients, a major goal of genetic counseling is to facilitate patient education and informed choices about whether to undergo genetic testing. Models of genetic counseling practice, such as the Reciprocal-Engagement Model (Veach et al., 2007), also strongly support the importance of patient education and promotion of patient autonomy as tenets of genetic counseling. Informed choice and autonomy are particularly critical when genetic tests are predictive for moderate to highly penetrant conditions or when there is data to suggest that a high percentage of patients choose to decline a genetic test. This chapter will review key considerations before genetic testing, with a focus on the informed consent process that is typically included in clinical genetic testing as a way to operationalize these two key tenets.

History of Informed Consent in Medicine

Informed consent arose during the 1900s as a response to the medical paternalism of the past, where physicians typically did not involve patients in medical decision making but rather simply told them what procedures would be performed, sometimes even overriding a patient's preference. It also arose in response to past research abuses (e.g., Nazi experimentation and the Tuskegee syphilis experiment). Informed consent is meant to promote a focus on trust and respect within the researcher–participant or provider–client relationship.

Several key principles underlie informed consent and apply to both research and clinical informed consents: (a) the right to self-determination—respect for persons (autonomy), which often is translated into the right to promote one's well-being in a way that is based on personal values and preferences, and (b) voluntariness, including a lack of coercion and deception (Beauchamp, 2011; Junkerman et al., 2008). To be able to promote one's personal values and interests, consent for a procedure or, in this case, a genetic test means the clinician or researcher must disclose appropriate information and the patient or participant must have the ability to understand it (Beauchamp, 2011; Bester et al., 2016). For those who desire more detailed background about informed consent in the broader medical and research context, please see Dankar et al. (2019).

It is important to understand some basics about research consent in order to understand informed consent within a clinical context. Research informed consent became relevant in the 1950s with the Nuremberg Code, which arose in response to the 1947 Nuremberg trials that examined atrocious human experimentation in Nazi Germany. The principles elaborated upon in the Nuremberg Code (1947) and the 1964 Declaration of Helsinki (updated in 2013; World Medical Association, 2013) emphasize voluntariness and awareness of risks and benefits, both of which are critical concepts in informed consent for both research and clinical care (Shuster, 1997). In the United States, the Belmont Report (National Commission for the Protection of Human Subjects of Biomedical and Behavioral Research, 1979) and more recent version of the "Common Rule" (Protection of Human Subjects, 2018) further the focus on beneficence (promoting good outcomes/benefits), justice, and autonomy, which frequently are operationalized in the research informed consent process.

In clinical care, one of the earliest cases to establish the legal duties of medical informed consent was *Schloendorff v. Society of New York Hospital* (1914), which established that performing a medical procedure (in this case surgical removal of a tumor) without patient consent constituted medical battery. Next, in *Salgo v. Leland Stanford Jr. University Board of Trustees* (1957), a patient sued his physician and the hospital that performed an aortogram that left him with permanent lower extremity paralysis under the premise that he was not appropriately apprised of the details and risks of the procedure. Prior to *Salgo*, it was not unusual for physicians to perform medical procedures without informing patients about specific risks. The *Salgo* ruling stressed that there is a legal duty not only to share the risks associated with any procedure but also to ensure patient understanding. Another critical legal precedent in understanding the current state of informed consent is *Canterbury v. Spence* (1972) which was the first case ruling to specifically lay out types of information that should be included in informed consent (Murray, 2012). Additionally, this ruling moved from a standard describing what a "typical practitioner" might include in the consent process (sometimes called the "medical standard" or "professional community standard"), often defined by local practice and/or professional guidelines (Junkerman et al., 2008), toward the notion of the "reasonable patient" standard for informed consent. The reasonable patient standard focuses on the amount and type of information that an average or typical patient would desire and expect to know to make an informed choice about whether or not to proceed with a medical treatment or intervention (Beauchamp, 2011; Junkerman et al., 2008; Main et al., 2016; Spatz et al., 2016). Regardless of which informational standard is considered, medical or reasonable patient, both remain somewhat subjective, as neither lays out clearly or consistently how a provider would operationalize the consent concepts in a consistent manner. A third approach, promoted by Jonsen and colleagues, is a more "subjective standard" that focuses on tailoring the information and discussion directly to the patient; it requires careful active listening to both the content and emotion that patients express (Jonsen et al., 2022); this model more closely mirrors the common approach taken in genetic counseling settings. Even further along this spectrum is a standard recently upheld in a United Kingdom legal case (*Montgomery v. Lanarkshire Health Board*, 2015), which held that "rather than being a matter for clinical judgment to be assessed by professional medical opinion, a patient should be told whatever they want to know, not what the doctor thinks they should be told" (Chan et al., 2017).

Finally, the informed consent process assumes a competent adult (with decisional capacity) who has an understanding of the options and related outcomes and can voluntarily voice their choice and its underlying reasoning (Barstow et al., 2018; Horton & Lucassen, 2019). For adult genetics patients, if they have intellectual disability, neurologic impairment, or dementia, then decisional capacity may be impaired. In some, this may be a transient lack of capacity (e.g., a person with an active psychiatric illness that could be resolved with medication), or it may be permanent. It may also be something they have had throughout their adult life (intellectual disability) or one that they acquire later in adulthood (e.g., dementia, a traumatic brain injury). When the patient does not have decisional capacity, surrogate decision making is required. Ideally there should be a person who is designated by the patient as the appropriate medical decision maker through an advance directive, or in some cases through legal conservatorship or guardianship. Surrogate decision makers for adult patients are often encouraged to focus on making decisions through "substituted judgment," which posits that they should make the decision based on the previously expressed views and values of the patient. Surrogate decisions can be made based on explicit communication from the patient, for example, through prior conversations or documents such as an advance directive; when these are unavailable, they can be made through inference based on the patient's prior actions and broader values and preferences. However, recent thinking acknowledges both that people's personal views evolve over time and that it is challenging to relay preferences for the range of potential future medical decisions that may occur. Based on this, some bioethicists propose using narrative approaches to decision making, focused on hearing the individual's values and life history; this demonstrates respect for persons by considering what matters to them contextually within the process of surrogate decision making (Torke et al., 2008).

There are two additional points about consent in adult patients that healthcare providers should be aware of. First, while many cultures strive to promote an individualistic conception of autonomy in decision making, it is critical to remember that a significant percentage of patients may want their family or a healthcare provider to be informed or even make the decision for them (Deem & Stokes, 2018; Levinson et al., 2005; Tariman et al., 2010) and that this is an appropriate assertion of their autonomy. There may also be cultural variation in terms of preferences for protecting patients from potentially upsetting information and norms against discussing specific health information that are worth considering as part of the informed consent process (Deem & Stokes, 2018). Second, in the event of a true emergency (which is unlikely when considering consent for genetic testing), there are provisions such that in time-sensitive situations where the patient does not have capacity and is without surrogates and where a "reasonable person" would consent, there can be an emergency privilege to waive the requirement for informed consent.

Children are a special case for informed consent. They may have an age-dependent ability (often loosely regarded as after age 7) to assent or dissent to a procedure but will not yet achieve decision-making capacity for several more years. Parents or guardians serve as surrogate medical decision makers under the premise that parents are broadly granted decisional authority for the health, protection, and general welfare of their children. From an ethical standpoint, parents generally make decisions based on the "best interests" principle, since a child does not yet have expressed values and interests; instead, these decisions usually focus on what a reasonable person might decide and/or on the parental perception of what is best for the child and their family. There is also the assumption that frequently the interests of parents and children align (Committee on Bioethics, 2016; Weithorn, 2020). The legal age of consent for medical procedures is generally considered to be the age of majority, which is 18 years old across most countries. In part, as a result of the United Nations Convention on the Rights of the Child (CRC; 1989), in some countries there are specific regulations that entitle children to make some or all medical decisions before reaching the age of majority (European Union Agency for Fundamental Rights, 2017). Additionally, most countries and states also have a legal process to declare a minor emancipated (e.g., active military service, being married, or living independently and being self-supporting); emancipation grants the rights of adulthood including ability to consent for medical procedures. Furthermore, minors over 14 years of age can, in some cases, be declared "mature minors" by a court or medical professional (U.S. state laws vary) and thus be allowed to make independent medical decisions. Because these laws vary by country and state/province, it is important to be familiar with any relevant laws in the jurisdiction where care is being provided (Committee on Bioethics, 2016; Weithorn, 2020).

In summary, informed consent is not only a legal concept, which may include a process that often ends in formal documentation, such as a signature on a consent form, aimed at reducing legal liability, but also a robust ethical concept. While the focus of informed consent is usually centered on respect for persons and promoting patient autonomy, clinicians and researchers must also remember that beneficence (doing good) and nonmaleficence (avoiding harm) are important principles to uphold (Bester et al., 2016). It is worth noting that some states have genetics-specific informed consent laws that must be attended to in genetic counseling. These may provide provisions for the content that must be included as part of the informed consent process, the manner in which it is documented, or the persons who are authorized to obtain it (Spector-Bagdady et al., 2018).

Approaches to Obtaining Informed Consent

There are a number of different approaches to informed consent; many are derived from a research setting approach but are applicable in clinical consent as well in the sense that they are meant to promote autonomy and to protect the person providing consent. An earlier volume of Jonsen et al. (1997, p. 53) says the following about informed consent in a clinical setting:

> The patient understands the information, assesses the treatment choices, and expresses a preference for one of the options proposed by the physician. As an ethical basis for the

> patient-physician relationship, informed consent refers to an encounter characterized by mutual participation, respect, and shared decision making. Informed consent should not designate a mechanical recitation of facts or a pro forma signature on a piece of paper. The phrase "I consented the patient," used too frequently by young clinicians, reveals a casual attitude towards informed consent.

These statements highlight that informed consent should strive to be a bidirectional conversation, rather than a unilateral information delivery process, unless the patient prefers otherwise.

Traditional approaches to informed consent typically focus on a single medical issue, present one or more options for medical management (treatment, surveillance, or diagnosis), and may include a fairly comprehensive conversation about the potential risks and benefits of the various approaches. More traditional medical models may also include a physician recommendation on the course of action (while genetic counselors more frequently avoid overt recommendations, depending on the medical specialty). From a general medical perspective, these approaches often involve sharing information about the diagnosis and natural history, the prognosis, treatment options with associated benefits and risks/burdens, and the likely impact of the various outcomes (Junkerman et al., 2008). While many medical risks often center on physical impact (e.g., risk of death, risk of complications), most genetic tests have very minimal physical risks and instead have emotional, financial, familial, and reproductive implications. Importantly, the degree of risk (and certainty or uncertainty about it) should play a role in how a clinician defines and enacts the informed consent process (Junkerman et al., 2008; Whitney et al., 2004). For example, those genetic testing decisions that have a lower risk (e.g., confirmation of a clinical diagnosis, prediction of a treatable condition with high penetrance, or a noninvasive screening test) may have a "lower bar" for the depth of content and discussion that is shared or for the degree of decisional capacity that is required. In contrast, those decisions with higher risk (testing for a fully penetrant condition with no clinically useful treatments available, such as a neurodegenerative condition; conditions where patients make a wide range of decisions about whether or not to test) may require a "higher bar" for consent.

In the early 1990s, in recognition of the increasing availability of expanding genetic testing options (e.g., carrier screening tests) and the already-documented "information overload" that could happen from genetic counseling, Elias and Annas (1994) proposed the "generic consent" approach. Grounded in the concepts that govern how consent is approached for things such as a general physical examination or a broad medical test like a complete blood count or general blood chemistries (which can detect a wide range of conditions of varying implications), this approach was based on the notion that most patients would benefit from a streamlined approach that focused on "broader concepts and common denominator issues" (Elias & Annas, 1994, p. 1612). The idea was that by covering high-level topics (e.g., test limitations, next steps after various test results) and allowing patients to request specific details as desired, patients could focus on making a meaningful decision rather than becoming caught up in details that may ultimately have limited meaning. Two points are key in understanding this concept of "generic consent": First, a patient can at any time request additional details, and second, the majority of details would be provided upon receiving results, when one could focus on a specific outcome and tailor information to the patient in a meaningful manner (Elias & Annas, 1994).

Building on the concept of generic consent, recognizing that genetic research and testing were expanding rapidly, and often examining a wide range of areas (including potentially unknown or unexpected areas), broad consent approaches were proposed (see Grady et al., 2015 for a comprehensive summary). Developed primarily for research, broad consent allows research participants to provide consent to participate in a research study that may include future research and potential return of results in unspecified areas. While these are controversial—some experts worry that this type of approach removes autonomy from the hands of research participants (Sheehan, 2011)—broad consent approaches often allow categorical opt-out of specific categories of research that the participant was not interested in, and they maintain a governance organization that oversees approval of future research to be conducted. Empiric data, summarized in part in Garrison et al. (2016), suggests that a majority of U.S.-based research participants welcome these broad consent approaches and often prefer them over a "study by study" consent approach. However, early data from Europe (Gaskell et al., 2013) suggests that there may be country-specific differences in support for broad consent approaches.

Finally, the concept of staged consents, sometimes called tiered consent (Bunnik et al., 2013) or dynamic consent (Teare et al., 2021), has been proposed to address concerns over information overload and its potential impact on decision making. This is especially true for genetic testing such as exome/genome sequencing where there are potentially test results that would be related to the testing indication, optional tests across a diverse range of areas (e.g., carrier results, pharmacogenomics, secondary findings), and truly incidental findings, as well as a range of uncertainty for some types of results (genes or variants of uncertain significance) that would be relevant parts of a consent discussion. The strength of these approaches is that they can focus on fewer issues at a time by stretching out the consent process to address individual decisions one at a time, rather than asking patients to make decisions about all the options at a single time point. At least in theory, this should allow patients and research participants to focus on and comprehend relevant issues, and it may be especially important for vulnerable populations (Tiffin, 2018) and those populations with which researchers or clinicians wish to maintain ongoing engagement (Teare et al., 2021). However, these approaches can be logistically complicated and may involve additional time and visits, or IT support, that make them more challenging to implement in typical clinical practice (Appelbaum et al., 2015; Bunnik et al., 2013; Tabor et al., 2017; Teare et al., 2021; Yu et al., 2013).

One last point that is worth considering regarding approaches to informed consent: While often conflated, there is a difference between "obtaining informed consent" and facilitating shared decision making (SDM). While both overlap in allowing patients/research subjects to autonomously authorize or decline a medical or research decision, they differ in key ways (Childress & Childress, 2020; Whitney et al., 2004, 2008). On one level, informed consent is a legal duty, with the potential for significant variation in how it is enacted. In some cases, a "simple" informed consent process can occur when the primary goal is patient authorization for a procedure where there are no reasonable choices between which to decide. For example, a patient with a clinical diagnosis of a genetic condition is offered a genetic test to confirm the diagnosis and identify the causal variant to allow for family cascade testing. This sort of testing would not usually require a complex decision and has lower risks, and a patient could consent or decline to undergo genetic testing likely without a lengthy discussion. In contrast, and likely in response to the abbreviated and noninteractive "consenting" that evolved in the 1980s, SDM is an ethical approach to complex consent situations that takes a more value-neutral approach and recognizes that both the provider and patient have important information and personal values and preferences to bring to the decision-making process (Whitney et al., 2004). An example of a situation where SDM would be particularly relevant is predictive testing for an adult-onset condition, particularly those where medical treatment or surveillance is ineffective and/or where there is wide variance in whether patients decide to undergo genetic testing. In these cases, it is critical to help patients clarify values and pair them with the appropriate choice, thus allowing informed choice to occur. Genetic counseling has evolved toward making SDM the "standard" approach (even though it may not always be needed in every situation) when working with a patient who is providing consent to undergo a genetic test (Elwyn et al., 1999). This has been in part because the "nondirectiveness" ethos of genetic counseling melds nicely with the emphasis on patient values and preferences in SDM.

Informed Consent as Part of the Pretest Genetic Counseling Process

The NSGC Code of Ethics, most recently updated in 2017 (National Society of Genetic Counselors, 2018; Senter et al., 2018), has several important reminders about the obligations of genetic counselors. As stated in Section II of the Code of Ethics, "The counselor-client relationship is based on values of care and respect for the client's autonomy" (National Society of Genetic Counselors, 2018, p. 7). Much of Section II focuses on areas relevant to informed consent in the pretest genetic counseling context, most specifically the role of genetic counselors to "enable their clients to make informed decisions, free of coercion, by providing or illuminating the necessary facts, and clarifying the alternatives and anticipated consequences" (National Society of Genetic Counselors, 2018, p. 7). Historically, the strong focus on informed consent in genetic counseling was both a response to eugenics, ensuring that patients and families approached genetic testing as voluntary, and in recognition of the differences in how individuals and families consider risk and interpret difference and disability (Parens, 2015). But what does it mean to integrate these concepts into genetic counseling practice?

Preparing for the Informed Consent Process

To appropriately facilitate informed consent and decision making, the first step is that a genetic counselor must themselves understand the medical information and options to be disclosed, so that they can ultimately be able to frame and interpret this information for the patient. Often, clarifying one's understanding of the medical context, including all options and their repercussions, will help elucidate any ethical issues that could arise (Jonsen et al., 2022), as well as help the genetic counselor frame the informed consent discussion. Initial considerations should include the following: (a) Is it a diagnostic or predictive test? (b) Is it performed prior to conception, prenatally, in childhood, or in adulthood? (c) Based on the available personal and medical history, how likely is a positive test result, and what other potential results may be generated from the various test options (e.g., secondary or incidental findings on an exome or broad gene panel test)? (d) What risks (physical, emotional, social, and financial) are associated, and how does this influence where you "set the bar" for what consent should entail and the degree of decisional capacity required (Junkerman et al., 2008)? Equally important is to consider how certain or uncertain the available medical information is and to what degree the potential genetic testing might impact these certainties (Horton & Lucassen, 2019). When thinking about how to frame these issues, Sudore reminds clinicians, "What matters most to patients is not the treatment, but the outcome of the treatment" (Institute of Medicine, 2015, p. 57). An analogy in genetic counseling would be to focus a prenatal genetic counseling discussion on describing an invasive procedure and its risks (e.g., amniocentesis) without first having an understanding of the patient's values around identifying a pregnancy with aneuploidy or losing a pregnancy to miscarriage and their perceptions of how that information would impact their pregnancy management.

Step 2 in the process, often done subconsciously, is to identify the proper decision maker and whether they have decision-making capacity. When testing an adult through either diagnostic or predictive testing, this is generally considered to be the adult themselves, unless they do not have decision-making capacity. When testing a person who does not have their own decision-making capacity (whether a child with developing autonomy or an adult with diminished decision-making capacity), identifying the appropriate surrogate decision maker and the basis upon which surrogate decision making will occur, along with issues of assent and involvement of the individual, are also important. When focusing on informed consent for childhood genetic testing, parents (or a court-ordered guardian) are typically considered the surrogate decision maker unless an adolescent is considered emancipated or a "mature minor" (Hickey, 2007). There are several professional guidelines on genetic testing in childhood that lay out recommendations for which tests parents should be considered able to consent for and which should be deferred so as to preserve the child's future autonomous choice (Borry et al., 2009; Botkin et al., 2015; Canadian Paediatric Society, n.d.; de Wert et al., 2021; Ross et al., 2013; Royal College of Physicians et al., 2022; Vears et al., 2020).

The Education Component

Since the beginning of genetic counseling, the education components of the informed consent process have been seen as critical. However, as Kessler (1997) cautions, the genetic counselor should be wary of falling into the trap of prioritizing information (the "teaching model" of genetic counseling) over the counseling aspects of the genetic counseling process. An important first step to providing education to a patient is to consider the patient's prior knowledge. Some examples of questions to ask oneself include: (a) What does the patient/family say that they want to know? (b) What is their prior knowledge about the condition, its lived experience, and potential treatments? (c) What patient characteristics could influence their desire for information (locus of control, sense of efficacy, informational desires, etc.), and how can these be assessed? (d) What is the patient's perception of risk?

Next, a genetic counselor will need to consider which pieces of information are critical to helping a patient make an informed decision. This typically focuses on procedure/process, risks, and potential benefits. But it can be complicated to determine what qualifies as a relevant risk or benefit when discussing a decision to undergo genetic testing. In medical informed consent, risk and benefit primarily include physical risks (e.g., of a complication from a procedure) or benefits (reduction in morbidity or mortality or changes to medical management, such as screening or targeted therapies, to address future risks). For genetic testing, risks include physical risks (which are often minimal from collection approaches that include blood draw or saliva/buccal swab), potential implications on emotions and life planning for both the individual and family, and potential privacy and discrimination risks. Psychological benefits might include the end to a diagnostic odyssey, a reduction in anxiety, and personal utility through life planning or reproductive planning to the individual and family.

Early approaches to genetic counseling prioritized significant informational content, and people discussed "fully informed consent" as a goal to strive for. Studies in other areas of medicine (e.g., Koenig, 2014; Lantos, 1993) suggest that patients range significantly in how much and what information they desire, from "all the information" to no information beyond their provider's recommendation; they also vary in their desires for format and frequency. As Tobias and Souhami (1993, p. 1200) state, "No sensible doctor makes full disclosure to every patient. This would be a recipe for needless cruelty and distress." More recent studies (Joseph et al., 2017) suggest that too much information overwhelms patients and inhibits recall and decision making. Certainly, some people are information seekers ("monitors"), while others are more likely to become emotionally overwhelmed and confused by too much information. This overload has been loosely correlated with education and income level, trust in the quality of information, and some aspects of literacy (Kim et al., 2007).

What information is relevant to informed consent?

How do we define "adequate" information that will meet the needs of most patients? This is a critical question, and the core set of information that would allow a patient to make an adequately informed decision has not been well defined within the genetic counseling literature.

As an example, early studies addressing expanded carrier screening suggested that core concepts desired by patients included the "value and purpose of testing," recurrence risk, options and next steps if found to be at risk, and the natural history of the condition for which they were at risk (Ormond et al., 2007, 2009). Other studies suggested that it is critical to define testing and screening clearly so as to differentiate the test from others that are being discussed (e.g., differentiating carrier screening from other prenatal testing options, such as tests that identify aneuploidies).

More recently, the CADRe (Consent and Disclosure Recommendations) Workgroup within the Clinical Genome (ClinGen) project examined how professionals define the core concepts of informed consent. A literature review summarized both clinical and research informed consent for genetic testing and resulted in a list of 77 concepts across five categories: (a) scope of the test, (b) description of the test and logistics, (c) confidentiality and privacy, (d) potential benefits, and (e) potential risks. Through a consensus process (Ormond et al., 2021) and follow-up national survey of U.S.-based genetic counselors and medical geneticists (Hallquist et al., 2022), the CADRe Workgroup identified a draft list of concepts that might be considered core educational concepts that would allow a "typical" patient to make an informed decision. They included the following: (a) the voluntariness of genetic testing; (b) the purpose of the testing and what the test will include (e.g., a panel, exome); (c) what results will (generally) be returned; (d) what other types of results, such as secondary findings, are available and their options for choice; (e) how prognosis and management may be impacted by potential results; (f) family implications of genetic testing (health risks, emotions, relationships) and potential for result sharing; (g) test limitations, including "no answers"; and (h) to whom the results will be reported (Ormond et al., 2021).

The survey data suggested that these concepts are a good starting place but that specific genes/disorders and testing indications may require unique additional concepts. For example, predictive genetic testing, but not clinical confirmations, may require some discussion of potential stigma and discrimination, as well as the state and national laws that may protect against discrimination (e.g., the Genetic Information Nondiscrimination Act). Other scenarios may have testing-specific points that regularly warrant discussion, such as issues regarding who the most useful person to test is for informative genetic testing results, issues that arise if family testing (e.g., a trio exome) is happening, and issues focused on secondary and incidental results in broader genomic tests such as exome or genome testing (Hallquist et al., 2023). In contrast, while some patients may wish to know these answers to make an informed choice, concepts that were uniformly ranked low included general genetics principles ("what is DNA," "everyone has mutations"), logistical and technical data (e.g., what lab will run the sample, how the sample is run, will it be used for quality control testing, for how long and where will the sample be kept, what happens to the data/reports if a patient dies, who can request reports at that time, how often will reanalysis occur, and who can request "raw data" and how), physical risks of getting the sample, and principles that may be more relevant to research (e.g., where is data entered/shared, is aggregate data entered into public databases).

Conveying information

Once the patient's prior knowledge has been assessed and the critical content has been determined, the genetic counselor must determine in what manner to convey the information. There are many excellent resources on how best to provide the educational aspects of genetic counseling (e.g., Smith & Pollin, 2011), and thus we will mention it only briefly here. One should, broadly, take into account considerations of adult learning theory; literacy, health literacy, and numeracy; language and cultural aspects relevant to the patient;[1] risk communication and framing; and health promotion models, as well as the

[1] For further discussion of cultural responsiveness and linguistic competence in genetic counseling, see Chapter 29 by Nancy Warren in this volume.

expressed patient preferences. Genetic counselors must balance a desire for organization and logical flow of content with flexibility to answer questions and address the patient's agenda. Since informed decisions are based on having accurate and relevant information upon which to base the decision, genetic counselors must also consider simply informing a person about relevant facts is different than knowing that they understand the information (Hammami et al., 2014). They must find practical ways to assess understanding, for example, the "teach back" approach (Glaser et al., 2020), and to identify and correct misconceptions.

Children should be given information at a developmentally appropriate level and involved in decision-making discussions and providing assent to the extent that is feasible for their age and maturity Regardless of legal status, adolescents have developing decisional capacity, and genetic counselors should strive to involve them actively in the informed consent process at levels appropriate for their development and maturity. While some adolescents' cognitive abilities may be similar to adults' by around age 14 to 15, other issues will impact decision-making processes, including psychological factors that impact risk perception, and social and contextual factors (Diekema, 2020; Jeremic et al., 2016).[2]

Conclusion

Informed consent is an important ethical and legal principle, one that is foundational to the practice of genetic counseling. It requires identifying the appropriate decision maker, determining what the risks and benefits of a particular genetic test are, and tailoring that information to meet the individual's informational needs, sometimes using an SDM approach.

References

Appelbaum, P. S., Fyer, A., Klitzman, R. L., Martinez, J., Parens, E., Zhang, Y., & Chung, W. K. (2015). Researchers' views on informed consent for return of secondary results in genomic research. *Genetics in Medicine*, *17*, 644–650. https://doi.org/10.1038/gim.2014.163

Barstow, C., Shahan, B., & Roberts, M. (2018, July 1). *Evaluating medical decision making capacity in practice.* https://www.aafp.org/afp/2018/0701/p40.html

Beauchamp, T. L. (2011). Informed consent: Its history, meaning, and present challenges. *Cambridge Quarterly of Healthcare Ethics*, *20*(4), 515–523.

Bernhardt, B. A., Biesecker, B. B., & Mastromarino, C. L. (2000). Goals, benefits, and outcomes of genetic counseling: Client and genetic counselor assessment. *American Journal of Medical Genetics*, *94*(3), 189–197.

Bester, J., Cole, C. M., & Kodish, E. (2016). The limits of informed consent for an overwhelmed patient: Clinicians' role in protecting patients and preventing overwhelm. *AMA Journal of Ethics*, *18*(9), 869–886.

[2] For further discussion of genetic counseling approaches for adolescents and young adults, see Chapter 14 by Melanie F. Myers and Wendy R. Uhlman in this volume.

Borry, P., Evers-Kiebooms, G., Cornel, M. C., Clarke, A., Dierickx, K., & Public and Professional Policy Committee (PPPC) of the European Society of Human Genetics (ESHG). (2009). Genetic testing in asymptomatic minors: Background considerations towards ESHG Recommendations. *European Journal of Human Genetics, 17*(6), 711–719.

Botkin, J. R., Belmont, J. W., Berg, J. S., Berkman, B. E., Bombard, Y., Holm, I. A., Levy, H. P., Ormond, K. E., Saal, H. M., Spinner, N. B., Wilfond, B. S., & McInerney, J. D. (2015). Points to consider: Ethical, legal, and psychosocial implications of genetic testing in children and adolescents. *American Journal of Human Genetics, 97*(1), 6–21.

Bunnik, E. M., Janssens, a. C. J. W., & Schermer, M. H. N. (2013). A tiered-layered-staged model for informed consent in personal genome testing. *European Journal of Human Genetics, 21*(6), 596–601.

Canadian Paediatric Society. (n.d.). *Genetic testing and screening in children*. https://cps.ca/en/documents/position/genetic-testing

Canterbury v. Spence, 464 F.2d 772 (D.C. Cir. 1972).

Chan, S. W., Tulloch, E., Cooper, E. S., Smith, A., Wojcik, W., & Norman, J. E. (2017). Montgomery and informed consent: Where are we now? *BMJ, 357*, j2224. https://www.bmj.com/content/357/bmj.j2224

Childress, J. F., & Childress, M. D. (2020). What does the evolution from informed consent to shared decision making teach us about authority in health care? *AMA Journal of Ethics, 22*(5), E423–E429.

Committee on Bioethics. (2016). Informed consent in decision making in pediatric practice. *Pediatrics, 138*(2), e20161484. https://doi.org/10.1542/peds.2016-1484

Dankar, F. K., Gergely, M., & Dankar, S. K. (2019). Informed consent in biomedical research. *Computational and Structural Biotechnology Journal, 17*, 463–474.

de Wert, G., Dondorp, W., Clarke, A., Dequeker, E. M. C., Cordier, C., Deans, Z., van El, C. G., Fellmann, F., Hastings, R., Hentze, S., Howard, H., Macek, M., Mendes, A., Patch, C., Rial-Sebbag, E., Stefansdottir, V., Cornel, M. C., Forzano, F., & European Society of Human Genetics. (2021). Opportunistic genomic screening. Recommendations of the European Society of Human Genetics. *European Journal of Human Genetics, 29*(3), 365–377.

Deem, M. J., & Stokes, F. (2018). Culture and consent in clinical care: A critical review of nursing and nursing ethics literature. *Annual Review of Nursing Research, 37*(1), 223–259.

Diekema, D. S. (2020). Adolescent brain development and medical decision making. *Pediatrics, 146*(Suppl. 1), S18–S24.

Elias, S., & Annas, G. J. (1994). Generic consent for genetic screening. *New England Journal of Medicine, 330*, 1611–1613.

Elwyn, G., Gray, J., & Clarke, A. (1999). Shared decision making and non-directiveness in genetic counselling. *Journal of Medical Genetics, 37*, 135–138.

European Union Agency for Fundamental Rights. (2017, November 14). *Consenting to medical treatment without parental consent*. https://fra.europa.eu/en/publication/2017/mapping-minimum-age-requirements-concerning-rights-child-eu/consenting-medical-treatment-without-parental-consent

Garrison, N. A., Sathe, N. A., Matheny Antommaria, A. H., Holm, I. A., Sanderson, S. C., Smith, M. E., McPheeters, M. L., & Clayton, E. W. (2016). A systematic literature review of individuals' perspectives on broad consent and data sharing in the United States. *Genetics in Medicine, 18*(7), 663–671. https://doi.org/10.1038/gim.2015.138

Gaskell, G., Gottweis, H., Starkbaum, J., Gerber, M. M., Broerse, J., Gottweis, U., Hobbs, A., Helén, I., Paschou, M., Snell, K., & Soulier, A. (2013). Publics and biobanks: Pan-European diversity and the challenge of responsible innovation. *European Journal of Human Genetics, 21*(1), 14–20.

Glaser, J., Nouri, S., Fernandez, A., Sudore, R. L., Schillinger, D., Klein-Fedyshin, M., & Schenker, Y. (2020). Interventions to improve patient comprehension in informed consent for medical and surgical procedures: An updated systematic review. *Medical Decision Making, 40*(2), 119–143.

Grady, C., Eckstein, L., Berkman, B., Brock, D., Cook-Deegan, R., Fullerton, S. M., Greely, H., Hansson, M. G., Hull, S., Kim, S., Lo, B., Pentz, R., Rodriguez, L., Weil, C., Wilfond, B. S., & Wendler, D. (2015). Broad consent for research with biological samples: Workshop conclusions. *American Journal of Bioethics, 15*(9), 34–42.

Hallquist, M. L. G., Borensztein, M. J., Coughlin II, C. R.s, Buchanan, A. H., Faucett, W. A., Peay, H. L., Smith, M. E., Tricou, E. P., Uhlmann, W. R., Wain, K. E., & Ormond, K. E. (2023). Defining the critical educational components of informed consent for genetic testing: Views of US-based genetic counselors and medical geneticists. *European Journal of Human Genetics, 31*, 1165–1174. https://doi.org/10.1038/s41431-023-01401-0

Hammami, M. M., Al-Gaai, E. A., Al-Jawarneh, Y., Amer, H., Hammami, M. B., Eissa, A., & Qadire, M. A. (2014). Patients' perceived purpose of clinical informed consent: Mill's individual autonomy model is preferred. *BMC Medical Ethics, 15*, 2.

Hickey, K. (2007). Minors' rights in medical decision making. *JONA'S Healthcare Law, Ethics and Regulation, 9*(3), 100–104; quiz 105–106.

Horton, R., & Lucassen, A. (2019). Consent and autonomy in the genomics era. *Current Genetic Medicine Reports, 7*(2), 85–91.

Institute of Medicine. (2015). *Informed consent and health literacy: Workshop summary*. The National Academies Press. https://doi.org/10.17226/19019

Jeremic, V., Sénécal, K., Borry, P., Chokoshvili, D., & Vears, D. F. (2016). Participation of children in medical decision making: Challenges and potential solutions. *Journal of Bioethical Inquiry, 13*(4), 525–534.

Jonsen, A. R., Siegler, M., & Winslade, W. J. (2022). *Clinical ethics: A practical approach to ethical decisions in clinical medicine* (9th ed.). McGraw Hill/Medical.

Jonsen, A. R., Seigler, M., Winslade, W. J., & Siegler, M. (1997). *Clinical ethics: A practical approach to ethical decisions in clinical medicine* (4th ed.). McGraw-Hill.

Joseph, G., Pasick, R. J., Schillinger, D., Luce, J., Guerra, C., & Cheng, J. K. Y. (2017). Erratum to: Information mismatch: Cancer risk counseling with diverse underserved patients (J Genet Counsel, 10.1007/s10897-017-0089-4). *Journal of Genetic Counseling, 26*(5), 1105.

Junkerman, C., Derse, A., & Schiedermayer, D. (2008). *Practical ethics for students, interns, and residents* (3rd ed.). University Publishing Group.

Kessler, S. (1997). Psychological aspects of genetic counseling. IX. Teaching and counseling. *Journal of Genetic Counseling, 6*(3), 287–295.

Kim, K., Lustria, M. L. A., Burke, D., & Kwon, N. (2007). Predictors of cancer information overload: Findings from a national survey. *Information Research, 12*(4), 12–14.

Koenig, B. A. (2014). Have we asked too much of consent? *Hastings Center Report, 44*(4), 33–34.

Lantos, J. (1993). Informed consent. The whole truth for patients? *Cancer, 72*(9 Suppl.), 2811–2815.

Levinson, W., Kao, A., Kuby, A., & Thisted, R. A. (2005). Not all patients want to participate in decision making. A national study of public preferences. *Journal of General Internal Medicine, 20*(6), 531–535.

Main, B. G., McNair, A., & Blazeby, J. M. (2016). Informed consent and the reasonable-patient standard [Review of *Informed Consent and the Reasonable-Patient Standard*]. *JAMA*, *316*(9), 992–993.

Montgomery v. Lanarkshire Health Board, UKSC 11 (2015).

Murray, B. (2012). Informed consent: What must a physician disclose to a patient? *AMA Journal of Ethics*, *14*(7), 563–566.

National Commission for the Protection of Human Subjects of Biomedical and Behavioral Research. (1979). *The Belmont report: Ethical principles and guidelines for the protection of human subjects of research.* U.S. Department of Health and Human Services. https://www.hhs.gov/ohrp/regulations-and-policy/belmont-report/read-the-belmont-report/index.html

National Society of Genetic Counselors. (2018). Code of ethics. *Journal of Genetic Counseling*, *27*(1), 6–8.

National Society of Genetic Counselors' Definition Task Force, Resta, R., Biesecker, B. B., Bennett, R. L., Blum, S., Hahn, S. E., Strecker, M. N., & Williams, J. L. (2006). A new definition of Genetic Counseling: National Society of Genetic Counselors' Task Force report. *Journal of Genetic Counseling*, *15*(2), 77–83.

Ormond, K. E., Banuvar, S., Daly, A., Iris, M., Minogue, J., & Elias, S. (2009). Information preferences of high literacy pregnant women regarding informed consent models for genetic carrier screening. *Patient Education and Counseling*, *75*(2), 244–250.

Ormond, K. E., Borensztein, M. J., Hallquist, M. L. G., Buchanan, A. H., Faucett, W. A., Peay, H. L., Smith, M. E., Tricou, E. P., Uhlmann, W. R., Wain, K. E., Coughlin, C. R., 2nd, & On Behalf of the Clinical Genome CADRe Workgroup. (2021). Defining the critical components of informed consent for genetic testing. *Journal of Personalized Medicine*, *11*(12), 1304–1316. https://doi.org/10.3390/jpm11121304

Ormond, K. E., Iris, M., Banuvar, S., Minogue, J., Annas, G. J., & Elias, S. (2007). What do patients prefer: Informed consent models for genetic carrier testing. *Journal of Genetic Counseling*, *16*(4), 539–550.

Parens, E. (2015). Drifting away from informed consent in the era of personalized medicine. *Hastings Center Report*, *45*(4), 16–20.

Protection of Human Subjects, 45 C.F.R. § 46. (2018). https://www.hhs.gov/ohrp/sites/default/files/ohrp/policy/ohrpregulations.pdf

Ross, L. F., Saal, H. M., David, K. L., & Anderson, R. R. (2013). Technical report: Ethical and policy issues in genetic testing and screening of children. *Genetics in Medicine*, *15*(3), 234–245.

Royal College of Physicians, Royal College of Pathologists, and British Society for Genetic Medicine. (2022). *Genetic testing in childhood. Guidance for clinical practice. Report of the Joint Committee on Genomics in Medicine.*

Salgo v. Leland Stanford Jr. University Board of Trustees. 154 Cal. App. 2d 560, 317 P.2d 170 (1957).

Schloendorff v. Society of New York Hospital, 211 N.Y. 125 (1914).

Senter, L., Bennett, R. L., Madeo, A. C., Noblin, S., Ormond, K. E., Schneider, K. W., Swan, K., Virani, A., & National Society of Genetic Counselors Code of Ethics Review Task Force. (2018). National Society of Genetic Counselors code of ethics: Explication of 2017 revisions. *Journal of Genetic Counseling*, *27*(1), 9–15.

Sheehan, M. (2011). Can broad consent be informed consent? *Public Health Ethics*, *4*(3), 226–235.

Shuster, E. (1997). Fifty years later: The significance of the Nuremberg Code. *New England Journal of Medicine, 337*(20), 1436–1440.

Smith, A. C. M., & Pollin, T. I. (2011). Patient education. In W. R. Uhlmann, J. L. Schuette, & B. M. Yashar (Eds.), *A guide to genetic counseling* (2nd ed., pp. 177–205). Wiley-Blackwell.

Spatz, E. S., Krumholz, H. M., & Moulton, B. W. (2016). Informed consent and the reasonable-patient standard—Reply. *JAMA*, 316(9), 993. https://doi.org/10.1001/jama.2016.10561

Spector-Bagdady, K., Prince, A. E. R., Yu, J.-H., & Appelbaum, P. S. (2018). Analysis of state laws on informed consent for clinical genetic testing in the era of genomic sequencing. *American Journal of Medical Genetics Part C: Seminars in Medical Genetics, 178*(1), 81–88.

Tabor, H. K., Jamal, S. M., Yu, J.-H., Crouch, J. M., Shankar, A. G., Dent, K. M., Anderson, N., Miller, D. A., Futral, B. T., & Bamshad, M. J. (2017). My46: A web-based tool for self-guided management of genomic test results in research and clinical settings. *Genetics in Medicine, 19*(4), 467–475.

Tariman, J. D., Berry, D. L., Cochrane, B., Doorenbos, A., & Schepp, K. (2010). Preferred and actual participation roles during health care decision making in persons with cancer: A systematic review. *Annals of Oncology, 21*(6), 1145–1151.

Teare, H. J. A., Prictor, M., & Kaye, J. (2021). Reflections on dynamic consent in biomedical research: The story so far. *European Journal of Human Genetics, 29*(4), 649–656.

Tiffin, N. (2018). Tiered informed consent: Respecting autonomy, agency and individuality in Africa. *BMJ Global Health, 3*(6), e001249.

Tobias, J. S., & Souhami, R. L. (1993). Fully informed consent can be needlessly cruel. *BMJ, 307*(6913), 1199–1201.

Torke, A. M., Alexander, G. C., & Lantos, J. (2008). Substituted judgment: The limitations of autonomy in surrogate decision making. *Journal of General Internal Medicine, 23*(9), 1514–1517.

United Nations Convention on the Rights of the Child. (1989, November). https://www.ohchr.org/en/professionalinterest/pages/crc.aspx

Veach, P. M., Bartels, D. M., & LeRoy, B. S. (2007). Coming full circle: A reciprocal-engagement model of genetic counseling practice. *Journal of Genetic Counseling, 16*(6), 713–728.

Vears, D. F., Ayres, S., Boyle, J., Mansour, J., & Newson, A. J. (2020). Human Genetics Society of Australasia position statement: Predictive and presymptomatic genetic testing in adults and children. *Twin Research and Human Genetics, 23*(3), 184–189.

Wang, C., Gonzalez, R., & Merajver, S. D. S. D. (2004). Assessment of genetic testing and related counseling services: Current research and future directions. *Social Science & Medicine, 58*(7), 1427–1442.

Weithorn, L. A. (2020). When does a minor's legal competence to make health care decisions matter? *Pediatrics, 146*(Suppl. 1), S25–S32.

Whitney, S. N., Holmes-Rovner, M., Brody, H., Schneider, C., Mccullough, L. B., Volk, R. J., & McGuire, A. L. (2008). Beyond shared decision making: An expanded typology of medical decisions. *Medical Decision Making, 28*, 699–705.

Whitney, S. N., McGuire, A. L., & McCullough, L. B. (2004). A typology of shared decision making, informed consent, and simple consent. *Annals of Internal Medicine, 140*(1), 54–59.

World Medical Association. (2013). World Medical Association Declaration of Helsinki: Ethical principles for medical research involving human subjects. *JAMA, 310*(20), 2191–2194.

Yu, J.-H., Jamal, S. M., Tabor, H. K., & Bamshad, M. J. (2013). Self-guided management of exome and whole-genome sequencing results: Changing the results return model. *Genetics in Medicine, 15*(9), 684–690.

CHAPTER 16

TESTING STRATEGIES

Navigating the Path of Genetic Testing

LEE A. ZELLMER AND EMILY G. FARROW

Introduction

Genetic testing has been an integral component of genetic counseling since its inception. Genetic counselors have traditionally been responsible for providing pretest counseling to discuss the risks and benefits of testing, assisting in the genetic testing process, interpreting laboratory results in the context of the patient and family, and providing posttest counseling. As genetic and genomic technologies have rapidly advanced, the demand for testing has also increased. Accordingly, the demands for genetic counseling have increased. In addition to traditional clinical counseling roles, genetic counselors are now fulfilling laboratory roles, both as analysts in genetic testing and in lab utilization (Cho & Guy, 2020; Hart et al., 2023). Irrespective of a genetic counselor's job title, staying abreast of genetic testing is imperative. This chapter provides an overview of genetic testing, a framework for evaluating genetic tests and laboratories, and a discussion on balancing testing options within the reality of financial constraints.

Genetic Variation and Evaluation

A newborn infant is transferred to the neonatal intensive care unit (NICU) with respiratory distress and hypotonia; an underlying genetic etiology is suspected. The NICU team orders a rapid short-read genome trio analysis, at a significant cost, but it is nondiagnostic. The NICU concludes that they have ruled out a genetic diagnosis for this infant because they have ordered the most comprehensive genetic test. However, this child has Prader-Willi Syndrome (PWS). What went wrong in the testing process?

This scenario plays out frequently in hospitals and clinics. The biggest test is ordered under the assumption that it will find everything, be more cost-effective, and reduce the time to diagnosis. However, every genetic test has limitations, and even with the current technology available, clinically there is no single test that can detect every type of genetic variation. Genetic counselors play a critical role in guiding genetic testing. In the scenario above, the infant had PWS, later determined to be due to an imprinting defect, a methylation change not detected by current short-read genome sequencing (GS). A thorough understanding of the molecular mechanisms of disease, associated disease categories, phenotypic characteristics and associated etiologies, and appropriate testing is critical for genetic testing, and genetic counselors are well poised to navigate testing options.

Through the efforts of the Human Genome Project, it is known that the human genome comprises roughly 3 billion base pairs, or 6 billion nucleotides (Collins et al., 2003). The genetic difference between any two individuals is roughly 0.5%; however, that 0.5% equates to roughly 16 million base pairs. Variation within the genome may be silent, protective, risk associated, or disease causing. The challenge, then, in genetic testing is differentiating normal variation from disease-associated alleles.

Genetic variation itself may be roughly divided into a few main categories: (a) sequence variation, (b) copy number variation, (c) structural variation, and (d) epigenetics or methylation. Sequence variation includes single nucleotide variants (SNVs), small insertions or deletions up to 100 nucleotides in length (insertion–deletion variants [INDELs]), and repeat expansions. Copy number variants (CNVs) include deletions and duplications greater than 100 nucleotides in length up to chromosomal aneuploidies. Structural variation includes translocations and inversions, and epigenetics encompasses expression of the genome, or methylation (Raje et al., 2014). Each of these types of variants have lab techniques that are best suited to detect them. Table 16.1 contains a summary of these techniques.

Sequence variation

SNVs refer to changes in the sequence of the genome wherein one nucleotide is changed, deleted, or duplicated. If present in the coding region of a gene, these variants may be silent and not alter the amino acid, or may change the resulting protein by either substituting one amino acid for another (missense variants) or introducing a premature stop codon (nonsense variants), which can lead to a functional but truncated protein or to the cell degrading a nonfunctional protein (nonsense-mediated decay; Cohn, 2024). If a single nucleotide is deleted or inserted in a coding region, it causes a change in the reading frame (frameshift variant), which alters all subsequent amino acids and frequently leads to a premature stop codon. SNVs may also impact splicing by altering a canonical splice site or through the creation of a novel intronic splice site. While INDELs result in a change in the copy number of a particular nucleotide or small number of nucleotides, they are typically included in the sequence variation category given their small size and effect on the gene product. Importantly, INDELs may or may not change the reading frame.

These relatively small variations in sequence impact the fewest number of nucleotides but occur the most frequently in the genome. SNVs are currently detected by two main laboratory methods, Sanger sequencing and next-generation sequencing (NGS). Sanger sequencing uses polymerase chain reaction (PCR) to amplify a specific region of the patient's genome using targeted primers and then forms the complementary strand using labeled nucleotides to determine the sequence of the target one base at a time (Sanger et al., 1977). It is extremely accurate but comparatively slow, expensive, and labor intensive. Another consideration of Sanger sequencing is a limited ability to detect low-level mosaicism, typically

Table 16.1 Common Testing Methodologies, Their Capabilities, and Their Limitations in Genetic Testing

Methodology	Capabilities	Limitations
Karyotype	Large CNVs, aneuploidy, structural rearrangements	Won't detect medium and small CNVs
FISH	Medium CNVs that are specifically targeted, good for recurrent CNV/familial testing	May miss CNVs that are smaller than typical recurrent CNVs, only for specified region
Genome-wide microarray	Large CNVs, medium CNVs	Won't show small (gene/exon-level) CNVs, won't show location of duplications
Exon-level microarray	Gene/exon-level CNVs	Not all relevant genes/exons covered, need to verify coverage for genes of high suspicion
MLPA/msMLPA	Small/exon-level CNVs, methylation disorders	Only for a single specified region
Sanger	SNVs for a single exon/gene	May miss mosaicism
TP-PCR	Repeat primed PCR to detect repeat expansions	Only detects the repeat size, not the repeat sequence motif
NGS panel	SNVs for multiple genes at once, may detect mosaicism with deep coverage, may also detect CNVs (if analyzed)	Short read length misses repeat expansions, poor coverage may miss variants, may miss noncoding SNVs, only the genes on the panel are sequenced/analyzed
Exome sequencing	SNVs for "all" genes, may detect mosaicism with deep coverage, may also detect CNVs (if analyzed)	Short read length misses repeat expansions, poor coverage may miss variants, may miss noncoding SNVs and noncoding genes
Short-read genome sequencing	Genome-wide SNV and CNV detection, including noncoding variants	Short read length may miss repeat expansions, may not have depth to detect mosaicism, coverage considerations remain
Long-read genome sequencing	SNVs with improved detection in complex genomic regions, expansions, methylation, CNVs, SVs, coding and noncoding variants	May not have depth to detect mosaicism, not widely available clinically, balanced structural rearrangements may not be detected

Note: CNV = copy number variant; FISH = fluorescence in situ hybridization; MLPA = multiplex ligation-dependent probe amplification; msMLPA = methylation-sensitive multiple ligation probe assay; NGS = next-generation sequencing; SNV = single nucleotide variant; SV = structural variant; TP-PCR = triplet repeat primed polymerase chain reaction.

only 10%. However, given its accuracy, Sanger sequencing is still considered a gold standard and is frequently used for orthogonal confirmation of variants identified through other testing mechanisms.

NGS has its own strengths and limitations. NGS was developed through the Human Genome Project in the early 2000s (Collins et al., 2003). In contrast to Sanger sequencing, NGS refers to technologies that sequence billions of DNA fragments simultaneously, allowing for multiple genomes to be sequenced at once (Behjati & Tarpey, 2013).

Historically this process was also referred to as massively parallel sequencing. Given the high throughput and continually decreasing sequencing costs, NGS has transformed clinical genetic testing. As a testament to the rapid change, in 2021 the American College of Medical Genetics and Genomics recommended exome sequencing (ES)/GS as a first- or second-tier test for children with intellectual disabilities, congenital anomalies, or developmental delay (Manickam et al., 2021). However, it is important to understand the process of NGS in order to recognize its current strengths and limitations. In short-read NGS, sample processing starts with fragmenting genomic DNA into short lengths, typically ~400 base pairs. After DNA fragmentation, the samples are taken through library preparation, where barcodes for identification and sequencing primers are added. In panel or ES, a subsequent step called enrichment must be completed. Enrichment refers to the selection of the genes and regions to sequence and the removal of nontargeted regions. ES refers to all the coding regions of the genome, which account for ~2% of the genome. After enrichment, a PCR amplification step is completed to amplify the targets for sequencing. Each short strand of DNA is then sequenced simultaneously, one base at a time, yielding "reads" that are most often 150 base pairs long. A computer then bioinformatically aligns each fragment to the reference genome and completes variant annotation, ultimately generating a list of variation from the reference. The number of times each individual nucleotide is sequenced is referred to as the coverage depth. Deep coverage of 100x or greater allows for better detection of low-level mosaic variants that would be missed by Sanger sequencing. However, targeted NGS invariably has gaps in coverage, and low or absent coverage can lead to false negatives. Regions that are GC rich are difficult to capture with short-read NGS and may need to be sequenced using alternative methods in order to detect variants (Seaby et al., 2016).

Short-read GS, as the name implies, differs from ES and panel sequencing in that the entire genome is sequenced. Each sample undergoes the same initial preparation, in that the genomic DNA is fragmented into short pieces of ~400 base pairs. After library preparation, the sample is ready for sequencing. The sample preparation can be completed relatively rapidly in the laboratory, which is one reason short-read GS is often utilized in rapid sequencing tests. Another consideration in short-read GS is the PCR amplification step is typically omitted, enabling the detection of a higher number of variants. PCR amplification has the potential to introduce sequencing bias as regions that are GC rich, highly repetitive, or highly homologous amplify poorly. Further, omitting PCR provides more even, balanced coverage throughout the genome (Zhou et al., 2022). The tradeoff compared to ES is in the number of nucleotides being sequenced, which generally means genomes have lower coverage than high-depth exomes or multigene panels. However, the coverage in short-read GS is more even with fewer gaps. In addition to the benefit of even coverage, short-read GS allows for the detection of intronic variants, variants in noncoding disease-associated genes, as well as novel gene discovery. Although sequencing prices continue to rapidly decline, short-read GS remains more expensive compared to ES (Ewans et al., 2022).

Both Sanger and targeted NGS testing (ES, multigene panels) use PCR to amplify the patient's DNA and therefore are at risk for allele dropout. Allele dropout occurs when one allele is preferentially amplified by the PCR step and therefore only one allele is sequenced. This can lead to a misinterpretation of the results, either a false negative (if a variant allele drops out) or, conversely, a variant may appear to be homozygous rather than heterozygous (if the reference allele drops out). Unless there are conveniently located heterozygous single nucleotide polymorphisms (SNPs) in the targeted sequence, allele dropout can be easily missed.

Also included in this category of variation are repeat expansions. The most common types of repeat expansion associated with disease are triplet repeats (three nucleotides), such as fragile X syndrome (Hunter et al., 1993), but repeats of different lengths, such as pentameric repeats, are increasingly being recognized (Corbett et al., 2019; Kurosaki & Ashizawa, 2022; Terasaki et al., 2021). Repetitive regions become unstable as they become larger and are then prone to further expansion. Repeats in the coding region generally only need a small expansion to disrupt the gene product, while repeats in regulatory or other noncoding regions may expand into the thousands in an affected individual. Repeat expansions are currently not detected by short-read panel or ES for two reasons. The PCR amplification of repetitive sequences utilized in NGS sample preparation performs poorly. Further, due to the DNA fragmentation in short-read NGS, a large expansion may consist of entire reads encompassing only the repeat sequence, which will therefore be aligned as additional copies of the reference sequence, leading to a false negative. However, progress continues to be made, with bioinformatic algorithms developed to estimate the repeat size at known disease-associated loci in short-read GS that do not contain PCR amplification (Rajan-Babu et al., 2021). In some cases, clinical laboratories offering short-read GS have validated these expansion algorithms as a screen for testing, with positive samples orthogonally confirmed. By far the most common method for evaluating a suspected repeat expansion disorder is to order targeted testing for the clinical differential. Triplet-primed PCR is the current gold standard, replacing Southern blot techniques. The limitation in all of these methods is that the expansion size will be an estimate and will not provide a complete sequence of the expanded allele (Spector et al., 2021).

While most diagnostic testing of single-gene disorders has moved to full gene sequencing, some laboratories continue to offer targeted panels, primarily as part of carrier screening. These panels only detect the presence of preselected, curated, and recurrent SNVs and will not detect anything else, as they most commonly utilize fragment analysis to detect a specific nucleotide change rather than sequencing.

Copy number and structural variation

CNVs are deletions or duplications resulting in extra or missing copies of DNA, which may impact exons, gene(s), or gene products. CNVs vary greatly in size, from single exons to entire chromosomes. The detection of CNVs has evolved over time and was transformed with the implementation of microarray comparative genomic hybridization (CGH; South et al., 2013). Array CGH uses oligo probes to bind DNA at specific locations and measures the comparative dose. Subsequent to array CGH, SNP arrays were introduced. SNP arrays utilize probes that are located at well-characterized SNPs, which allow for the determination of the genotype at that position, in addition to assessing for regions of homozygosity (Sheth, 2014). The lower size limit of CNVs detectable by microarray is dependent on the number and location of the oligo probes. Whole-genome array has probes spaced over the entire genome, while a more targeted exon-level array clusters the probes in the coding region of disease-associated genes to detect a CNV of a single exon. CNV detection relies on having a sufficient number of probes in the right regions, and deletions or duplications smaller than a single exon are difficult to detect using array technology. In addition, microarray cannot definitively identify the presence of gene fusions or the location and the orientation, tandem or inverted, of duplicated regions.

Techniques used to evaluate the presence of CNVs are broad and include karyotyping (chromosomes), fluorescence in situ hybridization (FISH), array CGH, multiplex ligation-dependent probe amplification (MLPA), and bioinformatic analysis of NGS data. While traditional cytogenetic studies easily detect aneuploidy and large deletions and duplications, smaller CNVs may be missed. In general, karyotype analysis has a limit of detection of 3 to 5 Mb for deletions and duplications (Wallace & Bean, 2020). Microarray CGH will detect aneuploidy, smaller CNVs, and regions of homozygosity. FISH analysis binds fluorescent probes to a targeted chromosomal region to detect copy number changes ("ACMG Updates Chromosomal Microarray Analysis Guidelines," 2022; Raca et al., 2023; Shao et al., 2021). This technique has the advantage of showing the chromosomal location of the CNV but is a targeted test rather than a general screening tool. FISH is especially useful at detecting recurrent CNVs, rearrangements such as chromosome translocations, and gene fusion events. FISH testing also has an advantage in that it can be completed rapidly, in less than 24 hours, and is cost efficient.

MLPA is another technique still used to detect intermediate-sized CNVs, as well as exon-level deletions or duplications. MLPA uses paired primers and measures the distance between them to look for losses or gains. Methylation-specific MLPA can also assess for changes in methylation patterns regardless of the presence or absence of an underlying deletion (Stuppia et al., 2012).

Recent advancements in CNV detection from short-read ES and GS are again transforming variant detection. In general, a reference of normal samples is used as a comparison for the patient sample to determine relative gains and losses. CNV detection from ES and GS has significant advantages in timing, overall costs, and diagnostic rates (Raca et al., 2023; Royer-Bertrand et al., 2021; Singh et al., 2021). Microarray testing alone has an established diagnostic rate of 10% to 15%, while ES and GS range from 30% to 40% (Ayaz et al., 2022; Huang et al., 2021; Soden et al., 2014; Thiffault et al., 2018). As a general rule, genetic testing is completed sequentially as part of lab utilization. Particularly in children, where there are often incomplete phenotypic disease presentations, determining which test to order first can be difficult. Combining CNV and SNV detection into a single test decreases the overall time for results, increases the diagnostic yield, and in an increasing number of cases leads to the detection of multiple diagnoses that may have been missed by the completion of a single test (Royer-Bertrand et al., 2021; Tilemis et al., 2023). A further advantage of CNV detection from GS is the ability to often detect the precise breakpoint of the copy number event (Raca et al., 2023). There are potential drawbacks to CNV detection from NGS. This approach can generate a significant number of artifacts, and this "noise" can result in a missed CNV. In addition, as it relies on NGS coverage data, areas of low coverage may not be able to be assessed. With short-read technology, NGS is not able to reliably detect gene fusions or the location of duplicated regions.

Epigenetics and methylation

Epigenetics broadly refers to the regulation of gene expression throughout the genome that does not alter the nucleotide sequence but rather modifies the structure of the nucleotide or DNA. Methylation is one type of epigenetic mechanism and is increasingly recognized as a mechanism of disease. In humans, the most common form of methylation occurs as the addition of a methyl group at the 5' carbon in cytosine, also referred to as 5mC (Cohn, 2024). Imprinting disorders are a class of disease associated with changes in methylation. Imprinting refers to specific parent-of-origin expression, that is, only maternal or only paternal. As previously mentioned, a classic example of an imprinted locus is the Prader-Willi/Angelman locus on chromosome 15. When maternal-only methylation is observed, meaning loss of expression of genes from the paternal chromosome, the patient will have a diagnosis of PWS. Conversely, at the same locus, when a paternal-only methylation pattern is observed, or loss of maternal expression, the patient will have a diagnosis of Angelman syndrome (Cohn, 2024).

Testing for disorders of methylation requires special consideration. Well-characterized syndromes, such as Prader-Willi/Angelman, Beckwith Wiedemann, and Silver-Russell, are routinely tested for using a locus-specific methylation-sensitive multiple ligation probe assay (msMLPA), which relies on the hybridization of probes within the targeted region that detect copy number, methylation status, and the parent of origin (Ma et al., 2023; Moelans et al., 2018). A caveat to msMLPA assays is that they only target a single locus at a time.

Although in some cases testing a single locus for methylation changes is warranted given the phenotypic presentation, disorders of methylation extend far broader than classic imprinting disorders. For example, methylation within a regulatory region can lead to gene silencing (Robertson, 2005). Methylation changes may also be used to clarify the impact of a variant of unknown significance identified by sequencing or copy number evaluation. Therefore, in some cases a more comprehensive approach may be beneficial, such as a genome-wide methylation array. Methylation-specific arrays, such as the EpiSign assay, can detect known methylation signatures across the genome and have been shown to have a diagnostic yield in one cohort of 18.7% (Kerkhof et al., 2024).

Standard short-read NGS (panel, exome, and genome) is not able to detect differences in methylation as the sequencing process results in the removal of 5mC. A separate assay, whole-genome bisulfite sequencing, can be completed with short-read sequencing to measure genome-wide methylation (Li & Tollefsbol, 2011). However, this assay is currently cost prohibitive and predominantly utilized in research testing. Genetic counselors must be aware that, despite ordering ES or GS, additional testing may be required.

Laboratory Stewardship

Given the complexity of genetic testing options and their respective strengths and weaknesses, genetic counselors are often recruited to assist providers with their test selection (Cho & Guy, 2020; Kotzer et al., 2014). The involvement of a genetic counselor in the laboratory has been shown to result in a change in order for approximately 30% of tests ordered by providers (Miller et al., 2014). Correct test-ordering efforts are often part of a larger test utilization management program, also referred to as laboratory stewardship. The purpose of laboratory stewardship, much like antibiotic stewardship, is to limit the inappropriate use of genetic testing, and it can take many approaches. The benefits of an effective laboratory stewardship program include a reduced time to diagnosis, a decrease in the incidence of missed diagnoses or misdiagnoses, increased confidence in the results of genetic testing, lower cost to the patient/payer, and more effective use of laboratory resources. Laboratory stewardship programs typically include one or more of the following techniques to optimize their test utilization.

Test selection management

Test selection management can take a variety of forms depending on the available resources and culture of the institution. Test formularies, which limit providers to a specific set of available tests, are another method to prevent inappropriate test ordering. Frequently a formulary is combined with a review committee, so that exceptions to the formulary can be granted for specific situations. Testing algorithms for common indications give guidance to the provider and decrease the overall number of tests required but may increase the time to diagnosis.

Ordering error management

This approach most commonly utilizes test order review, frequently by a genetic counselor, to ensure that a test ordered is appropriate for the indication and comprehensive enough to make or rule out a particular diagnosis. It takes specialized knowledge of medical genetics to recognize a typographical error in a typed order that changes the gene name to one that is for an entirely different disorder, as well as an understanding of the capabilities of each genetic test as described above, to prevent a costly genetic test from being inappropriately performed. Additionally, a laboratory genetic counselor's understanding of billing and reimbursement may be useful in directing a provider to a test that is more likely to be covered by a patient's insurance plan.

Reference laboratory management

A third approach to laboratory stewardship is to limit providers to reference laboratories that meet specific criteria established by the institution. A variety of factors can be considered when selecting which reference laboratories to use for genetic testing, as described in more detail in the following section.

Selecting a Reference Laboratory

Not all reference laboratories are created equal. There are significant differences in type of testing offered, technology used, pricing, turnaround times (TATs), reporting policies, and customer service. This section will describe the factors that should be considered when choosing which laboratory to use for a given genetic test. It is good practice to document the process of selecting reference laboratories. Figure 16.1 shows an example evaluation form for reference laboratories, highlighting areas to record. It's also important to review your selections regularly (e.g., on an annual basis).

Laboratory: ______________________

Review type: ☐ Initial ☐ Annual ☐ Other ______________

Accreditation/Certification	
CLIA number	
CLIA expiration date	
Accreditation body (CAP, COLA...)	
Accreditation expiration date	

Quality & Efficiency	
Onsite visit recommended (facility, equipment, personnel, policies, QA and QC records, etc.)	☐ Yes ☐ No
Scope of service • Genetics • General laboratory • Toxicology • Endocrinology • Other ______________	 ☐ Yes ☐ No ☐ Yes ☐ No ☐ Yes ☐ No ☐ Yes ☐ No ☐ Yes ☐ No
Customer service • Call-backs within 24 hours • Access to Medical/Technical Directors • Clearly defined instructions and policies related to specimen handling • Hours of operation: specify______________ • Frequency of test updates: specify______________	 ☐ Yes ☐ No ☐ Yes ☐ No ☐ Yes ☐ No
Specimen transportation frequency/convenience/cost • Courier • FedEx, etc. shipping costs included	 ☐ Yes ☐ No ☐ Yes ☐ No
Technical assistance and compatibility • Computer interface • Web-based ordering/resulting	 ☐ Yes ☐ No ☐ Yes ☐ No
Resulting and reporting (i.e. test method, frequency, clarity, etc.) completed in a timely fashion	☐ Yes ☐ No
Acceptable turnaround-times (refer to policy statement)	☐ Yes ☐ No
Pediatric reference ranges when appropriate	☐ Yes ☐ N/A
Pediatric specimen volumes when appropriate	☐ Yes ☐ N/A
FMV analysis required for high-volume procedures to high-volume laboratories	☐ Attached ☐ N/A

FIGURE 16.1 Example evaluation form for reference laboratories. CAP = College of American Pathologists; CLIA = Clinical Laboratory Improvement Amendments; COLA = Commission on Office Laboratory Accreditation; FMV = fair market value; QA = quality assurance; QC = quality control.

Certification and licensure

Clinical testing laboratories in the United States are regulated by both the College of American Pathology (CAP) and the Clinical Laboratory Improvement Amendments (CLIA). An important part of selecting a reference laboratory is to confirm that both of these entities have inspected and approved of the testing practices. Unless testing is being performed on a research basis, clinical testing should *never* be performed in a lab that is not CAP/CLIA approved.

Is a bad test worse than no test at all? If a provider can't (or shouldn't) trust the results of a test, then it is money, time, and effort wasted. The first consideration for testing should *always* be choosing a laboratory that is reliable and accurate. While CAP and CLIA assess a lab's technical quality, assessing a laboratory's variant interpretation quality is much more difficult. Some labs will reduce the number of variants of unknown significance that they report in order to not overwhelm the ordering provider. But what if one of those variants is subsequently reclassified to pathogenic? If a variant is not reported, ordering providers and genetic counselors cannot perform clinical correlation and monitor the variant in the literature themselves. In addition, many larger labs are leveraging artificial intelligence and natural language processing to help them complete analyses faster and cheaper (Birgmeier et al., 2020; Lee et al., 2024; Nykamp et al., 2017). However, these programs can and do miss identifying important information in the literature. They are tools and should not be expected to replace clinical experience and molecular expertise. One resource for assessing how a lab compares to others in variant classification is a tool called ClinVar Miner (https://clinvarminer.genetics.utah.edu/). It allows you to compare how a lab is categorizing its variant classifications against other labs and helps identify labs that routinely may overcall or undercall the pathogenicity of their variants.[1]

The price of a test should not be the only criterion used to select a reference laboratory. Prices of NGS testing have been steadily dropping over the last several years and are expected to continue to do so. However, the adage "you get what you pay for" may also be true when applied to genetic testing. There are numerous reference labs offering inexpensive tests, and some of these labs do not provide the same quality as their higher priced competitors. Hiring and retaining knowledgeable analysts incurs a significant cost, and laboratories, which must maintain their market, may be using cost-cutting methods that include personnel with less experience and/or expertise. However, if the quality between two laboratories is equivalent, then a laboratory that offers lower pricing and/or patient financial assistance programs may be a better fit for your institution and your patients' needs.

Many institutions strive to limit the overall number of reference laboratories they utilize due to the amount of time and effort it takes to maintain each contract. Depending on the institution, a Lab Service Agreement may need to be negotiated, purchase orders created, relationships with a sales representative established and maintained, and online accounts created for each laboratory utilized. There is a definite employee time advantage to selecting a lab with a large test menu, but there are points to consider using this approach. Some of the larger laboratories list tests on their menu that they do not actually perform; they simply pass the sample along to a subcontracted lab to complete. This is appealing to some institutions as they then have a "one-stop shop" and rely on the reference laboratory to evaluate their subcontractors. Other institutions would prefer to choose the most appropriate performing laboratory for a particular test themselves. These "pass-through" tests can be identified by checking the "performing location" section of the lab's online test directory. In reality, the types of technology used for genetic testing are so varied that no single lab offers

[1] Editors' note: For further discussion on variant interpretation, see Chapter 17 by Isabelle Thiffault and Carol J. Saunders in this volume.

every genetic test. Ultimately, the institution, which often includes a genetic counselor as part of the decision-making team, can either let the reference laboratory make the testing decisions on their behalf or choose to decide themselves.

Customer service

The relative importance of this criterion most likely depends on the amount of testing that will be sent. If testing volumes are low, a laboratory may only need to be contacted on a limited basis, and it may not matter how easy it is to reach a living person on the phone or receive a rapid reply to an email. But for regularly used labs, this issue becomes vital. How long does it take to find someone if you have a question about a result? Do they provide shipping and collection supplies? Are they kind and helpful to both you and your patients? Are their sales representatives knowledgeable about the tests they're selling? None of these intangibles affect the bottom line or the quality of the test, but should be considered in the context of other features being equal.

Turnaround times

Waiting for results can be difficult, especially in genetic testing. However, there are circumstances where a delay of even a few days can make a significant difference in a patient's outcome. Many times, faster tests are more expensive, and the need (or lack thereof) of faster results for clinical management must be weighed against cost. A laboratory should clearly state their established TAT and provide the percentage of tests that meet their stated times. The laboratory should also clarify how results are reported. In rapid testing, there are laboratories that will provide a verbal result before the formal written report. In other tests, results may be staggered, with SNV and CNV testing completed before the mitochondrial genome analysis. Each laboratory establishes their own TAT and reporting policies, and they will vary between sites. It is helpful to remember that the overall TAT is a direct reflection of the laboratories' testing volume, staffing, and instrumentation.

Reporting/recontacting policy

It does not matter if a test is of good quality and competitive pricing if you (or the ordering provider) cannot read and understand the report. This is of particular importance for genetic counselors, as they often interpret genetic test results for nongenetic providers and families. A good report should contain multiple patient identifiers, a summary result for quick reference, and detailed interpretation information about how they came to the conclusion that a test was diagnostic (or not). There should be a clear description of the methodology used that is in a large enough font to be readable, and there should be contact information clearly stated so that you can reach out with any questions. While it is accepted practice to omit benign or likely benign variants from a report, variants of unknown significance should be in the main body of the report, not listed in an addendum where they can be missed by a provider.

Lab policies vary regarding how/when/if they will recontact providers should the interpretation of a particular variant change. Some labs will issue an amended report automatically, while others will only reinterpret a test upon request. It is not uncommon for these reinterpretations to be completed at no charge for a single variant, but there will likely be a charge to reanalyze an entire data set such as a nondiagnostic exome. Until the legal system has issued guidelines for a lab's duty to reanalyze/recontact, these policies will continue to vary and should be investigated when choosing a new reference laboratory.

Privacy of sequence data

The Health Insurance Portability and Accountability Act (HIPAA) outlines 18 identifiers that it considers "protected health information" (PHI; United States, 1996). These identifiers must be removed from any data before it is transferred or sold to a third party. However, genomic data is not considered PHI under HIPAA. That means that a laboratory may remove demographic information from its genomic data and legally sell it to a third party. Many labs, as a mechanism to lower the cost of some of their tests, have partnered with industry to offer "sponsored" (i.e., free to the patient) genetic testing. In sponsored testing, the fiscal out-of-pocket cost may be low to zero; however, the sponsor will receive the genotype/phenotype information from the sponsored testing to use in their pharmaceutical research and development programs. Industry-sponsored testing provides many families with a mechanism to obtain testing. However, many patients are unaware of the inherently identifiable nature of genomic data and that there is no real way to deidentify it. Therefore, it is important that this information is conveyed to families during pretest counseling prior to using a sponsored test.

Beware of nepotism

Medical subspecialties are small communities, and it is not unusual for a provider to request a particular reference lab be used because "my colleague from institution X recommends it/works there and I trust them." In the current era of transparency this is a risky approach to take. Laboratory selection should be able to stand up to scrutiny by an administration, the patient/family, and the average person. One approach to mitigate potential conflicts of interest in testing is to have providers sign a disclosure form, detailing their request and rationale, which is routed to their institution's compliance team if they insist on using a reference lab that is not one of the institution-approved laboratories.

Emerging Technology

As noted in a previous section of this chapter, each genetic test has its own capabilities and limitations when it comes to detecting different types of genetic variation. Historically, this meant it frequently took multiple tests to diagnose or rule out a genetic cause for the patient's symptoms. However, technological advancements are changing this paradigm. In particular, two recent developments are once again transforming genetic testing.

Long-read NGS sequences DNA fragments that are greater than 13,000 base pairs in length, a stark contrast to the current read length of ~150 base pairs (Cohen et al., 2022; Groza et al., 2024). The significant increase in read length provides better alignment in repetitive regions, such as expansion disorders, and in complex regions. The increased alignment metrics in turn result in improved variant detection for SNVs and CNVs (Chen et al., 2023; Cohen et al., 2022). It also allows for the full sequencing of expansion disorders, enabling the precise numerical determination of the repeat, in addition to sequencing for potential interruptions within the repeat motif (Dolzhenko et al., 2024). The long-sequencing reads can provide allele phasing, without the inclusion of parents, which is particularly useful for singleton analyses where biological parents are unavailable for testing (Cohen et al., 2022; Kernohan & Boycott, 2024). Lastly, due to differences in how sequencing is completed, long-read sequencing is able to detect native methylation simultaneously with DNA sequencing (Cheung et al., 2023). Collectively, long-read genome testing allows for four separate clinical tests to be combined into a single assay.

Long-read platforms are also impacting the field of cytogenetics. Karyotyping provides single-cell resolution of chromosome number and structure; however, it is time intensive and requires highly trained laboratory personnel. Further, as previously stated, traditional karyotyping has an estimated limit of detection of 3 to 5 Mb for deletions and duplications (Wallace & Bean, 2020). A new technology, optimal genome mapping (OGM), labels ultralong pieces of DNA, greater than 150,000 base pairs, at a specific sequence motif that occurs approximately every 6,000 base pairs throughout the genome (Smith et al., 2023). By comparing the patient sample to a reference, the software is able to accurately detect structural variants, including balanced rearrangements and inversions, deletions, duplications, and aneuploidies. Implementation of OGM has been shown to increase efficiency in testing by increasing throughput and decreasing analysis time (Smith et al., 2023). Particularly in complex karyotypes, often detected in hematological specimens, the incorporation of OGM in addition to standard karyotype has been shown to add significant clinically relevant findings (Levy et al., 2024).

As with any test, although both long-read NGS and OGM have significant benefits, there are considerations in testing. Currently short-read NGS is more cost effective and has a higher throughput compared to long-read NGS. In laboratories that are sequencing thousands of samples a year, the limitation in sequencing capacity is significant. As a new technology, long-read sequencing is available on a limited basis, as laboratories and institutions must purchase new infrastructure to offer the test. OGM may have a higher throughput compared to karyotype analysis; however, it also has limitations in detection. An example often cited is the inability to detect Robertsonian translocations, or translocations between acrocentric chromosomes (Kernohan & Boycott, 2024). Perhaps most important, payers are often slow to adopt reimbursement for new technologies (Zion et al., 2023). Nonetheless, the continued development of new technologies will continue to improve genetic testing, increasing diagnosis rates and decreasing the overall time to diagnosis.

Navigating Testing Options

Genetic counselors are well poised to navigate the challenges of genetic testing, from both the laboratory utilization and patient perspective. After the clinical team has identified the need for testing, for outpatient genetic testing, a genetic counselor often is tasked with navigating insurance payers, institutional regulations, and patient preferences. In institutions with an established laboratory utilization process, many testing considerations may already have been made (i.e., which laboratory, what tests are allowed, etc.). Institutions that do not have a laboratory utilization team may still have a financial clearance team that will assist in determining testing costs for the patient and may provide preauthorization. It is important to remember that preauthorization does not equate to payment; it only states that the test is allowed. Additional resources, as previously mentioned, are that many commercial laboratories are able to offer testing at reduced to no cost or provide a maximum out-of-pocket cost to the family prior to commencing testing.

A common challenge in genetic testing is balancing the desire for a specific genetic test, perhaps GS as a first test instead of microarray. However, financial constraints may only allow for a conventional microarray. A genetic counselor may advocate for preferred testing directly with insurance, clearly outlining why a particular test was chosen, the benefits, and importantly how the test will impact medical management. In some cases, a stepwise testing approach may be necessary, that is, a microarray must be completed before additional testing will be approved. Genetic counselors can help by explaining the utility of testing, regardless of the timing.

In cases where families may be underinsured or have no insurance, there are often still options to pursue genetic testing. Many institutions have a patient assistance program, whereby the hospital has funding to offset testing for families that cannot afford it. In these programs, a genetic counselor will typically need to summarize why genetic testing is warranted, explain how it will impact medical management, and detail why the family qualifies for assistance. Commercial laboratories with sponsored testing may also be an appropriate solution. In these instances, pretest counseling should include not only a discussion of the potential risks and benefits of genetic testing but also a discussion of data privacy, supporting a family in making an informed decision. Data sharing is not inherently good or bad alone; however, it should be clear what data will be shared and how it will be utilized.

Financial constraints are not the only barrier to genetic testing. An often-overlooked challenge can be obtaining a sufficient sample to complete testing. This can be even further complicated for families that live in underserved or rural areas, far from testing laboratories. Many but not all tests can be completed with a buccal swab that can be mailed directly to patient homes. Karyotyping, long-read sequencing, and OGM all require a blood sample (Cohen et al., 2022; Kernohan & Boycott, 2024). A genetic counselor can help reconcile patient access and sample type to guide genetic testing.

Conclusion

Genetic testing has always played an integral role in the field of genetic counseling. The completion of the Human Genome Project and creation of NGS have led to exponential growth in diagnostic testing, ultimately leading to unprecedented gene–disease discovery, an increase in overall diagnostic rates, and a decrease in time to diagnosis. The rapid development of and changing field of genetic testing can be difficult for nonexperts. Genetic counselors play a vital role in identifying appropriate testing, pretest and posttest counseling, and return of results. Genetic testing technologies will continue to advance, replacing current testing algorithms and assays, inevitably making today's new tests obsolete. However, despite the changing field of testing, the need for genetic counselors will remain constant, providing patients and providers the education and guidance needed to navigate an ever-evolving field.

References

ACMG updates chromosomal microarray analysis guidelines. (2022). *American Journal of Medical Genetics Part A, 188*(2), 392–393. https://doi.org/10.1002/ajmg.a.62273

Ayaz, A., Gezdirici, A., Yilmaz Gulec, E., Ozalp, O., Koseoglu, A. H., Dogru, Z., & Yalcintepe, S. (2022). Diagnostic value of microarray method in autism spectrum disorder, intellectual disability, and multiple congenital anomalies and some candidate genes for autism: Experience of two centers. *Medeni Medical Journal, 37*(2), 180–193. https://doi.org/10.4274/MMJ.galenos.2022.70962

Behjati, S., & Tarpey, P. S. (2013). What is next generation sequencing? *Archives of Disease: Child Education and Practice Edition, 98*(6), 236–238. https://doi.org/10.1136/archdischild-2013-304340

Birgmeier, J., Haeussler, M., Deisseroth, C. A., Steinberg, E. H., Jagadeesh, K. A., Ratner, A. J., Guturu, H., Wenger, A. M., Diekhans, M. E., Stenson, P. D., Cooper, D. N., Re, C., Beggs, A. H., Bernstein, J. A., & Bejerano, G. (2020). AMELIE speeds Mendelian diagnosis by matching patient phenotype and genotype to primary literature. *Science Translational Medicine, 12*(544). https://doi.org/10.1126/scitranslmed.aau9113

Chen, X., Harting, J., Farrow, E., Thiffault, I., Kasperaviciute, D., Genomics England Research Consortium, Hoischen, A., Gilissen, C., Pastinen, T., & Eberle, M. A. (2023). Comprehensive SMN1 and SMN2 profiling for spinal muscular atrophy analysis using long-read PacBio HiFi sequencing. *American Journal of Human Genetics, 110*(2), 240–250. https://doi.org/10.1016/j.ajhg.2023.01.001

Cheung, W. A., Johnson, A. F., Rowell, W. J., Farrow, E., Hall, R., Cohen, A. S. A., Means, J. C., Zion, T. N., Portik, D. M., Saunders, C. T., Koseva, B., Bi, C., Truong, T. K., Schwendinger-Schreck, C., Yoo, B., Johnston, J. J., Gibson, M., Evrony, G., Rizzo, W. B., . . . Pastinen, T. (2023). Direct haplotype-resolved 5-base HiFi sequencing for genome-wide profiling of hypermethylation outliers in a rare disease cohort. *Nature Communications, 14*(1), 3090. https://doi.org/10.1038/s41467-023-38782-1

Cho, M. T., & Guy, C. (2020). Evolving roles of genetic counselors in the clinical laboratory. *Cold Spring Harbor Perspectives in Medicine, 10*(10). https://doi.org/10.1101/cshperspect.a036574

Cohen, A. S. A., Farrow, E. G., Abdelmoity, A. T., Alaimo, J. T., Amudhavalli, S. M., Anderson, J. T., Bansal, L., Bartik, L., Baybayan, P., Belden, B., Berrios, C. D., Biswell, R. L., Buczkowicz, P., Buske, O., Chakraborty, S., Cheung, W. A., Coffman, K. A., Cooper, A. M., Cross, L. A., . . . Pastinen, T. (2022). Genomic answers for children: Dynamic analyses of >1000 pediatric rare disease genomes. *Genetics in Medicine, 24*(6), 1336–1348. https://doi.org/10.1016/j.gim.2022.02.007

Cohn, R. D. (2024). *Thompson and Thompson genetics and genomics in medicine* (9th ed.). https://RX8KL6YF4X.search.serialssolutions.com/ejp/?libHash=RX8KL6YF4X#/search/?searchControl=title&searchType=title_code&criteria=TC_052471572

Collins, F. S., Morgan, M., & Patrinos, A. (2003). The Human Genome Project: Lessons from large-scale biology. *Science, 300*(5617), 286–290. https://doi.org/10.1126/science.1084564

Corbett, M. A., Kroes, T., Veneziano, L., Bennett, M. F., Florian, R., Schneider, A. L., Coppola, A., Licchetta, L., Franceschetti, S., Suppa, A., Wenger, A., Mei, D., Pendziwiat, M., Kaya, S., Delledonne, M., Straussberg, R., Xumerle, L., Regan, B., Crompton, D., . . . Gecz, J. (2019). Intronic ATTTC repeat expansions in STARD7 in familial adult myoclonic epilepsy linked to chromosome 2. *Nature Communications, 10*(1), 4920. https://doi.org/10.1038/s41467-019-12671-y

Dolzhenko, E., English, A., Dashnow, H., De Sena Brandine, G., Mokveld, T., Rowell, W. J., Karniski, C., Kronenberg, Z., Danzi, M. C., Cheung, W. A., Bi, C., Farrow, E., Wenger, A., Chua, K. P., Martinez-Cerdeno, V., Bartley, T. D., Jin, P., Nelson, D. L., Zuchner, S., . . . Eberle, M. A. (2024). Characterization and visualization of tandem repeats at genome scale. *Nature Biotechnology*. https://doi.org/10.1038/s41587-023-02057-3

Ewans, L. J., Minoche, A. E., Schofield, D., Shrestha, R., Puttick, C., Zhu, Y., Drew, A., Gayevskiy, V., Elakis, G., Walsh, C., Ades, L. C., Colley, A., Ellaway, C., Evans, C. A., Freckmann, M. L., Goodwin, L., Hackett, A., Kamien, B., Kirk, E. P., . . . Roscioli, T. (2022). Whole exome and genome sequencing in mendelian disorders: A diagnostic and health economic analysis. *European Journal of Human Genetics, 30*(10), 1121–1131. https://doi.org/10.1038/s41431-022-01162-2

Groza, C., Schwendinger-Schreck, C., Cheung, W. A., Farrow, E. G., Thiffault, I., Lake, J., Rizzo, W. B., Evrony, G., Curran, T., Bourque, G., & Pastinen, T. (2024). Pangenome graphs improve the analysis of structural variants in rare genetic diseases. *Nature Communications, 15*(1), 657. https://doi.org/10.1038/s41467-024-44980-2

Hart, T. R., Ahmed, S., Byrne, R., Sulmonte, L. A. G., Williams, L. M., & McWalter, K. (2023). Shifts in the genetic counseling workforce highlight a need for laboratory fieldwork experience for genetic counseling trainees. *Journal of Genetic Counseling, 32*(6), 1194–1199. https://doi.org/10.1002/jgc4.1817

Huang, H., Wang, Y., Zhang, M., Lin, N., An, G., He, D., Chen, M., Chen, L., & Xu, L. (2021). Diagnostic accuracy and value of chromosomal microarray analysis for chromosomal abnormalities in prenatal detection: A prospective clinical study. *Medicine (Baltimore), 100*(20), e25999. https://doi.org/10.1097/MD.0000000000025999

Hunter, J. E., Berry-Kravis, E., Hipp, H., & Todd, P. K. (1993). FMR1 disorders. In M. P. Adam, J. Feldman, G. M. Mirzaa, R. A. Pagon, S. E. Wallace, L. J. H. Bean, K. W. Gripp, & A. Amemiya (Eds.), *GeneReviews®*. University of Washington, Seattle. https://www.ncbi.nlm.nih.gov/pubmed/20301558

Kerkhof, J., Rastin, C., Levy, M. A., Relator, R., McConkey, H., Demain, L., Dominguez-Garrido, E., Kaat, L. D., Houge, S. D., DuPont, B. R., Fee, T., Fletcher, R. S., Gokhale, D., Haukanes, B. I., Henneman, P., Hilton, S., Hilton, B. A., Jenkinson, S., Lee, J. A., . . . Sadikovic, B. (2024). Diagnostic utility and reporting recommendations for clinical DNA methylation episignature testing in genetically undiagnosed rare diseases. *Genetics in Medicine, 26*(5), 101075. https://doi.org/10.1016/j.gim.2024.101075

Kernohan, K. D., & Boycott, K. M. (2024). The expanding diagnostic toolbox for rare genetic diseases. *Nature Reviews Genetics, 25*(6), 401–415. https://doi.org/10.1038/s41576-023-00683-w

Kotzer, K. E., Riley, J. D., Conta, J. H., Anderson, C. M., Schahl, K. A., & Goodenberger, M. L. (2014). Genetic testing utilization and the role of the laboratory genetic counselor. *Clinica Chimica Acta, 427*, 193–195. https://doi.org/10.1016/j.cca.2013.09.033

Kurosaki, T., & Ashizawa, T. (2022). The genetic and molecular features of the intronic pentanucleotide repeat expansion in spinocerebellar ataxia type 10. *Frontiers in Genetics*, *13*, 936869. https://doi.org/10.3389/fgene.2022.936869

Lee, B., Nasanovsky, L., Shen, L., Maglinte, D. T., Pan, Y., Gai, X., Schmidt, R. J., Raca, G., Biegel, J. A., Roytman, M., An, P., Saunders, C. J., Farrow, E. G., Shams, S., & Ji, J. (2024). Significance associated with phenotype score aids in variant prioritization for exome sequencing analysis. *Journal of Molecular Diagnostics*, *26*(5), 337–348. https://doi.org/10.1016/j.jmoldx.2024.01.009

Levy, B., Kanagal-Shamanna, R., Sahajpal, N. S., Neveling, K., Rack, K., Dewaele, B., Olde Weghuis, D., Stevens-Kroef, M., Puiggros, A., Mallo, M., Clifford, B., Mantere, T., Hoischen, A., Espinet, B., Kolhe, R., Sole, F., Raca, G., & Smith, A. C. (2024). A framework for the clinical implementation of optical genome mapping in hematologic malignancies. *American Journal of Hematology*, *99*(4), 642–661. https://doi.org/10.1002/ajh.27175

Li, Y., & Tollefsbol, T. O. (2011). DNA methylation detection: Bisulfite genomic sequencing analysis. *Methods in Molecular Biology*, *791*, 11–21. https://doi.org/10.1007/978-1-61779-316-5_2

Ma, V. K., Mao, R., Toth, J. N., Fulmer, M. L., Egense, A. S., & Shankar, S. P. (2023). Prader-Willi and Angelman syndromes: Mechanisms and management. *Application of Clinical Genetics*, *16*, 41–52. https://doi.org/10.2147/TACG.S372708

Manickam, K., McClain, M. R., Demmer, L. A., Biswas, S., Kearney, H. M., Malinowski, J., Massingham, L. J., Miller, D., Yu, T. W., Hisama, F. M., & ACMG Board of Directors. (2021). Exome and genome sequencing for pediatric patients with congenital anomalies or intellectual disability: An evidence-based clinical guideline of the American College of Medical Genetics and Genomics (ACMG). *Genetics in Medicine*, *23*(11), 2029–2037. https://doi.org/10.1038/s41436-021-01242-6

Miller, C. E., Krautscheid, P., Baldwin, E. E., Tvrdik, T., Openshaw, A. S., Hart, K., & Lagrave, D. (2014). Genetic counselor review of genetic test orders in a reference laboratory reduces unnecessary testing. *American Journal of Medical Genetics Part A*, *164A*(5), 1094–1101. https://doi.org/10.1002/ajmg.a.36453

Moelans, C. B., Atanesyan, L., Savola, S. P., & van Diest, P. J. (2018). Methylation-specific multiplex ligation-dependent probe amplification (MS-MLPA). *Methods in Molecular Biology*, *1708*, 537–549. https://doi.org/10.1007/978-1-4939-7481-8_27

Nykamp, K., Anderson, M., Powers, M., Garcia, J., Herrera, B., Ho, Y. Y., Kobayashi, Y., Patil, N., Thusberg, J., Westbrook, M., Invitae Clinical Genomics Group, & Topper, S. (2017). Sherloc: A comprehensive refinement of the ACMG-AMP variant classification criteria. *Genetics in Medicine*, *19*(10), 1105–1117. https://doi.org/10.1038/gim.2017.37

Raca, G., Astbury, C., Behlmann, A., De Castro, M. J., Hickey, S. E., Karaca, E., Lowther, C., Riggs, E. R., Seifert, B. A., Thorland, E. C., Deignan, J. L., & ACMG Laboratory Quality Assurance Committee. (2023). Points to consider in the detection of germline structural variants using next-generation sequencing: A statement of the American College of Medical Genetics and Genomics (ACMG). *Genetics in Medicine*, *25*(2), 100316. https://doi.org/10.1016/j.gim.2022.09.017

Rajan-Babu, I. S., Peng, J. J., Chiu, R., IMAGINE Study, CAUSES Study, Li, C., Mohajeri, A., Dolzhenko, E., Eberle, M. A., Birol, I., & Friedman, J. M. (2021). Genome-wide sequencing as a first-tier screening test for short tandem repeat expansions. *Genome Medicine*, *13*(1), 126. https://doi.org/10.1186/s13073-021-00932-9

Raje, N., Soden, S., Swanson, D., Ciaccio, C. E., Kingsmore, S. F., & Dinwiddie, D. L. (2014). Utility of next generation sequencing in clinical primary immunodeficiencies. *Current Allergy and Asthma Reports*, *14*(10), 468. https://doi.org/10.1007/s11882-014-0468-y

Robertson, K. D. (2005). DNA methylation and human disease. *Nature Reviews Genetics*, *6*(8), 597–610. https://doi.org/10.1038/nrg1655

Royer-Bertrand, B., Cisarova, K., Niel-Butschi, F., Mittaz-Crettol, L., Fodstad, H., & Superti-Furga, A. (2021). CNV detection from exome sequencing data in routine diagnostics of rare genetic disorders: Opportunities and limitations. *Genes (Basel)*, *12*(9). https://doi.org/10.3390/genes12091427

Sanger, F., Nicklen, S., & Coulson, A. R. (1977). DNA sequencing with chain-terminating inhibitors. *Proceedings of the National Academy of Sciences of the United States of America*, *74*(12), 5463–5467. https://doi.org/10.1073/pnas.74.12.5463

Seaby, E. G., Pengelly, R. J., & Ennis, S. (2016). Exome sequencing explained: A practical guide to its clinical application. *Briefings in Functional Genomics*, *15*(5), 374–384. https://doi.org/10.1093/bfgp/elv054

Shao, L., Akkari, Y., Cooley, L. D., Miller, D. T., Seifert, B. A., Wolff, D. J., Mikhail, F. M., & ACMG Laboratory Quality Assurance Committee. (2021). Chromosomal microarray analysis, including constitutional and neoplastic disease applications, 2021 revision: A technical standard of the American College of Medical Genetics and Genomics (ACMG). *Genetics in Medicine*, *23*(10), 1818–1829. https://doi.org/10.1038/s41436-021-01214-w

Sheth, J. (2014). Proceedings of the International Conference on Human Genetics and 39th Annual Meeting of Indian Society of Human Genetics. *Molecular Cytogenetics*, *7*(Suppl. 1), A1–P132. https://doi.org/10.1186/1755-8166-7-s1-a1

Singh, A. K., Olsen, M. F., Lavik, L. A. S., Vold, T., Drablos, F., & Sjursen, W. (2021). Detecting copy number variation in next generation sequencing data from diagnostic gene panels. *BMC Medical Genomics*, *14*(1), 214. https://doi.org/10.1186/s12920-021-01059-x

Smith, A. C., Hoischen, A., & Raca, G. (2023). Cytogenetics is a science, not a technique! Why optical genome mapping is so important to clinical genetic laboratories. *Cancers (Basel)*, *15*(22). https://doi.org/10.3390/cancers15225470

Soden, S. E., Saunders, C. J., Willig, L. K., Farrow, E. G., Smith, L. D., Petrikin, J. E., LePichon, J. B., Miller, N. A., Thiffault, I., Dinwiddie, D. L., Twist, G., Noll, A., Heese, B. A., Zellmer, L., Atherton, A. M., Abdelmoity, A. T., Safina, N., Nyp, S. S., Zuccarelli, B., . . . Kingsmore, S. F. (2014). Effectiveness of exome and genome sequencing guided by acuity of illness for diagnosis of neurodevelopmental disorders. *Science Translational Medicine*, *6*(265), 265ra168. https://doi.org/10.1126/scitranslmed.3010076

South, S. T., Lee, C., Lamb, A. N., Higgins, A. W., Kearney, H. M., & Working Group for the American College of Medical Genetics and Genomics Laboratory Quality Assurance Committee. (2013). ACMG Standards and Guidelines for constitutional cytogenomic microarray analysis, including postnatal and prenatal applications: Revision 2013. *Genetics in Medicine*, *15*(11), 901–909. https://doi.org/10.1038/gim.2013.129

Spector, E., Behlmann, A., Kronquist, K., Rose, N. C., Lyon, E., Reddi, H. V., & ACMG Laboratory Quality Assurance Committee. (2021). Laboratory testing for fragile X, 2021 revision: A technical standard of the American College of Medical Genetics and Genomics (ACMG). *Genetics in Medicine*, *23*(5), 799–812. https://doi.org/10.1038/s41436-021-01115-y

Stuppia, L., Antonucci, I., Palka, G., & Gatta, V. (2012). Use of the MLPA assay in the molecular diagnosis of gene copy number alterations in human genetic diseases. *International Journal of Molecular Sciences*, *13*(3), 3245–3276. https://doi.org/10.3390/ijms13033245

Terasaki, A., Nakamura, M., Urata, Y., Hiwatashi, H., Yokoyama, I., Yasuda, T., Onuma, T., Wada, K., Kaneko, S., Kan, R., Niwa, S. I., Hashimoto, O., Komure, O., Goto, Y. I., Yamagishi, Y., Nakano, M., Furusawa, Y., & Sano, A. (2021). DNA analysis of benign adult familial myoclonic epilepsy reveals associations between the pathogenic TTTCA repeat insertion in

SAMD12 and the nonpathogenic TTTTA repeat expansion in TNRC6A. *Journal of Human Genetics, 66*(4), 419–429. https://doi.org/10.1038/s10038-020-00855-0

Thiffault, I., Farrow, E., Zellmer, L., Berrios, C., Miller, N., Gibson, M., Caylor, R., Jenkins, J., Faller, D., Soden, S., & Saunders, C. (2018). Clinical genome sequencing in an unbiased pediatric cohort. *Genetics in Medicine, 21*(2), 303–310. https://doi.org/10.1038/s41436-018-0075-8

Tilemis, F. N., Marinakis, N. M., Veltra, D., Svingou, M., Kekou, K., Mitrakos, A., Tzetis, M., Kosma, K., Makrythanasis, P., Traeger-Synodinos, J., & Sofocleous, C. (2023). Germline CNV detection through whole-exome sequencing (WES) data analysis enhances resolution of rare genetic diseases. *Genes (Basel), 14*(7). https://doi.org/10.3390/genes14071490

United States. (1996). Health Insurance Portability and Accountability Act of 1996. Public Law 104–191. *US Statut Large, 110*, 1936–2103. https://www.ncbi.nlm.nih.gov/pubmed/16477734

Wallace, S. E., & Bean L. J. H. (2020, June 18). Educational materials—Genetic testing: Current approaches. In M. P. Adam, J. Feldman, G. M. Mirzaa, R. A. Pagon, S. E. Wallace, L. J. H. Bean, K. W. Gripp, & A. Amemiya (Eds.), *GeneReviews*®. University of Washington, Seattle. https://www.ncbi.nlm.nih.gov/books/NBK279899/

Zhou, G., Zhou, M., Zeng, F., Zhang, N., Sun, Y., Qiao, Z., Guo, X., Zhou, S., Yun, G., Xie, J., Wang, X., Liu, F., Fan, C., Wang, Y., Fang, Z., Tian, Z., Dai, W., Sun, J., Peng, Z., & Song, L. (2022). Performance characterization of PCR-free whole genome sequencing for clinical diagnosis. *Medicine (Baltimore), 101*(10), e28972. https://doi.org/10.1097/MD.0000000000028972

Zion, T. N., Berrios, C. D., Cohen, A. S. A., Bartik, L., Cross, L. A., Engleman, K. L., Fleming, E. A., Gadea, R. N., Hughes, S. S., Jenkins, J. L., Kussmann, J., Lawson, C., Schwager, C., Strenk, M. E., Welsh, H., Rush, E. T., Amudhavalli, S. M., Sullivan, B. R., Zhou, D., . . . Pastinen, T. (2023). Insurance denials and diagnostic rates in a pediatric genomic research cohort. *Genetics in Medicine, 25*(5), 100020. https://doi.org/10.1016/j.gim.2023.100020

CHAPTER 17

AFTER THE TEST
Interpreting a Clinical Report

ISABELLE THIFFAULT AND CAROL J. SAUNDERS

Introduction

Genetic testing has undergone a dramatic transformation with the implementation of next-generation sequencing (NGS). Initial testing methodologies, such as karyotype and single gene testing, provided valuable results but were limited in diagnostic yields. As technology has advanced, including the advent of NGS, genetic testing has become increasingly complex. As an example, exome sequencing (ES) and genome sequencing (GS) are now the recommended first-line tests for children with developmental delay (Manickam et al., 2021). It follows that with increasing test complexity there is also an increased interpretation burden. Clinical laboratories follow established guidelines for the interpretation of variants (Richards et al., 2015; Riggs et al., 2020). However, for a nonlaboratory clinician these frameworks may be difficult to understand and are prone to misuse (Berrios et al., 2021). Genetic counselors are often tasked with interpreting genetic test results for both clinicians and families. This chapter will provide a brief overview of genetic testing, examine interpretation guidelines, and provide a framework for genetic counselors on how to approach a negative test result.

Types of Genetic Tests

Many different methods are currently used in genetic testing laboratories, with the type of test governed by the type of variation being assessed. Such tests in general may be divided into those that detect structural variation (SV) or single nucleotide variation (SNV) and those, like NGS, that have recently developed dual capabilities.[1]

[1] Editors' note: For further discussion on genetic variation and testing, see Chapter 16 by Lee A. Zellmer and Emily G. Farrow in this volume.

SV has an important role in genetic disease and is defined as variation affecting more than 50 base pairs. This may include deletions, insertions, inversions, mobile element transpositions, translocations, tandem repeats, and copy number variants (CNVs). SVs may involve whole chromosomes, large segments including whole genes, or portions of genes, which may be detected using karyotype or array-comparative hybridization, depending on the resolution required. Such testing is often performed as a genome-wide interrogation, without a particular target in mind.

Another technique used for copy number testing of specific genes is multiple ligation probe assay (MLPA), which relies on hybridization of probes covering each exon and polymerase chain reaction (PCR), the results of which are normalized against a control. Methylation-sensitive MLPA is a comprehensive test for Prader-Willi/Angelman syndrome, allowing simultaneous detection of methylated and unmethylated DNA as well as copy number. As such, not only can it determine whether a 15q11.2 deletion is present but also, unlike fluorescence in situ hybridization, which only detects copy number, it can infer the parental origin based on the methylation pattern, thus determining whether the patient has Prader-Willi syndrome or Angelman syndrome. For this test, regardless of whether the clinical suspicion is Prader-Willi syndrome or Angelman syndrome, the same assay is run for each patient.

The expansion of simple sequence repeats is another important testing category that requires specific gene targeting. More than 50 diseases, most of which are primarily neurological, are caused by unstable expanded repeats of varying sizes. Expanded repeats are dynamic variations that often present with somatic and gonadal mosaicism and change size in successive generations, with growing repeat expansions resulting in more severe disease with earlier onset, a phenomenon known as anticipation. Moreover, depending on the size of the repeat expansion, the diseases can manifest with markedly varied phenotypes and age of onset (Kong et al., 2017; Zhou et al., 2022). Detection of expanded repeats is most commonly ascertained by PCR and fragment analysis, an example being CGG repeat analysis in *FMR1* for the detection of fragile X syndrome. There are versions of this test that detect abnormal methylation, and those that simply reveal abnormal copy number. Testing for other repeat expansion disorders relies on similar principles, with the gene target and expansion range varying according to the disease in question.

Variants affecting single nucleotides or small insertions/deletions (generally less than 25 base pairs) are, with few exceptions, tested by sequencing-based technologies. Sanger sequencing was the mainstay in the 1990s/2000s for testing everything from single genes to large panels of genes, with the list of targets governed by heterogeneity or lack thereof (Sanger et al., 1977). For example, achondroplasia is due to variation at a recurrent variant at a single codon, p.Gly308Arg, and 99% of affected individuals have this or a different nucleotide variant affecting the same position in *FGFR3* (Legare, 1998), which can be interrogated by a single targeted sequence reaction. Sanger sequencing remains an efficient option in cases where there is a specific target, such as familial testing where at-risk relatives are being tested for one or two variants of interest. By contrast, although cystic fibrosis is a single gene disorder and there is a panel of common *CFTR* variants accounting for most cases, there are over 1,500 pathogenic variants reported, necessitating full gene sequencing in some cases. Other conditions, such as nonspecific neurodevelopmental disorders, have an ever-expanding list of potential causative genes, requiring a much broader approach to diagnosis.

Broad testing approaches commonly include NGS-based techniques, which are now widely available clinically, including targeted panels as well as ES and GS. Briefly, ES requires a selection step, also called enrichment, to target the coding region, representing ~2% of the genome. The depth of coverage for an exome is not uniform; therefore, the analytical sensitivity of ES may be lower than some disease-targeted gene panels, which should ideally cover every nucleotide of interest and potentially at a higher level than ES. However, ES has a higher overall diagnostic yield compared to panel testing due to its broader coverage. GS, as its name implies, covers both coding and noncoding sequences, with several advantages: It requires no enrichment step prior to sequencing, which saves time and provides more even, albeit lower, coverage than ES. Despite obtaining more sequence than ES, it is debatable whether GS offers increased diagnostic yield since the added coverage is mostly in noncoding regions, which are largely uninterpretable in the clinical laboratory setting. In addition, GS coverage is lower overall than ES or NGS panels, limiting the sensitivity to detect mosaicism. Whereas exonic deletions are not detectable by Sanger sequencing, analysis of copy number variation is increasingly possible for both ES and GS.

The type of test, whether targeted panel, ES, or GS, determines the number of variants that will be generated, which range from ~150,000 for ES to 3.5 to 5 million for GS, depending on the reference and ethnicity of the individual being tested. However, it is important to realize that there is a high degree of interlaboratory variability in the upstream processes in terms of what is targeted, sequencing methodology, variant detection, annotation, filtering, interpretation, and reporting. Exomes are not all the same, and none of them are "whole"—there are regions that drop out due to sequence makeup or complexity. Additional enrichment for problem areas may be used to ameliorate this and will differ from lab to lab, resulting in variability in coverage.

How one defines the region analyzed is variable as well; while the exome is clearly defined as the coding exons of the genome, the analysis should also include splice junctions. The amount of intronic sequence analyzed is highly dependent on the laboratory; some labs may only report ±2 base pairs on either side of an exon, while other laboratories will analyze up to ±20 base pairs into the intronic regions. Other intronic or other noncoding regions are likely not analyzed unless a variant is within the targeted region and has been previously reported as pathogenic. This variability extends to synonymous variants as well, which do not change the amino acid codon but can potentially lead to aberrant splicing. While most pathogenic variants are thought to lie within the codon regions, for some conditions common intronic or noncoding variants are an important part of the variant spectrum. Examples include cystic fibrosis (Bergougnoux et al., 2019), retinopathies (Qian et al., 2021), primary carnitine deficiency (Ferdinandusse et al., 2019), and Leber congenital amaurosis (Perrault et al., 2021). Indeed, more than half of Leber congenital amaurosis cases are associated with a deep intronic variant, c.2991+1655A>G in *CEP290*, which is generally not captured by ES (Sheck et al., 2018; Valkenburg et al., 2018). In addition, some laboratories include the mitochondrial genome in their NGS analysis; for others, this is a separate test not captured by exome kits (Dinwiddie et al., 2013).

Regardless of all the upstream variability involved, variant analysis critically involves filtering and prioritization of variants. The decision of which variants to include for consideration as well as the interpretation process itself remains highly subjective. Variant calling, interpretation software, and professional interpretation are highly variable from laboratory to laboratory, resulting in differences in what is reported and how it is described in the clinical context. For instance, some laboratories do not report variants of uncertain significance or secondary/unanticipated findings for ES unless specifically requested. Standards and guidelines to address many of these points are lacking. To date, there are no recommended guidelines for bioinformatic algorithms, interpretation software, and types of variants that should be included in clinical testing reports.

The American College of Medical Genetics and Genomics (ACMG) published a revision of technical standards and guidance for the clinical use of NGS-based techniques in 2021 (Rehder et al., 2021). While this document is intended to promote quality detection, interpretation, and reporting of variants by NGS, the adherence to these recommendations is voluntary. For example, it is suggested that the targeted regions should minimally include all coding exons with sufficient intronic coverage to allow the analysis of positions of the donor site (−1 to −16 base pairs) and acceptor site (+1 to + 5 base pairs). Moreover, it is recommended that laboratories design additional target probes or provide Sanger sequencing to ensure proper coverage of regions with known recurrent pathogenic variants. Genomic regions with technical difficulty may be excluded from analysis to avoid reporting false-positive or false-negative calls. However, clinically relevant genomic regions should be considered for testing by a second testing type (orthogonal methodology) if unreliably assessed by NGS. If not, disclosures are needed at reporting. A nondiagnostic result by NGS should not be considered definitive. Healthcare providers should interact with the laboratory, provide detailed phenotypic information, and consider reanalysis in a timely manner. It is important for clinicians to recognize the limitations of any test ordered, and the ordering provider should understand the reporting policy of the laboratory.

Understanding Variant Interpretation

Understanding test results in the era of NGS is intuitively more complicated, and the sheer number of variants generated necessitated guidelines for a more standardized approach to sequence variant interpretation as well as the nomenclature used to describe pathogenicity. To address this problem, the ACMG and the Association for Molecular Pathology (AMP) published guidelines in 2015 that provide a more structured approach for sequence variant interpretation (Richards et al., 2015). Prior to the ACMG/AMP guidelines, clinical laboratories each had their own criteria for variant classification and applied varying terminology to describe pathogenicity, breeding interlaboratory discordance of up to 60% for the interpretation of the same variant (Pepin et al., 2016).

These guidelines only apply to genes with well-established associations with Mendelian conditions with relatively high penetrance; they are not intended for the interpretation of complex traits, mitochondrial variants, or pharmacogenetic variants. Although clinicians do not need to understand the criteria in detail, it is helpful to understand the framework that laboratories are using to classify individual variants in reporting. In this way, clinicians, particularly genetic counselors, can better understand why a particular variant was classified and what limitations there were in classification and may assist in gathering additional information.

Assessing variant pathogenicity

Leveraging the current guidelines, variants are broadly categorized according to a five-tier system describing pathogenicity: pathogenic (P), likely pathogenic (LP), variant of uncertain significance (VUS), likely benign (LB), or benign (B) (Richards et al., 2015). The terms LP and LB are intended to indicate at least 90% certainty for a variant to be pathogenic or benign, respectively. The guidelines provide a framework to classify variants within these five classes based on the combination of weighted evidence defined by criteria that broadly fall into the following categories of evidence types: population data, allelic evidence and cosegregation data, computational and predictive criteria, functional studies, and "other." Each piece of evidence, whether for or against pathogenicity, is assigned a measure of strength and a point system: supportive (P), moderate (M), strong (S), very strong (VS), or standalone. Each individual criterion (PVS1, PS1, PS2, PS3, PS4, PM1, PM2, PM3, PM4, PM5, PM6, PP1, PP2, PP3, PP4, PP5, BA1, BS1, BS2, BS3, BS4, BP1, BP2, BP3, BP4, BP5, BP6, BP7) is assigned a point system that is modified based on the strength of the data (Richards et al., 2015). Collectively the points awarded for each variant are combined to determine the classification of a variant. The guidelines continue to be revised; however, the basic tenets of gathering evidence systematically for variant interpretation remain the same.

Five criteria fall under the population data category (Table 17.1). The only standalone evidence available relates to population data and may be applied as benign criteria when the minor allele frequency (MAF) exceeds 5%, meaning the variant is observed in greater than 5% of the population, provided it is not a founder allele. A variant with a MAF greater than

Table 17.1 Criteria for Variant Interpretation

Evidence category	ACMG criteria[a]	Description
Population data	PS4, PM2, BA1, BS1	Criteria that evaluate enrichment in affected individuals and allele frequency in control populations
Allelic evidence and segregation data	PS2, PM6, PP1 and BS4, BP2, BP5	Criteria that evaluate inheritance patterns and occurrence of variant in affected/unaffected individuals
Variant impact (predicted null)	PVS1	Loss-of-function variant (premature stop, frameshift, canonical splice variant, small deletion, etc.)
Functional analyses	PS1, PS3, PM1, PM3, PM4, PM5, PP2, PP3, BS3, BP1, BP3, BP4, BP7	Criteria that evaluate the functional consequence of each variant, from in vitro/animal models to predictive algorithms
Phenotypic characteristics	PP4	Patient's phenotype is highly specific for a specific disorder

Note: ACMG = American College of Medical Genetics and Genomics; AMP = Association for Molecular Pathology.

[a] A detailed description of the ACMG interpretation criteria and the pathogenicity calculation can be found in the ACMG and AMP sequence variant interpretation guidelines (Richards et al., 2015).

expected for the disorder but less than 5% is considered to have strong evidence for a benign classification. Establishing B/LB variants is important, as laboratories will not include them in clinical reports as a general rule. Conversely, if a variant is absent in control populations, this is evidence for supporting pathogenicity. The remaining population criteria assess the presence of a variant in unaffected individuals or enrichment in affected individuals compared to population controls, both of which ideally depend on the population controls being well phenotyped (Richards et al., 2015).

In light of the subjective nature of population frequencies, disease-specific guidelines have been developed to supplement general interpretation guidelines (Gelb et al., 2018; Hall et al., 2018; Lee et al., 2018; Oza et al., 2018; Patel et al., 2021). These guidelines are created by Clinical Genome Resource (ClinGen) expert panels, panels of disease experts that have revised interpretation criteria for specific diseases, such as RASopathy (Variant Curation Expert Panels [VCEPs], https://clinicalgenome.org/docs/clingen-variant-curation-expert-panel-vcep-protocol/). In these revised guidelines, as an example, in the absence of case-control studies for rare disorders, they specify proband counts for evaluating enrichment in disease populations, allowing modifications of the strength of evidence. ClinGen expert panel interpretation guidelines are available on the ClinGen website and updated by each panel (https://www.clinicalgenome.org/affiliation/).

Of course, the familial context of a variant is important in clinical genetics, and there are multiple criteria relevant to allelic evidence and cosegregation data. In evaluating inheritance, careful judgment must be applied, particularly if the gene or disease is known to have incomplete penetrance or variable expressivity, or carrier(s) were not well clinically evaluated. The presence of a de novo variant is considered strong evidence in situations where parents are unaffected, relationships have been confirmed, and the variant is in a gene associated with a specific phenotype exhibited by the patient. The strength of this is downgraded to moderate or supportive in cases of less specific or highly heterogeneous phenotypes, and not used at all if the phenotype is inconsistent. It is worth noting that a variant may appear de novo, but if parentage has not been confirmed, then the points awarded are decreased.

New standards for evaluating constitutional CNV were published in 2019 (Riggs et al., 2020), which encourage the same five-tier classification system used in sequence variant interpretation, employ a semiquantitative point-based system, and recommend "uncoupling" variant interpretation from the potential implications for a specific individual. For example, the deletion of an autosomal recessive gene is pathogenic, although not diagnostic without a second pathogenic variant. The point-based system roughly corresponds to the strength categories in the sequencing guidelines: 0.90 or higher is very strong, 0.45 is strong, 0.30 is moderate, and 0.15 is supporting evidence. Importantly, they defer to sequence variant interpretation guidelines for small, intragenic deletions. In this vein, it is recognized that the deletion of a single gene where haploinsufficiency is the known mechanism is sufficient to be called pathogenic regardless of whether the specific event has been previously reported.

Both sets of guidelines provide rules for combining evidence to reach a given classification. For example, for sequence variant interpretation, a de novo (parentage-confirmed) nonsense variant, absent in population databases, for a gene like *ZEB2*, which conveys a recognizable and specific phenotype of Mowat-Wilson syndrome, due to haploinsufficiency, is easily pathogenic. The same variant can be interpreted as likely pathogenic even without parental samples, given the type of variant. However, a rare missense variant, even if affecting a highly conserved amino acid predicted to be deleterious by in silico tools, will remain a VUS without additional evidence, such as the variant lying in a known functional domain, familial studies to prove it arose as a *de novo* event, or segregation with disease.

Mitochondrial variant guidelines

Additional standards were published for evaluating variation in the mitochondrial genome (McCormick et al., 2020). Mitochondrial DNA (mtDNA) variant pathogenicity interpretation has special considerations given unique features of the mtDNA genome, including maternal inheritance; variant heteroplasmy, or number of mitochondria with a variant; threshold effect; absence of splicing and nonsense mediated decay; and contextual effects of haplogroups. The McCormick document expands on specific guidance related to mtDNA, including mtDNA annotations, standardized naming/nomenclature, reporting level of heteroplasmy/threshold, utilization of mtDNA genomic databases, computational algorithms, and scoring functional data, while remaining consistent with ACMG/AMP variant interpretation guidelines. ACMG criteria were reviewed for relevance to the mitochondrial genome (McCormick et al., 2020). Minimal modifications were made to the rules regarding de novo variants, but close attention must be paid to the testing method, the tissues tested, and the level of heteroplasmy. Given the lack of specificity of most mitochondrial variants, de novo variants should be modified to moderate strength. Functional studies were specifically addressed, citing transmitochondrial cybrid studies as the only functional data acceptable for evidence of pathogenicity. Biochemical studies to assess electron transport chain and oxidative phosphorylation function may be performed in patient cell lines but support a mitochondrial defect, not the specific mtDNA variant in question. Furthermore, biochemical defect/enzymatic deficiency (less than 20% of normal activity of controls) should be correlated to the level of heteroplasmy. In addition, several factors must be considered when utilizing data from a database for purposes of mtDNA variant curation:

- Caution must be used when considering mtDNA sequences generated from ES or GS as it may contain nuclear DNA mitochondrial pseudogenes. With regard to the mitochondrial genome, the quality and nature of sequence databases are not "equal."
- Several mitochondrial haplogroups are underrepresented.
- Low or absent variant allele frequencies are expected in control datasets with a few exceptions, one example being a common pathogenic variant, m.11778G>A, with a frequency above 1%, associated with Leber hereditary optic neuropathy.
- In most control data sets, heteroplasmy is not reported.

Another significant difference is due to the quantitative nature of mtDNA inheritance. Healthy or mildly affected individuals are expected to have low or undetectable heteroplasmy levels in various tissues. To simplify the "weight" accorded to segregation studies, the expert panel proposed that the above criteria in five or more maternal family members are moderate evidence for pathogenicity and in two to four maternal family members are supporting evidence for pathogenicity. While the above specifications generally hold true, this rule cannot be applied when a variant is not known to have variable heteroplasmy levels across tissues and maternal family members or if present at homoplasmy in all family members.

As such, lack of mtDNA variant segregation in affected matrilineal family members and variable heteroplasmy levels are evidence for benign classification. Moreover, the features of mitochondrial disease are nonspecific and exhibit variable expressivity. Therefore, to meet enrichment or phenotypic criteria, the proband must have a recurrent pathogenic mtDNA variant. In this regard, it is recognized that expertise directly influences variant assessment of the mtDNA genome.

Efforts to Reduce Discrepancy

Although the ACMG/AMP guidelines represent a major step forward to the standardization of variant classification, several factors still contribute to differences in variant interpretation. The rules for variant interpretation are highly nuanced and continually evolving, combining available evidence, which differs according to internal data and case-specific details. In addition, there is a degree of subjectivity encountered for some criteria, which will foster differences between curators based on expertise and experience. One study found that the criterion of a patient's phenotype is highly specific for a gene with a single etiology to be the most problematic in terms of consistency of application due to subjectivity in deciding the specificity of the phenotype in question (Amendola et al., 2016). In addition, the application of criteria likely differs according to the expertise of the individual user and is subject to human error. For some criteria, such as cosegregation data, the strength of evidence may be modified at the curator's discretion, which will differ according to human judgment. As a result, variant interpretation still differs between different laboratories and even between different curators within the same laboratory. In addition to having differences related to curator-level subjectivity, laboratories may use internally modified versions of the guidelines, which results in further discrepancy (Nykamp et al., 2017).

To utilize the full potential of NGS, precise variant classification and interpretation are essential for the diagnosis of patients and the implementation of appropriate management, genetic counseling, and potential therapy. To decrease some of the subjectivity, Amendola et al. recommended the following: (a) developing disease-specific allele frequency thresholds to enable lowering of the standalone benign criteria from an MAF of greater than 5% to disease-appropriate values; (b) establishing a resource of all genes to define whether loss of function is a known mechanism of disease (ClinGen dosage, https://search.clinicalgenome.org/kb/gene-dosage); (c) providing recommendations for which in silico prediction tools are best in practice; (d) defining what "well established" functional data apply and when strength should be decreased; (e) developing quantitative thresholds of evidence for and against segregation of different strengths; and (f) promoting the development of software tools that automate computable aspects of the ACMG/AMP guidelines (Amendola et al., 2016).

To address variability in the use of criteria related to the consideration of functional data, the ClinGen clinical validity framework offers guidance, giving more weight to in vivo data (model systems) compared to in vitro (function and functional alteration) experimental data (Kanavy et al., 2019; Strande et al., 2017). Furthermore, VCEPs published guidance related to experimental evidence, both in vivo and in vitro, for specific genes to reduce inconsistencies in clinical interpretation. In addition, they established criteria for evaluating and scoring functional studies based on disease mechanism, general class of assay, and the characteristics of specific assays. Such VCEP-approved assays are intended to standardize curation and improve consistency in variant interpretation. Integration of VCEP-approved assays or robust functional analysis into routine clinical laboratory tests would be ideal but challenging. Some of these challenges include the requirement of specialized expertise, billing cost, and collaboration with research laboratories. Knowledge of the mechanism of disease is essential, and experiments can only be designed if the pathway or structural effect is known, as is the case for ciliopathies, channelopathies, and mitochondrial disorders. Such knowledge is obviously not available for every gene or variant.

Another significant contribution from the VCEPs is the resolution of conflicting interpretations for variants with multiple submissions in ClinVar, which requires expert review to adjudicate. ClinVar is a freely available database that catalogs clinical classification of variants for diseases with supporting evidence, submitted by laboratories from around the world (Landrum et al., 2020). Differences in variant interpretations between clinical laboratories often occur due to variability in algorithms used for weighing evidence or differences in available evidence, such as internal variants reported, segregation studies performed, allele frequencies, and other data that may be stored in proprietary databases such as phenotypic descriptions. One report predating ClinVar found that 33% of interpretation differences between clinical laboratories were due to lack of access to privately held data (Pepin et al., 2016). To help users navigate ClinVar assertions, variant records are weighted by level of review supporting the interpretation, using a star system to provide graphical representation of the review status (Harrison et al., 2019). Variants with practice guideline–level assertions have four stars. Those curated by ClinGen expert panels have three stars. Two stars are assigned to variants with two or more independent submitters providing assertion criteria with consistent interpretation. The assignment of one star is given in two situations: (a) two or more independent submitters provided assertion criteria/evidence but conflicting interpretation and (b) only one submitter provided assertion criteria/evidence and interpretation.

ClinVar has been recognized by the U.S. Food and Drug Administration (FDA) since 2018 as a public human genetic variant database to support regulatory review of genetic and genomic tests (https://clinicalgenome.org/docs/fda-recognizes-clingen-assertions-in-clinvar-frequently-asked-questions/; https://www.fda.gov/media/119313/download). This FDA recognition program aims to improve access to privately held genetic data by encouraging laboratories to submit genetic variant data to publicly accessible databases, which are expected to contribute to the advancement of precision medicine. The FDA recognition supports that the genetic variant information in the ClinGen consortium's ClinGen Expert Curated Human Genetic Data, which is funded by the National Institutes of Health, is a valid source of scientific evidence that can be used to support the clinical validity of genetic testing and can improve patient care. To promote transparency, the record page of a variant reviewed by an expert panel includes interpretation status, evidence details, publications reviewed, links to relevant external databases, and the ClinGen VCEP page. To date, over 1,901,396 variants have been submitted to ClinVar (https://www.ncbi.nlm.nih.gov/clinvar/submitters/). However, there are only 663 records with practice guidelines (four stars) and 12,622 records from expert panels (three stars), leaving much work to be done in this effort.

Addressing Uncertainty

Although significant progress in developing bioinformatic prediction tools and data sharing has been achieved, challenges in variant interpretation still impede the diagnostic rate for rare genetic disorders. The clinical significance of reported variants can range from pathogenic to benign, but in many cases, the interpretation lies firmly in the middle in VUS territory—a highly unsatisfying answer for all parties involved as the uncertainty creates confusion and cannot be used for guiding management. Conservatism is preferred over false pathogenicity assignments, which can have adverse consequences for patient care, genetic counseling, and recurrence risk assessment. With few exceptions, a novel missense variant will be classified as a VUS if it cannot be shown to be de novo since, unlike a loss-of-function variant, the functional significance is often not predictable. Exceptions include when the gene is well characterized and known to have a functional domain and when different pathogenic variants affecting the same residue have been reported. Additional data that may help upgrade the variant to likely pathogenic include familial studies to show phasing, segregation, or proving a variant arose de novo. Further, more detailed patient phenotyping including imaging or laboratory studies is helpful when there is a finding such as a biochemical profile, enzyme test, or flow cytometry marker specifically ascribed to the gene of interest, in which case phenotypic criteria may be modified from supportive to moderate criteria and used in combination with other criteria to bring the variant to LP. Communication between the laboratory and healthcare providers, often genetic counselors, regarding the outcomes of such follow-up studies is highly important to capture the information and upgrade the variant interpretation as appropriate. The identification of additional patients harboring the variant in question may also result in reclassification; this may seem like a long shot but is made possible through data-sharing efforts such as ClinVar. In many cases, communication with the submitting laboratory yields useful information that assists in rare disease diagnosis.

In addition to discrepancy resolution for interpretations of individual variants, ClinGen has many expert teams engaged to evaluate the clinical validity of gene–disease relationships. Gene curations performed using ClinGen's standardized scoring procedure can help to clarify and strengthen the content of gene panels and enhance symptom-driven analysis. An entire class of uncertainty centers around variants in genes of uncertain significance (GUSs), which have insufficient evidence for a gene–disease association and, if reported, are automatically classified as VUSs as the application of ACMG interpretation criteria is restricted to genes with well-established associations. However, new disease–gene assertions are being made at an impressive rate, with around 40 OMIM entries cataloging new disease-associated genes per month (https://omim.org/statistics/update). The evidence behind such assertions must be thoroughly assessed to ensure accurate interpretation of genomic testing for the patient. ClinGen has guidelines for vetting such gene–disease assertions, which use scoring methods to weigh genetic and experimental data such as pathway, expression, functional studies, and animal models in the literature to classify assertions in a semiquantitative manner into one of six categories: definitive, strong, moderate, limited, disputed, or refuted (Strande et al., 2017). Regarding genes with less defined disease relationships, laboratories may differ in whether to include a variant in such a gene.

Although it is assumed that pathogenic variants associated with monogenic disorders are rare or private and highly penetrant, the clinical spectrum and penetrance are often limited by published data. Currently a little less than 50% of OMIM genes have been curated by ClinGen working groups (https://search.clinicalgenome.org/kb/reports/stats). Many genes associated with intellectual disability and autism spectrum disorders lack OMIM accession numbers, highlighting a specific need for focus in this area (Thiffault et al., 2018). The goal is to find a balance between the number of VUSs reported and not missing a potential diagnosis, particularly given the possibility that a VUS/GUS may by diagnostic. In some situations, not reporting VUSs/GUSs increases the risk of false-negative diagnoses and may limit access to further genetic testing, given potential insurance constraints.

Considerations for a Negative Result: What May Be Missed

Patients suspected to have a genetic disease may search for a diagnosis for years and spend thousands of dollars on testing only to have a negative or uncertain result. Depending on symptoms, family history, and overall level of suspicion, roughly 50% of patients will have a negative result. While some cases may be due to nongenetic causes such as infections or other environmental components, no test is perfect, and it is important to consider why variants may be missed:

- The wrong test may have been performed for the variant in question. As discussed earlier, some disorders require specific methods or targeted approaches that would not be captured by NGS or microarray, such as methylation disorders (Prader-Willi/Angelman, Beckwith-Wiedemann syndrome, Silver-Russell syndrome) or triplet repeat expansions (fragile X syndrome, myotonic dystrophy, spinocerebellar ataxias, Friedreich's ataxia, Huntington's disease, and others). Another example is missing a deletion in a patient not tested for copy number changes. If tested by array, the deletion must be in the detectable size range. Some deletions are in the size range that falls between what is detectable by sequencing (~25 base pairs or less) and microarray, which is variable according to probe density and reporting practice. Only recently have laboratories started doing copy number from NGS (Truty et al., 2019).
- The correct test was performed but the variant was not detected (false negative). Examples include allele dropout in testing that relies on PCR, where an allele does not amplify and is lost, which can happen when variants interfere with primer binding. There are also structural complexes that preclude accurate PCR and Sanger sequencing (Saunders et al., 2010). For NGS-based sequencing, there are difficult regions of the genome to sequence, such as homopolymers or regions with high homology to other sequences in the genome, as is the case with pseudogenes. There are many examples of disorders impacted by homology, including common diseases such as spinal muscular atrophy, congenital adrenal hyperplasia, and autosomal recessive polycystic kidney disease. Such regions also affect microarray analysis. An undetectable variant could also relate to test design, such as insufficient probe density on array, or a method

failure, such as the bioinformatic pipeline failing to call a variant by NGS or annotating it incorrectly. The variant could also be present at a level not detectable by the method, such as a mosaic or heteroplasmic variant. The variant may not be detectable in blood, as some are only present in certain tissues, as in the case of overgrowth conditions, segmental neurofibromatosis, mitochondrial disorders, and others.

- The variant was detectable but was not reported. There are many potential reasons for this, including the variant falling outside the reportable region, such as a deep intronic variant or other noncoding region. Even if sequenced, as previously mentioned, laboratories limit the flanking intronic regions reported, and this varies greatly by lab, ranging from ±2 to 20 or more nucleotides in the intronic region flanking a coding exon. Synonymous variants also may not be reported by the lab; these are variants that change the nucleotide but not the amino acid codon, which often have no impact on protein function but in some cases affect splicing. In the case of ES or GS where the patient's phenotype is used to guide analysis and reporting, the gene may be judged to be unrelated to the reason for referral and variants omitted by the reporting lab. For example, a VUS in a gene associated with seizures detected in an infant referred for failure to thrive may not be reported; however, this variant would likely be reported on reanalysis with new symptoms of seizures. If the variant in question is pathogenic and not related to the present symptoms, whether it is reported depends on individual laboratory policy, which varies greatly between labs. Some laboratories do not report VUSs unless requested; the reporting of GUSs is similarly variable.

Following Up: After a Negative or Uncertain Test Result

If genetic testing failed to provide a diagnosis for the patient, the next steps vary according to situation and can be challenging for genetic counselors to navigate. A logical first step is to carefully review all previous test results. Strategies for next steps can be broken down into negative results with no variants reported and reports disclosing a VUS or GUS.

Negative results with no reported variants

For negative results, testing should be reviewed for completeness. Keep in mind what each testing methodology does and does not detect as described earlier—all testing has limitations.

- For some indications, the tissue type and depth of coverage are very important; the affected tissue may be needed, requiring a tissue biopsy. Some testing indications, such as overgrowth syndromes, require especially high depth of coverage not offered by routine testing, given the high incidence of mosaicism.
- If only a subset of genes was sequenced as a panel, consider broader testing such as ES/GS. One consideration is that many panels are bioinformatically created from ES, and resequencing may not be required.

- If ES/GS has been completed, were parental samples included? If available, parental samples are very helpful for highlighting de novo events, particularly missense variants in genes that may have been otherwise overlooked due to an atypical presentation. Sometimes when reevaluated, a variant previously overlooked due to lack of phenotypic correlation is relevant due to phenotypic expansion.
- The reporting policy of the laboratory should be reviewed. Were VUSs and GUSs included? If not, are they available by request?
- If ES/GS was done over 2 years ago, consider resequencing or requesting bioinformatic repipelining for new gene and variant annotations.
- If deletion/duplication has not been performed, consider CNV analysis to detect intragenic events.
- Metabolomic or methylome testing may be considered, as appropriate (Almontashiri et al., 2020; Liu et al., 2021; Schenkel et al., 2021).
- If clinical testing has been exhausted, alternative options may be considered. Consider offering enrollment in an appropriate research study, where newer methods, such as long-read sequencing, may be explored. Although research studies may provide additional options, it is important to remember that many individuals may not qualify for research given regulations for consent, and this can be limiting.

Negative results with a VUS or GUS

For results where a VUS or GUS was disclosed, the variants should be carefully evaluated. This encompasses microarray results, and considerations for CNVs include following:

- Deletions may be noted that were not known to be disease associated at the time but may contain regions currently known to be haploinsufficient. Intervals should be examined in ClinGen for genes with high pLi, meaning they are intolerant to loss-of-function variation; candidates should be evaluated for disease associations in the literature. Public databases provide a gene's pLi score by comparing the observed number of loss-of-function variants within the database to the expected number, based on genetic equilibrium (Tanner et al., 2022). Additional publicly available resources that can be helpful are Decipher and the UCSC Genome Brower.
- Duplications should be evaluated on a case-by-case basis for their potential to be inverted and disrupting haploinsufficient gene(s). If there is a compelling candidate, breakpoints can be sequenced by a second method, such as Sanger sequencing.
- Was there a VUS call on array, deleting an autosomal recessive gene of potential interest for the patient? If so, was the other allele sequenced?

Sequence variants should also be reevaluated. Performing a literature search for updates can often be helpful for both gene- and variant-level data. Candidate variants should be investigated as appropriate. Follow-up recommendations should also be reviewed. The following questions should be considered: Were segregation or parental studies recommended? Were they completed? Is there a biochemical or other test that may help with interpretation?

Evaluating new depositions into ClinVar may facilitate the identification of additional patients with a particular variant. Individual laboratories may be contacted for clinical context and available data; if identified in the de novo state in an affected individual, then this information is useful for interpretation. The testing laboratory may contact ClinVar; however, in the interim genetic counselors may also reach out to laboratories for additional information on individual submissions.

GUSs are often entered into GeneMatcher, a matchmaking service that helps clinicians, laboratory directors, and researchers find additional individuals to gather evidence for gene–disease associations and genotype–phenotype correlations by the testing laboratory. GeneMatcher is a resource that can be used by clinicians, genetic counselors, researchers, and families to facilitate gene discovery. The publication of such findings is of the utmost importance to the genetics community.

Research partnerships can be useful. In some cases, it may be possible to find a researcher with interest in the gene or variant in question who may be able to design an animal or cellular model for further evaluation.

Increasingly, testing laboratories have a lab utilization team, with genetic counselors. It can be particularly helpful for patient-facing genetic counselors to contact laboratory-based peers to discuss specific cases and results.

Reinterpretation of Clinical Results

The utility of doing a formal reinterpretation hinges largely on previous findings (e.g., VUS/GUS), how much time has elapsed since the original analysis, and whether additional samples such as those from parents and/or siblings are available for segregation studies. In the United States, a current procedural terminology (CPT) billing code for insurance does exist for the reanalysis of existing data; however, individual laboratories will have their own policies on the time required before a reanalysis can be requested and the associated cost. The availability of new data, whether it is variant or gene specific, may help prove a gene–disease association in the case of a GUS, which requires the identification of additional individuals harboring variants in the same GUS.

Sometimes a genetic finding is judged to be not clinically relevant for a patient because of a perceived lack of phenotypic overlap. Indeed, the early literature was populated with reports of patients ascertained by a specific set of clinical criteria and tested for the relevant gene(s). With ES/GS widely in use in the clinic, the reverse approach is often applied, where broad testing is performed and not directed or limited to a specific subset of genes. With this may come surprising diagnoses; that is, patients with atypical features are found to have a pathogenic variant in a gene that was not on the differential. As a result, there is a growing recognition of phenotypic expansion for many disorders. Such observations of expanded phenotypes are important to report in the literature for the broader genetics community (Gannamani et al., 2021; Weerakkody et al., 2016; Yu & Zhang, 2015). In addition, patients may develop additional phenotypic features that warrant evaluation for relevance of previously detected variants.

Patient-Centered Interpretation

Optimal clinical evaluation (e.g., physical, biochemical, histopathological, imaging, etc.) and familial history are often essential to achieve a molecular diagnosis, which is important for establishing prognosis, necessary follow-up, treatment, and genetic counseling. A pathogenic variant does not necessarily mean a diagnosis for the individual, since elements such as inheritance pattern of the gene in question, incomplete penetrance, and age of onset factor in. Incomplete penetrance and variable expressivity are encountered frequently in the diagnostic setting and may complicate interpretation, particularly when a child is diagnosed with an autosomal dominant condition and parental testing reveals an unexpected heterozygosity in a parent who does not qualify as having the diagnosis. Similarly, a child with developmental delay found to have a pathogenic *BRCA1* variant has an increased lifetime risk of cancer, but this finding is not diagnostic in this setting. In addition, a heterozygous pathogenic deletion including an autosomal recessive gene indicates only carrier status unless there is a second pathogenic allele. If the individual shows signs of the disease in question, then the finding may be diagnostic and sequencing the other allele is necessary. Array guidelines address this situation; whereas the deletion of a recessive gene previously would be classified as VUS or other if not diagnostic for the patient, the guidelines recommend uncoupling the interpretation of the variant from the patient's clinical status.

Barriers to Obtaining a Diagnostic Result

Rare diseases by nature have few or no other patients with a specific variant, variant type, or gene association. Many pathogenic variants are private variants that have never been previously reported; the chance of finding another patient with the exact variant may be unlikely, particularly in the absence of data sharing. Many pathogenic variants are de novo, particularly for neurodevelopmental disorders, and as mentioned, this is a highly weighted criterion for variant interpretation. When parental samples are unavailable, there is often insufficient evidence to reach pathogenicity when de novo status is unknown. The availability of other family members to be tested for segregation studies may also be limiting. Lack of available relevant functional studies to assess variant pathogenicity is also problematic. A general lack of knowledge of the potential phenotypes and the variant spectrum as well as important protein domains, particularly for genes with new disease associations, limits accurate variant interpretation. Indeed, many reanalyzes resulting in new diagnoses are due to new gene–disease associations or updated information/knowledge about variant interpretation or inheritance (Shashi et al., 2019; Tan et al., 2020; Wright et al., 2018). Finally, disparities in access to genetic testing are associated with reduced diagnostic rates, particularly for underrepresented minorities (Bonkowsky et al., 2018; Clarke et al., 2021; Edwards et al., 2020; Landry & Rehm, 2018). Most (greater than 70%) large-scale genetic studies focus on populations of European ancestry (Martin et al., 2019). This is exacerbated for diseases such as hearing loss and cardiomyopathy, which do not have reduced reproductive fitness and have fewer observations of de novo variants for evidence of pathogenicity. Furthermore, these diseases have a high burden of missense variants, which are difficult to interpret without multiple case observations and/or functional studies to implicate the variants in disease. Thus, these disorders are likely to suffer more significantly from a poor ethnicity representation (Clarke et al., 2021; Landry & Rehm, 2018).

New Technology

Advances in sequencing have changed the approach to diagnosing rare disease, in both clinical and research environments. Despite these advances, the rate of diagnosis remains ~30%, partially due to the technical limitations of current or short-read sequencing methods to detect certain types of variants such as SVs, repetitive elements, guanine-cytosine–rich content, or sequences with multiple homologous elements. Long-read or third-generation sequencing offers advantages over short-read sequencing, as the long-read sequencing reads, which are ~15,000 base pairs in length, are better able to detect SVs, repeat expansions, and mapping certainty across problematic regions such as those with high homology (Borras et al., 2017; Corbett et al., 2019; Frans et al., 2018; Florian et al., 2019; Hiatt et al., 2021; Ishiura et al., 2018; Miao et al., 2018; Miller et al., 2021; Su et al., 2021). In addition, it allows variant phasing and the potential for de novo assembly (Amarasinghe et al., 2020). Furthermore, long-read sequencing is completed without the use of PCR amplification, reducing amplification bias while preserving methylation modifications, allowing for the capture of sequencing and methylation in a single assay. It is important to note that the output of long-read sequencing differs greatly from short-read sequencing, requiring tailored analysis tools (Amarasinghe et al., 2020; Jiang et al., 2021; Senol Cali et al., 2019). Despite the fast-paced development of such applications, the scalability, comparably higher cost, and lower throughput currently limit their use clinically.

The role of new tools to assess functional significance of VUSs

The resolution of a VUS remains a difficult task for researchers, laboratories, clinicians including genetic counselors, and families. While the assays needed to fully resolve each VUS are not currently available, new tools are being developed and may provide resolution in the future. It is helpful for clinicians to be aware of developing methods to assist in functional studies. Two emerging approaches for evaluating the functional consequences of a variant are briefly described below as examples of the types of assays that can be leveraged.

Traditional experimental assays that measure the variant impact on protein function, expression, and/or localization lack the throughput needed and remain expensive. Multiplexed assays of variant effects (MAVEs), such as deep mutational scanning (DMS), resolve this bottleneck by measuring the effects of thousands of variants on a particular function or cellular property simultaneously (Gasperini et al., 2016; Weile & Roth, 2018). MAVEs have shown utility for several types of variation, particularly in regulatory/noncoding regions, in numerous genes. However, disease-related proteins have multiple functions, and, generally, no single large-scale variant effect data set can capture all of them. Thus, multiple distinct

MAVEs might be needed to accurately stratify variants by their impact on the biochemical or cellular activity of interest (Esposito et al., 2019; Gasperini et al., 2016).

CRISPR (clustered regularly interspaced short palindromic repeats)–based tools offer several options to mutagenesis of in vivo and in vitro models. CRISPR-based tools may be used to identify variations that confer drug response or resistance and for the mouse knock-in model of human diseases, where a specific variant or human sequence is inserted to study the effect in the mouse. The scope of base editing tools has exponentially broadened, allowing higher efficiency, specificity, and accessibility to complex regions. CRISPR base editing in patients' cells has been recently applied to characterize variants' impact on protein function and pathogenicity (Cuella-Martin et al., 2021; Hanna et al., 2021). It is anticipated that CRISPR base editing screens will enable the discovery of gene function or cellular phenotypes, expediting variant characterization, and thus VUS reclassification. It is anticipated that these tools, in addition to novel patient-derived assays, will continue to be developed, providing a much-needed functional assay for interpretation (McQuerry et al., 2022).

Conclusion

In summary, variant interpretation remains an evolving field, continually changing to keep pace with technological advances. As genetic testing is increasingly utilized, genetic counselors are playing critical roles in the interpretation of clinical testing results, for both ordering providers and families. While the laboratory is responsible for providing the interpretation and results for genetic testing, genetic counselors should broadly be aware of how variant interpretation is completed in order to understand the testing. Further, a general knowledge of variant interpretation can assist genetic counselors in partnering with the testing laboratory. Genetic counselors play a key role in genetic testing, and the need will only continue to increase.

References

Almontashiri, N. A. M., Zha, L., Young, K., Law, T., Kellogg, M. D., Bodamer, O. A., & Peake, R. W. A. (2020). Clinical validation of targeted and untargeted metabolomics testing for genetic disorders: A 3 year comparative study. *Scientific Reports*, *10*(1), 9382. https://doi.org/10.1038/s41598-020-66401-2

Amarasinghe, S. L., Su, S., Dong, X., Zappia, L., Ritchie, M. E., & Gouil, Q. (2020). Opportunities and challenges in long-read sequencing data analysis. *Genome Biology*, *21*(1), 30. https://doi.org/10.1186/s13059-020-1935-5

Amendola, L. M., Jarvik, G. P., Leo, M. C., McLaughlin, H. M., Akkari, Y., Amaral, M. D., Berg, J. S., Biswas, S., Bowling, K. M., Conlin, L. K., Cooper, G. M., Dorschner, M. O., Dulik, M. C., Ghazani, A. A., Ghosh, R., Green, R. C., Hart, R., Horton, C., Johnston, J. J., . . . Rehm, H. L. (2016). Performance of ACMG-AMP variant-interpretation guidelines among nine laboratories in the clinical sequencing exploratory research consortium. *American Journal of Human Genetics*, *98*(6), 1067–1076. https://doi.org/10.1016/j.ajhg.2016.03.024

Bergougnoux, A., Deletang, K., Pommier, A., Varilh, J., Houriez, F., Altieri, J. P., Koenig, M., Ferec, C., Claustres, M., Lalau, G., Bienvenu, T., Audrezet, M. P., Pagin, A., Girodon, E., Raynal, C., & Taulan-Cadars, M. (2019). Functional characterization and phenotypic spectrum of three recurrent disease-causing deep intronic variants of the CFTR gene. *Journal of Cystic Fibrosis*, *18*(4), 468–475. https://doi.org/10.1016/j.jcf.2018.10.012

Berrios, C., Hurley, E. A., Willig, L., Thiffault, I., Saunders, C., Pastinen, T., Goggin, K., & Farrow, E. (2021). Challenges in genetic testing: Clinician variant interpretation processes and the impact on clinical care. *Genetics in Medicine*, *23*(12), 2289–2299. https://doi.org/10.1038/s41436-021-01267-x

Bonkowsky, J. L., Wilkes, J., Bardsley, T., Urbik, V. M., & Stoddard, G. (2018). Association of diagnosis of leukodystrophy with race and ethnicity among pediatric and adolescent patients. *JAMA Network Open*, *1*(7), e185031. https://doi.org/10.1001/jamanetworkopen.2018.5031

Borras, D. M., Vossen, R., Liem, M., Buermans, H. P. J., Dauwerse, H., van Heusden, D., Gansevoort, R. T., den Dunnen, J. T., Janssen, B., Peters, D. J. M., Losekoot, M., & Anvar, S. Y. (2017). Detecting PKD1 variants in polycystic kidney disease patients by single-molecule long-read sequencing. *Human Mutation*, *38*(7), 870–879. https://doi.org/10.1002/humu.23223

Clarke, S. L., Assimes, T. L., & Tcheandjieu, C. (2021). The propagation of racial disparities in cardiovascular genomics research. *Circulation: Genomic and Precision Medicine*, *14*(5), e003178. https://doi.org/10.1161/CIRCGEN.121.003178

Corbett, M. A., Kroes, T., Veneziano, L., Bennett, M. F., Florian, R., Schneider, A. L., Coppola, A., Licchetta, L., Franceschetti, S., Suppa, A., Wenger, A., Mei, D., Pendziwiat, M., Kaya, S., Delledonne, M., Straussberg, R., Xumerle, L., Regan, B., Crompton, D., . . . Gecz, J. (2019). Intronic ATTTC repeat expansions in STARD7 in familial adult myoclonic epilepsy linked to chromosome 2. *Nature Communications*, *10*(1), 4920. https://doi.org/10.1038/s41467-019-12671-y

Cuella-Martin, R., Hayward, S. B., Fan, X., Chen, X., Huang, J. W., Taglialatela, A., Leuzzi, G., Zhao, J., Rabadan, R., Lu, C., Shen, Y., & Ciccia, A. (2021). Functional interrogation of DNA damage response variants with base editing screens. *Cell*, *184*(4), 1081–1097.e1019. https://doi.org/10.1016/j.cell.2021.01.041

Dinwiddie, D. L., Smith, L. D., Miller, N. A., Atherton, A. M., Farrow, E. G., Strenk, M. E., Soden, S. E., Saunders, C. J., & Kingsmore, S. F. (2013). Diagnosis of mitochondrial disorders by concomitant next-generation sequencing of the exome and mitochondrial genome. *Genomics*, *102*(3), 148–156. https://doi.org/10.1016/j.ygeno.2013.04.013

Edwards, T. L., Breeyear, J., Piekos, J. A., & Velez Edwards, D. R. (2020). Equity in health: Consideration of race and ethnicity in precision medicine. *Trends in Genetics*, *36*(11), 807–809. https://doi.org/10.1016/j.tig.2020.07.001

Esposito, D., Weile, J., Shendure, J., Starita, L. M., Papenfuss, A. T., Roth, F. P., Fowler, D. M., & Rubin, A. F. (2019). MaveDB: An open-source platform to distribute and interpret data from multiplexed assays of variant effect. *Genome Biology*, *20*(1), 223. https://doi.org/10.1186/s13059-019-1845-6

Ferdinandusse, S., Te Brinke, H., Ruiter, J. P. N., Haasjes, J., Oostheim, W., van Lenthe, H., Lodewijk, I., Ebberink, M. S., Wanders, R. J. A., Vaz, F. M., & Waterham, H. R. (2019). A mutation creating an upstream translation initiation codon in SLC22A5 5'UTR is a frequent cause of primary carnitine deficiency. *Human Mutation*, *40*(10), 1899–1904. https://doi.org/10.1002/humu.23839

Florian, R. T., Kraft, F., Leitao, E., Kaya, S., Klebe, S., Magnin, E., van Rootselaar, A. F., Buratti, J., Kuhnel, T., Schroder, C., Giesselmann, S., Tschernoster, N., Altmueller, J., Lamiral, A.,

Keren, B., Nava, C., Bouteiller, D., Forlani, S., Jornea, L., . . . Depienne, C. (2019). Unstable TTTTA/TTTCA expansions in MARCH6 are associated with familial adult myoclonic epilepsy type 3. *Nature Communications*, *10*(1), 4919. https://doi.org/10.1038/s41467-019-12763-9

Frans, G., Meert, W., Van der Werff Ten Bosch, J., Meyts, I., Bossuyt, X., Vermeesch, J. R., & Hestand, M. S. (2018). Conventional and single-molecule targeted sequencing method for specific variant detection in IKBKG while bypassing the IKBKGP1 pseudogene. *The Journal of Molecular Diagnostics: JMD*, *20*(2), 195–202. https://doi.org/10.1016/j.jmoldx.2017.10.005

Gannamani, R., van der Veen, S., van Egmond, M., de Koning, T. J., & Tijssen, M. A. J. (2021). Challenges in clinicogenetic correlations: One phenotype—many genes. *Movement Disorders Clinical Practice*, *8*(3), 311–321. https://doi.org/10.1002/mdc3.13163

Gasperini, M., Starita, L., & Shendure, J. (2016). The power of multiplexed functional analysis of genetic variants. *Nature Protocols*, *11*(10), 1782–1787. https://doi.org/10.1038/nprot.2016.135

Gelb, B. D., Cave, H., Dillon, M. W., Gripp, K. W., Lee, J. A., Mason-Suares, H., Rauen, K. A., Williams, B., Zenker, M., Vincent, L. M., & ClinGen RASopathy Working Group. (2018). ClinGen's RASopathy Expert Panel consensus methods for variant interpretation. *Genetics in Medicine*, *20*(11), 1334–1345. https://doi.org/10.1038/gim.2018.3

Hall, C. L., Sutanto, H., Dalageorgou, C., McKenna, W. J., Syrris, P., & Futema, M. (2018). Frequency of genetic variants associated with arrhythmogenic right ventricular cardiomyopathy in the genome aggregation database. *European Journal of Human Genetics*, *26*(9), 1312–1318. https://doi.org/10.1038/s41431-018-0169-4

Hanna, R. E., Hegde, M., Fagre, C. R., DeWeirdt, P. C., Sangree, A. K., Szegletes, Z., Griffith, A., Feeley, M. N., Sanson, K. R., Baidi, Y., Koblan, L. W., Liu, D. R., Neal, J. T., & Doench, J. G. (2021). Massively parallel assessment of human variants with base editor screens. *Cell*, *184*(4), 1064–1080.e1020. https://doi.org/10.1016/j.cell.2021.01.012

Harrison, S. M., Biesecker, L. G., & Rehm, H. L. (2019). Overview of specifications to the ACMG/AMP variant interpretation guidelines. *Current Protocols in Human Genetics*, *103*(1), e93. https://doi.org/10.1002/cphg.93

Hiatt, S. M., Lawlor, J. M. J., Handley, L. H., Ramaker, R. C., Rogers, B. B., Partridge, E. C., Boston, L. B., Williams, M., Plott, C. B., Jenkins, J., Gray, D. E., Holt, J. M., Bowling, K. M., Bebin, E. M., Grimwood, J., Schmutz, J., & Cooper, G. M. (2021). Long-read genome sequencing for the molecular diagnosis of neurodevelopmental disorders. *HGG Advances*, 2(2). https://doi.org/10.1016/j.xhgg.2021.100023

Ishiura, H., Doi, K., Mitsui, J., Yoshimura, J., Matsukawa, M. K., Fujiyama, A., Toyoshima, Y., Kakita, A., Takahashi, H., Suzuki, Y., Sugano, S., Qu, W., Ichikawa, K., Yurino, H., Higasa, K., Shibata, S., Mitsue, A., Tanaka, M., Ichikawa, Y., . . . Tsuji, S. (2018). Expansions of intronic TTTCA and TTTTA repeats in benign adult familial myoclonic epilepsy. *Nature Genetics*, *50*(4), 581–590. https://doi.org/10.1038/s41588-018-0067-2

Jiang, T., Liu, S., Cao, S., Liu, Y., Cui, Z., Wang, Y., & Guo, H. (2021). Long-read sequencing settings for efficient structural variation detection based on comprehensive evaluation. *BMC Bioinformatics*, *22*(1), 552. https://doi.org/10.1186/s12859-021-04422-y

Kanavy, D. M., McNulty, S. M., Jairath, M. K., Brnich, S. E., Bizon, C., Powell, B. C., & Berg, J. S. (2019). Comparative analysis of functional assay evidence use by ClinGen Variant Curation Expert Panels. *Genome Medicine*, *11*(1), 77. https://doi.org/10.1186/s13073-019-0683-1

Kong, H. E., Zhao, J., Xu, S., Jin, P., & Jin, Y. (2017). Fragile X-associated tremor/ataxia syndrome: From molecular pathogenesis to development of therapeutics. *Frontiers in Cellular Neuroscience*, *11*, 128. https://doi.org/10.3389/fncel.2017.00128

Landrum, M. J., Chitipiralla, S., Brown, G. R., Chen, C., Gu, B., Hart, J., Hoffman, D., Jang, W., Kaur, K., Liu, C., Lyoshin, V., Maddipatla, Z., Maiti, R., Mitchell, J., O'Leary, N., Riley,

G. R., Shi, W., Zhou, G., Schneider, V., . . . Kattman, B. L. (2020). ClinVar: Improvements to accessing data. *Nucleic Acids Research*, *48*(D1), D835–D844. https://doi.org/10.1093/nar/gkz972

Landry, L. G., & Rehm, H. L. (2018). Association of racial/ethnic categories with the ability of genetic tests to detect a cause of cardiomyopathy. *JAMA Cardiology*, *3*(4), 341–345. https://doi.org/10.1001/jamacardio.2017.5333

Lee, K., Krempely, K., Roberts, M. E., Anderson, M. J., Carneiro, F., Chao, E., Dixon, K., Figueiredo, J., Ghosh, R., Huntsman, D., Kaurah, P., Kesserwan, C., Landrith, T., Li, S., Mensenkamp, A. R., Oliveira, C., Pardo, C., Pesaran, T., Richardson, M., . . . Karam, R. (2018). Specifications of the ACMG/AMP variant curation guidelines for the analysis of germline CDH1 sequence variants. *Human Mutation*, *39*(11), 1553–1568. https://doi.org/10.1002/humu.23650

Legare, J. M. (1998). Achondroplasia. In M. P. Adam, J. Feldman, G. M. Mirzaa, R. A. Pagon, S. E. Wallace, L. J. H. Bean, K. W. Gripp, & A. Amemiya (Eds.), *GeneReviews®* [Internet]. University of Washington, Seattle. https://www.ncbi.nlm.nih.gov/sites/books/NBK1152/

Liu, N., Xiao, J., Gijavanekar, C., Pappan, K. L., Glinton, K. E., Shayota, B. J., Kennedy, A. D., Sun, Q., Sutton, V. R., & Elsea, S. H. (2021). Comparison of untargeted metabolomic profiling vs traditional metabolic screening to identify inborn errors of metabolism. *JAMA Network Open*, *4*(7), e2114155. https://doi.org/10.1001/jamanetworkopen.2021.14155

Manickam, K., McClain, M. R., Demmer, L. A., Biswas, S., Kearney, H. M., Malinowski, J., Massingham, L. J., Miller, D., Yu, T. W., Hisama, F. M., & ACMG Board of Directors. (2021). Exome and genome sequencing for pediatric patients with congenital anomalies or intellectual disability: An evidence-based clinical guideline of the American College of Medical Genetics and Genomics (ACMG). *Genetics in Medicine*, *23*(11), 2029–2037. https://doi.org/10.1038/s41436-021-01242-6

Martin, A. R., Kanai, M., Kamatani, Y., Okada, Y., Neale, B. M., & Daly, M. J. (2019). Clinical use of current polygenic risk scores may exacerbate health disparities. *Nature Genetics*, *51*(4), 584–591. https://doi.org/10.1038/s41588-019-0379-x

McCormick, E. M., Lott, M. T., Dulik, M. C., Shen, L., Attimonelli, M., Vitale, O., Karaa, A., Bai, R., Pineda-Alvarez, D. E., Singh, L. N., Stanley, C. M., Wong, S., Bhardwaj, A., Merkurjev, D., Mao, R., Sondheimer, N., Zhang, S., Procaccio, V., Wallace, D. C., . . . Falk, M. J. (2020). Specifications of the ACMG/AMP standards and guidelines for mitochondrial DNA variant interpretation. *Human Mutation*, *41*(12), 2028–2057. https://doi.org/10.1002/humu.24107

McQuerry, J. A., McLaird, M., Hartin, S. N., Means, J. C., Johnston, J., Pastinen, T., & Younger, S. T. (2022). Massively parallel identification of functionally consequential noncoding genetic variants in undiagnosed rare disease patients. *Scientific Reports*, *12*(1), 7576. https://doi.org/10.1038/s41598-022-11589-8

Miao, H., Zhou, J., Yang, Q., Liang, F., Wang, D., Ma, N., Gao, B., Du, J., Lin, G., Wang, K., & Zhang, Q. (2018). Long-read sequencing identified a causal structural variant in an exome-negative case and enabled preimplantation genetic diagnosis. *Hereditas*, *155*, 32. https://doi.org/10.1186/s41065-018-0069-1

Miller, D. E., Sulovari, A., Wang, T., Loucks, H., Hoekzema, K., Munson, K. M., Lewis, A. P., Fuerte, E. P. A., Paschal, C. R., Walsh, T., Thies, J., Bennett, J. T., Glass, I., Dipple, K. M., Patterson, K., Bonkowski, E. S., Nelson, Z., Squire, A., Sikes, M., . . . Eichler, E. E. (2021). Targeted long-read sequencing identifies missing disease-causing variation. *American Journal of Human Genetics*, *108*(8), 1436–1449. https://doi.org/10.1016/j.ajhg.2021.06.006

Nykamp, K., Anderson, M., Powers, M., Garcia, J., Herrera, B., Ho, Y. Y., Kobayashi, Y., Patil, N., Thusberg, J., Westbrook, M., Invitae Clinical Genomics Group, & Topper, S. (2017).

Sherloc: A comprehensive refinement of the ACMG-AMP variant classification criteria. *Genetics in Medicine*, *19*(10), 1105–1117. https://doi.org/10.1038/gim.2017.37

Oza, A. M., DiStefano, M. T., Hemphill, S. E., Cushman, B. J., Grant, A. R., Siegert, R. K., Shen, J., Chapin, A., Boczek, N. J., Schimmenti, L. A., Murry, J. B., Hasadsri, L., Nara, K., Kenna, M., Booth, K. T., Azaiez, H., Griffith, A., Avraham, K. B., Kremer, H., . . . ClinGen Hearing Loss Clinical Domain Working Group. (2018). Expert specification of the ACMG/AMP variant interpretation guidelines for genetic hearing loss. *Human Mutation*, *39*(11), 1593–1613. https://doi.org/10.1002/humu.23630

Patel, M. J., DiStefano, M. T., Oza, A. M., Hughes, M. Y., Wilcox, E. H., Hemphill, S. E., Cushman, B. J., Grant, A. R., Siegert, R. K., Shen, J., Chapin, A., Boczek, N. J., Schimmenti, L. A., Nara, K., Kenna, M., Azaiez, H., Booth, K. T., Avraham, K. B., Kremer, H., . . . ClinGen Hearing Loss Clinical Domain Working Group. (2021). Disease-specific ACMG/AMP guidelines improve sequence variant interpretation for hearing loss. *Genetics in Medicine*, *23*(11), 2208–2212. https://doi.org/10.1038/s41436-021-01254-2

Pepin, M. G., Murray, M. L., Bailey, S., Leistritz-Kessler, D., Schwarze, U., & Byers, P. H. (2016). The challenge of comprehensive and consistent sequence variant interpretation between clinical laboratories. *Genetics in Medicine*, *18*(1), 20–24. https://doi.org/10.1038/gim.2015.31

Perrault, I., Hanein, S., Gerard, X., Mounguengue, N., Bouyakoub, R., Zarhrate, M., Fourrage, C., Jabot-Hanin, F., Bocquet, B., Meunier, I., Zanlonghi, X., Kaplan, J., & Rozet, J. M. (2021). Whole locus sequencing identifies a prevalent founder deep intronic RPGRIP1 pathologic variant in the French Leber congenital amaurosis cohort. *Genes (Basel)*, *12*(2), 1–15. https://doi.org/10.3390/genes12020287

Qian, X., Wang, J., Wang, M., Igelman, A. D., Jones, K. D., Li, Y., Wang, K., Goetz, K. E., Birch, D. G., Yang, P., Pennesi, M. E., & Chen, R. (2021). Identification of deep-intronic splice mutations in a large cohort of patients with inherited retinal diseases. *Frontiers in Genetics*, *12*, 647400. https://doi.org/10.3389/fgene.2021.647400

Rehder, C., Bean, L. J. H., Bick, D., Chao, E., Chung, W., Das, S., O'Daniel, J., Rehm, H., Shashi, V., Vincent, L. M., & ACMG Laboratory Quality Assurance Committee. (2021). Next-generation sequencing for constitutional variants in the clinical laboratory, 2021 revision: A technical standard of the American College of Medical Genetics and Genomics (ACMG). *Genetics in Medicine*, *23*(8), 1399–1415. https://doi.org/10.1038/s41436-021-01139-4

Richards, S., Aziz, N., Bale, S., Bick, D., Das, S., Gastier-Foster, J., Grody, W. W., Hegde, M., Lyon, E., Spector, E., Voelkerding, K., Rehm, H. L., & ACMG Laboratory Quality Assurance. (2015). Standards and guidelines for the interpretation of sequence variants: A joint consensus recommendation of the American College of Medical Genetics and Genomics and the Association for Molecular Pathology. *Genetics in Medicine*, *17*(5), 405–424. https://doi.org/10.1038/gim.2015.30

Riggs, E. R., Andersen, E. F., Cherry, A. M., Kantarci, S., Kearney, H., Patel, A., Raca, G., Ritter, D. I., South, S. T., Thorland, E. C., Pineda-Alvarez, D., Aradhya, S., & Martin, C. L. (2020). Technical standards for the interpretation and reporting of constitutional copy-number variants: A joint consensus recommendation of the American College of Medical Genetics and Genomics (ACMG) and the Clinical Genome Resource (ClinGen). *Genetics in Medicine*, *22*(2), 245–257. https://doi.org/10.1038/s41436-019-0686-8

Sanger, F., Nicklen, S., & Coulson, A. R. (1977). DNA sequencing with chain-terminating inhibitors. *Proceedings of the National Academy of Sciences of the United States of America*, *74*(12), 5463–5467. https://doi.org/10.1073/pnas.74.12.5463

Saunders, C. J., Friez, M. J., Patterson, M., Nzabi, M., Zhao, W., & Bi, C. (2010). Allele drop-out in the MECP2 gene due to G-quadruplex and i-motif sequences when using polymerase chain reaction-based diagnosis for Rett syndrome. *Genetic Testing and Molecular Biomarkers*, *14*(2), 241–247. https://doi.org/10.1089/gtmb.2009.0178

Schenkel, L. C., Aref-Eshghi, E., Rooney, K., Kerkhof, J., Levy, M. A., McConkey, H., Rogers, R. C., Phelan, K., Sarasua, S. M., Jain, L., Pauly, R., Boccuto, L., DuPont, B., Cappuccio, G., Brunetti-Pierri, N., Schwartz, C. E., & Sadikovic, B. (2021). DNA methylation episignature is associated with two molecularly and phenotypically distinct clinical subtypes of Phelan-McDermid syndrome. *Clinical Epigenetics*, *13*(1), 2. https://doi.org/10.1186/s13148-020-00990-7

Senol Cali, D., Kim, J. S., Ghose, S., Alkan, C., & Mutlu, O. (2019). Nanopore sequencing technology and tools for genome assembly: Computational analysis of the current state, bottlenecks and future directions. *Briefings in Bioinformatics*, *20*(4), 1542–1559. https://doi.org/10.1093/bib/bby017

Shashi, V., Schoch, K., Spillmann, R., Cope, H., Tan, Q. K., Walley, N., Pena, L., McConkie-Rosell, A., Jiang, Y. H., Stong, N., Need, A. C., Goldstein, D. B., & Undiagnosed Diseases Network. (2019). A comprehensive iterative approach is highly effective in diagnosing individuals who are exome negative. *Genetics in Medicine*, *21*(1), 161–172. https://doi.org/10.1038/s41436-018-0044-2

Sheck, L., Davies, W. I. L., Moradi, P., Robson, A. G., Kumaran, N., Liasis, A. C., Webster, A. R., Moore, A. T., & Michaelides, M. (2018). Leber congenital amaurosis associated with mutations in CEP290, clinical phenotype, and natural history in preparation for trials of novel therapies. *Ophthalmology*, *125*(6), 894–903. https://doi.org/10.1016/j.ophtha.2017.12.013

Strande, N. T., Riggs, E. R., Buchanan, A. H., Ceyhan-Birsoy, O., DiStefano, M., Dwight, S. S., Goldstein, J., Ghosh, R., Seifert, B. A., Sneddon, T. P., Wright, M. W., Milko, L. V., Cherry, J. M., Giovanni, M. A., Murray, M. F., O'Daniel, J. M., Ramos, E. M., Santani, A. B., Scott, A. F., . . . Berg, J. S. (2017). Evaluating the clinical validity of gene-disease associations: An evidence-based framework developed by the Clinical Genome Resource. *American Journal of Human Genetics*, *100*(6), 895–906. https://doi.org/10.1016/j.ajhg.2017.04.015

Su, Y., Fan, L., Shi, C., Wang, T., Zheng, H., Luo, H., Zhang, S., Hu, Z., Fan, Y., Dong, Y., Yang, J., Mao, C., & Xu, Y. (2021). Deciphering neurodegenerative diseases using long-read sequencing. *Neurology*, *97*(9), 423–433. https://doi.org/10.1212/WNL.0000000000012466

Tan, N. B., Stapleton, R., Stark, Z., Delatycki, M. B., Yeung, A., Hunter, M. F., Amor, D. J., Brown, N. J., Stutterd, C. A., McGillivray, G., Yap, P., Regan, M., Chong, B., Fanjul Fernandez, M., Marum, J., Phelan, D., Pais, L. S., White, S. M., Lunke, S., & Tan, T. Y. (2020). Evaluating systematic reanalysis of clinical genomic data in rare disease from single center experience and literature review. *Molecular Genetics & Genomic Medicine*, *8*(11), e1508. https://doi.org/10.1002/mgg3.1508

Tanner, A., Chan, H. W., Schiff, E., Mahroo, O. A., & Pulido, J. S. (2022). Exploring the mutational landscape of genes associated with inherited retinal disease using large genomic datasets: Identifying loss of function intolerance and outlying propensities for missense changes. *BMJ Open Ophthalmology*, *7*(1), 1–8. https://doi.org/10.1136/bmjophth-2022-001079

Thiffault, I., Cadieux-Dion, M., Farrow, E., Caylor, R., Miller, N., Soden, S., & Saunders, C. (2018). On the verge of diagnosis: Detection, reporting, and investigation of de novo variants in novel genes identified by clinical sequencing. *Human Mutation*, *39*(11), 1505–1516. https://doi.org/10.1002/humu.23646

Truty, R., Paul, J., Kennemer, M., Lincoln, S. E., Olivares, E., Nussbaum, R. L., & Aradhya, S. (2019). Prevalence and properties of intragenic copy-number variation in Mendelian disease genes. *Genetics in Medicine*, *21*(1), 114–123. https://doi.org/10.1038/s41436-018-0033-5

Valkenburg, D., van Cauwenbergh, C., Lorenz, B., van Genderen, M. M., Bertelsen, M., Pott, J. R., Coppieters, F., de Zaeytijd, J., Thiadens, A., Klaver, C. C. W., Kroes, H. Y., van Schooneveld, M. J., Preising, M., Hoyng, C. B., Leroy, B. P., van den Born, L. I., & Collin, R. W. J. (2018). Clinical characterization of 66 patients with congenital retinal disease due to the deep-intronic c.2991+1655A>G mutation in CEP290. *Investigative Ophthalmology and Visual Science*, *59*(11), 4384–4391. https://doi.org/10.1167/iovs.18-24817

Weerakkody, R. A., Vandrovcova, J., Kanonidou, C., Mueller, M., Gampawar, P., Ibrahim, Y., Norsworthy, P., Biggs, J., Abdullah, A., Ross, D., Black, H. A., Ferguson, D., Cheshire, N. J., Kazkaz, H., Grahame, R., Ghali, N., Vandersteen, A., Pope, F. M., & Aitman, T. J. (2016). Targeted next-generation sequencing makes new molecular diagnoses and expands genotype-phenotype relationship in Ehlers-Danlos syndrome. *Genetics in Medicine*, *18*(11), 1119–1127. https://doi.org/10.1038/gim.2016.14

Weile, J., & Roth, F. P. (2018). Multiplexed assays of variant effects contribute to a growing genotype-phenotype atlas. *Human Genetics*, *137*(9), 665–678. https://doi.org/10.1007/s00439-018-1916-x

Wright, C. F., McRae, J. F., Clayton, S., Gallone, G., Aitken, S., FitzGerald, T. W., Jones, P., Prigmore, E., Rajan, D., Lord, J., Sifrim, A., Kelsell, R., Parker, M. J., Barrett, J. C., Hurles, M. E., FitzPatrick, D. R., Firth, H. V., & Deciphering Developmental Disorders Study. (2018). Making new genetic diagnoses with old data: Iterative reanalysis and reporting from genome-wide data in 1,133 families with developmental disorders. *Genetics in Medicine*, *20*(10), 1216–1223. https://doi.org/10.1038/gim.2017.246

Yu, H., & Zhang, V. W. (2015). Precision medicine for continuing phenotype expansion of human genetic diseases. *Biomedical Research International*, *2015*, 745043. https://doi.org/10.1155/2015/745043

Zhou, Z. D., Jankovic, J., Ashizawa, T., & Tan, E. K. (2022). Neurodegenerative diseases associated with non-coding CGG tandem repeat expansions. *Nature Reviews Neurology*, *18*, 145–157. https://doi.org/10.1038/s41582-021-00612-7

CHAPTER 18

GENETIC COUNSELOR LIABILITY AND LICENSURE IN THE GENOMICS ERA

SUSAN M. WOLF, GARY E. MARCHANT, HANNAH M. OLIASON, AND BONNIE S. LEROY

Introduction

The increasing importance of genetics and genomics in medicine raises complex issues concerning the evolving standard of care for genetics professionals and potential liability of genetic counselors. Genetic counseling practitioners may not be fully familiar with the issues raised by rapidly evolving genomic tests such as exome and genome sequencing, polygenic risk scores, cutting-edge research analyses yielding results shared with patient-participants, and direct-to-consumer (DTC) analyses. Even genetic counselors comfortable with these and other emerging technologies may (like other genetics professionals) face uncertainty about the relevant standard of care in cutting-edge domains such as the potential duty to recontact patients when variant interpretations change due to progress in understanding.

Because genetic counselors often face front-line responsibility for explaining how genetics plays a role in health and disease, obtaining consent for testing, and communicating genetic and genomic analyses and results to patients and research participants and their families, they shoulder an extraordinary burden at a time of rapid technological advance. Not only patients and families but also colleagues turn to genetic counselors for education and advice. Additionally, in many states genetic counselors are licensed and with this license may come the authority to order appropriate testing for patients and families who are at risk for genetic disorders (Abacan et al., 2019). All of this is in the context of a major transition in health care with the emergence of telemedicine.

As genomics is changing the landscape of genetic counseling practice, it is also changing liability. The most common forms of liability for health professionals are malpractice and negligence. Both are customarily governed by state law rather than federal law and thus may vary somewhat from state to state. Many genetic counselors work for companies where they provide services online to patients in multiple states. For those genetic counselors, they may hold a license in multiple states and will be held to the law in those states. In general, malpractice claims allege the existence of a clinician–patient relationship creating a duty of care, breach of the applicable standard of care, and that this breach caused harm to the patient compensable in money damages. Negligence generally claims that the professional failed to exercise due care under the circumstances and that this failure caused compensable harm. While distinguishing malpractice from general negligence may be challenging at times, state law may impose different rules depending on which cause of action is alleged, such as whether the standard of care is based on professional custom (medical malpractice) or considerations of reasonableness (negligence), and differing time limits (such as statutes of limitations) for bringing the lawsuit.

As the more familiar territory of genetics gives way to the greater complexity of genomics, the risk of liability for genetic counselors is increasing. Evolving technology and approaches to variant interpretation and reinterpretation may leave genetic counselors operating in some spheres without clinical practice guidelines or definitive guidance. If the goal of malpractice and negligence liability is to promote quality care and provide compensation for patients injured due to unreasonable breaches of quality, then defining what constitutes quality care in the evolving landscape of genomics is essential. In domains of continuing uncertainty about still-emerging quality standards, a responsible approach to developing standards is needed.

By explicating the relevant law and emerging issues, this chapter aims to help genetic counselors anticipate key issues that are emerging and manage their liability exposure. The first part will discuss the law that governs liability of genetic counselors. The second part will discuss genetic counselor licensure as a mechanism for promoting standards of care. The third part will discuss current and emerging liability issues and potential causes of action. The fourth part will address strategies for managing liability exposure.

What Law Governs Liability of a Genetic Counselor?

The two primary sources of liability for genetic counselors are negligence and malpractice. Both negligence and malpractice sound in tort, an area of law providing redress for those injured or wronged by another, by awarding money damages to restore the victim(s) to their prior state, deter negligence, and encourage due care (Schmerler, 2008). Negligence occurs when a person fails to comply with the standard of care to protect a person from harm. Malpractice is professional negligence, and in the context of medicine, is called "medical malpractice" (Schmerler, 2008).

There are important distinctions between malpractice and negligence. For example, statutes of limitation and repose—which are largely determined by state law—can impose different time limits on plaintiffs seeking to bring a lawsuit, depending on whether they are making medical malpractice or negligence claims. It is not uncommon for plaintiffs to sue for malpractice and, in the alternative, negligence, although some states allow only malpractice and not ordinary negligence arising from clinical care (see, e.g., Foulkes et al.,

2020; *Flythe v. Davis*, 2011; *Johnson v. Botsford Gen. Hosp.*, 2008). Negligence claims can provide an avenue of recourse for those harmed in the course of their medical care but who are barred from bringing a medical malpractice claim by statutes of limitation. In addition, negligence claims arise more commonly in research settings when participants cannot bring malpractice claims.

The main source of liability for genetic counselors derives from medical malpractice suits, which hold medical providers liable for breach of the applicable standards of care. The plaintiff has the burden of proof to establish three basic elements: (a) the existence of a duty, (b) breach of that duty, and (c) causation of compensable damages (Schmerler, 2008). The existence of a duty is relatively easy to establish if there is a patient–provider relationship such as that between a genetic counselor and their patient.

For purposes of determining whether a breach occurred, courts look to the standard of care, though this can be difficult to ascertain in fast-moving fields such as genetics and genomics. In the majority of states, the medical malpractice standard of care is based on a national standard, but in a sizeable minority of states, the standard of care is based on the locality rule, that is, the standard in that locality (Lewis et al., 2007). When states rely on national or local custom, they are determining the standard of care based on what a similarly trained professional would do in that same situation. However, a growing number, but still a minority, of states now apply a "reasonableness" standard, in which liability is based on the overall reasonableness of the medical professional's actions and custom is just one factor (Lewis et al., 2007).

In determining the standard of care, state courts typically hear testimony from expert witnesses, who may refer to professional society practice guidelines and ethics codes. It is important to note that practice guidelines in emerging fields may lag behind technology. Some authorities have suggested the use of provisional standards (such as use of clinical practice advisory documents) until rigorous and evidence-based clinical practice guidelines can be formulated (Burke et al., 2019).

Lastly, the breach itself must have caused compensable damages. Damages sought in a genetic counseling malpractice suit might include past and future medical expenses and emotional damages resulting from the breach (Pergament & Ilijic, 2014).

Genetic Counselor Licensure and Scope of Practice

States vary in whether they require licensure of genetic counselors (National Society of Genetic Counselors [NSGC], 2020b). Licensure requirements can be helpful in indicating the relevant training, scope of practice, standard of care, and continuing education expected. Licensure can thus set a baseline for what is required of genetic counselors to enter the profession and embark on patient care. In addition, states may require that the licensee earn a specific number of continuing education credits prior to license renewal, to promote competence ("Genetic counselor licensure," 2016, p. 9).

As of 2020, 26 states have statutes licensing genetic counselors, and three states license genetic counselors through rulemaking (NSGC, 2020b). Many of these laws are based on the

NSGC Model Legislative Provisions (NSGC, 2020a). The NSGC encourages the expansion of state licensure of genetic counselors to promote uniformity of regulation across states. States that license genetic counselors require applicants to have a current American Board of Genetic Counseling (ABGC) certification and to have graduated from a master's degree program accredited by the Accreditation Council for Genetic Counseling (ABGC, n.d.-c). It is important to note that the ABGC was established in 1993 and offered the first genetic counseling certification exam in 1996 (ABGC, n.d.-a). Prior to 1996, genetic counselors were certified by the American Board of Medical Genetics (ABMG) (ABGC, n.d.-a).[1] The ABGC began accrediting graduate programs in 1995 (ABGC, n.d.-a).[2] Genetic counselors who graduated before 1995 mostly graduated from master's degree genetic counseling programs, but some early genetic counselors came to the profession with other degrees. Any practicing genetic counselor who had been certified by the ABMG prior to 1996 was offered the opportunity to be grandfathered into the ABGC and encouraged to voluntarily recertify with the ABGC (ABGC, n.d.-a, n.d.-b). Those certified by the ABGC in 1996 or later must maintain certification either through continuing education credits or by taking the ABGC recertification exam once every 5 years (ABGC, n.d.-b).

State licensure laws help delineate the scope of practice for genetic counselors, such as the authority to order genetic tests and whether physician oversight is required. Some states allow genetic counselors to order genetic tests independently, others require a "collaborative agreement" between a genetic counselor and a physician, and still others forbid genetic counselors from ordering genetic tests. The NSGC's Model Legislative Provisions define a "collaborative agreement" as "a written document that memorializes a relationship between a genetic counselor and a physician and that authorizes a genetic counselor to perform the functions specified [e.g., ordering genetic tests] . . . as applied to the practice of genetic counseling" (NSGC, 2020a, Definitions section). Louisiana, Ohio, and Washington have specified that ordering genetic tests requires a collaborative agreement (see La. Stat., 2018; Ohio Rev., 2012; Wash. Admin., 2010). By contrast, genetic counselors in Pennsylvania are prohibited from ordering genetic tests (Pa. Stat., 2012).

Disciplinary actions are separate from malpractice litigation. Professional licensure requirements customarily provide that complaints may be brought to a state licensing or practice board and disciplinary actions instituted to hold professionals responsible for breach of standards. Disciplinary actions thus present another mechanism to hold genetic counselors accountable for a breach of guidelines and ethics standards. Such actions help "correct people who lack the necessary skills or are practicing outside their scope of practice" ("Genetic counselor licensure," 2016, p. 9). NSGC's Model Legislative Provisions encourage creation of a state genetic counselors licensing board to "conduct hearings, fine, censure, revoke, suspend or deny a license, place on probation, reprimand or otherwise discipline licensees for violations of the ethics of the rule of the board" (NSGC, 2020a, Duties, Functions, and Responsibilities of the Board section). This authority may alternatively be exercised by a state medical board. In Arkansas, for example, the State Medical Board has

[1] Editors' note: While at the time of these events the organization was the ABMG, it is now the American Board of Medical Genetics and Genomics (ABMGG).

[2] Editors' note: The Accreditation Council for Genetic Counseling was formed in 2012 after separating from the ABGC and is responsible for genetic counseling program accreditation.

the authority to hold hearings and deny, suspend, revoke, or refuse to renew a license or "may reprimand, censure, place on probation, or otherwise discipline" a licensed genetic counselor (Ark. Code Ann., 2019, Section I).

Federal efforts to provide Medicare and Medicaid payment for genetic counseling may encourage more states to consider licensure. Congressional enactment of H.R. 3235, the Access to Genetic Counselor Services Act of 2019, would recognize genetic counselors as "health-care providers" and enable such payment (Access to Genetic Counselor Services Act of 2019, 2019). Although a large number of organizations have supported H.R. 3235, the American College of Medical Genetics and Genomics (ACMG) has opposed the bill as written, citing concerns that it "would permit genetic counselors to practice medicine" by reimbursing them for "ordering medical tests; including genetic testing" (Gregg & Muenke, 2020, p. 1; see also Ray, 2020). The ACMG has advocated amending H.R. 3235 to require collaborative agreements, stating that its "proposed amendments to HR 3235 would not . . . preclude genetic counselors from ordering genetic testing" but rather "encourage continuation of the collaborative environments that most benefit patients . . . [and] the addition of brief language to support such collaborative relationships" (ACMG Member Informational Session, 2020). The ACMG has engaged in similar lobbying efforts at the state level, citing concerns that some proposed state licensure laws would permit genetic counselors to engage in the practice of medicine (Ray, 2021). Enactment of H.R. 3235 could encourage states that do not yet license genetic counselors to do so, recognizing genetic counseling as a domain of clinical practice warranting a framework for licensure and discipline to promote quality assurance.

Ultimately, the goal of licensure is to ensure competence and quality while encouraging uniformity of regulation across states. Although licensure creates a baseline set of requirements to show competence, meeting those requirements does not by itself show that a genetic counselor met the standard of care in a malpractice lawsuit. Even licensed clinicians can breach the relevant standard of care.

Current and Emerging Liability Issues

Reported malpractice cases involving genetics and genomics are not yet common but are gradually increasing. One study found 12 or fewer cases reported per year, and not all of these cases name genetic counselors as defendants (Marchant et al., 2020). While new technologies may enlarge the scope of potential claims, a number of factors may deter plaintiffs from filing suit. Some cases may be blocked by statutes of limitation, may be subject to mandatory arbitration, or may settle for confidential amounts (Marchant & Lindor, 2018). Nonetheless, genetic counselors and other genetics professionals are wise to consider the breadth of claims that can be brought, especially in the transition from genetics to genomics in clinical care, with an associated increase in the volume and complexity of data.

Prenatal causes of action

Prenatal causes of action make up a large portion of genetic counselors' liability risk, as "persons at risk for bearing children with a genetic disease may have their reproductive lives determined by information presented by a genetic counselor" (Reilly, 1975, p. 641). There are four primary prenatal causes of action: wrongful birth, wrongful life, wrongful conception, and wrongful termination of pregnancy.

Damages sought in prenatal causes of action might include the cost of raising and caring for a child with a genetic condition versus a healthy child. Parents may also attempt to recover damages for emotional distress, though courts are generally more reluctant to award such damages due to the difficulty of quantifying emotional distress.

Wrongful birth

Actions for wrongful birth are brought when a provider allegedly fails to predict, diagnose, or discover a genetic disorder through prenatal testing or counseling, thereby depriving the parents of the opportunity to decide whether to continue or terminate the pregnancy based on a known genetic risk. The parents must demonstrate that but for the genetic counselor's failure to properly predict, diagnose, or inform the parents of their future child's genetic risk, the mother would have avoided or terminated the pregnancy.

The states are split on whether they recognize wrongful birth causes of action (see *Plowman v. Fort Madison Cmty. Hosp.*, 2017). A number of states have abolished such claims by legislation over the past decade because of the relationship of the claims to abortion (see generally, Harris, 2014; Hegeman, 2020). The theory of damages in wrongful birth actions is that the parents were "wrongfully deprived of the ability to avoid or terminate the pregnancy to prevent the birth of a child with the defect or disease" (Zittler, 2019, I.C.§5). Parents may also try to recover emotional damages caused by wrongful birth. This may or may not be permitted based on the jurisdiction; for example, the D.C. Circuit Court of Appeals has held that there is no cause of action for negligent infliction of emotional distress resulting from a wrongful birth (*Cauman v. George Washington University*, 1993). Other jurisdictions do recognize general damages for emotional distress based on wrongful birth claims (see, e.g., *Wuth ex rel. Kessler v. Laboratory Corp. of Am.*, 2015, recognizing damages for emotional distress and mental anguish arising from wrongful birth in the state of Washington).

The Florida case of *Estrada v. University of South Florida Board of Trustees* (2007) exemplifies wrongful birth claims. The parents' first child was born with genetically based disabilities and had been under the care of a geneticist who failed to detect Smith-Lemli-Opitz syndrome. Moreover, the geneticist advised the parents that they did not have an elevated risk of having another child with this condition. The parents alleged that but for the geneticist's failure to detect Smith-Lemli-Opitz syndrome in their first child, they would have understood the risk of their second child having the disorder, tested for the disorder prior to birth, and terminated the pregnancy when the results showed the presence of the syndrome. The jury awarded the parents more than $20 million.

In *Naccash v. Burger* (1982), parents sued their physician for wrongful birth after their child was born with Tay-Sachs disease. The father was tested for Tay-Sachs disease, but due to mishandling and mislabeling of the father's blood sample, the test produced a false negative. The child was then born with Tay-Sachs disease and died at age 2. The Supreme Court of Virginia held that the parents had a cause of action for wrongful birth. The court reasoned that the parents were owed a duty of reasonable care in the handling of the blood drawn for the test. The mishandling and mislabeling of the blood sample constituted negligence, and there was a clear causal connection between the father's negative Tay-Sachs test and the parents' decision to give birth to their child. The court held that the parents were entitled to recover damages for the cost of their child's care during her life as well as for emotional distress. Moreover, since the technician was acting within the scope of their employment when they erroneously labeled the sample, the physician could be found liable as the technician's supervisor.

Wrongful life

Wrongful life actions are brought by parents on behalf of a disabled child, suing the physician or hospital for negligent genetic testing or counseling. Wrongful life claims are not recognized in most states and have been a source of significant controversy. This is largely because the primary question in wrongful life actions is whether the child would have been better off not having been born. Most courts refuse to evaluate claims "requiring the calculation of damages based on comparisons of the value of life with a disability and the value of non-existence" (Pergament & Ilijic, 2014, p. 1444). For example, the court in *Becker v. Schwartz* (1978) said, "Whether it is better never to have been born at all than to have been born with even gross deficiencies is a mystery more properly to be left to the philosophers and the theologians." Other jurisdictions have echoed this sentiment (see, e.g., *John v. De Vivo*, 2020, holding that an infant has no claim for wrongful life in the state of New York).

In *Turpin v. Sortini* (1982), parents sued medical providers on behalf of their deaf child, alleging that the providers failed to inform them of the possibility of the hereditary condition. The Supreme Court of California held that the child could not recover general damages but could recover special damages, such as those necessary to treat her deafness. The court reasoned that recovery of general damages should be denied because

> (1) it is simply impossible to determine in any rational or reasoned fashion whether the plaintiff has in fact suffered an injury in being born impaired rather than not being born, and (2) even if it were possible to overcome the first hurdle, it would be impossible to assess general damages in any fair, nonspeculative manner.

In *Ermoian v. Desert Hospital* (2007), a California court elaborated that the "'resulting injury' in a wrongful life action is not the plaintiff's disease or birth defects, but the birth of the plaintiff with the defect. . . . In essence, injury occurs when never being born, or nonexistence, is preferable to existence in the plaintiff's diseased state."

In *Harbeson v. Parke-Davis, Inc.* (1983), however, the Washington Supreme Court recognized a wrongful life action on the basis that "it would be illogical and anomalous to permit only parents, and not the child, to recover for the cost of the child's own medical care." The court stated:

> The child's need for medical care and other special costs . . . will not miraculously disappear when the child attains his majority. In many cases, the burden of those expenses will fall on the child's parents or the state. Rather than allowing this to occur by refusing to recognize the cause of action, we prefer to place the burden of those costs on the party whose negligence was in fact a proximate cause of the child's continuing need for such special medical care and training.

Wrongful life lawsuits may be brought when the statute of limitations has run on the parents' wrongful birth lawsuit—because wrongful life lawsuits are brought on behalf of the affected child, the statute of limitations for that claim does not start to run until the child has reached the age of majority (Stein, 2020; *Procanik by Procanik v. Cillo*, 1984). As state law governs wrongful life claims, genetic counselors should understand where their state stands on these controversial claims.

Wrongful conception

Wrongful conception actions are brought by parents alleging that they would have avoided conception if they had received proper and nonnegligent counseling. Wrongful conception is distinct from wrongful birth, as the alleged negligence occurs not during the course of pregnancy but before a child is even conceived. For example, parents may undergo testing prior to conception to determine if they carry genetic disorders that would put their child-to-be at risk (Zittler, 2019). The claim "is that a physician or other healthcare provider did not cause the damage or disease in the fetus, but their negligence caused a loss of opportunity to prevent conception . . . of an infant with a genetic abnormality" (Pergament & Ilijic, 2014, p. 1445).

In *Gallagher v. Duke University* (1988), parents were successful in proving a cause of action for medical malpractice based on wrongful conception. The parents' first child died of severe congenital disabilities, but a cytogeneticist determined that the child's disorder had no genetic basis. The parents were advised that, based on the tests conducted by the cytogeneticist, their risk of having another affected child was not elevated and that the parents need not undergo genetic testing. The parents had a second child who was born with severe birth anomalies similar to those affecting their first child. The cytogeneticist then discovered that he had missed a genetic abnormality in the first child's test. A later test of the parents revealed that the father carried a genetic abnormality that he passed down to both children. The court found that the cytogeneticist breached the standard of care and proximately caused the conception and birth of the second child with serious disabilities. As such, they awarded damages to the parents for the cost of raising that child.

Similar cases in which failure to diagnose a first-born child results in the birth of a second-born child with the same genetic abnormality continue to emerge. In *Blouin v. Koster* (2016), for example, parents alleged that they would not have conceived their children had they known they were carriers for cystic fibrosis and, moreover, would not have conceived their second-born child had the defendants timely diagnosed their first-born child.

Wrongful termination of pregnancy

Lastly, prenatal causes of action may include wrongful termination of a pregnancy due to negligent genetic counseling. In *Alger v. Strong Memorial Hospital* (2014), a patient and her husband sued several individuals and entities, including a genetic counselor, seeking damages for physical and emotional injuries due to the patient's decision to terminate her pregnancy as a result of the defendants' alleged negligence in performing prenatal diagnostic tests and advising them regarding the results of such tests. The jury found that the genetic counselor was not negligent, and although they found several of the other defendants negligent, they determined such negligence was not a proximate cause of the plaintiffs' injuries.

Similarly, in *Martinez v. Long Island Jewish Hillside Medical Center* (1987), the patient sued genetic counselors and a medical center after terminating her pregnancy due to defendants' erroneous advice that her child would be born with microcephaly or anencephaly. The patient claimed that she "suffered mental anguish and depression from her awareness that, as a result of defendants' negligence, she had needlessly committed an act in violation of her deep-seated convictions." The court determined that plaintiff was entitled to sue the defendants for breach of the standard of care and could seek damages for emotional distress.

Causes of action related to other genomic testing

Apart from prenatal causes of action, genetic counselors can be sued for a range of actions related to genetic or genomic testing. These include failure to order the testing, ordering excessively broad testing or tests with inadequate coverage, negligent choice of specific tests or panels, incorrect interpretation of clinical laboratory reports, and incorrect variant calls or test interpretation. Some of these causes of action can only be brought against genetic counselors in states where the genetic counselor is in the position of ordering testing. There, failure to select the appropriate test from the appropriate laboratory could result in a liability risk. A publication from the NSGC in 2017 notes close to 50,000 different tests available for over 10,000 conditions (NSGC, 2017). The complexity of tests available will continue to grow.

Failure to test

Failure to test will most often occur due to a provider's failure to recognize risk in a patient. For example, a provider may fail to test a patient who is the only affected person in their otherwise healthy family, resulting in a failure to diagnose their condition and identify other family members who could be at risk (Marchant et al., 2020). However, genetic counselors will be liable for failure to test only when it breaches the standard of care.

In *Cohen v. Rashba* (2005), a patient's surviving spouse sued the patient's surgeon for wrongful death after the surgeon failed to order testing to detect risk of ovarian cancer and perform prophylactic surgery to prevent the development of cancer. The patient was diagnosed with breast cancer and inquired about removing her ovaries to prevent ovarian cancer. The surgeon allegedly stated that surgery was not necessary and neither referred the patient for genetic counseling nor ordered any tests. Less than 2 years later, the plaintiff was diagnosed with ovarian cancer and ultimately died. The jury found that the surgeon was not negligent and awarded no damages to the plaintiff.

Failure to test can also be part of a suit for medical malpractice in prenatal care. For example, in *Reed v. Campagnolo* (1993), parents sued two physicians for failing to conduct prenatal alpha-fetoprotein (AFP) tests. They claimed the tests would have shown severe genetic anomalies in the fetus and resulted in the mother terminating her pregnancy. In another medical malpractice lawsuit, a couple in which the mother was a known carrier of Canavan disease sued a genetic counselor who had advised that the father need not be genetically tested because his risk of also being a carrier was so low. He turned out to be a carrier and they gave birth to a child with Canavan disease (Miller & Zois, n.d.-b).

Overtesting and inadequate coverage

In some cases, patients may be harmed by overtesting, when it leads to additional testing or medical procedures that are unwarranted. Genetic counselors should be wary of ordering excessively broad testing. "A major challenge already confronting those who employ sequencing as a diagnostic test is determining the appropriate breadth of testing to implement" (Marchant et al., 2020, p. 13). Claims can arise if a genetic counselor is accused of ordering testing that is "too broad and encompasses too many genes, leading to spurious, irrelevant findings" (Marchant et al., 2020, p. 14). Pursuing those extra findings may itself cause harm and prove iatrogenic.

In addition, broad panels or large-scale genomic sequencing may provide less coverage of genomic domains that later prove relevant to diagnosis or treatment. Targeted panels, while narrower in scope, can provide greater coverage when testing for a specific gene (Marchant et al., 2020). Thus, genetic counselors should consider both appropriate scope and analytic coverage when choosing what tests to order.

Negligent choice of specific tests or panels

In addition to overtesting and inadequate information, the transition from genetics to genomics heightens risk of liability for negligent choice of specific tests or panels. Genetic counselors may face liability if they recommend an inferior panel for an individual patient that misses important genetic variants that would have been detected if a better panel had been recommended (Marchant et al., 2020). However, to succeed on a claim for negligent choice of a specific panel, the plaintiff must show that

> (1) an alternative gene panel was available and would have been utilized by the patient, (2) that this alternative panel would have disclosed information that would have resulted in a better outcome for the plaintiff, and (3) the physician should have had some reason to suspect that the alternative gene panel would have produced a superior result. (Marchant et al., 2020, p. 21)

A recent medical malpractice lawsuit alleged that a physician relied on an inadequate gene panel in concluding that a couple was not at risk of delivering a child with a serious genetic risk. The physician ordered a genetic carrier screening panel from a commercial vendor for both parents, and the results showed "that the woman was a carrier of Canavan disease and the man was a carrier of cystic fibrosis, Smith-Lemi-Opitz Syndrome, and alpha-1 antitrypsin deficiency" (Miller & Zois, n.d.-a). Because these are all recessive conditions and there were no overlaps in the genes for which the parents had pathogenic variants, the physician assured the couple that they were not at risk of having children with serious genetic conditions. The couple subsequently gave birth to three children, the last of whom was diagnosed with Canavan disease. It turned out the father had a less common variant of the Canavan gene that was not included in the commercial screening panel. The couple sued the physician for negligence in providing advice and violation of informed consent based on the failure to explain that the panel only tested for common variants (*Anonymous v. Greater Washington Maternal Fetal Medicine & Genetics*, 2019).

Incorrect interpretation of clinical laboratory reports

Liability can also arise from incorrectly interpreting a clinical laboratory report of a patient's genetic test results. In *Cooke-Moore v. Curry Community Health, Inc.* (2017), a plaintiff sought genetic testing for cancer due to her family history. She "contended that her physicians erroneously told her that she carried the *MLH1* gene mutation and Lynch syndrome, which indicate an increased risk of colorectal, uterine, ovarian, and other cancers". She also "claimed that she was told that she carried the *BRCA1* gene," indicating an elevated risk of breast and ovarian cancer. As a result, the plaintiff underwent a hysterectomy and double mastectomy. She discovered the mistake in reading the clinical laboratory report in her medical file after the surgeries. The case settled, with compensation to the plaintiff.

Incorrect interpretation of clinical laboratory reports may become increasingly prevalent with the rise of more complex genomic testing and sequencing in clinical care. The risk of such error suggests that genetic counselors interpreting and communicating genomic results to patients should be well versed in technological advancements and genomic variant interpretation.

Incorrect variant calls or test interpretation

Genetic counselors can also be held liable for incorrect variant calls and test interpretation. Although variant interpretations are initially reported by clinical testing laboratories, many genetic counselors report seeking additional evidence to support a laboratory's variant classification, or even reaching a different conclusion as to the correct variant classification (Richards et al., 2015; Wain et al., 2020). As such, genetic counselors may be held liable for their own incorrect variant calls and test interpretations, despite the fact that clinical testing laboratories make the initial call.

The liability risk is exacerbated by divergence across reference databases in their classification of variants as pathogenic, likely pathogenic, or variants of uncertain significance (VUSs) (Marchant et al., 2020). In addition, the ancestral background of an individual can make a difference as to the correct variant interpretation. Genetic counselors may thus need to consider disagreement across reference databases and a patient's ancestral background when interpreting genetic variants.

An important emerging test modality generates polygenic risk scores, which quantify genetic contributions in the prediction of disease risks (Janssens, 2019). Polygenic risk scores analyze an individual's relative risk for a disease compared to others with a different genetic constitution (National Human Genome Research Institute, 2020). Because the majority of genomic studies to date have examined individuals of European ancestry, such scores may be less useful for non-European ancestry populations (National Human Genome Research Institute, 2020). This increases the risk of test misinterpretation as applied to patients with non-European ancestry.

A successful malpractice claim relating to incorrect variant calls and test interpretation could result in significant damages. If a gene variant is identified as harmless when it is actually pathogenic, and the patient takes action in reliance on that erroneous interpretation, the patient could endure lasting and serious harm. The doctor in *Gallagher v. Duke University* (1988) performed a chromosome analysis on a child who exhibited multiple congenital anomalies and died just 3 weeks after birth. The erroneous results of this analysis were not discovered until the parents gave birth to their second child with congenital anomalies similar to those of the first child. The parents alleged that but for the doctor's incorrect interpretation of test results, they would not have conceived their second child. Conversely, if a gene variant is identified as pathogenic when it is harmless, the patient could undergo unnecessary testing and procedures that are not only costly but also potentially iatrogenic.

Causes of action related to mishandling the results of testing

Once testing has occurred, genetic counselors have duties to properly handle and communicate results. Failure to fulfill those duties as well as other related duties could result in liability.

Failure to properly communicate results

Failure to communicate results properly (or failure to communicate the results at all) can result in liability. Problems may be most likely to occur in communicating with the patient, but failure to communicate properly with the patient's physician may be a source of liability as well. In *Molloy v. Meier* (2004), a 3-year-old child underwent chromosomal testing after her doctor noticed developmental delay. The doctor reported the test results to the child's family as "negative." However, the parents were under the erroneous impression that their child underwent chromosomal testing *and* testing for fragile X syndrome (FXS), due to the fact that the doctor discussed the possibility of Fragile X testing at a previous appointment. The child was later diagnosed with FXS after the mother gave birth to a second child with similar developmental delays who tested positive for FXS. The Supreme Court of Minnesota found sufficient evidence to submit the negligence claim against the doctors to a jury to determine whether they failed to meet the standard of care.

Failure to communicate results to the patient effectively may also occur due to the difficulty of communicating genetic analysis in terms understandable to a layperson. This problem is compounded in genomic testing, as patients may be presented with complex information involving a substantial number of gene variants. In addition, communicating relevant sources of uncertainty in genomic sequencing can be challenging.

Failure to communicate with the patient's doctor can also create liability. An example would be failing to communicate the results of pharmacogenomic (PGx) testing. For example:

> If a patient has a bad reaction to a drug (or failure of drug effectiveness) that could have been prevented by PGx-based prescribing, by either prescribing a different dose or a different drug to a genetically at-risk patient, there may be a malpractice lawsuit. (Marchant et al., 2020, p. 25)

The reality that physicians vary in their understanding of genetics and genomics means that the genetic counselor may face challenges communicating effectively to a physician unfamiliar with the testing and the significance of the results (Fuchs, 2010).

Although cases have also been brought for failure to communicate results to family members (see, e.g., *Mydske v. University of Washington*, 1988), this is a complex area of law and ethics. While failure to communicate the heritability of a disorder and to encourage the patient to offer this information to relevant family members could result in liability, legal authorities have also recognized that a patient's test results constitute personal health information protected by privacy law. Relevant law includes the federal Health Insurance Portability and Accountability Act (HIPAA), when HIPAA-covered entities are involved, although HIPAA recognizes some exceptions (Marchant et al., 2020; Wolf et al., 2008). In general, clinicians are not obligated to breach patient confidentiality to warn relatives directly, though they may be obligated to alert patients to the heritability of a pathogenic variant and encourage patient disclosure to relatives (Rothstein, 2018). Full discussion of a duty or privilege to warn relatives is beyond the scope of this chapter. (For more on this topic, see, e.g., Marchant et al., 2011; Perry et al., 2020; Rothstein, 2018; Wolf et al., 2015).

Failure to offer, communicate, or appropriately manage incidental and secondary findings

Incidental or secondary findings can arise in either clinical or research testing. Commentators may distinguish between incidental and secondary findings based on whether the additional findings are sought intentionally (secondary findings) or discovered without deliberate search (incidental findings) (Presidential Commission for the Study of Bioethical Issues, 2013). In the context of clinical testing, results beyond those sought to resolve the diagnostic, predictive, or treatment question at hand are considered incidental or secondary findings. In clinical genomic sequencing, there has been considerable debate over whether to routinely seek secondary findings and offer them to the patient. In 2013, the ACMG recommended routine analysis of 56 additional genes (subsequently updated)—selected for pathogenicity and clinical actionability—whenever clinical sequencing is undertaken in order to offer the findings to patients and their clinicians (Green et al., 2013; Kalia et al., 2017; Wolf, 2017). However, this recommendation generated extensive debate (e.g., McGuire et al., 2013; Wolf, 2017; Wolf et al., 2013) and the ACMG subsequently recommended that adult patients have the opportunity to decline this additional analysis (ACMG, 2015).

Whether or not secondary findings are deliberately sought as the ACMG recommends, incidental findings can arise in genetic or genomic testing. "In clinical care, liability can result from a failure to analyze and communicate genomic incidental findings, from incorrect analysis of incidental findings (including a false positive), or from miscommunication of incidental findings" (Marchant et al., 2020, p. 26). The transition from genetic to genomic sequencing in clinical care may generate more incidental findings due to the broader scope of genomic sequencing, the progression in understanding of gene–disease associations, and the increasing amount of information that can be gleaned from a genomic test (Clayton et al., 2013). Thus, genetic counselors are likely to face a growing set of issues regarding their obligations to disclose incidental or secondary findings.

Genetic counselors may also be faced with incidental or secondary findings discovered through a patient's participation in genetic or genomic research. This is a complex domain, as the question of researchers' obligation to communicate incidental or secondary findings to the research participant or their clinician is an evolving one (Wolf, 2013; Wolf et al., 2008, 2012; Fabsitz et al., 2010). Moreover, research findings may not have been generated or validated in a laboratory that is compliant with the Clinical Laboratory Improvement Amendments (CLIA), and thus will likely require such validation before clinical use (Evans & Wolf, 2019; Wolf & Evans, 2018). In addition, a full clinical evaluation may be needed, including consideration of family history. Genetic counselors and other clinicians thus face duties to handle responsibly incidental or secondary findings from research. As Marchant et al. (2020) describe:

> Once the laboratory has reported an incidental finding with health implications for the patient, the clinician is obligated to offer disclosure of that finding to the patient and obligated to manage the finding in keeping with the standard of care (either directly or through appropriate referral). (p. 27)

Failure to update variant interpretation and recontact

Our understanding of the role that many genetic variants play in disease and health is dynamic in nature and subject to rapid change. A variant may be reported out with an uncertain significance and within months it may be reinterpreted as pathogenic or likely pathogenic in nature. This potential for rapid changes in knowledge raises the question of when genetic counselors have the duty to contact a patient with new information about the interpretation of a genetic variant. This is distinct from the clear duty to recontact patients to correct a laboratory result or interpretation that was erroneous when rendered. If the test result and variant interpretation were correct when rendered but subsequent progress yields a change in understanding, do clinicians have a duty to recontact the patient, and if so, what are the limits on that duty?

This has been much debated, in part due to the case of *Belser v. Quest Diagnostics* (2020), which held that a clinical diagnostics service testing laboratory did not violate CLIA requirements by failing to update a variant interpretation. (See also *Williams v. Quest Diagnostics*, 2018.) The court reasoned that "CLIA Section 493.129(k) applies to situations where the lab detects an 'error' in its original report," but there is no "error" if the original classification of "variant of unknown significance" was reasonable at the time the report was made. The debate is not fully resolved, and questions remain about the duty to update variant classifications and recontact patients. However, courts are more likely to find a duty when the clinician–patient relationship is ongoing. Indeed, courts have recognized a duty to recontact (a) "when a physician administers a procedure or treatment that requires an established follow-up procedure or test" and (b) "when a patient is being treated with a drug or device prescribed by the physician, and the physician learns of new risks associated with that treatment, such as a new warning issued by the [Food and Drug Administration]" (Marchant et al., 2020, p. 29). Consulting professional guidelines in this evolving domain may prove helpful (see, e.g., Berliner et al., 2013; Bombard et al., 2019; Carrieri et al., 2019; David et al., 2019; Deignan et al., 2019).

Failure to properly handle results from direct-to-consumer testing

While genetic and genomic testing in conventional clinical contexts may expose genetic counselors to potential liability, the rise of DTC testing services raises additional concerns. Although some genetic counselors may be employed by DTC companies to offer counseling to customers, we focus here on genetic counselors in clinical settings who may encounter a patient with DTC results. People may purchase DTC testing for a variety of reasons, such as curiosity about their health, efforts to understand a health condition, ascertaining risk of future health conditions, or informing their reproductive decision making. Individuals may then present their results to a genetic counselor and other clinicians. State and federal regulation of DTC company testing, including regulation by the federal Food and Drug Administration (FDA), is evolving and complex (Majumder et al., 2021). As the FDA itself has recognized, not all DTC tests are equally accurate (FDA, 2018). However, simply ignoring DTC test results could risk liability if those results reveal a variant relevant to health or medical care and ignoring that result eventuates in harm (Marchant et al., 2020). At the same time, relying on a DTC result without validation can be perilous. Best practice is likely to require validation of the DTC test result in a CLIA-compliant clinical laboratory before relying on the result in providing health advice (Marchant et al., 2020).

Managing Liability Exposure

Genetic counselors can take steps to manage their liability exposure. They can make sure they have malpractice insurance—through their institution, privately, or both. They should check these insurance policies to ascertain limits on their coverage.

In addition, genetic counselors should be cognizant of licensure and continuing education requirements in their state: "It will be important to demonstrate that your skills and knowledge (1) at least meet a minimum standard by having certification and a valid license if available and (2) are up to date through continuing education credits" (Schmerler, 2008, p. 99). Licensure and continuing education requirements may be used by courts to help determine the standard of care in a malpractice lawsuit.

Genetic counselors should also consult clinical practice guidelines and other guidance from professional societies such as the NSGC (Marchant et al., 2020). Such guidelines inform the relevant standards of care in genetic counseling. Genetic counselors may also choose to take an active role in promulgating sound practice guidelines through the NSGC and other bodies.

Genetic counselors can also manage liability exposure by ensuring sound communication with patients and documentation throughout the counseling process. To meet the standard of care:

> There must be clear evidence that the patient had knowledge of the risk, appreciated and understood the nature of the risk, and voluntarily chose to incur the risk. Documentation of an informed consent process goes a long way to satisfy the requirements. (Schmerler, 2008, pp. 100–101)

In addition, genetic counselors should discuss the limitations of genetic and genomic tests with their patients. Rapid advances in genomic testing and sequencing require a sophisticated understanding by genetic counselors of the strengths and limitations of different testing and sequencing approaches and the ability to communicate the relevant information. The patient should have enough information to make an informed choice about whether to rely on the data from genomic tests and how to use the information. The patient should also be warned that the interpretation of their test results could change over time as more information is collected about different gene variants.

Genetic counselors must also bear in mind that failure to update a patient can result in liability in some circumstances. "If a provider discovers that the previous information communicated to the patient was erroneous at the time of the communication, the provider should notify the patient of the corrected information as soon as possible" (Marchant et al., 2020, p. 31). Genetic counselors should make reasonable efforts to contact patients if they later discover that, based on new evidence, their original analysis was faulty at the time it was made. Even if the analysis was correct at the time counseling occurred, a genetic counselor may be liable if they discover new information implicating a former patient's health and fail to make a reasonable effort to communicate that information (Marchant et al., 2020).

Lastly, genetic counselors should be cautious with regard to DTC testing services. If a patient requests interpretation of their DTC test results, then the genetic counselor should make a reasonable effort to review, validate, and contextualize such results in a clinical evaluation. Liability may arise for failure to adequately review or counsel a patient regarding DTC test results if the patient seeks advice on their results and is later harmed by the genetic counselor's lack of guidance (Marchant et al., 2020).

Conclusion

Rapidly evolving technology, integration of genomics into clinical care, and progress in genomic knowledge all create new potential avenues of liability for genetic counselors. Genetic counselors should not be found liable if their actions conform to the standard of care, but such standards may be difficult to establish in a rapidly changing field like genetics and genomics. Consulting practice guidelines may be helpful. State licensure frameworks can also help clarify the standard of care.

Genetic counselors are crucial professionals involved in the delivery of genetic and genomic services. For both patients and clinicians, genetic counselors can serve as translators of complex genetics and genomics information, as well as advocates for the appropriate use of this powerful set of technologies. Like all clinicians, genetic counselors face potential liability for malpractice or negligence. However, genetic counselors can take steps to manage and reduce their liability exposure. Most importantly, genetic counselors can help lead the successful and informed integration of genetics and genomics into clinical care while advocating for appropriate ethical and legal standards.

Acknowledgments

Preparation of this chapter was supported in part by NIH/NHGRI/NCI #R01HG008605 on "LawSeq^{SM}: Building a Sound Legal Foundation for Translating Genomics into Clinical

Application" (Wolf, Clayton, Lawrenz, Principal Investigators). Thanks to Meredith Gingold and Aron Mozes for excellent research assistance. The content provided in this chapter reflects legal analysis through November 2020 and its discussion of the law was current as of that date. The chapter's discussion does not constitute legal advice.

References

Abacan, M., Alsubaie, L., Barlow-Stewart, K., Caanen, B., Cordier, C., Courtney, E., Davoine, E., Edwards, J., Elackatt, N. J., Gardiner, K., Guan, Y., Huang, L., Malmgren, C. I., Kejriwal, S., Kim, H. J., Lambert, D., Lantigua-Cruz, P. A., Lee, J. M. H., Lodahl, M., . . . Wicklund, C. (2019). The global state of the genetic counseling profession. *European Journal of Human Genetics*, *27*(2), 183–197. https://doi.org/10.1038/s41431-018-0252-x

Access to Genetic Counselor Services Act of 2019, H.R. 3235, 116th Cong. (2019). https://www.congress.gov/bill/116th-congress/house-bill/3235/all-actions

ACMG Member Informational Session: Understanding the details of ACMG's position on HR 3235. (2020, October 23). https://www.acmgeducation.net/Public/Catalog/Details.aspx?id=ckf9vrWXStFoBMcPqo4L9Q%3D%3D&returnurl=%2fUsers%2fUserOnlineCourse.aspx%3fLearningActivityID%3dckf9vrWXStFoBMcPqo4L9Q%253d%253d.

Alger v. Strong Memorial Hospital, 980 N.Y.S.2d 200 (N.Y. App. Div. 2014).

American Board of Genetic Counseling. (n.d.-a). *ABGC restructuring committee*. https://www.abgc.net/about-abgc/detailed-history/

American Board of Genetic Counseling. (n.d.-b). *Getting recertified*. https://www.abgc.net/for-diplomates/get-recertified/

American Board of Genetic Counseling. (n.d.-c). *State licensure*. https://www.abgc.net/research-resources/state-licensure/

American College of Medical Genetics and Genomics. (2015). ACMG policy statement: Updated recommendations regarding analysis and reporting of secondary findings in clinical genome-scale sequencing. *Genetics in Medicine*, *17*(1), 68–69.

Ark. Code Ann. §§ 17.95.1104, 17.95.1109 (2019).

Becker v. Schwartz, 386 N.E.2d 807 (N.Y. 1978).

Belser v. Quest Diagnostics, Inc., No. 3:16-0972-MBS, 2020 WL 6526084 (D.S.C. Nov. 5, 2020).

Berliner, J. L., Fay, A. M., Cummings, S. A., Burnett, B., & Tillmanns, T. (2013). NSGC practice guideline: Risk assessment and genetic counseling for hereditary breast and ovarian cancer. *Journal of Genetic Counseling*, *22*(2), 155–163.

Blouin v. Koster, No. PC-2015-3817, 2016 WL 3976926 (R.I. Super. July 19, 2016).

Bombard, Y., Brothers, K. B., Fitzgerald-Butt, S., Garrison, N. A., Jamal, L., James, C. A., Jarvik G. P., McCormick, J. B., Nelson, T. N., Ormond, K. E., Rehm, H. L., Richer, J., Souzeau, E., Vassy, J. L., Wagner, J. K., & Levy H. P. (2019). The responsibility to recontact research participants after reinterpretation of genetic and genomic research results. *American Journal of Human Genetics*, *104*(4), 578–595.

Burke, W., Clayton, E. W., Wolf, S. M., Berry, S. A., Evans, B. J., Evans, J. P., Hall, R., Korngiebel, D., Laberge, A., LeRoy, B. S., & McGuire, A. L. (2019). Improving recommendations for genomic medicine: Building an evolutionary process from clinical practice advisory documents to guidelines. *Genetics in Medicine*, *21*(7), 2431–2438.

Carrieri, D., Howard, H. C., Benjamin, C., Clarke, A. J., Dheensa, S., Doheny, S., Hawkins, N., Halbersma-Konings, T. F., Jackson, L., Kayserili, H., Kelly, S. E., Lucassen, A. M.,

Mendes, Á., Rial-Sebbag, E., Stefánsdóttir, V., Turnpenny, P. D., van El, C. G., van Langen, I., Cornel, M. C., & Forzano, F. (2019). Recontacting patients in clinical genetics services: Recommendations of the European Society of Human Genetics. *European Journal of Human Genetics, 27*(2), 169–182.

Cauman v. George Washington University, 630 A.2d 1104 (D.C. 1993).

Clayton, E. W., Haga, S., Kuszler, P., Bane, E., Shutske, K., & Burke, W. (2013). Managing incidental genomic findings: Legal obligations of clinicians. *Genetics in Medicine, 15*(8), 624–629.

Cohen v. Rashba, No. CV2000-00584, 2005 WL 4044514 (Sup. Ct. Mass. Jan. 10, 2005).

Cooke-Moore v. Curry Community Health, Inc., No. 17CV46203, 2018 WL 4999015 (Or. Cir. Apr. 1, 2018).

David, K. L., Best, R. G., Brenman, L. M., Bush, L., Deignan, J. L., Flannery, D., Hoffman, J. D., Holm, I., Miller, D. T., O'Leary, J., & Pyeritz, R. E., ACMG Social Ethical Legal Issues Committee. (2019). Patient re-contact after revision of genomic test results: Points to consider—A statement of the American College of Medical Genetics and Genomics (ACMG). *Genetics in Medicine, 21*(4), 769–771.

Deignan, J. L., Chung, W. K., Kearney, H. M., Monaghan, K. G., Rehder, C. W., Chao, E. C., ACMG Laboratory Quality Assurance Committee. (2019). Points to consider in the reevaluation and reanalysis of genomic tests results: A statement of the American College of Medical Genetics and Genomics (ACMG). *Genetics in Medicine, 21*(6), 1267–1270.

Ermoian v. Desert Hospital, 61 Cal. Rptr.3d 754 (Cal. Dist. Ct. App. 2007).

Estrada v. University of South Florida Board of Trustees, No. 06-000625, 2007 WL 2491545 (Fla. Cir. Ct. July 24, 2007).

Evans, B. J., & Wolf, S. M. (2019). A Faustian bargain that imperils people's rights to see their own personal information. *Florida Law Review, 71*(5), 1281–1345.

Fabsitz, R. R., McGuire, A., Sharp, R. S., Puggal, M., Beskow, L. M., Biesecker, L. G., Bookman, E., Burke, W., Burchard, E. G., Church, G., Clayton, E. W., Eckfeldt, J. H., Fernandez, C. V., Fisher, R., Fullerton, S. M., Gabriel, S., Gachupin, F., James, C., Jarvik, G. P., . . . Burke, G. L. (2010). Ethical and practical guidelines for reporting genetic research results to study participants: Updated guidelines from a National Heart, Lung, and Blood Institute Working Group. *Circulation: Cardiovascular Genetics, 3*(6), 574–580.

Flythe v. Davis, No. 4:10-CV-00126-BO, 2011 WL 1870229, at *3 (E.D.N.C., May 16, 2011).

Food and Drug Administration. (2018, October 31). *The FDA warns against the use of many genetic tests with unapproved claims to predict patient response to specific medications: FDA safety communication.* https://www.fda.gov/medical-devices/safety-communications/fda-warns-against-use-many-genetic-tests-unapproved-claims-predict-patient-response-specific

Foulkes, A. L., Roberts, J. L., Appelbaum, P. S., Chung, W. K., Clayton, E. W., Evans, B., & Marchant, G. E. (2020). Can clinical genetics laboratories be sued for medical malpractice? *Annals of Health Law and Life Sciences, 29*(1), 153–171.

Fuchs, S. A. (2010). Will the FDA's 2010 warfarin label changes finally provide the legal impetus for warfarin pharmacogenetic testing? *North Carolina Journal of Law & Technology, 12*(1), 99–157.

Gallagher v. Duke University, 852 F.2d 773 (4th Cir. 1988).

Genetic counselor licensure proponents call for more states to adopt licensing laws: Benefits of licensure extend to geneticists, counselors, and patients. (2016). *American Journal of Medical Genetics, 170A*(1), 8–9.

Green, R. C., Berg, J. S., Grody, W. W., Kalia, S. S., Korf, B. R., Martin, C. L., McGuire, A., Nussbaum, R. L., O'Daniel, J. M., Ormond, K. E., Rehm, H. L., Watson, M. S., Williams, M. S., & Biesecker, L. G. (2013). ACMG recommendations for reporting of incidental findings in clinical exome and genome sequencing. *Genetics in Medicine, 15*(7), 565–574.

Gregg, A. R., & Muenke, M. (2020, January 9). H.R. 3235—Access to Genetic Counselor Services Act of 2019. https://www.acmg.net/PDFLibrary/ACMG_Letter_HR3235_Jan2020.pdf

Harbeson v. Parke-Davis, Inc., 656 P.2d 483 (Wash. 1983), *aff'd*, 746 F.2d 517 (9th Cir. 1984).

Harris, C. (2014). Statutory prohibitions on wrongful birth claims & their dangerous effects on parents. *Boston College Journal of Law and Social Justice, 34*(2), 365–396.

Hegeman, R. (2020, September 16). *Kansas court hears arguments over 'wrongful birth' law*. Associated Press. https://www.usnews.com/news/us/articles/2020-09-16/kansas-court-hears-arguments-over-wrongful-birth-law

Janssens, A. (2019). Validity of polygenic risk scores: Are we measuring what we think we are? *Human Molecular Genetics, 28*(R2), R143–R150. https://doi.org/10.1093/hmg/ddz205.

John v. De Vivo, 117 N.Y.S.3d 230 (N.Y. App. Div. 1st Dept. 2020).

Johnson v. Botsford Gen. Hosp., 748 N.W.2d 907, 910-11 (Mich. Ct. App. 2008) (quoting Bryant v. Oakpointe Villa Nursing Ctr., Inc., 684 N.W.2d 864, 871 (Mich. 2004)).

Kalia, S. S., Adelman, K., Bale, S. J., Chung, W. K., Eng, C., Evans, J. P., Herman, G. E., Hufnagel, S. B., Klein, T. E., Korf, B. R., McKelvey, K. D., Ormond, K. E., Richards, S., Vlangos, C. N., Watson, M., Martin, C. L., & Miller, D. T. (2017). Recommendations for reporting of secondary findings in clinical exome and genome sequencing, 2016 update (ACMG SF v2.0): A policy statement of the American College of Medical Genetics and Genomics. *Genetics in Medicine, 19*(2), 249–255.

La. Stat. Ann. § 37:1360.103 (2018). Collaborative practice agreement; requirements. http://legis.la.gov/legis/Law.aspx?d=1108929

Lewis, M. H., Gohagan, J. K., & Merenstein, D. J. (2007). The locality rule and the physician's dilemma: Local medical practices vs the national standard of care. *JAMA, 297*(23), 2633–2637.

Majumder, M. A., Guerrini, C. J., & McGuire, A. L. (2021). Direct-to-consumer genetic testing: Value and risk. *Annual Review of Medicine, 72*, 151–166.

Marchant, G., Barnes, M., Evans, J. P., LeRoy, B., & Wolf, S. M. (2020). From genetics to genomics: Facing the liability implications in clinical care. *Journal of Law, Medicine & Ethics, 48*(1), 11–43.

Marchant, G. E., Campos-Outcalt, D. E., & Lindor, R. A. (2011). Physician liability: The next big thing for personalized medicine? *Personalized Medicine, 8*(4), 457–467.

Marchant, G. E., & Lindor, R. A. (2018). Genomic malpractice: An emerging tide or gentle ripple? *Food and Drug Law Journal, 73*(1), 1–37.

Martinez v. Long Island Jewish Hillside Medical Center, 512 N.E.2d 538 (N.Y. 1987).

McGuire, A. L., Joffe, S., Koenig, B. A., Biesecker, B. B., McCullough, L. B., Blumenthal-Barby, J. S., Caulfield, T., Terry, S. F., & Green, R. C. (2013). Ethics and genomic incidental findings. *Science, 340*(6136), 1047–1048.

Miller & Zois. (n.d.-a). *Canavan disease genetic counseling lawsuit*. https://malpracticecases.millerandzois.com/canavan-disease-lawsuit.html

Miller & Zois. (n.d.-b). *Genetic counseling negligence lawsuit*. https://www.millerandzois.com/medical-malpractice/maryland-malpractice-lawsuits/genetic-counseling-negligence-lawsuit/

Molloy v. Meier, 679 N.W.2d 711 (Minn. 2004).

Mydske v. University of Washington, No. 84-2-04702-0, 1988 WL 365445 (King Cty. Super. Ct. Wash. 1988).

Naccash v. Burger, 223 Va. 406 (1982).

National Human Genome Research Institute. (2020, August 11). *Polygenic risk scores*. https://www.genome.gov/Health/Genomics-and-Medicine/Polygenic-risk-scores

National Society of Genetic Counselors. (2017). *Genetic testing resource*. https://www.nsgc.org/Portals/0/Docs/About/Genetic%20Testing%20Resource%20-%20Final.pdf?ver=TpsDLkLv-JGHXLtwDcfpuA%3d%3d

National Society of Genetic Counselors. (2020a). *Policy & publications: Model legislative provisions*. https://www.nsgc.org/Policy-Research-and-Publications/State-Licensure-for-Genetic-Counselors/Model-Legislative-Provisions

National Society of Genetic Counselors. (2020b). *Policy & publications: States issuing licenses for genetic counselors*. https://www.nsgc.org/Policy-Research-and-Publications/State-Licensure-for-Genetic-Counselors/States-Issuing-Licenses

Ohio Rev. Code Ann. § 4778.11 (2012). Authorized activities for licensees. https://codes.ohio.gov/orc/4778

Pa. Stat. and Cons. Stat. § 271.10c (West 2012). Genetic counselor. https://codes.findlaw.com/pa/title-63-ps-professions-and-occupations-state-licensed/pa-st-sect-63-271-10c.html

Pergament, D., & Ilijic, K. (2014). The legal past, present and future of prenatal genetic testing: Professional liability and other legal challenges affecting patient access to services. *Journal of Clinical Medicine*, *3*(4), 1437–1465.

Perry, T. J., Patton, S. I., Farmer, M. B., Hurst, C. B., McGwin, G., & Robin, N. H. (2020). The duty to warn at-risk relatives: The experience of genetic counselors and medical geneticists. *American Journal of Medical Genetics*, *182*(2), 314–321.

Plowman v. Fort Madison Cmty. Hosp., 896 N.W.2d 393 (Iowa 2017).

Presidential Commission for the Study of Bioethical Issues. (2013). *Anticipate and communicate: Ethical management of incidental and secondary findings in the clinical, research, and direct-to-consumer contexts*. https://bioethicsarchive.georgetown.edu/pcsbi/sites/default/files/FINALAnticipateCommunicate_PCSBI_0.pdf

Procanik by Procanik v. Cillo, 478 A.2d 755 (N.J. 1984).

Ray, T. (2020, February 11). *Genetic counselors Medicare payment bill gaining support despite 'scope of practice' disagreement*. https://www.genomeweb.com/policy-legislation/genetic-counselors-medicare-payment-bill-gaining-support-despite-scope-practice

Ray, T. (2021, February 24). *ACMG lobbying state legislatures on genetic counselors' scope of practice draws criticism*. https://www.genomeweb.com/policy-legislation/acmg-lobbying-state-legislatures-genetic-counselors-scope-practice-draws#.Y_uj6nbMKUk

Reed v. Campagnolo, 332 Md. 226 (1993).

Reilly, P. R. (1975). Genetic counseling and the law. *Houston Law Review*, *12*(3), 640–660.

Richards, S., Aziz, N., Bale, S., Bick, D., Das, S., Gastier-Foster, J., Grody, W. W., Hegde, M., Lyon, E., Spector, E., Voelkerding, K., & Rehm, H. L. (2015). Standards and guidelines for the interpretation of sequence variants: A joint consensus recommendation of the American College of Medical Genetics and Genomics and the Association for Molecular Pathology. *Genetics in Medicine*, *17*(5), 405–423.

Rothstein, M. A. (2018). Reconsidering the duty to warn genetically at-risk relatives. *Genetics in Medicine*, *20*(3), 285–290.

Schmerler, S. (2008). *Lessons learned: Risk management issues in genetic counseling*. Springer.

Stein, J. A. (2020). *Personal injury damages* (Vol. 2, § 12:8, 3rd ed.). Thomson Reuters.

Turpin v. Sortini, 31 Cal. 3d 220 (1982).
Wain, K. E., Azzariti, D. R., Goldstein, J. L., Johnson, A. K., Krautscheid, P., Lepore, B., O'Daniel, J. M., Ritter, D., Savatt, J. M., Riggs, E. R., & Martin, C. L. (2020). Variant interpretation is a component of clinical practice among genetic counselors in multiple specialties. *Genetics in Medicine*, *22*(4), 785–792.
Wash. Admin. Code § 246-825-030 (2010). Collaborative agreement. https://app.leg.wa.gov/wac/default.aspx?cite=246-825-030
Williams v. Quest Diagnostics, Inc., 353 F. Supp. 3d 432 (D.S.C. 2018).
Wolf, S. M. (2013). Return of individual research results and incidental findings: Facing the challenges of translational science. *Annual Review of Genomics and Human Genetics*, *14*, 557–577.
Wolf, S. M. (2017). The continuing evolution of standards for genomic sequencing in clinical care: Restoring patient choice. *Journal of Law, Medicine & Ethics*, *45*(3), 333–340.
Wolf, S. M., Annas, G. J., & Elias, S. (2013). Patient autonomy and incidental findings in clinical genomics. *Science*, *340*(6136), 1049–1050.
Wolf, S. M., Branum, R., Koenig, B. A., Petersen, G. M., Berry, S. A., Beskow, L. M., Daly, M. B., Fernandez, C. V., Green, R. C., LeRoy, B. S., Lindor, N. M., O'Rourke, P. P., Breitkopf, C. R., Rothstein, M. A., Van Ness, B., & Wilfond, B. S. (2015). Returning a research participant's genomic results to relative: Analysis and recommendations. *Journal of Law, Medicine & Ethics*, *43*(3), 440–463.
Wolf, S. M., Crock, B. N., Van Ness, B., Lawrenz, F., Kahn, J. P., Beskow, L. M., Cho, M. K., Christman, M. F., Green, R. C., Hall, R., Illes, J., Keane, M., Knoppers, B. M., Koenig, B. A., Kohane, I. S., LeRoy, B., Maschke, K. J., McGeveran, W., Ossorio, P., . . . Wolf, W. A. (2012). Managing research results and incidental findings in genomic research involving biobanks & archived datasets. *Genetics in Medicine*, *14*(4), 361–384.
Wolf, S. M., & Evans, B. J. (2018). Return of results and data to study participants. *Science*, *362*(6411), 159–160.
Wolf, S. M., Lawrenz, F. P., Nelson, C. A., Kahn, J. P., Cho, M. K., Clayton, E. W., Fletcher, J. G., Georgieff, M. K., Hammerschmidt, D., Hudson, K., Illes, J., Kapur, V., Keane, M. A., Koenig, B. A., LeRoy, B. S., McFarland, E. G., Paradise, J., Parker, L. S., Terry, S. F., . . . Wilfond, B. S. (2008). Managing incidental findings in human subjects research: Analysis and recommendations. *Journal of Law, Medicine & Ethics*, *36*(2), 219–248.
Wuth ex rel. Kessler v. Laboratory Corp. of Am., 359 P.3d 841 (Wash. App. Div. 1 2015).
Zittler, J. M. (2019). Malpractice liability in genetic counseling. In *American Jurisprudence Proof of Facts* (Vol. 105, 3rd ed., p. 483). Lawyers Cooperative Publishing.

CHAPTER 19

FAMILY HISTORY IN CONTEMPORARY GENETICS

DEBRA L. COLLINS AND DEVIN M. COX

Introduction

Family history plays a critical role in assessing the risk of inherited medical conditions including single gene disorders as well as more complex or multifactorial conditions. Historically, the multigeneration family history, referred to by genetics professionals as a pedigree, was the main method of determining inheritance and recurrence risk. Prior to the discovery of the underlying genetic mechanism for many diseases, the pedigree was the primary way to assess potential at-risk family members based on the perceived inheritance pattern within the family. When testing first became available for many genes, it was cost and time prohibitive to test individual genes, making it vitally important to assess the family history pedigree and determine the most likely familial condition before clinical testing. With new genetic testing methods, such as next-generation sequencing panel testing, exome sequencing, and genome testing, genetic testing has become more cost effective and available, with the pedigree utilized to determine the extent and type of genetic testing.

A thorough family history can demonstrate the genetic variation of familial diseases, identify genotype–phenotype correlations, and enhance the ability to predict those at risk of developing an inherited medical condition. Correlating family history with test results may help guide management and preventative measures including increased surveillance of newly identified family members. Obtaining, analyzing, and interpreting a family medical history has been called the "cheapest genetic test" (Guttmacher et al., 2004) as this seemingly simple tool provides a wealth of information about potential genetic and environmental influences. Eliciting a three-generation family history (including first-, second-, and third-degree relatives) can reveal potential inheritance patterns or indicate multiple genetic conditions in the family. Genetic conditions often affect multiple body systems, have several clinical features (with major and subtle expression), and show variation in clinical expression including age of onset and severity.

Box 19.1 Pedigrees

Pedigrees enable clinicians to:

- establish the pattern of inheritance
- determine inheritance risks
- make a medical diagnosis
- conduct a risk assessment
- identify at-risk family members
- decide on testing strategies
- develop patient rapport
- explore patient and family understanding
- manage/recommend interventions
- analyze personal and familial psychosocial elements
- assess potential relevance of variant(s) of uncertain clinical significance
- consider if multiple genetic conditions could be occurring simultaneously

Family medical history is often solicited prior to a clinical genetics visit through patient questionnaires or electronic medical record tools. This information is refined through additional targeted inquiries during the clinic visit. Reviewing the family medical history is an opportunity to establish rapport with patients, which enhances counseling as well as follow-up discussions about services, screenings, and referrals. After genetic testing, a critical review of the pedigree contributes to variant interpretation, helps estimate risks, and guides management.

The Ongoing Value of Pedigree Analysis

Interpretation of the family medical history is an ongoing and valuable part of a genetic counseling evaluation at all ages and in all clinics. A pedigree is a tool to visually assess multiple pieces of information at a glance and may suggest an underlying inheritance pattern including which side of the family a condition may be arising from. This may determine the extent of genetic testing recommendations. If testing is unavailable, then the pedigree analysis may suggest risks for extended family members. The pedigree can show the variability of a condition within a family, provide an opportunity for psychosocial interactions with patients, and be a visual aid to explain inheritance (Box 19.1).

Important Considerations in Pedigree Construction

Several published guidelines provide standards on representing a family medical history as a pedigree, including traditional nomenclature (squares and circles), documenting complex family structures, and inclusive symbols to recognize the wide variety of family relationships and nuances (Bennett, 1999; Bennett et al., 2022).

Family history information can be collected by the completion of a previsit family medical information form. When available, patients can enter this information online. Patients often need to contact other family members to gather the most accurate details of their family medical history. All family history information, family genetic test results, and sometimes photos of family members contribute to a comprehensive assessment and discussion using the most accurate information. The pedigree is an active document; assessments and recommendations may need to be modified when new family health information is updated.

Proband

The process of creating a pedigree begins with indicating the proband or the person who first established care in a genetic clinic. The symbol for the proband is drawn as a circle (identifying as female), square (identifying as male), or diamond (nonbinary, gender diverse, or sex/gender unknown/unspecified) and denoted with an arrow; this allows all providers or reviewers to quickly establish relationships between members of the pedigree. The information documented on the proband differs by the clinic, age, or reason for the clinic visit (Box 19.2). Information can be obtained in advance through a medical records review and edited in the pedigree. Confirmation of information with the proband is an opportunity for the genetic counselor to establish rapport and use counseling skills and strategies for eliciting sensitive information (see Building Rapport During the Pedigree Construction Process for further details).

Family members

Pedigrees use visual symbols for quick assessment of the conditions in the proband and family members. These symbols vary with conditions, medical evaluation, and the

Box 19.2 Documentation for Proband Based on Reason for Referral[a]

- Prenatal/prepregnancy: pregnancy history including pregnancy loss and infertility, maternal age, ultrasound findings, teratogen exposure, noninvasive prenatal screening, anomalous maternal serum screening
- Pediatric/newborn/adolescent clinic: positive newborn screening test (e.g., phenylketonuria), congenital anomaly, developmental delay, intellectual delay, dysmorphic features including appropriate measurements, vision/hearing limitations, major surgeries
- Adult clinics: congenital anomaly, developmental/intellectual disability, dysmorphic features, age of diagnosis of disease, imaging related to disease (echocardiogram, positron emission tomography scan, computed tomography, magnetic resonance imaging, etc.), diagnostic evaluations related to disease (electrocardiography, colonoscopy, etc.), relevant blood work (hormone levels, etc.), relevant surgical history (hysterectomy, cardiac ablation, etc.)

[a] While not exhaustive, examples were obtained from Pletcher et al. (2007).

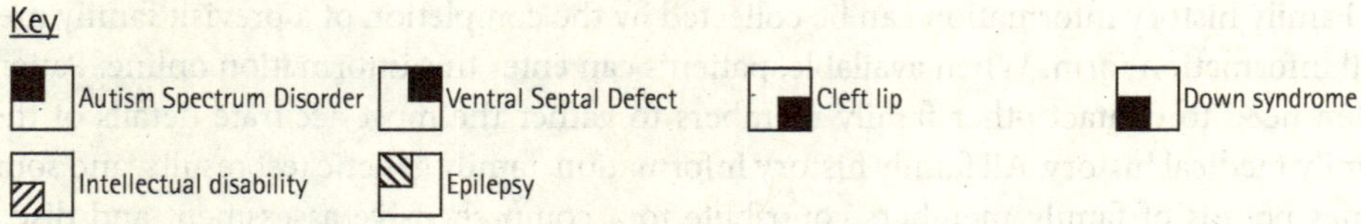

FIGURE 19.1 Example of pedigree symbols and key.

diagnosis of concern. If there are multiple features or conditions, the symbol may be divided into quadrants. The pedigree should provide a key to the symbols used (Figure 19.1). Information can be reviewed and updated periodically. After the proband's personal medical history is documented, the pedigree is expanded to include first-, second-, and third-degree relatives.

Not all family members' medical information needs to be documented; see Box 19.3 for examples of potentially relevant information to assess during a pedigree. It is important to document information that alters the assessment of the final pedigree, including adoption into or out of the family, ages of deceased individuals, individuals who have transitioned/are transitioning from their biological sex, twins or multiples including zygosity, infertility, multiple miscarriages, and pregnancies achieved with donor eggs/sperm or surrogates. The interpretation of the pedigree and evaluation of inheritance risks are influenced by these scenarios.

All biological siblings, including both maternal and paternal half-siblings, should be documented. It is important to accurately record sibling relationships, including full or half-siblings versus step-siblings, which will allow for an adjustment of pedigree analysis and recommendations. As patients may not always understand the genetic implications of full, half-, or step-siblings, it is vital to clarify these relationships. Similarly, as a general rule, only biologically related relatives should be included. Unique situations, such as when a relative could be documented on both sides of the family, may be challenging; for example, if two sisters have children with brothers from another family, their children will be double first cousins, which challenges the interpretation of inheritance patterns of traits in the family (Figure 19.2).

Box 19.3 Family Medical Information Needed for a Genetic Evaluation

- Maternal and paternal relatives—current age, age at death, cause of death, ancestry
- Diagnosis/genetic conditions—clinical symptoms, age of diagnosis
- Genetic test results for family members
- Sudden death in someone who seemed healthy
- Three or more pregnancy losses, stillbirth, infertility
- Oncology specific—primary site for cancer, bilateral tumor occurrence/paired organs/multifocal
- Occurrence of a condition in the less-often-affected sex (e.g., male breast cancer)
- Serious, chronic, recurrent illnesses or anomalies (e.g., birth defects, intellectual disability, autism, etc.)

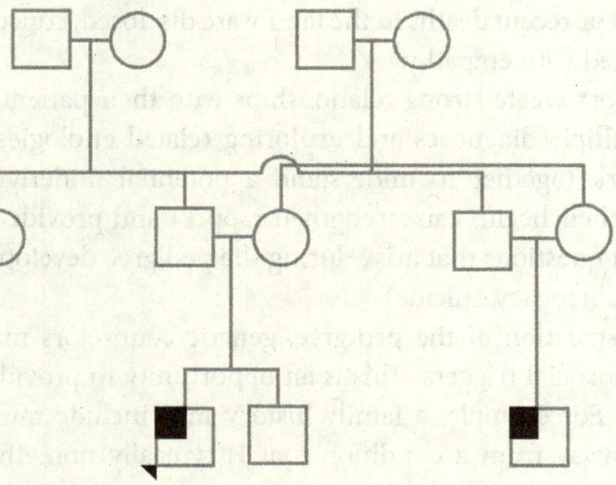

FIGURE 19.2 Example of documenting double first cousins, relationship line jumping from left of pedigree to right.

Ancestry and consanguinity

Maternal and paternal ancestry, noting Ashkenazi Jewish or other ancestry with known founder variants, should be recorded. Ancestry and ethnicity information formerly directed testing options offered, as these groups were perceived to have different genetic risks. We now recognize the genetic intermingling of all individuals, regardless of ancestry; however, this information can still be potentially useful in clarifying founder risks. Consanguinity, when blood relatives have children together, is another important but potentially sensitive issue. It is important to clarify that consanguinity refers to blood relationships, not marriage or legal relationships. In a pediatric clinic, one approach is to ask parents, "Is there any chance you and your partner are related by blood?" This question might be posed later in the construction of a pedigree, which allows the genetic counselor an opportunity to develop rapport and determine the best way to approach the question. Consanguinity is documented in a pedigree by connecting the symbols for the two blood relatives by a double line.

Building Rapport During the Pedigree Construction Process

Genetic counseling sessions are enhanced by good patient rapport. One easy and rewarding way to build rapport and provide psychosocial support is through the creation, interpretation, and analysis of the pedigree. The questions asked about family history demonstrate genuine interest in the patient and their family. This can allow patients to feel more open and perceive that a genetic counselor is a partner in their diagnostic and testing odyssey. Soliciting information on each individual family member can produce unique anecdotes and stories that help genetic counselors and their patients connect on a more personal level.

When tragic events or recent deaths in the family are disclosed, concern for their family loss can be acknowledged with empathy.

Genetic counselors create strong relationships with their patients through recognizing concern about multiple diagnoses and exploring related etiologies. The patient and the counselor can work together to understand a potential underlying condition. Patient discussions about their health can strengthen rapport and provide clues to address other potentially difficult questions that arise during the pedigree development process (e.g., infertility, adoption, surrogacy, suicide).

During the construction of the pedigree, genetic counselors may uncover previously unexpressed psychosocial triggers. This is an opportunity to provide more advanced psychosocial support. For example, a family history may include multiple family members who have passed away from a condition that is typically nonlethal. This may underlie your patient's frustration with physicians and the appointment. A patient may feel that extra appointments and evaluations or other barriers prevented early diagnosis and care. Acknowledging these concerns and the severity in their family is important to help the patient feel that the counselor is an ally who understands their situation. See Chapter 6—"New Perspectives in Psychosocial Genetic Counseling" in this volume for further details on psychosocial aspects of genetic counseling.

Pedigree drawing programs

Many pedigree drawing programs are available for purchase or subscription. Others are accessible through laboratories or genetic testing services with proprietary online pedigree drawing programs. The programs have similar features for adding the proband and extended family members, with a key to describe the symbols used. Some may include a digital preclinic questionnaire for patients to complete.

Standardized pedigree shapes and symbols provide a valuable way to share information between genetics professionals and to add extended family members. These standard ways of presenting pedigrees continue to evolve as complex family structures and recognition of appropriate gender and biological sex designations are acknowledged (Bennet et al., 2022).

Targeted pedigree questions

Once a likely or suspected diagnosis in the family has been identified, genetic counselors can explore more specific questions to assess the range of clinical presentations in the family. Targeted pedigree questions prior to genetic testing help distinguish between differential diagnoses and guide genetic testing strategies (Box 19.4). For example, another family member may be identified as the more appropriate family member to test first. More specific targeted information may also be solicited after the results of genetic testing to identify manifestations of a specific genetic variant in the family. Posttest evaluation of the pedigree may retrospectively identify additional members to test and evaluate and be used to explore the gene variant classification (to determine variant of uncertain clinical significance

Box 19.4 Pedigree Questions Tailored to a Suspected Diagnosis

- Consider what the pedigree would look like if your patient *did* have the suspected diagnosis (inheritance pattern, reduced/full penetrance, de novo variant).
- Ask specifically about potentially affected family members if an inheritance pattern is suspected (e.g., children of individual suspected of having an autosomal dominant condition).
- Discuss features of the suspected diagnosis that the family may not realize are relevant (e.g., tremors/ataxia in families with fragile X syndrome).
- Determine if the patient or family members have had or need evaluations for signs or symptoms of the suspected diagnosis (e.g., echocardiogram or evaluations for autism).
- Assess if the patient or family members have symptoms indicative of undiagnosed features of the suspected diagnosis (e.g., uncontrollable blood pressure and unexplained fight-or-flight response associated with pheochromocytomas).
- Confirm and review genetic testing on extended family members, noting variants of uncertain significance (which may have been reclassified) and the number of genes tested. Establish if a variant is from the suspected side of the family. Assess whether a "negative" genetic test included the gene(s) associated with the suspected or likely diagnosis.

versus a pathogenic/likely pathogenic variant). An explanation of the reasoning behind the targeted questioning helps clarify the questions and solicit clearer responses from the patient and family.

Pedigree analysis with noninformative genetic test results

Genetic counselors have the unique skill set to provide additional risk and screening information to patients who receive negative test results, or when no genetic testing is available. If the family history is concerning, then patients can return to explore new advances in genetic testing and gain knowledge about specific genes.

In prenatal clinics, risk counseling incorporates empiric risk for a recurrence of the identified congenital anomaly in another family member; these risks are based on the degree of relationship (e.g., cleft palate). In pediatric clinics, test results may be reinterpreted as a child ages and develops additional features. In hereditary cancer clinics, even when a pathogenic variant is not identified by genetic testing, patients may be referred for high-risk screenings and surveillance based on the family history of cancer. Similarly, in cardiology clinics, screening and surveillance recommendations are also based on the family history of cardiac conditions.

Pedigree analysis for variants of unknown significance

In clinical testing, many variants are not easily characterized. The challenges in interpretation may be due to a lack of published cases, limitations of a laboratory's database, or the specific molecular change, for example. These variant changes are reported as variants of uncertain (or unknown) significance (VUS). The likelihood of finding a VUS can depend on the rarity of the indication for testing. As more information becomes known and data are shared, the VUS may be later reinterpreted as likely benign or as pathogenic. How much weight is placed clinically on a VUS depends on how closely linked the gene of interest is to the indication for testing and the clinical presentation.

A VUS result requires careful interpretation and communication with patients, explaining the variant change as well as the likelihood of reclassification and reinterpretation of the result after more research, published data, knowledge of gene structure and function, and technology evolve. It is estimated that up to 90% of VUSs will be reclassified as benign or likely benign (negative results) (Mersch et al., 2018). When clinicians suspect that a VUS contributes to a clinical diagnosis, various tools help with potential reclassification, including online gene databases, laboratory collaborations, and evaluation of additional affected family members in the pedigree (Richards et al., 2015). Additional in-depth bioinformatics analyses may be pursued by genetic testing laboratories to help resolve interpretation of test results. See Chapter 17—"After the Test: Interpreting a Clinical Report" in this volume for further details on VUS.

Inheritance patterns in pedigree analysis

A fundamental knowledge of Mendelian genetics and the concepts of dominant and recessive traits is required in clinical genetics. Mendelian genetics explains the observed patterns of many genetic conditions, based on clinical characteristics as well as molecular analyses. Understanding Mendelian principles helps diagnose and screen for symptoms needing surveillance, management, and treatment. The inheritance pattern can also help identify risk for other family members.

For many conditions, the pattern of Mendelian inheritance was historically established through published individual or family cases from worldwide research in the medical literature. Over the last 55 years or so, this information from peer-reviewed biomedical literature has been collected in Dr. Victor A. McKusick's *Mendelian Inheritance in Man* in 12 print editions from 1966 to 1998 and which then transitioned after 1995 to Online Mendelian Inheritance in Man (OMIM), a continuously updated catalog of human genes and genetic disorders and traits (https://www.ncbi.nlm.nih.gov/omim). Through this compilation of literature and case/family studies, some conditions were found to be inherited in more than one way, following autosomal recessive or dominant patterns (genes on the autosomal chromosomes), as well as X-linked patterns, or other genetic mechanisms. We now recognize epigenetic factors, contiguous gene syndromes, and other molecular mechanisms that affect inheritance patterns. Of note, few conditions are associated with genes on the Y chromosome. The Clinical Genome Resource (ClinGen) is also helpful to establish gene–disease validity through curation committees and standardized assessments (https://clinicalgenome.org).

Genetic conditions may be influenced by a number of different mechanisms, including gene variants, imprinting, skewed X chromosome inactivation, inversion of gene sequences, mitochondrial inheritance, dual/triple diagnoses, variable expressivity, and reduced penetrance. More recently, genome-wide association studies have led to the development of polygenic risk scores, which utilize multiple single nucleotide polymorphisms with either increased or decreased risk for a condition along with other more typical risk models to create a personalized risk score. See Chapter 20—"Common and Complex Traits: Considerations for Genetic Counseling" in this volume for further details on polygenic risk scores. This approach differs from traditional Mendelian inheritance interpretations as multiple genetic changes with small impacts combine to provide insight into the risk for a condition and can influence screening recommendations. While non-Mendelian complex inheritance patterns may be challenging to identify through pedigree analysis alone, it is still important to take a detailed family history.

Case Examples

Efficiently documenting an accurate family history, while building rapport, is a skill genetic counselors build through practice. Examining case examples can help illustrate the complexities and nuances of taking and analyzing a pedigree. Each case below represents a specific mode of inheritance and genetic counseling concepts. After a summary of the inheritance pattern for each case, recommended questions are provided for the proband and family members, including questions related to ancestry and/or consanguinity. The pedigree example for each case illustrates possible responses to these questions. Each case concludes with an analysis of the pedigree and additional counseling considerations.

Autosomal dominant inheritance

Genetic counselors frequently encounter families that believe a parent's condition will *always* be passed to a child. Analysis of their family pedigree helps them understand autosomal dominant inheritance and concepts such as variable expressivity, penetrance, and de novo variation (Box 19.5). Basic genetic concepts adapted to each individual or family are invaluable, such as a short explanation of inheritance outlining that there is a 50% chance that a child will get any given gene from a parent (not 100%). This can also be presented as a 1 in 2 (50%) chance. An important caveat is that this does not mean that if the first child has the condition, then the next child will not have it, as there is a 1 in 2 or 50% chance with *each* pregnancy. The use of visual aids, as exhibited in Figure 19.3, may be helpful to clearly illustrate inheritance patterns during a counseling session.

Box 19.5 Characteristics of Autosomal Dominant Inheritance

- Vertical transmission through two or more generations
- Biological males and females equally affected
- Biological male-to-male transmission

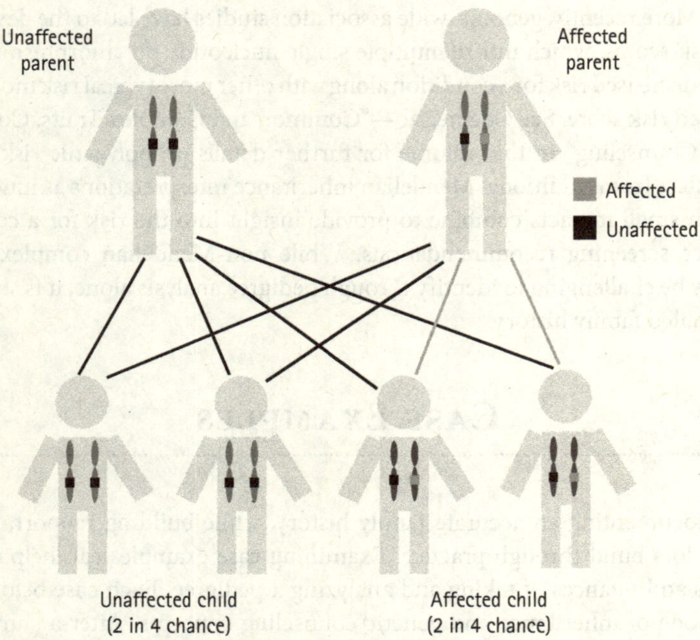

FIGURE 19.3 Example of autosomal dominant inheritance.

Many conditions do not present in an expected Mendelian fashion. Family histories can be complicated by the occurrence of a new de novo variant, gonadal mosaicism, misattributed paternity, conception via artificial insemination by donor, conception via surrogate or donor egg, variable expression, incomplete penetrance, and other factors. Various alternative conception methods and relationships/partnerships are important to keep in mind to ensure an accurate family history.

Not everyone who has a pathogenic variant in an autosomal dominant gene expresses the phenotype or expresses it in the same way. There are various factors that contribute to nonpenetrance, including how clinical expression is defined, modifying genes, genes more likely to be expressed in one sex, and the age of an individual. An individual may be found through molecular analysis to have a pathogenic variant but not necessarily manifest the condition, or to manifest the condition in a nontypical manner. For many dominant traits, the degree of penetrance that has been observed is documented in the literature by the percentage of persons with the feature being considered. As genetic testing continues to become more accessible and available, many genetic syndromes have some degree of variable expressivity or reduced penetrance that was previously unrecognized. Autosomal dominant conditions often have multiple reported features, and those with the condition can differ in which of those features they express. It is also worth acknowledging the potential for ascertainment bias in many genetic studies (Ranola et al., 2019).

Case example: Hereditary breast and ovarian cancer

A 29-year-old female is seeking genetic counseling for a family history of ovarian cancer. What are the targeted pedigree questions you may want/need to ask during the appointment? What records can you try to obtain prior to the visit? In this case example, the patient called to make her own appointment and no further information is available prior to the appointment. For the patient's responses, refer to the pedigree in Figure 19.4.

Proband pedigree considerations. When taking a pedigree for an autosomal dominant condition, in this case a potential hereditary cancer syndrome, it is important to establish what, if any, features of that condition a patient exhibits. When possible, information on the proband should be gathered from their chart and confirmed during the appointment. If patients indicate they have a personal history of cancer, then the type of cancer and their age of diagnosis is always important to document. Depending on the type of cancer, it may also be prudent to inquire about the extent of surgery or treatment. This might determine remaining organs at increased risk or potential treatment-related cancer risks. Asking about non-cancer-related surgeries can also be important to establish risk. When possible, these questions should be asked without using medical terms to lessen potential confusion (e.g., stomach removal versus gastrectomy). Eliciting the proband's cancer screening history is important to determine if they have had any prior concerns on screening or noncancerous findings indicative of a potential hereditary cancer syndrome (e.g., polyps on colonoscopy). Other questions for the proband should include any additional medical issues that could be related to the dominant condition of interest (e.g., autism with *PTEN*). Some examples of proband questions for this case include:

- Do you have a personal history of cancer?
- How old were you when you were diagnosed? Did you require surgery, chemotherapy, or radiation?
- Are your ovaries and uterus intact?
- Have you had any past breast exams or imaging?
  - o Were any of these considered abnormal (e.g., lump felt on exam, fibrocystic breast disease)?
- Have you ever had a colonoscopy screening?
  - o Have you ever had any colon polyps? Approximate lifetime number of colon polyps?
- Do you have any other major medical issues?

Family pedigree considerations. After you have addressed the proband, additional family members in the pedigree should be considered. When possible, the age, living/deceased status, and any diagnosis of cancer should be documented for every individual. More directed questions regarding symptoms of the autosomal dominant condition may need to be asked. In this case, the assessment is for hereditary breast and ovarian cancer syndromes, and therefore, documenting if female relatives have their ovaries and uterus intact when possible is useful for analysis. There may be multiple opportunities to provide psychosocial support during this step of the pedigree, such as when discussing deceased relatives or relatives currently diagnosed with cancer and undergoing treatments. When documenting family members who have been diagnosed with cancer, it can be important to ask if the individual had any other cancers in their lifetime. Patients may be focused on the last cancer and forget their family member's previous cancer history.

When adding family members to the pedigree, as previously explained, it is important to clarify biological relationships, such as full versus half-siblings, as patients may not understand the implications to the family history. When inquiring about aunts and uncles, it is important to ask only about parents' siblings to ensure patients are not confused by relatives who have married into the family. Similarly, patients may not understand the concept of first cousins; sometimes asking about the children of aunts/uncles is a more direct way to gather this information.

Including three generations is standard for pedigrees; however, based on the patient's responses, you may find it necessary or useful to attempt to go further back in the family history. Going beyond the typical three generations can be difficult for patients, and it can be helpful to explain that this is additional information beyond the basics typically asked of patients but could be very useful in the assessment. When attempting to go beyond the standard three generations, it is important to document not only those diagnosed with cancer but also those who were *not* diagnosed with cancer. It can be beneficial at the end of the family history to give patients a final opportunity to include additional family members. These could be individuals they didn't think of the first time through, or they could be individuals beyond the typical three generations that are asked for during the appointment. The following are examples of family member questions for this case:

- Do you have any children? Siblings?
  - o Are you full siblings? Or: Do you share the same mother and father with your siblings?
  - o Have any of your nieces/nephews been diagnosed with cancer? Or: Have any of your sibling's children been diagnosed with cancer?
- Are your parents still living?
- Did your mother have any siblings?
- Have any of your first cousins been diagnosed with cancer? Or: Have any of your aunts/uncles' children been diagnosed with cancer?
- Are your mother's parents still living?
- Do you know if any of your maternal grandmother's siblings were diagnosed with cancer?
  - o How many brothers and sisters did she have in total?
  - o Did your maternal grandmother's parents have any known cancer history?
- Are there any other cancer diagnoses in the family? Is there anyone else that we didn't talk about that we should have?

Ancestry pedigree considerations. Typically, one of the last steps of a pedigree is to document ancestry and, if indicated, any potential consanguinity. For hereditary cancer syndrome pedigrees, ancestry information could potentially indicate a founder variant within the family. Some patients have a hard time answering ancestry questions, and it can be helpful to provide examples (e.g., Europe, Africa, Asia, etc.) or to use the term "family line" instead of "ancestry." Some examples of ancestry questions for this case include:

- Where would you say your mother's family ancestry (family line) originally comes from?
- Do they have any known Jewish ancestry?

Pedigree analysis and counseling considerations. In the case example, the three-generation family history revealed that the patient's mother was diagnosed with ovarian cancer. Her mother had relatives on one side of her family with colon and uterine cancer under the age of 50 and on the other side with breast, pancreas, and prostate cancer. The patient is a candidate for genetic testing.

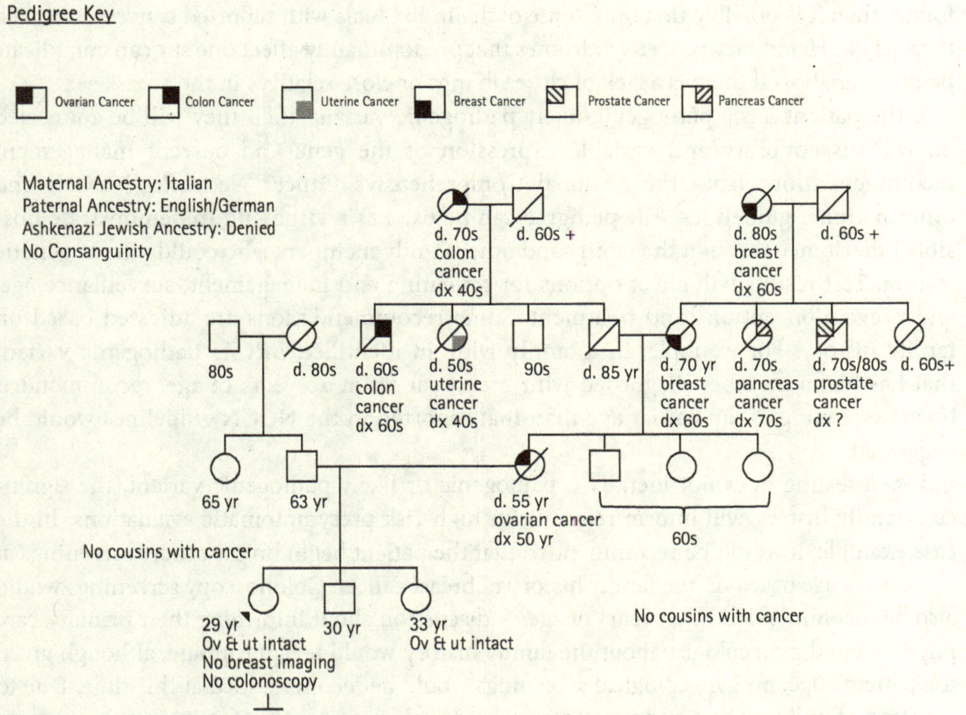

FIGURE 19.4 Pedigree for autosomal dominant case example.

Given the various types of cancers present in the family, genetic testing should include a large panel of genes associated with increased susceptibly to breast, ovarian, pancreatic, colon, stomach, and other cancers based on the family history of multiple cancers. Comprehensive testing is also recommended as multiple hereditary cancer syndromes can present similarly in a pedigree; a family history with a pathogenic *BRCA2* variant can look the same as one with a pathogenic *PALB2* variant. Utilizing the pedigree can help determine the minimum amount of genetic testing to offer to the patient. It is important to note that the amount and options of testing offered to patients may vary by clinic or genetic counselor; some clinics have standard panels and choices they offer all patients, some genetic counselors always choose a large multicancer panel test regardless of family history, and some genetic counselors tailor the testing options to offer testing only for the most appropriate genes based on the family history. There is no right or wrong approach; these differences instead reflect different viewpoints regarding genetic testing.

When reviewing the pedigree, it is important to recognize that most hereditary cancer syndromes demonstrate reduced penetrance; not every individual who inherits the pathogenic variant will develop cancer in their lifetime. In the case example, the patient's maternal grandfather may have had a hereditary cancer syndrome but never developed cancer. His side of the family should not be dismissed simply because he did not develop cancer. Family members may have passed away before cancers had a chance to develop (e.g., a family member passed away in an accident in their 30s). Cancers can also occur in family members unaffected by the known family pathogenic variant. In the case example, if a variant was found, then it is possible that only some of the individuals with reported cancers inherited the variant. Hereditary cancer syndromes that predominantly affect one sex can complicate pedigree analysis if there is a lack of close siblings or close relatives in the at-risk sex.

If the patient has a pathogenic/likely pathogenic variant, then they will be counseled on the susceptibility and variable expression of the gene and current management recommendations from the National Comprehensive Cancer Network (NCCN) and other national guidelines. The pedigree can be used as a visual aid to demonstrate possible inheritance through the family and other family members who could pursue genetic testing. Test results will affect options for screening and management, surveillance age, and prevention options and treatment. Some recommendations are adjusted based on family history. For example, in a family with an identified *BRCA1* pathogenic variant that has had a member diagnosed with breast cancer at 20 years of age, recommended breast screenings at an earlier age than that reported in the NCCN guidelines would be suggested.

When testing does not identify a pathogenic or likely pathogenic variant, the significant family history will inform referrals for high-risk presymptomatic evaluations. In the case example, it would be recommended that the patient begin breast cancer screenings at 40 years of age based on the family history of breast cancer. Colonoscopy screenings would also be recommended by 45 years of age. A discussion about informing their primary care physician and gynecologist about the family history would be appropriate, although given the patient's age, no gynecological screenings would be recommended at this time. Due to the strong family history, additional testing and evaluation of other family members would be recommended as it is possible the patient did not inherit a familial variant. Future repeat testing or reanalysis based on new discoveries would be relevant to address.

Autosomal recessive inheritance

Autosomal recessive conditions are those in which an affected person has two pathogenic variants in the same gene—one inherited from each parent. An individual with one pathogenic variant in an autosomal recessive gene, described as a carrier, will typically not manifest features of the condition. As gene carriers are much more frequent in the general population than affected individuals with the condition, it is often rare to have a family history of the condition. Further, most individuals do not know they are a carrier for an autosomal recessive condition. However, some carriers of autosomal recessive conditions have mild expression of the condition and are considered manifesting carriers. There are also some conditions that follow both an autosomal dominant and recessive pattern of inheritance (e.g., Fanconi anemia is an autosomal recessive disorder with adult carriers having an autosomal dominant cancer risk, or constitutional mismatch repair syndrome and Lynch syndrome in adults). Box 19.6 outlines features of autosomal recessive inheritance.

Genetic counseling for parents of a child with an autosomal recessive condition includes a discussion of possible outcomes in subsequent pregnancies. Each child will have a 1 in 4 (or 25%) chance of inheriting both pathogenic variants and expressing the condition, a 1 in 2 (or 50%) chance of being a carrier for the condition, and a 1 in 4 (or 25%) chance of not inheriting either pathogenic variant (Figure 19.5).

Box 19.6 Characteristics of Autosomal Recessive Inheritance

- Biological males and females equally affected
- Horizontal pattern/sibship affected (parents unaffected)
- Often young age of onset
- More uniform expression in affected persons
- Typically, complete penetrance, common with metabolic/enzyme conditions
- Usually only one generation affected
- Common ancestry/founder populations/consanguinity

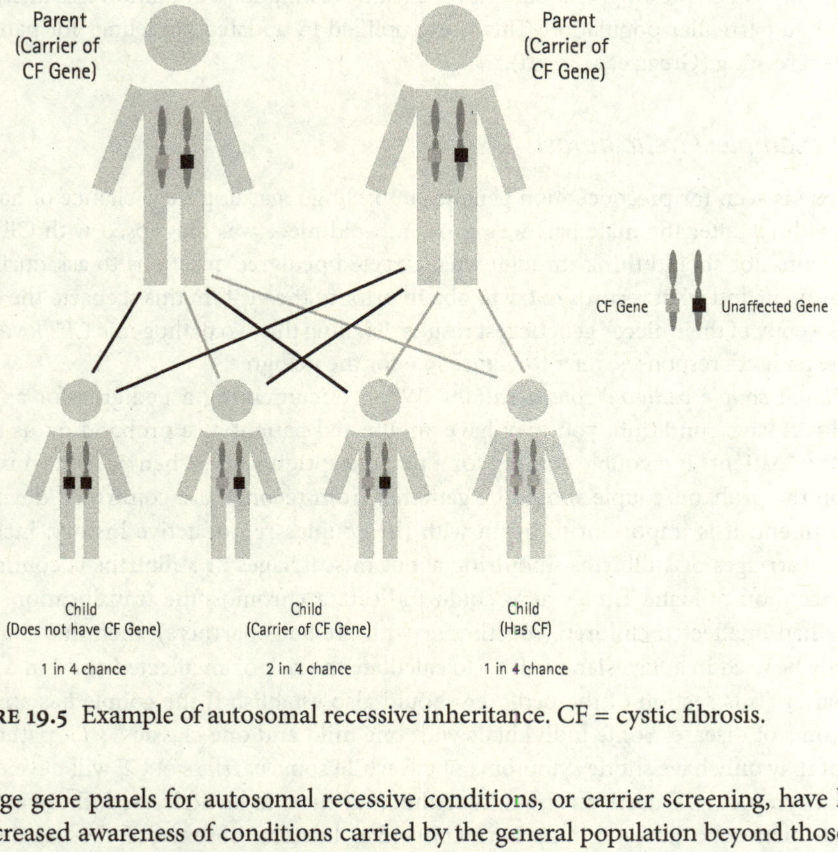

FIGURE 19.5 Example of autosomal recessive inheritance. CF = cystic fibrosis.

Large gene panels for autosomal recessive conditions, or carrier screening, have led to an increased awareness of conditions carried by the general population beyond those previously known. Some autosomal recessive conditions have a higher carrier frequency in specific populations due to founder variants in people who historically were geographically, culturally, or religiously isolated from other populations. If both partners are from the same founder group, there is a higher probability of each one carrying a pathogenic variant in the same gene. For example, Tay-Sachs disease is more common in Ashkenazi Jewish families; the *HEXA* pathogenic variant carrier rate of 1 in 27 in Ashkenazi Jewish individuals is approximately 10 times higher than the carrier rate of 1 in 350 in non–Ashkenazi Jewish individuals. Individuals with Northern European ancestry have a higher cystic fibrosis (CF) carrier rate of approximately 1 in 25 for a pathogenic variant in the *CFTR* gene and an incidence of CF of approximately 1 in 2,500 individuals. Individuals with African ancestry have a higher incidence of sickle cell anemia with approximately 1 in 13 persons carrying a pathogenic variant. Other ancestry groups such as French Canadian, Mediterranean, Finnish, or Cajun populations have higher incidences of specific genetic conditions. If an individual is from one of these founder populations, then they may have a higher probability of having one of these conditions in their family.

The world is increasingly more diverse and multicultural as people of many religions, languages, and economic and cultural groups live in closer proximity; therefore, it is important to consider all conditions in all populations. For instance, Black Americans have CF, Latina/Hispanic individuals have Tay-Sachs disease, and White individuals have sickle cell disease. Therefore, while ancestry or country-of-origin information may be useful when considering genetic testing, it should never exclude testing for a condition less likely to be found in a particular population. This is exemplified in updated guidelines for panethnic carrier screening (Gregg et al., 2021).

Case example: Cystic fibrosis

A couple is seen for preconception genetic counseling regarding their chance of having a child with CF after the male partner's 10-month-old niece was diagnosed with CF. A genetic counselor should think through what targeted pedigree questions to ask during the appointment and what records to try to obtain prior to the visit. In this scenario the couple brings a copy of their niece's genetic test results detailing the two pathogenic *CFTR* variants. For the patient's responses, refer to Figure 19.6 for the pedigree.

Proband/couple pedigree considerations. When documenting a pedigree for an autosomal recessive condition, you may have an affected patient as a proband or, as in this case, the "patient" is a couple coming for a preconception visit. When possible, information on the proband/couple should be gathered from records and confirmed during the appointment. It is important to begin with the couple's reproductive history, including any miscarriages or stillbirths. Inquiring about miscarriages or stillbirths is common in preconception/prenatal clinics as it could indicate a chromosome translocation. If the couple had unaffected children (together or with previous partners), then this could potentially be used in a Bayesian analysis to calculate the risk of an affected child in a future pregnancy. This section of the pedigree should also establish if the couple has any mild symptoms of disease. Some individuals with one mild and one classic *CFTR* pathogenic variant may only have subtle symptoms of CF, while some carriers of CF will develop significant symptoms. Questions about infertility may need to be addressed; those assigned male at birth who have CF may have congenital bilateral absence of the vas deferens (CBAVD), which is associated with infertility (see Pedigree Analysis below). Discussing infertility can be difficult for some patients and asking the couple instead of singling out the male partner can lead to a more open discussion. As carrier screening is widely available, clinically and through DTC testing, it is important to directly ask if the couple has pursued any previous screenings or genetic testing. Examples of pedigree questions for this case include:

- Have you had any previous pregnancies, miscarriages, or stillbirths?
- Do either of you have any major medical concerns? Any problems with your lungs, gastrointestinal (GI) system, or pancreas?

- Have either of you experienced infertility?
- Have either of you pursued carrier screening or genetic testing previously?

Family pedigree considerations. After addressing the proband/couple, the next step is to elicit information about family members in the pedigree, including their age, living/deceased status, and if they've been diagnosed with CF. More directed questions regarding symptoms of the autosomal recessive condition/carrier status may need to be asked. In this case, discussing the affected family member in greater detail will be important in the analysis and counseling considerations. As seen in the previous case example, when discussing family members, it is important to note full versus half-siblings and biological versus nonbiological relatives (for question examples see autosomal dominant case example). As the proband is a couple, it is important to document both partners' immediate families. For autosomal recessive conditions, nonbiological relatives who are parents of children who are affected may need to be documented to establish their genetic testing history or variants. Establishing how the diagnosis was made in the family and the extent of symptoms in the affected family member is important for pedigree analysis but also for counseling considerations. Understanding how individuals are diagnosed (e.g., newborn screening, chloride sweat test, etc.) and treated for the condition can facilitate communication and rapport building with the patients. This section of the pedigree importantly allows for additional psychosocial support for the family members. The following are examples of family member questions for this case:

- How many brothers and sisters do you have?
- Have either of your siblings had any lung, GI, pancreas, or infertility problems?
- Have any of your siblings or their partners pursued genetic testing?
- Which of your siblings has a child diagnosed with CF? How many children do they have in total?
- Does your niece currently have any symptoms or health concerns?
- How was your niece diagnosed?
- What types of genetic testing have been pursued for your niece?

Ancestry pedigree considerations. Typically, one of the last steps of a pedigree is to document ancestry and any potential consanguinity. It is important to document ancestry when available, to determine whether additional carrier screening may be appropriate, following current American College of Medical Genetics and Genomics (ACMG) screening recommendations. For autosomal recessive conditions it is important to establish any possibility for consanguinity, remembering to be culturally sensitive. Waiting until the end of the pedigree allows for rapport and trust to be built with the couple, allowing for a more open conversation about consanguinity. During ancestry questions, should the couple establish that their families are from the same region, it may be prudent to ask additional follow-up questions to assess for the presence of unknown consanguinity. Examples of consanguinity questions for this case include:

- Is there any way the two of you could be related by blood?
- If your families have lived in the same small town for generations, is it possible you have common family members?

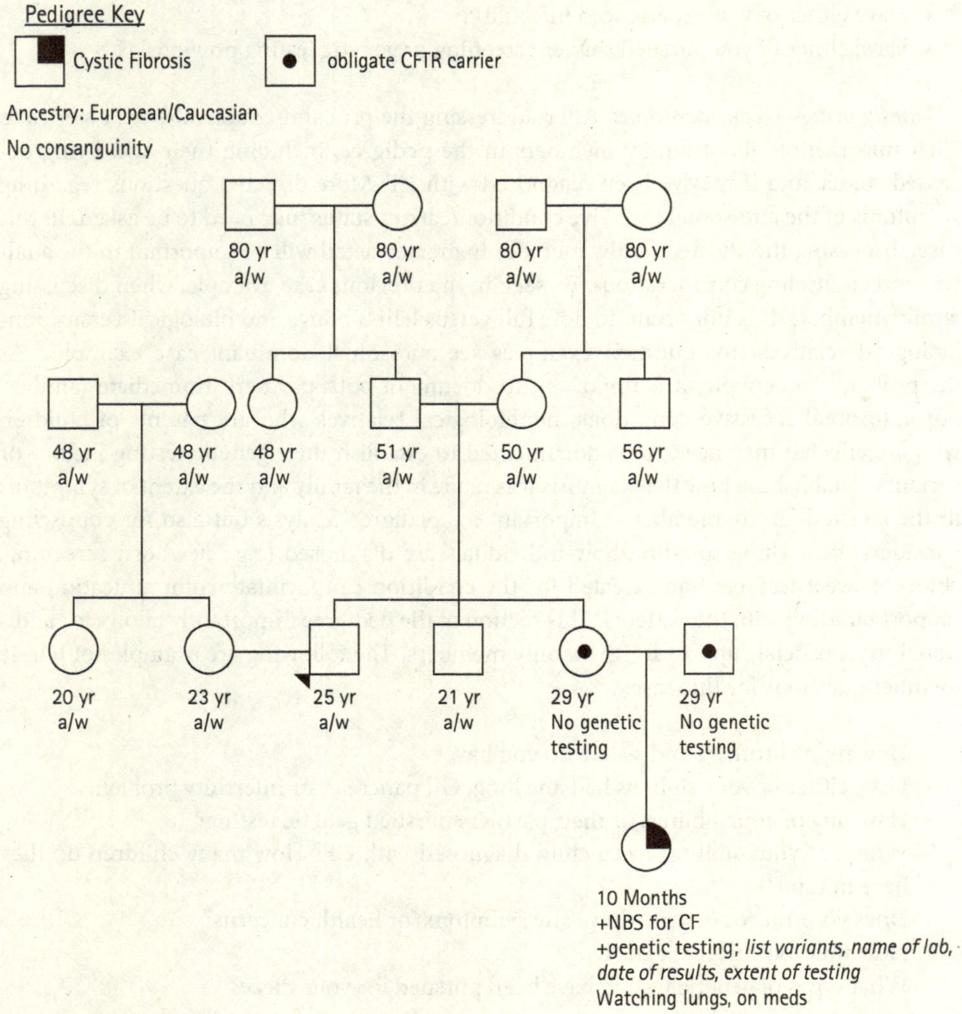

FIGURE 19.6 Pedigree for autosomal recessive case example. a/w = alive and well; CF = cystic fibrosis; NBS = newborn screening.

Pedigree analysis and counseling considerations. Prior to the appointment, it may be appropriate to calculate the chance of the couple having a child with CF, using known population carrier rates (Box 19.7). This calculation indicated a risk of less than 1% for having a child with CF even if the couple has had no carrier screening.

In the case example, the couple brought in a copy of the niece's genetic test results, which indicates she is homozygous for the ΔF508 variant; this is the most common CF variant and is included in carrier screening panels. Carrier screening for CF varies by laboratory. If instead the patient's niece had a variant not included in the ACMG recommended minimum 23 *CFTR* variants, then part of the discussion would be to review appropriate carrier testing choices (Deignan et al., 2020). Another consideration is to evaluate the genotype–phenotype association and whether a variant is considered less severe (for example, the R117H variant can lead to nonclassic CF or CBAVD when inherited with a known severe variant).

Box 19.7 Autosomal Recessive Risk Calculation Using the Hardy-Weinberg Equation

This equation allows the use of disease incidence of cystic fibrosis (CF) to calculate a population carrier frequency.

$$p+q=1 \qquad p^2+2pq+q^2=1$$

$$\text{incidence rate of CF in Caucasian population is } q^2=\frac{1}{2500}$$

$$\text{therefore } q=\frac{1}{50}=.02 \text{ and } p=.08$$

$$\text{incidence rate of CF carriers is } 2pq=2\times.08\times.02=.0392 \text{ or approximately } \frac{1}{25}$$

- The chance the male partner is a carrier for CF is 1 in 2 or 50% as the sister is an obligate carrier.
- The female partner's carrier risk is 1 in 25 or 4% (the approximate population carrier rate).
- If both partners are carriers, then each pregnancy would have a 1 in 4 or 25% chance of receiving both CF variants (one from each parent).
- These risks combined are $\frac{1}{2} \times \frac{1}{25} \times \frac{1}{4} = \frac{1}{200}$ (or less than 1%) chance to have a child with CF.

After analyzing the pedigree and niece's test report, standard carrier screening would be appropriate for this couple. There are no other obvious concerns in the family history to indicate that additional testing should be discussed. Counseling should include assessing the couple's desire to pursue carrier screening as they currently have less than a 1% chance of having a pregnancy affected by CF. Visual aids such as Punnett squares or autosomal recessive inheritance images can help in this discussion by allowing patients to visualize potential outcomes for future pregnancies.

Should the couple choose to pursue carrier screening, then one option is to test in a sequential manner. In this approach one partner is screened, and should the test result reveal a pathogenic variant, then the other partner is tested. Alternatively, testing could be conducted concurrently with both partners screened at the same time. The amount of testing desired should be discussed; the couple could decide to do a large carrier screening panel for multiple autosomal recessive conditions or choose to focus on their CF status. The ACMG practice guidelines regarding carrier screening outline important information (Gregg et al., 2021). If only the male partner pursued testing and was positive for the ΔF508 variant, then the couple's risk of having an affected child would be $1 \times \frac{1}{25} \times \frac{1}{4} = \frac{1}{100}$ or approximately a 1% chance. This could be an important point to address during the discussion regarding the desire to pursue carrier screening.

X-linked inheritance

X-linked syndromes are conditions associated with variants on the X chromosome that are often severe in males. This is because, unlike females, males have only one X chromosome, and when a pathogenic variant is present, it is hemizygous. In contrast, females have two X

Box 19.8 Characteristics of X-Linked Inheritance

- No male-to-male transmission
- Phenotype depends on whether "recessive" or "dominant."
  - X-linked dominant—both biological males and females are affected; all daughters of affected males are affected and 1 in 2 of children of affected females are affected. Depending on the severity of the condition, some conditions may be presumed to be lethal in males, leading to multiple miscarriages or pregnancy losses.
  - X-linked recessive—biological males are more severely affected, while biological females may manifest milder symptoms.

chromosomes; a female may have one copy of the pathogenic variant but not be clinically affected due to the presence of a second unaffected X chromosome.

Counseling a female who has a pathogenic variant for an X-linked condition includes discussing the 1 in 2 (or 50%) chance of passing the pathogenic variant to each child. Of these children, a male is likely to develop the condition, while female children will have more varying degrees of symptoms. All daughters of a male with an X-linked condition will inherit the pathogenic variant, while sons will inherit their father's Y chromosome. Due to X-inactivation (the Lyon hypothesis), females have mosaicism for the expressed X chromosome. This can cause differences in expression in various tissues, leading to the expression of X chromosome pathogenic variants in some but not all tissues.

While some X-linked conditions will cause the same symptoms in both sexes (e.g., X-linked hypophosphatemia), other X-linked conditions are more often or only seen in affected females. It is presumed that these X-linked conditions cause such severe symptoms in males who have only one X chromosome (hemizygous) that they may not survive. An example of this is incontinentia pigmenti (IP), a condition that segregates as an X-linked disorder and is usually lethal prenatally in males (Smahi et al., 2000). In affected females it causes highly variable abnormalities of the skin, hair, nails, teeth, eyes, and central nervous system.

Counseling for X-linked conditions may require a more in-depth explanation due to the different expression in males and females; visual aids may be helpful to show how genes are passed down in families on the X chromosome, depending on whether a biological male or female has the gene (Box 19.8).

Case example: Duchenne/Becker muscular dystrophy

A couple is seeking genetic counseling for a family history of Becker muscular dystrophy (BMD). Their son has been diagnosed with BMD. The mother's father and paternal cousin have also been diagnosed with muscular dystrophy. They would like to know the chance that their daughters will have a child with BMD. It is important to consider targeted pedigree questions to ask during the appointment and the records to obtain prior to the visit. In this case the couple sent copies of their son's genetic test results confirming his diagnosis of BMD. For the patient's responses, refer to the pedigree in Figure 19.7.

Proband pedigree considerations. When documenting a pedigree for an X-linked condition, a genetic counselor should first establish the extent of disease in the proband,

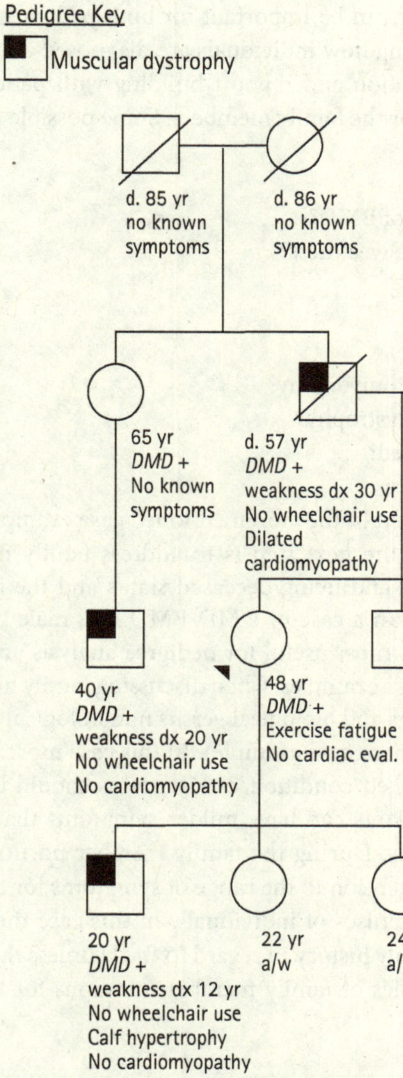

FIGURE 19.7 Pedigree for X-linked case example. a/w = alive and well; DMD = Duchenne muscular dystrophy.

including which features they do or do not express. When possible, information on the proband/couple should be gathered from records and confirmed during the appointment. The current case is regarding Duchenne muscular dystrophy (DMD)/BMD, and establishing the extent of disease is important as dystrophinopathies can vary in degree of symptoms, even within the same family. Some family members may have the more classic DMD, requiring wheelchair assistance before 13 years of age, while others may have the milder BMD, defined by wheelchair dependency after 16 years of age. It is believed that variants within the *DMD* gene that preserve the reading frame will more often be associated with milder symptoms, but this should still be correlated with clinical features and molecular test results. Determining how the diagnosis was established in the family and the extent of symptoms in the affected family member can be important for both pedigree analysis and counseling considerations. Understanding how individuals are diagnosed and treated for the condition may facilitate communication and rapport building with patients and allows for additional psychosocial support for the family members. Some possible proband questions for this case are:

- Can you describe your son's symptoms of BMD?
- At what age did he begin to have muscle weakness?
- Does he require a wheelchair?
- Does he develop cramps after exercise?
- Are his calf muscles larger than typical?
- Has he had his heart examined for cardiomyopathy?
- How was he diagnosed with muscular dystrophy?
- How much genetic testing has he pursued?

Family pedigree considerations. As described in the aforementioned case examples, after gathering information about the proband, the next step is to address family members in the pedigree and inquire about their age and living/deceased status and the presence of any features of the condition of interest. In a case of DMD/BMD in a male proband, documenting the maternal family history is most useful for pedigree analysis and counseling considerations. As seen in the other case examples, when discussing family members, it is important to note full versus half-siblings and biological versus nonbiological relatives (for question examples see autosomal dominant case example). In this case more directed questions regarding symptoms of the X-linked condition/carrier status should be asked of female relatives. Women with *DMD* variants can have milder symptoms than males, such as muscle weakness or cardiomyopathy. During the family member portion of the pedigree, it is important to pay particular attention to the range of symptoms for the muscular dystrophy in the family and testing statuses of individuals. In this case there is no need to document the proband's father's family history in regard to BMD unless the couple indicates additional concerns. Some examples of family member questions for this case include:

- Have you (mother) had any muscle weakness or symptoms of muscular dystrophy?
- Have you (mother) had your creatine phosphokinase levels checked?
- Have you (mother) pursued genetic testing?
- Have you (mother) had your heart examined?

Pedigree analysis and counseling considerations. BMD is an X-linked condition; each of the children has a 1 in 2 (50%) chance of inheriting the X chromosome with the pathogenic *DMD* variant. Most females with a pathogenic *DMD* variant will have no or mild signs or symptoms. While the couple came in to discuss future grandchildren, a conversation about health screenings for the female partner regarding potential muscle weakness and cardiac status is appropriate. It is possible that they are unaware that females can have symptoms of muscular dystrophy.

Without genetic testing, each of the daughters has a 1 in 2 chance of inheriting the familial *DMD* variant. With each pregnancy, carriers have a 1 in 2 chance of passing on the variant and a 1 in 2 chance of having a biological male child. Therefore, the couple has a $\frac{1}{2} \times \frac{1}{2} \times \frac{1}{2} = \frac{1}{8}$ or 12.5% chance of having an affected male grandson.

Counseling should include discussing the daughters' desire to pursue evaluations or genetic testing and recommending they have their own genetic counseling appointments, at an appropriate age, to discuss the full implications for them and their future families.

Dual or triple diagnoses inheritance

With the increased availability of genetic testing, the ability to interpret more nuanced forms of genetic information has added complexities, leading to a greater understanding of milder forms of conditions that can now be identified from genetic testing. Individuals who have multiple genetic diagnoses potentially leading to blended phenotypes have also been discovered. The blending of multiple conditions would have in the past confounded genetic evaluations, which may have incorrectly attributed all the features to a single condition. Research shows that up to 5% of those pursuing exome sequencing have multiple diagnoses (Posey et al., 2017).

Case example: Coffin-Siris and KBG syndrome

A 6-year-old male with developmental delay, intellectual disability, short stature, sparse scalp hair growth, delayed bone age, and seizures presents to a pediatric genetic clinic for evaluation. Targeted pedigree questions for the appointment and the records to obtain prior to the visit should be determined. In this case, the patient had all previous evaluations at your facility, and you can confirm his symptoms and the severity prior to the appointment. Parental responses are shown in the pedigree in Figure 19.8.

Proband pedigree considerations. When taking a pedigree for a proband who appears to have multiple diagnoses or a blended phenotype, it is important to establish all features that could be associated with a genetic condition (e.g., congenital anomalies, developmental or intellectual delays, behavioral problems, medical conditions). When possible, information on the proband should be gathered from their chart and confirmed during the appointment. More targeted questions may be asked to gain additional details regarding the extent of a given symptom. During the appointment, a dysmorphology exam will be pursued and additional features should be documented. In the case, during the evaluation by the clinical geneticist, it is noted that the child has a coarse round face, low-set prominent ears, strabismus, bushy eyebrows, large mouth, fused incisors, and prominent finger pads. Proband questions for this case include:

- Which milestones has your son struggled with, for example, feeding himself, speaking?
- Do you feel his seizures are well controlled with his medication? How many seizures did he have prior to medication compared to after medication?

Family pedigree considerations. After you have addressed the proband, the next step is to address family members in the pedigree. Every individual will need their age, living/deceased status, and any features of a genetic syndrome they may exhibit documented, paying particular attention to the symptoms of the proband. When asking adults about learning or

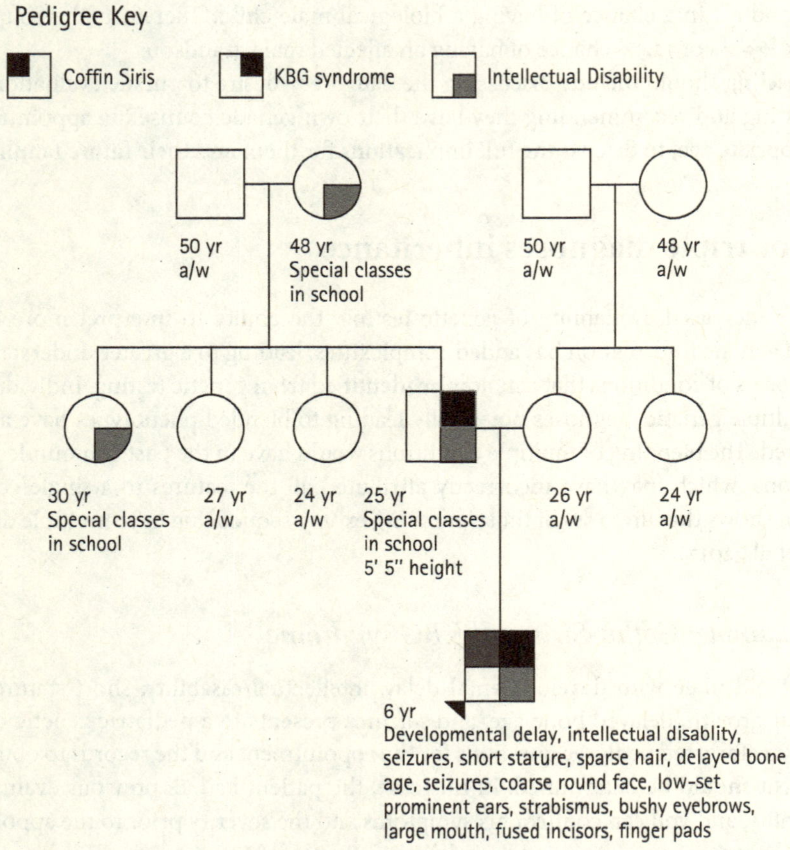

FIGURE 19.8 Pedigree for blended phenotype case example. a/w = alive and well.

developmental disabilities, some individuals may be uncomfortable admitting to any form of intellectual disability. Asking individuals if they had any difficulties in school may be an easier way for them to disclose that they have learning problems. In the case example, the child is documented to have short stature, and ascertaining parental heights can help determine whether the child's height is within the expected range. The father is noted to have a shorter height than average. When parents are at the appointment, the presence of any congenital anomalies or dysmorphic features in them may be evaluated by the geneticist. Several possible family member questions for this case are:

- Do you have any other children?
- Did either of you (parents) have any delays in meeting your milestones as children?
- Did you have any difficulties in school?
- Did either of you (parents) have any birth defects that you were born with?
- Do you have any seizure disorders or sparse hair growth?

Ancestry pedigree considerations. Typically, one of the last steps of a pedigree is to document ancestry. In this case, as the condition of interest is not known, it could be important to document ancestry to determine the potential for a founder variant (for examples of ancestry questions see the autosomal dominant case example). As autosomal recessive conditions are possible for this case, it is important to assess for the possibility for consanguinity (for examples of consanguinity questions see the autosomal recessive case example). *Pedigree analysis and counseling considerations.* Due to the patient's constellation of symptoms, trio exome sequencing is ordered. Trio sequencing includes sending in a sample of the affected individual and both biological parents to determine inheritance and de novo status. Testing revealed that the patient has pathogenic variants in genes for both Coffin-Siris syndrome and KBG syndrome. The testing revealed that the KBG syndrome is paternally inherited while the Coffin-Siris variant was found to be de novo, or a new variant not present in either parent. As the father also has the KBG syndrome pathogenic variant, he will need evaluations for health issues related to this condition.

Given the information found from testing, additional targeted pedigree questions can now be asked of the father and his side of the family regarding specific features of KBG syndrome. For instance, has anyone in your (father) family had a flattened head as an infant or required a helmet to reshape their skull? Does anyone have larger, jagged, or crowded teeth? The geneticist may also perform an examination of the father to determine what features of KBG syndrome he may have.

Counseling will be complicated and involve discussing both genes with the parents. The use of visual aids can be helpful in explaining genetic information in complex cases. The genetic counseling discussion should include the 1 in 2 (or 50%) recurrence chance of having another child with KBG (an autosomal dominant syndrome). Since the pathogenic variant for Coffin-Siris syndrome is de novo, the recurrence risk is low, but testing in future pregnancies is an option due to the possibility of gonadal mosaicism. As it is unlikely for both pathogenic variants to be inherited by a future child, the counseling session may include that the current blended features seen in their son are not likely to present again in a future child. Explanation should include the features of both Coffin-Siris and KBG syndromes and how features present in both syndromes may manifest in their son.

Additional factors influencing inheritance and pedigree analysis

There are many other considerations in addition to the classic dominant, recessive, or X-linked inheritance. When evaluating a pedigree, it is important to consider factors such as heterogeneity, variability of expression, variant detection rate, the full range of clinical features, sex differences in expression, parent of origin, and even health history of miscarriages and pregnancy history. Other considerations include mitochondrial inheritance, chromosomal translocations, imprinting disorders, and epigenetic factors.

Mitochondrial conditions can be caused by nuclear or mitochondrial DNA pathogenic variants. At fertilization, only maternally derived mitochondria are passed to children; therefore, all children of an affected mother are at risk of being affected. No children of affected males will be affected (Figure 19.9). Mitochondrial inheritance is further complicated as each mitochondrion has multiple copies of its DNA and a maternal egg stores multiple mitochondria. Each egg includes a random sampling of a mother's mitochondria. When the mother has a mixture of affected and unaffected mitochondria (referred to as heteroplasmy), her children could inherit a range of affected versus unaffected mitochondria, leading to the potential for large variability of expression.

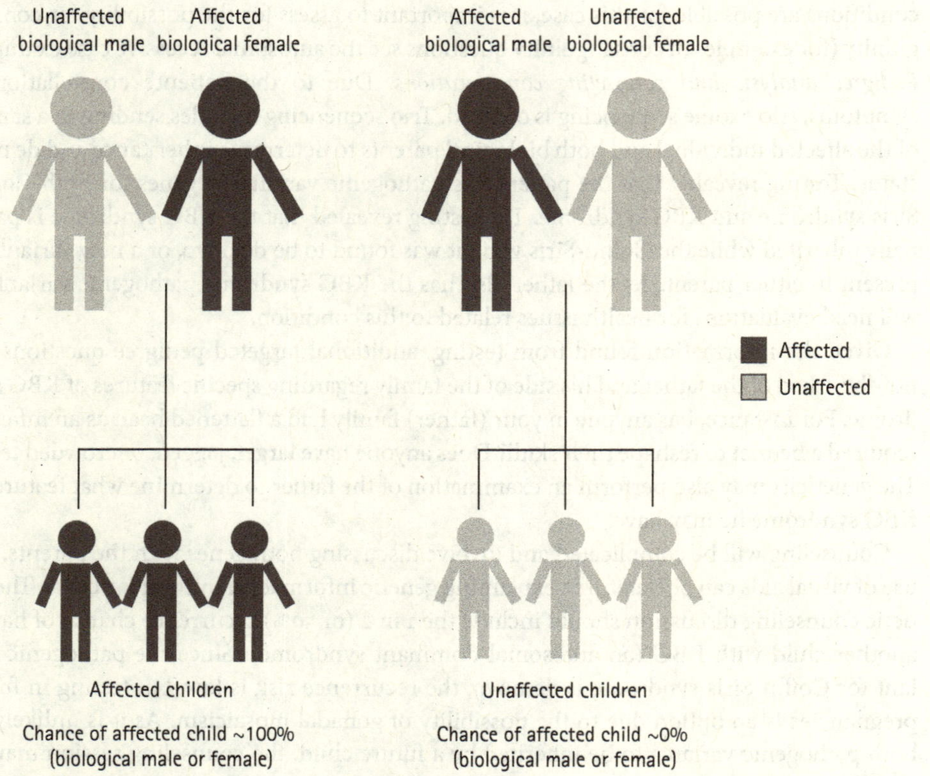

FIGURE 19.9 Example of mitochondrial inheritance.

Chromosomal anomalies may also be transmitted in families. One common type of chromosome anomaly is a chromosome translocation. Translocations occur when pieces of chromosomes are exchanged; these exchanged pieces are balanced when the amount of genetic material for each chromosome remains the same. However, this exchange of genetic material can disrupt gene functioning when there is missing genetic material or cause new hybrid genes when two genes are fused or spliced together. For example, some genes for renal cancer are located on the short arm (p arm) of chromosome 3. A chromosomal translocation involving chromosome 3 may lead to gene fusions during mitosis, causing an increased risk for kidney cancer (Haas & Nathanson, 2014). Balanced translocations can lead to multiple miscarriages as pregnancies with an unbalanced mix of chromosomes may not survive, while those that do survive may have multiple congenital anomalies or a chromosomal syndrome. When eliciting a family history, it is important to inquire about a history of multiple miscarriages in the family, infertility, or children with physical/developmental anomalies (see the autosomal recessive case for an example).

Imprinting is a process where certain genes on the maternal and paternal chromosomes are "imprinted" or silenced, which leads to exclusive expression of specific genes from only one parent. The expression depends on the parent of origin. In maternal imprinting, the allele of a particular gene inherited from the mother is transcriptionally silent and the paternally inherited allele is active. The opposite happens with paternal imprinting; the paternally inherited allele is silenced and the maternally inherited allele is active. Imprinting is reset in meiosis. Disruptions in imprinting occur in genetic conditions such as Prader-Willi syndrome and Angelman syndrome. Because the process of imprinting can silence a variant given the parent of origin, inheritance patterns may not be as obvious. They may even appear to "skip" generations when the variants are passed by the parent that has imprinted or silenced it.

Case example: Mitochondrial inheritance

A 36-year-old female would like to know the chance of her children developing progressive external ophthalmoplegia (PEO). One of her brothers, her sister, and her sister's son were recently clinically diagnosed with PEO. As described in the prior case examples, it is important to think through what targeted pedigree questions to ask during the appointment and the records to obtain prior to the visit. In this case the patient brings a copy of her brother's genetic test results to her appointment. For the patient's responses, refer to the pedigree in Figure 19.10.

Proband pedigree considerations. When taking a pedigree for a proband with a concern for a mitochondrial syndrome, it is important to establish all features that could be associated with the condition and their severity. When possible, information on the proband should be gathered from their chart and confirmed during the appointment. More targeted questions may be asked to gain additional details regarding the extent of a given symptom. During the appointment, a dysmorphology exam will typically be performed and additional symptoms should be documented. In the case, during the evaluation by the clinical geneticist, it is noted that the patient has mild ptosis and a weak grip. A few possible questions to ask the proband are:

- Do you have any major medical issues?
- Have you previously noticed that your eyelids have a slight droop?
- Do you have any problems with exercise fatigue?
- Do you have any problems with your eyesight or heart?

Family pedigree considerations. Information to document for family members in the pedigree includes their age, living/deceased status, and any features of a genetic syndrome they may exhibit, paying particular attention to the symptoms of the proband. For patients concerned about a hereditary mitochondrial syndrome, more in-depth questions for potentially affected relatives should be asked. In the case the patient brought a copy of her brother's genetic test results, confirming a deletion of mitochondrial DNA consistent with a diagnosis of PEO. Since the brother has a variant in the mitochondrial DNA, all the patient's siblings and maternal family members should be closely evaluated for even mild symptoms. Establishing who has a confirmed genetic diagnosis can be useful to correlate the disease spectrum in the family. A few examples of family member questions for this case include:

- Who was the first person to receive the diagnosis of PEO?
  - o Do they have any other symptoms?
  - o Did they pursue genetic testing?
- Has anyone else pursued genetic testing?

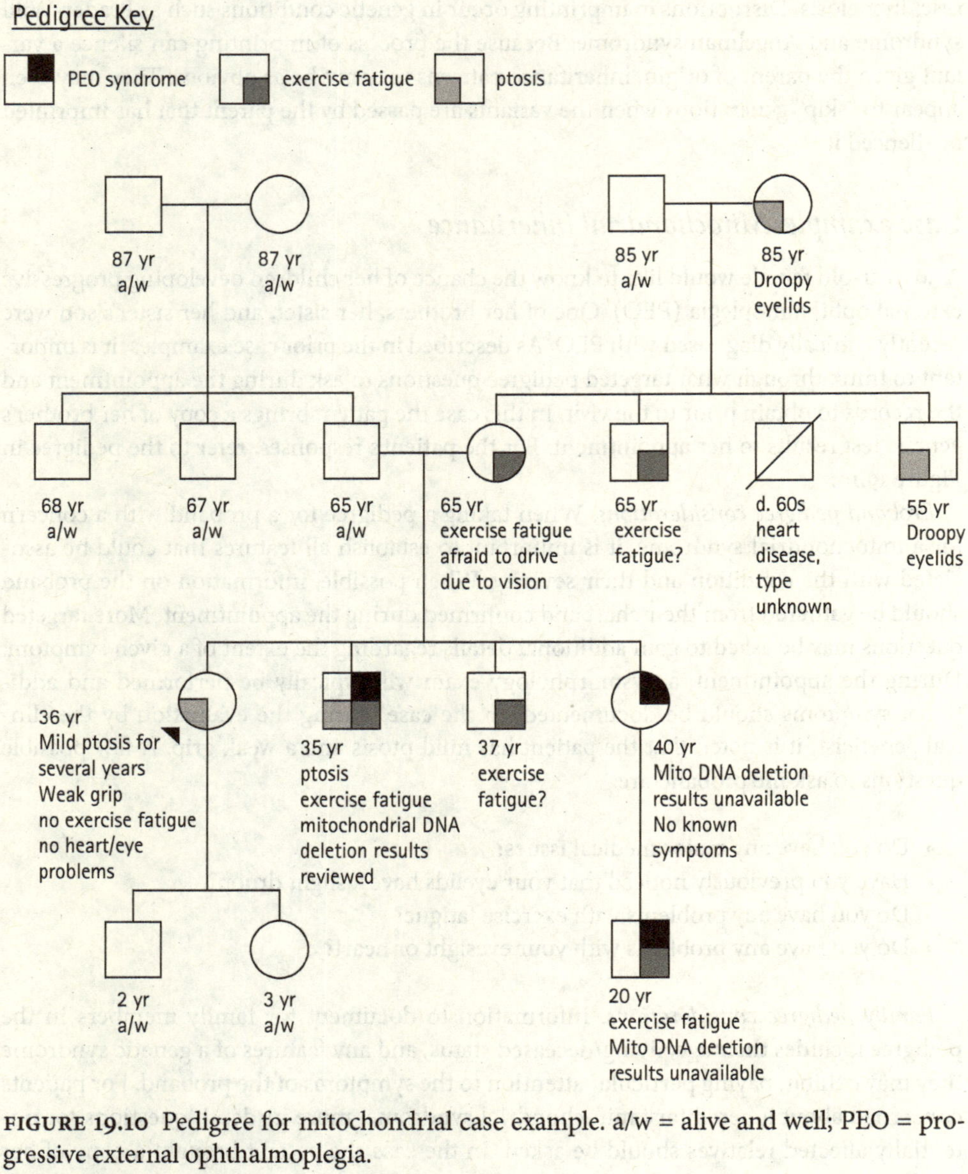

FIGURE 19.10 Pedigree for mitochondrial case example. a/w = alive and well; PEO = progressive external ophthalmoplegia.

Pedigree analysis and counseling considerations. Since PEO syndrome can be caused by pathogenic variants in either mitochondrial or nuclear DNA, it is important to determine what mode of inheritance to suspect in this family. The brother's genetic test results report a mitochondrial DNA deletion. This is also seen via the genetic testing of affected family members in the pedigree.

The family should be provided with an explanation of mitochondria, including their location and function, to help them understand why the syndrome can have such a variable presentation in different members of the family.

Explanations should include maternal inheritance of mitochondrial DNA and that prognosis is difficult to predict due to heteroplasmy. It can be helpful to use the pedigree as a visual aid when discussing inheritance patterns or varying degrees of symptoms. Visual aids can also be used to discuss the concept of heteroplasmy; it is quite likely that the patient's mother has a mixture of affected and unaffected mitochondrial DNA, and this could explain why family members have differing degrees of symptoms.

While the patient came to the clinic to discuss her children, genetic testing would first be offered to the patient. This explanation should include potential difficulties in testing adults for mitochondrial disorders as deletions may not always be present in a blood sample, and testing additional tissues, such as urine or a muscle biopsy, might be indicated.

If the patient is interested in having additional children, then the discussion could include the option of an ovum donor through in vitro fertilization. For those living in the United Kingdom, the option of a mitochondrial replacement could be discussed as well (this technology is not currently legal in the United States or Canada).

Conclusion

Pedigree analysis and evaluation of a family medical history in genetic counseling are evolving with the rapid development of genetic testing technologies, online pedigree tools, and other resources. An accurate family history not only guides genetic testing but also increasingly aids in the interpretation of complex genetic testing results. Unlike other specialties, in genetics, the family unit is often "the patient" as genetic conditions may impact multiple members within the same family. Understanding the patient's family medical history through analysis of their pedigree, and appropriate use of standard symbols, is a foundation for developing a relationship with the patient and their family members. Discussing family history, addressing concerns within the family, and determining family members' risks are at the heart of genetic counseling. Pedigrees are an integral part of that process as they allow genetic counselors to establish rapport, visually assess inheritance patterns, and determine additional family members who may benefit from assessment.

Family History/Pedigree Tools and Resources

- *How to Draw Your Family Tree*, National Society of Genetic Counselors http://www.aboutgeneticcounselors.com/Resources-to-Help-You/Post/how-to-draw-your-family-tree. Describes how to construct a family tree.
- *My Family Health Portrait*, Office of the Surgeon General https://phgkb.cdc.gov/FHH/html/index.html. A free online family health history collection tool to share family health history information and assess risk for certain conditions. This tool allows an individual to enter, print, and update their family health history.
- *Family Health History*, Center for Disease Control and Prevention's Office of Public Health Genomics https://www.cdc.gov/family-health-history/?CDC_AAref_Val=https://www.cdc.gov/genomics/famhistory/. Includes links to publications, reports, and tools for recording family health information.

- *Collecting a Family History*, American Medical Association https://www.ama-assn.org/delivering-care/precision-medicine/collecting-family-history. Provides family history tools, questionnaires, and forms for collecting medical information.
- *Obtaining an Older Patient's Medical History*, National Institute on Aging https://www.nia.nih.gov/health/obtaining-older-patients-medical-history. Offers suggestions on how to obtain a health history from older individuals.
- *Does It Run in the Family?*, Genetic Alliance http://familyhealthhistory.org/. Explains the "why" and "how" behind collecting family health history information, tips for talking to family members, examples of conditions that can run in the family, and hints for health. The booklet can be customizable with personal health stories, photos, and health condition information.
- *Family History*, MedlinePlus http://medlineplus.gov/familyhistory.html. Describes the importance of family history information and provides links to several resources for family health history.
- *Online Pedigree Tool*, Progeny https://pedigree.progenygenetics.com/. A pedigree software drawing program.

Acknowledgments

We would like to thank Cam Clark for her work in creating Figures 19.3, 19.5 and 19.9.

References

Bennett, R. L. (1999). *The practical guide to the genetic family history*. John Wiley & Sons.

Bennett, R. L., French, K. S., Resta, R. G., & Austin, J. (2022). Practice resource-focused revision: Standardized pedigree nomenclature update centered on sex and gender inclusivity: A practice resource of the National Society of Genetic Counselors. *Journal of Genetic Counseling, 31*(6), 1238–1248.https://doi.org/10.1002/jgc4.1621

Deignan, J. L., Astbury, C., Cutting, G. R., Del Gaudio, D., Gregg, A. R., Grody, W. W., Monaghan, K. G., Richards, S., & ACMG Laboratory Quality Assurance Committee. (2020). CFTR variant testing: A technical standard of the American College of Medical Genetics and Genomics (ACMG). *Genetics in Medicine, 22*(8), 1288–1295. https://doi.org/10.1038/s41436-020-0822-5

Gregg, A. R., Aarabi, M., Klugman, S., Leach, N. T., Bashford, M. T., Goldwaser, T., Chen, E., Sparks, T. N., Reddi, H. V., Rajkovic, A., Dungan, J. S., & ACMG Professional Practice and Guidelines Committee. (2021). Screening for autosomal recessive and X-linked conditions during pregnancy and preconception: A practice resource of the American College of Medical Genetics and Genomics (ACMG). *Genetics in Medicine, 23*(10), 1793–1806. https://doi.org/10.1038/s41436-021-01203-z

Guttmacher, A. E., Collins, F. S., & Carmona, R. H. (2004). The family history—more important than ever. *New England Journal of Medicine, 351*(22), 2333–2336.

Haas, N. B., & Nathanson, K. L. (2014). Hereditary kidney cancer syndromes. *Advances in Chronic Kidney Disease, 21*(1), 81–90. https://doi.org/10.1053/j.ackd.2013.10.001

Mersch, J., Brown, N., Pirzadeh-Miller, S., Mundt, E., Cox, H. C., Brown, K., Aston, M., Esterling, L., Manley, S., & Ross, T. (2018). Prevalence of variant reclassification following hereditary cancer genetic testing. *JAMA*, *320*(12), 1266–1274. https://doi.org/10.1001/jama.2018.13152.

Pletcher, B. A., Toriello, H. V., Noblin, S. J., Seaver, L. H., Driscoll, D. A., Bennett R. L., & Gross, S. J. (2007). Indications for genetic referral: A guide for healthcare providers. *Genetics in Medicine*, *9*, 385–389. doi.org/10.1097/GIM.0b013e318064e70c

Posey, J. E., Harel, T., Liu, P., Rosenfeld, J. A., James, R. A., Akdemir, C., Walkiewicz, M., Bi, W., Xiao, R., Ding, Y., Xia, F., Beaudet, A. L., Muzny, D. M., Gibbs, R. A., Boerwinkle, E., Eng, C. M., Sutton, V. R., Shaw, C. A., Plon, S. E., Yan, Y., & Lupski, J. R. (2017). Resolution of disease phenotypes resulting from multilocus genomic variation. *New England Journal of Medicine*, *376*(1), 21–31. https://doi.org/10.1056/NEJMoa1516767

Ranola, J. M. O., Tsai, G. J., & Shirts, B. H. (2019). Exploring the effect of ascertainment bias on genetic studies that use clinical pedigrees. *European Journal of Human Genetics*, *27*(12), 1800–1807. https://doi.org/10.1038/s41431-019-0467-5

Richards, S., Aziz, N., Bale, S., Bick, D., Das, S., Gastier-Foster, J., Grody, W. W., Hegde, M., Lyon, E., Spector, E., Voelkerding, K., Rehm, H. L., & ACMG Laboratory Quality Assurance Committee. (2015). Standards and guidelines for the interpretation of sequence variants: A joint consensus recommendation of the American College of Medical Genetics and Genomics and the Association for Molecular Pathology. *Genetics in Medicine*, *17*(5), 405–424. https://doi.org/10.1038/gim.2015.30

Smahi, A., Courtois, G., Vabres, P., Yamaoka, S., Heuertz, S., Munnich, A., Israël, A., Heiss, N. S., Klauck, S. M., Kioschis, P., Wiemann, S., Poustka, A., Esposito, T., Bardaro, T., Gianfrancesco, F., Ciccodicola, A., D'Urso, M., Woffendin, H., Jakins, T., . . . Nelson, D. L. (2000). Genomic rearrangement in NEMO impairs NF-kappaB activation and is a cause of incontinentia pigmenti. The International Incontinentia Pigmenti (IP) Consortium. *Nature*, *405*(6785), 466–472. https://doi.org/10.1038/35013114

CHAPTER 20

COMMON AND COMPLEX TRAITS

Considerations for Genetic Counseling

ELEANOR FEINGOLD

Definitions and Genetic Models

The defining feature of complex traits is the contribution of multiple genetic, environmental, and behavioral factors to the etiology. Such traits can be early or late onset (including congenital), but clearly late-onset traits have more opportunity to be influenced by complex life history factors. Historically, "complex" has also meant "unknowable," but contemporary scientific knowledge often includes knowledge of one or more specific factors that contribute to the etiology. A classic example is Alzheimer's disease (Kamboh, 2021). Genotype at the *APOE* locus is well established to have a major effect on risk, but there is a great deal of risk it does not explain; there are other genetic factors (even within the same gene) that have an effect, there are monogenic early-onset forms of the disease, and there are lifestyle/behavioral factors including exercise and education that have a significant explanatory effect. Moreover, current understanding of the molecular mechanisms for the *APOE* effect and other effects is still unclear. This partially understood interplay of multiple factors is what makes Alzheimer's disease a classically complex trait.

There are several traditional mathematical and molecular models that have been used to characterize complex traits (described below), though it is rare for a trait to follow one of these models precisely. It is likely that most traits include elements of all of these models, and in fact the models are not entirely distinct from each other. It is also important to note that there is some interplay between disease models and disease definitions. It is common to redefine certain cases of a disease as a "monogenic subtype," for example, a single-gene cancer syndrome or an early-onset Alzheimer's disease phenotype, or as a "phenocopy" (environmental version of a genetic disorder). In that case, the model for the remaining cases changes. Similarly, inclusion of subclinical versions of a phenotype may change the appropriate model for that phenotype. For example, the model for an addiction disorder may look very different if any use of the substance is included in the case definition.

Ultimately, there is no universal definition of a complex trait. All traits have complexities, even the most Mendelian ones. At one end of the spectrum (admittedly oversimplified), phenylketonuria is only a disease in the presence of an environmental effect (exposure to phenylalanine) and a behavioral effect (failure to adhere to the necessary diet). At the other end of the spectrum, breast cancer and Alzheimer's disease have monogenic forms, environmental forms, and complex gene-by-environment interaction forms. Arguably, from a genetic counseling point of view, one standard definition is not necessary—complexity is simply a measure of how difficult it is to communicate about the disease etiology and risks with patients and with the public.

Polygenic model

The classical polygenic model is defined as a very large number of genetic factors with each additively contributing a small amount to risk, leading to a Gaussian distribution of "risk level" for individuals. Individuals are then affected with a disease or trait if their risk level exceeds some threshold in that distribution. The classical polygenic model does not include environmental factors, but from a mathematical point of view it can easily include numerous small additive environmental factors as well. It is not possible to cite examples of a purely polygenic trait; even with environmental factors included, the polygenic model is hypothetical. Traits may exhibit polygenic contributions to risk but will always have larger discrete genetic or environmental risk factors as well and most likely interacting (nonadditive) components.

Oligogenic model

Oligogenic inheritance refers to a somewhat more realistic model in which there is a small number of major genes that contribute to disease risk, generally in addition to polygenic contributions. As in the polygenic model, environmental effects are not part of the classical definition of the model but are easily incorporated. Examples of at least approximately oligogenic traits abound, including Alzheimer's disease (Kamboh, 2021), Hirschsprung disease (Karim et al., 2021), cleft lip and palate (Leslie, 2021), and many cancers.

Modifier and interaction models

Modifier models generally assume one or more major genetic effects, which are then modified by additional genes or environmental factors. The epidemiological definition of a modifier is that the effect of the primary gene on risk differs depending on the individual's genotype at the modifying locus or on exposure to an environmental factor. Interaction is a related term that is often preferred by geneticists because it connotes biological interaction among the factors as opposed to a purely statistical relationship. The term "digenic model" can be used if precisely two genes are involved. If there is one major gene and one major environmental/behavioral factor, then we generally describe it as a gene-by-environment interaction model. For example, variants at the nicotinic receptor gene confer major susceptibility to nicotine addiction (Lee et al., 2018), but only in the presence of exposure to nicotine. Similarly, interaction between blood coagulation genes and pharmaceutical estrogen is well established (J. Kim et al., 2022); risk genes for clotting magnify the clotting risk due to estrogen in a manner that is beyond additive. Interaction is somewhat difficult to identify in human studies as large sample sizes are needed, but it can be more easily studied in animal models. For example, the interacting effect of prenatal stress and genes on neurodevelopmental disorders has been studied in mice (Papale et al., 2021), where the prenatal stress can be experimentally induced and measured. Most of the traits listed above as oligogenic examples include interaction and modifier effects as well.

Extreme heterogeneity

An important model that was not part of the classical genetics literature is that of extreme heterogeneity—a trait or disease that can be caused by any of a large number of private or semiprivate pathogenic variants in different individuals. As with the above models, this is unlikely to be a pure model for any trait and can also include major genes or environmental factors both additively and interactively. The current understanding of autism has significant resonance with this model (Waye & Cheng, 2018), as does congenital heart disease (Geddes et al., 2019). In both cases hundreds if not thousands of pathogenic variants have been identified, most present in only a small number of affected individuals. Note that the issue of disease definition is particularly pertinent here: Is a trait that has 100 distinct causes really one trait or 100 traits? Evolving understanding of certain traits and improved molecular diagnosis can change these definitions over time.

Epidemiology and Basic Science of Complex Traits

Scientific understanding of the role of genetics in complex disease started in the premolecular era with studies of concordance rates between twins and other relative pairs. Terminology for this study type includes concordance rates, twin studies, heritability, segregation analysis, and path analysis. These studies, which do not genotype individuals, compare correlation between relatives that is expected under a particular genetic model with what is observed in data. A high estimate of heritability was generally interpreted as evidence of a genetic effect for the trait. However, some such results were misleading, as a heritability estimate is essentially an estimate of correlation between relatives and will generally include both genetic and environmental/behavioral reasons for that correlation. For example, a simple estimate of the heritability of breast cancer based on sibling pairs would include effects of shared genetics but also of shared diet, similarity in reproductive history due to shared socioeconomic status, and so forth. More sophisticated versions of these methods can incorporate a small number of distinct environmental and genetic effects, and lack of fit of the simple models can then be interpreted as evidence of even more complex inheritance (e.g., Juo et al., 1998; Weissbecker et al., 1993). These historical approaches are still a useful baseline for establishing potential genetic effects as a preliminary to genotyping studies or when genotype data are unavailable (e.g., Weinberg et al., 2013).

The next generation of inquiry into complex traits was gene discovery using linkage analysis, which involved genotyping families in which a disease was seen segregating and testing for cosegregation of disease with genetic markers. Linkage analysis was first performed at specific loci and then expanded to genome-wide panels when those became available. Linkage analysis was successful in discovering genes for many Mendelian disorders but had limited success for complex disease because it requires making specific assumptions about the trait model and is easily stymied by low-level complexity such as genetic heterogeneity or phenocopies. For example, the *BRCA1* gene was discovered via linkage analysis, but only after the insight that early-onset breast cancer cases might be the most likely to be genetic and linkage was applied only to the earliest onset families (Hall et al., 1990). In theory, linkage analysis could be used more broadly for complex disorders, but collecting the requisite enormous numbers of affected families has proved to be daunting.

The insight that collecting individuals is far easier than collecting families (Risch & Merikangas, 1996) ushered in the next generation of gene discovery—association studies. An association study collects unrelated individuals with phenotypic information. This often means cases and controls, but any standard epidemiological study design can be used. The researcher then tests for association between the trait and genotype frequencies at markers. Such studies can have enormous statistical power to detect genes as compared to linkage analysis, especially given that thousands or even tens of thousands of participants can be enrolled relatively easily compared to the effort required to recruit families. Genetic association studies were also initially performed at small numbers of markers or genes, which is now generally described as a candidate gene study. Later association studies were performed genome-wide using genotyping chips, a technological breakthrough that was critical to advancing genomic studies (Broman & Feingold, 2004). These studies were termed genome-wide associate studies (GWAS).

The primary (and extremely important) limitation to association studies is the potential for false-positive results due to confounding variables. In particular, the effects of population differences, generally termed population stratification, can have an enormous effect on genetic association studies. If one's sample is anything short of purely ethnically homogeneous, any trait that has a different frequency in different ancestral subgroups will appear to be associated with any genetic marker whose frequency differs between those subgroups. One early paper discussing this issue (Knowler et al., 1988) described an association between diabetes mellitus and the *Gm* locus in an admixed group of Pima Indians and then demonstrated quite clearly that the association was due to population admixture rather than a causal effect of the locus. This issue was ignored or forgotten (by some) and rediscovered a number of times but became critically important in the GWAS era. When the entire genome is assayed, such spurious associations are not just a potential problem but are essentially guaranteed to happen. Ultimately, the stratification issue for GWAS was broadly recognized (e.g., Freedman et al., 2004). It was eventually, though not entirely, mitigated when methods were developed for using the genome-wide data from chips to control for ancestry differences in subpopulations (e.g., Price et al., 2006).

Once the population stratification problem was (relatively) solved, GWAS became the main tool for gene discovery in humans. GWAS using chips were successful at finding common variants (minor allele frequency greater than 2% or 5%) associated with many diseases. Early successes included age-related macular degeneration (Klein et al., 2005) and type 2 diabetes (Diabetes Genetics Initiative of Broad Institute of Harvard and MIT, Lund University, and Novartis Institutes of BioMedical Research et al., 2007). However, GWAS turned out to be disappointing in several important ways. First, the identified loci are rarely causal, and in fact, it can be rather difficult to interpret associations and identify potentially functional loci. Because of linkage disequilibrium (ancestral correlation among nearby loci), associations may extend over fairly broad regions encompassing many genes. In addition, most GWAS loci are not in genes at all, but in intergenic regions. Intergenic associations are presumed likely to have regulatory effects, but the state of knowledge of those regions and those effects is limited. Finally, loci that are identified by GWAS, functional or not, almost always have relatively small effect size due to the intrinsic complexity of the traits and thus have questionable individual clinical utility. These limitations were highly frustrating to early GWAS proponents, who were hoping for quick clinical applications. However, the real benefit of GWAS turned out to be more in the realm of basic science, with the clinical value following. That is, a GWAS association may not identify a functional variant, but it may well identify a likely functional gene, which can lead to a better understanding of the disease process and/or to a drug target.

One limitation of GWAS research has been the predominance of populations of European ancestry being studied. Even more fundamentally, the chips themselves were developed to assay genetic variation in European ancestry populations. This situation has been gradually improving, but the state of knowledge for non-European populations still lags far behind (Hindorff et al., 2018).

Contemporary GWAS can be performed either with chips or with genome sequencing (Wheeler et al., 2008). Both technologies allow genome-wide genotyping of individuals, which can then be used in GWAS analyses to discover risk genes for traits and diseases. The primary difference between the two technologies is that sequencing produces genotype data at potentially almost every locus on the genome, so that rare variants can be directly studied. In theory, this allows better detection of causal variants. Sequencing also helps with the European bias of the assay somewhat, although there are still problems due to the ancestry of the reference sequences. In practice, success of sequencing studies in finding new variants beyond those discovered in GWAS has been limited, largely because sequencing is significantly more expensive than chips and thus sequencing studies have had much smaller sample sizes than chip-based GWAS.

In addition to technological advances such as chips and sequencing methods, two social changes were also key to making GWAS successful. One was the development of large national and international consortia. Once it became apparent that success in finding genes for complex diseases required enormous sample sizes, investigators, who were initially protective of their own data, found their way into data-sharing consortia given that this approach was the primary path to scientific discovery (e.g., Lango Allen et al., 2010). The other critical change, driven by national and international policy, was the development of large public databases to provide the infrastructure for gene discovery. These include the original human genome sequence (Lander et al., 2001), the HapMap database (International HapMap Consortium, 2003), and numerous more recent resources.

Because of the limited ability of all of the aforementioned methods to pinpoint causal variants, gene discovery continues to rely heavily on functional studies to establish or even suggest causality. Traditionally, this required experimental approaches such as animal or cell line knockout studies. For example, Musunuru et al. (2010) used knockdown and viral overexpression studies in mouse liver to demonstrate mechanisms for expression of the *SORT1* gene and their relevance to low-density lipoprotein cholesterol. More recently, many such experiments use gene editing to increase efficiency and test more candidates. Even with gene editing, however, these experiments are extremely costly and are limited by the fact that they can mostly be performed in cell lines, which may not represent the natural target cell for the disease. More recently, bioinformatic approaches that rely on established experimental data sets have become quite useful as an alternative. These include genome-wide transcriptome or chromatin data in dozens of different human tissue types. Methods and databases for functional studies are evolving rapidly but are reviewed and summarized relatively regularly (e.g., Cano-Gamez & Trynka, 2020; Claussnitzer et al., 2020).

Throughout the history described above, there has been an ongoing discussion of the importance of phenotype definition. For example, in autism, should one carefully phenotype individuals and try to identify homogeneous subtypes in the hope that they will share genetic causes, or is it better to expend those resources to collect more study subjects and perform a large heterogeneous study? This question is more economic than biological. But there are also important biological questions. Clinical definitions of disease are typically historical and not necessarily biologically well founded. In theory, gene discovery should work best with low-level biological phenotypes, sometimes known as endophenotypes. Endophenotypes are quantitative phenotypes such as enzyme levels that may underlie a clinical disease. The use of endophenotypes has been particularly prevalent in psychiatry. For example, Lowe et al. (2015) used social responsiveness, a quantitative endophenotype for autism, to discover two regions on chromosome 8 that may be related to autism. The counterargument to the use of endophenotypes is that it is possible to discover genes that are related to the endophenotype but not necessarily to the meaningful clinical phenotype. For example, if one is interested in bone health in older adults, is it more meaningful to find genes for bone density, for change in bone density with time, for a clinical diagnosis of osteoporosis, or perhaps even for the occurrence of fracture?

The current state of gene discovery for complex traits is one of steady increases in incremental knowledge based on all of the study types described above. In addition, newer study types such as those based on electronic medical records are expected to accelerate the growth in knowledge (Pendergrass & Crawford, 2019). New associated loci are constantly being identified, but proof of causality remains difficult as functional studies are both challenging and expensive. Building true understanding of all factors influencing a complex trait and how they interact biologically is a distant aspirational challenge. For most complex traits we are not yet even close to fully explaining all of the observed heritability. On the other hand, as discussed in the following section, complete information and proof of causality are not necessarily needed to make clinical use of the information generated by these studies.

Risk Prediction for Complex Traits

The discovery methods outlined above all lead to partial information about disease etiology, which can be used to predict disease risk with varying levels of certainty. There are enormous and important questions about the practicality and ethics of doing disease prediction based on such partial information (discussed further below), but the general methods that are available can be categorized as follows.

Population recurrence risk estimation

In the absence of any specific risk information, individuals can be provided with risk numbers based purely on population frequency of a trait, perhaps in a particular ethnic or age group. For example, the frequency of various birth defects can be found in data from the National Birth Defects Prevention Network (Mai et al., 2019). Similarly, an individual who has had a child with a particular genetic disorder can be provided with a population-based empiric recurrence risk that does not depend on individual risk factors (Agopian et al., 2018). The primary disadvantage of these methods is that no information specific to the individual is incorporated into the risk estimate.

Epidemiological models

For some disorders there are epidemiological models that expand on population risks by predicting risk based on multiple individual factors such as age, sex, parity, and perhaps one or two specific genotypes. The longest history of this can be found in breast cancer, where a number of different models exist that are applicable to different populations and that incorporate differing factors. Breast cancer models were reviewed by G. Kim and Bahl (2021). For example, the Breast Cancer Risk Assessment Tool uses reproductive history, family history of breast cancer, and other factors to predict risk of developing breast cancer. The tool has been validated in several different ethnic groups. However, it is inappropriate for women who are known to carry a *BRCA1* pathogenic variant, because it does not take that information into account. The type of information needed for these epidemiological models is available for a number of other traits (e.g., Alzheimer's disease) but may not be considered clinically useful unless there is an intervention that can be offered to at-risk individuals. However, as seen in breast cancer, the availability of the risk prediction tool can actually spur the development of such interventions.

Genetic testing and sequencing

When there are one or more loci strongly implicated for a particular disease, genetic tests may be offered. These are sometimes combined with epidemiological data to produce a risk estimate, but more often results are interpreted deterministically—whether or not the individual has a known disease-causing variant. In the context of complex disease, this approach is only useful for Mendelian subtypes, for example, *BRCA1*-related breast cancer. Some of these tests, particularly in cancer, simultaneously genotype or sequence moderately large panels of known variants. Even though no quantitative risk estimate is produced, the interpretation and communication of results can be quite difficult, especially when there are variants of unknown significance. There is an extensive literature on the issues around communicating these types of results (e.g., Gustavsson et al., 2020; Medendorp et al., 2020).

Using genome or exome sequencing in clinical settings is similar but multiplies the communication challenges and ethical quandaries.

Polygenic risk scores

A more recent risk prediction paradigm is the polygenic risk score (PRS). A PRS uses genome-wide association data to predict disease outcome based on multiple loci (anywhere from tens to millions) across the genome. These models are naïve or anonymous predictors, in the sense that no biological information about the genes is needed or used—the prediction is based on purely statistical results from a mathematical (usually regression) model. The theoretical benefit of PRS is that it can harness a single full-genome scan based on either sequence or chip data to provide an individual with risk estimates for a variety of diseases. The prediction does not require much knowledge about the biology of the disease or the markers used in the model, making it possible to predict risk even for disorders that are not well understood biologically. There are, of course, many corresponding concerns and drawbacks, discussed below. Development of PRSs has grown exponentially over the past few years, with models developed for almost every trait imaginable. For example, a PubMed search for papers with the words "polygenic," "risk," and "cancer" in the title yields 21 references in 2019, 39 in 2020, and 70 in 2021.

PRS models have been shown to be moderately predictive in many cases. Examples include breast cancer (Yiangou et al., 2021), hypertension (Vaura et al., 2021), and cardiovascular disease (Trinder et al., 2022). The best PRS models also include or separately account for discrete known risk genes or environmental factors in addition to the polygenes. Numerous examples have shown that the polygenic risk adds substantial information beyond that of the known genes. For example, Fahed et al. (2020) used over 80,000 samples from the UK biobank and case-control studies to study polygenic risk and monogenic risk for familial hypercholesterolemia, hereditary breast and ovarian cancer, and Lynch syndrome. They found that incorporation of the polygenic risk increased predictive power substantially beyond the monogenic risk information. For example, individuals with risk genotypes at major loci but low PRS had only average population risk overall. This type of result is of significant interest in terms of the basic science of disease—what is the biological mechanism by which a major gene effect is mediated back down to "normal" by polygenes? It also raises very important clinical questions—should an at-risk individual whose PRS brings them back down to average risk still receive the high-risk intervention? Fahed et al. (2020) discuss potential applications for the diseases they studied from the timing of lipid therapy to major decisions such as prophylactic mastectomy. Despite the significant statistical predictive power, the use of PRS models in clinical settings is controversial for a number of reasons. There needs to be an appropriate intervention—a clinical action that would result from a high (or low) risk score—and then the predictive power needs to be large enough to change that recommended clinical intervention.

The most important limitation of PRS models (though true to some extent of all risk models) is that they are specific to the population in which they were developed. Application of PRS models to a group or individual with a different ancestry, age, sex, or even environmental exposure is generally completely inappropriate. Specifically, most PRS models were initially developed in populations of European ancestry and are not applicable to individuals from African or Asian populations or even many subpopulations of European ancestry. This is a serious issue for the clinical application of PRS models and cannot be overemphasized. They can *only* be applied to the correct population, and sometimes it is not clear what that population is if patients may come from a slightly different subgroup (say, Southern European ancestry when the model was developed in the United Kingdom). Example publications in which cross-ethnic applicability is discussed include Hoang et al. (2021) and Evans et al. (2022). James et al. (2021) make an even broader analysis of how racial and ethnic categories are used in breast cancer screening.

In addition to the specific scientific limitations described above, there are significant ethical concerns surrounding clinical use of PRS models, including the potential for eugenic uses, stigmatization, inequities in application and access (Martin et al., 2019), and emotional distress due to poor communication of results. All of these are risks in the use of any disease predictor, but they are exacerbated with PRS because of the potential for multiple PRSs to be calculated for an individual in a primary care or population screening setting or even a direct-to-consumer setting. The International Common Disease Alliance recently created a PRS Task Force, which published an extensive review of the potential benefits and risks of using PRS in the clinic (Adeyemo et al., 2021). This review paints an overall fairly positive picture of the potential for clinical use of PRS but describes important safeguards and further research that are necessary. In contrast, a recent editorial from the Executive Committee of the European Society of Human Genetics unequivocally brands the use of PRS in preimplantation genetic testing as "an unproven, unethical practice" (Forzano et al., 2021, p. 493), and Palk et al. (2019) discuss specific concerns regarding the use of PRS in psychiatry.

The Future of Risk Prediction

All of the risk prediction paradigms discussed will continue to improve as our basic scientific knowledge of disease etiology improves. In addition, that increasing scientific knowledge will add to the already significant list of potential interventions that can be offered based on genomic information. We are poised for a massive increase in the use of these tools in both clinical and consumer settings. This makes it all the more critical to continue to take on the scientific and ethical challenges surrounding these methods.

For complex traits in particular, when prediction is based on statistical/epidemiological correlations rather than biology, application to populations other than the one in which the model was developed will continue to be highly questionable. The PRS is the apotheosis of this problem, in that the very mathematics behind the development of the score assumes a specific and homogeneous population. Development of risk scores for more varied populations, as well as a better understanding of the limits of the models, will be important areas for future scientific work.

Another technical issue that deserves further attention is calibrating the sensitivity and specificity of the tests, perhaps based on the setting in which the test will be used. PRSs in particular are often developed by basic scientists, but careful attention to where to place low-/medium-/high-risk cutoffs requires clinical consideration. For rare diseases, these models can suffer from the same issue as any diagnostic test—if the test is not extremely specific, false positives can be far more numerous than true positives in a population-based setting.

Another key issue for future work is that of practical interventions, both developing interventions and continuing the ethical discussion of when it might be appropriate to provide information without an available intervention. In addition, situations in which the only intervention is behavioral (e.g., warning patients that they are at high risk for cardiovascular disease and encouraging a healthy diet) are quite common, but the historic failure of such interventions suggests that further work is needed in risk communication science.

Other issues on the social science side include communication of results more generally, in particular communication of uncertainty, the psychological impacts of genetic information, stigmatization effects, and equitable access effects. All of these areas would benefit from both ethical discussion and qualitative and quantitative research.

Finally, there is a need for further discussion of the differences among settings in which the models may be used. Much of the current literature focuses on clinical settings, but that may well not be the major use case for personal genomic information in the future. All of the scientific and social issues described above have different implications in a direct-to-consumer setting, a public health population screening setting, a primary care setting, or a clinical setting in which individuals are already known to have familial or genetic risk. The trend toward more and more direct-to-consumer options makes this discussion of setting critical as we think about appropriate future uses of these risk prediction methods.

References

Adeyemo, A., Balaconis, M. K., Darnes, D. R., Fatumo, S., Granados Moreno, P., Hodonsky, C. J., Inouye, M., Kanai, M., Kato, K., Knoppers, B. M., Lewis, A. C. F., Martin, A. R., McCarthy, M. I., Meyer, M. N., Okada, Y., Richards, J. B., Richter, L., Ripatti, S., Rotimi, C. N., . . . Polygenic Risk Score Task Force of the International Common Disease Association. (2021). Responsible use of polygenic risk scores in the clinic: Potential benefits, risks and gaps. *Nature Medicine*, *27*(11), 1876–1884. https://doi.org/10.1038/s41591-021-01549-6

Agopian, A. J., Salemi, J. L., Tanner, J. P., & Kirby, R. S. (2018). Using birth defects surveillance programs for population-based estimation of sibling recurrence risks. *Birth Defects Research*, *110*(19), 1383–1387. https://doi.org/10.1002/bdr2.1387

Broman, K. W., & Feingold, E. (2004). SNPs made routine. *Nature Methods*, *1*(2), 104–105. https://doi.org/10.1038/nmeth1104-104

Cano-Gamez, E., & Trynka, G. (2020). From GWAS to function: Using functional genomics to identify the mechanisms underlying complex diseases. *Frontiers in Genetics*, *11*, 424. https://doi.org/10.3389/fgene.2020.00424

Claussnitzer, M., Cho, J. H., Collins, R., Cox, N. J., Dermitzakis, E. T., Hurles, M. E., Kathiresan, S., Kenny, E. E., Lindgren, C. M., MacArthur, D. G., North, K. N., Plon, S. E., Rehm, H. L., Risch, N., Rotimi, C. N., Shendure, J., Soranzo, N., & McCarthy, M. I. (2020). A brief history of human disease genetics. *Nature*, *577*(7789), 179–189. https://doi.org/10.1038/s41586-019-1879-7

Diabetes Genetics Initiative of Broad Institute of Harvard and MIT, Lund University, and Novartis Institutes of BioMedical Research, Saxena, R., Voight, B. F., Lyssenko, V., Burtt, N. P., de Bakker, P. I., Chen, H., Roix, J. J., Kathiresan, S., Hirschhorn, J. N., Daly, M. J., Hughes, T. E., Groop, L., Altshuler, D., Almgren, P., Florez, J. C., Meyer, J., . . . Purcell, S. (2007).

Genome-wide association analysis identifies loci for type 2 diabetes and triglyceride levels. *Science*, *316*(5829), 1331–1336. https://doi.org/10.1126/science.1142358

Evans, D. G., van Veen, E. M., Byers, H., Roberts, E., Howell, A., Howell, S. J., Harkness, E. F., Brentnall, A., Cuzick, J., & Newman, W. G. (2022). The importance of ethnicity: Are breast cancer polygenic risk scores ready for women who are not of White European origin? *International Journal of Cancer*, *150*(1), 73–79. https://doi.org/10.1002/ijc.33782

Fahed, A. C., Wang, M., Homburger, J. R., Patel, A. P., Bick, A. G., Neben, C. L., Lai, C., Brockman, D., Philippakis, A., Ellinor, P. T., Cassa, C. A., Lebo, M., Ng, K., Lander, E. S., Zhou, A. Y., Kathiresan, S., & Khera, A. V. (2020). Polygenic background modifies penetrance of monogenic variants for tier 1 genomic conditions. *Nature Communications*, *11*(1), 3635. https://doi.org/10.1038/s41467-020-17374-3

Forzano, F., Antonova, O., Clarke, A., de Wert, G., Hentze, S., Jamshidi, Y., Moreau, Y., Perola, M., Prokopenko, I., Read, A., Reymond, A., Stefansdottir, V., van El, C., Genuardi, M., Executive Committee of the European Society of Human Genetics and the Public and Professional Policy Committee of the European Society of Human Genetics. (2021). The use of polygenic risk scores in pre-implantation genetic testing: an unproven, unethical practice. *European Journal of Human Genetics*, *30*, 493–495. https://doi.org/10.1038/s41431-021-01000-x

Freedman, M. L., Reich, D., Penney, K. L., McDonald, G. J., Mignault, A. A., Patterson, N., Gabriel, S. B., Topol, E. J., Smoller, J. W., Pato, C. N., Pato, M. T., Petryshen, T. L., Kolonel, L. N., Lander, E. S., Sklar, P., Henderson, B., Hirschhorn, J. N., & Altshuler, D. (2004). Assessing the impact of population stratification on genetic association studies. *Nature Genetics*, *36*(4), 388–393. https://doi.org/10.1038/ng1333

Geddes, G. C., Syverson, E., & Earing, M. G. (2019). Three year experience of a clinical cardiovascular genetics program for infants with congenital heart disease. *Congenital Heart Disease*, *14*(5), 832–837. https://doi.org/10.1111/chd.12817

Gustavsson, E., Galvis, G., & Juth, N. (2020). Genetic testing for breast cancer risk, from BRCA1/2 to a seven gene panel: An ethical analysis. *BMC Medical Ethics*, *21*(1), 102. https://doi.org/10.1186/s12910-020-00545-8

Hall, J. M., Lee, M. K., Newman, B., Morrow, J. E., Anderson, L. A., Huey, B., & King, M. C. (1990). Linkage of early-onset familial breast cancer to chromosome 17q21. *Science*, *250*(4988), 1684–1689. https://doi.org/10.1126/science.2270482

Hindorff, L. A., Bonham, V. L., Brody, L. C., Ginoza, M. E. C., Hutter, C. M., Manolio, T. A., & Green, E. D. (2018). Prioritizing diversity in human genomics research. *Nature Reviews Genetics*, *19*(3), 175–185. https://doi.org/10.1038/nrg.2017.89

Hoang, T., Nguyen Ngoc, Q., Lee, J., Lee, E. K., Hwangbo, Y., & Kim, J. (2021). Evaluation of modifiable factors and polygenic risk score in thyroid cancer. *Endocrine Related Cancer*, *28*(7), 481–494. https://doi.org/10.1530/ERC-21-0078

International HapMap Consortium. (2003). The International HapMap Project. *Nature*, *426*(6968), 789–796. https://doi.org/10.1038/nature02168

James, J. E., Riddle, L., Koenig, B. A., & Joseph, G. (2021). The limits of personalization in precision medicine: Polygenic risk scores and racial categorization in a precision breast cancer screening trial. *PLoS One*, *16*(10), e0258571. https://doi.org/10.1371/journal.pone.0258571

Juo, S. H., Beaty, T. H., Xu, J., Prenger, V. L., Coresh, J., & Kwiterovich, P. O., Jr. (1998). Segregation analysis of two-locus models regulating apolipoprotein-A1 levels. *Genetic Epidemiology*, *15*(1), 73–86. https://doi.org/10.1002/(SICI)1098-2272(1998)15:1<73::AID-GEPI6>3.0.CO;2-5

Kamboh, M. I. (2021). Genomics and functional genomics of Alzheimer's disease. *Neurotherapeutics*, *19*, 152–172. https://doi.org/10.1007/s13311-021-01152-0

Karim, A., Tang, C. S., & Tam, P. K. (2021). The emerging genetic landscape of Hirschsprung disease and its potential clinical applications. *Frontiers in Pediatrics, 9*, 638093. https://doi.org/10.3389/fped.2021.638093

Kim, G., & Bahl, M. (2021). Assessing risk of breast cancer: A review of risk prediction models. *Journal of Breast Imaging, 3*(2), 144–155. https://doi.org/10.1093/jbi/wbab001

Kim, J., Bhupathiraju, S. N., Harrington, L. B., Hagan, K. A., Lindstrom, S., Manson, J. E., Kraft, P., & Kabrhel, C. (2022). Oral postmenopausal hormone therapy and genetic risk on venous thromboembolism: Gene-hormone interaction results from a large prospective cohort study. *Menopause, 29*, 293–303. https://doi.org/10.1097/GME.0000000000001924

Klein, R. J., Zeiss, C., Chew, E. Y., Tsai, J. Y., Sackler, R. S., Haynes, C., Henning, A. K., SanGiovanni, J. P., Mane, S. M., Mayne, S. T., Bracken, M. B., Ferris, F. L., Ott, J., Barnstable, C., & Hoh, J. (2005). Complement factor H polymorphism in age-related macular degeneration. *Science, 308*(5720), 385–389. https://doi.org/10.1126/science.1109557

Knowler, W. C., Williams, R. C., Pettitt, D. J., & Steinberg, A. G. (1988). Gm3;5,13,14 and type 2 diabetes mellitus: An association in American Indians with genetic admixture. *American Journal of Human Genetics, 43*(4), 520–526. https://www.ncbi.nlm.nih.gov/pubmed/3177389

Lander, E. S., Linton, L. M., Birren, B., Nusbaum, C., Zody, M. C., Baldwin, J., Devon, K., Dewar, K., Doyle, M., FitzHugh, W., Funke, R., Gage, D., Harris, K., Heaford, A., Howland, J., Kann, L., Lehoczky, J., LeVine, R., McEwan, P., . . . International Human Genome Sequencing Consortium. (2001). Initial sequencing and analysis of the human genome. *Nature, 409*(6822), 860–921. https://doi.org/10.1038/35057062

Lango Allen, H., Estrada, K., Lettre, G., Berndt, S. I., Weedon, M. N., Rivadeneira, F., Willer, C. J., Jackson, A. U., Vedantam, S., Raychaudhuri, S., Ferreira, T., Wood, A. R., Weyant, R. J., Segre, A. V., Speliotes, E. K., Wheeler, E., Soranzo, N., Park, J. H., Yang, J., . . . Hirschhorn, J. N. (2010). Hundreds of variants clustered in genomic loci and biological pathways affect human height. *Nature, 467*(7317), 832–838. https://doi.org/10.1038/nature09410

Lee, S. H., Ahn, W. Y., Seweryn, M., & Sadee, W. (2018). Combined genetic influence of the nicotinic receptor gene cluster CHRNA5/A3/B4 on nicotine dependence. *BMC Genomics, 19*(1), 826. https://doi.org/10.1186/s12864-018-5219-3

Leslie, E. J. (2021). Genetic models and approaches to study orofacial clefts. *Oral Diseases, 28*, 1327–1338. https://doi.org/10.1111/odi.14109

Lowe, J. K., Werling, D. M., Constantino, J. N., Cantor, R. M., & Geschwind, D. H. (2015). Social responsiveness, an autism endophenotype: Genomewide significant linkage to two regions on chromosome 8. *American Journal of Psychiatry, 172*(3), 266–275. https://doi.org/10.1176/appi.ajp.2014.14050576

Mai, C. T., Isenburg, J. L., Canfield, M. A., Meyer, R. E., Correa, A., Alverson, C. J., Lupo, P. J., Riehle-Colarusso, T., Cho, S. J., Aggarwal, D., Kirby, R. S., & National Birth Defects Prevention Network. (2019). National population-based estimates for major birth defects, 2010–2014. *Birth Defects Research, 111*(18), 1420–1435. https://doi.org/10.1002/bdr2.1589

Martin, A. R., Kanai, M., Kamatani, Y., Okada, Y., Neale, B. M., & Daly, M. J. (2019). Clinical use of current polygenic risk scores may exacerbate health disparities. *Nature Genetics, 51*(4), 584–591. https://doi.org/10.1038/s41588-019-0379-x

Medendorp, N. M., van Maarschalkerweerd, P. E. A., Murugesu, L., Daams, J. G., Smets, E. M. A., & Hillen, M. A. (2020). The impact of communicating uncertain test results in cancer genetic counseling: A systematic mixed studies review. *Patient Education Counseling, 103*(9), 1692–1708. https://doi.org/10.1016/j.pec.2020.03.015

Musunuru, K., Strong, A., Frank-Kamenetsky, M., Lee, N. E., Ahfeldt, T., Sachs, K. V., Li, X., Li, H., Kuperwasser, N., Ruda, V. M., Pirruccello, J. P., Muchmore, B., Prokunina-Olsson, L.,

Hall, J. L., Schadt, E. E., Morales, C. R., Lund-Katz, S., Phillips, M. C., Wong, J., . . . Rader, D. J. (2010). From noncoding variant to phenotype via SORT1 at the 1p13 cholesterol locus. *Nature, 466*(7307), 714–719. https://doi.org/10.1038/nature09266
Palk, A. C., Dalvie, S., de Vries, J., Martin, A. R., & Stein, D. J. (2019). Potential use of clinical polygenic risk scores in psychiatry—Ethical implications and communicating high polygenic risk. *Philosophy, Ethics, and Humanities in Medicine, 14*(1), 4. https://doi.org/10.1186/s13010-019-0073-8
Papale, L. A., Madrid, A., Zhang, Q., Chen, K., Sak, L., Keles, S., & Alisch, R. S. (2021). Gene by environment interaction mouse model reveals a functional role for 5-hydroxymethylcytosine in neurodevelopmental disorders. *Genome Research, 32*, 266–279. https://doi.org/10.1101/gr.276137.121
Pendergrass, S. A., & Crawford, D. C. (2019). Using electronic health records to generate phenotypes for research. *Current Protocols in Human Genetics, 100*(1), e80. https://doi.org/10.1002/cphg.80
Price, A. L., Patterson, N. J., Plenge, R. M., Weinblatt, M. E., Shadick, N. A., & Reich, D. (2006). Principal components analysis corrects for stratification in genome-wide association studies. *Nature Genetics, 38*(8), 904–909. https://doi.org/10.1038/ng1847
Risch, N., & Merikangas, K. (1996). The future of genetic studies of complex human diseases. *Science, 273*(5281), 1516–1517. https://doi.org/10.1126/science.273.5281.1516
Trinder, M., Vikulova, D., Pimstone, S., Mancini, G. B. J., & Brunham, L. R. (2022). Polygenic architecture and cardiovascular risk of familial combined hyperlipidemia. *Atherosclerosis, 340*, 35–43. https://doi.org/10.1016/j.atherosclerosis.2021.11.032
Vaura, F., Kauko, A., Suvila, K., Havulinna, A. S., Mars, N., Salomaa, V., FinnGen, Cheng, S., & Niiranen, T. (2021). Polygenic risk scores predict hypertension onset and cardiovascular risk. *Hypertension, 77*(4), 1119–1127. https://doi.org/10.1161/HYPERTENSION AHA.120.16471
Waye, M. M. Y., & Cheng, H. Y. (2018). Genetics and epigenetics of autism: A review. *Psychiatry and Clinical Neurosciences, 72*(4), 228–244. https://doi.org/10.1111/pcn.12606
Weinberg, S. M., Parsons, T. E., Marazita, M. L., & Maher, B. S. (2013). Heritability of face shape in twins: A preliminary study using 3D stereophotogrammetry and geometric morphometrics. *Dentistry 3000, 1*(1). https://doi.org/10.5195/d3000.2013.14
Weissbecker, K. A., Wolf, B., Eaves, L. J., Marazita, M. L., & Nance, W. E. (1993). Combined pedigree and twin family study to determine the sources of variation in serum biotinidase activity: The usefulness of multiple study designs. *American Journal of Medical Genetics, 47*(2), 231–240. https://doi.org/10.1002/ajmg.1320470218
Wheeler, D. A., Srinivasan, M., Egholm, M., Shen, Y., Chen, L., McGuire, A., He, W., Chen, Y. J., Makhijani, V., Roth, G. T., Gomes, X., Tartaro, K., Niazi, F., Turcotte, C. L., Irzyk, G. P., Lupski, J. R., Chinault, C., Song, X. Z., Liu, Y., . . . Rothberg, J. M. (2008). The complete genome of an individual by massively parallel DNA sequencing. *Nature, 452*(7189), 872–876. https://doi.org/10.1038/nature06884
Yiangou, K., Kyriacou, K., Kakouri, E., Marcou, Y., Panayiotidis, M. I., Loizidou, M. A., Hadjisavvas, A., & Michailidou, K. (2021). Combination of a 15-SNP polygenic risk score and classical risk factors for the prediction of breast cancer risk in Cypriot women. *Cancers (Basel), 13*, 4568. https://doi.org/10.3390/cancers13184568

CHAPTER 21

RISK ASSESSMENT OF SECONDARY FINDINGS

ERIC T. RUSH

Introduction

Secondary findings encompass likely pathogenic (LP) and pathogenic (P) variants detected on genomic testing that are unrelated to the original indication for testing. For consistency of terminology, the term "secondary findings" will be used in this chapter as this is currently the preferred term, although the term "incidental findings" has frequently been used (ACMG Board of Directors, 2015). Disclosure of secondary findings is a relatively recent challenge given the emergence of next-generation sequencing and has become a practical consideration more frequently given the ubiquity of exome sequencing (ES) and genome sequencing (GS).

The historical approach to genetic testing was more targeted out of necessity. It was simply too difficult to test for more than one gene (or at most a very few genes) at one time. This approach, while laborious, ensured that results of testing would be applicable to the underlying indication. The expansion of genetic testing to curated panels increased our burden of variant interpretation, but since the majority were directed toward a phenotype or disease state group, the burden of secondary findings was still relatively low.

The introduction of clinical ES and GS greatly increased overall diagnostic yield but increased the challenge of secondary findings, which in turn needed to be appropriately managed. Further proliferation of ES and GS into other clinical specialties makes this process even more challenging and underscores the need for practical guidelines.

A uniform approach to secondary findings in pre- and posttest counseling and subsequent medical management has been helpful in this process. That current recommendations have been amended several times over only a few years reinforces that this is an iterative process that will continue. Readers are strongly encouraged to refer to the current literature to familiarize themselves with any updates to current recommendations that have been released subsequent to the publication of this text.

Recent Guidelines for Disclosure and Management of Secondary Findings

Prior to the publication of the original guidelines for secondary findings, clinicians did not have clear guidelines for the reporting of secondary findings, although ethically it had been argued that some obligation did exist to return secondary findings that were "firmly associated with high risk of diseases with specific strategies that ameliorate expected morbidity and mortality" (J. P. Evans & Rothschild, 2012, p. 358). The difficulty in the construction of any guidelines is in the details, most significantly in what constitutes a condition with high risk that also has viable strategies for amelioration. Given that truly objective classification of potentially high-risk conditions does not exist, current guidance has been based on expert consensus instead. The first expert working group was convened in 2012 by the American College of Medical Genetics and Genomics (ACMG) and worked from a previously established list of genes (Green et al., 2012) and narrowed this list to 56 genes, which formed the initial set of recommendations we will refer to retroactively as the ACMG Secondary Findings version 1.0 (SF v1.0).

While consideration was given to inclusion of all secondary findings, the working group ultimately decided instead to include a minimum list of genes in which reporting was likely to have medical benefit for individuals and families (Green et al., 2013). Consideration of epidemiology was given by the working group, and while many genes included in the list are still by definition rare, a strong trend exists in favoring less rare conditions.

Specific recommendations given in ACMG SF v1.0 that bear mention include, first, the decision to include only pathogenic variants for a secondary finding, whereas variants of uncertain significance are reported for primary findings. Second, responsibility for pre- and posttest counseling is assigned to the ordering clinician. Third, comprehensive genetic testing such as ES and GS should only be obtained by clinicians who are familiar with the benefits and limitations. Fourth, while adult-onset disorders are generally not evaluated for minors, it was suggested that these usual guidelines be relaxed for secondary findings given that the benefits for early diagnosis of family members would outweigh the damage of early disclosure to the minor patient.

Philosophically, the ACMG Working Group on Incidental Findings in Clinical Exome and Genome Sequencing noted a range of opinions. It was acknowledged that difficult choices needed to be made, and although overall consensus was reached on a minimum list of genes to include, this was not a truly evidence-based process and disagreement existed among members of the working group. It was also acknowledged that there are inherent limitations of the evaluation and interpretation of secondary findings, as they are by definition secondary. For this reason, they should not be used in an exclusionary manner as a "screening test." Patient preference was discussed as a part of this working group; the group ultimately decided against recommending that patients be able to opt out of receiving a secondary finding but acknowledged that this may "be seen to violate existing ethical norms" (Green et al., 2013, p. 568). The working group felt that the fiduciary duty to prevent harm in patients outweighed the removal of patient autonomy and right not to know damaging information. It should be noted that this opinion was immediately controversial and current practice for most genetics professionals includes the ability to opt out of secondary findings in the pretest counseling phase of ES and GS.

If we can summarize the overall nature of discussion in the working group, two main clusters of opinion were identified, both of which continue to inform our thoughts about genetic testing in general and secondary findings specifically. Genetic libertarians felt that individuals had the right to full and complete disclosure of all possible risks and that secondary findings should be interpreted more broadly as to what constitutes a high-risk gene and which variants should be reported (i.e., variants of uncertain significance). The counterpoint is argued by genetic empiricists who warn against sharing variants with insufficient evidence of benefit and underscore the psychological burden of awaiting a disease process that may never present. Broad agreement has been reached among both groups regarding the need for continued curation of the genes included in SF guidelines and the importance of informed consent (Scheuner at al., 2015).

Initially, an annual review of these guidelines was proposed, but it was not until 2017 that the first revision was published. This revision updated the gene list to include *ATP7B*, *BMPR1A*, *SMAD4*, and *OTC* and to remove *MYLK* (Kalia et al., 2017). More important were revisions to the spirit of the recommendations. First, criteria for acceptability of intervention were established, acknowledging that the burden of treatment or surveillance is an important factor in selection of appropriate genes for inclusion or exclusion. Notably, the 2015 ACMG guidelines for interpretation of variants was published prior to the publication of the SF v2.0 (Richards et al., 2015). The inclusion of the LP category that is now utilized routinely in variant interpretation is acknowledged in SF v2.0, but ultimately it was decided to continue to use the terminology of known pathogenic (KP) or expected pathogenic (EP) variants. It was immediately unclear whether KP and EP corresponded cleanly to P and LP, which created ambiguity. This issue was expertly communicated by a member of the original working group along with a strong recommendation that the guidelines be further updated to harmonize the terminology used with current ACMG guidelines for variant interpretation (Biesecker, 2017). Readers are encouraged to review this short communication as it succinctly summarizes many of the current challenges in communication of secondary findings. Notably, the ACMG Secondary Findings Working Group reconvened in 2020 both to create updates to the policies surrounding reporting of secondary findings and to update the list of actionable genes based on criteria previously established and new criteria that are now integrated into these guidelines. The policy document resulting from this effort clarifies and expands several questions and considerations from earlier iterations of this policy (Miller, Lee, Abul-Husn et al., 2021). This version of the SF clarified that the list of genes is considered to be a minimum list, not a comprehensive one. It also reiterated that the SF list was not intended to provide carrier screening for recessive conditions but that an additional working group has been established to explore the possibility of this being part of future recommendations (ACMG Board of Directors, 2019). Several ethical considerations have been clarified. For the sake of this text, the key considerations would be to utilize an "opt out" versus an "opt in" strategy for SF, consideration of adult-onset conditions in pediatric patients, the importance of clear and complete communication in the risk and benefits of ES/GS, and consideration of individual clinical context when discussing SF that may include incomplete or unknown penetrance. An important change in this policy is aligning the language of LP and P with the ACMG/Association for Molecular Pathology guidelines for variant classification.

The ACMG SF v3.0 list was published in 2021 and, aside from the addition of specific genes, also groups genes into four categories: genes related to cancer phenotypes, genes related to cardiovascular phenotypes, genes related to inborn errors of metabolism phenotypes, and genes related to miscellaneous phenotypes (Miller, Lee, Chung et al., 2021). This policy statement also recommends the inclusion of 14 additional genes for return as secondary findings: *PALB2*, *MAX*, *TMEM127*, *CASQ*, *TRDN*, *FLNC*, *TTN*, *BTD*, *GAA*, *HFE*, *ACVRL1*, *ENG*, *HNF1A*, and *RPE65*. The ACMG SF v.3.1 list for reporting of secondary findings was published in 2022 and expands this further, recommending inclusion of *BAG3*, *DES*, *RBM20*, *TNNC1*, and *TTR* (Miller et al., 2022). In 2023 an additional three genes were added to the ACMG SF v3.2: *CALM1*, *CALM2*, and *CALM3* (Miller et al., 2023).

Applying Secondary Findings to Risk Assessment and Clinical Management

A number of factors come into play for risk assessment and clinical management for individuals who have secondary findings identified on ES/GS. Some of these factors are intrinsic to the variant itself, including issues of variable expressivity and incomplete penetrance, and some of these factors are extrinsic to the variant, including the palatability of surveillance.

Managing secondary findings starts during the consultation as a part of pretest counseling. When making recommendations for ES or GS, clinicians must discuss several important elements and limitations of the testing, including yield, expected burden of variants of uncertain significance, costs, and privacy considerations. Along with this discussion, it is important to acknowledge the current SF recommendations, and these should be integrated into other portions of the discussion as an inherent part of the informed consent process. Patients and clinicians are often not aware that a formal list of secondary findings exists, although when explained, my experience is that most do intuitively grasp the concept that there may be important findings within comprehensive genetic testing such as ES/GS that do not relate to the indications. Some patients may wish to receive secondary findings, often with the thought that any health information is likely to be helpful. Other patients may wish to opt out of secondary findings, and more frequently those patients may have personal philosophical or religious reasons for doing so. It is my opinion that if patients are appropriately counseled prior to testing, the decision to either receive or to opt out of secondary findings is acceptable based on the concept of self-determination.

Discussion of penetrance and variability can be challenging, but these concepts are very important for patients to understand. As the ACMG SF recommendations have expanded, incomplete penetrance has become extremely common. This is particularly true for patients with hereditary malignancy syndromes, in which incomplete penetrance is the general rule. This is even true in conditions like Li-Fraumeni syndrome, which is often perceived to be one of the most severe hereditary malignancy syndromes, but even in this condition, approximately 10% of patients will escape malignancy by age 60. It is also true in hereditary breast and ovarian cancer caused by *BRCA1* and *BRCA2*, a predisposition that has decidedly entered the public consciousness and in which the public may assume a more deterministic, even fatalistic outcome, when in reality people with pathogenic variants in these genes can and do escape malignancy. Genetic cardiovascular disorders are somewhat different in that many may show complete or essentially complete penetrance. Loeys-Dietz syndrome is a good example of a condition where penetrance is likely to be complete. However, significant variability in the presentation of Loeys-Dietz still exists, with some patients presenting early in adulthood and others not presenting until middle age. Other cardiovascular disorders such as long QT syndrome show both incomplete penetrance and variability in expression, with 25% of patients possessing a pathogenic variant lacking a prolonged QT interval and the remaining 75% presenting in one of several ways at a variety of ages.

There is also a tendency for patients to understand the results of genetic testing in a very deterministic fashion; therefore, in addition to understanding the concepts of penetrance and variability, it is important for patients to have a basic understanding of the probabilistic way in which genetics professionals consume the information derived from genetic testing. In the subsequent discussion of individual genes and disorders, probabilities are given where they are known and applicable. It is not practically possible or advised to discuss specific probabilities for individual disorders during pretest counseling, but the concept that the risk of a pathogenic variant confers a probability of risk for but not a guarantee of disease should be introduced. Should secondary findings result from ES/GS, it is appropriate to discuss specific probabilities of disease during a posttest counseling session.

As a practical matter, the types of variants included in the ACMG SF recommendations are relatively narrow compared to the approximately 20,000 human genes. Per the framework established in SF v3.0, we will categorize these 81 genes into four categories:

- Genes related to cancer phenotypes
- Genes related to cardiovascular phenotypes
- Genes related to inborn errors of metabolism phenotypes
- Genes related to miscellaneous phenotypes

Table 21.1 organizes the list of 81 genes according to this nosology.

Genes Related to Cancer Phenotypes

1. Hereditary breast and ovarian cancer (HBOC) caused by *BRCA1* and *BRCA2* are the prototypes of hereditary predisposition to breast and ovarian cancer. Pathogenic variants in the *BRCA1* gene confer a 46% to 87% risk of breast cancer and a 39% to 63% risk of ovarian cancer. Pathogenic variants in the *BRCA2* gene confer a 38% to 84% risk of breast cancer and a 16.5% to 27% risk of ovarian cancer (Mavaddat et al., 2013). Both are inherited in an autosomal dominant manner. It is also known that pathogenic variants in *BRCA1* or *BRCA2* confer a risk for prostate cancer, male breast cancer, and pancreatic cancer, with pathogenic variants in *BRCA2* conferring a higher risk than *BRCA1* (van Asperen et al., 2005). The approach to *BRCA1*- and *BRCA2*-related HBOC includes surveillance, which is recommended in women generally starting at age 25, but even earlier surveillance may be required if particularly early onset of disease is present in the family. Risk reduction surgery may be

Table 21.1 Genes Included in ACMG SF v3.2, Associated Phenotype, and Inheritance Pattern

Gene (OMIM)	Phenotype (OMIM)	Inheritance pattern
Genes related to cancer phenotypes		
APC (MIM 611731)	Adenomatous polyposis coli (MIM 175100)	AD
BRCA1 (MIM 113705)	Breast-ovarian cancer, familial 1 (MIM 604370)	AD
BRCA2 (MIM 600185)	Breast-ovarian cancer, familial 2 (MIM 612555)	AD
PALB2 (MIM 601355)	Susceptibility to breast cancer (MIM 114480)	AD
MEN1 (MIM 613733)	Multiple endocrine neoplasia, type 1 (MIM 131100)	AD
RET (MIM 164761)	Familial medullary thyroid carcinoma (MIM 155240)	AD
	Multiple endocrine neoplasia, type 2a (MIM 171400)	AD
	Multiple endocrine neoplasia, type 2b (MIM 162300)	AD
BMPR1A (MIM 601299)	Juvenile polyposis syndrome (MIM 174900)	AD
SMAD4 (MIM 600993)		
TP53 (MIM 191170)	Li-Fraumeni syndrome 1 (MIM 151623)	AD
MLH1 (MIM 120436)	Lynch syndrome (MIM 120435)	AD
MSH2 (MIM 609309)		
MSH6 (MIM 600678)		
PMS2 (MIM 600259)		
MUTYH (MIM 604933)	MYH-associated polyposis (MIM 608456)	AR
NF2 (MIM 607379)	Neurofibromatosis, type 2 (MIM 101000)	AD
SDHD (MIM 602690)	Paragangliomas 1 (MIM 168000)	AD
SDHAF2 (MIM 613019)	Paragangliomas 2 (MIM 601650)	AD
SDHC (MIM 602413)	Paragangliomas 3 (MIM 605373)	AD
SDHB (MIM 185470)	Paragangliomas 4 (MIM 115310)	AD
MAX (MIM 154950)	Susceptibility to pheochromocytoma (MIM 171300)	AD
TMEM127 (MIM 613403)	Susceptibility to pheochromocytoma (MIM 171300)	AD
STK11 (MIM 602216)	Peutz-Jeghers syndrome (MIM 175200)	AD
PTEN (MIM 601728)	PTEN hamartoma tumor syndrome (MIM 153480)	AD
RB1 (MIM 614041)	Retinoblastoma (MIM 180200)	AD
TSC1 (MIM 605284)	Tuberous sclerosis 1 (MIM 191100)	AD
TSC2 (MIM 191092)	Tuberous sclerosis 2 (MIM 613254)	AD
VHL (MIM 608537)	Von Hippel-Lindau syndrome (MIM 193300)	AD
WT1 (MIM 607102)	Wilms tumor (MIM 194070)	AD
Genes related to cardiovascular phenotypes		
MYH11 (MIM 160745)	Aortic aneurysm, familial thoracic 4 (MIM 132900)	AD
ACTA2 (MIM 102620)	Aortic aneurysm, familial thoracic 6 (MIM 611788)	AD
TMEM43 (MIM 612048)	Arrhythmogenic right ventricular cardiomyopathy, type 5 (MIM 604400)	AD
DSP (MIM 125647)	Arrhythmogenic right ventricular cardiomyopathy, type 8 (MIM 607450)	AD
PKP2 (MIM 602861)	Arrhythmogenic right ventricular cardiomyopathy, type 9 (MIM 609040)	AD
DSG2 (MIM 125671)	Arrhythmogenic right ventricular cardiomyopathy, type 10 (MIM 610193)	AD
DSC2 (MIM 125645)	Arrhythmogenic right ventricular cardiomyopathy, type 11 (MIM 610476)	AD, AR

Table 21.1 Continued

Gene (OMIM)	Phenotype (OMIM)	Inheritance pattern
SCN5A (MIM 600163)	Brugada syndrome 1 (MIM 601144)	AD
	Long QT syndrome 3 (MIM 603830)	AD
CALM1 (MIM 114180)	Long QT syndrome 14 (MIM 616247)	AD
CALM2 (MIM 114182)	Long QT syndrome 15 (MIM 616249)	AD
CALM3 (MIM 114183)	Long QT syndrome 16 (MIM 618782)	AD
RYR2 (MIM 180902)	Catecholaminergic polymorphic ventricular tachycardia, 1 (MIM 604772)	AD
CASQ (MIM 114251)	Catecholaminergic polymorphic ventricular tachycardia, 2 (MIM 611938)	AR
TRDN (MIM 603283)	Cardiac arrythmia syndrome with or without skeletal muscle weakness (MIM 615441)	AR
LMNA (MIM 150330)	Dilated cardiomyopathy 1A (MIM 115200)	AD
MYBPC3 (MIM 600958)	Dilated cardiomyopathy 1MM (MIM 615396)	AD
	Familial hypertrophic cardiomyopathy 4 (MIM 115197)	AD, AR
FLNC (MIM 102565)	Dilated cardiomyopathy	AD
TTN (MIM 188840)	Dilated cardiomyopathy 1G (MIM 604145)	AD
BAG3 (MIM 603883)	Dilated cardiomyopathy 1HH (MIM 613881)	AD
DES (MIM 125660)	Dilated cardiomyopathy 1I (OMIM 604765)	AD
RBM20 (MIM 613171)	Dilated cardiomyopathy 1DD (OMIM 613172)	AD
TNNC1 (MIM 191040)	Dilated cardiomyopathy 1Z (OMIM 611879)	AD
COL3A1 (MIM 120180)	Ehlers-Danlos syndrome, vascular type (MIM 130050)	AD
LDLR (MIM 606945)	Familial hypercholesterolemia, type 1 (MIM 143890)	AD
APOB (MIM 107730)	Familial hypercholesterolemia, type 2 (MIM 144010)	AD
PCSK9 (MIM 607786)	Hypercholesterolemia, autosomal dominant, 3 (MIM 603776)	AD
MYH7 (MIM 160760)	Familial hypertrophic cardiomyopathy 1 (MIM 192600)	AD, DD
TPM1 (MIM 191010)	Familial hypertrophic cardiomyopathy 3 (MIM 115196)	AD
PRKAG2 (MIM 602743)	Familial hypertrophic cardiomyopathy 6 (MIM 600858)	AD
TNNI3 (MIM 191044)	Familial hypertrophic cardiomyopathy 7 (MIM 613690)	AD
	Dilated cardiomyopathy 1FF (MIM 611880)	AD
MYL3 (MIM 160790)	Familial hypertrophic cardiomyopathy 8 (MIM 608751)	AD, AR
MYL2 (MIM 160781)	Familial hypertrophic cardiomyopathy 10 (MIM 608758)	AD
ACTC1 (MIM 102540)	Familial hypertrophic cardiomyopathy 11 (MIM 612098)	AD
TNNT2 (MIM 191045)	Dilated cardiomyopathy 1D (MIM 601494)	AD
	Hypertrophic cardiomyopathy (MIM 115195)	
TGFBR1 (MIM 190181)	Loeys-Dietz syndrome, type 1A (MIM 609192)	AD
	Loeys-Dietz syndrome, type 2A (MIM 608967)	AD
TGFBR2 (MIM 190182)	Loeys-Dietz syndrome, type 1B (MIM 610168)	AD
	Loeys-Dietz syndrome, type 2B (MIM 610380)	AD
SMAD3 (MIM 603109)	Loeys-Dietz syndrome, type 3 (MIM 613795)	AD
KCNQ1 (MIM 607542)	Long QT syndrome 1 (MIM 192500)	AD
KCNH2 (MIM 152427)	Long QT syndrome 2 (MIM 613688)	AD
FBN1 (MIM 134797)	Marfan syndrome (MIM 154700)	AD

(continued)

Table 21.1 Continued

Gene (OMIM)	Phenotype (OMIM)	Inheritance pattern
Genes related to inborn errors of metabolism phenotypes		
BTD (MIM 609019)	Biotinidase deficiency (MIM 253260)	AR
GLA (MIM 300644)	Fabry disease (MIM 301500)	XL
OTC (MIM 300461)	Ornithine transcarbamoylase deficiency (MIM 311250)	XL
GAA (MIM 606800)	GSD II/Pompe disease (MIM 232300)	AR
Genes related to miscellaneous phenotypes		
HFE (MIM 613609)	Hemochromatosis (MIM 235200)	AR
ACVRL1 (MIM 601284)	Hereditary hemorrhagic telangiectasia, 2 (MIM 600376)	AD
ENG (MIM 131195)	Hereditary hemorrhagic telangiectasia, 1 (MIM 187300)	AD
RYR1 (MIM 180901)	Malignant hyperthermia, 1 (MIM 145600)	AD
CACNA1S (MIM 114208)	Malignant hyperthermia, 5 (MIM 145600)	AD
HNF1A (MIM 142410)	Maturity-onset diabetes of the young, 3 (MIM 600496)	AD
RPE65 (MIM 180069)	RPE65-related retinopathy (MIM 613794)	AR
ATP7B (MIM 606882)	Wilson disease (MIM 277900)	AR
TTR (MIM 176300)	Hereditary *TTR* amyloidosis (MIM 105210)	AD

Note: Mendelian Inheritance in Man (MIM) numbers included for genes and phenotypes for reference (https://www.omim.org). AD = autosomal dominant; AR = autosomal recessive; DD = digenic dominant; OMIM = Online Mendelian Inheritance in Man; XL = X-linked.

considered for women who are found to have a pathogenic variant in *BRCA1* or *BRCA2*, which may include prophylactic bilateral mastectomy and oophorectomy (Rebbeck et al., 2002).

2. *PALB2*-related breast cancer susceptibility was described in the latter part of the 2000s and has been increasingly well characterized since that time. It is known that breast cancer is the highest risk for patients who are heterozygous for a pathogenic *PALB2* variant, reaching approximately 53% by age 80. Other malignancies are reported in excess but at much lower absolute values compared to *BRCA1*- and *BRCA2*-related HBOC, including a 5% risk of ovarian cancer, a 0.9% risk of male breast cancer, and a 2% to 3% risk of pancreatic cancer (Yang et al., 2020). Based on this knowledge, it has been suggested that surveillance and mitigation strategies used in *BRCA1/BRCA2* HBOC could be reasonably utilized in *PALB2*-related breast cancer susceptibility and that treatment strategies might also be similar.
3. Li-Fraumeni syndrome (LFS) can present with a wide variety of malignancies, although a handful of cancer types predominate: soft tissue sarcoma, osteosarcoma, adrenocortical carcinoma, breast cancer, and central nervous system (CNS) cancer (Mai et al., 2012). Hematologic and gastrointestinal malignancies can also be seen (Bougeard et al., 2015). Penetrance is high, with greater than 70% of women and greater than 90% of men with a LFS pathogenic variant in *TP53* experiencing at least

one lifetime episode of malignancy (Mai et al., 2016). Surveillance for this condition is intense and commences early in life, with affected children requiring surveillance for CNS and adrenocortical malignancies. Adults with LFS require annual brain magnetic resonance imaging (MRI), whole-body MRI, and endoscopy every 2 to 5 years. Women with LFS require greater intensity of breast cancer surveillance starting at age 20 (Kratz et al., 2015).

4. *APC*-related familial adenomatous polyposis (FAP) is a condition in which innumerable adenomatous polyps develop in the colon. These polyps typically develop in childhood and adolescence, with a typical diagnosis of colon cancer in the fourth decade of life (Gupta et al., 2019). FAP is inherited in an autosomal dominant manner and is highly penetrant, with inevitable development of colon cancer if left untreated. Individuals with FAP are also at increased risk for cancer of the small bowel, pancreas, thyroid, liver, bile duct, and stomach (Giardiello et al., 1993; Kadmon et al., 2001). Prophylactic colectomy is the preferred surgical treatment due to the 100% risk of colon cancer. Periodic upper endoscopy and thyroid ultrasound are also part of surveillance in individuals with FAP.
5. Lynch syndrome is a relatively common condition that increases the risk for several cancers including colon, endometrial, gastric, and ovarian (Bonadona et al., 2011). Five genes are known to be associated with Lynch syndrome, of which four are included in the ACMG SF recommendations (*MLH1*, *MSH2*, *MSH6*, and *PMS2*). Penetrance is incomplete in Lynch syndrome, and the risks for malignancy are higher in individuals who have pathogenic variants in *MLH1* and *MSH2* compared to *MSH6* and *PMS2* (Giardiello et al., 2014). Surveillance for colon cancer in Lynch syndrome is recommended every 1 to 2 years starting between age 20 and 25 years. Screening for endometrial, ovarian, and gastric cancers has been met with more controversy (Provenzale et al., 2016).
6. *MUTYH*-related polyposis presents with significant polyposis, although the overall polyp burden is often less than what may be seen in *APC*-related polyposis. Individuals with *MUTYH*-related polyposis have an approximately 80% to 90% lifetime risk of colon cancer, with the average age of diagnosis being somewhat later than in APC-related polyposis (Lubbe et al., 2009). Extracolonic malignancies may occur in the duodenum, ovary, and bladder. *MUTYH*-related polyposis is inherited in an autosomal recessive manner, and although the risk is not entirely clear, it is believed that people who are heterozygous for a pathogenic variant in *MUTYH* may be at modestly increased risk for colon cancer (Win et al., 2014). Surveillance includes management of polyp burden and ultimately colectomy if this is no longer possible (Sampson & Jones, 2009). Endoscopic surveillance and removal of duodenal polyps is also recommended in individuals with *MUTYH*-related polyposis.
7. Juvenile polyposis syndrome (JPS) features hamartomatous polyps. The term "juvenile" in the description of this disorder is misleading, as it is the hamartomatous polyps themselves that are considered juvenile. The polyp burden varies greatly, with some individuals only experiencing a handful of polyps, while others may have dozens of polyps. The overall risk of malignancy in JPS may be lower than for other polyposis syndromes, with one recent case series reporting 14% of individuals with a history of cancer (Latchford et al., 2012), and colon cancer being the most common malignancy. Gastric cancer can also be seen in individuals with a history of gastric

polyps (Brosens et al., 2007). This condition is inherited in an autosomal dominant manner, and variants in two genes (*BMPR1A* and *SMAD4*) are known to be causative (Honda et al., 2013). Both are included in the ACMG SF recommendations. It should be noted that variants in *BMPR1A* cause only JPS, while most individuals with JPS due to variants in *SMAD4* also have features of hereditary hemorrhagic telangiectasia.

8. Peutz-Jeghers syndrome (PJS) predisposes individuals to hamartomatous polyps similar to JPS but has a difference in polyp pathology. Individuals with PJS also have pigmented macules on mucocutaneous regions like the lips and buccal mucosa (Kidambi et al., 2019). Individuals with PJS have an approximately 40% lifetime risk of colorectal cancer and increased risk for gastric cancer, small bowel cancer, breast cancer, ovarian cancer, and testicular cancer (Syngal et al., 2015). PJS is inherited in an autosomal dominant manner, and variants in *STK11* are the only known cause. Polyps in PJS can develop early in life, which is reflected by guidelines that suggest upper endoscopy and colonoscopy beginning at 8 years of age, breast cancer screening starting at age 25, and testicular cancer screening starting at birth.
9. Multiple endocrine neoplasias (MENs) and familial medullary thyroid carcinoma (FMTC) are divided into MEN1 and MEN2, with MEN2 being further divided into MEN2A and MEN2B. MEN1 has the classic triad of parathyroid tumors, pituitary tumors, and pancreatic endocrine tumors. Carcinoid tumors and adrenocortical tumors can also be seen. In contrast to most of the other cancer predisposition conditions in this section, tumors in MEN1 do not tend to be malignant, but they are often hormone secreting and can still cause local mass effect. MEN1 is inherited in an autosomal dominant manner, and variants in *MEN1* are the only known cause of MEN1. Functional parathyroid tumors are essentially inevitable in individuals with MEN1 by age 50. Approximately 30% to 40% of individuals with MEN1 will develop pituitary tumors, with prolactinoma being the most common type. Pancreatic endocrine tumors are present in 70% to 95% of individuals with MEN1, and the majority either are non–hormone secreting or are gastrin secreting (Thakker et al., 2012). Surveillance for MEN1 commences at age 5 and increases in intensity through childhood and early adulthood. The treatment of MEN1 relies on a combination of surgical removal of tumors and medical management of the effects of excess hormone production (Brandi et al., 2001). MEN2A is characterized by the triad of medullary thyroid carcinoma (MTC), pheochromocytoma, and parathyroid tumor. Nearly all individuals with MEN2A will develop MTC, about half will develop pheochromocytoma, and 20% to 30% will develop parathyroid tumors (Neumann et al., 2019). Since FMTC is defined by the presence of MTC in four or more family members without history of pheochromocytoma or parathyroid pathology, it should be seen as a subtype of MEN2A (Kloos et al., 2009). Individuals with MEN2B have a virtually 100% risk of developing MTC, and in some cases the risk is manifest at a very young age. These individuals also will have a distinctive appearance, with mucosal neuromas and an asthenic build. The risk of parathyroid disease is low in MEN2B, while the risk of pheochromocytoma is similar to that of MEN2A (Castinetti et al., 2019). MEN2A, MEN2B, and FMTC are all inherited in an autosomal dominant manner, and variants in *RET* are the only known cause of these conditions. Surveillance in MEN2 is largely based on the behavior of the individual variant, with the highest

risk variants requiring thyroidectomy in the first year of life and screening for pheochromocytoma starting at age 8 years, and the lowest risk variants allowing for thyroidectomy after age 5 years with screening for pheochromocytoma and parathyroid disease starting at age 20 years.

10. Hereditary paraganglioma (PGL) and pheochromocytoma (PCC) are characterized by the presence of PGLs and/or PCCs (PGLs confined to the adrenal gland). These tumors often secrete catecholamines, and catecholamine excess may cause PGLs/PCCs to become symptomatic. PGLs located in the head and neck are less likely to secrete catecholamines, but due to their proximity to key neurovascular structures, they may become symptomatic due to mass effect alone. In rare cases, head and neck PGLs may metastasize (Lenders et al., 2014). There are currently seven genes that are known to be associated with hereditary PGL and PCC, of which four (*SDHAF2*, *SDHB*, *SDHD*, and *SDHC*) were included in the original ACMG SF v1.0, and an additional two (*MAX* and *TMEM127*) were added in ACMG SF v3.0. Hereditary PGL and PCC caused by *SDHB*, *SHDC*, and *TMEM127* are inherited in an autosomal dominant manner. Hereditary PGL and PCC caused by *SDHAF2* and *SDHD* are autosomal dominant with paternal imprinting. Male individuals who have inherited such a variant from their biological mothers will themselves not be at risk, but should they pass a pathogenic variant in *SHDAF2* or *SDHD* to one of their children, those children would be at risk for development of PGL and PCC. The mode of inheritance of *MAX*-related PCC is not completely understood and may be autosomal dominant or may show paternal imprinting as well. Penetrance is incomplete, likely between 25% and 50%, and the risk for those with heterozygous pathogenic variants in *MAX* and *TMEM127* appears to be mostly PCC, with lower risk of extra-adrenal involvement (Andrews et al., 2018; Bausch et al., 2017). Surveillance typically commences in childhood and utilizes a combination of biochemical and imaging modalities. Treatment of PGL and PCC requires both medical and surgical interventions (Muth et al., 2019).
11. Von Hippel-Lindau syndrome (VHL) is associated with an increased risk for a number of tumors including hemangioblastomas (of the brain, retina, and spinal cord), renal cell carcinoma, PCCs, and pancreatic neuroendocrine tumors (Binderup et al., 2016). Penetrance is virtually complete, although both the age and location of the first tumor diagnosis vary greatly. VHL is inherited in an autosomal dominant manner, and approximately 80% of individuals with VHL have an affected parent (van Leeuwaarde et al., 2018). Surveillance of VHL starts in childhood and utilizes both biochemical and imaging modalities. Treatment of VHL-related tumors is primarily surgical, and much progress has been made in recent years in reducing damage to adjacent normal tissue when resecting tumors.
12. Tuberous sclerosis complex (TSC) is classically characterized by the presence of central nervous system findings such as cortical tubers, cortical dysplasia, and subependymal giant cell astrocytomas (SEGAs) and specific skin findings such as facial angiofibromas, hypopigmented macules, and connective tissue nevi. Individuals with TSC also may have cardiac rhabdomyomas, renal angiomyolipomas, and lymphangioleiomyomatosis (Northrup & Krueger, 2013). TSC is inherited in an autosomal dominant manner and should be considered to be fully penetrant, but involvement may not be obvious. It is not an uncommon occurrence for an asymptomatic

parent of a symptomatic patient to have radiological evidence of TSC, and this significant variability in presentation should be a part of counseling for this condition. Individuals with TSC require lifelong surveillance, which includes monitoring for neoplastic processes but also assessing for neurodevelopmental complications and seizure disorders (Krueger & Northrup, 2013).

13. *RB1*-related retinoblastoma is commonly diagnosed when leukocoria (a white pupil) is noticed in a child. Retinoblastoma is an ocular malignancy that typically occurs in infants and young children. About 60% of affected individuals have unilateral retinoblastoma, and about 40% have bilateral retinoblastoma. The pineal gland may also be involved, and if a pineoblastoma is seen along with bilateral retinoblastoma, it is known as trilateral disease. *RB1*-related retinoblastoma is inherited in an autosomal dominant manner. The penetrance of retinoblastoma in individuals with pathogenic *RB1* variants is generally complete, although in a small number of families, lower penetrance variants have been identified (Dommering et al., 2014). Individuals with pathogenic variants in *RB1* are also at risk for osteosarcomas, soft tissue sarcomas, and melanomas (Kleinerman et al., 2012). Surveillance includes an aggressive schedule of eye examinations in the first few months of life, continuing on a less intensive basis thereafter. Treatment of retinoblastoma has traditionally involved enucleation of the affected eye(s), but newer options are available that can preserve sight in some cases.
14. Neurofibromatosis type 2 (NF2) may be considered something of a misnomer, as it differs greatly from neurofibromatosis type 1. Individuals with NF2 classically present with bilateral vestibular schwannomas and may present with symptoms of hearing loss, tinnitus, or vertigo. Individuals may also present with meningioma, cataract, or neuropathy. NF2 is inherited in an autosomal dominant manner and is caused exclusively by variants in the *NF2* gene (D. G. Evans et al., 1992). Penetrance is complete, and although NF2 has been traditionally considered to be an adult-onset condition, childhood onset of disease is increasingly recognized, particularly with neuropathies such as facial palsy (Ruggieri et al., 2018). Surveillance for CNS lesions using MRI is recommended starting around age 10 years. Hearing assessment and eye examination are also considered to be part of surveillance for NF2, although they are also part of normal preventive healthcare. Treatment of schwannomas is primarily surgical in nature, although recent progress has been made in medical therapies for *NF2*-related schwannomas (Halliday et al., 2018).
15. *WT1*-related disorder includes variable findings of childhood-onset Wilms tumor, progressive glomerulopathy, and disorder of sex development. Individuals may also have other anomalies of the kidney and urinary tract structure. *WT1*-related disorder is inherited in an autosomal dominant manner, and penetrance is as high as 90% but is not complete (Lehnhardt et al., 2015). Comprehensive surveillance and management are critical for individuals with *WT1*-related disorder, and surveillance for Wilms tumor requires imaging every 3 months until age 7 years (Gariépy-Assal et al., 2018).
16. *PTEN* hamartoma tumor syndrome includes several overlapping phenotypes. In the context of secondary findings, we are mostly concerned with the Cowden syndrome (CS) phenotype. Individuals with CS have a high risk of breast, nonmedullary thyroid, renal, and endometrial cancer. Individuals with CS often have additional

mucocutaneous lesions, colorectal cancer, and macrocephaly. *PTEN*-related disorders are inherited in an autosomal dominant manner, and penetrance is not complete, although it is believed that more than 90% of individuals will have some manifestations of disease by adulthood (Eng, 2000). The lifetime risk of breast cancer is approximately 85%, the risk of thyroid cancer is 35%, the risk of renal cancer is 35%, and the risk of endometrial cancer is 28%. The risk of colorectal cancer is lower at 9% (Tan et al., 2012). All individuals with a pathogenic *PTEN* variant should have annual thyroid imaging and skin examination. As individuals age, additional evaluations are recommended, including breast cancer and endometrial cancer screening in biological females at age 30, colonoscopy at age 35, and renal imaging at age 40.

Genes Related to Cardiovascular Phenotypes

1. Hereditable thoracic aortic disease refers to the condition unified by a high risk of thoracic aortic aneurysm and dissection (TAAD), but it does not meet clinical criteria for a known syndrome such as Marfan syndrome or Loeys-Dietz syndrome. Thus far, 16 genes have been associated with TAAD, but only *ACTA2* and *MYH11* are included in the SF v3.1 guidelines. Of note, *MYLK* was included in the SF v1.0 guidelines but was subsequently removed. TAAD due to *ACTA2* and *MYH11* is inherited in an autosomal dominant manner with incomplete penetrance and variable expressivity. The estimated cumulative risk of aortic dissection or repair of aneurysm for individuals with a pathogenic *ACTA2* variant is 76% by age 85 (Regalado et al., 2014). Similar estimates are not available for individuals with a pathogenic *MYH11* variant, although the age of onset of disease is thought to be somewhat later (mid 40s versus early 30s) for *MYH11* disease (Pannu et al., 2007). Serial (usually annual) imaging is the mainstay of surveillance for individuals with TAAD. More intensive monitoring is typically recommended if the rate of aortic diameter increase exceeds 0.5 cm per year or when the aortic root diameter is greater than 4.0 cm. The aortic diameter at which prophylactic repair is indicated depends partly on the affected gene. In the case of *ACTA2*-related TAAD, repair at a maximum of 4.5 cm is recommended (Regalado et al., 2015).
2. Arrhythmogenic right ventricular cardiomyopathy (ARVC) is a condition that results from the myocardial tissue of the right ventricle being replaced with fibrofatty tissue. This phenomenon results in predisposition to ventricular tachycardia and can result in sudden cardiac death. Thirteen genes are known to be responsible for ARVC, with five genes being included in the ACMG SF v3.0 (*TMEM43*, *DSP*, *PKP2*, *DSG2*, and *DSC2*). The diagnostic criteria for ARVC utilizes imaging findings, electrocardiogram (ECG) findings, and family history to categorize individuals with definite, borderline, and possible diagnosis (Marcus et al., 2010). Inheritance pattern is most frequently autosomal dominant, although autosomal recessive inheritance has been seen with *DSC2*-related disease (Heuser et al., 2006). Penetrance for AVRC is likely to be relatively low, although knowledge is somewhat limited. In one series,

324 out of 385 (68%) family members of an affected patient who themselves had a pathogenic variant were asymptomatic, and most of those individuals did not meet criteria for diagnosis of ARVC (Groeneweg et al., 2015). Individuals with a pathogenic variant predisposing to ARVC who are asymptomatic should have annual surveillance to assess for onset of cardiac involvement starting at 10 years of age (Charron et al., 2010).

3. Familial dilated cardiomyopathy (DCM) is characterized by enlargement of the left ventricle resulting in systolic dysfunction such that the ejection fraction is less than 50%. There are currently approximately 30 genes that have been implicated in this condition (Hershberger et al., 2013), and there is significant allelic heterogeneity with DCM and other forms of cardiomyopathy. The eight genes that are associated with DCM and included in the ACMG SF v3.1 (*TNNT2*, *LMNA*, *FLNC*, *TTN*, *BAG3*, *DES*, *RBM20*, and *TNNC1*) are inherited in an autosomal dominant manner (Morales & Hershberger, 2015). However, DCM is genetically heterogeneous, and these eight genes together only account for between 29% and 32% of the DCM disease burden (Hershberger & Jordan, 2007). Penetrance in DCM as a class varies; in one study of individuals with *LMNA*-related DCM it was estimated to be 85% (Hasselberg et al., 2018), and in another study in individuals with *TNNT2*-related disease penetrance was complete in a small cohort (Mogensen et al., 2004). Individuals with a pathogenic variant in a known DCM gene found as a secondary finding should have cardiac phenotyping performed. If abnormal, the patient should be managed per existing DCM guidelines. If normal, periodic cardiac evaluations are appropriate (Hershberger et al., 2018).
4. Brugada syndrome presents with high risk for ventricular arrhythmias and features specific ECG findings (ST-segment elevations in leads V1 to V3 on ECG). Individuals with Brugada syndrome may have a history of ventricular fibrillation, ventricular tachycardia, and unexplained syncope and may have a family history of the same including sudden cardiac death. Brugada syndrome is inherited in an autosomal dominant manner. Penetrance is incomplete, with approximately 20% to 30% of individuals with Brugada syndrome having characteristic ECG changes at rest but a much higher percentage having characteristic ECG changes with provocative testing (Benito et al., 2009). *SCN5A* is the most common single cause of Brugada syndrome and is the only one of the 23 genes known to cause Brugada syndrome that is included in the ACMG SF v3.0. Management of Brugada syndrome includes identification of individuals who are at risk for complications, avoidance of stimuli that can predispose to characteristic ECG changes, and potentially use of implantable cardiac defibrillators (ICDs; Antzelevitch et al., 2002).
5. Long QT syndrome (LQTS), as the name implies, is a cardiac arrhythmia syndrome characterized by prolongation of the QT interval on ECG. This can predispose affected individuals to ventricular arrhythmias, particularly polymorphic ventricular tachycardia, known colloquially as torsades de pointes given its striking appearance on ECG (Sharma et al., 2020). Individuals with LQTS most commonly will present with syncope, which may be associated with exercise or stress in some cases. Sudden cardiac death may also occur in LQTS and may provide a helpful clue when collecting a family history. LQTS is inherited in an autosomal dominant manner and is incompletely penetrant—approximately 25% of people who have a pathogenic variant in one of the several LQTS genes do not have prolongation of their QT

interval (Goldenberg et al., 2011). The vast majority of LQTS is caused by variants in the *KCNH2*, *KCNQ1*, and *SCN5A* genes, which are included in the ACMG SF recommendations. Management of LQTS includes treatment with beta blockade medications and in some cases ICDs. In the ACMG SF v3.2 three genes associated with LQTS were added, *CALM1*, *CALM2*, and *CALM3*, given their classification of having definitive evidence for being disease-causing genes, with similar prevalence and penetrance to other LQTS genes (Adler et al., 2020; Miller et al., 2023).

6. Hypertrophic cardiomyopathy (HCM) is one of the most common genetic heart diseases and is diagnosed when unexplained left ventricular hypertrophy is identified. As the disease progresses, individuals with HCM may develop arrhythmias, left ventricular outflow obstruction, and in some instances sudden cardiac death (Elliott et al., 2014). HCM is most commonly inherited in an autosomal dominant manner (with autosomal recessive inheritance in some cases, and an even smaller subset with observed digenic dominant inheritance), and although a large number of genes have been implicated in its etiology, a smaller number are included in the ACMG SF recommendations (*MYBPC3*, *MYH7*, *TPM1*, *TNNI3*, *TNNT2*, *ACTC1*, *MYL2*, *PRKAG2*, and *MYL3*), which together account for greater than 90% of HCM. Penetrance in HCM varies by the affected gene and the specific nature of the identified variant but is generally incomplete and increases with age (Sabater-Molina et al., 2017). Individuals known to have a pathogenic variant in a gene associated with HCM should have periodic echocardiography and ECG.
7. Vascular Ehlers-Danlos syndrome (vEDS) is a connective tissue disorder most notably characterized by significant vascular fragility, which can result in arterial rupture or dissection, most commonly occurring in large or medium-sized arteries in the thorax, abdomen, head, and neck. Uterine or intestinal rupture can also be seen in vEDS (Malfait et al., 2017). vEDS is inherited in an autosomal dominant manner, and penetrance should be considered to be complete, although there is considerable phenotypic variability. Pathogenic variants in *COL3A1* are the only known cause of vEDS. Surveillance in vEDS has been controversial in the past, given that traditional forms of angiography confer significant risk. Modern imaging techniques such as computed tomography or magnetic resonance angiography are significantly safer and are commonly used to assess for occult dissection or aneurysms (Chu et al., 2014). Surgical intervention for arterial dissection or organ rupture can be lifesaving, but the decision on how to proceed for elective procedures is much more difficult, with need for frank discussion of risks versus benefits.
8. Marfan syndrome is often used as a prototype for genetic connective tissue disorders. Individuals with Marfan syndrome present variably with cardiovascular findings including aortic dilation and mitral valve prolapse, ocular findings such as myopia or ectopia lentis, and skeletal findings such as dolichostenomelia (long and slender limbs as compared to the trunk), scoliosis, and pectus excavatum/carinatum (Loeys et al., 2010). Individuals with Marfan syndrome are at risk for aortic aneurysm and dissection, which can be associated with considerable mortality. Marfan syndrome is caused by pathogenic variants in the *FBN1* gene and is inherited in an autosomal dominant manner. Although considerable phenotypic variability is present, Marfan syndrome should be considered to be completely penetrant. Surveillance for progression of aortic pathology has been shown to be highly effective, as it is understood that the risk of dissection increases with aortic root size and acceleration of dilation.

Once thresholds (typically 5.0 cm or 0.5 cm/year) for intervention have been met, individuals are referred for aortic root surgery as the morbidity and mortality are considerably lower when performed nonemergently (Dietz, 2001).

9. Loeys-Dietz syndrome (LDS) is a relatively recently described connective tissue disorder that is associated with arterial aneurysms, dissections, and tortuosity. Individuals with LDS may have skeletal findings such as asthenic habitus, scoliosis, and pectus abnormalities, which significantly overlap those of Marfan syndrome, and indeed prior to the initial description of LDS in 2005, individuals were likely misdiagnosed as having Marfan syndrome (Loeys et al., 2005). Dissection of the aorta and other major arteries are the main cause of mortality in individuals with LDS. LDS is inherited in an autosomal dominant manner, and penetrance, if not complete, is quite high. Currently, five genes are known to be associated with LDS, and three of those genes (*TGFBR1*, *TGFBR2*, and *SMAD3*) are included in the ACMG SF recommendations. Considerable phenotypic variability is noted in individuals with LDS. Surveillance for LDS involves periodic vascular imaging and evaluation of skeletal manifestations such as scoliosis. Management of vascular manifestations of LDS overlaps that of Marfan syndrome, but given the overall more severe clinical course of LDS, a lower aortic diameter threshold is used when making the decision for surgical repair (MacCarrick et al., 2014).
10. Familial hypercholesterolemia (FH) is a relatively common genetic condition that results in severe elevation of low-density lipoprotein (LDL) cholesterol and development of premature atherosclerotic disease, which may manifest as coronary artery disease/myocardial infarction or cerebrovascular disease (Nordestgaard et al., 2013). Individuals with FH may also exhibit xanthomas, which are yellow-colored lesions that can develop on the tendons. FH can be inherited in both an autosomal dominant and autosomal recessive manner, and pathogenic variants in *LDLR* and *APOE* are responsible for between 60% and 85% of FH. Pathogenic variants in *PCSK9* account for less than 1% of FH. Those individuals with autosomal dominant disease typically develop atherosclerotic disease in middle age, whereas those with autosomal recessive disease develop atherosclerotic disease by early adulthood (Harada-Shiba et al., 2012). Individuals with FH may require multiple medical therapies to achieve a normal LDL cholesterol level, and these may include HMG-CoA reductase inhibitors and PCSK9 inhibitors (Ison et al., 1993). Some individuals, especially those with homozygous FH, may still require more invasive therapies such as LDL apheresis.
11. Catecholaminergic polymorphic ventricular tachycardia (CPVT) is a unique arrhythmia syndrome that occurs at times of increased catecholamine production such as strong emotional response or exercise. Most commonly, these events of ventricular tachycardia will result in syncope and can self-terminate. Family history of sudden cardiac death or syncope may be helpful in the diagnosis (Priori et al., 2013). CPVT can be inherited in an autosomal dominant or autosomal recessive manner. *RYR2* was included in the ACMG SF v1.0 and is inherited in an autosomal dominant manner. *TRDN* was added in the ACMG SF v3.0, is inherited in an autosomal recessive manner, and can also feature a skeletal myopathic phenotype. *CASQ2* is also included in the ACMG SF recommendations and is generally considered to show autosomal recessive inheritance; however, some patients who are heterozygous

for *CASQ2* variants have shown a CPVT phenotype (Wilde et al., 2022). Whether this represents an occult second pathogenic variant or true potential for autosomal dominance inheritance is unknown. Penetrance has been estimated at 83% in *RYR2*-related CPVT (Napolitano et al., 2022). It is believed that patients with biallelic *CASQ2* pathogenic variants have complete or near-complete penetrance. The penetrance of *TRDN*-related CPVT is as yet unknown. About 30% of individuals with CPVT will experience at least one episode of cardiac arrest. Management is primarily pharmacologic, and follow-up is important to ensure adequate treatment.

Genes Related to Inborn Errors of Metabolism Phenotypes

1. Biotinidase deficiency is an inborn error of metabolism with neurocutaneous manifestations. Untreated patients may present with seizures, hypotonia, developmental delay, optic atrophy, hearing loss, alopecia, and an eczema-like skin rash. There is a broad spectrum of disease, and there is noted to be a partial biotinidase deficiency phenotype that can present later in childhood or in rare cases in adulthood (Canda et al., 2020). It is inherited in an autosomal recessive manner and is caused by biallelic variants in the *BTD* gene. There are five variants that account for the majority of symptomatic disease. The prevalence of biotinidase deficiency is believed to be approximately 1:60,000, and this accounts for both partial and profound disease (Küry et al., 2016). The treatment of biotinidase deficiency is lifelong supplementation with biotin and is associated with significant improvement in patients with symptomatic disease (Wolf, 2012). Prior to inclusion of this disorder on state newborn screening panels, patients were generally detected after they became symptomatic, and incomplete resolution of presenting signs and symptoms was common (Wolf, 2015). Now that individuals are detected on newborn screening while asymptomatic, biotin supplementation can be commenced, and as long as they are compliant with therapy, it is expected that individuals with biotinidase deficiency will remain asymptomatic for their entire lives (Wolf, 2000).
2. Fabry disease is a multisystemic lysosomal storage disease that in its classic form can present with episodes of severe pain in the extremities (acroparesthesias), angiokeratomas, abnormal sweating, and corneal opacities. As the disease progresses, individuals can experience end-stage renal disease, left ventricular hypertrophy, and strokes. Cardiac and renal variant Fabry disease are well described. Fabry disease is inherited in an X-linked manner, and pathogenic variants in *GLA* are the only known cause of Fabry disease. Fabry disease in males who are hemizygous for a pathogenic variant is completely penetrant. Heterozygous females can show a range of presentations, from asymptomatic to as severe as affected males, but on balance females show less severe disease than males (Deegan et al., 2006). Surveillance includes annual evaluation of cardiac and renal function and periodic brain imaging. Treatment includes use of enzyme replacement therapy, medical treatment of acroparesthesias, and preservation of renal function (Felis et al., 2019).

3. Ornithine transcarbamylase (OTC) deficiency is an inborn error of metabolism and the most common of the urea cycle disorders. Urea cycle disorders are defined by impairment in the metabolism of ammonia into urea. Individuals with OTC deficiency can have varying levels of hyperammonia, which can present with vomiting, mental status changes, headaches, and seizures and in extreme cases may mimic a diagnosis of cerebral palsy (Tuchman et al., 2008). OTC deficiency is an X-linked disorder, and variants in *OTC* are the only known cause of this condition. Penetrance for OTC deficiency is complete in males, who are hemizygous for *OTC* pathogenic variants. Penetrance is incomplete for heterozygous females but is likely higher than previously thought as clinical variability is significant, with some individuals having neonatal presentation of symptoms and some individuals having mild symptoms that may result in self-restriction of protein (McCullough et al., 2000). Individuals with OTC deficiency require lifelong management with dietary protein restriction and in many cases nitrogen scavengers. In both cases, management seeks to maintain normal plasma ammonia levels.
4. Pompe disease is an inborn error of metabolism affecting glycogen metabolism primarily within cardiac and skeletal muscle. The two classic presentations of Pompe disease are infantile onset and late onset. Patients with infantile-onset Pompe disease will typically present with muscle weakness, motor delay, cardiomyopathy, and respiratory insufficiency. Patients with late-onset disease will tend to present with muscle weakness, respiratory insufficiency, and sleep disturbances. Late-onset Pompe disease is somewhat of a misnomer, as patients may also present from as early as later infancy to as late as middle age (Marques et al., 2022). Pompe disease is inherited in an autosomal recessive manner and is caused by biallelic variants in the *GAA* gene, which encodes for the acid alpha-glucosidase enzyme. The incidence of Pompe disease is believed to be around 1:40,000. Pompe disease is included on newborn screening in some but not all states in the United States (Leslie & Bailey, 2007). Treatment of Pompe disease is partly supportive and partly proactive. Those with cardiomyopathy require management by a cardiologist familiar with the unique needs of individuals with this condition. Also, physical therapy is often required to maintain function and to avoid complications such as contractures (Davison, 2020). Patients with Pompe disease also benefit from enzyme replacement therapy, which has been shown to alter the natural history of patients with both infantile- and late-onset disease, although the extent of that is less well understood in patients with late-onset disease (Sarah et al., 2022).

Genes Related to Miscellaneous Phenotypes

1. Hereditary hemochromatosis is a relatively common genetic condition that causes excessive iron absorption from the intestine that can result in iron overload and end-organ damage. Excess iron is stored in predictable places, including the liver, joints, pancreas, and heart. Patients with this condition may eventually present with weakness, lethargy, arthritis, type 2 diabetes, and heart failure. Hemochromatosis is inherited in an autosomal recessive manner and is caused by specific biallelic variants

in the *HFE* gene. Heterozygosity for either the p.His64Asp or the p.Cys282Tyr variants is common and is not associated with increased risk of iron overload (Barton & Edwards, 2000). Either homozygosity for the p.His64Asp allele or compound heterozygosity for the p.His64Asp and p.Cys282Tyr alleles is associated with a low risk of iron overload. Therefore, the decision for inclusion in SF v3.0 recommends only reporting out the p.Cys282Tyr variant, as while it is still incompletely penetrant, that penetrance is estimated to be as high as 35% (Grosse et al., 2018). Treatment for hereditary hemochromatosis includes monitoring for biochemical and clinical signs of iron overload and periodic phlebotomy to reduce iron overload and the risk of end-organ damage. This strategy has proved to be highly effective (Rombout-Sestrienkova et al., 2016).

2 Hereditary hemorrhagic telangiectasia (HTT) is a condition characterized by arteriovenous malformations (AVMs) in internal organs and cutaneously. Classically, patients with HTT present with recurrent epistaxis in childhood. Cutaneous AVMs can be seen on the lips and inside of the mouth. AVMs are also commonly found in the liver, lungs, gastrointestinal (GI) tract, and brain (McDonald & Stevenson, 2000). Patients can experience significant GI bleeding, heart failure, stroke, or cerebral abscess as complications of this condition. The vast majority of HHT is caused by pathogenic variants in one of two genes: *ACVRL1* and *ENG*, which are responsible for 52% and 44% of cases, respectively; are both inherited in an autosomal dominant manner; and were first included as secondary findings in SF v3.0. A third gene, *SMAD4*, is responsible for approximately 1% of HHT cases and also is associated with juvenile polyposis (McDonald et al., 2020). *SMAD4* is not included in the current guidelines. The incidence of HHT is believed to be between 1:5,000 and 1:10,000. The management of HHT includes control of epistaxis, management of GI bleeding, screening for AVMs with appropriate medical or surgical management (Faughnan et al., 2020), and medical management of bleeding with antiangiogenic and antifibrinolytic agents (Hammill et al., 2021).

3. Malignant hyperthermia susceptibility (MHS) is a condition that can present when certain anesthetic medications such as halogenated ethers and succinylcholine are used. Affected individuals will experience increased metabolic activity in the skeletal muscle, which results in lactic acidosis and excess heat production and can be life-threatening (Rosenberg et al., 2015). MHS is inherited in an autosomal dominant manner, and pathogenic variants in *RYR1* and *CACNA1S* are thought to be responsible for 50% to 60% of the total disease burden. Penetrance for *RYR1*-related MHS has been estimated at 40% (Ibarra Moreno et al., 2019). Individuals who are known to have MHS should avoid halogenated ethers and succinylcholine and are also advised to avoid extremes of heat.

4. Maturity-onset diabetes of the young (MODY) is a group of conditions that cause diabetes mellitus in patients typically in adolescence or early adulthood. It behaves more like type 2 diabetes given that patients with MODY generally continue to produce some insulin and do not as a rule go into diabetic ketoacidosis. However, patients also generally do not have risk factors for type 2 diabetes such as advanced age and obesity (Naylor et al., 2018). The incidence of MODY as a group is likely at least 1:1,000, with one estimate suggesting that 2.5% of all diabetes could be attributed to MODY (Shepherd et al., 2016). In practice, these conditions are almost certainly

underdiagnosed and are treated as typical type 1 or type 2 diabetes. Although some 14 genes have been implicated in MODY, only *HNF1A*-related MODY (MODY3) is included in the SF recommendations. There are two reasons for this. First, *GCK*-related MODY (MODY2) and *HNF1A*-related MODY are responsible for approximately 70% of the disease burden. Second, unlike *GCK*-related MODY, which does not typically require treatment, *HNF1A*-related MODY does require treatment and is known to be exquisitely sensitive to sulfonylurea medications, which are both inexpensive and widely available (Tosur & Philipson, 2022).

5. *RPE65*-related retinopathy refers to a type of autosomal recessive early-onset severe retinal dystrophy that generally presents within the first 5 years of life and results in progressive visual loss such that most individuals are legally blind by young adulthood. Individuals with this condition may also develop cataracts and keratoconus. Most also have significant myopia (Chao et al., 2019). While the genetics of retinal dystrophies are extraordinarily complex, only RPE-related disease is included in SF v3.1. The reason for this is that unlike other forms of retinal dystrophy, a specific treatment exists for this form. Voretigene neparvovec-rzyl was approved by the Food and Drug Administration in the United States in 2017 and is indicated for patients with confirmed biallelic *RPE65*-associated retinal dystrophy (Maguire et al., 2021). It should be noted that the inclusion of this condition in the SF v3.0 represented a response to a specific therapy that made diagnosis of this condition actionable.
6. Wilson disease is a disorder of copper metabolism resulting from pathogenic variants in the *ATP7B* gene. Individuals may present with signs and symptoms of Wilson disease at any point between early childhood and middle age. There are three main categories of findings: hepatic, neurologic, and psychiatric. Hepatic findings can include hepatitis and acute or chronic liver failure. Neurologic findings can include movement disorders and dystonic findings. Psychiatric findings can include depression and personality changes (Roberts & Schilsky, 2008). Wilson disease is inherited in an autosomal recessive manner, and penetrance is incomplete (Roberts, 2018). Surveillance involves evaluation of liver function and assessment for CNS structural alterations. Treatment involves copper chelating agents, dietary copper restriction, zinc therapy, and in rare cases liver transplant (Saroli Palumbo & Schilsky, 2019).
7. Hereditary *TTR*-related amyloidosis is a condition caused by buildup of amyloid protein deposits in end organs with clinical manifestations including cardiomyopathy, sensorimotor neuropathy, and nephropathy (Gościniak et al., 2022). Hereditary *TTR*-related amyloidosis is caused by pathogenic variants in the *TTR* gene and is inherited in an autosomal dominant manner, and like many autosomal dominant conditions, penetrance is incomplete and there is considerable phenotypic variability (Saito et al., 2021). However, it is known that *TTR*-related amyloidosis can occur in people without a pathogenic variant in the *TTR* gene, but such patients tend to have more limited end-organ involvement and present at an earlier age. Although hereditary *TTR*-related amyloidosis is relatively rare in the general population with a prevalence estimated to be approximately 1:100,000, there are certain populations within Portugal, Sweden, and Japan and in Black Americans where the prevalence is strikingly higher (Caponetti et al., 2021). The inclusion of this condition occurred in SF v3.1 in response to several targeted therapies that aim to either stabilize the TTR tetramer or silence the *TTR* gene (Tschöpe & Elsanhoury, 2022).

Conclusion

The ACMG SF v3.2 represents meaningful progress over previous guidelines both in the addition of several meaningful genes and in some evolution in the reporting philosophy of secondary findings. However, it is equally clear that these are imperfect guidelines that are products of their time. Genetics professionals have become more comfortable with the idea of counseling individuals and their family members about the risk of secondary findings, but recent initiatives to create molecular diagnostic panels for population screening that deliberately include the 81 genes contained within ACMG v3.2 challenge the paradigm as purely secondary findings. The ACMG has reiterated that the policy was not intended for population screening (ACMG Board of Directors, 2019), but this has been challenged by other members of the community who point out that the intent of individuals who choose to pursue proactive analysis of these genes is likely similar to individuals who choose to have the results of analysis of those same genes disclosed on ES or GS (Nussbaum et al., 2019). As ES and GS continue to move into mainstream medicine, evolution of these guidelines will be crucial to maximizing their utility and clarity.

References

ACMG Board of Directors. (2015). ACMG policy statement: Updated recommendations regarding analysis and reporting of secondary findings in clinical genome-scale sequencing. *Genetics in Medicine*, *17*(1), 68–69. https://doi.org/10.1038/gim.2014.151

ACMG Board of Directors. (2019). The use of ACMG secondary findings recommendations for general population screening: A policy statement of the American College of Medical Genetics and Genomics (ACMG). *Genetics in Medicine*, *21*(7), 1467–1468. https://doi.org/10.1038/s41436-019-0502-5

Adler, A., Novelli, V., Amin, A. S., Abiusi, E., Care, M., Nannenberg, E. A., Feilotter, H., Amenta, S., Mazza, D., Bikker, H., Sturm, A. C., Garcia, J., Ackerman, M. J., Hershberger, R. E., Perez, M. V., Zareba, W., Ware, J. S., Wilde, A. A. M., & Gollob, M. H. (2020). An international, multicentered, evidence-based reappraisal of genes reported to cause congenital long QT syndrome. *Circulation*, *141*(6), 418–428. https://doi.org/10.1161/CIRCULATIONAHA.119.043132

Andrews, K. A., Ascher, D. B., Pires, D. E. V., Barnes, D. R., Vialard, L., Casey, R. T., Bradshaw, N., Adlard, J., Aylwin, S., Brennan, P., Brewer, C., Cole, T., Cook, J. A., Davidson, R., Donaldson, A., Fryer, A., Greenhalgh, L., Hodgson, S. V., Irving, R., & Lalloo, F. (2018). Tumour risks and genotype-phenotype correlations associated with germline variants in succinate dehydrogenase subunit genes SDHB, SDHC and SDHD. *Journal of Medical Genetics*, *55*(6), 384–394. https://doi.org/10.1136/jmedgenet-2017-105127

Antzelevitch, C., Brugada, P., Brugada, J., Brugada, R., Shimizu, W., Gussak, I., & Perez Riera, A. R. (2002). Brugada syndrome: A decade of progress. *Circulation Research*, *91*(12), 1114–1118. https://doi.org/10.1161/01.res.0000046046.53721.90

Barton, J. C., & Edwards, C. Q. (2000). *HFE-related* hemochromatosis. In M. P. Adam, J. Feldman, G. M. Mirzaa, R. A. Pagon, S. E. Wallace, & A. Amemiya (Eds.), *GeneReviews®*. University of Washington, Seattle.

Bausch, B., Schiavi, F., Ni, Y., Welander, J., Patocs, A., Ngeow, J., Wellner, U., Malinoc, A., Taschin, E., Barbon, G., Lanza, V., Söderkvist, P., Stenman, A., Larsson, C., Svahn, F., Chen, J. L., Marquard, J., Fraenkel, M., Walter, M. A., Peczkowska, M., . . . European-American-Asian Pheochromocytoma-Paraganglioma Registry Study Group. (2017). Clinical characterization of the pheochromocytoma and paraganglioma susceptibility genes SDHA, TMEM127, MAX, and SDHAF2 for gene-informed prevention. *JAMA Oncology*, *3*(9), 1204–1212. https://doi.org/10.1001/jamaoncol.2017.0223

Benito, B., Brugada, J., Brugada, R., & Brugada, P. (2009). Brugada syndrome. *Revista espanola de cardiologia*, *62*(11), 1297–1315. https://doi.org/10.1016/s1885-5857(09)73357-2

Biesecker, L. G. (2017). ACMG secondary findings 2.0. *Genetics in Medicine*, *19*(5), 604. https://doi.org/10.1038/gim.2017.27

Binderup, M. L., Budtz-Jørgensen, E., & Bisgaard, M. L. (2016). Risk of new tumors in von Hippel-Lindau patients depends on age and genotype. *Genetics in Medicine*, *18*(1), 89–97. https://doi.org/10.1038/gim.2015.44

Bonadona, V., Bonaïti, B., Olschwang, S., Grandjouan, S., Huiart, L., Longy, M., Guimbaud, R., Buecher, B., Bignon, Y. J., Caron, O., Colas, C., Noguès, C., Lejeune-Dumoulin, S., Olivier-Faivre, L., Polycarpe-Osaer, F., Nguyen, T. D., Desseigne, F., Saurin, J. C., Berthet, P., Leroux, D., . . . French Cancer Genetics Network (2011). Cancer risks associated with germline mutations in MLH1, MSH2, and MSH6 genes in Lynch syndrome. *JAMA*, *305*(22), 2304–2310. https://doi.org/10.1001/jama.2011.743

Bougeard, G., Renaux-Petel, M., Flaman, J. M., Charbonnier, C., Fermey, P., Belotti, M., Gauthier-Villars, M., Stoppa-Lyonnet, D., Consolino, E., Brugières, L., Caron, O., Benusiglio, P. R., Bressac-de Paillerets, B., Bonadona, V., Bonaïti-Pellié, C., Tinat, J., Baert-Desurmont, S., & Frebourg, T. (2015). Revisiting Li-Fraumeni syndrome from TP53 mutation carriers. *Journal of Clinical Oncology*, *33*(21), 2345–2352. https://doi.org/10.1200/JCO.2014.59.5728

Brandi, M. L., Gagel, R. F., Angeli, A., Bilezikian, J. P., Beck-Peccoz, P., Bordi, C., Conte-Devolx, B., Falchetti, A., Gheri, R. G., Libroia, A., Lips, C. J., Lombardi, G., Mannelli, M., Pacini, F., Ponder, B. A., Raue, F., Skogseid, B., Tamburrano, G., Thakker, R. V., Thompson, N. W., . . . Marx, S. J. (2001). Guidelines for diagnosis and therapy of MEN type 1 and type 2. *Journal of Clinical Endocrinology and Metabolism*, *86*(12), 5658–5671. https://doi.org/10.1210/jcem.86.12.8070

Brosens, L. A., van Hattem, A., Hylind, L. M., Iacobuzio-Donahue, C., Romans, K. E., Axilbund, J., Cruz-Correa, M., Tersmette, A. C., Offerhaus, G. J., & Giardiello, F. M. (2007). Risk of colorectal cancer in juvenile polyposis. *Gut*, *56*(7), 965–967. https://doi.org/10.1136/gut.2006.116913

Canda, E., Kalkan Uçar, S., & Çoker, M. (2020). Biotinidase deficiency: Prevalence, impact and management strategies. *Pediatric Health, Medicine and Therapeutics*, *11*, 127–133. https://doi.org/10.2147/PHMT.S198656

Caponetti, A. G., Rapezzi, C., Gagliardi, C., Milandri, A., Dispenzieri, A., Kristen, A. V., Wixner, J., Maurer, M. S., Garcia-Pavia, P., Tournev, I., Planté-Bordeneuve, V., Chapman, D., Amass, L., & THAOS Investigators. (2021). Sex-related risk of cardiac involvement in hereditary transthyretin amyloidosis: Insights from THAOS. *JACC Heart Failure*, *9*(10), 736–746. https://doi.org/10.1016/j.jchf.2021.05.005

Castinetti, F., Waguespack, S. G., Machens, A., Uchino, S., Hasse-Lazar, K., Sanso, G., Else, T., Dvorakova, S., Qi, X. P., Elisei, R., Maia, A. L., Glod, J., Lourenço, D. M., Valdes, N., Mathiesen, J., Wohllk, N., Bandgar, T. R., Drui, D., Korbonits, M., & Druce, M. R. (2019). Natural history, treatment, and long-term follow up of patients with multiple endocrine neoplasia type 2B: An international, multicentre, retrospective study. *Lancet Diabetes & Endocrinology*, *7*(3), 213–220. https://doi.org/10.1016/s2213-8587(18)30336-x

Chao, D. L., Burr, A., & Pennesi, M. (2019). *RPE65*-related leber congenital amaurosis/early-onset severe retinal dystrophy. In M. P. Adam, J. Feldman, G. M. Mirzaa, R. A. Pagon, S. E. Wallace, & A. Amemiya (Eds.), *GeneReviews*®. University of Washington, Seattle.

Charron, P., Arad, M., Arbustini, E., Basso, C., Bilinska, Z., Elliott, P., Helio, T., Keren, A., McKenna, W. J., Monserrat, L., Pankuweit, S., Perrot, A., Rapezzi, C., Ristic, A., Seggewiss, H., van Langen, I., Tavazzi, L., & European Society of Cardiology Working Group on Myocardial and Pericardial Diseases. (2010). Genetic counselling and testing in cardiomyopathies: A position statement of the European Society of Cardiology Working Group on Myocardial and Pericardial Diseases *European Heart Journal*, *31*(22), 2715–2726. https://doi.org/10.1093/eurheartj/ehq271

Chu, L. C., Johnson, P. T., Dietz, H. C., & Fishman, E. K. (2014). CT angiographic evaluation of genetic vascular disease: Role in detection, staging, and management of complex vascular pathologic conditions. *AJR American Journal of Roentgenology*, *202*(5), 1120–1129. https://doi.org/10.2214/AJR.13.11485

Davison, J. E. (2020). Advances in diagnosis and management of Pompe disease. *Journal of Mother and Child*, *24*(2), 3–8. https://doi.org/10.34763/jmotherandchild.20202402si.2001.000002

Deegan, P. B., Baehner, A. F., Barba Romero, M. A., Hughes, D. A., Kampmann, C., Beck, M., & European FOS Investigators. (2006). Natural history of Fabry disease in females in the Fabry Outcome Survey. *Journal of Medical Genetics*, *43*(4), 347–352. https://doi.org/10.1136/jmg.2005.036327

Dietz, H. (2001). *FBN1*-related Marfan syndrome. In M. P. Adam, J. Feldman, G. M. Mirzaa, R. A. Pagon, S. E. Wallace, & A. Amemiya (Eds.), *GeneReviews*®. University of Washington, Seattle.

Dommering, C. J., Mol, B. M., Moll, A. C., Burton, M., Cloos, J., Dorsman, J. C., Meijers-Heijboer, H., & van der Hout, A. H. (2014). RB1 mutation spectrum in a comprehensive nationwide cohort of retinoblastoma patients. *Journal of Medical Genetics*, *51*(6), 366–374. https://doi.org/10.1136/jmedgenet-2014-102264

Elliott, P. M., Anastasakis, A., Borger, M. A., Borggrefe, M., Cecchi, F., Charron, P., Hagege, A. A., Lafont, A., Limongelli, G., Mahrholdt, H., McKenna, W. J., Mogensen, J., Nihoyannopoulos, P., Nistri, S., Pieper, P. G., Pieske, B., Rapezzi, C., Rutten, F. H., Tillmanns, C., . . . Watkins, H. (2014). 2014 ESC Guidelines on diagnosis and management of hypertrophic cardiomyopathy: The Task Force for the Diagnosis and Management of Hypertrophic Cardiomyopathy of the European Society of Cardiology (ESC). *European Heart Journal*, *35*(39), 2733–2779. https://doi.org/10.1093/eurheartj/ehu284

Eng, C. (2000). Will the real Cowden syndrome please stand up: Revised diagnostic criteria. *Journal of Medical Genetics*, *37*(11), 828–830. https://doi.org/10.1136/jmg.37.11.828

Evans, D. G., Huson, S. M., Donnai, D., Neary, W., Blair, V., Newton, V., & Harris, R. (1992). A clinical study of type 2 neurofibromatosis. *Quarterly Journal of Medicine*, *84*(304), 603–618.

Evans, J. P., & Rothschild, B. B. (2012). Return of results: Not that complicated? *Genetics in Medicine*, *14*(4), 358–360. https://doi.org/10.1038/gim.2012.8

Faughnan, M. E., Mager, J. J., Hetts, S. W., Palda, V. A., Lang-Robertson, K., Buscarini, E., Deslandres, E., Kasthuri, R. S., Lausman, A., Poetker, D., Ratjen, F., Chesnutt, M. S., Clancy, M., Whitehead, K. J., Al-Samkari, H., Chakinala, M., Conrad, M., Cortes, D., Crocione, C., Darling, J., . . . Zarrabeitia, R. (2020). Second International Guidelines for the Diagnosis and Management of Hereditary Hemorrhagic Telangiectasia. *Annals of Internal Medicine, 173*(12), 989–1001. https://doi.org/10.7326/M20-1443

Felis, A., Whitlow, M., Kraus, A., Warnock, D. G., & Wallace, E. (2019). Current and investigational therapeutics for Fabry disease. *Kidney International Reports, 5*(4), 407–413. https://doi.org/10.1016/j.ekir.2019.11.013

Gariépy-Assal, L., Gilbert, R. D., Žiaugra, A., & Foster, B. J. (2018). Management of Denys-Drash syndrome: A case series based on an international survey. *Clinical Nephrology: Case Studies, 6*, 36–44. https://doi.org/10.5414/CNCS109515

Giardiello, F. M., Allen, J. I., Axilbund, J. E., Boland, C. R., Burke, C. A., Burt, R. W., Church, J. M., Dominitz, J. A., Johnson, D. A., Kaltenbach, T., Levin, T. R., Lieberman, D. A., Robertson, D. J., Syngal, S., & Rex, D. K. (2014). Guidelines on genetic evaluation and management of Lynch syndrome: A consensus statement by the US Multi-society Task Force on Colorectal Cancer. *American Journal of Gastroenterology, 109*(8), 1159–1179. https://doi.org/10.1038/ajg.2014.186

Giardiello, F. M., Offerhaus, G. J., Lee, D. H., Krush, A. J., Tersmette, A. C., Booker, S. V., Kelley, N. C., & Hamilton, S. R. (1993). Increased risk of thyroid and pancreatic carcinoma in familial adenomatous polyposis. *Gut, 34*(10), 1394–1396. https://doi.org/10.1136/gut.34.10.1394

Goldenberg, I., Horr, S., Moss, A. J., Lopes, C. M., Barsheshet, A., McNitt, S., Zareba, W., Andrews, M. L., Robinson, J. L., Locati, E. H., Ackerman, M. J., Benhorin, J., Kaufman, E. S., Napolitano, C., Platonov, P. G., Priori, S. G., Qi, M., Schwartz, P. J., Shimizu, W., Towbin, J. A., . . . Zhang, L. (2011). Risk for life-threatening cardiac events in patients with genotype-confirmed long-QT syndrome and normal-range corrected QT intervals. *Journal of the American College of Cardiology, 57*(1), 51–59. https://doi.org/10.1016/j.jacc.2010.07.038

Gościniak, P., Baron, T., Milczarek, S., Kostkiewicz, M., & Machaliński, B. (2022). Updates for the diagnosis and management of cardiac amyloidosis. *Advances in Clinical and Experimental Medicine, 31*(2), 175–185. https://doi.org/10.17219/acem/142252

Green, R. C., Berg, J. S., Berry, G. T., Biesecker, L. G., Dimmock, D. P., Evans, J. P., Grody, W. W., Hegde, M. R., Kalia, S., Korf, B. R., Krantz, I., McGuire, A. L., Miller, D. T., Murray, M. F., Nussbaum, R. L., Plon, S. E., Rehm, H. L., & Jacob, H. J. (2012). Exploring concordance and discordance for return of incidental findings from clinical sequencing. *Genetics in Medicine, 14*(4), 405–410. https://doi.org/10.1038/gim.2012.21

Green, R. C., Berg, J. S., Grody, W. W., Kalia, S. S., Korf, B. R., Martin, C. L., McGuire, A. L., Nussbaum, R. L., O'Daniel, J. M., Ormond, K. E., Rehm, H. L., Watson, M. S., Williams, M. S., & Biesecker, L. G. (2013). ACMG recommendations for reporting of incidental findings in clinical exome and genome sequencing. *Genetics in Medicine, 15*(7), 565–574. https://doi.org/10.1038/gim.2013.73

Groeneweg, J. A., Bhonsale, A., James, C. A., te Riele, A. S., Dooijes, D., Tichnell, C., Murray, B., Wiesfeld, A. C., Sawant, A. C., Kassamali, B., Atsma, D. E., Volders, P. G., de Groot, N. M., de Boer, K., Zimmerman, S. L., Kamel, I. R., van der Heijden, J. F., Russell, S. D., Jan Cramer, M., Tedford, R. J., . . . Calkins, H. (2015). Clinical presentation, long-term follow-up, and outcomes of 1001 arrhythmogenic right ventricular dysplasia/cardiomyopathy patients and family members. *Circulation: Cardiovascular Genetics, 8*(3), 437–446. https://doi.org/10.1161/CIRCGENETICS.114.001003

Grosse, S. D., Gurrin, L. C., Bertalli, N. A., & Allen, K. J. (2018). Clinical penetrance in hereditary hemochromatosis: Estimates of the cumulative incidence of severe liver disease among HFE C282Y homozygotes. *Genetics in Medicine, 20*(4), 383–389. https://doi.org/10.1038/gim.2017.121

Gupta, S., Provenzale, D., Llor, X., Halverson, A. L., Grady, W., Chung, D. C., Haraldsdottir, S., Markowitz, A. J., Slavin, T. P., Jr., Hampel, H., Ness, R. M., Weiss, J. M., Ahnen, D. J., Chen, L., Cooper, G., Early, D. S., Giardiello, F. M., Hall, M. J., Hamilton, S. R., & Kanth, P. (2019). NCCN guidelines insights: Genetic/familial high-risk assessment: Colorectal, version 2.2019. *Journal of the National Comprehensive Cancer Network*, *17*(9), 1032–1041. https://doi.org/10.6004/jnccn.2019.0044

Halliday, J., Rutherford, S. A., McCabe, M. G., & Evans, D. G. (2018). An update on the diagnosis and treatment of vestibular schwannoma. *Expert Review of Neurotherapeutics*, *18*(1), 29–39. https://doi.org/10.1080/14737175.2018.1399795

Hammill, A. M., Wusik, K., & Kasthuri, R. S. (2021). Hereditary hemorrhagic telangiectasia (HHT): A practical guide to management. *Hematology: American Society of Hematology Education Program*, *2021*(1), 469–477. https://doi.org/10.1182/hematology.2021000281

Harada-Shiba, M., Arai, H., Oikawa, S., Ohta, T., Okada, T., Okamura, T., Nohara, A., Bujo, H., Yokote, K., Wakatsuki, A., Ishibashi, S., & Yamashita, S. (2012). Guidelines for the management of familial hypercholesterolemia. *Journal of Atherosclerosis and Thrombosis*, *19*(12), 1043–1060. https://doi.org/10.5551/jat.14621

Hasselberg, N. E., Haland, T. F., Saberniak, J., Brekke, P. H., Berge, K. E., Leren, T. P., Edvardsen, T., & Haugaa, K. H. (2018). Lamin A/C cardiomyopathy: Young onset, high penetrance, and frequent need for heart transplantation. *European Heart Journal*, *39*(10), 853–860. https://doi.org/10.1093/eurheartj/ehx596

Hershberger, R. E., Givertz, M. M., Ho, C. Y., Judge, D. P., Kantor, P. F., McBride, K. L., Morales, A., Taylor, M. R. G., Vatta, M., Ware, S. M., & ACMG Professional Practice and Guidelines Committee. (2018). Genetic evaluation of cardiomyopathy: A clinical practice resource of the American College of Medical Genetics and Genomics (ACMG). *Genetics in Medicine*, *20*(9), 899–909. https://doi.org/10.1038/s41436-018-0039-z

Hershberger, R. E., Hedges, D. J., & Morales, A. (2013). Dilated cardiomyopathy: The complexity of a diverse genetic architecture. *Nature Reviews Cardiology*, *10*(9), 531–547. https://doi.org/10.1038/nrcardio.2013.105

Hershberger, R. E., & Jordan, E. (2007). Dilated cardiomyopathy overview. In M. P. Adam, J. Feldman, G. M. Mirzaa, R. A. Pagon, S. E. Wallace, & A. Amemiya (Eds.), *GeneReviews®*. University of Washington, Seattle.

Heuser, A., Plovie, E. R., Ellinor, P. T., Grossmann, K. S., Shin, J. T., Wichter, T., Basson, C. T., Lerman, B. B., Sasse-Klaassen, S., Thierfelder, L., MacRae, C. A., & Gerull, B. (2006). Mutant desmocollin-2 causes arrhythmogenic right ventricular cardiomyopathy. *American Journal of Human Genetics*, *79*(6), 1081–1088. https://doi.org/10.1086/509044

Honda, Y., Sato, Y., Yokoyama, J., Kobayashi, M., Narisawa, R., Kawauchi, Y., Hoshi, T., Yajima, K., Kanda, T., Ajioka, Y., Hatakeyama, K., & Aoyagi, Y. (2013). Familial juvenile polyposis syndrome with a novel SMAD4 germline mutation *Clinical Journal of Gastroenterology*, *6*(5), 361–367. https://doi.org/10.1007/s12328-013-0413-y

Ibarra Moreno, C. A., Hu, S., Kraeva, N., Schuster, F., Johannsen, S., Rueffert, H., Klingler, W., Heytens, L., & Riazi, S. (2019). An assessment of penetrance and clinical expression of malignant hyperthermia in individuals carrying diagnostic ryanodine receptor 1 gene mutations. *Anesthesiology*, *131*(5), 983–991. https://doi.org/10.1097/ALN.0000000000002813

Ison, H. E., Clarke, S. L., & Knowles, J. W. (1993). Familial hypercholesterolemia. In M. P. Adam, J. Feldman, G. M. Mirzaa, R. A. Pagon, S. E. Wallace, & A. Amemiya (Eds.), *GeneReviews®*. [Internet]. University of Washington, Seattle; 1993–2025. https://www.ncbi.nlm.nih.gov/pubmed/24404629

Kadmon, M., Tandara, A., & Herfarth, C. (2001). Duodenal adenomatosis in familial adenomatous polyposis coli. A review of the literature and results from the Heidelberg Polyposis Register. *International Journal of Colorectal Disease, 16*(2), 63–75. https://doi.org/10.1007/s003840100290

Kalia, S. S., Adelman, K., Bale, S. J., Chung, W. K., Eng, C., Evans, J. P., Herman, G. E., Hufnagel, S. B., Klein, T. E., Korf, B. R., McKelvey, K. D., Ormond, K. E., Richards, C. S., Vlangos, C. N., Watson, M., Martin, C. L., & Miller, D. T. (2016). Recommendations for reporting of secondary findings in clinical exome and genome sequencing, 2016 update (ACMG SF v2.0): A policy statement of the American College of Medical Genetics and Genomics. *Genetics in Medicine, 19*(2), 249–255. https://doi.org/10.1038/gim.2016.190

Kidambi, T. D., Kohli, D. R., Samadder, N. J., & Singh, A. (2019). Hereditary polyposis syndromes. *Current Treatment Options in Gastroenterology, 17*(4), 650–665. https://doi.org/10.1007/s11938-019-00251-4

Kleinerman, R. A., Yu, C. L., Little, M. P., Li, Y., Abramson, D., Seddon, J., & Tucker, M. A. (2012). Variation of second cancer risk by family history of retinoblastoma among long-term survivors *Journal of Clinical Oncology, 30*(9), 950–957. https://doi.org/10.1200/JCO.2011.37.0239

Kloos, R. T., Eng, C., Evans, D. B., Francis, G. L., Gagel, R. F., Gharib, H., Moley, J. F., Pacini, F., Ringel, M. D., Schlumberger, M., & Wells, S. A., Jr. (2009). Medullary thyroid cancer: Management guidelines of the American Thyroid Association. *Thyroid, 19*(6), 565–612. https://doi.org/10.1089/thy.2008.0403

Kratz, C. P., Achatz, M. I., Brugières, L., Frebourg, T., Garber, J. E., Greer, M. C., Hansford, J. R., Janeway, K. A., Kohlmann, W. K., McGee, R., Mullighan, C. G., Onel, K., Pajtler, K. W., Pfister, S. M., Savage, S. A., Schiffman, J. D., Schneider, K. A., Strong, L. C., Evans, D. G. R., Wasserman, J. D., . . . Malkin, D. (2017). Cancer screening recommendations for individuals with Li-Fraumeni syndrome. *Clinical Cancer Research, 23*(11), e38–e45. https://doi.org/10.1158/1078-0432.CCR-17-0408

Krueger, D. A., & Northrup, H., on behalf of the International Tuberous Sclerosis Complex Consensus Group. (2013). Tuberous sclerosis complex surveillance and management: Recommendations of the 2012 International Tuberous Sclerosis Complex Consensus Conference. *Pediatric Neurology, 49*(4), 255–265. https://doi.org/10.1016/j.pediatrneurol.2013.08.002

Küry, S., Ramaekers, V., Bézieau, S., & Wolf, B. (2016). Clinical utility gene card for: Biotinidase deficiency-update 2015. *European Journal of Human Genetics, 24*(7). https://doi.org/10.1038/ejhg.2015.246

Latchford, A. R., Neale, K., Phillips, R. K. S., & Clark, S. K. (2012). Juvenile polyposis syndrome. *Diseases of the Colon & Rectum, 55*(10), 1038–1043. https://doi.org/10.1097/dcr.0b013e31826278b3

Lehnhardt, A., Karnatz, C., Ahlenstiel-Grunow, T., Benz, K., Benz, M. R., Budde, K., Büscher, A. K., Fehr, T., Feldkötter, M., Graf, N., Höcker, B., Jungraithmayr, T., Klaus, G., Koehler, B., Konrad, M., Kranz, B., Montoya, C. R., Müller, D., Neuhaus, T. J., Oh, J., . . . Kemper, M. J. (2015). Clinical and molecular characterization of patients with heterozygous mutations in Wilms tumor suppressor gene 1. *Clinical Journal of the American Society of Nephrology, 10*(5), 825–831. https://doi.org/10.2215/CJN.10141014

Lenders, J. W. M., Duh, Q.-Y., Eisenhofer, G., Gimenez-Roqueplo, A.-P., Grebe, S. K. G., Murad, M. H., Naruse, M., Pacak, K., & Young, W. F. (2014). Pheochromocytoma and paraganglioma: An Endocrine Society clinical practice guideline. *Journal of Clinical Endocrinology & Metabolism, 99*(6), 1915–1942. https://doi.org/10.1210/jc.2014-1498

Leslie, N., & Bailey, L. (2007). Pompe disease. In M. P. Adam, J. Feldman, G. M. Mirzaa, R. A. Pagon, S. E. Wallace, & A. Amemiya (Eds.), *GeneReviews®*. University of Washington, Seattle.

Loeys, B. L., Chen, J., Neptune, E. R., Judge, D. P., Podowski, M., Holm, T., Meyers, J., Leitch, C. C., Katsanis, N., Sharifi, N., Xu, F. L., Myers, L. A., Spevak, P. J., Cameron, D. E., De Backer, J., Hellemans, J., Chen, Y., Davis, E. C., Webb, C. L., Kress, W., . . . Dietz, H. C. (2005). A syndrome of altered cardiovascular, craniofacial, neurocognitive and skeletal development caused by mutations in TGFBR1 or TGFBR2. *Nature Genetics, 37*(3), 275–281. https://doi.org/10.1038/ng1511

Loeys, B. L., Dietz, H. C., Braverman, A. C., Callewaert, B. L., De Backer, J., Devereux, R. B., Hilhorst-Hofstee, Y., Jondeau, G., Faivre, L., Milewicz, D. M., Pyeritz, R. E., Sponseller, P. D., Wordsworth, P., & De Paepe, A. M. (2010). The revised Ghent nosology for the Marfan syndrome. *Journal of Medical Genetics, 47*(7), 476–485. https://doi.org/10.1136/jmg.2009.072785

Lubbe, S. J., Di Bernardo, M. C., Chandler, I. P., & Houlston, R. S. (2009). Clinical implications of the colorectal cancer risk associated with MUTYH mutation. *Journal of Clinical Oncology, 27*(24), 3975–3980. https://doi.org/10.1200/JCO.2008.21.6853

MacCarrick, G., Black, J. H., 3rd, Bowdin, S., et al. (2014). Loeys-Dietz syndrome: A primer for diagnosis and management. *Genetics in Medicine, 16*(8), 576–587. https://doi.org/10.1038/gim.2014.11

Maguire, A. M., Bennett, J., Aleman, E. M., Leroy, B. P., & Aleman, T. S. (2021). Clinical perspective: Treating RPE65-associated retinal dystrophy. *Molecular Therapy, 29*(2), 442–463. https://doi.org/10.1016/j.ymthe.2020.11.029

Mai, P. L., Best, A. F., Peters, J. A., DeCastro, R. M., Khincha, P. P., Loud, J. T., Bremer, R. C., Rosenberg, P. S., & Savage, S. A. (2016). Risks of first and subsequent cancers among TP53 mutation carriers in the National Cancer Institute Li-Fraumeni syndrome cohort. *Cancer, 122*(23), 3673–3681. https://doi.org/10.1002/cncr.30248

Mai, P. L., Malkin, D., Garber, J. E., Schiffman, J. D., Weitzel, J. N., Strong, L. C., Wyss, O., Locke, L., Means, V., Achatz, M. I., Hainaut, P., Frebourg, T., Evans, D. G., Bleiker, E., Patenaude, A., Schneider, K., Wilfond, B., Peters, J. A., Hwang, P. M., Ford, J., . . . Savage, S. A. (2012). Li-Fraumeni syndrome: Report of a clinical research workshop and creation of a research consortium. *Cancer Genetics, 205*(10), 479–487. https://doi.org/10.1016/j.cancergen.2012.06.008

Malfait, F., Francomano, C., Byers, P., Belmont, J., Berglund, B., Black, J., Bloom, L., Bowen, J. M., Brady, A. F., Burrows, N. P., Castori, M., Cohen, H., Colombi, M., Demirdas, S., De Backer, J., De Paepe, A., Fournel-Gigleux, S., Frank, M., Ghali, N., Giunta, C., . . . Tinkle, B. (2017). The 2017 international classification of the Ehlers-Danlos syndromes. *American Journal of Medical Genetics Part C: Seminars in Medical Genetics, 175*(1), 8–26. https://doi.org/10.1002/ajmg.c.31552

Marcus, F. I., McKenna, W. J., Sherrill, D., Basso, C., Bauce, B., Bluemke, D. A., Calkins, H., Corrado, D., Cox, M. G., Daubert, J. P., Fontaine, G., Gear, K., Hauer, R., Nava, A., Picard, M. H., Protonotarios, N., Saffitz, J. E., Sanborn, D. M., Steinberg, J. S., Tandri, H., . . . Zareba, W. (2010). Diagnosis of arrhythmogenic right ventricular cardiomyopathy/dysplasia: Proposed modification of the Task Force criteria. *European Heart Journal, 31*(7), 806–814. https://doi.org/10.1093/eurheartj/ehq025

Marques, J. S. (2022). The clinical management of Pompe disease: A pediatric perspective. *Children (Basel, Switzerland), 9*(9), 1404. https://doi.org/10.3390/children9091404

Mavaddat, N., Peock, S., Frost, D., Ellis, S., Platte, R., Fineberg, E., Evans, D. G., Izatt, L., Eeles, R. A., Adlard, J., Davidson, R., Eccles, D., Cole, T., Cook, J., Brewer, C., Tischkowitz, M.,

Douglas, F., Hodgson, S., Walker, L., Porteous, M. E., . . . EMBRACE. (2013). Cancer risks for BRCA1 and BRCA2 mutation carriers: Results from prospective analysis of EMBRACE. *Journal of the National Cancer Institute*, *105*(11), 812–822. https://doi.org/10.1093/jnci/djt095

McCullough, B. A., Yudkoff, M., Batshaw, M. L., Wilson, J. M., Raper, S. E., & Tuchman, M. (2000). Genotype spectrum of ornithine transcarbamylase deficiency: Correlation with the clinical and biochemical phenotype. *American Journal of Medical Genetics*, *93*(4), 313–319. https://doi.org/10.1002/1096-8628(20000814)93:4<313::aid-ajmg11>3.0.co;2-m

McDonald, J., Bayrak-Toydemir, P., DeMille, D., Wooderchak-Donahue, W., & Whitehead, K. (2020). Curaçao diagnostic criteria for hereditary hemorrhagic telangiectasia is highly predictive of a pathogenic variant in ENG or ACVRL1 (HHT1 and HHT2). *Genetics in Medicine*, *22*(7), 1201–1205. https://doi.org/10.1038/s41436-020-0775-8

McDonald, J., & Stevenson, D. A. (2000). Hereditary hemorrhagic telangiectasia. In M. P. Adam, J. Feldman, G. M. Mirzaa, R. A. Pagon, S. E. Wallace, & A. Amemiya (Eds.), *GeneReviews®*. University of Washington, Seattle.

Miller, D. T., Lee, K., Abul-Husn, N. S., Amendola, L. M., Brothers, K., Chung, W. K., Gollob, M. H., Gordon, A. S., Harrison, S. M., Hershberger, R. E., Klein, T. E., Richards, C. S., Stewart, D. R., & Martin, C. L. (2022). ACMG SF v3.1 list for reporting of secondary findings in clinical exome and genome sequencing: A policy statement of the American College of Medical Genetics and Genomics (ACMG). *Genetics in Medicine*, *24*(7), 1407–1414. https://doi.org/10.1016/j.gim.2022.04.006

Miller, D. T., Lee, K., Abul-Husn, N. S., Amendola, L. M., Brothers, K., Chung, W. K., Gollob, M. H., Gordon, A. S., Harrison, S. M., Hershberger, R. E., Klein, T. E., Richards, C. S., Stewart, D. R., Martin, C. L., & ACMG Secondary Findings Working Group. (2023). ACMG SF v3.2 list for reporting of secondary findings in clinical exome and genome sequencing: A policy statement of the American College of Medical Genetics and Genomics (ACMG). *Genetics in Medicine*, *25*(8), 100866. https://doi.org/10.1016/j.gim.2023.100866

Miller, D. T., Lee, K., Chung, W. K., Gordon, A. S., Herman, G. E., Klein, T. E., Stewart, D. R., Amendola, L. M., Adelman, K., Bale, S. J., Gollob, M. H., Harrison, S. M., Hershberger, R. E., McKelvey, K., Richards, C. S., Vlangos, C. N., Watson, M. S., & Martin, C. L. (2021). ACMG SF v3.0 list for reporting of secondary findings in clinical exome and genome sequencing: A policy statement of the American College of Medical Genetics and Genomics (ACMG). *Genetics in Medicine*, *23*(8), 1582–1584. https://doi.org/10.1038/s41436-021-01172-3

Miller, D. T., Lee, K., Gordon, A. S., Amendola, L. M., Adelman, K., Bale, S. J., Chung, W. K., Gollob, M. H., Harrison, S. M., Herman, G. E., Hershberger, R. E., Klein, T. E., McKelvey, K., Richards, C. S., Vlangos, C. N., Stewart, D. R., Watson, M. S., & Martin, C. L. (2021). Recommendations for reporting of secondary findings in clinical exome and genome sequencing, 2021 update: A policy statement of the American College of Medical Genetics and Genomics (ACMG). *Genetics in Medicine*, *23*(8), 1391–1398. https://doi.org/10.1038/s41436-021-01171-4

Mogensen, J., Murphy, R. T., Shaw, T., Bahl, A., Redwood, C., Watkins, H., Burke, M., Elliott, P. M., & McKenna, W. J. (2004). Severe disease expression of cardiac troponin C and T mutations in patients with idiopathic dilated cardiomyopathy *Journal of the American College of Cardiology*, *44*(10), 2033–2040. https://doi.org/10.1016/j.jacc.2004.08.027

Morales, A., & Hershberger, R. E. (2015). The rationale and timing of molecular genetic testing for dilated cardiomyopathy. *Canadian Journal of Cardiology*, *31*, 1309–1312.

Muth, A., Crona, J., Gimm, O., Elmgren, A., Filipsson, K., Stenmark Askmalm, M., Sandstedt, J., Tengvar, M., & Tham, E. (2018). Genetic testing and surveillance guidelines in hereditary pheochromocytoma and paraganglioma *Journal of Internal Medicine, 285*(2), 187–204. https://doi.org/10.1111/joim.12869

Napolitano, C., Mazzanti, A., Bloise, R., & Priori, S. G. (2004) Catecholaminergic polymorphic ventricular tachycardia. In M. P. Adam, J. Feldman, G. M. Mirzaa, R. A. Pagon, S. E. Wallace, & A. Amemiya (Eds.), *GeneReviews*® [Internet]. University of Washington, Seattle; 1993–2025. PMID: 20301466.

Naylor, R., Knight Johnson, A., & del Gaudio, D. (2018). Maturity-onset diabetes of the young overview. In M. P. Adam, J. Feldman, G. M. Mirzaa, R. A. Pagon, S. E. Wallace, & A. Amemiya (Eds.), *GeneReviews*®. University of Washington, Seattle.

Neumann, H. P. H., Young, W. F., Jr., & Eng, C. (2019). Pheochromocytoma and paraganglioma. *New England Journal of Medicine, 381*(6), 552–565. https://doi.org/10.1056/NEJMra1806651

Nordestgaard, B. G., Chapman, M. J., Humphries, S. E., Ginsberg, H. N., Masana, L., Descamps, O. S., Wiklund, O., Hegele, R. A., Raal, F. J., Defesche, J. C., Wiegman, A., Santos, R. D., Watts, G. F., Parhofer, K. G., Hovingh, G. K., Kovanen, P. T., Boileau, C., Averna, M., Borén, J., Bruckert, E., . . . European Atherosclerosis Society Consensus Panel. (2013). Familial hypercholesterolaemia is underdiagnosed and undertreated in the general population: Guidance for clinicians to prevent coronary heart disease: Consensus statement of the European Atherosclerosis Society. *European Heart Journal, 34*(45), 3478–3490. https://doi.org/10.1093/eurheartj/eht273

Northrup, H., & Krueger, D. A., on behalf of the International Tuberous Sclerosis Complex Consensus Group. (2013). Tuberous sclerosis complex diagnostic criteria update: Recommendations of the 2012 International Tuberous Sclerosis Complex Consensus Conference. *Pediatric Neurology, 49*(4), 243–254. https://doi.org/10.1016/j.pediatrneurol.2013.08.001

Nussbaum, R. L., Haverfield, E., Esplin, E. D., & Aradhya, S. (2019). Response to "The use of ACMG secondary findings recommendations for general population screening: A policy statement of the American College of Medical Genetics and Genomics (ACMG)." *Genetics in Medicine, 21*(12), 2836–2837. https://doi.org/10.1038/s41436-019-0572-4

Pannu, H., Tran-Fadulu, V., Papke, C. L., Scherer, S., Liu, Y., Presley, C., Guo, D., Estrera, A. L., Safi, H. J., Brasier, A. R., Vick, G. W., Marian, A. J., Raman, C. S., Buja, L. M., & Milewicz, D. M. (2007). MYH11 mutations result in a distinct vascular pathology driven by insulin-like growth factor 1 and angiotensin II. *Human Molecular Genetics, 16*(20), 2453–2462. https://doi.org/10.1093/hmg/ddm201

Priori, S. G., Wilde, A. A., Horie, M., Cho, Y., Behr, E. R., Berul, C., Blom, N., Brugada, J., Chiang, C. E., Huikuri, H., Kannankeril, P., Krahn, A., Leenhardt, A., Moss, A., Schwartz, P. J., Shimizu, W., Tomaselli, G., & Tracy, C. (2013). Executive summary: HRS/EHRA/APHRS expert consensus statement on the diagnosis and management of patients with inherited primary arrhythmia syndromes *Heart Rhythm, 10*(12), e85–e108. https://doi.org/10.1016/j.hrthm.2013.07.021

Provenzale, D., Gupta, S., Ahnen, D. J., Bray, T., Cannon, J. A., Cooper, G., David, D. S., Early, D. S., Erwin, D., Ford, J. M., Giardiello, F. M., Grady, W., Halverson, A. L., Hamilton, S. R., Hampel, H., Ismail, M. K., Klapman, J. B., Larson, D. W., Lazenby, A. J., & Lynch, P. M. (2016). Genetic/familial high-risk assessment: Colorectal version 1.2016, NCCN Clinical Practice Guidelines in Oncology. *Journal of the National Comprehensive Cancer Network, 14*(8), 1010–1030. https://doi.org/10.6004/jnccn.2016.0108

Rebbeck, T. R., Lynch, H. T., Neuhausen, S. L., Narod, S. A., Van't Veer, L., Garber, J. E., Evans, G., Isaacs, C., Daly, M. B., Matloff, E., Olopade, O. I., Weber, B. L., & Prevention and Observation of Surgical End Points Study Group. (2002). Prophylactic oophorectomy in carriers of BRCA1 or BRCA2 mutations *New England Journal of Medicine, 346*(21), 1616–1622. https://doi.org/10.1056/NEJMoa012158.

Regalado, E. S., Guo, D. C., Estrera, A. L., Buja, L. M., & Milewicz, D. M. (2014). Acute aortic dissections with pregnancy in women with ACTA2 mutations. *American Journal of Medical Genetics Part A, 164A*(1), 106–112. https://doi.org/10.1002/ajmg.a.36208

Regalado, E. S., Guo, D. C., Prakash, S., Bensend, T. A., Flynn, K., Estrera, A., Safi, H., Liang, D., Hyland, J., Child, A., Arno, G., Boileau, C., Jondeau, G., Braverman, A., Moran, R., Morisaki, T., Morisaki, H., Montalcino Aortic Consortium, Pyeritz, R., Coselli, J., . . . Milewicz, D. M. (2015). Aortic disease presentation and outcome associated with ACTA2 mutations. *Circulation: Cardiovascular Genetics, 8*(3), 457–464. https://doi.org/10.1161/CIRCGENETICS.114.000943

Richards, S., Aziz, N., Bale, S., Bick, D., Das, S., Gastier-Foster, J., Grody, W. W., Hegde, M., Lyon, E., Spector, E., Voelkerding, K., Rehm, H. L., & ACMG Laboratory Quality Assurance Committee. (2015). Standards and guidelines for the interpretation of sequence variants: A joint consensus recommendation of the American College of Medical Genetics and Genomics and the Association for Molecular Pathology. *Genetics in Medicine, 17*(5), 405–424. https://doi.org/10.1038/gim.2015.30

Roberts, E. A. (2018). Update on the diagnosis and management of Wilson disease. *Current Gastroenterology Reports, 20*(12), 56. https://doi.org/10.1007/s11894-018-0660-7

Roberts, E. A., & Schilsky, M. L. (2008). Diagnosis and treatment of Wilson disease: An update. *Hepatology (Baltimore, Md.), 47*(6), 2089–2111. https://doi.org/10.1002/hep.22261

Rombout-Sestrienkova, E., van Kraaij, M. G., & Koek, G. H. (2016). How we manage patients with hereditary haemochromatosis. *British Journal of Haematology, 175*(5), 759–770. https://doi.org/10.1111/bjh.14376

Rosenberg, H., Pollock, N., Schiemann, A., Bulger, T., & Stowell, K. (2015). Malignant hyperthermia: A review. *Orphanet Journal of Rare Diseases, 10*, 93. https://doi.org/10.1186/s13023-015-0310-1

Ruggieri, M., Praticò, A. D., Serra, A., Maiolino, L., Cocuzza, S., Di Mauro, P., Licciardello, L., Milone, P., Privitera, G., Belfiore, G., Di Pietro, M., Di Raimondo, F., Romano, A., Chiarenza, A., Muglia, M., Polizzi, A., & Evans, D. G. (2016). Childhood neurofibromatosis type 2 (NF2) and related disorders: From bench to bedside and biologically targeted therapies [Neurofibromatosi tipo 2 (NF2) e sindromi correlate in età infantile: dalla biologia molecolare alla pratica clinica e nuove terapie con farmaci biologici]. *Acta otorhinolaryngologica Italica: organo ufficiale della Societa italiana di otorinolaringologia e chirurgia cervico-facciale, 36*(5), 345–367. https://doi.org/10.14639/0392-100X-1093

Sabater-Molina, M., Saura, D., García-Molina Sáez, E., González-Carrillo, J., Polo, L., Pérez-Sánchez, I., Olmo, M. D. C., Oliva-Sandoval, M. J., Barriales-Villa, R., Carbonell, P., Pascual-Figal, D., & Gimeno, J. R. (2017). A novel founder mutation in MYBPC3: Phenotypic comparison with the most prevalent MYBPC3 mutation in Spain. *Revista espanola de cardiologia (English ed.), 70*(2), 105–114. https://doi.org/10.1016/j.rec.2016.06.020

Saito, Y., Nakamura, K., & Ito, H. (2021). Molecular mechanisms of cardiac amyloidosis. *International Journal of Molecular Sciences, 23*(1), 25. https://doi.org/10.3390/ijms23010025

Sampson, J. R., & Jones, N. (2009). MUTYH-associated polyposis. *Best Practice & Research: Clinical Gastroenterology, 23*(2), 209–218. https://doi.org/10.1016/j.bpg.2009.03.006

Sarah, B., Giovanna, B., Emanuela, K., Nadi, N., Josè, V., & Alberto, P. (2022). Clinical efficacy of the enzyme replacement therapy in patients with late-onset Pompe disease: A systematic review and a meta-analysis. *Journal of Neurology*, *269*(2), 733–741. https://doi.org/10.1007/s00415-021-10526-5

Saroli Palumbo, C., & Schilsky, M. L. (2019). Clinical practice guidelines in Wilson disease. *Annals of Translational Medicine*, *7*(Suppl. 2), S65. https://doi.org/10.21037/atm.2018.12.53

Scheuner, M. T., Peredo, J., Benkendorf, J., Bowdish, B., Feldman, G., Fleisher, L., Mulvihill, J. J., Watson, M., Herman, G. E., & Evans, J. (2015). Reporting genomic secondary findings: ACMG members weigh in. *Genetics in Medicine*, *17*(1), 27–35. https://doi.org/10.1038/gim.2014.165.

Sharma, N., Cortez, D., Disori, K., Imundo, J. R., & Beck, M. (2020). A review of long QT syndrome: Everything a hospitalist should know. *Hospital Pediatrics*, *10*(4), 369–375. https://doi.org/10.1542/hpeds.2019-0139

Shepherd, M., Shields, B., Hammersley, S., Hudson, M., McDonald, T. J., Colclough, K., Oram, R. A., Knight, B., Hyde, C., Cox, J., Mallam, K., Moudiotis, C., Smith, R., Fraser, B., Robertson, S., Greene, S., Ellard, S., Pearson, E. R., Hattersley, A. T., & UNITED Team. (2016). Systematic population screening, using biomarkers and genetic testing, identifies 2.5% of the U.K. Pediatric diabetes population with monogenic diabetes. *Diabetes Care*, *39*(11), 1879–1888. https://doi.org/10.2337/dc16-0645

Syngal, S., Brand, R. E., Church, J. M., Giardiello, F. M., Hampel, H. L., Burt, R. W., & American College of Gastroenterology. (2015). ACG clinical guideline: Genetic testing and management of hereditary gastrointestinal cancer syndromes. *American Journal of Gastroenterology*, *110*(2), 223–263. https://doi.org/10.1038/ajg.2014.435

Tan, M. H., Mester, J. L., Ngeow, J., Rybicki, L. A., Orloff, M. S., & Eng, C. (2012). Lifetime cancer risks in individuals with germline PTEN mutations. *Clinical Cancer Research*, *18*(2), 400–407. https://doi.org/10.1158/1078-0432.CCR-11-2283

Thakker, R. V., Newey, P. J., Walls, G. V., Bilezikian, J., Dralle, H., Ebeling, P. R., Melmed, S., Sakurai, A., Tonelli, F., Brandi, M. L., & Endocrine Society. (2012). Clinical practice guidelines for multiple endocrine neoplasia type 1 (MEN1). *Journal of Clinical Endocrinology and Metabolism*, *97*(9), 2990–3011. https://doi.org/10.1210/jc.2012-1230

Tosur, M., & Philipson, L. H. (2022). Precision diabetes: Lessons learned from maturity-onset diabetes of the young (MODY). *Journal of Diabetes Investigation*, *13*(9), 1465–1471. https://doi.org/10.1111/jdi.1386

Tschöpe, C., & Elsanhoury, A. (2022). Treatment of transthyretin amyloid cardiomyopathy: The current options, the future, and the challenges. *Journal of Clinical Medicine*, *11*(8), 2148. https://doi.org/10.3390/jcm11082148

Tuchman, M., Lee, B., Lichter-Konecki, U., Summar, M. L., Yudkoff, M., Cederbaum, S. D., Kerr, D. S., Diaz, G. A., Seashore, M. R., Lee, H. S., McCarter, R. J., Krischer, J. P., Batshaw, M. L., & Additional members of Urea Cycle Disorders Consortium of the Rare Diseases Clinical Research Network. (2008). Cross-sectional multicenter study of patients with urea cycle disorders in the United States. *Molecular Genetics and Metabolism*, *94*(4), 397–402. https://doi.org/10.1016/j.ymgme.2008.05.004

van Asperen, C. J., Brohet, R. M., Meijers-Heijboer, E. J., Hoogerbrugge, N., Verhoef, S., Vasen, H. F., Ausems, M. G., Menko, F. H., Gomez Garcia, E. B., Klijn, J. G., Hogervorst, F. B., van Houwelingen, J. C., van't Veer, L. J., Rookus, M. A., van Leeuwen, F. E., & Netherlands Collaborative Group on Hereditary Breast Cancer (HEBON). (2005). Cancer risks in BRCA2 families: Estimates for sites other than breast and ovary. *Journal of Medical Genetics*, *42*(9), 711–719. https://doi.org/10.1136/jmg.2004.028829

van Leeuwaarde, R. S., Ahmad, S., Links, T. P., & Giles, R. H. (2018). Von Hippel-Lindau syndrome. In M. P. Adam, J. Feldman, G. M. Mirzaa, R. A. Pagon, S. E. Wallace, & A. Amemiya (Eds.), *GeneReviews®*. University of Washington, Seattle.

Wilde, A. A. M., Semsarian, C., Márquez, M. F., Sepehri Shamloo, A., Ackerman, M. J., Ashley, E. A., Sternick, E. B., Barajas-Martinez, H., Behr, E. R., Bezzina, C. R., Breckpot, J., Charron, P., Chockalingam, P., Crotti, L., Gollob, M. H., Lubitz, S., Makita, N., Ohno, S., Ortiz-Genga, M., Sacilotto, L., . . . Deneke, T. (2022). European Heart Rhythm Association (EHRA)/Heart Rhythm Society (HRS)/Asia Pacific Heart Rhythm Society (APHRS)/Latin American Heart Rhythm Society (LAHRS) expert consensus statement on the state of genetic testing for cardiac diseases. *Heart Rhythm*, *19*(7), e1–e60. https://doi.org/10.1016/j.hrthm.2022.03.1225

Win, A. K., Dowty, J. G., Cleary, S. P., Kim, H., Buchanan, D. D., Young, J. P., Clendenning, M., Rosty, C., MacInnis, R. J., Giles, G. G., Boussioutas, A., Macrae, F. A., Parry, S., Goldblatt, J., Baron, J. A., Burnett, T., Le Marchand, L., Newcomb, P. A., Haile, R. W., Hopper, J. L., . . . Jenkins, M. A. (2014). Risk of colorectal cancer for carriers of mutations in MUTYH, with and without a family history of cancer. *Gastroenterology*, *146*(5), 1208–11.e115. https://doi.org/10.1053/j.gastro.2014.01.022

Wolf, B. (2000). Biotinidase deficiency. In M. P. Adam, J. Feldman, G. M. Mirzaa, R. A. Pagon, S. E. Wallace, & A. Amemiya (Eds.), *GeneReviews®*. University of Washington, Seattle.

Wolf, B. (2012). Biotinidase deficiency: "If you have to have an inherited metabolic disease, this is the one to have." *Genetics in Medicine*, *14*(6), 565–575. https://doi.org/10.1038/gim.2011.6

Wolf, B. (2015). Biotinidase deficiency should be considered in individuals exhibiting myelopathy with or without and vision loss. *Molecular Genetics and Metabolism*, *116*(3), 113–118. https://doi.org/10.1016/j.ymgme.2015.08.012

Yang, X., Leslie, G., Doroszuk, A., Schneider, S., Allen, J., Decker, B., Dunning, A. M., Redman, J., Scarth, J., Plaskocinska, I., Luccarini, C., Shah, M., Pooley, K., Dorling, L., Lee, A., Adank, M. A., Adlard, J., Aittomäki, K., Andrulis, I. L., Ang, P., . . . Tischkowitz, M. (2020). Cancer risks associated with germline *PALB2* pathogenic variants: An international study of 524 families. *Journal of Clinical Oncology*, *38*(7), 674–685. https://doi.org/10.1200/JCO.19.01907

CHAPTER 22

GENETICS AND GENETIC COUNSELING IN THE INTERNET AGE

LAUREN GALLAGHER AND LESLIE ORDAL

Introduction

The rapid growth of genetic and genomic technologies, especially over the past 30 years, has led to the profession of genetic counseling being defined partly by its constant need to evolve and adapt. Over a similar time period, society and culture have been shaped by the explosion of the internet and on-demand access to information. While the genetic testing landscape continuously changes and shifts, so does the amount and accessibility of information available to both providers and patients. Clinicians can access tools and knowledge with a speed only dreamed of before the widespread adoption of broadband internet. Patients are increasingly informed, with many having done their own internet-based research—or even genetic testing—prior to their appointments. Genetic counselors can now take advantage of advances in virtual care, artificial intelligence (AI)–powered technologies, and online networking to improve their practice. This chapter will provide an overview of the changes to genetic counseling practice and patient care driven by the incorporation of the internet into everyday communication and culture.

Access to Genetic Information

Patient access to genetic information

Over the past two decades, the availability and accessibility of health-related information online has expanded. The internet allows people to access information that was previously only found in the medical literature conveniently, inexpensively, and anonymously. Early concerns with the use of the internet in the healthcare context included concerns that patients would access information from unreliable sources and use it as a substitute for seeking medical attention; however, most credible health organizations nowadays have a strong online presence, producing trustworthy and accurate health-related information. This has dramatically changed the healthcare landscape, where patients have increasingly become proactive partners in the management of their health (Schaffer et al., 2008).

Higher education level and income, previous experience with the internet, younger age, and having a diagnostic label to search are all positive influencers of health-related internet use (Bansil et al., 2006; Roche & Skinner, 2009; Schaffer et al., 2008). Interestingly, factors impacting the understanding of content, such as literacy and language, are larger barriers than lack of access to computers or the internet (Schaffer et al., 2008). Studies exploring the use of the internet related to genetic services have found that patient and family motivations for going online are to get information in lay terms, prepare for a genetics clinic visit, learn about genetic testing options, obtain diagnostic and prognostic information, and learn about support services, treatment/management options, and research opportunities (Morgan et al., 2014; Roche & Skinner, 2009; Taylor et al., 2001).

The widespread availability of health information online has impacted patient–provider relationships in many ways. It leads to improved patient comprehension of genetic information and has the potential to give patients a greater sense of autonomy and confidence when making decisions (Baker et al., 2003; Broom, 2005). Information learned online can provide patients with a foundation of knowledge upon which they can build following their interaction with their healthcare provider. (Bansil et al., 2006). Patients and their families also make valuable contributions to our understanding of genetic disease by sharing their lived experiences online and, in doing so, provide valuable information and serve as advocates. While the impacts of this have been positive for the most part, this new responsibility can also lead to information overload and place pressure on families to advocate (Skinner & Schaffer, 2006).

Clinicians should also be aware of the potential for the rapid spread of misinformation via the internet, particularly on social media. Many clinicians may be surprised to find that a treatment or test they view as beneficial may be represented very differently by patients online (Savas et al., 2014). While it is critical not to disregard the patient experience, it is important to know that the information from the top hits on Google searches may be completely different from prevailing clinical beliefs. This may consist of unintentional misunderstanding of clinical research posted on message boards but could also encompass pseudoscience and outright fraud (Dijkstra et al., 2018). The potential for a mismatch between patient and provider attitudes as a result of information found on the internet can affect trust and rapport in the clinical setting. Being aware of potentially pervasive misinformation found online can aid genetic counselors in acknowledging potential patient concerns as well as facilitating an informed discussion of the issues with their patients.

As patients arrive at appointments with more knowledge as well as self-sourced results, genetic counselors may at times see their role shift from "information provider" to "information curator," helping patients sort through and critically assess the information they have found on their own. This requires genetic counselors to stay abreast of developments not only in the traditional space of clinician-ordered testing but also in the less regulated realm of direct-to-consumer (DTC) and patient-initiated testing.

Patient access to genetic testing

Once available only through healthcare providers, genetic testing can now be ordered directly by patients, usually via the internet. Initially focused on ancestry testing, these DTC tests now encompass carrier screening, predisposition to developing multifactorial diseases, and even entertainment, as in the case of one test that predicts wine preference (Chen, 2017). As of early 2019, more than 26 million people had taken a DTC genetic ancestry test (Regalado, 2019), with the total number of DTC tests undoubtedly much higher. DTC testing's enormous popularity has led to an explosion in the number of companies selling such tests, with growth only occasionally held in check by regulation as governments struggle to keep pace with new advances and market offerings (Kalokairinou et al., 2018).[1]

For the genetic counselor, DTC tests add another potential layer of complexity to the patient encounter. It is increasingly common for patients to have done their own genetic testing long before ever setting foot in a genetics clinic, and they may have questions about their results they wish to review. This adds additional time to the consult and demands new strategies for accepting, triaging, and managing referrals for the indication of review of DTC results. One study of Australian genetic counselors found that referrals related to DTC genetic testing were often related to results with little clinical importance, such as variants in *MTHFR*. About half of genetic counselors in the study reported that both the patient and the referring provider had misunderstood the meaning of the DTC test results (Millward et al., 2020). Clearly, there is a need for genetic counselors in the landscape of DTC genetic testing, though challenges present in identifying lower priority referrals and balancing them with existing and possibly more time-sensitive cases.

Significant implications for genetic counseling practice arise from the varying quality and oversight among DTC genetic testing companies. In many jurisdictions, DTC tests are not subject to the same regulations as clinical genetic tests and errors have been reported, including false-positive results indicating the presence of a pathogenic mutation. In one study, 40% of pathogenic mutations found through DTC testing turned out to be false positives (Tandy-Connor et al., 2018). While some DTC genetic test companies employ a molecular geneticist to oversee testing and have certified genetic counselors on staff to advise in product development and communication of results, others provide scant guidance about how to proceed even in the case of pathogenic variants with life-altering medical management, such as the identification of a pathogenic variant in *BRCA1* or *TP53* (de Pauw et al., 2020). In fact, many DTC genetic test companies lack Clinical Laboratory Improvement Amendments or College of American Pathologists certification, compounding concerns about test validity (MedlinePlus, n.d.). Genetic counselors must now educate themselves about the claims, validity, and methodology behind the DTC test results their patients present and be ready to help patients understand the mismatch between what is written on the reports and the potential gravity of the results. Additionally, any pathogenic variants discovered through DTC testing ideally should be confirmed by clinical genetic testing before any changes to medical management are made.

[1] Editors' note: For further discussion on DTC genetic testing, see Chapter 11 by Anne E. Greb in this volume.

Patients who are avid knowledge seekers may go further with their DTC results and submit them for analysis to a third-party company that interprets raw data not included on original reports. These interpretations often rely on publicly available databases such as SNPedia, with clinical validity not always established (Badalato et al., 2017). While some consumers may consult third-party raw data interpretation tools purely out of curiosity, using such results for clinical guidance could have life-altering implications, for example, if a third-party tool suggested a change in medication dosage based on single nucleotide polymorphisms associated with drug metabolism. Genetic counselors and other healthcare providers should also be aware that, at least in the United States, uptake of DTC testing is highest among White consumers; companies who use consumer data to update their reporting algorithms are therefore at risk of exacerbating bias already present due to the prevalence of samples from White individuals in genetic research (Bentley et al., 2017).

In response to many of the challenges presented by DTC genetic testing, a few companies have begun to offer what has been termed "patient-initiated testing," or PIT. These are usually well-known clinical labs offering patients the ability to self-pay for a genetic test, which is ordered with the oversight of a physician (and sometimes a genetic counselor) working for the company or through a contract with an independent practice (Allyse et al., 2018). The stated goal for PIT is to allow for patient autonomy—and often faster access to testing—while ensuring that the test ordered is appropriate and adheres to stricter quality measures than typically seen in DTC genetic testing. At the time this chapter is being written, PIT has been available in a limited fashion for a limited time (Ashford, 2019), and it remains to be seen if it is an effective solution to the desire for individual and on-demand access to genetic testing while delivering clinical-quality results and guidance. Additionally, the self-pay model effectively limits access to PIT to wealthier patients, potentially exacerbating current disparities in access to genetics services (Yip et al., 2019).

The rapid growth of DTC genetic testing and other changes to the genetic testing landscape may make keeping up with new advancements appear to be a formidable task. In a recent survey of genetic counselors, most (approximately 90%) agreed that genetic counselors should be involved in the DTC genetic testing process. Less than a third, however, felt confident about providing genetic counseling related to these tests (Hsieh et al., 2020). Nonetheless, staying informed about new developments in this area is in many ways the same as the constant continuing education that is integral to the practice of the genetic counselor. Information is readily available through journals, conference proceedings, and other traditional sources of clinical knowledge, with social media now offering an even broader pool of resources and access to experts (see section on Social Media and Genetic Counselors).

Impact on Genetic Counseling Practice

Telegenetics and virtual care

Telemedicine broadly refers to the use of telecommunications technologies to support long-distance healthcare. Over 20 years have passed since telemedicine was first piloted in a genetics setting (Gray et al., 2000). In the early days, the primary appeal of telegenetics was to increase access to genetics services for patients living in rural and remote areas, reducing travel and related costs and increasing reach. Recent growth in the medical genetics field including genetic testing has led to an increased demand for genetic counseling services (Hoskevec et al., 2017). In addition, genetic counselors are increasingly accepting positions outside of patient-facing roles, which places additional pressure on genetic counselors who are providing patient care (Hoskevec et al., 2017). The desire to expand genetic counseling services to meet demand has strengthened the appeal of telegenetics as an alternate model of service delivery to increase clinic efficiency, reduce clinic costs, and overcome geographical barriers to recruitment (Weissman et al., 2018). Moreover, high patient satisfaction with telegenetics has been well documented for several indications (Abrams & Geier, 2006; d'Agincourt-Canning & McGillivray, 2008; Hopper et al., 2011).

Telegenetics can be delivered in a variety of modalities. The most commonly used modality for delivering telegenetics service is live video conferencing, which allows real-time interaction between the genetic counselor and patient in lieu of meeting in person; other modalities such as the transfer of information and images (store-and-forward), remote patient monitoring, and mobile health are less popular and less commonly used in genetics (Terry et al., 2019; Vrečar et al., 2017). In exploring the telegenetics landscape in several U.S. states, Terry et al. (2019) surveyed several self-identified telegenetics programs and found that many of them report being capable of providing video appointments to patients at home and report patient access and convenience to be their biggest successes.

Telegenetics also offers several potential benefits to genetic counselors. Traditionally, genetic counselors have been restricted to work in larger cities, where genetics clinics are located. The availability and adoption of telegenetics modalities in patient care have opened up more opportunities for genetic counselors to work remotely, offering them greater career flexibility. Genetic counselors working in telegenetics report that being involved in an innovative method of healthcare delivery that offers greater patient satisfaction and the ability to work from home with more flexible hours are the appealing aspects of telegenetics; the downsides are challenges in providing psychosocial counseling (e.g., difficulty reading nonverbal cues, establishing rapport, etc.) and limited social interaction with colleagues (Zierhut et al., 2018).

Despite all the potential and promise of telegenetics, until recently, few genetic counselors reported routinely using it in practice. Barriers to the integration of telegenetics include issues with billing and licensure, technology-related access difficulties, limited ability to perform a comprehensive physical exam, and practical and administrative constraints (e.g., sending testing requisitions via mail; Burgess et al., 2016; Zierhut et al., 2018). While some academic medical centers used telegenetics, virtual care was adopted more quickly by private practice, with companies such as GeneMatters, Grey Genetics, Genome Medical, Informed DNA, and Metis Genetics emerging to offer remote service delivery.

In the spring of 2020, the COVID-19 pandemic was experienced worldwide, forcing genetics clinics to quickly adapt to continue to meet the needs of their patients during the crisis. Many genetic counselors were forced to work from home, and only urgent indications were prioritized for in-person genetic counseling. This provided the impetus for governments, insurers, and academic health centers to address the long-standing barriers with telemedicine, resolving some of the issues with billing, exploring varied comprehensive virtual care platforms that allow more connected care, and solving a number of the practical challenges. While published literature is only beginning to emerge that describes this shift to virtual care at the time of the writing of this chapter, the speed and magnitude of the adaptation were remarkable. As benefits were realized and challenges solved, the scales tipped in favor of telemedicine for the provision of genetic counseling. Whether the popularity and sustainability of telemedicine will persist post-COVID-19 remains to be seen.

Tools to support practice

Technological solutions are now available to help support nearly every aspect of the genetic counseling process, including family history and medical record collection, risk assessment, education, decision support, family communication, and connecting patients to support networks. Family history and risk assessment software have been around for nearly 30 years but have become increasingly automated and comprehensive; many are capable of electronic medical record integration and offer additional functionalities such as the ability to track genetic tests and generate standard consult letters (Gordon et al., 2018). While these tools are most commonly used in cancer genetics, they are also becoming available to support nongenetics providers in the collection of family history information and risk analysis to help determine patients for whom a referral to genetics is indicated. Many genetics clinics have developed educational videos and e-learning modules designed for both patients and providers to provide standardized information in advance of an appointment and help increase the appropriateness of referrals. Interactive, online decision aids are also gaining popularity in genetic counseling for their ability to provide accurate information and decision support as potential alternatives to pretest genetic counseling (Adam et al., 2018). While genetic counselors often assist patients in communicating risks to relatives through the use of educational letters, platforms such as the University of California, San Francisco's Kintalk (https://www.kintalk.com) are now available to help with this task. Furthermore, patient advocacy groups have moved online, allowing the connection of families with similar conditions from across the world, and online portals such as MyGene2 (https://www.mygene2.org) are now available to facilitate connections for rare disease. These tools are increasingly used in genetic counseling to help optimize referrals and maximize efficiency, allowing genetic counselors to apply their skills where they are most needed.

Artificial Intelligence-powered technologies

AI involves the use of computer programs and technology to perform tasks that usually require human intelligence and is being applied in many industries to improve performance and efficiency and reduce cost. Many people consider AI to be futuristic, without realizing how commonly they encounter it in their daily lives (Kearney et al., 2020). Healthcare applications of AI have existed for years but are increasing in sophistication, offering greater promise to transform healthcare delivery and systems. AI technology is already being weaved into the genetic counseling process, with applications available to aid with information gathering and pedigree construction, risk assessment, diagnostic evaluation, decision support, and genetic testing. While much hype surrounds the potential for AI technology in genetics, many fears and limitations remain.

The earliest example of AI used a rules-based algorithm to program a computer to perform a series of tasks (Kearney et al., 2020). Examples of this in genetic counseling include pedigree construction software and risk assessment programs. The widespread use of these tools in genetic counseling has increased the efficiency with which genetic counselors practice.

A comprehensive genetics assessment that carefully describes a patient's physical features to establish a diagnosis is time-consuming and requires a great deal of expertise. Machine learning technology lends itself well to medical diagnostics, where computers can be programmed to recognize diagnoses based on images, and is currently used across several medical disciplines, including genetics. AI tools have existed to help with the genetics evaluation since SYNDROC, a microcomputer that could establish a differential diagnosis for dysmorphic syndromes, was described in 1985 (Schorderet & Aebischer, 1985). In recent years, more advanced diagnostic algorithms, such as FDNA's Face2Gene (https://www.face2gene.com), have leveraged deep learning and computer vision technologies to analyze patient photos and determine a prioritized differential diagnosis. Similar diagnostic tools are now publicly available, for example, ThinkGenetic's SymptomMatcher (https://www.thinkgenetic.com), which allows a person to enter their symptoms to determine if they may have an underlying genetic diagnosis. These technologies offer increasing promise to support clinicians in establishing a diagnosis with greater efficiency and precision and in decreasing the time to diagnosis for patients.

Machine learning has arguably the greatest potential in genomics, where it is used to overcome the limitations of both human intelligence and statistical methods in the performance of more complex tasks (Libbrecht & Noble, 2015). Genomic applications of AI offer much promise with activities such as variant calling, genome annotation, variant classification, and genotype–phenotype mapping (Dias & Torkamani, 2019) and are currently being used in the bioinformatics pipelines of some commercial genetic testing laboratories (Gordon et al., 2018).

Natural language processing technologies such as chatbots, designed to simulate human conversation, are also becoming increasingly prevalent in genetics. Similar to voice-activated home assistants, chatbots can recognize human speech and be programmed with a series of responses. Invitae offers a virtual care platform guided by a genetics information assistant named Gia to take patients through the genetic testing process, covering topics such as consent, pretest and posttest counseling, education, test ordering, and possible results (https://www.invitae.com). Other examples of genetic chatbots include Gene, which guides users through the ThinkGenetic SymptomMatcher program, and Dokbot, from ItRunsInMyFamily, which collects family history information so that cancer risk assessment modeling can be performed. Incorporating chatbots into tasks such as information gathering and education may help genetic counselors meet the increasing demand for their services, freeing up their time to focus on the more complex aspects of their work.

Kearney et al. (2020) designed a framework for the assignment of computer versus clinician tasks in the future. They describe the possible use of this technology throughout the genetic counseling process while emphasizing the importance of the clinician's critical thinking and counseling skills in the review and assessment of information and provision of personalized care and support (Kearney et al., 2020). While this offers the potential for genetic counselors to focus their time and energy on higher impact parts of the job, a cautious approach should be taken as these technologies continue to shape our practice.

Education and professional development

The widespread and on-demand nature of the internet has increased opportunities for genetic counselors to further their education and professional skills, whether seeking continuing education credits or obtaining advanced degrees. The first fully online genetic counseling program in the United States received accreditation in 2018, with several other programs operating in hybrid models that incorporate a range of online elements (Boise State University, 2018). Online opportunities to obtain advanced degrees or training are now available; for example, the University of British Columbia now offers a graduate certificate in genomic counseling and variant interpretation, the requirements for which can be fully obtained online. With the COVID-19 pandemic and concerns mounting about global warming, virtual conferences will likely become more mainstream. For example, the European Society of Human Genetics hosted a successful "live from your living room" virtual conference in June 2020. While genetic counselors used to rely almost solely on conference attendance for continuing education, other opportunities such as webinars are increasing in number and popularity. See Chapter 2—"The Development of Education for Genetic Counselors" in this volume for further details on genetic counseling education.

Social Media and Genetic Counselors

One of the most powerful tools for genetic counselors is social media. Among the multitude of platforms, Twitter[2] has emerged over the past decade as a popular one for genetic counselors and other healthcare professionals to keep up with current events and engage in networking. Twitter users "follow" others with similar interests and see their "tweets" in a central feed; they can also label and access genetic-specific content through the use of hashtags. At the time this chapter was written, the predominant hashtag for genetic counseling on Twitter was #GeneChat, with other specialty-specific hashtags also in use (such as #cardiogen for cardiac genetics). The rapidly changing nature of social media and technology makes it impossible to future-proof these suggestions, and readers are encouraged to search or ask colleagues for the most up-to-date hashtags if needed. Content on Twitter under the #GeneChat hashtag includes notifications about new journal articles, opinions about issues related to the profession, and even requests for very specific information in near real time, such as inquiries about the existence of testing or other resources for an upcoming patient. LinkedIn's newsfeed function also serves as a forum for genetic counselors to post content and engage with each other professionally and makes similar use of hashtags.

The utility of maintaining a social media presence is still largely anecdotal due to its recent emergence, but clinicians in other fields have demonstrated its value through

[2] Editors' Note: While at the time of writing this platform was known as Twitter, it is now referred to as X.

projects such as a themed journal issue sourced entirely via calls for submissions posted on Twitter (Chisolm, 2015) or acknowledgment of formal collaborations that began as an exchange of messages. Evidence of its incorporation into clinical practice and teaching has begun to appear in the form of commentaries, opinion pieces, and academic journal clubs taking place on Twitter (Topf & Hiremath, 2015), as well as requests for talks on the topic at professional conferences (Ordal, 2019). With the rapid growth of social media uptake among clinicians, there is likely to be more research on its effectiveness as a networking, information-gathering, and teaching tool.

The public nature of social media platforms, which makes them quite useful for connecting and sharing information with fellow clinicians, also means they are accessible to patients, the media, and other unintended recipients. Although no formal guideline exists specifically for social media use among genetic counselors, guidelines from other healthcare professions as well as a basic knowledge of what can be considered "identifying" information are helpful in using social media platforms efficiently and ethically (Choo et al., 2015). Obvious identifiers like name and date of birth should never be used publicly, but even more passive references to the date and time of appointment can be identifying. Sharing an anecdote that references a patient seen today or yesterday morning becomes even riskier in a public venue where all messages have a timestamp.

Genetic counselors may find themselves followed by their own patients or receiving requests from patients to connect on social media. Engaging with patients outside of the clinical sphere may impact patient–provider dynamics, create risks to privacy, and cause other harms, as well as violate hospital or other workplace policies governing social media usage by employees (Surani et al., 2017). Many genetic counselors maintain separate professional and personal social media presences, with the latter locked and requiring approval to view. Genetic counselors using social media under their professional identity should be mindful that they become a face for the entire profession and can influence public perceptions, though this also represents an opportunity to make the profession more visible and approachable to patients (Gallagher et al., 2016).

CONCLUSION

In less than 30 years, the internet has evolved from dial-up modems and basic email capabilities to an inexhaustible and instantaneous source of information. Clinicians and patients alike have incorporated the internet into their daily lives, in ways both mundane and potentially life changing. For the contemporary genetic counselor, the internet is an essential tool for clinical practice and a new source of professional challenges and ethical dilemmas. Significant advances in genetic testing have occurred alongside the growth of the internet, transforming the roles of genetic counselors in ways scarcely dreamed of when the profession was new. With all of the challenges of such rapid growth come new opportunities for career advancement and diversification and further democratization of access to genetic and genomic services. With further careful and considerate use of the internet in professional practice, genetic counseling is poised to continue its broad expansion into new roles and improved patient care.

References

Abrams, D. J., & Geier, M. R. (2006). A comparison of patient satisfaction with telehealth and on-site consultations: A pilot study for prenatal genetic counseling. *Journal of Genetic Counseling, 15*(3), 199–205.

Adam, S., Birch, P. H., Coe, R. R., Bansback, N., Jones, A. L., Connolly, M. B., Demos, M. K., Toyota, E. B., Farrer, M. J., & Friedman, J. M. (2018). Assessing an interactive online tool to support parents' genomic testing decisions. *Journal of Genetic Counseling, 28*(1), 10–17. https://doi.org/10.1007/s10897-018-0281-1

Allyse, M. A., Robinson, D. H., Ferber, M. J., & Sharp, R. R. (2018). Direct-to-consumer testing 2.0: Emerging models of direct-to-consumer genetic testing. *Mayo Clinic Proceedings, 93*(1), 113–120.

Ashford, M. (2019, July 26). *Invitae reflects on consumer-initiated test pilot, plans improvements to counseling outreach.* https://www.genomeweb.com/inherited-disease/invitae-reflects-consumer-initiated-test-pilot-plans-improvements-counseling

Badalato, L., Kalokairinou, L., & Borry, P. (2017). Third party interpretation of raw genetic data: An ethical exploration. *European Journal of Human Genetics, 25*(11), 1189–1194.

Baker, L., Wagner, T. H., Singer, S., & Bundorf, M. K. (2003). Use of the internet and e-mail for health care information: Results from a national survey. *JAMA, 289*(18), 2400–2406.

Bansil, P., Keenan, N. L., Zlot, A. I., & Gilliland, J. C. (2006). Health-related information on the web: Results from the HealthStyles Survey, 2002–2003. *Preventing Chronic Disease, 3*(2), A36.

Bentley, A. R., Callier, S., & Rotimi, C. N. (2017). Diversity and inclusion in genomic research: Why the uneven progress? *Journal of Community Genetics, 8*(4), 255–266.

Boise State University. (2018, October 24). *Boise State launches first fully online genetic counseling graduate program* [Press release]. https://www.boisestate.edu/news/2018/10/24/boise-state-launches-first-fully-online-genetic-counseling-graduate-program/

Broom, A. (2005). Virtually He@ Lthy: The impact of internet use on disease experience and the doctor-patient relationship. *Qualitative Health Research, 15*(3), 325–345.

Burgess, K. R., Carmany, E. P., & Trepanier, A. M. (2016). A comparison of telephone genetic counseling and in-person genetic counseling from the genetic counselor's perspective. *Journal of Genetic Counseling, 25*(1), 112–126.

Chen, A. (2017, November 20). *I paid $300 for DNA-based fitness advice and all I got was junk science.* The Verge. https://www.theverge.com/2017/11/20/16613650/helix-dna-testing-kit-fitness-genes-results-dnafit

Chisolm, M. S. (2015). Social media in medicine: The volume that Twitter built. *International Review of Psychiatry, 27*(2), 83–84.

Choo, E. K., Ranney, M. L., Chan, T. M., Trueger, N. S., Walsh, A. E., Tegtmeyer, K., McNamara, S. O., Choi, R. Y., & Carroll, C. L. (2015). Twitter as a tool for communication and knowledge exchange in academic medicine: A guide for skeptics and novices. *Medical Teacher, 37*(5), 411–416.

d'Agincourt-Canning, L., & McGillivray, B. (2008). Evaluation of genetic counseling for hereditary cancer by videoconference in British Columbia. *BC Med, 50*(10), 554–559. https://pdfs.semanticscholar.org/834f/71d69abb6e74f555c4dd56e8e0dd93d44a31.pdf

de Pauw, A., Schwartz, M., Colas, C., Golmard, L., & Stoppa-Lyonnet, D. (2020). Direct-to-consumer misleading information on cancer risks calls for an urgent clarification of health genetic testing performed by commercial companies. *European Journal of Cancer, 132*, 100–103.

Dias, R., & Torkamani, A. (2019). Artificial intelligence in clinical and genomic diagnostics. *Genome Medicine, 11*(1), 70.

Dijkstra, S., Kok, G., Ledford, J. G., Sandalova, E., & Stevelink, R. (2018). Possibilities and pitfalls of social media for translational medicine. *Frontiers of Medicine*, 5, 345.

Gallagher, L., McCuaig, J., Benoit, L., & Davies, C. (2016). It's time for the genetic counseling profession to embrace social media. *Journal of Genetic Counseling, 25*(6), 1338–1341.

Gordon, E. S., Babu, D., & Laney, D. A. (2018). The future is now: Technology's impact on the practice of genetic counseling. *American Journal of Medical Genetics Part C: Seminars in Medical Genetics, 178*(1), 15–23.

Gray, J., Brain, K., Iredale, R., Alderman, J., France, E., & Hughes, H. (2000). A pilot study of telegenetics. *Journal of Telemedicine and Telecare, 6*(4), 245–247.

Hopper, B., Buckman, M., & Edwards, M. (2011). Evaluation of satisfaction of parents with the use of videoconferencing for a pediatric genetic consultation. *Twin Research and Human Genetics, 14*(4), 343–346.

Hoskevec, J. M., Bennett, R. L., Carey, M. E., DaVanzo, J. E., Dougherty, M., Hahn, S. E., LeRoy, B. S., O'Neal, S., Richardson, J. G., & Wicklund, C. A. (2018). Projecting the supply and demand for certified genetic counselors: A workforce study. *Journal of Genetic Counseling, 27*, 16–20.

Hsieh, V., Braid, T., Gordon, E., & Hercher, L. (2020). Direct-to-consumer genetic testing companies tell their customers to "see a genetic counselor." How do genetic counselors feel about direct-to-consumer genetic testing? *Journal of Genetic Counseling, 86*, 359.

Kalokairinou, L., Howard, H. C., Slokenberga, S., Fisher, E., Flatscher-Thöni, M., Hartlev, M., van Hellemondt, R., Juškevičius, J., Kapelenska-Pregowska, J., Kováč, P., Lovrečić, L., Nys, H., de Paor, A., Phillips, A., Prudil, L., Rial-Sebbag, E., Romeo Casabona, C. M., Sándor, J., Schuster, . . . Borry, P. (2018). Legislation of direct-to-consumer genetic testing in Europe: A fragmented regulatory landscape. *Journal of Community Genetics, 9*(2), 117–132. https://doi.org/10.1007/s12687-017-0344-2

Kearney, E., Wojcik, A., & Babu, D. (2020). Artificial intelligence in genetic services delivery: Utopia or apocalypse? *Journal of Genetic Counseling, 29*(1), 8–17.

Libbrecht, M. W., & Noble, W. S. (2015). Machine learning applications in genetics and genomics. *Nature Reviews Genetics, 16*(6), 321–332.

MedlinePlus. (n.d.). *How can consumers be sure a genetic test is valid and useful?* https://medlineplus.gov/genetics/understanding/testing/validtest/

Millward, M., Tiller, J., Bogwitz, M., Kincaid, H., Taylor, S., Trainer, A. H., & Lacaze, P. (2020). Impact of direct-to-consumer genetic testing on Australian clinical genetics services. *European Journal of Medical Genetics, 63*(9), 103968.

Morgan, T., Schmidt, J., Haakonsen, C., Lewis, J., Della Rocca, M., Morrison, S., Biesecker, B., & Kaphingst, K. A. (2014). Using the internet to seek information about genetic and rare diseases: A case study comparing data from 2006 and 2011. *JMIR Research Protocols, 3*(1), e10.

Ordal, L. (2019). Social media for genetic counselors: Network, advance your career, and avoid common pitfalls. In *Hamilton Regional Genetic Counselling Conference* [Conference presentation], Hamilton, ON, Canada.

Regalado, A. (2019, February 11). More than 26 million people have taken an at-home ancestry test. *MIT Technology Review*. https://www.technologyreview.com/2019/02/11/103446/more-than-26-million-people-have-taken-an-at-home-ancestry-test/2

Roche, M. I., & Skinner, D. (2009). How parents search, interpret, and evaluate genetic information obtained from the internet. *Journal of Genetic Counseling, 18*(2), 119–129.

Savas, J. A., Huang, K. E., Moradi Tuchayi, S., & Feldman, S. R. (2014). Understanding the influence of social media in medicine: Lesson learned from Facebook. *Dermatology Online Journal*, *20*(9). https://www.ncbi.nlm.nih.gov/pubmed/25244178

Schaffer, R., Kuczynski, K., & Skinner, D. (2008). Producing genetic knowledge and citizenship through the internet: Mothers, pediatric genetics, and cybermedicine. *Sociology of Health & Illness*, *30*(1), 145–159.

Schorderet, D., & Aebischer, P. (1985). SYNDROC: Microcomputer based differential diagnosis of malformation patterns. *Archives of Disease in Childhood*, *60*(3), 248–251.

Skinner, D., & Schaffer, R. (2006). Families and genetic diagnoses in the genomic and internet age. *Infants & Young Children*, *19*(1), 16–24. https://doi.org/10.1097/00001163-200601000-00003

Surani, Z., Hirani, R., Elias, A., Quisenberry, L., Varon, J., Surani, S., & Surani, S. (2017). Social media usage among health care providers. *BMC Research Notes*, *10*(1), 654.

Tandy-Connor, S., Guiltinan, J., Krempely, K., LaDuca, H., Reineke, P., Gutierrez, S., Gray, P., & Tippin Davis, B. (2018). False-positive results released by direct-to-consumer genetic tests highlight the importance of clinical confirmation testing for appropriate patient care. *Genetics in Medicine*, *20*(12), 1515–1521.

Taylor, M. R., Alman, A., & Manchester, D. K. (2001). Use of the internet by patients and their families to obtain genetics-related information. *Mayo Clinic Proceedings*, *76*(8), 772–776.

Terry, A. B., Wylie, A., Raspa, M., Vogel, B., Sanghavi, K., Djurdjinovic, L., Caggana, M., & Bodurtha, J. (2019). Clinical models of telehealth in genetics: A regional telegenetics landscape. *Journal of Genetic Counseling*, *28*(3), 673–691.

Topf, J. M., & Hiremath, S. (2015). Social media, medicine and the modern journal club. *International Review of Psychiatry*, *27*(2), 147–154.

Vrečar, I., Hristovski, D., & Peterlin, B. (2017). Telegenetics: An update on availability and use of telemedicine in clinical genetics service. *Journal of Medical Systems*, *41*(2), 21.

Weissman, S. M., Zellmer, K., Gill, N., & Wham, D. (2018). Implementing a virtual health telemedicine program in a community setting. *Journal of Genetic Counseling*, *27*(2), 323–325.

Yip, C. H., Evans, D. G., Agarwal, G., Buccimazza, I., Kwong, A., Morant, R., Prakash, I., Song, C. Y., Taib, N. A., Tausch, C., Ung, O., & Meterissian, S. (2019). Global disparities in breast cancer genetics testing, counselling and management. *World Journal of Surgery*, *43*(5), 1264–1270.

Zierhut, H. A., MacFarlane, I. M., Ahmed, Z., & Davies, J. (2018). Genetic counselors' experiences and interest in telegenetics and remote counseling. *Journal of Genetic Counseling*, *27*(2), 329–338.

PART V

NORMATIVE CONCEPTS AND ETHICAL ISSUES IN GENETIC COUNSELING

CHAPTER 23

NONDIRECTIVENESS IN GENETIC COUNSELING

Conceptual and Normative Dimensions

MICHAEL J. DEEM

Introduction: The Many Notions of Nondirectiveness

When one considers the ethics of genetic counseling, the concept of nondirectiveness is likely to come first to mind. Historically, genetic counseling has placed a strong emphasis on taking a nondirective approach to providing the results of genetic tests to patients and assisting them in making decisions in light of this information.[1] Yet, despite this broad familiarity with the idea of nondirectiveness within genetic counseling and the central role that it has seemingly played in guiding the practice of genetic counseling from the earliest phases of its professionalization, debate persists among genetic counselors and ethicists over what precisely the term "nondirectiveness" means, what exactly it demands of genetic counselors, when a "nondirective approach" is appropriate in practice, and whether alternative counseling techniques might be more appropriate for facilitating informed decision making and attending to patients' psychosocial well-being.

A survey of the genetic counseling literature shows how differently nondirectiveness has been conceived—historically and presently—among genetic counselors and ethicists. Broadly speaking, nondirectiveness has been understood minimally to require that genetic

[1] The convention of characterizing the recipients of genetic counseling services as "clients" rather than as "patients" remains commonplace in the field and in the literature. I will opt for referring to the recipients of genetic counseling services as "patients" throughout this chapter, given much of the field's focus on counseling individuals (including providing care for psychosocial well-being) within healthcare or health-related contexts, and given the many genetic counseling contexts that are directly involved with or ancillary to health care. This is not to suggest that all genetic counseling services are oriented toward these goals but rather that the term "patient" generally is an appropriate term for referring to recipients of such services.

counselors educate and guide their patients in a manner that is free from bias or coercion, enabling patients to make decisions consistent with their own beliefs, preferences, and values (Baumiller et al., 1996; Fraser, 1974; Stoll & Jackson, 2020). However, while widely accepted as far as it goes, this conception does little more than restate the general requirements of an even more familiar ethical principle, namely, respect for patient autonomy. Beyond this very general notion of autonomy promotion, there is considerable ambiguity and even confusion surrounding the meaning and role of "nondirectiveness." Consider, for example, a published summary of the qualitative results of a focus group study of practicing genetic counselors' perspectives on the place of nondirectiveness within the profession (Weil et al., 2006). In this single publication, nondirectiveness is variously characterized as a "guiding principle," a "guideline," an "ethical stance," a "central tenet," the field's "central ethos," a "value-laden approach" to counseling, a "goal at which to strive," and a "model" of counseling. Despite this conceptional and terminological ambiguity, genetic counselors generally give continued, albeit qualified, support for adherence to nondirectiveness in practice (Bartels et al., 1997; Conrad & Stanley, 2015; Weil et al., 2006; Wertz & Fletcher, 1988).

Among the various and nonequivalent characterizations of nondirectiveness within the genetic counseling literature, there is a discernable focus on the normative character of the concept. For example, nondirectiveness has been characterized as a "central tenet" of genetic counseling (Fine, 1993, p. 101), as the "most universally espoused norm in genetic counseling literature" (Bartels et al., 1997, p. 173), and as a "guiding principle" of genetic counseling (Weil, 2003, p. 199). These characterizations point to something *normative* about nondirectiveness; that is, nondirectiveness *requires* or *demands* something, ethically speaking, of genetic counselors. It is widely viewed as an integral component of respect and support for patient autonomy within genetic counseling contexts, especially in cases where decisions and actions are highly personal or may affect the interests and well-being of family members (Bosk, 1993; Conrad & Stanley, 2015; LeRoy, 1993). This suggests that nondirectiveness continues to play some role in guiding genetic counselors' interaction with patients, as a *norm* of the profession.[2]

[2] Some genetic counselors have characterized nondirectiveness as the "central ethos of genetic counseling" (Weil, 2003, p. 199; Weil et al., 2006), as "the most defining feature of genetic counseling" (Walker, 2009, p. 10), and, even less clearly, as a "counseling technique" (Resta, 2021, p. 15). It seems that such characterizations maintain tacitly a connection between nondirectiveness in genetic counseling and nondirective Rogerian psychotherapy, from which genetic counseling loosely adopted the term "nondirectiveness." But these characterizations appear to neglect the rather significant distinction between genetic counseling's *facilitating* a patient's autonomous healthcare decision through the provision and elucidation of information that a patient does not already possess and Rogerian psychotherapy's *removing* obstacles to patients' motivation to actualize their own latent potential for freedom and healing. So, while it may make sense to describe the ethos and defining feature of Rogerian psychotherapy as "nondirectiveness," genetic counseling involves significantly active roles for genetic counselors in providing information, delineating outcomes, and setting boundaries for discourse with patients. Moreover, as a form of healthcare provision, genetic counseling signals to patients that there are discreet goals (e.g., health, well-being, mitigation of risk of harm) toward which the field aims. In contrast, Rogerian psychotherapy signals no such pre-established, specified goals in the clinical encounter. For these reasons (and perhaps more), it would be appropriate for genetic counseling to shed conceptions of nondirectiveness as an "ethos," a "technique," or a "defining feature," as simply a residual holdover from Rogerian psychotherapy.

In this chapter, I clarify the conceptual and normative dimensions of nondirectiveness, with a particular aim to arrive at a plausible conception of the norm that does justice both to the moral intuitions that animated genetic counseling acceptance of this norm and to the most salient features of clinical encounters between genetic counselors and patients. To accomplish this aim, I present two main arguments. First, I assess the strengths and weaknesses of what I am calling "autonomy-based" conceptions of nondirectiveness, which Seymour Kessler and Jon Weil develop in their important work on the ethics and practice of genetic counseling. Kessler and Weil reject the traditional conception of the norm of nondirectiveness, which requires that genetic counselors remain "value neutral" in their communication with patients about diagnostic information, risk assessment, and available treatment modalities. Kessler and Weil recast the norm of nondirectiveness in terms of response to patients' psychosocial needs and enhancing their autonomy. While I am sympathetic to their efforts to rethink nondirectiveness, I argue that their conception of nondirectiveness fails to provide adequate guidance for the protection and promotion of autonomy in genetic counseling contexts. More importantly, their respective conceptions leave genetic counselors with less, not more, clarity about the role that nondirectiveness should play in their practice. Second, I begin the positive task of identifying which features of genetic counseling might ground a *special* duty to safeguard patient decision making beyond prohibiting direct coercion, manipulation, and undue influence—actions that are considered to be ethically problematic in most clinical contexts. In other words, if nondirectiveness is a specifiable norm within genetic counseling, then its prescriptions must likewise be more specific than those that fall under our broad notions of the principle of respect for patient autonomy. I identify two such grounding features, which obtain commonly—but not exclusively—in genetic counseling encounters, namely, epistemic dependence and patient trust, which are typically present to a degree higher in genetic counseling than most other clinical contexts. I argue that nondirectiveness is best understood conceptually as a formal constraint on the interactions between genetic counselors and patients that aims at augmenting patients' decisional authority while restricting counselors from exploiting their discretionary authority in the facilitation of patient decisions. Understood in this way, the norm of nondirectiveness retains the prohibitive profile of the traditional value-neutral conception, avoids the problem of indeterminacy that Kessler's and Weil's autonomy-based conceptions of nondirectiveness face, and affirms the profession's aim of facilitating informed decisions that patients recognize as genuinely their own.

Value Neutrality: Noble Goal or Unfortunate Overcorrection?

Historically, debates over the role of nondirectiveness in genetic counseling practice tended to focus on whether the norm requires that a genetic counselor refrain from bringing their own ethical commitments into a counseling encounter. For convenience, let us call the view that nondirectiveness prohibits genetic counselors from bringing their own ethical commitments to bear on conversations with patients the "value-neutral conception" of nondirectiveness. The value-neutral conception was the result of several historical and normative factors during the early developmental phases of the genetic counseling profession. Genetic counselors and clinical geneticists consciously sought to disassociate their practice from earlier forms of applied genetics that aimed to reduce and prevent incidences of genetically linked disorders within the population. In the wake of the demise of social eugenics programs, genetic counseling initially oriented itself toward communicating and clarifying diagnostic information and risk assessments regarding occurrence or reoccurrence of genetic or chromosomal abnormalities (Fine, 1993; Resta, 1997; Sorenson, 1993; Stern, 2012; Walker, 2009).[3] Therapeutic decisions were largely left to the patient, in part due to lingering concern to avoid any semblance of eugenic coercion in the fledgling practice. However, the absence at the time of treatments for many diagnosable genetic disorders and the only prevention for such disorders in most cases being elective abortion also contributed to a reluctance on the part of genetic counselors to provide recommendations to patients.

Genetic counseling's emergence as a profession also coincided with increased concern within the broader medical community about the potential and actual harms of medical paternalism and lack of protection for human subjects participating in medical research. Medical research in the United States was just coming to terms with the gross abuses of the Tuskegee syphilis study, and the World Medical Association Declaration of Helsinki raised international concern about undue paternalism in both clinical care and research. This intensified concern over protecting the autonomy of patients and research participants, coupled with the conscious distancing from eugenics programs, served as the backdrop to genetic counseling's early lurch toward value neutrality.

Historical accounts aside, genetic counseling maintained an uneasy commitment to keeping "values" out of genetic counseling practice. Some genetic counselors and ethicists have contended that value neutrality was always an impossible goal to achieve in genetic counseling, arguing that the offer or recommendation of particular kinds of genetic screening or testing for medically labeled groups (e.g., prenatal genetic screening for women of "advanced maternal age") is itself a value-laden practice. This is because the offer or recommendation of screening or testing in a healthcare context may suggest to patients either that the conditions that these tools detect are *bad* or *to be avoided* or that these services should be regarded as *beneficial* for the patient. Such offers, these commentators suggest, may tacitly recommend that testing *ought* to be done and that patients *should* factor positive diagnostic results into their decision making (Clarke, 1991, 1997; Lippman, 1991).[4] Moreover, these commentators note that genetic counseling is structured and governed by a very specific value—namely, the value of *patient autonomy*—so there can be no pretense of

[3] For a historical retelling of genetic counseling's emergence after, and conscientious differentiation from, social eugenics programs, see Chapter 1 in this volume by Devon Stillwell.

[4] Additionally, the earliest contexts of genetic counseling took place within prenatal care. Insofar as elective abortion was an option that genetic counselors might present to patients in light of abnormal screening or testing results, the profession may have conveyed initially that it endorsed a specific value judgment, namely, that abortion after diagnosis of a genetically linked condition is *morally permissible*. This, in part, led to concerns that genetic counseling as a profession risked embodying bias toward disability (and thus indirectly toward persons living with disability). For more on disability critiques of genetic counseling and potential stigmatization of individuals with disability, see Chapter 31 by Elizabeth Dietz and Joel Michael Reynolds and Chapter 32 by Angus Clarke in this volume.

value neutrality with respect to the structure or to the practice (Sorenson, 1993; Wachbroit & Wasserman, 1995).

Other commentators have characterized value neutrality primarily as a constraint on the counselor's interaction with patients. Traditionally, the demands of value neutrality in genetic counseling have been taken to extend beyond the prohibition of coercion or undue influence. Value neutrality has been thought also to require that genetic counselors refrain from guiding patients through the ethical terrain of decision making, as well as from providing advice or recommending specific goals to patients, even if such advice or guidance was expressly requested or thought by the genetic counselor to be in the patient's best interest (Bernhardt, 1997; Davis, 2010; Weil, 2003).[5] The value-neutral conception of nondirectiveness has been roundly criticized for a number of reasons. First, aspiring to value neutrality in practice effectively reduces the counselor's role to that of mere "fact provider" or "information provider" (Bosk, 1993, p. 34), placing the full burden of ethical deliberation and decision making on the patient. Second, a value-neutral approach to counseling restricts the genetic counselor's ability to attend to patients' psychosocial needs and provide what many take to be critical guidance for patients who struggle with reaching a decision after a positive diagnosis or troubling risk assessment (Caplan, 1993; Oduncu, 2002; Weil, 2000; White, 1999). Several empirical studies of genetic counselors' attitudes toward value neutrality indicate that counselors frequently feel that value neutrality is not always appropriate, especially when patients struggle with decisions and appeal for guidance, or when the counselor feels that a particular decision may not be in a patient's best interest (Bartels et al., 1997; Burke & Kolker, 1994; Michie et al., 1997; Weil et al., 2006; Williams et al., 2002). Third, as genetic counseling is further integrated into healthcare contexts in which there are specified goals of care—for example, pediatrics or oncology—it may be inappropriate for the genetic counselor to abscond from clarifying how a genetic diagnosis might affect clinical care or recommending courses of action consonant with patients' current medical management in such contexts (Walker, 2009).

It is little surprise, then, that the genetic counseling literature presently reflects the view that value neutrality is neither a feasible nor a desirable constraint on genetic counseling practice. However, the rejection of value neutrality raises several questions about the broader concept of nondirectiveness. While nondirectiveness has historically been closely associated with value neutrality, does the former conceptually entail the latter? If so, then a rejection of value neutrality is also a rejection of nondirectiveness. But if nondirectiveness does not entail value neutrality, what constraints does nondirectiveness place on genetic counseling practice, particularly with respect to advising patients and promoting particular values and therapeutic goals? One influential approach to answering these questions has been offered by Kessler and Weil. In elucidating the concept of nondirectiveness, each shifts away from concerns over the appropriateness of expressing value judgments and offering

[5] Some characterize value neutrality as a "morally neutral attitude about the particular choices [patients] may eventually make" (Yarborough et al., 1989, p. 140) or a "morally neutral posture overall" (Gervais, 1993, p. 119). When conceived as a constraint not on the genetic counselors' *interactions* with patients but on genetic counselors' attitudes or stances toward patients' deliberations and decisions, value neutrality is clearly an unrealistic goal of practice. It is one thing to constrain a counselor's behavior during counseling; it is quite another to constrain the content of a genetic counselor's psychological states during counseling.

advice and toward shaping and developing counseling techniques that effectively promote patient autonomy.

Autonomy-Based Conceptions of Nondirectiveness

Expressing dissatisfaction with the traditional value-neutral conception of nondirectiveness, Kessler (1997, 2001) and Weil (2000, 2003) have developed alternative conceptions of nondirectiveness that highlight the positive responsibilities connected to support and respect for patient autonomy. In contrast to value-neutral conceptions of nondirectiveness, which specify what genetics counselors ought *not* to do, Kessler's and Weil's positive conceptions of nondirectiveness urge counselors to utilize their extensive knowledge, experience, and counseling skills to promote informed decision making, offer sound clinical and personal advice to patients, and attend to patients' psychosocial well-being. Kessler and Weil contend that their positive conceptions avoid many of the practical difficulties that confront the value-neutral conception of nondirectiveness, while still respecting and promoting patient autonomy.

Kessler takes aim at the prohibitive nature of the value-neutral conception of nondirectiveness. His main contention is that the value-neutral approach is too restrictive on counseling techniques and impedes rather than enhances patients' ability to reach their own decisions. The genetic counselor's effort to remain value neutral in communication with patients, Kessler (1997) contends, "does not necessarily give [patients] a way of thinking about the information they receive," and it "tends to emphasize the professional's authority and knowledge, factors which tend to foster psychological passivity in [patients]" (p. 167). He views value neutrality as an obstacle to patients' deliberation and action, and he claims that it "interferes with their evaluative processes and self-directiveness and tends to increase their dependency on professional advice" (Kessler, 1997, p. 167). Thus, according to Kessler, value neutrality ends up working against the very goals it is supposed to achieve. He takes these points to support a view of nondirectiveness that does not restrict the counselor from actively guiding patients toward a decision. He proposes the following alternative to the value-neutral conception: "[Nondirectiveness] refers to any procedure used in genetic services that promotes the autonomy and self-directedness of the [patient]" (Kessler, 2001, p. 188). Let us call this the "autonomy-based conception" of nondirectiveness.

Kessler's autonomy-based conception of nondirectiveness retains genetic counseling's traditional commitment to ensuring that a patient's decision is informed, voluntary, and reflective of the patient's own values. But, in framing nondirectiveness in terms of autonomy promotion, Kessler pivots away from the question of what a genetic counselor should refrain from doing (e.g., providing advice or expressing value judgments) and toward the question of how the counselor can best support and promote autonomous decision making in patients. As Kessler (1997) puts it: "By themselves disparate behaviors, such as giving directions, conveying information, making health-promoting suggestions, giving 'bad' news, giving advice, and expressing one's biases, are neither directive nor [non] directive. With the introduction of deception and coercive techniques, these activities become directive" (p. 167). Kessler envisages a more active and advisory role for genetic counselors than that of mere information providers, freeing them to attend to patients' psychosocial well-being and to address directly the ethically salient features of counseling encounters. Rather than avoid responding to deeply personal or ethical concerns patients might raise—including queries about what the counselor might do if in the same position as the patient—the genetic counselor might discern appropriate ways to express attitudes and views about the patient's worries, available treatment modalities, and the practical and normative implications of particular decisions. Kessler (1997) contends that this approach to counseling will provide patients with "greater control over their lives and decisions" than will a value-neutral approach (p. 167).

Now, on any plausible interpretation of the principle of respect for patient autonomy, intentional deception and withholding of information pertinent to patient decision making are morally problematic. So too are tactics that involve direct coercion, such as threats to patient interests, aggressive persuasion, or undue influence toward a particular outcome. It is not clear, then, what requirements Kessler's autonomy-based conception of nondirectiveness imposes on genetic counseling beyond *those already recognized* as entailed by the principle of respect for autonomy. Indeterminacy, it seems, is the tradeoff for Kessler's insistence that genetic counselors deploy the full scope of their counseling competencies.

Weil (2003), who is broadly sympathetic to Kessler's view, seems to detect as much. He suggests that genetic counseling should retain the normative commitments of the autonomy-based conception but drop the term "nondirectiveness" from its lexicon. Drawing directly from Kessler, but without using the term, Weil (2003) suggests that a "guiding principle for genetic counseling should be to promote the autonomy and self-directiveness of the [patient]" (p. 204). Weil (2003) suggests that this reformulation of Kessler's proposal "loses nothing in terms of its contribution to a discussion of genetic counseling," yet it carries the advantage of avoiding the "inhibiting" connotations historically associated with the term "nondirectiveness" (p. 204). Weil suggests that the central ethical concern of genetic counseling should be the development of effective counseling techniques for the promotion of patient autonomy and self-directed choice. But Weil goes further, recommending that nondirectiveness be replaced as the central guiding norm of genetic counseling practice by the following principle: "The central ethos of genetic counseling should be to bring the psychosocial component into every aspect of the work" (Weil, 2003, p. 207). This approach, which Weil calls "psychosocial genetic counseling," involves tailoring the counseling strategy to the needs, hopes, and preferences of the individual patient and determining what kind and degree of counseling intervention is needed according to such factors as the medical context in which a genetic counseling referral is made, the patient's psychological and emotional response to referral, and the subsequent presentation and receipt of genetic services.

Weil's approach certainly permits considerable flexibility with respect to which counseling techniques counselors choose to employ, how genetic counselors address the psychosocial well-being of patients, and the manner in which they respond to the particularities of counseling contexts. Further, Weil's approach sanctions the development and deployment of a range of techniques that promote patient autonomy without the burden of second-guessing the appropriateness of offering advice or recommending specific treatment modalities to patients.

A Norm or an Approach?

While Kessler's and Weil's autonomy-based conceptions of nondirectiveness bear many attractive features, they face their own set of difficulties. First, consider again Kessler's characterization of nondirectiveness: Nondirectiveness refers to any procedure used in genetic services that promotes the autonomy and self-directedness of the patient. This characterization seems to entail that traditionally distinct genetic counseling norms, such as respect for patient privacy and protection of patient confidentiality, count as instances of nondirectiveness. This is because these norms have traditionally been understood as specifications of the broader principle of respect for patient autonomy, each promoting and protecting patient autonomy within a different area of genetic counseling. Nondirectiveness is but one norm governing interactions between genetic counselors and patients, while norms of respect for privacy and protection of confidentiality typically govern quite different activities—data storage and sharing and medical record keeping, for example. By characterizing *any* procedure that promotes autonomy as an instance of nondirectiveness, Kessler's account blurs the conceptual and practical lines between distinct norms of genetic counseling specifically and clinical care more generally.

This leads us to a second problem with Kessler's conception of nondirectiveness. Kessler's view appears to collapse nondirectiveness into the broader ethical principle of respect for patient autonomy. The result is a conception of nondirectiveness that is too indeterminate to guide genetic counselors' interaction with their patients. To see that this is the case, let us consider the role subsidiary norms play in the application of general ethical principles to the contexts in which they are invoked. General ethical principles, such as the principle of respect for patient autonomy or the principle of beneficence, lack the specificity needed to serve as guides for practical deliberation and judgment in light of the facts of particular cases. While general ethical principles serve to provide a normative framework for ethical deliberation, more specific norms are needed to guide and evaluate actions.

Many philosophers and bioethicists thus formulate subsidiary norms within these frameworks to move from general ethical principles to particular ethical judgments about these cases (Audi, 2004; O'Neill, 2001). To show how this move might be made within genetic counseling without raising a worry about question begging, let us consider a medical context far removed from the domain of genetic counseling: determining what is a just allocation of organs for transplantation. Ruth Macklin (2015) argues that judgments about the ethical allocation of organs for transplantation require guidance from norms of greater specificity than the principle of justice. To determine what a just allocation scheme for organ transplantation would look like, we might appeal to subsidiary norms such as the norm of first come first served, the norm of fair innings (organs should be allotted to younger patients prior to older patients), or the norm of urgent need (allocation should be ordered according to who will deteriorate or die first if the organ is not allocated to them). These norms are purportedly based on the broad principle of justice, and they provide more specific guidance for moving from the principle to particular ethical judgments about allocation of transplantable organs. This case brings an important aspect of the formulation of subsidiary norms into relief: It need not be the case that the ground of each of these aforementioned norms is present in every case of organ allocation. We can imagine a case in which, say, two patients require immediate heart transplantation for survival, but only one heart is available. Without the transplant, each is expected to die at roughly the same point in time. In this case, the facts that ground a norm of urgent need are not present (though perhaps grounds for other subsidiary norms are present—e.g., one patient is an adolescent and the other, an octogenarian). The application of the subsidiary norm of urgent need thus varies according to the specific facts of a given case (e.g., age of eligible organ recipients, degree of scarcity, severity of need). Generalizing from Macklin's example, we see that subsidiary norms have variable applicability across cases in which their base principle is invoked. Thus, whether a subsidiary norm obtains depends not just on whether the general principle on which it is based applies, but also on whether the facts that ground a duty to adhere to the norm are present.

Returning to the norm of nondirectiveness, it seems that it is best characterized as a subsidiary norm whose basis is the general principle of respect for patient autonomy, rather than as a principle or "central tenet" of genetic counseling. Recall that the value-neutral conception of nondirectiveness, while susceptible to many of the critiques issued by Kessler and Weil, also takes the shape of a subsidiary norm, providing guidance for identifying genetic counseling techniques that inappropriately impinge on patient autonomy. While I am broadly sympathetic to these critiques of this conception of nondirectiveness, the alternative autonomy-based conception loses the specificity we desire of subsidiary norms. An unfortunate consequence of defining the norm of nondirectiveness in terms of the more general principle of respect for patient autonomy, then, is the loss of action guidance beyond broad duties that are inferable from the principle itself.

The principle of respect for patient autonomy states a very broad, general requirement for genetic counseling practice. To be sure, it is not so broad as to preclude any derivation of duties or specification of act types that violate it. For example, we can plausibly take counseling tactics that involve coercion, manipulation, or deception as violations of the principle. And these are precisely the sorts of actions that Kessler identifies as running afoul of nondirectiveness. But beyond serving as a starting point for determining which act types are ethically problematic, the principle of respect for patient autonomy provides little direct action guidance for the genetic counselor. It is difficult to see how additional requirements or constraints on genetic counseling practice can be derived strictly on the basis of Kessler's conception of nondirectiveness. The autonomy-based conception, thus, seems to have the unfortunate effect of rendering the norm too indeterminate to provide specific guidance within the counselor's interaction with patients. The foregoing considerations also bear on Weil's proposal that nondirectiveness be supplanted as the central tenet of genetic counseling. While Weil wishes to shed the label "nondirectiveness," he retains the content of Kessler's autonomy-based conception of nondirectiveness, thereby inheriting the same indeterminacy problem.

We have seen that subsidiary norms are formulated on the basis of general ethical principles in response to the particular facts of the contexts in which the principles are invoked. We have also seen that subsidiary norms are variably applicable in these contexts; we might have two cases in which we invoke the principle of respect for patient autonomy, but divergent features of these cases may result in our relying on different subsidiary norms to move from the principle to a particular ethical judgment. This is no less true of genetic counseling cases. For example, the norm of respecting patient confidentiality, but likely not the norm of nondirectiveness, would apply to cases where a patient's genetic information is sought by a third party to whom disclosure by the counselor has not been authorized. While both norms are unified by, and formed on the basis of, the principle of respect for patient autonomy, the determination of which subsidiary norms to apply is in large part determined by the features of the cases to which we direct our ethical analysis. It is not clear, then, what it would mean for nondirectiveness—or any subsidiary norm, for that matter—to be the "central tenet" or "ethos" of genetic counseling.[6] And this is one of the key insights at which Weil arrives in his analysis of nondirectiveness. While he does not utilize the language of subsidiary norms, his psychosocial approach to counseling implies that the norm of nondirectiveness is *but one* subsidiary norm governing the practice of genetic counseling.

Nondirectiveness as a Formal Constraint on Genetic Counseling Practice

Recall that the traditional justification for the norm of nondirectiveness in genetic counseling is that adherence to this norm is one way in which counselors respect and promote patient autonomy in decision making. If nondirectiveness is subsidiary to the principle of respect for patient autonomy, as I have argued above, then we might ask what the scope of the norm is. We have already seen that its scope is narrower than that of the principle of respect for patient autonomy; there are domains within genetic counseling where the norm need not be invoked (e.g., maintaining confidentiality of medical records, protecting patient privacy). Given that the concept of nondirectiveness is linked to the facilitation of patient decisions, it is reasonable to take its scope to extend to genetic counseling scenarios involving decision making. This conclusion must be stated here provisionally, however, for we still must identify which particular facts ground a duty of nondirectiveness as well as determine whether this ground is always present in such scenarios.

Nondirectiveness is meant to serve as a safeguard against counseling techniques that impair or interdict patients' autonomous decision making. An assumption that underlies the perceived need for this safeguard is that the exercise of patient autonomy is somehow rendered vulnerable within the interaction between genetic counselors and their patients. It is widely acknowledged among philosophers and bioethicists that situations in which individuals are in a heightened state of vulnerability to harm or impaired agency demand some sort of moral response (Hurst, 2008; Rogers et al., 2012; Straehle, 2016). This response might be directed toward the remediation or mitigation of the sources of vulnerability, or it might be aimed at constraining certain actions that exacerbate vulnerability. We can view nondirectiveness as a moral response of the latter sort since it is meant to constrain actions that increase or exploit the vulnerability of patients in genetic counseling contexts. To be sure, our capacity for making our own decisions and acting in accordance with them is vulnerable to myriad interpersonal and social factors in our everyday lives, be it aggressive consumer marketing, the pressures of social conformity, or strong familial expectations

[6] It may even be that the claim that nondirectiveness has historically been taken to be the central ethos of genetic counseling is false, as Biesecker (2003) contends.

for our practical lives. But we generally do not think that such autonomy-compromising factors warrant a special moral response along the lines of nondirectiveness. What, then, are the interpersonal conditions of genetic counseling that constitute sources of patient vulnerability in decision making, such that a special moral response is required by the genetic counselor? Here I identify two, epistemic dependence and patient trust, which seem to be present in most, if not all, genetic counseling scenarios involving patient decision making.

Genetic counseling often involves the presentation and clarification of technical diagnostic, risk, or therapeutic information in the service of placing patients in positions to make informed decisions. These decisions regard a wide range of outcomes, from treatment and management modalities, to commencement and continuation of medical surveillance, to disclosure of genetic information within families. Information about genetic and chromosomal abnormalities, gene–disease associations, and genetic risk assessment is typically highly complex, placing patients in an epistemic dependency relation to the counselor. The patient is thus in a position of significant reliance on the genetic counselor's competence, ability, and willingness to present and elucidate that information in such a way that the patient can make an informed, autonomous decision. Empirical studies of genetic literacy in the general population bear out the degree to which patients are epistemically dependent on the genetic counselor. Several studies show that despite the general public's awareness of the proliferation and clinical application of genetic technologies, its understanding of genetic concepts and information, genetic risk, and clinical management of genetically linked disorders remains low (Haga et al., 2013; Lanie et al., 2004; Lea et al., 2011; Syurina et al., 2011). Thus, a significant knowledge and power differential between genetic counselors and their patients typically occurs within genetic counseling contexts. This differential may undermine a patient's autonomy in decision making, since the high degree of epistemic dependence on the genetic counselor renders vulnerable patients' ability to make decisions that are informed and voluntary. Patients may perceive themselves as incapable of processing and acting on complex diagnostic information or risk assessments. This might further lead to patients experiencing the debilitating effects of self-doubt and self-distrust regarding their capacity to deliberate and reach an appropriate decision. Moreover, in recognizing the genetic counselor's epistemic authority within the domain of genetic counseling, patients may feel inclined or even compelled to cede their decision-making authority to the counselor.

Does this show, then, that the kind of vulnerability to which epistemic dependence gives rise in genetic counseling demands a special safeguard for patient autonomy? Some philosophers argue that the abdication of decision-making authority in clinical contexts need not undermine a patient's autonomy. For example, James Childress (1993) suggests that patients may choose "to yield to their physicians when medical treatment is proposed," but "if a person autonomously chooses to yield first-order decision making . . . that person has exercised what may be called second-order autonomy" (p. 13). No special safeguard for patient autonomy beyond duties to refrain from coercion, manipulation, and undue influence seems called for in such scenarios. Would this also, then, be the case for a patient who yields decision-making authority to the genetic counselor? There are reasons against reaching this conclusion, when we consider the degree to which a patient is epistemically dependent on a genetic counselor.

When we consider epistemic dependence within genetic counseling, and especially in conjunction with a second feature of counselor–patient interaction that places patient autonomy at risk, it is evident that the ground of a special duty to safeguard patient autonomy is typically present in counseling scenarios where patients must make decisions about the genetic information they receive. This second feature, to which I now turn, is patient trust. In her now-classic article on the nature of trust, Annette Baier (1986) warns that "exploitation and conspiracy, as much as justice and fellowship, thrive better in an atmosphere of trust" (p. 231–232). While trust enables us to build interpersonal relationships that importantly contribute to our well-being, it also opens us up to the risk of being disappointed, betrayed, or exploited. There are two salient features of the trust relation that I wish to focus on here. First, trust involves an attitude of optimism on the part of one who trusts toward the competence of the one trusted to perform the expected task or fulfill the expected role (Jones, 1996; McLeod, 2002). Second, trust involves an expectation that the trusted one is committed to fulfilling that role (Hawley, 2014). Naturally, patients trust that genetic counselors possess a sufficient degree of competence with respect to understanding and effectively communicating information about genetic diagnosis, genetic risk, and available options for treatment. And patients trust that the counselor will fulfill the roles and duties associated with their professional identity, particularly those that govern interaction with patients. Many of these duties overlap with those associated with other professional roles in healthcare, including positive duties of fidelity and truth telling and prohibitive duties to refrain from coercion, manipulation, or withholding information that will impact decisions about medical management. But what professional aims are specific to the genetic counseling profession such that patients would expect the counselor to fulfill them? The NSGC Code of Ethics states seven such aims, ranging from the explanation of services that genetic counselors provide to the protection of patient confidentiality. Two in particular are relevant to counselor–patient interaction and patient decision making: "Respect their patients' beliefs, inclinations, circumstances, feelings, family relationships and cultural traditions" and "Enable their patients to make informed decisions, free of coercion, by providing or illuminating the necessary facts, and clarifying the alternatives and anticipated consequences" (National Society of Genetic Counselors, 2017). We can plausibly infer that, according to these stated aims, the primary goal of counselor–patient interaction is an informed decision that is expressive of the patient's *own* commitments and values and that does not necessarily depend on the genetic counselors' beliefs, attitudes, or feelings about how the patient should respond to genetic information. Thus, patient trust in genetic counseling (ideally) involves the expectation that the counselor will facilitate decisions that bear these *formal* features.

Patients grant to the genetic counselor discretionary authority in guiding the process through which these features are expected to obtain, rendering the former vulnerable to potential deviation from that process at the hands of the latter. Genetic counselors, then, have a duty to attend to this form of patient vulnerability by safeguarding the process from inappropriate deviations from the expected outcome. Together, then, epistemic dependence and trust in genetic counseling render a patient's capacity to make and act upon autonomous decisions vulnerable. Where does this leave us with respect to the question of the nature and scope of nondirectiveness in genetic counseling? We have seen that patients are vulnerable in virtue of both their epistemic dependence on the expertise of the genetic counselor and the trust they place in the genetic counselor's commitment to the stated goals of the profession. Strong epistemic dependence places the patient at risk of developing an overly deferential stance toward, and of ceding decisional authority to, the genetic counselor. The discretionary authority that the patient grants to the genetic counselor renders the patient vulnerable to the manner in which the counselor guides the process of decision making. Jointly, epistemic dependence and trust engender a special kind of vulnerability, constituting the ground of a duty to safeguard patient autonomy through this process. And, traditionally, that safeguard has been understood to be nondirectiveness.

The norm of nondirectiveness, then, should not be understood as a *contentual* constraint on the facilitation of the patient's autonomous decisions. While the value-neutral conception of nondirectiveness correctly views the norm as a constraint, it focuses only on the *content* of the communication between counselor and patient, thereby failing to attend to the ways in which the very features of genetic counseling contexts might undermine patient autonomy. Perhaps a more fruitful way of conceiving of nondirectiveness is to understand it as a *formal* constraint on the process of facilitating autonomous decision making. In addition to serving as a corrective to the value-neutral conception, conceiving nondirectiveness as a formal constraint provides the norm with the specificity that Kessler's and Weil's autonomy-based conceptions lack. Corresponding to epistemic dependence, nondirectiveness prohibits counselors from acceding to patients' decisional authority. And corresponding to patient trust, nondirectiveness prohibits counselors from abusing their discretionary authority and failing to facilitate informed decisions that the patient regards as truly their own.

We can now see that the scope of nondirectiveness extends to those genetic counseling scenarios in which patient decision making is among the primary aims. This is because the ground of the duty to adhere to nondirectiveness—epistemic dependence and patient trust—is present in virtually all of these scenarios. The ubiquity of this ground, however, does not entail that nondirectiveness carries a presumptive priority above other norms of genetic counseling, nor does it imply that other principles or norms are less important than the norm of nondirectiveness. Because nondirectiveness is only a formal constraint on counselor–patient interaction—though, as we have seen, a morally important one—it is compatible with views such as Kessler's and Weil's that emphasize positive duties toward patients, and even with recent views that healthcare provision is contrained by human goods such as health and preservation of life (Curlin & Tollefsen, 2021).

One might object that characterizing nondirectiveness in this formal way, with little constraint placed on the content of genetic counseling communication, evades the very purpose of the norm—to protect and promote patient autonomy. But this objection may rest on a thin conception of autonomy as nothing more than freedom from constraints or external influences on choice. Indeed, the value-neutral conception of autonomy seems largely to rest on this notion of autonomy. However, in our practical lives, our values, preferences, and interests are strongly shaped by our social environments, so much so that the idea of a pure, unadulterated "choice" originating solely in the individual chooser seems mythic. Feminist reflections on autonomy have led to a more realistic picture of autonomy as a capacity that emerges in individuals through the social and cultural scaffolding provided through relationships (Deem & Stokes, 2018; MacKenzie, 2014; MacKenzie & Stoljar, 2000). On such relational conceptions of autonomy, the marks of autonomous decision making are not necessarily freedom from external influence or even adoption of others' decisions for oneself, but rather the degree to which an individual recognizes one's decision as truly one's own, regardless of the source(s) of the content of that decision.[7]

[7] Many of the concerns that Resta (2021) raises focus on this traditional, individualist conception of autonomy. Were genetic counseling to shift toward a more relational conception of autonomy, such concerns would likely dissipate.

Presently, there remain characterizations of autonomy in the genetic counseling literature that rest primarily on freedom from constraint in one's choices (e.g., Resta, 2021). However, there is emerging support for genetic counseling adopting a more relational conception of autonomy (e.g., Jamal et al., 2020), which arguably aligns better with approaches to genetic counseling that emphasize empathetic responsiveness and attending to the psychosocial needs of patients.[8] Furthermore, nondirectiveness, when understood as a formal rather than contentual constraint on genetic counseling practice, can be part of such broader, relational approaches to information provision, addressing the psychosocial and affective needs of patients and, depending on context, providing advice and guidance toward shared therapeutic goals.

Conclusion

Among the historical factors that led genetic counseling practice to adopt the concept of nondirectiveness in its earliest development, the concern of the profession to protect and promote patient autonomy was a significant reason for it. Dominant conceptions of nondirectiveness, including value-neutral and autonomy-based conceptions, aim to do justice to this original concern. However, as I argued above, neither provides adequate normative guidance to genetic counseling practice. Moreover, neither straightforwardly identifies what features of genetic counseling might ground a norm to protect autonomy beyond the broadly applicable principle of respect for autonomy, familiar to any clinician.

When nondirectiveness is conceptualized as a formal constraint on the facilitation of informed decisions by patients, protecting patient autonomy in genetic counseling involves avoiding the exploitation of the vulnerability that patients experience through their relations of epistemic dependency on and trust in genetic counselors. While the norm does not prevent genetic counselors from responding to the unique psychosocial and ethical features of each counseling encounter, it prohibits abuse of the discretionary authority invested in them by patients in virtue of their professional identities. In this way, the norm of nondirectiveness can play a significant role in promoting patient autonomy without posing obstacles to the deployment of those distinguishing skills and competencies of the genetic counseling profession.

Interestingly, nondirectiveness, so conceived, need not be seen as unique to genetic counseling among the healthcare professions. The commonly existing grounds giving rise to epistemic dependency and trust within genetic counseling—opacity of information, uncertainty of outcome and risk, complexity and variability of testing and sequencing modalities, and/or potential for error in interpretation—can certainly be present in other complex areas of healthcare. This could, then, ground norms similar to nondirectiveness in other clinical domains within which these factors obtain. However, arguably, these conditions are present more acutely (currently) in genetic counseling contexts, which likely accounts for the field's somewhat unique focus on this norm. Perhaps this is why the field at its inception

[8] For more on empathetic responsiveness and psychosocial counseling, see Chapter 4 in this volume by Robin E. Grubs and Maria Piantanida and Chapter 6 by Jon Weil, respectively.

committed, and continues presently to commit, to some notion that nondirectiveness generally is an appropriate ethical commitment for genetic counseling.

Acknowledgments

Portions of this chapter originally appeared in Deem (2017). I am grateful to Routledge for permission to include and revise that material here.

References

Audi, R. (2004). *The good in the right: A theory of intuition and intrinsic value.* Princeton University Press.

Baier, A. (1986). Trust and anti-trust. *Ethics, 96*(2), 231–260.

Bartels, D. M., LeRoy, B. S., McCarthy, P., & Caplan, A. L (1997). Nondirectiveness in genetic counseling: A survey of practitioners. *American Journal of Medical Genetics, 72*(2), 172–179.

Baumiller, R. C., Cunningham, G., Fisher, N., Fox, L., Henderson, M., Lebel, R., McGrath, G., Pelias, M. Z., Porter, I., Seydel, F., & Roper Wilson, N. (1996). Code of ethical principles for genetics professionals: An explication. *American Journal of Medical Genetics, 65*, 179–183.

Bernhardt, B. A. (1997). Empirical evidence that genetic counseling is directive: Where do we go from here? *American Journal of Human Genetics, 60*(1), 17–20.

Biesecker, B. B. (2003). Back to the future of genetic counseling: Commentary on "psychosocial genetic counseling in the post-nondirective era." *Journal of Genetic Counseling, 12*(3), 213–217.

Bosk, C. L. (1993). The workplace ideology of genetic counselors. In D. Bartels, B. Leroy, & A. Caplan (Eds.), *Prescribing our future: Ethical challenges in genetic counseling* (pp. 25–38). Aldine de Gruyter.

Burke, M., & Kolker, A. (1994). Directiveness in prenatal genetic counseling. *Women & Health, 22*(2), 31–53.

Caplan, A. L. (1993). Neutrality is not morality: The ethics of genetic counseling. In D. Bartels, B. Leroy, & A. Caplan (Eds.), *Prescribing our future: Ethical challenges in genetic counseling* (pp. 149–165). Aldine de Gruyter.

Childress, J. F. (1993). The place of autonomy in bioethics. *Hastings Center Report, 20*(1), 12–17.

Clarke, A. J. (1991). Is non-directive genetic counseling possible? *The Lancet, 338*, 998–1001.

Clarke, A. J. (1997). The process of genetic counseling: Beyond non-directiveness. In P. S. Harper & A. J. Clarke (Eds.), *Genetics, society, and clinical practice* (pp. 179–200). Oxford BIOS.

Conrad, D., & Stanley, C. S. (2015). The (micro) array of options for prenatal testing. In J. L. Berliner (Ed.), *Ethical dilemmas in genetics and genetic counseling: Principles through case scenarios* (pp. 20–60). Oxford University Press.

Curlin, F., & Tollefsen, C. (2021). *The way of medicine: Ethics and the healing profession.* University of Notre Dame Press.

Davis, D. S. (2010). *Genetic dilemmas: Parental choices and children's futures* (2nd ed.). Oxford University Press.

Deem, M. J. (2017). Vulnerability in genetic counseling and the ground of nondirectiveness. In C. Straehle (Ed.), *Vulnerability, autonomy, and applied ethics* (pp. 138–156). Routledge.

Deem, M. J., & Stokes, F. (2018). Culture and consent in clinical care: A critical review of the nursing and nursing ethics literature. *Annual Review of Nursing Research, 37*(1), 223–259.

Fine, B. A. (1993). The evolution of nondirectiveness in genetic counseling and the implications of the human genome project. In D. Bartels, B. Leroy, & A. Caplan (Eds.), *Prescribing our future: Ethical challenges in genetic counseling* (pp. 101–117). Aldine de Gruyter.

Fraser, F. C. (1974). Genetic counseling. *American Journal of Human Genetics, 26*(5), 636–659.

Gervais, K. G. (1993). Objectivity, value neutrality, and nondirectiveness in genetic counseling. In D. Bartels, B. Leroy, & A. Caplan (Eds.), *Prescribing our future: Ethical challenges in genetic counseling* (pp. 119–130). Aldine de Gruyter.

Haga, S. B., Barry, W. T., Mills, R., Ginsburg, G. S., Svetkey, L., Sullivan, J., & Willard, H. F. (2013). Public knowledge of and attitudes toward genetics and genetic testing. *Genetic Testing and Molecular Biomarkers, 17*(4), 327–335.

Hawley, K. (2014). Trust, distrust, and commitment. *Noûs, 48*(1), 1–20.

Hurst, S. A. (2008). Vulnerability in research and health care: Describing the elephant in the room? *Bioethics, 22*(3), 191–202.

Jamal, L., Schupmann, W., & Berkman, B. E. (2020). An ethical framework for genetic counseling in the genomic era. *Journal of Genetic Counseling, 29*(5), 718–727.

Jones, K. (1996). Trust as an affective attitude. *Ethics, 107*(1), 4–25.

Kessler, S. (1997). Psychological aspects of genetic counseling: XI. Nondirectiveness revisited. *American Journal of Medical Genetics, 72*(2), 164–171.

Kessler, S. (2001). Psychological aspects of genetic counseling: XIV. Nondirectiveness and counseling skills. *Genetic Testing, 5*(3), 187–191.

Lanie, A. D., Epstein, J., Toby, S., Jane, P., Kardia, S. L. R., Anderson, E. S., Feldbaum, M., & Petty, E. M. (2004). Exploring the public understanding of basic genetic concepts. *Journal of Genetic Counseling, 13*(4), 305–320.

Lea, D. H., Kaphingst, K. A., Bowen, D., Lipkus, I., & Hadley, D. W. (2011). Communicating genetic and genomic information: Health literacy and numeracy considerations. *Public Health Genomics, 14*(4–5), 279–289.

LeRoy, B. S. (1993). When theory meets practice: Challenges to the field of genetic counseling. In D. Bartels, B. Leroy, & A. Caplan (Eds.), *Prescribing our future: Ethical challenges in genetic counseling* (pp. 39–57). Aldine de Gruyter.

Lippman, A. (1991). The genetic construction of prenatal testing: Choice, consent, or conformity for women? *American Journal of Law & Medicine, 17*(1–2), 15–50.

Mackenzie, C. (2014). Three dimensions of autonomy: A relational analysis. In A. Veltman & M. Piper (Eds.), *Autonomy, oppression, and gender* (pp. 15–41). Oxford University Press.

Mackenzie, C., & Stoljar, N. (Eds.). (2000). *Relational autonomy: Feminist perspectives on autonomy, agency, and the social self.* Oxford University Press.

Macklin, R. (2015). Can one do good medical ethics without principles? *Journal of Medical Ethics, 41*, 75–78.

McLeod, C. (2002). *Self-trust and reproductive autonomy*. MIT Press.

Michie, S., Bron, F., Bobrow, M., & Marteau, T. M. (1997). Nondirectiveness in genetic counseling: An empirical study. *American Journal of Human Genetics, 60*(1), 40–47.

National Society of Genetic Counselors. (2017, April). *NSG code of ethics*. https://www.nsgc.org/Portals/0/NSGC%20Code%20of%20Ethics%20%28New%20Logo%29.pdf

Oduncu, F. S. (2002). The role of non-directiveness in genetic counseling. *Medicine, Health Care and Philosophy, 5*, 53–63.

O'Neill, O. (2001). Practical principles and practical judgment. *Hastings Center Report, 31*(4), 15–23.

Resta, R. G. (1997). Eugenics and nondirectiveness in genetic counseling. *Journal of Genetic Counseling, 6*(2), 255–258.

Resta, R. G. (2021). Complicated shadows: The limitations of autonomy in genetic counseling. In B. Leroy, P. McCarthy, & N. Callanan (Eds.), *Genetic counseling practice: Advanced concepts and skills* (2nd ed., pp. 9–24). Wiley-Blackwell.

Rogers, W., MacKenzie, C., & Dodds, S. (2012). Why bioethics needs a concept of vulnerability. *International Journal of Feminist Bioethics*, 5, 11–38.

Sorenson, J. R. (1993). Genetic counseling: Values that have mattered. In D. Bartels, B. Leroy, & A. Caplan (Eds.), *Prescribing our future: Ethical challenges in genetic counseling* (pp. 3–14). Aldine de Gruyter.

Stern, A. M. (2012). *Telling genes: The story of genetic counseling in America*. Johns Hopkins University Press.

Stoll, K., & Jackson, J. (2020). Supporting patient autonomy and informed decision-making in prenatal genetic testing. *Cold Spring Habor Perspectives in Medicine, 10*, a036509.

Straehle, C. (2016). Vulnerability, health agency and capability to health. *Bioethics, 30*(1), 34–40.

Syurina, E. V., Brankovic, I., Probst-Hensch, N., & Brand, A. (2011). Genome-based health literacy: A new challenge for public health genomics. *Public Health Genetics, 14*(4–5), 201–210.

Wachbroit, R., & Wasserman, D. (1995). Patient autonomy and value-neutrality in nondirective genetic counseling. *Stanford Law & Policy Review, 6*(2), 103–111.

Walker, A. P. (2009). The practice of genetic counseling. In R. Uhlmann, J. L. Schuette, & B. M. Yashar (Eds.), *A guide to genetic counseling* (2nd ed., pp. 1–36). Wiley-Blackwell.

Weil, J. (2000). *Psychosocial genetic counseling*. Oxford University Press.

Weil, J. (2003). Psychosocial genetic counseling in the post-nondirective era: A point of view. *Journal of Genetic Counseling, 12*(3), 199–211.

Weil, J., Ormond, K., Peters, J., Peters, K., Bowles Biesecker, B., & Leroy, B. (2006). The relationship of nondirectiveness to genetic counseling: Report of a workshop at the 2003 NSGC Annual Education Conference. *Journal of Genetic Counseling, 15*(2), 85–93.

Wertz, D. C., & Fletcher, J. C. (1988). Attitudes of genetic counselors: A multinational study. *American Journal of Human Genetics, 42*(4), 592–600.

White, M. T. (1999). Making responsible decisions: An interpretive ethic for genetic decision making. *Hastings Center Report, 29*(1), 14–21.

Williams, C., Anderson, P., & Farsides, B. (2002). Is nondirectiveness possible within the context of antenatal screening and testing? *Social Science & Medicine, 54*(3), 339–347.

Yarborough, M., Scott, J. A., & Dixon, L. K. (1989). The role of beneficence in clinical genetics: Non-directive counseling reconsidered. *Theoretical Medicine, 10*(2), 139–149.

CHAPTER 24

COMMUNICATING FAMILY INFORMATION IN GENETIC COUNSELING

An Ethical Perspective

SAMANTHA J. LEONARD AND AINSLEY J. NEWSON

Introduction

Healthcare has traditionally had at its core the notion of a professional–patient relationship bound by a duty of confidentiality. Maintaining confidentiality is, on the face of it, justifiable on both ethical and pragmatic grounds. Ethically, protecting confidentiality is considered to be paramount to respecting patient autonomy—it is for a patient to decide with whom their health information should be shared (Kottow, 1986). Pragmatically, a healthcare professional needs to be trusted so that the patient divulges their health history, to facilitate diagnosis and ongoing management.

A health professional's[1] duty to protect confidentiality may, however, come into conflict when keeping medical information confidential could harm another person. Examples that have formed the basis for much ethical discussion in medicine include circumstances where a patient with an infectious disease refuses to self-isolate or where a patient threatens violence against a specific person. Clinical genetics also poses interesting challenges for information sharing and presumptions of confidentiality, as it is by its very nature familial (Duncan & Newson, 2006). A patient[2] has inherited their genes from their parents and shares them with their siblings and other family members.

[1] Throughout this chapter, we use the terms "health professional" and (less frequently) "genetic health professional." We have chosen these terms because genetic (and genomic) information is now requested or ordered by many health professionals, including genetic counselors and clinical geneticists. And while we have focused on the ethical issues as they arise in a genetic counseling context, we also recognize that the same kinds of issues will increasingly also arise in other healthcare contexts.

[2] The term "patient" is used in this introduction to denote a person seeking care in relation to a genetic condition. We note and accept that not everyone seeking care in this context will be unwell

Genetic counselors have long recognized the so-called "sociality" of genetic information (Rehmann-Sutter, 2009). It can lead to knowledge that is important to more than one person, be it current and future offspring (forward sociality) or one's relatives (lateral sociality). In the context of the genetics clinic, relatives are inextricably linked to patient assessment, for example, the recording of a family pedigree to inform diagnosis, variant interpretation, and prognostication.

Many patients receiving genetic test results will have relatives who may also have (or be at risk of developing) the condition being discussed. In some cases, the condition is well known within the family, but in other cases the patient may be the proband—the index case—and their relatives may not yet be aware of their own risk.[3] The questions then arise of whether and how these relatives should be informed of that risk and who should take responsibility to ensure the communication occurs.

Ideally, information will be freely and accurately shared within a family, and studies suggest that probands are generally keen to help (Heaton & Chico, 2016). But even when a proband is willing to share or where processes are in place to enable clinic-led dissemination, information is sometimes not passed on or may be conveyed or understood inaccurately. Multiple barriers exist that can make communicating genetic risk within families difficult, although this is not to discount that facilitators exist too (Wilson & Etchegary, 2010).[4] Instances where a healthcare professional has not passed on information have been the subject of legal proceedings in several countries. We discuss this further below.

As genetic and genomic testing become integrated into other clinical specialties, genetic conditions will continue to bring significant communication challenges for both probands and healthcare providers. Additionally, nongenetics healthcare professionals are beginning to be confronted with these issues for the first time. Some may feel unsure about their responsibilities to encourage or enact communication to at-risk family members. Probands also may feel unsure what their obligations are or uncomfortable about carrying them out. When potentially important information has implications for relatives, ethical issues arise.

In this chapter, we outline the ethical aspects underlying communicating family information in genetic counseling. We begin by describing three case studies that together exemplify some of the ways in which ethical issues in family communication can arise. After describing a taxonomy of nondisclosure, we then briefly consider whether novel methods of genomic sequencing can resolve existing communication dilemmas. Next, we discuss relevant legal cases and regulatory guidance. These preliminary analyses allow us to articulate

and that terms such as "client" or "consult" are also used. Later in this chapter, we shift our language to "proband" or "index patient" to describe a person who is the first in their family to receive information that will be relevant to other genetically related family members.

[3] Sometimes relatives can be particularly important for finalizing a diagnosis, for example, to clarify the pathogenicity of a variant by seeing whether all family members possessing it show signs of the condition.

[4] These include factors relating to the condition (e.g., whether it can be prevented and how penetrant the gene is), factors relating to the individuals involved (e.g., emotions and coping), and the nature of the family unit (e.g., proximity, social closeness). Communication is also mediated by wider social factors such as gender roles and concerns about discrimination (B. J. Wilson & Etchegary, 2010).

the ethical questions that arise. From here, we turn to consider some of the models for conceptualizing and managing communication of genetic information in families. While we have deliberately chosen not to endorse any particular model, we go on to describe some overarching points for consideration, which can inform how family communication can best be approached in practice.

Case Studies and a Taxonomy of Nondisclosure

While the majority of patients pass relevant information to family members (e.g., Hunter et al., 2023), we also know that successful family communication of genetic information does not always occur. Studies show the majority of genetic health professionals have experienced at least one case of familial non-disclosure over their career (e.g., Falk et al., 2003). We also know some of the reasons why communication of genetic information to at-risk family members does not occur. These include knowledge-based issues (e.g., a lack of understanding of the risk to the family), perceived irrelevance of the information (including disbelief that pathogenic variants cause disease), emotions and feelings such as reticence over passing negative information on, and fear over how the conversation will go. There are also reasons having to do with family dynamics, including conflict, family "rules" (or wider cultural norms) about who should disclose, not being able to find the right time, not being close to the at-risk relatives, and concern about revealing an absence of genetic kinship, such as misattributed paternity (Arribas-Ayllon et al., 2011; Chivers Seymour et al., 2010; Weaver, 2016). More practically, probands may also encounter barriers such as not having contact details. Box 24.1 provides three such examples of nondisclosure.

As others have done (e.g., Chico, 2012; Clarke et al., 2005; Parker & Lucassen, 2018), we will refer to instances where genetic information is not passed on to at-risk family members as *nondisclosure*. But what are the kinds of nondisclosure? Perhaps the most prevalent partition is between *active* and *passive* nondisclosure (Leonard & Newson, 2010). For the purposes of this chapter, we define three main types of nondisclosure: active, passive, and unwitting—although, as we explain below, we will not discuss the latter in detail. In all of these instances, there are genetic relatives who are also at risk but are unaware of this risk. In Table 24.1, active and passive forms of nondisclosure are integrated with the case studies described in Box 24.1.

Active nondisclosure

As the name implies, active nondisclosure involves an intentional behavior on behalf of a proband. We have previously defined active nondisclosure as occurring when "a family member has explicitly or actively refused to pass on information to a relative" (Leonard & Newson, 2010, p. 199). There is a clear refusal to disclose genetic information to a genetic relative who may benefit from receiving that information. While clearly recognizable as

Box 24.1 Family Communication: Three Case Studies

The following scenarios illustrate some of the ways in which ethical issues in family communication can arise.

Case 1: Disclosing a recessive condition

A and B come to the genetics clinic because their child has been diagnosed with spinal muscular atrophy. They opt not to have testing themselves but are almost certain to be carriers. They are counseled that their siblings may also be carriers. A and B explain that they feel this information is private and that they do not intend to share it with their families. The geneticist has not been provided with any contact details for the family.

Case 2: Warning a sister about a *BRCA1* pathogenic variant

C presents to the genetics clinic with a personal history of bilateral breast cancer that has occurred at the ages of 38 and 45 years. In addition, her mother died at age 80 with breast cancer. Suspecting a pathogenic variant, the geneticist requests/orders a cancer multigene panel test. This confirms a pathogenic variant in the *BRCA1* gene. The geneticist advises that at-risk family members should be informed of the possibility of having the same variant and the attendant increased cancer risks. C informs her geneticist that she is estranged from her sister and does not intend to contact her to share this news.

Some time later D, who is C's sister, comes to the same genetics clinic seeking carrier screening for cystic fibrosis (as her partner is a known carrier). D is not aware of her sister's clinical history, nor of the presence of the pathogenic *BRCA1* variant in the family. However, on taking the family history, the genetics professional recognizes the family relationship. But based on the family history as D tells it, testing for the *BRCA1* pathogenic variant would not be suggested. What should the professional do? (case adapted from Parker & Lucassen, 2018).

Case 3: Disseminating a diagnosis of Lynch syndrome

E comes to the genetics clinic following a diagnosis of multiple polyps and bowel cancer. He is informed that he is a carrier of a Lynch syndrome pathogenic variant and that other family members may also carry this variant. He states that he will let his family know. Months later, a family member comes to the clinic. It is clear that this family member has not been given any information and that other members of the family have also not been informed of their risk.

Table 24.1 Nondisclosure

	Definition	Case study
Active nondisclosure	"a family member has explicitly or actively refused to pass on information to a relative" (Leonard & Newson, 2010, p. 199)	• A and B's child with spinal muscular atrophy: A and B refuse to disclose, and the genetics professional has no obvious way of contacting relatives. • C's *BRCA1* diagnosis: C refuses to disclose to her sister D, but the same genetics professional is in contact with D.
Passive nondisclosure	"a proband has not passed on genetic information to family members, despite the best of intentions" (Leonard & Newson, 2010, p. 199)	• E's Lynch syndrome diagnosis: E is aware that this is important information for the family and expresses the intention to pass it on.

nondisclosure, it is thought that such active refusals occur in less than 1% of clinical genetics consultations (Clarke et al., 2005).

Passive nondisclosure

Passive nondisclosure occurs "when it becomes apparent that a proband has not passed on genetic information to family members, despite the best of intentions" (Leonard & Newson, 2010, p. 199). It can thus arise even where a proband initially appears enthusiastic about disclosure. Passive nondisclosure is known to occur in clinical practice and is attributed to reasons such as the patient not finding the right time or experiencing problems of coping or feeling overwhelmed in light of their diagnosis (Parker & Lucassen, 2018; Wiseman et al., 2010). This is also likely to be a more difficult, even intractable form of nondisclosure, because the absence of a refusal can leave health professionals less certain of grounds for intervention, or perhaps even uncertain as to whether nondisclosure occurred.

Unwitting nondisclosure

Unwitting nondisclosure, as described by Parker and Lucassen (2018), occurs when "a patient is unaware . . . that there are relatives who might benefit" (p. 956) and so does not disclose the information to them. This type of nondisclosure may have different ethical implications from active and passive nondisclosure, as it may be difficult to discuss or ascribe duties or responsibilities when the proband is not in a position to know they can benefit others. As such, we will not consider it further in this chapter.

From Genetics to Genomics: Do Developments in DNA Testing Technologies Resolve Family Communication Dilemmas?

When we first wrote about ethics and family communication in genetics (Leonard & Newson, 2010), not only did people generally need to be informed by another family member about their genetic risk in order to access genetic testing, but also in most cases they needed an affected relative to have been tested and a pathogenic variant identified to undergo testing themselves. In the intervening period, gene testing technologies and the clinical and commercial contexts in which they are deployed have significantly changed. High-throughput, next-generation DNA sequencing methods have become far more widely used, overtaking Sanger sequencing for testing in probands. Patients regularly undergo gene testing using multiple gene panels or through exome or genome sequencing. Individuals are also accessing their genetic information through commercial direct-to-consumer providers outside of the traditional professional–patient context.

With the advent of genomics, do family members still need to rely on being informed of genetic risks? Contemporary DNA sequencing technologies mean that accessing our genomes has never been easier or cheaper. This, some may claim, means that the dilemma of family communication will be limited to a small subset of patients (such as those living with a rare condition) or disappear altogether. Family members could simply obtain their own information, as and when they wish to. This view is, however, premature, for at least six reasons.

First, the situation in which every person has ready access to their genome data remains some time away. Concerns around financial cost, variant interpretation, overdiagnosis, and subsequent overtreatment mean genome-wide sequencing is not currently routinely offered to everyone (Murray, 2018). And if genome testing is available only on a user-pays basis (as will be the case in many healthcare systems), then serious existing disparities in socioeconomic status and health literacy (as well as a lack of public funds to support testing in many countries) will mean that individual genome sequencing remains out of reach for the majority, and is likely to be so for some time to come.

Second, as Parker and Lucassen (2018) point out, we still need information about a person's family history to interpret the information obtained from sequencing, such as novel or rare variants. While this is a slightly different point—one that focuses on the use of family information to clarify a proband's result rather than using a proband's result to care for their family members—this feature could be said to give rise to an obligation, based on reciprocity, for a proband to share the eventual results. Third, as genomics increasingly enters mainstream medicine, dilemmas about communicating genetic information in families may arise more frequently (Wouters et al., 2016).

Fourth, as genomic sequencing begins to offer greater prediction of future health, disclosure dilemmas will increasingly be about predictive rather than diagnostic information (Rothstein, 2018). Fifth, unless genome sequencing becomes entirely routine, in most cases people will still only come to know about the existence of a risk because of their family relationships. Information about a genetic condition in the family would also remain important in guiding testing modality—genome sequencing, even if freely available to all, would be of limited use in some conditions that may require different molecular testing approaches, such as disorders of methylation. And finally, sixth, while direct-to-consumer providers have wasted no time in allowing people to access their genomes, they have historically been slower in drawing on the strong existing evidence base to facilitate their customers' communication with their families about their results (Middleton, 2012; Middleton et al., 2017).

Thus, as advances in genomics continue to occur, healthcare professionals will likely continue to confront family communication challenges (Mendes et al., 2018). Indeed, some applications of genomic testing may actually exacerbate family communication dilemmas (Parker & Lucassen, 2018). If more people have genomic testing, then more diagnoses will be made, and the interests of more genetic relatives will need to be considered. While this may not apply to situations such as the return of polygenic scores (as these will be highly specific to an individual), rapid mainstreaming of genomic testing will undoubtedly generate situations where family communication is advisable.

Legal and Regulatory Consideration of the Dimensions of Family Communication

Just as innovations in genomic sequencing cannot resolve ethical dilemmas in family communication, neither can law or regulation. While a full examination of global laws, legal cases, regulations, and professional guidelines regarding communicating familial genetic information is beyond the scope of this chapter, it is important to note that the responsibilities and permitted actions for both professionals and probands vary in different healthcare settings (Godard et al., 2006).[5] Additionally, even when specific laws or regulations are in place, ethical uncertainties may remain regarding whether, or how, a legal duty or permissibility to share or disclose genetic information will activate. Relevant dimensions include whether genetic information is routinely shared, whose responsibility it is to pass on genetic information to at-risk family members, and what options are legally permissible when it becomes apparent that nondisclosure has occurred.

Taking all of this into consideration, we can discern at least three legal questions, all of which sit above a background issue, namely, the value of individual health privacy and professional obligations to uphold confidentiality (de Paor, 2018). First, what professional liabilities may arise in this area? This can go two ways: Some genetics professionals may be concerned about liability that follows a breach of confidentiality; others may be concerned over liability from a failure to disclose genetic information to a relative (Chico, 2016).

Second, there is the related question over whether there is (or should be) a legal "duty to warn" about genetic risk (Falk et al., 2003; Lacroix et al., 2008; Mitchell et al., 2016; Offit et al., 2004; Rothstein, 2018). Such a duty has been considered in case law in several countries. In the United States, two state appellate court decisions, *Pate v. Threlkel* (1995) and *Safer v. Estate of Pack* (1996), considered instances where relatives were not warned of their genetic risk. Each held that the health professional (in these cases, a physician) did have a duty to warn at-risk genetic relatives when the proband was their patient. In *Pate*, however, the duty was satisfied by telling the proband of the risk to relatives, including that the proband should inform them of the risk in the family. *Safer* went further, claiming that relevant health professionals may have a need to go further and contact relatives directly themselves.

As Rothstein (2018) points out, these cases do not prove a general duty to warn or that such a duty (if it exists) would apply to all health professionals. They have also now been superseded by a statute (the Health Insurance Portability and Accountability Act Privacy Rule), the interpretation of which suggests that there is permission, but not a duty, for health professionals or patients to notify genetic relatives about genetic risk when necessary (Henrikson et al., 2020; Rothstein, 2018). Such a disclosure would need to meet numerous requirements, including that there is no agreed-upon restriction on disclosure and

[5] There are calls for more and clearer policy and guidelines relating to family communication of genetic and genomic information, especially in countries where there is currently no clear guidance (Mendes et al., 2024; Phillips et al., 2024, 2025). Healthcare providers should always check latest guidelines applicable to their region, as new regulations or legal cases may arise that are not discussed in this chapter.

that (unless the patient specifically consents) the communication could only be to another health provider and not to a relative directly (Henrikson et al., 2020; Rothstein, 2018).

This permission to disclose in the absence of a duty, subject to a regulated process, is also the status quo in some Australian healthcare settings. A federal regulatory regime is in place to facilitate disclosure of genetic information by health professionals without consent (Otlowski, 2013, 2015). This is applicable to health professionals who are bound by federal privacy law, with mirroring regulation to cover all health professionals in the state of New South Wales. A notable feature of the regime in Australia is that it provides health professionals with a route to enable disclosure without breaching statutory privacy provisions, while at the same time not imposing a duty to warn. However, Australia's lack of national consistency in regulation remains problematic (McWhirter et al., 2019). Additionally, the regime may be judged as not going far enough from the perspective of a relative who is harmed through nondisclosure (Otlowski, 2013).

In the United Kingdom, *ABC v. St George's Healthcare Trust & Others* (2020) considered whether there is a legal duty to warn genetic relatives in the face of active nondisclosure. The daughter (ABC) of a man with a clinical diagnosis of Huntington's disease asked the court to determine whether her father's medical team should have disclosed his diagnosis to her. The man, who was under the care of forensic psychiatrists, had explicitly refused that his diagnosis be disclosed to his daughter. ABC discovered this information inadvertently and subsequently received a positive result on a predictive genetic test. By this time, she had also had a child of her own. She claimed that had she known of her own prognosis, she would have chosen not to continue the pregnancy, on the basis that she would be unable to parent the child until it reached adulthood.

ABC's case reached the High Court of England and Wales. On the facts, the judge ruled that she was unconvinced ABC would have had a termination of pregnancy and, as such, the legal requirement of causation was not met. But the judgment also makes clear that health professionals do have a duty—arguably a novel duty (Foster & Gilbar, 2021)—to undertake a detailed and careful balancing exercise to consider a patient's interest in confidentiality against the interests of any genetic relatives (with whom the health professionals have a "proximal" relationship) in being informed. Notably, this is a duty to weigh in the balance rather than a freestanding duty to consider relatives. If the reasoning handed down in *ABC* is more widely followed, then, where health professionals consider that a proximal relative's interests (such as an interest in knowing about a serious genetic condition) should be prioritized over those of a patient, a breach of confidentiality to disclose will be unlikely to generate legal liability. It is also a duty limited to proximal relatives. While ABC met this proximal requirement, it was held that the medical team had carried out the balancing exercise appropriately and, as such, no duty had been breached in this case (Foster & Gilbar, 2021; Lucassen, 2020; Middleton et al., 2020). This judgment thus brings the law in England and Wales into line with relevant professional guidelines (Joint Committee on Genomics in Medicine, 2019; Middleton et al., 2020) as well as academic literature that argues in favor of such a balancing approach (Dove et al., 2019).

A third question is, if a legal duty exists, on whom should this legal duty rest? Several jurisdictions have introduced laws to manage family communication and nondisclosure and have placed certain responsibilities on health professionals or patients (Forrest et al., 2007; Godard et al., 2006). In France, for example, a 2011 law places the main responsibility to disclose on the proband, although health professionals are also required to undertake "indirect disclosure" when a proband refuses to disclose or when the proband authorizes them to disclose (d'Audiffret Van Haecke & de Montgolfier, 2018; Derbez et al., 2019). While laws like these can provide clear direction, evidence also suggests that health professionals may not always know exactly how to use and apply relevant guidelines or laws (e.g., Meggiolaro et al., 2020). They also remain uncomfortable about contacting relatives (Chico, 2019) and continue to use a variety of approaches to encourage the patient to contact their relatives themselves.

Ethics and Family Communication of Genetic Information

As the preceding sections demonstrate, the dynamics and dimensions of family communication of genetic information are complex, and consequently, a range of ethical questions, concepts, and principles are relevant. In this section, we describe four key ethical questions that arise when we think about family communication of genetic information.

An interest in knowing?

First, we need to ask whether genetic relatives have an interest in knowing or a right to know that they are at risk of developing, or passing on, a genetic condition. The answer to this question will have a clinical dimension—for example, the inheritance pattern of the condition, the penetrance of the particular variant, and the actionability of the information. It also has an ethical dimension: Is this information something that genetic relatives would reasonably have an interest in, and what should we do about those who may not want to know?

It is reasonable to suggest that genetic relatives have an interest in knowing they may develop, or pass on, a genetic condition. Many genetic conditions allow steps to be taken, such as preventive or early intervention measures (e.g., screening) or enabling reproductive choice. A claim (although subject to contention) could also be made that such knowledge is intrinsically valuable regardless of whether it is actioned or actionable. While not all relatives will go on to confirm a genetic risk, enabling a relative to weigh this option themselves therefore appears reasonable.

This interest in knowing should also, however, be moderated by a consideration of any harms that may arise from the knowledge that one is at risk. When family members are aware of a risk, they sometimes choose not to find out their status. Husted (1997) highlights that the "right not to know" one's genetic information has two aspects: the right not to know one's variant status and the right not to know that a condition is in the family at all. Both have been discussed at length in the literature (e.g., MacDougall, 2004; Rhodes, 1998; Takala, 1999; Wilson, 2005) and the right not to know can also be given by patients as a reason for non-disclosure (Murphy et al., 2024). Overall, there is some consensus that there is a right not to know one's variant status, although some frame this as a preference rather than a "right," and also argue that choosing not to know about actionable genetic information may not be upholding certain substantive notions of autonomy (Dive, 2021).[6] However, others have noted that these richer notions of autonomy are not typically reflected in law and that there may not be legal recourse for those told about genetic risk against their wishes (Chico, 2012).

The second aspect—a right to complete genetic ignorance—is more difficult to uphold. How can this be discerned in advance without disclosing the information? From a practical ethics perspective, genetics professionals should facilitate any approach to at-risk relatives with a sensitivity to genetic ignorance, striking a balance between encouraging a relative to present for testing and providing information they wish they had not been told. This will influence modes and methods of communication, including counseling probands about communication and the wording of family letters (Dheensa et al., 2018; Mendes et al., 2016; van den Heuvel et al., 2019).

Is the information individual or familial?

A second and parallel consideration is whether the information about genetic risk "belongs" to the proband or the family. This is not (or not only) about legal ownership—as the legal ownership of genetic information and samples is itself a complex question (Montgomery, 2017). Rather, it is a question about the level that genetic information should best be perceived at, namely, the individual or the family. This question has also been discussed in a rich literature. Skene (1998) was among the first to address this problem, dichotomizing the more general information that there is a genetic condition in the family, which should be sensitively disseminated to genetic relatives, and a proband's identity and variant status, which should, so far as possible, remain confidential. This approach has since been endorsed and expanded by others (Lucassen & Gilbar, 2018; Parker & Lucassen, 2018; Phillips et al., 2025). On this family-level view, a relative who coincidentally presents to a genetics department could be informed that records showed a family genetic risk, and what gene and health risks were involved. The disclosure could also be less specific, such as a medical team encouraging a genetic relative to seek advice about their family history and symptoms that are known to them (Lucassen & Gilbar, 2018).

Lucassen and Clarke (2022) have written about actively informing relatives that they are at risk of a hereditary condition without disclosing the medical details of the index patient. They have also discussed the notion that laboratory-generated genetic information is shared and familial and can be separated from individual health status. This approach, which they describe as a nuanced disclosure, could potentially have allowed the doctors in the *ABC* case (outlined above) to divulge information about the risk of a hereditary

[6] Briefly, a substantive approach to autonomy highlights the importance of critical reflection, being sensitive to social context and our relationships with each other, as well as acting authentically. It emphasizes normative competence, which describes people's ability to evaluate their choices in light of their higher order values. It is not merely whether a person has options to choose between, but whether they have reflected on them and determined that they align with higher order desires and values (such as self-understanding; Dive & Newson, 2018). This can be contrasted with more simplistic notions of autonomy that focus on information provision and an absence of coercion.

condition to the daughter of a patient with Huntington's disease without going into detail about her father's specific condition (Lucassen & Clarke, 2022).

Some have also argued for a family approach to genetic information, supported by the ethical concepts of relational autonomy and communitarianism (Bell & Bennett, 2001; Dove et al., 2017; Gilbar, 2007). Relational autonomy recognizes relationships and the impact these can have on decision making, both positive and negative.[7] This is mirrored in Parker and Lucassen's "joint account" model, which holds that information from testing should be routinely shared among those who share genes unless there is a strong reason for not doing so (Parker & Lucassen, 2004). This approach, which has been endorsed by patients (Dheensa et al., 2016), shifts the emphasis toward the family without completely deviating from traditional frameworks of confidentiality in medical practice. However, in this model the family members must still rely on the decision-making processes of individual health professionals, who must make judgments as to what constitutes a "strong reason" for not sharing information. In practice, it may be easier to invoke "strong reasons" for keeping information from family members than risk facing claims of breach of confidentiality. In addition, those who are most vociferously opposed to sharing might be those considered to be at most risk of harm by breaching confidentiality, which would then render the approach ineffective in practice for protecting family members.

Who should disclose genetic risk?

Third is a question about responsibility for the task of disclosure. If we accept that making genetic risk information available to relatives is important, then who should facilitate this—the health professional, proband, or both? And who should hold ethical (or perhaps legal) responsibility to ensure this occurs? There will likely be both practical and regulatory nuances that inform an answer to this question. For example, a health professional may simply have no way of contacting at-risk genetic relatives, or legal regulations may preclude health professionals from approaching people who are not their patients. But setting those considerations to one side, debate is ongoing regarding who should facilitate the communication of genetic information to family members.

The prevailing view is that probands are the ones who should be supported to disseminate the information to their at-risk genetic relatives (Mendes et al., 2024). Pragmatically, probands (or their carers) will usually have the necessary contact details and the appropriate understanding of how best to approach each relative. This is supported by various national guidelines, many of which place responsibility for informing relatives primarily in the hands of patients (Phillips et al., 2021). Philosophers have also offered an ethical justification for probands having a moral responsibility to disclose, for example, Kilbride's work on the principle of rescue (Kilbride, 2018). This responsibility, Kilbride argues, has nothing to do with family obligation but rather the fact that the proband knows about this possible risk, that it could have serious health impacts, and that telling the at-risk relative has a low cost. On a more practical level, it can also be argued that probands can also be

[7] Editors' note: For discussion of relational autonomy and its implications for genetic counseling, see Chapter 23 by Michael J. Deem in this volume.

appropriately supported through this process, including maintaining regular contact with genetic counselors and using standard letters.

Nevertheless, as outlined above, probands may not find this process easy. They may experience practical and emotional barriers to communication, including a lack of counseling experience, a lack of familiarity with genetic terminology, a lack of regular contact, or more complex issues such as family estrangement. And while active nondisclosure can be identified fairly easily, passive failures to communicate may not always come to light. As a result, some models of managing family communication draw on these concerns about ineffectiveness and responsibilization (i.e., probands being made to assume responsibility to oversee family communication) to propose a more active role for the healthcare professional.

Professional-led family communication has been argued for in various ways. One involves looking at the modes of contact, such as advocating for direct (i.e., healthcare-mediated/assisted) rather than proband- or family-mediated contact (Newson & Humphries, 2005). This model also has evidence of public (Andersson et al., 2020), patient (Tiller et al., 2025), and clinical (Stott et al., 2025) support, although a systematic review suggests that probands are keen to undertake family communication themselves with support from professionals (van den Heuvel et al., 2019). Others have suggested that health professionals could move away from nondirectiveness and take a more active role in shaping probands' preferences. This could include using a "moral accountability nudge" to frame options where communication occurs while not mentioning noncommunication (Wouters et al., 2016). Practically, this would involve working through which relatives to contact while at the same time identifying and discussing barriers to communication. It would then be up to the proband to decide whether they or the professional contacts relatives (Wouters et al., 2016). Some have gone further, arguing that health professionals have a duty (or at least a responsibility) to make information available to at-risk family members to support both individual empowerment and population health (Grill & Rosen, 2020).

How should nondisclosure be managed?

A fourth question arises when attempts to disclose genetic risk have not been successful. In other words, what should a genetic counselor do when a proband refuses to, or otherwise fails to, disclose a genetic risk to a family member? This scenario gives rise to some of the classic ethical and legal issues in family communication (van den Heuvel et al., 2021). Should a proband's confidentiality be breached to warn genetic relatives? Is such warning of genetic relatives permissible, or obligatory? Or is it beyond reasonable expectations of duty, both practically and ethically? This dilemma has been framed in various ways in the literature. At a general level, it can be described as a tension between wanting to respect the respective interests of both the proband and their genetic relatives, while mitigating harm to all parties.

If this question of managing active nondisclosure is considered in line with the traditional tenets of medical ethics and law, then there is a rebuttable presumption of proband confidentiality. This presumption is based in the importance of autonomy, privacy, and trust and helps to help facilitate full disclosure of health information by patients. But, as we have seen, it also comes into conflict with a desire to benefit genetic relatives and protect them from harm. The health professional thus needs to weigh the benefits and harms of a discretionary breach of confidentiality. As has been described above, discretionary breaches of confidentiality are countenanced or sanctioned in some jurisdictions and supported by some professional guidelines. It also mirrors issues arising in other areas of medicine, such as managing disclosure of diagnoses of infectious or sexually transmitted diseases.

However, a discretionary breach approach has several drawbacks (Chico, 2016). One is that, as mentioned, healthcare professionals do not feel confident in breaching confidentiality in cases such as the ones we outline above (Chico, 2019; Clarke et al., 2005; Falk et al., 2003). It may also lead to inconsistency of practice; some may choose to breach while others may not. A breach of confidentiality could also lead to professional or legal sanctions, although (as noted above) there could also be legal and professional consequences for *not* breaching confidentiality. But perhaps most importantly, it overlooks the familial nature of genetic information.[8]

One way to keep the dilemma of whether to breach confidentiality at bay might be to conceive of genetic information as familial, as discussed above. Or, if genetic information remains conceptually individual, a "fair warning" model could be adopted (Leonard & Newson, 2010). This approach maintains a distinction between individual and family genetic information but also aims to protect family members. A proband would be counseled about the importance of alerting genetic relatives, who would be identified prior to testing. The test consent process would incorporate the proband's agreement to relatives being informed about any identified familial risk, and the test would not proceed unless this is agreed to. The activity of informing would be assigned to either the proband or the clinical service. In this way, it is clear to the proband that there are limits to confidentiality while maintaining trust. It also mitigates dilemmas for genetic counselors.

Of course, if a proband has or intends to withhold relevant information from at-risk family members and none of these approaches have been used, then the decision becomes whether to breach confidentiality. The decision in the *ABC* case is instructive here, with its emphasis on undertaking a detailed and careful balancing of the proband's interest in confidentiality with the interests of relatives, although the relatives in that case also needed a "proximal" relationship with the proband's healthcare team.

Returning to the Case Studies

In the first case (see Box 24.1), the clinical geneticist has concerns that specific relatives may carry a genetic variant, which, if they were aware of it, could alter their reproductive decisions. Without this information, they may go on to have children with a serious

[8] There is ongoing debate regarding genetic exceptionalism, that is, whether genetic information is distinct from other kinds of health information and as such deserves exceptional treatment in ethics, law, or regulation. We recognize this debate and contend that there will be some kinds of genetic information that are exceptional, while others (especially diagnostic genomic testing in specialized areas such as neonatal intensive care) may begin to look more like other kinds of diagnostic tests. A full discussion of whether and how genetic exceptionalism influences ethical issues in family communication is important yet is beyond the scope of this chapter.

progressive condition, which may go unrecognized for some years, denying them the opportunity of early intervention. Their opportunity to consider alternative reproductive options has also been denied to them. However, there are three potential factors weighing against the healthcare professional communicating information to the family—A and B's refusal to disclose information, the lack of a readily available means of contacting at-risk relatives, and the fact that the health of the relatives themselves is not in question, but rather the health of potential future offspring.

Various authors have pondered the question of whether there is a degree of probability or its potential mitigation that might be relevant in determining whether to contact relatives directly in the case of proband refusal to disclose (e.g., Steel, 2009). There is debate over whether the responsibility of the healthcare professional (from an ethical perspective at least) ends with informing the proband or whether there is a need to take further steps. Additionally, the question of the potential harm of communicating familial genetic information to unsuspecting relatives has been raised (Steel, 2009). But at the same time, the issue of not unreasonably burdening the health professional with the expectation that exceptional measures will be necessary to track down relatives against the will of a proband should be considered. So, the actual questions posed to the healthcare professional are whether they should breach confidentiality in this case and, even if they should, whether it is possible to get a hold of these relatives without the proband's cooperation.

In the second case, the health professional does have a professional duty to D, which is put directly into conflict with their duty to C, as C and D are patients at the same genetics clinic. Can a health professional have a professional duty that is specific to one person, even if relatives are patients too? Here there is a direct health risk to D, and there is already contact with her. The professional is faced with a health risk to a known and readily contactable individual, where steps are available to mitigate the risks, all of which could be considered to weigh in favor of disclosure.

In the third case, E expresses willingness to communicate with relatives, but it becomes apparent that this has not been done effectively (passive nondisclosure; see Table 24.1). The question that this raises for health professionals is whether there is a way of avoiding this situation, so that any relative who is willing to engage in communication to relatives is assisted in such a way that passive nondisclosure is reduced or eliminated. We will return to this point in the next section, where we also consider some of the overarching ethical aspects of family communication. We then provide some practical measures and tools that may be drawn on in cases like these.

Ethically Promoting Family Communication

Families and their attendant interests, preferences, and duties are complex. As the discussion in this chapter so far has shown, family communication of genetic information is similarly multifaceted. There are several ways in which genetic information is, and is not, passed on. There are multiple stakeholders. There may be nascent professional duties, although on whom they fall will vary with circumstances and where a health professional lives and practices. Ultimately, family communication of genetic information will be framed to some extent by the context in which the consultation is taking place—the local legal and professional guidance that exists, as well as the context of the specific family in which a genetic risk has been identified. In this penultimate section, we broaden our focus to look at ethics and the communication of genetic information in families in a more overarching way, before turning to some pragmatic suggestions to ethically promote family communication.

Nondisclosure can be considered as an instance where communication has failed.[9] When a proband refuses, or otherwise does not transmit genomic information, the health professional faces a dilemma regarding whether to intervene and, if so, how. Traditionally, nondisclosure has tended to be framed as a dilemma between alternatives: Do we respect confidentiality or breach it? Do we say it is out of professionals' hands, or do we enforce a duty to warn? These framings have also led to a tendency within the literature to write about family communication and nondisclosure in terms of professional duties (Wouters et al., 2016). Yet as the above discussion illustrates, the shared nature of genetic information challenges these dichotomous and legalistic ways of framing dilemmas of family communication. A focus on any professional duty to warn may clash with predominant values in genetic counseling, such as nondirectiveness (Hodgson & Gaff, 2013).[10] Furthermore, an approach based on confidentiality dilemmas will justify disclosure in only a limited set of circumstances, precluding the opportunity for many at-risk family members to decide whether they want to know their risk (Gilbar, 2007).

Focusing on confidentiality and limited professional duties to disclose also exemplifies liberal individualism (Gilbar, 2007). Pitting professionals against probands, and probands against their families, could end up creating greater tensions, leading to harm. As such, the literature on family communication is changing emphasis to focus on "family communication" rather than the punitive moniker of "nondisclosure" (Wilson & Etchegary, 2010). This emphasis on family communication is being discussed as it relates to both probands and families more broadly.

Regarding a positive approach to family communication that focuses on probands, Rehmann-Sutter (2009) emphasizes the importance of recognizing patient agency in the process of family communication. It is important to recognize a proband's sense of self and autonomy, while also helping them to find a course of action to communicate genetic information that is both practical for them and in line with their values. Weaver (2016) similarly calls for an approach that draws on an ethics of care "grounded in voice and relationships, recognizing the importance of a patient's being listened to carefully and heard with respect" (p. 185).

Regarding families, Doukas and Berg (2001) offer an ethical framing of the fair warning model discussed above, which they call the "family covenant." This covenant, which is defined consensually before testing, balances a proband's autonomy with the potential benefit to genetic relatives. Davey et al. (2006) advocate for "familial comity," which denotes

[9] This issue will arise most often in those settings where genetic health professionals are not tasked (whether legally or due to professional standards) with routinely managing and overseeing family communication.

[10] Editors' note: For a discussion of the various conceptions of nondirectiveness in genetic counseling, see Chapter 23 by Michael J. Deem in this volume.

"considerate behavior towards others" and calls for the implications of genetic information for relatives to be routinely considered in practice. Gilbar (2007) and Mendes et al. (2018) argue for family-centered approaches, which explicitly account for familial relationships and make the family the "unit" that is cared for. Others, such as Chico (2016), argue for a "culture of sharing" in genetics and claim that sharing can occur while still upholding the core justificatory bases for confidentiality, namely, full disclosure and trust from patients, albeit a different kind of trust. In these approaches, all stakeholders deliberate on communication and work together to address conflict.

Taken together, these ideas suggest a move toward a more proactive, positive, and facilitative approach, one that aims to recognize and involve health professionals, probands, and their genetic relatives, as noted in the counseling literature (Hodgson & Gaff, 2013; McClellan et al., 2013; Mendes et al., 2016). Both the proband's perspective regarding interpersonal relationships in the family and the information needs of family members are accounted for, as is the impact that the quality of communication or the event of nondisclosure can have. How probands reach their decision is important, as are other factors about their lives, as well as the imputed perspectives of at-risk relatives. Time pressures can also be considered, such as whether disclosure needs to happen imminently.

These approaches, however, may not suggest concrete options in practice and so may generate uncertainty for health professionals regardless of legal, regulatory, or professional oversight. It may therefore be helpful to consider some general considerations (Box 24.2) to assist genetics professionals in navigating family communication. With these points, our hope is that whatever ethical or legal constraints health professionals find themselves facing, they will have some means to deliberate and manage these issues. We have also discussed here the benefits of a more holistic approach to managing genetic information within families. However, we recognize that this will also likely require additional resources to operationalize, especially with the mainstreaming of genomics (Phillips et al., 2025). Health professionals may require education, including developing mediation skills. Resources such as clinic time will also need to be dedicated (Mendes et al., 2024; Phillips et al., 2025).

Conclusion

Contributing to the ethical communication of familial genetic and genomic information is an important aspect of genetic counseling practice. Ensuring that appropriate communication occurs is motivated by the goal of ensuring that any genetic relative who may develop, or have a future child with, a serious genetic condition will have the opportunity to make decisions about testing and further intervention, if they wish to. But even stating this stipulation gives rise to multiple considerations. There are ethical considerations of autonomy, privacy, familial obligations, and professionalism. There are legal considerations around possible duties, on whom they may fall, and how they may be discharged. The relevant stakeholders include genetic counselors, probands, and genetic relatives. Information could be passed on by the counselor, another health professional, or the proband. Disclosure could be permissible or mandated. None of these issues are resolved by the move from genetic to genomic technologies.

Box 24.2 Tools to Assist Health Professionals Navigate Family Communication

1. Be aware of the possibility of both active and passive nondisclosure, even when probands express understanding of familial risk and a willingness to communicate.
2. Engage the idea of family communication and the familial nature of genetic information early in the process. Reassuring probands and engaging with them regarding how to share may help to limit instances of nondisclosure (Black et al., 2013).
3. Offer to help the proband with communication and be available to answer relatives' questions, which may assist with clearer and more accurate communication (Black et al., 2013; Mendes et al., 2016). Such guidance may also increase patients' willingness to reach out to more distant family members (Black et al., 2013).
4. Be prepared: Even when a proband gives consent to undergo testing but declares their intention to not share information, it is important to discuss the potential relevance of findings for family members prior to testing, as well as the clinic's approach to family communication (e.g., patient or family-mediated, direct contact) and the support available to the proband. Doing so can help to keep lines of communication open after testing.
5. Undertake regular discussion: When communication is difficult and a risk of (active or passive) nondisclosure is apparent, health professionals can work as a team to consider the relative risks and benefits of different courses of action or inaction (Steel, 2009).
6. Consult relevant regulations or guidelines, which outline the position of pertinent national and/or professional societies (Middleton et al., 2020; Steel, 2009).
7. Seek additional support, such as clinical ethics consultation, where it is available. Clinical ethics support services, especially those that are patient facing, can help health professionals consider specific dilemmas in family communication.
8. Document the decision made: Noting the discussions and thought processes when making plans around managing family communication may not only help with that reflection process but also be of value if a case is subsequently subject to external review (Middleton et al., 2020).

In this chapter, we have discussed these issues and shown how they can be grouped into key legal and ethical questions. Ultimately, recognition of the potential for active or passive nondisclosure and the difficulties that patients may face in communicating information (Mendes et al., 2016), as well as early and active engagement of the proband with the notion of familial risk and the importance of sharing information, may help to emphasize the familial nature of genetic information, improve communication, and diminish the risk of a breakdown in family communication.

References

ABC v. St George's Healthcare Trust and Others (2020) EWHC 455.

Andersson, A., Hawranek, C., Ofverholm, A., Ehrencrona, H., Grill, K., Hajdarevic, S., Melin, B., Tham, E., Hellquist, B. N., & Rosén, A. (2020). Public support for healthcare-mediated disclosure of hereditary cancer risk information: Results from a population-based survey in Sweden. *Hereditary Cancer in Clinical Practice, 18*, 18. https://doi.org/10.1186/s13053-020-00151-0

Arribas-Ayllon, M., Featherstone, K., & Atkinson, P. (2011). The practical ethics of genetic responsibility: Non-disclosure and the autonomy of affect. *Social Theory & Health, 9*(1), 3–23.

Bell, D., & Bennett, B. (2001). Genetic secrets and the family. *Medical Law Review*, *9*(2), 130–161.

Black, L., McClellan, K. A., Avard, D., & Knoppers, B. M. (2013). Intrafamilial disclosure of risk for hereditary breast and ovarian cancer: Points to consider. *Journal of Community Genetics*, *4*(2), 203–214.

Chico, V. (2012). Known unknowns and unknown unknowns: The potential and the limits of autonomy in non-disclosure of genetic risk. *Journal of Professional Negligence*, *3*, 162–181.

Chico, V. (2016). Non-disclosure of genetic risks: The case for developing legal wrongs. *Medical Law International*, *16*(1–2), 3–26.

Chico, V. (2019). Reasonable expectations of privacy in non-disclosure of familial genetic risk: What is it reasonable to expect? *European Journal of Medical Genetics*, *62*(5), 308–315.

Chivers Seymour, K., Addington-Hall, J., Lucassen, A. M., & Foster, C. L. (2010). What facilitates or impedes family communication following genetic testing for cancer risk? A systematic review and meta-synthesis of primary qualitative research. *Journal of Genetic Counseling*, *19*(4), 330–342.

Clarke, A., Richards, M., Kerzin-Storrar, L., Halliday, J., Young, M. A., Simpson, S. A., Featherstone, K., Forrest, K., Lucassen, A., Morrison, P. J., Quarrell, O. W. J., & Stewart, H. (2005). Genetic professionals' reports of nondisclosure of genetic risk information within families. *European Journal of Human Genetics*, *13*(5), 556–562.

d'Audiffret Van Haecke, D., & de Montgolfier, S. (2018). Genetic diseases and information to relatives: Practical and ethical issues for professionals after introduction of a legal framework in France. *European Journal of Human Genetics*, *26*(6), 786–795.

Davey, A., Newson, A. J., & O'Leary, P. (2006). Communication of genetic information within families: The case for familial comity. *Journal of Bioethical Inquiry*, *3*, 161–166.

de Paor, A. (2018). Genetic risks and doctors' disclosure obligations—Revisiting the duty of confidentiality. *European Journal of Health Law*, *25*, 365–388.

Derbez, B., de Pauw, A., Stoppa-Lyonnet, D., Galacteros, F., & de Montgolfier, S. (2019). Familial disclosure by genetic healthcare professionals: A useful but sparingly used legal provision in France. *Journal of Medical Ethics*, *45*(12), 811–816.

Dheensa, S., Fenwick, A., & Lucassen, A. (2016). "Is this knowledge mine and nobody else's? I don't feel that." Patient views about consent, confidentiality and information-sharing in genetic medicine. *Journal of Medical Ethics*, *42*(3), 174–179.

Dheensa, S., Lucassen, A., & Fenwick, A. (2018). Limitations and pitfalls of using family letters to communicate genetic risk: A qualitative study with patients and healthcare professionals. *Journal of Genetic Counseling*, *27*(3), 689–701.

Dive, L. (2021). From a right to a preference: Rethinking the right to genomic ignorance. *Journal of Medicine and Philosophy*, *46*(5), 605–629.

Dive, L., & Newson, A. J. (2018). Reconceptualizing autonomy for bioethics. *Kennedy Institute Ethics Journal*, *28*(2), 171–203.

Doukas, D. J., & Berg, J. W. (2001). The family covenant and genetic testing. *American Journal of Bioethics*, *1*(3), 3–10.

Dove, E. S., Chico, V., Fay, M., Laurie, G., Lucassen, A. M., & Postan, E. (2019). Familial genetic risks: How can we better navigate patient confidentiality and appropriate risk disclosure to relatives? *Journal of Medical Ethics*, *45*(8), 504–507.

Dove, E. S., Kelly, S. E., Lucivero, F., Machirori, M., Dheensa, S., & Prainsack, B. (2017). Beyond individualism: Is there a place for relational autonomy in clinical practice and research? *Clinical Ethics*, *12*(3), 150–165.

Duncan, R. E., & Newson, A. J. (2006). Clinical genetics and the problem with unqualified confidentiality. *American Journal of Bioethics, 6*(2), 41–43.

Falk, M. J., Dugan, R. B., O'Riordan, M. A., Matthews, A. L., & Robin, N. H. (2003). Medical geneticists' duty to warn at-risk relatives for genetic disease. *American Journal of Medical Genetics Part A, 120A*(3), 374–380.

Forrest, L. E., Delatycki, M. B., Skene, L., & Aitken, M. (2007). Communicating genetic information in families—A review of guidelines and position papers. *European Journal of Human Genetics, 15*(6), 612–618.

Foster, C., & Gilbar, R. (2021). Is there a new duty to warn family members in English medical law? ABC V St George's Healthcare NHS Trust and Others [2020] EWHC 4551. *Medical Law Review, 29*(2), 359–372.

Gilbar, R. (2007). Communicating genetic information in the family: The familial relationship as the forgotten factor. *Journal of Medical Ethics, 33*(7), 390–393.

Godard, B., Hurlimann, T., Letendre, M., Egalite, N., & INHERIT BRCAs. (2006). Guidelines for disclosing genetic information to family members: From development to use. *Familial Cancer, 5*(1), 103–116.

Grill, K., & Rosen, A. (2020). Healthcare professionals' responsibility for informing relatives at risk of hereditary disease. *Journal of Medical Ethics, 47*, e12. https://doi.org/10.1136/medethics-2020-106236

Heaton, T. J., & Chico, V. (2016). Attitudes towards the sharing of genetic information with at-risk relatives: Results of a quantitative survey. *Human Genetics, 135*(1), 109–120.

Henrikson, N. B., Wagner, J. K., Hampel, H., DeVore, C., Shridhar, N., Williams, J. L., Donohue, K. E., Kullo, I., & Prince, A. E. R. (2020). What guidance does HIPAA offer to providers considering familial risk notification and cascade genetic testing? *Journal of Law and the Biosciences, 7*(1), lsaa071. https://doi.org/10.1093/jlb/lsaa071

Hodgson, J., & Gaff, C. (2013). Enhancing family communication about genetics: Ethical and professional dilemmas. *Journal of Genetic Counseling, 22*(1), 16–21.

Hunter, J. E., Riddle, L., Joseph, G., Amendola, L. M., Gilmore, M. J., Zepp, J. M., Shuster, E., Bulkley, J. E., Muessig, K. R., Anderson, K. P., Goddard, K. A.B., Wilfond, B. S., Leo, M. C., & CHARM study team. (2023). Most people share genetic test results with relatives even if the findings are normal: Family communication in a diverse population. *Genetics in Medicine, 25*(11), 100923.

Husted, J. (1997). Autonomy and a right not to know. In R. F. Chadwick, M. Levitt, & D. Shickle (Eds.), *The right to know and the right not to know* (pp. 55–68). Avebury.

Joint Committee on Genomics in Medicine. (2019). *Consent and confidentiality in genomic medicine*. https://www.rcplondon.ac.uk/projects/outputs/consent-and-confidentiality-genomic-medicine

Kilbride, M. K. (2018). Genetic privacy, disease prevention, and the principle of rescue. *Hastings Center Report, 48*(3), 10–17.

Kottow, M. H. (1986). Medical confidentiality: An intransigent and absolute obligation. *Journal of Medical Ethics, 12*(3), 117–122.

Lacroix, M., Nycum, G., Godard, B., & Knoppers, B. M. (2008). Should physicians warn patients' relatives of genetic risks? *Canadian Medical Association Journal, 178*(5), 593–595.

Leonard, S. J., & Newson, A. J. (2010). Ethical perspectives. In C. L. Gaff & C. L. Bylund (Eds.), *Family communication about genetics: Theory and practice* (pp. 199–214). Oxford University Press.

Lucassen, A. (2020, March 2). *ABC v St George's: exercising judgment without fear*. BioNews. https://www.bionews.org.uk/page_148351

Lucassen, A., & Clarke, A. (2022). In the family: Access to, and communication of, familial information in clinical practice. *Human Genetics*, *141*(5), 1053–1058.

Lucassen, A., & Gilbar, R. (2018). Disclosure of genetic information to relatives: Balancing confidentiality and relatives' interests. *Journal of Medical Genetics*, *55*(4), 285–286.

MacDougall, R. (2004). Rethinking the "right not to know." *Monash Bioethics Review*, *23*(1), 22–36.

McClellan, K. A., Kleiderman, E., Black, L., Bouchard, K., Dorval, M., Simard, J., Knoppers, B. M., & Avard, D. (2013). Exploring resources for intrafamilial communication of cancer genetic risk: We still need to talk. *European Journal of Human Genetics*, *21*(9), 903–910.

McWhirter, R., Johnston, C., & Burke, J. (2019). Disclosure of genetic results to at-risk relatives without consent: Issues for health care professionals in Australia. *Journal of Law and Medicine*, *27*(1), 108–121.

Meggiolaro, N., Barlow-Stewart, K., Dunlop, K., Newson, A. J., & Fleming, J. (2020). Disclosure to genetic relatives without consent—Australian genetic professionals' awareness of the health privacy law. *BMC Medical Ethics*, *21*(1), 13. https://doi.org/10.1186/s12910-020-0451-1

Mendes, A., Metcalfe, A., Paneque, M., Sousa, L., Clarke, A. J., & Sequeiros, J. (2018). Communication of information about genetic risks: Putting families at the center. *Family Process*, *57*(3), 836–846.

Mendes, Á., Paneque, M., & Sequeiros, J. (2024). Disclosure of genetic risk to family members: A qualitative study on healthcare professionals' perceived roles and responsibilities. *European Journal of Medical Genetics*, *68*, 104931.

Mendes, A., Paneque, M., Sousa, L., Clarke, A., & Sequeiros, J. (2016). How communication of genetic information within the family is addressed in genetic counselling: A systematic review of research evidence. *European Journal of Human Genetics*, *24*(3), 315–325.

Middleton, A. (2012). Communication about DTC testing: Commentary on a "family experience of personal genomics." *Journal of Genetic Counseling*, *21*(3), 392–398.

Middleton, A., Mendes, A., Benjamin, C. M., & Howard, H. C. (2017). Direct-to-consumer genetic testing: Where and how does genetic counseling fit? *Journal of Personalized Medicine*, *14*(3), 249–257.

Middleton, A., Patch, C., Roberts, J., Milne, R., Costa, A., Robarts, L., & Autornu, J. (2020). Professional duties are now considered legal duties of care within genomic medicine. *European Journal of Human Genetics*, *28*(10), 1301–1304.

Mitchell, C., Ploem, M. C., Hennekam, R. C., & Kaye, J. (2016). A duty to warn relatives in clinical genetics: Arguably "fair just and reasonable" in English law? *Tottel's Journal of Professional Negligence*, *32*(2), 120–136.

Montgomery, J. (2017). Data sharing and the idea of ownership. *New Bioethics*, *23*(1), 81–86.

Murphy, C., Sturm, S., McKenna, M. J., & Ormond, K. E. (2024). The right not to know: Non-disclosure of primary genetic test results and genetic counselors' response. *Journal of Genetic Counseling*, *33*(4), 875–887.

Murray, M. F. (2018). The path to routine genomic screening in health care. *Annals of Internal Medicine*, *169*(6), 407–408.

Newson, A. J., & Humphries, S. E. (2005). Cascade testing in familial hypercholesterolaemia: How should family members be contacted? *European Journal of Human Genetics*, *13*(4), 401–408.

Offit, K., Groeger, E., Turner, S., Wadsworth, E. A., & Weiser, M. A. (2004). The "duty to warn" a patient's family members about hereditary disease risks. *JAMA*, *292*(12), 1469–1473.

Otlowski, M. (2013). Australian law reforms enabling disclosure of genetic information to genetic relatives by health practitioners. *Journal of Law and Medicine*, *21*, 217–234.

Otlowski, M. F. (2015). Disclosing genetic information to at-risk relatives: New Australian privacy principles, but uniformity still elusive. *Medical Journal of Australia, 202*(6), 335–337.
Parker, M., & Lucassen, A. (2018). Using a genetic test result in the care of family members: How does the duty of confidentiality apply? *European Journal of Human Genetics, 26*(7), 955–959.
Parker, M., & Lucassen, A. M. (2004). Genetic information: A joint account? *BMJ, 329*(7458), 165–167.
Pate v. Threlkel 661 So. 2d 278, 282 (Fla. 1995).
Phillips, A., Borry, P., Van Hoyweghen, I., & Vears, D. F. (2021). Disclosure of genetic information to family members: A systematic review of normative documents. *Genetics in Medicine, 23*(11), 2038–2046.
Phillips, A., Van Steijvoort, E., Siermann, M., Kuiper, J. M. L., Mendes, Á., de Montgolfier, S., Petersen, H. V., Rosén, A., Van Esch, H., Pasquier, L., Vears, D. F., Patch, C., Van Hoof, W., Newson, A. J., Bulk, S., van El, C., Dancet, E., Rial-Sebbag, E., Mitchell, C., & Borry, P. (2025). Genomic findings with familial implications: agenda setting in light of mainstreaming. *Open Research Europe, 5*, 4.
Phillips, A., Vears, D. F., Van Hoyweghen, I., & Borry, P. (2024). Clinician perspectives on policy approaches to genetic risk disclosure in families. *Familial Cancer, 23*(2), 177–186.
Rehmann-Sutter, C. (2009). Allowing agency: An ethical model for communicating personal genetic information. In H. Müller (Ed.), *Disclosure dilemmas: Ethics of genetic prognosis after the "right to know/not to know" debate* (pp. 231–259). Routledge.
Rhodes, R. (1998). Genetic links, family ties, and social bonds: Rights and responsibilities in the face of genetic knowledge. *Journal of Medicine and Philosophy, 23*(1), 10–30.
Rothstein, M. A. (2018). Reconsidering the duty to warn genetically at-risk relatives. *Genetics in Medicine, 20*(3), 285–290.
Safer v. Estate of Pack 677 A. 2d 1188, 1192-1193 (N.J. Super. Ct. App. Div.).
Skene, L. (1998). Patients' rights or family responsibilities? Two approaches to genetic testing. *Medical Law Review, 6*(1), 1–41.
Steel, M. (2009). Responsibility towards relatives. In H. Müller (Ed.), *Disclosure dilemmas: Ethics of genetic prognosis after the "right to know/not to know" debate* (pp. 153–165). Routledge.
Stott, A., Madelli, E. O., Boughtwood, T., Nowak, K. J., Otlowski, M., & Tiller, J. (2025). Health professionals contacting patients' relatives directly about genetic risk (with patient consent): Current clinical practice and perspectives. *European Journal of Human Genetics, 33*(4), 476–484.
Takala, T. (1999). The right to genetic ignorance confirmed. *Bioethics, 13*(3–4), 288–293.
Tiller, J., Finlay, K., Madelli, E. O., Monnik, M., Jackson, M. R., Poplawski, N., Boughtwood, T., Nowak, K. J., & Otlowski, M. (2025). Patients' perspectives regarding health professionals contacting their relatives about genetic risk directly (with patient consent). *European Journal of Human Genetics, 33*(4), 485–495.
van den Heuvel, L. M., Maeckelberghe, E. L. M., Ploem, M. C., & Christiaans, I. A. (2021). A genetic researcher's devil's dilemma: Warn relatives about their genetic risk or respect confidentiality agreements with research participants? *BMC Medical Ethics, 22*(1), 155.
van den Heuvel, L. M., Smets, E. M. A., van Tintelen, J. P., & Christiaans, I. (2019). How to inform relatives at risk of hereditary diseases? A mixed-methods systematic review on patient attitudes. *Journal of Genetic Counseling, 28*(5), 1042–1058.
Weaver, M. (2016). The double helix: Applying an ethic of care to the duty to warn genetic relatives of genetic information. *Bioethics, 30*(3), 181–187.
Wilson, B. J., & Etchegary, H. (2010). Family communication of genomic information. In K. B. Tercyak (Ed.), *Handbook of genomics and the family* (pp. 163–189). Springer.

Wilson, J. (2005). To know or not to know? Genetic ignorance, autonomy and paternalism. *Bioethics, 19*(5–6), 492–504.

Wiseman, M., Dancyger, C., & Michie, S. (2010). Communicating genetic risk information within families: A review. *Familial Cancer*, 9(4), 691–703.

Wouters, R. H., Bijlsma, R. M., Ausems, M. G., van Delden, J. J., Voest, E. E., & Bredenoord, A. L. (2016). Am I my family's keeper? Disclosure dilemmas in next-generation sequencing. *Human Mutation, 37*(12), 1257–1262.

CHAPTER 25

GENETIC COUNSELORS' PERSONAL REACTIONS AND THE ETHICAL IMPLICATIONS FOR GENETIC COUNSELING PRACTICE

PATRICIA MCCARTHY VEACH AND
KRISTA REDLINGER-GROSSE

Introduction

GENETIC counseling is a profession that requires its practitioners to have both deep and extensive biomedical knowledge and strong intra- and interpersonal skills. Genetic counseling practice is a dynamic process in which genetic counselors' knowledge, skills (e.g., communication), and individual and cultural characteristics (e.g., empathy) interact with those of their patients (Abrams & Kessler, 2002; Marks, 1993, 2003; McCarthy & Leroy, 2012; McCarthy Veach et al., 2002, 2007; Weil, 2003). Genetic counselors must strive to develop and maintain an accurate awareness of their unique set of characteristics and the potential impact on genetic counseling processes and outcomes. As Pirzadeh et al. (2007) noted, "When genetic counselors provide clinical service, who they are may play as important a role as what they know" (p. 763).

Seymour Kessler's writings serve to illuminate key aspects of "the inner life" of genetic counselors (cf. Abrams & Kessler, 2002). Inner life refers to a counselor's personal "psychological world" (Abrams & Kessler, 2002, p. 5). Abrams and Kessler (2002) note, "The two worlds—the scientific and the psychological—follow their own kind of logic, sometimes converging and often diverging along differing paths. The interior psychological world does not always show the linearity and structure we experience in the scientific domain of genetic counseling" (p. 5).

Kessler was among the first individuals to write about the importance of genetic counselors engaging in self-reflection (cf. Kessler, 1979) to recognize and address their inner life and its effects on practice. His work contributed to the development of a current model of genetic counseling practice, the Reciprocal-Engagement Model (REM) (McCarthy Veach et al., 2007). The REM emphasizes genetic counselor self-awareness/reflective practice (e.g., "genetic counselors are reflective practitioners, who are self-aware, ethical, objective to the extent possible, and open and responsive to feedback," McCarthy Veach et al., 2007, p. 721; and "genetic counselors assess and address relevant patient psychosocial factors and they are aware of and manage their own psychosocial histories within an individualized process," McCarthy Veach et al., 2007, p. 725).[1]

The Accreditation Council of Genetic Counseling (ACGC) practice-based competencies require entry-level genetic counselors to "demonstrate a self-reflective, evidence-based and current approach to genetic counseling practice" (ACGC, 2019, p. 2). Similarly, the 2017 NSGC Code of Ethics (National Society of Genetic Counselors [NSGC], 2018) identifies several aspects of genetic counselor professional conduct that imply the necessity of self-reflection. These include being "aware of the ethical implications of their professional actions"; recognizing "the limits of their own knowledge, expertise, and competence"; acknowledging "circumstances that may interfere with or influence professional judgment or objectivity"; being "responsible for their own physical and emotional health as it impacts their professional judgment and performance, including seeking professional support, as needed"; providing "genetic counseling services to their clients within their scope of practice regardless of personal interests or biases"; and referring "clients to an alternate genetic counselor or other qualified professional when situations arise in which a genetic counselor's personal values, attitudes and beliefs may impede his or her ability to counsel a client" (NSGC, 2018, pp. 6–7).

As self-reflective practice is fundamental in supporting many aspects of genetic counseling practice and counselor competencies, we begin this chapter by briefly defining "self-reflection." The importance of self-reflective practice is evident in the next sections in which we discuss theory and research on common genetic counselor reactions of countertransference, moral distress, and compassion fatigue. We end the chapter by suggesting strategies for recognizing and managing these types of reactions. The strategies are intended to help genetic counselors to maintain a standard of patient care as well as their own professional vitality and efficacy.

Self-Reflection

Self-reflection, in the context of a health profession like genetic counseling, is a cognitive skill that involves processing one's experiences as a practitioner (Lowe et al., 2007), especially challenging experiences. Self-reflection generally involves deliberate, persistent, and careful consideration of any belief or supposed form of knowledge in light of the grounds supporting it and the further consequences to which it leads (Dewey, 1933). Reiser (2021) notes that "reflection is not simply thinking, or ruminating without purpose. Reflection is

[1] Editors' note: For more on the Reciprocal-Engagement Model, see Chapter 5 by Patricia McCarthy Veach and Bonnie S. LeRoy in this volume.

a process characterized by deliberate, active seeking of growth and development involving both one's professional and personal selves, often including self-examination and subsequent changes in one's beliefs, actions, and perspectives" (p. 351).

Self-reflection is *valuable* to the extent that it improves the quality of the reflective outcome. Reflective outcomes vary and may include, for instance, revised beliefs, rejection of certain beliefs, and/or justification of certain beliefs. Research indicates that self-reflective practice allows practitioners to better distinguish between empathy and countertransference (Silverman, 2008). Research further demonstrates that self-reflection contributes to successful ethical decisions. Practitioners who intentionally evaluate value conflicts are better able to both identify and set aside their values in favor of clients' values (Deming et al., 2007).

Studies of genetic counselors' characteristics and experiences support the importance of self-reflection. For instance, an investigation of practicing genetic counselors revealed that self-reflection is an essential skill for promoting awareness of their thoughts, feelings, and actions and for promoting their sense of meaning and purpose (Wells et al., 2016). Miranda et al. (2016) found that master genetic counselor clinicians shared a common characteristic of engaging in self-reflection about their professional and personal life experiences. Their participants described self-reflection as "a willingness and openness to continuously engage in a process of critical analysis of one's thoughts and/or behaviors in order to understand motives and continually 'self-evaluate'" (Miranda et al., 2016, p. 772).

Zahm et al. (2016) interviewed clinical genetic counselors at varying stages of professional experience (novice, experienced, seasoned). A prevalent theme across professional levels was the critical role self-reflection played in their professional development. Wells et al. (2016), in their study of genetic counselors' experiences of meaning, postulated that practicing self-reflection might lessen genetic counselor experiences of compassion fatigue and burnout. Findings from studies consistently suggest that "A commitment to lifelong learning and self-reflective practice . . . greatly enhance [a genetic counselor's] ability to develop professionally" (McCarthy Veach et al., 2018, p. 359).

Countertransference

> Genetic counselor: *I think countertransference can be productive if a person is aware of it in the moment. I often have patients whose situations cause me strong emotions. . . . [R]ealizing that countertransference is present can actually lead to a really productive conversation even though it can be extremely uncomfortable.* (Reeder et al., 2017, p. 942)

Genetic counselor countertransference refers to "conscious and unconscious emotions, fantasies, behaviors, perceptions and psychological defenses the genetic counselor experiences as a response to any aspect of the genetic counseling situation" (Redlinger-Grosse, 2021, p. 154). Given the challenging interpersonal work genetic counselors perform in the context of complex genetic information and decision making, countertransference is a dynamic that inevitably arises during the genetic counseling process (Reeder et al., 2017). Countertransference is ubiquitous in healthcare relationships. As an emergency room physician notes, "No manual can prepare us fully for patients who reject help, tug on our heartstrings, revive our deepest memories, or elicit fear, pity or shock, and disbelief. . . . as such emotions will be present, and need to be acknowledged and managed, so we offer our patients, the best care possible" (Moukaddam et al., 2016, p. 95).

Recognition of countertransference elements that emerge for genetic counselors is critical to providing patients with a standard of care. The range of issues and emotions that can elicit countertransference is undeniably broad. The literature provides examples of common triggers for countertransference in genetic counseling that include patient characteristics; disease, disability, and loss; diversity issues; and challenging genetic counseling situations such as patient anger (e.g., Redlinger-Grosse, 2021; Reeder et al., 2017; Schema, 2021; Schema et al., 2015).

Kessler (1992) identified two general types of genetic counselor countertransference: projective and associative countertransference. *Projective countertransference* occurs when the genetic counselor overidentifies with some characteristic(s) of the patient or aspects of the patient's experience (e.g., the patient and genetic counselor both lost a mother to breast cancer) and mistakenly replaces the patient's feelings with their own. Relatedly, genetic counselors experience *associative countertransference* when something about the patient's situation prompts the counselors to become immersed in/distracted by their own inner experience (e.g., worrying about their own ovarian cancer risk as they hear about the patient's ovarian cancer diagnosis). As a consequence, the counselor has difficulty focusing on the patient and the patient's individual needs. While associative countertransference may be triggered by projective identification, an awareness exists that the genetic counselor's feelings and reactions differ from those of the patient. Thus, associative countertransference may be somewhat easier for a genetic counselor to anticipate, recognize, and manage.

Reeder et al. (2017) surveyed genetic counselors about their countertransference experiences and found evidence of both projective and associative countertransference. Prevalent triggers included similarity to the patient, medical/genetic similarity, angry patients, patient behaviors that differ from the genetic counselor's expectations, and delivering bad news. Additional sources of countertransference include grief/loss, diverse or differing cultural influences, disability experiences, family dynamics, and medical diagnoses (e.g., Ali & Bellcross, 2021; Redlinger-Grosse, 2021; Warren, 2021). Several genetic counselors have shared moving accounts of personal life experiences that affected their responses to patient issues arising in their genetic counseling practice (e.g., Anonymous, 2008; Bellcross, 2012; Clark, 2010, 2012; Hyatt, 2012; Keilman, 2002). A pivotal reflection point for these authors is distinguishing between empathy and countertransference in their genetic counseling practice. The authors describe an ongoing deliberate practice of asking themselves in the moment whose feelings and needs they are serving—the patient's or their own. This question helps them to remain grounded in empathy while setting aside their countertransference reactions. In other words, the genetic counselor takes a step back to think about the source of their feelings and reactions to the patient's situation. This allows the counselor to distinguish between empathy and countertransference.

A genetic counselor's awareness and management of countertransference influence its impact on the patient and, potentially, genetic counseling outcomes. When recognized and managed appropriately, countertransference may increase empathy and strengthen the patient–counselor relationship, as well as the meaning and connection genetic counselors find in their work. For instance, as McCarthy Veach et al. (2018) note regarding genetic counselor countertransference:

> One possible positive consequence of countertransference is that the triggering of experiences from your past might give you increased empathy for patients (to the extent that your experiences are similar to theirs).... [Of note,] however, there is always the risk that you may listen less carefully to patients and instead impose your experience on them. (p. 335)

Self-reflection remains central to this process, helping genetic counselors anticipate their countertransference reactions and notice when countertransference is occurring in the moment. Awareness can be fostered through an understanding of one's countertransference triggers, emotional attunement to feelings prior to or during sessions such as frustration or sadness (Kessler, 1992; Reeder et al., 2017), and recognition of behaviors such as an increase in self-disclosure or loss of neutrality (Hofsess & Tracey, 2010).

In contrast, unmanaged countertransference may have deleterious effects on session processes and outcomes, due to, for example, a reduction of counselor empathy, withdrawal and disengagement in the session, unhealthy boundaries, and/or inadequate follow-up (Kessler, 1992; Likhite, 2000; Nathan et al., 2018; Reeder et al., 2017; VandenLangenberg et al., 2012). The effects of unmanaged countertransference on the genetic counselor may include placing them at increased risk of moral distress and compassion fatigue and ethically questionable practices such as boundary violations.

Moral Distress

> Genetic counselor: *When you cannot give them concrete information to go on . . . [y]ou just kind of feel helpless that no matter how much research you do you still cannot clarify the situation for them and they are looking to you for support and for information. . . . I guess feeling helpless is probably the biggest thing of just not being able to provide what they need.* (Bernhardt et al., 2010, p. 292)

Moral distress is a prevalent topic in the healthcare literature, although there is not a universally agreed-upon definition (Dean et al., 2020; Morley et al., 2019). Morley et al. (2019) conducted a systematic literature review and narrative synthesis of 34 papers from nursing, medicine, social work, and education "to explore the necessary and sufficient conditions required to define moral distress" (p. 646). Based on their analysis, they concluded:

> Moral distress is said to occur when one has made a moral judgement but is unable to act upon it. . . . We suggest the combination of (1) the experience of a moral event, (2) the experience of "psychological distress" and (3) a direct causal relation between (1) and (2) together are necessary and sufficient conditions for moral distress. (Morley et al., 2019, p. 646).

Dean et al. (2020) draw distinctions among moral dilemmas, moral distress, and moral injury to characterize their potential contributions to physician distress. They assert that interventions aimed at reducing or addressing clinician distress may be best viewed as a continuum "that begins with moral dilemma and progresses through moral distress, moral injury" (Dean et al., 2020, p. 924). They define moral dilemmas as situations in which "more than 1 answer is morally defensible, but none leads to an ideal outcome" (Dean et al., 2020, p. 923). Moral distress

> occurs when an individual believes he or she knows the right thing to do, but institutional or other constraints make it difficult to do what is right. . . . Moral distress happens at the intersection between the clinician's own moral framework, which remains intact, and the values of the health care system. (Dean et al., 2020, p. 923)

The authors assert that moral injury occurs when morally distressing situations lack "resolution with sufficient processing," resulting in moral residue, that is, "the unresolved emotional and psychological conflicts attendant to episodes of distress" (Dean et al., 2020, p. 923). Moral residue makes subsequent moral dilemmas or moral distress less tolerable, which increases the risk of moral injury.

> Moral injury implies an erosion of a person's moral framework as the result of a single egregious violation or persistent, repeated moral distresses. The accumulation of these incidents could drive clinicians to question their perceptions of medicine as a safe, benevolent profession and the belief that those working in it are trustworthy. (Dean et al., 2000, p. 923)

Within the genetic counseling literature, moral distress has been conceptualized as "the physical or emotional suffering that is experienced when constraints, either internal or external, prevent one from following the course of action that one believes is right" (Bernhardt et al., 2009, p. 527). Bernhardt et al. (2009) assert that it is critical to recognize and manage moral distress as unmanaged moral distress "may lead to a crisis of conscience and is associated with job dissatisfaction and attrition" (p. 527). They cautioned about the risk posed by unmanaged moral distress and suggested a general approach for minimizing this risk:

> Unless feelings are identified and accepted as normal, maladaptive behaviors are likely to follow that will interfere with the clinician being able to provide high quality and compassionate care that meets the needs and goals of both the patient and the clinician. The clinician therefore needs to become self-aware by reflecting on experienced emotions, examining belief systems and values, and understanding the connection between the emotions and behavior. (Bernhardt et al., 2010, p. 295)

Research has identified situations that elicit moral distress in genetic counselors as well as common emotional reactions to those situations. Bernhardt et al. (2010) interviewed genetic counselors and identified the following experiences as variously distressing for their participants: patient/family decisions, colleague behavior, and difficult patients, which included personal value conflicts, among others; giving bad news; end-of-life issues, which included a burden of professional responsibility, among others; unintended outcomes (e.g., patient dread); and injustice/humanity, which prompted compassion stress. Across these experiences, the counselors reported a range of emotions that varied in intensity. For instance, counselors mentioned feeling guilt, anger, confusion, helplessness, inadequacy, grief, embarrassment, resentment, frustration, abandonment, apprehension, rejection, and outrage.

Moral distress, as defined by Bernhardt et al. (2009), is evident in a series of studies of ethical and professional challenges genetic counselors encounter in clinical settings (Alliman et al., 2009; Bower et al., 2002; Gschmeidler & Flatscher-Thoeni, 2010; McCarthy

Veach et al., 2001) and in laboratory settings (Groepper et al., 2015). Major ethical challenges found in these studies include, among others, value conflicts between the genetic counselor and patients/family members, other professionals, and society; colleague errors; colleague misconduct; uncertainty; and dealing with intense emotions (either the patient's or one's own feelings). These challenges involve ethical considerations established by the genetic counseling profession, legal considerations, and a practitioner's personal values/beliefs, and they provoke emotional reactions similar to those described by Bernhardt et al. (2010). Participants in the studies recommended various strategies for addressing ethical and professional challenges. Their recommendations included consultation with a colleague and setting aside personal beliefs. Arguably, self-reflection is a key component of these strategies, helping genetic counselors act in ways that align with ethical and legal guidelines.

Compassion Fatigue

> Genetic counselor: . . . *I do find days where I feel like I want to care more about my patients but just don't have the energy. I do my job and go through the motions but more days I feel like I don't really "feel" for my patients as much as I might have in the past. There are days when I really connect with a patient but those are the days when I take their concerns home with me and dwell on them so that's not great either.* (Lee et al., 2015, p. 366)

Exposure to patient suffering in genetic counseling work can exact a heavy toll—personally and professionally. When unmanaged, the cost can be a reduction in the genetic counselor's capacity for empathy and/or interest in engaging empathically (Figley, 2002). Described most commonly in healthcare professionals who help others in distress, compassion fatigue is "an extreme state of tension and preoccupation with the suffering of those being helped to the degree that it is traumatizing for the helper" (Figley, 2002, as cited in Injeyan et al., 2011, p. 526). While related to burnout, compassion fatigue differs in that it tends to be immediate and intense, can result from a single episode or event, and is specific to the helping professions. Burnout, which occurs in all professions, tends to be more chronic, develop over time in a cumulative manner, and have more systemic or institutional origins such as work overload and real or perceived inability of a worker to change the situation (Dexter et al., 2003).

Compassion fatigue is prevalent in genetic counseling. Udipi et al. (2008) surveyed 222 genetic counselors and found that 73% were at moderate to high risk for compassion fatigue. Lee et al. (2015) surveyed 402 genetic counselors and found that 61% were at high risk for compassion fatigue, with another 39% at average risk. Thus, genetic counselors are at substantial risk for experiencing compassion fatigue at some point in their work. Studies examining who and what place genetic counselors at risk for compassion fatigue have identified a host of factors, including personality/temperament traits such as perfectionism and low dispositional optimism (Benoit et al., 2007; Injeyan et al., 2011) and trait anxiety (Lee et al., 2015); low or absent social support and inadequate/unsupportive work environment (Udipi et al., 2008); low emotional intelligence (Zeidner et al., 2013); having an external locus of control (Injeyan et al., 2011); and burnout (Dexter et al., 2003; Johnstone et al., 2016).

Benoit et al. (2007) conducted a focus group with 12 practicing genetic counselors. Their participants described unique aspects of the genetic counseling process they believed contribute to compassion fatigue. These aspects include the short-term nature of the relationship, the intensity of encounters, and the fact that most people do not necessarily want to see a genetic counselor. Their participants described triggers for compassion fatigue that included giving bad news and an inability to prevent patient suffering. Of note, similar triggers have been identified in countertransference and moral distress research, suggesting the interrelated nature of these dynamics.

The impact of unrecognized and unmanaged compassion fatigue is far-reaching. For the genetic counselor, there are physical and psychological effects including exhaustion, sluggishness, and mood changes that can involve sadness, anger, and irritability (Figley, 2002). Professionally, compassion fatigue can lead to reduced work satisfaction and increased job turnover (Alkema et al., 2008; Sprang et al., 2007). Ultimately, patient care may suffer from the genetic counselor's reduced ability for and/or desire to engage empathically (Benoit et al., 2007). As with other dynamics (countertransference, moral distress), the impact of compassion fatigue depends in large part on its recognition and management. Once again, self-reflection is essential for recognizing this dynamic. Effective management involves self-care, increased professional education and conversations on compassion fatigue, and collegial supports (e.g., peer consultation; Alkema et al., 2008; Benoit et al., 2007; Dreher et al., 2019; Figley, 2002). These strategies and others are described in more detail in the next section.

Recognition and Management Strategies

A number of strategies may promote genetic counselor self-awareness and management of countertransference, moral distress, and compassion fatigue. These include individual behaviors on the part of the genetic counselor, group strategies, and efforts by the genetic counseling profession. These types of strategies may also increase genetic counselor resilience in the face of challenging professional experiences (Bernhardt et al., 2010). While mitigating factors (e.g., organizational/institutional constraints) may render some strategies more or less feasible for individual counselors, the following strategies have been shown to be generally efficacious.

Make time to practice intentional self-reflection

Self-reflection is key to self-awareness. Benefits of self-reflection include serving as ongoing motivation to continue one's practice that derives from reflecting on one's successes, achievements, and mistakes (Morgan et al., 2006); increasing the likelihood that one's professional experiences enhance behavior/professional development (Lowe et al., 2007; Reiser, 2021); and preventing stagnation (Ronnestad & Skovholt, 2001). Some of Miranda and colleagues' (2016) master genetic counselor clinicians noted that self-reflection serves as a coping strategy for managing emotional distress.

Practice mindfulness

Bernhardt et al. (2010) suggest activities such as mindfulness meditation (p. 295). They describe mindfulness as self-monitoring, remaining open to new experiences and perspectives, and fostering a sense of curiosity (e.g., about patients' lives/experiences). Silver et al. (2018) found that genetic counselors who practiced mindfulness had increased empathy and less compassion fatigue.

Engage in reflective writing

Bernhardt et al. (2010) recommend reflective writing activities such as "writing a brief narrative about a specific patient care experience, with a focus on the clinician reacting to the situation and then sharing it and working with a group of colleagues" (p.295).

Engage in strategic self-questioning

> Truth walks towards us on the paths of our questions. . . . As soon as you think you have the answer you have closed the path and may miss vital new information. Wait awhile in the stillness, and do not rush to conclusions, no matter how uncomfortable the unknowing. (Winspear, 2003, p. 32)

General questions genetic counselors could ask themselves about their practice include: What happened in the situation(s)? How was I feeling then? What am I feeling now? What thoughts did I have at the time? What thoughts do I have now about the situation? What did I do then? What do I think was prompting my reactions at the time? Have I ever felt this way before? What can I do to further understand the situation and my reactions? How will I recognize and manage similar situations in the future? Reeder et al. (2017) similarly recommended three key questions for genetic counselor reflection about countertransference experiences: "What is (was) my reaction (feelings, thoughts, actions?); Why am I reacting (did I react) that way?; and Where did my reaction come from?" (p. 945).

Maintain wellness through self-care activities

Wellness is "a way of life oriented toward optimal health and well-being in which the body, mind, and spirit are integrated by the individual to live more fully within the human and natural community" (Myers et al., 2000, as cited in Santana, 2017, p. 49). Myers et al. (2000) created a wellness wheel depicting dimensions of individual wellness. Four of these dimensions are physical, emotional, cognitive, and interpersonal. Other authors have identified self-care strategies that promote individual wellness. Self-care is "a set of purposeful behavioral strategies that promote the well-being of the self but also help to reduce stress and overcome challenges that enable the worker to engage effectively with their clients" (Acker, 2018, p. 715). Venart et al. (2007) described a number of self-care strategies for promoting wellness:

- *Physical wellness strategies* include adequate sleep, nutrition, and physical exercise; engaging in calming behaviors (e.g., monitoring and deepening one's breathing throughout the workday, meditation, massage, progressive muscle relaxation); and grounding one's self through the senses (paying attention to body signals at all times; pp. 52–53).
- *Emotional wellness strategies* include tuning into emotion—instead of escapist activities (e.g., computer games, drinking, surfing the internet), spend quiet time alone, engage in conversation, watch an inspiring film, or read a good book; playing with a pet or spending time with children; using self-reflection to consider one's work and personal reactions to it; and expressing emotions—research shows that writing/journaling about one's deepest thoughts and feelings can reduce depression and anxiety symptoms (pp. 53–55).
- *Cognitive wellness strategies* include cultivating healthy thinking patterns (e.g., recognize and avoid catastrophic or black-and-white thinking, recognize small victories and nuances of gray, refute the cognitive errors that fuel workaholism); acknowledging what one does not know, admitting mistakes, and giving oneself credit for what one does know; remaining curious rather than fearful of new experiences and ambiguous situations; savoring/celebrating small victories in one's professional development and service provision (pp. 55–58).
- *Interpersonal wellness strategies* include spending time with family and friends, especially those with whom there is a high quality of support; considering personal therapy for reducing physical and emotional distress; and engaging in peer consultation/supervision/support (pp. 58–62).

Seek personal counseling/psychotherapy

Counseling/therapy can help genetic counselors deepen their awareness of the origins of countertransference, value conflicts that lead to moral distress, and the type of fatigue that arises from compassionate empathic engagement with patients. Personal counseling can also provide support and guidance as genetic counselors identify and practice ways to manage these dynamics effectively.

Participate in ongoing supervision/consultation

A number of researchers recommend lifelong participation in formal or informal peer group supervision meetings as well as consultation with colleagues or mentors (e.g., Bernhardt et al., 2010; Kennedy, 2000a, 2000b; Lewis et al., 2017; Miranda et al., 2016; Zahm et al., 2008, 2016).

Provide training in self-reflective practice

Genetic counseling training programs and continuing education efforts should encourage ongoing development of self-reflection skills. As Pirzadeh et al. (2007) concluded, "Genetic counseling students and genetic counselors should be trained as reflective practitioners, engaging in continual self-scrutiny of their personal values and how they potentially affect their service provision" (p. 772).

Closing Thoughts

We have a few final thoughts about the dynamics described in this chapter. Genetic counselors should *not* have as their goal the elimination of countertransference, moral distress, and compassion fatigue. These dynamics are inherent to genetic counseling practice and to the caring and compassionate individuals who constitute the genetic counseling profession. Rather, through self-reflective practice, genetic counselors can learn to manage and embrace personal and professional challenges as bringing richness to their work. The content presented in this chapter suggests that genetic counselors bring themselves (flaws and all) to every genetic counseling experience.

References

Abrams, L. J., & Kessler, S. (2002). The inner world of the genetic counselor. *Journal of Genetic Counseling, 11*, 5–17.

Accreditation Council for Genetic Counseling. (2019). *Practice based competencies for genetic counselors*. https://www.gceducation.org/practice-based- competencies/

Acker, G. A. (2018). Self-care practices among social workers: Do they predict job satisfaction and turnover intention? *Social Work in Mental Health, 16*, 713–727.

Ali, N., & Bellcross, C. (2021). A genetic counselor's guide to understanding grief. In B. S. LeRoy, P. McCarthy Veach, & N. P. Callanan (Eds.), *Genetic counseling practice: Advanced concepts and skills* (2nd ed., pp. 79–108). John Wiley & Sons.

Alkema, K., Linton, J., & Davies, R. (2008). A study of the relationship between self-care, compassion satisfaction, compassion fatigue, and burnout among hospice professionals. *Journal of Social Work in End of Life and Palliative Care, 4*, 101–119.

Alliman, S., McCarthy Veach, P., Bartels, D. M., Lian, F., James, C., & LeRoy, B. S. (2009). A comparative analysis of ethical and professional challenges experienced by Australian and US genetic counselors. *Journal of Genetic Counseling, 18*, 379–394.

Anonymous. (2008). My story: A genetic counselor's journey from provider to patient: A mother's story. *Journal of Genetic Counseling, 17*, 412–418.

Bellcross, C. (2012). A genetic counselor's story of birth, grief, and survival. *Journal of Genetic Counseling, 21*, 169–172.

Benoit, L. G., Veach, P. M., & LeRoy, B. S. (2007). When you care enough to do your very best: Genetic counselor experiences of compassion fatigue. *Journal of Genetic Counseling, 16*, 299–312.

Bernhardt, B. A., Rushton, C. H., Carrese, J., Pyeritz, R. E., Kolodner, K., & Geller, G. (2009). Distress and burnout among genetic service providers. *Genetics in Medicine, 11*, 527–535.

Bernhardt, B. A., Silver, R., Rushton, C. H., Micco, E., & Geller, G. (2010). What keeps you up at night? Genetics professionals' distressing experiences in patient care. *Genetics in Medicine, 12*, 289–297.

Bower, M., McCarthy Veach, P., Bartels, D. M., & LeRoy, B. S. (2002). A survey of genetic counselors' strategies for addressing ethical and professional challenges in practice. *Journal of Genetic Counseling, 11*, 163–186.

Clark, K. (2010). Life as a pregnant genetic counselor. *Journal of Genetic Counseling, 19*, 235–237.

Clark, K. (2012). Life as a pregnant genetic counselor: Take two. *Journal of Genetic Counseling, 21*, 27–30.

Dean, W., Talbot, S. G., & Caplan, A. (2020). Clarifying the language of clinician distress. *JAMA, 323*, 923–924.

Deming, N., Fryer-Edwards, K., Dudzinski, D., Starks, H., Culver, J., Hopley, E., Robins, L., & Burke, W. (2007). Incorporating principles and practical wisdom in research ethics education: A preliminary study. *Academic Medicine, 82*, 18–23.

Dewey, J. (1933). *How we think: A restatement of the relation of reflective thinking to the education process*. D.C. Health.

Dexter, N., Mahoney, S. K., Schrag Wangh, K., & Rintell, D. (2003). Burnout in genetic counselors. *Journal of Genetic Counseling, 12*, 563–564.

Dreher, M., Hughes, R., Handley, P., & Tavokoli, A. (2019). Improving retention among certified nursing assistants through compassion fatigue awareness and self-care skills education. *Journal of Holistic Nursing, 37*, 296–308.

Figley, C. R. (2002). Compassion fatigue: Psychotherapists' chronic lack of self care. *Journal of Clinical Psychology, 58*, 1433–1441.

Groepper, D., McCarthy Veach, P., LeRoy, B. S., & Bower, M. (2015). Who are laboratory genetic counselors and what ethical and professional challenges do they encounter? *Journal of Genetic Counseling, 24*, 580–596.

Gschmeidler, B., & Flatscher-Thoeni, M. (2010). Ethical and professional challenges of genetic counseling—The case of Austria. *Journal of Genetic Counseling, 22*, 741–752.

Hofsess, C. D., & Tracey, T. J. (2010). Countertransference as a prototype: The development of a measure. *Journal of Counseling Psychology, 57*, 52–67.

Hyatt, J. (2012). Countertransference in the genetic counseling setting: One counselor's personal journey. *Journal of Genetic Counseling, 21*(2), 197–198.

Injeyan, M. C., Shuman, C., Shugar, A., Chitayat, D., Atenafu, E. G., & Kaiser, A. (2011). Personality traits associated with genetic counselor compassion fatigue: The roles of dispositional optimism and locus of control. *Journal of Genetic Counseling, 20*, 526–540.

Johnstone, B., Kaiser, A., Injeyan, M. C., Sappleton, K., Chitayat, D., Stephens, D., & Shuman, C. (2016). The relationship between burnout and occupational stress in genetic counselors. *Journal of Genetic Counseling, 25*, 731–741.

Keilman, K. (2002). Genetic counselor or patient—Who am I today? *Journal of Genetic Counseling, 11*(4), 389–392.

Kennedy, A. L. (2000a). A leader-led supervision group as a model for practicing genetic counselors. *Journal of Genetic Counseling, 9*(5), 391–397.

Kennedy, A. L. (2000b). Supervision for practicing genetic counselors: An overview of models. *Journal of Genetic Counseling, 9*, 379–390.

Kessler, S. (1979). The psychological foundations of genetic counseling. In S. Kessler (Ed.), *Genetic counseling: Psychological dimensions* (pp. 17–34). Elsevier.

Kessler, S. (1992). Psychological aspects of genetic counseling. VIII. Suffering and countertransference. *Journal of Genetic Counseling, 1*, 303–308.

Lee, W., McCarthy Veach, P., MacFarlane, I. M., & LeRoy, B. S. (2015). Who is at risk for compassion fatigue? An investigation of genetic counselor demographics, anxiety, compassion satisfaction, and burnout. *Journal of Genetic Counseling, 24*, 358–370.

Lewis, K. L., Erby, L. A. H., Bernger, A. L., Reed, K., Johnson, M., Adcock, J. Y., & Weaver, M. A. (2017). The dynamics of a genetic counseling peer supervision group. *Journal of Genetic Counseling, 26*, 532–540.

Likhite, M. L. (2000). The interface between countertransference and projective identification in a case presented to peer supervision. *Journal of Genetic Counseling, 9*, 417–424.

Lowe, M., Rappolt, S., Jaglal, S., & MacDonals, G. (2007). The role of reflection in implementing learning from continuing education into practice. *Journal of Continuing Education in the Health Professions, 27*, 143–148.

Marks, J. H. (1993). The training of genetic counselors: Origins of a psychosocial model. In D. M. Bartels, B. S. LeRoy, & A. L. Caplan (Eds.), *Prescribing our future: Ethical challenges in genetic counseling* (pp. 15–24). Aldine de Gruyter.

Marks, J. H. (2003). The importance of genetic counseling: 2003 ASHG award for excellence in human genetics education. *American Journal of Human Genetics, 74*, 395–396.

McCarthy Veach, P., Bartels, D. M., & LeRoy, B. S. (2001). Ethical and professional challenges posed by patients with genetic concerns: A report of focus group discussions with genetic counselors, physicians, and nurses. *Journal of Genetic Counseling, 10*, 97–120.

McCarthy Veach, P., Bartels, D. M., & LeRoy, B. S. (2002). Commentary: Genetic counseling—A profession in search of itself. *Journal of Genetic Counseling, 11*, 187–191.

McCarthy Veach, P., Bartels, D. M., & LeRoy, B. S. (2007). Coming full circle: A Reciprocal-Engagement Model of genetic counseling practice. *Journal of Genetic Counseling, 16*, 713–728.

McCarthy Veach, P., & LeRoy, B. (2012). Defining moments in genetic counselor professional development: One decade later. *Journal of Genetic Counseling, 21*, 162–166.

McCarthy Veach, P., LeRoy, B. S., & Callanan, N. P. (2018). *Facilitating the genetic counseling process: Practice-based skills* (2nd ed.). Springer.

Miranda, C., McCarthy Veach, P., Martyr, M. A., & LeRoy, B. S. (2016). Portrait of the master genetic counselor clinician: A qualitative investigation of expertise in genetic counseling. *Journal of Genetic Counseling, 25*, 767–785.

Morgan, J., Rawlinson, M., & Weaver, M. (2006). Facilitating online reflective learning for health and social care professionals. *Open Learning: The Journal of Open and Distance Learning, 21*, 167–176.

Morley, G., Ives, J., Bradbury-Jones, C., & Irvine, F. (2019). What is "moral distress"? A narrative synthesis of the literature. *Nursing Ethics, 26*, 646–662.

Moukaddam, N., Tucci, V., Galwankar, S., & Shah, A. (2016). In the blink of an eye: Instant countertransference and its application in modern healthcare. *Journal of Emergencies, Trauma, and Shock, 9*(3), 95–96.

Myers, J. E., Sweeney, T. J., & Witmer, J. M. (2000). The wheel of wellness counseling for wellness: A holistic model for treatment planning. *Journal of Counseling and Development, 78*, 251.

Nathan, M. L., Ormond, K. E., Dial, C. M., Gamma, A., & Lunn, M. R. (2018). Genetic counselors' and genetic counseling students' implicit and explicit attitudes toward homosexuality. *Journal of Genetic Counseling, 28*(1), 91–101.

National Society of Genetic Counselors. (2018). National Society of Genetic Counselors code of ethics. *Journal of Genetic Counseling, 27*, 6–8.

Pirzadeh, S. M., McCarthy Veach, P., Bartels, D. M., Kao, J., & LeRoy, B. S. (2007). A national survey of genetic counselors' personal values. *Journal of Genetic Counseling*, *16*, 763–773.

Redlinger-Grosse, K. (2021). Countertransference: Making the unconscious conscious. In B. S. LeRoy, P. McCarthy Veach, & N. P. Callanan (Eds.), *Genetic counseling practice: Advanced concepts and skills* (2nd ed., pp. 153–176). John Wiley & Sons.

Reeder, R., McCarthy Veach, P., MacFarlane, I. M., & LeRoy, B. S. (2017). Characterizing clinical genetic counselors' countertransference experiences: An exploratory study. *Journal of Genetic Counseling*, *26*, 934–947.

Reiser, C. A. (2021). "Oh the places you'll go!" The genetic counselor professional development journey. In B. S. LeRoy, P. McCarthy Veach, & N. P. Callanan (Eds.), *Genetic counseling practice: Advanced concepts and skills* (2nd ed., pp. 341–364). John Wiley & Sons.

Ronnestad, M. H., & Skovholt, T. M. (2001). Learning arenas for professional development . . . *Professional Psychology: Research and Practice*, *32*, 181–187.

Santana, M. (2017). *Development and validation of a self-care scale for clinical and counseling doctoral students* (Publication No. 1692) [Doctoral dissertation, University of Wisconsin, Milwaukee]. *UW Milwaukee Electronic Theses and Dissertations*. https://dc.uwm.edu/etd/1692

Schema, L. (2021). Patient anger: Insights and strategies. In B. S. LeRoy, P. McCarthy Veach, & N. P. Callanan (Eds.), *Genetic counseling practice: Advanced concepts and skills* (2nd ed., pp. 109–130). John Wiley & Sons.

Schema, L., McLaughlin, M., Veach, P. M., & LeRoy, B. S. (2015). Clearing the air: A qualitative investigation of genetic counselors' experiences of counselor-focused patient anger. *Journal of Genetic Counseling*, *24*, 717–731.

Silver, J., Caleshu, C., Casson-Parkin, S., & Ormond, K. (2018). Mindfulness among genetic counselors is associated with increased empathy and work engagement and decreased burnout and compassion fatigue. *Journal of Genetic Counseling*, *27*, 1175–1186.

Silverman, E. (2008). Ongoing self-reflection. *American Journal of Speech Pathology*, *17*, 92.

Sprang, G., Clark, J., & White-Woosley, A. (2007). Compassion fatigue, compassion satisfaction, and burnout: Factors impacting a professional's quality of life. *Journal of Loss and Trauma: International Perspectives on Stress & Coping*, *12*, 259–280.

Udipi, S., Veach, P. M., Kao, J., & LeRoy, B. S. (2008). The psychic costs of empathic engagement: Personal and demographic predictors of genetic counselor compassion fatigue. *Journal of Genetic Counseling*, *17*, 459–471.

VandenLangenberg, E., McCarthy Veach, P., LeRoy, B. S., & Glessner, H. D. (2012). Gay, lesbian, and bisexual patients' recommendations for genetic counselors: A qualitative investigation. *Journal of Genetic Counseling*, *21*(5), 741–747.

Venart, E., Vassos, S., & Pitcher-Heft, H. (2007). What individual counselors can do to sustain wellness. *Journal of Humanistic Counseling, Education and Development*, *46*, 50–65.

Warren, N. S. (2021). Cultural competency and genetic counseling: Key concepts. In B. S. LeRoy, P. McCarthy Veach, & N. P. Callanan (Eds.), *Genetic counseling practice: Advanced concepts and skills* (2nd ed., pp. 219–246). John Wiley & Sons.

Weil, J. (2003). Psychosocial genetic counseling in the post-nondirective era: A point of view. *Journal of Genetic Counseling*, *12*, 199–212.

Wells, D. M., McCarthy Veach, P., Martyr, M. A., & LeRoy, B. S. (2016). Development, experience, and expression of meaning in genetic counselors' lives: An exploratory analysis. *Journal of Genetic Counseling*, *25*, 799–817.

Winspear, J. (2003). *Maisie Dobbs*. Penguin Books.

Zahm, K. W., McCarthy Veach, P., & LeRoy, B. S. (2008). An investigation of genetic counselor experience in peer group supervision. *Journal of Genetic Counseling*, *17*, 220–233.

Zahm, K. W., Veach, P. M., Martyr, M. A., & LeRoy, B. S. (2016). From novice to seasoned practitioner: A qualitative investigation of genetic counselor professional development. *Journal of Genetic Counseling*, *25*, 818–834.

Zeidner, M., Hadar, D., Matthews, G., & Roberts, R. D. (2013). Personal factors related to compassion fatigue in health professionals. *Anxiety Stress Coping*, *26*, 595–609.

CHAPTER 26

ETHICAL AND SOCIAL ISSUES CONNECTED TO GENETIC TESTING OF FETUSES, INFANTS, AND CHILDREN

DENA S. DAVIS

INTRODUCTION

What kind of knowledge is genetic knowledge?

THERE is a difference between knowledge and information. Information is organized data. Information tells us, for example, that children born with an extra chromosome 21 will exhibit some cluster of characteristics that we term trisomy 21, or Down syndrome (DS), and that those characteristics always include some degree of intellectual limitation. New or prospective parents receiving that information may find it useful, but without more context, this information does not rise to the level of knowledge. Information can only be acted on appropriately when it is appropriated by someone and becomes knowledgeable. Knowledge in this instance would include awareness of other families' experience with children who have DS, an assessment of one's own strengths and weaknesses, family support, societal support, claims of the family's other children, and so on. Knowledge would also include an understanding of what information we cannot have: Children with DS exhibit a wide spectrum of physical and mental challenges, and there is no way of knowing how affected a child will be until after it is born.

Genetic testing can give us information. To know if and when genetic testing is ethically appropriate, we need to know who is asking for the information, how they intend to use it, and if the information they want will yield the knowledge they seek. For example, many people erroneously think that genetics is always 100% predictive (so-called *genetic determinism*), whereas in fact most genes merely confer higher or lower risk. Having a *BRCA* pathogenic variant confers a higher risk for breast and ovarian cancer than in the general population, but it is by no means inevitable, even if people do not take means to avoid it.

And not having a *BRCA* pathogenic variant does not mean one is "home free" and will never develop breast and ovarian cancer.

Is genetic information special?

For decades, perhaps centuries, before the Human Genome Project was completed in 2003, people have treated genetic information with heightened concern (sometimes referred to as *genetic exceptionalism*; Murray, 2019). There are varied reasons for this. If a disease is thought to "run in the family," family members may go to great lengths to keep it secret, for fear of damaging the marriage prospects of the younger generation, or simply to avoid being stigmatized. People may fear negative consequences for their ability to obtain health, life, disability, or long-term care insurance or fear employment discrimination. Many people believe that carrier status is deleterious to one's health, which is rarely the case, or that genetic predispositions are more penetrant than they actually are; this misinformation can have a negative impact on the status of the person involved.

Few genetic diseases are completely penetrant, meaning that someone with the variant will always have the disease. Achondroplasia is an example of a dominant disorder that shows complete penetrance when a person has the most common pathogenic variant. Tay-Sachs disease (TSD) is an example of a recessive disease that demonstrates complete penetrance; if a person has two copies of a pathogenic variant, then they will inevitably have the disease. However, as noted above, many genetic variants convey higher or lower risk, rather than certainty. And even genes that are completely penetrant may still have variable expressivity; for example, individuals with osteogenesis imperfecta have a wide range of fracture phenotypes, even within families.

Now that we can quickly and inexpensively map a person's entire genetic blueprint, concerns about genetic privacy have grown exponentially. Discovering at least some facts about one's genome can often be helpful, but the benefits must be weighed against the risks of misuse, loss of privacy, and one's own anxieties and sense of self. Individuals must weigh these risks for themselves. When it comes to fetuses, infants, and children, however, adults must make those decisions for them. This raises several ethical questions surrounding the genetic testing of children.

Should Infants, Children, and Adolescents Receive Genetic Testing?

When a competent adult makes decisions about medical care, including genetic testing, informed consent is the core ethical concept upon which these decisions are based. Authentic informed consent includes an understanding of the pros and cons of the proposed course of action, including its foreseeable consequences, and how those align with the person's individual situation and values. The emphasis on informed consent rests on the primacy given to the principle of respect for autonomy, that is, respecting the right of every adult to decide for themselves what care is right for them (within the range of reasonable medical options).

With children, however, the situation is a great deal more complicated, as children themselves range from newborns to sophisticated older adolescents. As I have argued elsewhere, even embryos and fetuses have certain rights to future privacy and autonomy, rights that should be respected in the present (Davis, 2001).

Parents are assumed to be the best decision makers for their children; they typically know their own children the best and have their interests most in mind. According to the American Academy of Pediatrics (AAP), "Parental decision-making should best be understood as parents' responsibility to support the interests of their child and to preserve family relationships, rather than being focused on their [the parents'] rights to express their own autonomous choices" (AAP Committee on Bioethics, 2016, p. 3). Thus, when the patient is a child, the emphasis on autonomy shifts to an emphasis on beneficence. The medical profession recognizes the difference between making decisions for oneself and for others by noting that parents cannot give *consent* for their children's care; rather, they give *permission*. Children who are old enough to participate in decision making are said to give their *assent* to testing or treatment. The AAP urges physicians to involve pediatric patients in decision making at appropriate developmental levels (AAP Committee on Bioethics, 1995).[1]

With respect to predictive (rather than diagnostic) genetic testing, the watchwords should be *caution* and *conservatism*. Unlike interventions such as childhood vaccines, there is little medical or societal consensus on the benefits of genetic testing when there is no appropriate clinical response to a detected variant. Because information, once obtained, cannot be erased or unlearned, genetic testing of minors should only be done when the benefits to them are clear and when the testing cannot wait until they are of age to make their own decisions. For this reason, Botkin and colleagues (2015) highlight the following aspect of the 1995 joint report of the American Society for Human Genetics (ASHG) and the American College of Medical Genetics and Genomics (ACMG): "In the absence of timely medical benefits to the child, or the expressed wishes of adolescents, testing should be deferred until adulthood, particularly for adult-onset conditions or for carrier status for reproductive decision-making" (Botkin et al., 2015, p. 7). The 2013 joint policy recommendations of the AAP Committee on Bioethics and the ACMG Social, Ethical, and Legal Issues Committee state, "Predictive genetic testing for adult-onset conditions generally should be deferred unless an intervention initiated in childhood may reduce morbidity or mortality," and "the AAP and ACMG do not support routine carrier testing in minors when such testing does not provide health benefits in childhood" (AAP Committee on Bioethics et al., 2013, p. 621). In other words, since benefit to the child is the reigning criterion, balanced against the child's own right to make decisions once they become an adult, there is little justification for testing children for genetic information for which no action is indicated. To cite Kodish, a "robust" rule is that "genetic testing should be permitted no earlier than the age of first possible onset of the disease," as it is at that age that surveillance would begin (Kodish, 1999, p. 393).

For a short period of time this policy represented a broad consensus (Borry et al., 2006; Garrett et al., 2019; Hardart & Chung, 2014). I suspect, however, that the consensus was not

[1] Editors' note: This statement was reaffirmed by the AAP in 2006. The AAP issued a new statement, "Pediatric Decision Making: Consensus Recommendations," in August 2023 (Salter et al., 2023).

all that deep, because it did not hold for very long. In the next two decades, that consensus came under attack, and there was more support for allowing parents to have children tested even for conditions that were not medically actionable in childhood (Hardart & Chung, 2014; Lucassen et al., 2014). I believe that there were several reasons for this.

First, the original recommendations went against broadly accepted social norms on the role and force of parental authority (Strong et al., 2014). Those societal norms had fallen to the moral panic and "genetic determinism" that followed the advent of the Human Genome Project, with the tremendous, almost mythic, power given to genetic knowledge (Sabatello & Jeungst, 2019). Over time, that knowledge began to seem more mundane, as people were giving each other direct-to-consumer (DTC) genetic testing kits as holiday gifts, and physicians and genetic counselors were displaced from their role as gatekeepers to the magic kingdom of genetic knowledge. Second, going along with this trend, empirical research seems to corroborate that children are not usually harmed by being tested (Strong et al., 2014).

Third, a more family-centered approach to decision making echoed the general swing from a predominantly individualistic, autonomy-oriented ethics to a more familial, communitarian one (Botkin et al., 2015; Hardart & Chung, 2014). Given that the main objection to genetic testing of children for nonmedically actionable information had been the rather theoretical argument of the child's future autonomy—that is, their right to decide for themselves whether or not to test when they come of age (Davis, 2001)—it is perhaps not surprising that the consensus began to crumble, faced with families' proclaimed interest in knowing the information *now*.

A fourth reason is that the original policy recommendations of the 1995 ASHG and ACMG joint report, while "influential," were often "over-interpreted" in a stricter manner than had been intended (Botkin et al., 2015, p. 7). Thus, the original recommendations against childhood testing became something of a misrepresentation of the ethical concerns, inviting pushback. Finally, as the focus on single-gene testing gave way to a concern with genome sequencing, some commentators began to argue that the policy against predictive childhood testing was either overly simplistic or a poor fit (Garrett et al., 2019).

In 2013, two sets of recommendations for genetic testing were released, both of which impacted clinical and ethical perspectives on the genetic testing of children. The first was the aforementioned joint statement of the ACMG and AAP (AAP Committee on Bioethics et al., 2013). It addressed the standard question of whether it was appropriate to test children in high-risk families for pathogenic variants for which there was no intervention during childhood. The recommendations reaffirmed that nonmedically actionable predictive genetic testing of children "generally should be deferred" but also acknowledged circumstances in which it might be appropriate, for example, to relieve "significant psychosocial burden" (AAP Committee on Bioethics et al., 2013, p. 621). The second recommendation was issued solely by the ACMG, and it addressed the relatively new question of the return of results from clinical exome- and genome-wide sequencing that are not related to the reason for the ordering of the testing but may have "medical value or utility," often termed "incidental" or "secondary" findings (Green et al., 2013, p. 2). The topic of returning secondary findings in pediatrics specifically, and in clinical genetics generally, is beyond the scope of this chapter.[2] However, as mentioned above, it appears that the

[2] Editors' note: For further discussion on secondary findings, see Chapter 21 by Eric T. Rush in this volume.

emergence of the issue of managing secondary findings was one of the factors that softened the original consensus. The ACMG/AAP continued to put the child's interests front and center, whereas the ACMG recommendation "also considered the potential health benefit to . . . family members as a factor in deciding which results to seek and disclose" (Clayton et al., 2014, p. 6).

Following this trend, a 2015 policy statement by the ASHG softened somewhat the earlier consensus, offering the following recommendations: (a) parents should be encouraged to defer predictive testing for adult-onset conditions until adulthood or older adolescence, (b) adolescents should be encouraged to defer predictive testing because of the possible impact of that information at "formative life stages," and (c) providers should explore the reasons that parents or teens are interested in such testing, so that any decisions are deliberative in nature (Botkin et al., 2015, p. 8).

However, as Garrett et al. (2019) point out, a number of position statements from professional organizations reiterated the consensus. For example, the National Society of Genetic Counselors' position statement regarding the genetic testing of minors for adult-onset conditions recommends

> deferring predictive genetic testing of minors for adult-onset conditions when results will not impact childhood medical management or significantly benefit the child. Predictive testing should optimally be deferred until the individual has the capacity to weigh the associated risks, benefits, and limitations of this information, taking his/her circumstances, preferences, and beliefs into account to preserve his/her autonomy and right to an open future. (National Society of Genetic Counselors, 2018)

Furthermore, Fenwick et al. (2017) summarized the "status quo" by saying that the earlier recommendations against testing that has no childhood benefit "are well-established and have not changed significantly" (p. 244).

The most obvious reason to seek medically relevant genetic information is if it can produce knowledge with "actionable" consequences for someone's health. Diagnostic testing can help rule out or pinpoint the reason for troubling symptoms. For example, genetic testing for human leukocyte antigens can be used to rule out celiac disease. Sometimes it can be useful to discover a genetic disease even before symptoms begin. The Cystic Fibrosis Foundation (2023) supports newborn screening for the disease because taking steps very early in a child's life can lead to better outcomes.

However, not all types of genetic information are medically actionable, and even when they are, appropriate actions may not happen until the person becomes an adult. There are three types of genetic information that require no medical action during childhood. First, there may be no preventative intervention for a genetic disease. An example of that is Huntingdon's disease (HD). HD is a degenerative neurological disease that causes deterioration in a person's physical, mental, and emotional capacities, leading to death within 10 to 30 years of diagnosis. The first symptoms can be unaccustomed clumsiness or unusual mood swings and irritability. HD is an "adult-onset disease"; symptoms typically arise in one's late 30s or 40s. HD is an autosomal dominant genetic disease; if a person has it, each of that person's children has a 50% chance of having it as well. Furthermore, it is a condition that demonstrates high penetrance, meaning that if one has a HD pathogenic expansion, then one is predicted to develop the disease. Currently, there is, unfortunately, no medical intervention to change the course of the disease, and therefore little justification for testing children. Because it is a dominant disease, people usually know when it runs in their family, and they may decide to find out their status for reproductive decision making or for planning their lives. But many adults at risk for HD decide against getting tested (Anderson et al., 2019).

Second, some information may indeed have an appropriate medical response, but not until the child is at least 18. A *BRCA1/2* pathogenic variant is one such instance. Every person has *BRCA1* and *BRCA2* genes, which normally play a role in blocking tumor production. But if a person has a pathogenic variant in one or both of these genes, then they are at a higher risk than the general population to develop cancers of the breast, ovaries, or prostate, as well as some less common cancers. The person is also more likely to develop these cancers at a younger age. There is no way to directly change the deleterious workings of these variants. Medical intervention focuses on early screening and possibly risk-reducing surgery. However, there is no current recommendation to screen people below the age of 25 unless there is a family history that would indicate an earlier age to start screening, and therefore, in most circumstances, there is no medical need to discover a child's genetic status before the age of 18 (Johns Hopkins Medicine, 2023).

Third, when a child is a carrier for a recessive genetic disease, such as TSD or cystic fibrosis, there are few or no medical implications for that child, at any point in their life. People may use information about their carrier status to choose a spouse or to avoid having a child with the disease if their spouse is also a carrier. These are reproductive decisions appropriate to adults; therefore, there is no ethically defensible reason to test children for their carrier status. When a person is tested as an adult, they can control who else has access to the information. But when children are tested, their parents presumably know the results and can also share those with anyone they wish. This abrogates these children's privacy and developing autonomy.

I believe that the trend toward a more family-centered approach to predictive genetic testing of children is ill-conceived. First, arguments based on the lack of evidence of harm fail to address the difference between being *harmed* and being *wronged*. Most people would agree that one can be wronged without being harmed. In a classic example from the law of torts, imagine a patient who is induced to agree to an operation, because the physician withholds from the patient the information that the operation is exceedingly risky and that they have never performed it before. Fortunately for them both, the operation is a complete success. The patient has not been harmed, but clearly they have been wronged. In the same way, a person can be wronged by not having the choice to decide for themselves whether to undergo a genetic test, even if they have not been harmed (e.g., by discrimination or psychological distress).

Second, the arguments for the child's right to decide for themself usually rest on the fact that many adults decide not to be tested for diseases such as HD (Clayton et al., 2014). Thus, not testing children is glossed as a person's "right not to know" (Berkman & Hull, 2014). The right not to know is certainly important, but that is only part of the story. A person also has the right to decide with whom they will share information, even if they themself choose to know it. Privacy within the family is as important as privacy between the family unit and the outside world. Especially with information that is relevant for reproductive decisions (such as carrier status for recessive conditions), a person has the same interest in controlling that information as they do in controlling information about their sex life, use of contraceptives, and other private matters. The decision of how much to share with the parents ought to be left to the person or couple themselves, and that choice should not be preempted (Davis, 2001).

Imagine a parent who barges into a genetic counselor's office and demands to know the results of a test recently taken by their 18-year-old child. Or imagine a parent who comes into the office, dragging their 18-year-old, and demanding that the young adult be tested against their wishes. Does anyone believe that the parent's interests ought to prevail? I think not. And yet, if the parent is allowed to test a toddler for an adult-onset genetic condition that requires no medical intervention until adulthood, the parent is essentially accomplishing the same result.

The main arguments in favor of allowing parents to test children for adult-onset or carrier conditions for which there is no appropriate medical intervention during childhood rest on claims about avoiding harm to the parents or other siblings and about parental autonomy (Allain, 2014). The current guidelines, however, already take into account the possibility of "disabling" parental anxiety as an exception to the default position against childhood testing. The argument for parental autonomy misunderstands the meaning of autonomy. One does not have "autonomy" over others. As mentioned above, the reason parents are the usual medical decision makers for their children is based on beneficence (the children's well-being), not on parental autonomy.

It is certainly true that, for most medical conditions until at least the teenage years, there is little question that parental knowledge is generally in the child's best interest. If a child has asthma, needs glasses, or has a genetic condition that can be addressed during childhood, parental knowledge is crucial to the child's well-being. The relatively recent advent of genetic testing has inserted a new factor: information about the future for which there is nothing to be done in the present. In such cases, it is no longer obvious that parental knowledge is in the best interests of the child.

Do Fetuses, Infants, and Children Have Privacy and Autonomy?

As children grow and develop, they become increasingly able to participate in decisions about their health. Children who grow up in families affected by genetic disease may have had life experiences that help to prepare them for this kind of decision (Kodish, 1999). The concept of "assent" captures the idea that children can have a role in healthcare decisions appropriate to their age and maturity, balanced against the seriousness of the decision and its possible consequences (AAP Committee on Bioethics, 1995). However, there is a common view that babies and young children, not to mention fetuses, have no interests in autonomy or privacy that need to be taken into account. I believe that that view is mistaken. It is certainly true that a newborn *now* has neither privacy nor autonomy, but a newborn does have an important interest in preserving the autonomy and privacy that it *will* have in the future. In the same way that one preserves for an infant *now* a trust fund that it will only inherit when it achieves majority, one preserves for the child now a "trust fund" of possible decisions that it will make for itself when it is of age. Just as an adult has the right to decide whether or not to be tested for a genetic condition, so the fetus, baby, or child has the right to have that decision preserved for it, when it becomes an adult. This right is part of a constellation famously parsed by legal philosopher Joel Feinberg (1980) as "rights-in-trust," which are "rights that are to be *saved* for the child until he is an adult" (p. 125). Other examples in this constellation are the right to freedom of religion; the right to choose whether, when, and to whom one marries; and so on. Children cannot act on or express those rights now, but it would be wrong for parents to foreclose their ability to make at least some of the most significant life choices in adulthood. These rights, taken together, are famously characterized by Feinberg (1980) as "the child's right to an open future" (p. 125). Of course, a child's rights, now or in the future, must be balanced against the possible benefits of testing or the harm of not testing. But, in the cases under discussion, the benefits are few or none, and the decisions can be left until adulthood or at least late adolescence (Kodish, 1999).

Garrett and colleagues (2019) argue for demoting this "right" to an "interest," one among a number of interests that "should be evaluated" when making decisions for children. They claim that all children are subject to parental decision making that shapes or even curtails future choices and that "the idea of a right to an open future is thus impractical, ambiguous, and ripe for misinterpretation" (Garrett et al., 2019, p. 10). Interestingly, many of the "interests" they name could and probably should be better described as "rights," for example, to be "adequately nourished and sheltered" or to have "protection from physical or mental abuse." Certainly, these are among the rights of the child enumerated in the 1989 United Nations Convention on the Rights of the Child (United Nations, 1989).

Genetic specialists go to great lengths to protect the rights of adults to make the decision for themselves whether to get tested and to have the confidentiality of the resultant information protected. But when there is no current benefit to the child, testing the child at the parents' behest effectively takes the decision away from the adult the child *will become*.

A good example of this problem is the discovery of the gene for TSD. Just as HD has become a paradigm for autosomal dominant disorders, TSD is a paradigm case of recessive disorders (other examples are sickle cell disease and cystic fibrosis). TSD is a neurological disease in which children appear to be healthy when born but soon show signs of neurological degeneration and typically die before their fifth year. Like a number of recessive conditions, TSD is commonly, but not exclusively, concentrated in certain ethnic populations. In the general population, one in 300 individuals is a carrier of a TSD pathogenic variant; among Ashkenazi Jewish, Acadian, and Cajun populations, it is closer to one in 30. Since intramarriage within populations at significant carrier risk is more likely to bring together a couple of whom both are carriers of recessive pathogenic variants in the same gene, this is a source of concern for genetics specialists. In any couple in which both prospective parents are carriers for a recessive pathogenic variant in the same gene, the chance of having an affected child is 25% in each pregnancy. The chances of having a child who is a carrier but unaffected is 50%, and the chance of having a child with no copy of the pathogenic variant is 25%.

Once it became possible to test for TSD in the 1970s, the Ashkenazi Jewish community embraced various strategies to avoid having affected children, to the point where there are now currently almost no Jewish babies born with TSD in North America. This resounding success is the result of tremendous group pressure and the normalization of a group's preferred form of carrier testing. In Orthodox groups that practice arranged courtship, young people are tested for an array of "Jewish genetic diseases" but are not told the results; instead, they are given an ID number. When a match is contemplated, the ID numbers are compared, and the parents are told whether or not this is an acceptable pairing. The young people themselves are not told which of the relevant variants they carry (Glausiusz, 2013). Among non-Orthodox and secular Jews, testing often occurs in Jewish day schools and is offered throughout the community. The proselytization for testing is relentless. Some rabbis are on record as not being willing to marry people who have not been tested (Rochman, 2017). Given the intense focus on avoiding TSD in this community, a young couple might be especially concerned to guard their marital privacy while making reproductive decisions.

There are a number of ways in which parents might find out the carrier status of their children. Parents who know they are carriers and who use amniocentesis or chorionic villus sampling to determine whether their fetus is affected will often be told also whether the fetus is a carrier. Preimplantation genetic diagnosis (PGD) is available for TSD and many other genetic diseases. A couple at risk for having an affected child may have the option to use in vitro fertilization (IVF) and PGD to avoid implantation of any embryos that have two copies of the pathogenic variant. Thus, various prenatal genetic techniques aimed at determining whether an embryo or fetus has a recessive condition (two copies of the pathogenic recessive variant) will also reveal whether the embryo or fetus is a carrier (has one copy of the pathogenic recessive variant). Parents have the legal right to this information in many jurisdictions, which at this point is in the pregnant patient's own medical record, but there are policies that could be put in place to discourage at least the routine disclosure of these results. As part of the initial genetic counseling, parents could be encouraged to consider how private this information seems to them and, by extension, whether they should respect that same privacy for their unborn child. Another way in which parents could discover the carrier status of their children is if they discover their own carrier status after they have had one or more (healthy) children, and they bring the whole family in to be tested. Despite the policies discussed above, geneticists may accede to family wishes in these scenarios. It is also possible that parents could use DTC testing to discover their child's carrier status. Although most DTC companies will not knowingly test children, nor test one person's DNA at the behest of another, there seems to be little provision to prevent a parent from sending in a child's saliva sample and claiming it for their own.

Confidentiality

It is difficult to talk about confidentiality in the relationship between the genetic specialist and a young child, much less genetic specialist and fetus, since confidentiality implies a relationship in which one person shares private information with another on the basis of trust. And yet, if this *voluntary* sharing of private information is not possible, it becomes much more important for the professional to guard the privacy of those whose personal information is mined without their knowledge or consent. Such is the case when healthcare professionals are asked to discover and/or to disclose genetic information about children or fetuses when discovery and disclosure are not necessary for the child's health and welfare.

However odd it may sound to speak of the privacy of a fetus, it is conceptually no different than speaking of the privacy of a young child. A fetus—at least assuming its parents intend to carry it to term—will become that small child, and then a teen, and finally an adult. The argument for protecting its privacy now—to preserve its right to privacy in the future—is the same. Analogously, one can argue that depriving a fetus of proper nutrition (again, on the assumption that one expects it to eventually be born) is no different ethically than depriving a child (Murray, 1996). In both cases, the concern is for the child's future.

In the bulk of what has been written on privacy and confidentiality issues in genetics, the concern has been for the deleterious consequences of having one's genetic status known to possible employers and insurance carriers. But there are also important privacy issues to be considered within families. Bok (1989) describes confidentiality as resting on three premises: individual autonomy over personal information, respect for relationships among human beings and for intimacy, and the moral obligation engendered by making a promise of silence. The third premise cannot concern us here, as one cannot make a promise of secrecy to a small child, let alone an embryo or fetus. But the first two premises do speak to this issue. The child will grow up to be an adult. Respecting them now as a potential adult means respecting their right and ability when they reach that state to have control over information personal to them. Likewise, respecting their capacity as an adult to form intimate relationships (including sexual and reproductive partnerships) means respecting and protecting their ability now to decide when and with whom certain secrets will be shared.

In Western religious heritage, the concept of a new couple forming a partnership distinct and separate from their families of origin is as old as the Book of Genesis, which says, "[A] man leaves his father and his mother and cleaves to his wife, and they become one flesh." Choices and actions surrounding sex, marriage, and reproduction are perhaps the most jealously guarded zones of privacy in our culture. Parental knowledge of children's carrier status falls into a uniquely protected category because of the use to which this information is put, namely, to make reproductive decisions with one's partner. When, in Western culture, a couple unites, a new family is created. While the couple retains significant ties to their families of origin, certain bonds of loyalty and intimacy undergo a subtle but seismic shift. We acknowledge this in law and medicine by automatically shifting the privilege and burden of making decisions for incompetent patients to the spouse as the new next of kin, even if the marriage is only a day old. A common cause of relational strife is when couples disagree about how much of their "private business" to share with parents, or when in-laws are too intrusive and fail to respect the privacy and decision-making sphere of the new family.

Of all the decisions for the new couple to make, perhaps the most intimate, and the most intrinsic to their new status as "one flesh," are those connected with sexuality and parenthood. That is not to imply that the couple's parents have no interest in the matter. On the contrary, they are likely to have strong opinions and expectations about grandchildren, family size, behavior choices consonant with their religious and cultural traditions, and so on. But it is for the couple to decide together how their reproductive lives will be conducted, and ideally, they would decide together how much to bring their parents into that conversation. Whether the couple uses contraception, whether they hope for one child or eight, and whether they would consider abortion for fetal indications are all decisions that belong within the privacy of the couple.

An example of the practical implications of this issue comes from the documentary film *Sound and Fury* (Aronson & Weisberg, 2000). The story follows three generations of two families, joined by marriage, who have both deaf and hearing members. There are two brothers, one hearing and one deaf from birth, both of whose parents are hearing. The deaf brother married a deaf woman (both of whose parents are deaf), and they now have two deaf children; the family is deeply committed to the Deaf[3] community and has refused cochlear implants for their 5-year-old daughter, even though she wants them. The hearing brother married a hearing woman who also has deafness in her family tree; they have just given birth to fraternal twin boys, of whom one is hearing and the other deaf. This couple also has an older child who is hearing. Conflict arises because the hearing couple decides to get cochlear implants for the deaf twin. This decision causes a deep rift in the family. The Deaf grandparents say they feel "slapped in the face" and wonder if the hearing couple still considers them part of the family. They worry that the little boy will grow up estranged from his grandparents. The hearing grandparents passionately support the cochlear implant. Tellingly, the existence of the two children born hearing in the young couple's family did not cause any tension; the rift occurred only because of the young couple's decision to "convert" their deaf child into a member of the hearing world. Had the couple known their genetic risk for having a deaf child, they might have quietly decided to use IVF and PGD to avoid that possibility, but had their genetic blueprint been known to their parents, that decision would probably have caused even more family discord.

Western societies' legal systems, and the health professions in those societies, give great weight to the privacy of reproductive decisions. It would be highly unusual for a healthcare provider to share information about an adult's carrier status with the parents. Preserving privacy within families, thus, is an ongoing challenge and commitment for genetic counselors. For example, healthcare providers will rarely break confidentiality with a client by sharing their genetic test results with a sibling over the client's objections, no matter how beneficial to the sibling (Gallo et al., 2009). Acceding to a parental request for testing, or divulging results of a test that was performed for some other purpose, violates rights to privacy and autonomy that will be activated when the child reaches adulthood. The challenge, then, would be to show how it could be ethically acceptable to share that information with the parents of a minor child when it is information that requires a response only when the child becomes an adult.

Conclusion

Despite modest pushback, protection of the child's autonomy and confidentiality—whether parsed as rights or as interests—appears to continue as the foundation of genetic decision making. This may change in the future, however, as the focus shifts from single-gene testing to comprehensive exome and genome sequencing. It may also change if the proliferation of DTC sites and the sharing of genetic information through social media erode how society values genetic confidentiality.

[3] The usual convention is to use "deaf" to denote people who do not hear, while "Deaf" denotes nonhearing people who identify as part of a cultural/linguistic community. All Deaf people are deaf, but not all deaf people identify as Deaf.

References

Allain, D. C. (2014). Testing children for adult-onset disorders. In J. Berliner (Ed.), *Ethical dilemmas in genetics and genetic counseling: Principles through case scenarios* (pp. 96–117). Oxford University Press.

American Academy of Pediatrics Committee on Bioethics. (1995). Informed consent, parental permission, and assent in pediatric practice. *Pediatrics*, *95*(2), 314–317.

American Academy of Pediatrics Committee on Bioethics. (2016). Informed consent in decision-making in pediatric practice. *Pediatrics*, *138*(2), e20161484.

American Academy of Pediatrics Committee on Bioethics, Committee on Genetics, and American College of Medical Genetics and Genomics Social Ethical and Legal Issues Committee. (2013). Ethical and policy issues in genetic testing and screening of children. *Pediatrics*, *131*(3), 620–622.

Anderson, K. E., Eberly, S., Marder, K. S., Oakes, D., Kayson, E., Young A., & Shoulson, I., & PHAROS Investigators. (2019). The choice not to undergo genetic testing for Huntington disease: Results from the PHAROS study. *Clinical Genetics*, *96*(1), 28–34.

Aronson, J. (Director and Producer), & Weisberg, R. (Producer). (2000). *Sound and fury* [Film]. Aronson Films.

Berkman, B. E., & Hull, S. C. (2014). The "right not to know" in the genomic era: Time to break from tradition? *American Journal of Bioethics*, *14*(3), 28–30.

Bok, S. (1989). *Secrets*. Vintage Books.

Borry, P., Stultiens, L., Nys, H., Cassiman, J. J., & Dierickx, K. (2006). Presymptomatic and predictive genetic testing in minors: A systematic review of guidelines and position papers. *Clinical Genetics*, *70*(5), 374–381.

Botkin, J. R., Belmont, J. W., Berg, J. S., Berkman, B. E., Bombard, Y., Holm, I. A., Levy, H. P., Ormond, K. E., Saal, H. M., Spinner, N. B., Wilfond, B. S., & McInerney, J. D. (2015). Points to consider: Ethical, legal, and psychosocial implications of genetic testing in children and adolescents. *American Journal of Human Genetics*, *97*(1), 6–21.

Clayton, E. W., McCullough, L. B., Biesecker, L. G., Joffe, S., Ross, L. F., & Wolf, S. M. (2014). Addressing the ethical challenges in genetic testing and sequencing of children. *American Journal of Bioethics*, *14*(30), 3–9.

Cystic Fibrosis Foundation. (2023). *Newborn screening for CF*. https://www.cff.org/intro-cf/newborn-screening-cf

Davis, D. S. (2001). *Genetic dilemmas: Reproductive technology, genetic choices, and children's futures*. Oxford University Press.

Feinberg, J. (1980). The child's right to an open future. In W. Aiden & H. La Follette (Eds.), *Whose child? Children's rights, parental authority, and state power* (pp. 124–153). Littlefield & Adams.

Fenwick, A., Plantinga, M., Dheensa, S., & Lucassen, A. (2017). Predictive genetic testing of children for adult-onset conditions: Negotiating requests with parents. *Journal of Genetic Counseling*, *26*(2), 244–250.

Gallo, A. M., Angst, D. B., & Knafl, K. A. (2009). Disclosure of genetic information within families. *American Journal of Nursing*, *109*(4), 65–69.

Garrett, J. R., Lantos, J. D., Biesecker, L. G., Childerhose, J. E., Chung, Holm, I. A., Koenig, B. A., MacEwen, J. E., Wilfond, B. S., & Brothers, K. (2019). Rethinking the "open future" argument against predictive genetic testing of children. *Genetics in Medicine*, *21*(10), 2190–2198.

Glausiusz, J. (2013, November 12). Haredi love goes high-tech: No DNA testing, no wedding. *Haaretz*.

Green, R. C., Berg, J. S., Grody, W. W., Kalia, S. S., Korf, B. R., Martin, C. L., McGuire, A. L., Nussbaum, R. L., O'Daniel, J. M., Ormond, K. E., Rehm, H. L., Watson, M. S., Williams, M. S., Biesecker, L. G., & American College of Medical Genetics and Genomics (2013). ACMG recommendations for reporting of incidental findings in clinical exome and genome sequencing. *Genetics in Medicine, 15*(7), 565–574.

Hardart, G. E., & Chung, W. K. (2014). Genetic testing of children for diseases that have onset in adulthood: The limits of family interests. *Pediatrics, 134*(Suppl. 2), S104–S110.

Johns Hopkins Medicine. (2023). *Breast cancer*. https://www.hopkinsmedicine.org/health/conditions-and-diseases/breast-cancer

Kodish, E. (1999). Testing children for cancer genes: The rule of earliest onset. *Journal of Pediatrics, 135*(3), 390–395.

Lucassen, A., Widdershoven, G., Metselaar, S., Fenwick, A., & Parker, M. (2014). Genetic testing of children: The need for a family perspective. *American Journal of Bioethics, 14*(3), 26–28.

Murray, T. (1996). *The worth of a child*. University of California Press.

Murray, T. (2019). Is genetic exceptionalism past its sell-by date? On genomic diaries, context, and content. *American Journal of Bioethics, 19*(1), 13–15.

National Society of Genetic Counselors. (2018, April 12). *Genetic testing of minors for adult-onset conditions*. https://www.nsgc.org/POLICY/Position-Statements/Position-Statements/Post/genetic-testing-of-minors-for-adult-onset-conditions

Rochman, B. (2017, February 28). More than Tay-Sachs. *Tablet*.

Sabatello, M., & Jeungst, E. (2019). Genomic essentialism: Its provenance and trajectory as an anticipatory ethical concern. *Hastings Center Report, 49*(4), S10–S18.

Salter, E. K., Hester, D. M., Vinarcsik, L., Matheny Antommaria, A. H., Bester, J., Blustein, J., Wright Clayton, E., Diekema, D. S., Iltis, A. S., Kopelman, L. M., Malone, J. R., Mercurio, M. R., Navin, M. C., Talati Paquette, E., Mason Pope, T., Rhodes, R., & Ross, L. F. (2023). Pediatric decision making: Consensus recommendations. *Pediatrics, 152*(3), e2023061832.

Strong, K. A., Derse, A. R., Dimmock, D. P., Zusevics, K., Jeruzal, J., Worthey, E., Bick, D., Scharer, G., Kirschner, A. L., Spellecy, R., Farrell, M. H., Geurts, J., Veith, R., & May, T. (2014). In the absence of evidentiary harm, existing societal harms regarding parental authority should prevail. *American Journal of Bioethics, 14*(3), 24–26.

United Nations. (1990, March). *Convention on the rights of the child*. United Nations Treaty Collection. https://treaties.un.org/doc/source/publications/MTDSG/1989-english.pdf

CHAPTER 27

GENETIC COUNSELING AND THE PROBLEM OF EXPLOITATION

NAOMI SCHEINERMAN

Introduction

The 2017 National Society of Genetic Counselors (NSGC) Code of Ethics mentions "exploitation" twice. First, to ensure the "autonomy, individuality, welfare, and freedom in clinical and research interactions," genetic counselors should work to "avoid the exploitation of their clients for personal, professional, or institutional advantage, profit or interest" (NSGC, 2017, II.8). In the second, genetic counselors should "maintain appropriate boundaries to avoid exploitation in their relationships with trainees, employees, employers, and colleagues" (NSGC, 2017, III.5). And though the concern of "exploitation" features quite prominently in bioethics literature writ large, such as in matters of patient payment for participation in clinical research trials (Emanuel et al., 2015) and in international research on marginalized populations (Ballantyne, 2008; Panitch, 2013), the literature on genetic counseling is comparatively quiet as to how this concern becomes manifested, and ultimately avoided, within its domain.

This chapter gives an overview of what it means to exploit, what kind of wrong or harm exploitation is, why it is helpful to understand exploitation as an intrinsic problem in a profit-driven system and thus that it may actually be rather difficult *not* to exploit, and what the resulting responsibilities are of those in the system to at least mitigate its nefarious effects. I take the code's second reference to "exploitation" for granted, that like in any industry one should maintain noncoercive and nonabusive relationships with colleagues and coworkers, particularly in hierarchical systems wherein some have power over others. Instead, I expand on and describe a nonexploitative relationship between counselor and client wherein the concern of exploitation may be not only more prominent but also more difficult to identify and hence avoid.

Scholars often use the term "exploitation" rather widely to mean a variety of different kinds of moral considerations, from coercion to unfairness. While different formulations of exploitation range from more technical explanations of where profit in a capitalist system comes from to more normative ones of procedural injustice (like oppression), often when we think of exploitation, we think of taking advantage of another's precarious position due to power imbalances and limited options. In an exploitative relationship, one party depends on the other's knowledge, resources, influence, status, or skills for a needed benefit. Wage laborers in large corporations, for example, are also exploited because they have diminished bargaining power with their bosses, and as a result they have little say in their contract conditions including salary, time off, and benefits. As a result, they may be more inclined to engage in behavior they otherwise would not do and/or are in a state of unfair coercion. The concept therefore collides with many others in bioethics, including fairness, autonomy, consent, and vulnerability.

Exploitation is also perhaps a surprisingly challenging moral problem to evaluate the wrongness of given that the exploited, by definition, derive benefit, such as payment or social support, that they (often) could (or would) not otherwise receive. To be exploited can not only be definitionally unfair, and thus a kind of moral wrong, but also result in horrible feelings of degradation and violation, if not insurmountable debt. Just as in other problems of power, such as oppression and domination, there can be a range of experiences and intensities within this space.

In a clinical environment, often the practitioner holds more information, experience, and influence to determine medical treatment, and as a result, the patient is vulnerable to the guidance and permission of this authority figure to determine their medical care and thus welfare. The trajectory of the relationship is one that is often fraught with power imbalances, with one paying for the other's services, one to benefit financially and one who will suffer otherwise (Goodyear-Smith & Buetow, 2001). There may be exceptions to this, as there are many ways in which patients may have more power than clinicians, such as by holding influence or wealth, that create certain sway or political capital (see, e.g., Sointu, 2016). But that is not most people or most clinical interactions. For the majority, illness, or the potential for it, is a vulnerability. This can be seen especially for certain groups and populations (such as along racial, gender, sexuality, and ableist lines) that have been historically and/or chronically exploited within and by overlapping social and political systems (Evans et al., 2018). Compounding the situation is the element of profit and payment, especially in a U.S. healthcare environment where cost is high and outcomes are often unclear (Rosenthal, 2017). But even if it were possible to strip away these nefarious forms of discrimination, one would still be susceptible to exploitation given the structure of the system and the inborn power imbalances as well as the possible lack of alternative options.

Exploitation should thus be understood as a *systemic problem*: It is a definitional feature of any system based on profit. As a result, while genetic counselors may be complicit in a flawed system, it is not entirely clear how solely responsible they are for eliminating all its moral failings. But like in many areas, such as climate change and corrupt political systems, individual responsibility is diminished but not eliminated. Genetic counselors do indeed have a moral duty, more easily understood in the "maintenance of appropriate boundaries" in their relationships, but also in their interactions and information shared with patients. The goal of this chapter is to understand the conditions of exploitation in order to clearly track the more deleterious problems that can emerge from exploitative interactions. In what follows, I offer genetic counselors some thoughts on how to identify systemic and individual occurrences of exploitation and ways to understand their role in mitigating its worst effects. I begin by examining how exploitation is (or more often is not) discussed in the genetic counseling literature; how we should discuss the problem more generally, especially in relationship to the concepts of fairness, dignity, autonomy, and consent; and lastly how we should then apply this discussion to genetic counseling cases.

Genetic Counseling Literature on Exploitation

As introduced earlier, despite the references to exploitation in the 2017 NSGC Code of Ethics, the literature on genetic counseling ethics is relatively silent on the question of exploitation. In this section, I examine the lack of clarity around exploitation in genetic counseling, understanding how it is used in other domains of reproductive ethics, genetics research, clinical trials, participant payment, and consumer industry products (particularly genetic testing services). In these areas we see various avenues for how exploitation manifests, including taking advantage of one's vulnerable conditions, unfairness, use as a "means to an end," nonconsensual violations of autonomy, undue burden, and unequal distribution of benefits from a transaction. Those who are exploited may experience one or multiple forms of exploitation, and experiences are not universal but rather may depend on the situation. This section lays out the various uses to gain some traction on what the various situations may look like. The next section offers a closer examination into explicating each concern before connecting the discussion to the genetic counseling context through some case analyses.

First, the concern of exploitation is not as predominant in the field of genetic counseling ethics as compared with other cornerstone values of bioethics, such as autonomy, justice, and beneficence. It is not mentioned early in the field's existence in a report entitled "Screening and Counseling for Genetic Conditions: The Ethical, Social, and Legal Implications of Genetic Screening, Counseling, and Education Programs" by the President's Commission for the Study of Ethical Problems in Medicine and Biomedical and Behavioral Research (1983), nor in more recent totems of the genre, such as *Advanced Genetic Counseling: Theory and Practice* (Biesecker et al., 2019), *The Counselor and the Law: A Guide to Legal and Ethical Practice* (Wheeler & Bertram, 2015), and the more practice-oriented guide *Facilitating the Genetic Counseling Process* (Veach et al., 2018). In *Ethical Dilemmas in Genetics and Genetic Counseling: Principles Through Case Scenarios* (Berliner, 2015), exploitation is referenced only regarding surrogates.

The lack of a detailed exploration of counseling as nonexploitative in several important articles that have been published in the field reflects this broad neglect of in-depth examinations of exploitation (see Clarke & Wallgren-Pettersson, 2019; Schupmann et al., 2020). For example, in "Genetic Counseling, 2030: An On-Demand Service Tailored to the Needs of a Price Conscious, Genetically Literate, and Busy World," the authors make genetic counseling field predictions for the coming decade, particularly given rising costs of consumer technologies, but do not reference exploitation (Rashkin et al., 2019). In Veach et al. (2002), patient exploitation by other healthcare professionals is described as a kind of "professional misconduct" existing in "situations in which the professional must deal with intentional, improper behavior by other professionals" (p. 108). They cite the example of using a blood sample as part of a research study without patients' knowledge or consent. However, what kind of misconduct this is, beyond nonconsent, is unclear in their analysis.

When attention is paid to exploitation, it is often reflected in a desire to protect vulnerable populations. In "Racial and Ethnic Differences in Genetic Counseling Experiences and Outcomes in the United States: A Systematic Review," Southwick et al. (2020) make note of but do not expand upon the important ways that "investigations into the barriers to participation in research for minority communities have helped to understand how different communities perceive the limited benefits and potential harms of research, [and] how mistreatment and exploitation has influenced decision making" (p. 162). In *Genetic Counseling Research: A Practical Guide*, MacFarlane et al. (2014) argue that "Recruitment and interactions with vulnerable populations (e.g., pregnant women, minors, individuals with cognitive impairment) [should be] properly planned to minimize possible harms or exploitation" (p. 84). Similarly, Lydia Sinclair and Matthew Griffiths (1994) write:

> For people who are mentally handicapped there may be additional practical, emotional and medical problems. There is real concern about exploitation and a need to protect vulnerable people from harm and abuse. This must be balanced with a respect of autonomy, a wish for personal development, and a real need to establish and enable advocacy by and on behalf of people with a mental handicap. (p. 155)

This concern for the exploitation of vulnerable populations reflects a kind of ability to make freely or autonomous decisions and features much more prominently in domains adjacent to genetic counseling, such as gestational surrogacy and gamete donation (Ikemoto, 2009). The formulation of this worry is "taking advantage of one's circumstances." In these acts, a good or service is provided in exchange for payment. As a result, ethicists worry about the individuals "choosing" to engage in these exchanges only because they have no viable alternative source of monetary support. This concern has also been applied to the domain of sex work.[1] In this context, vulnerable populations are vulnerable precisely because they have less power and resources than potentially their clients or have no other job opportunity and therefore are more susceptible to engaging in behavior they otherwise would not have chosen for themselves given more free conditions.

Often this formulation of the concern of exploitation leads to policies aimed at eliminating the labor that is exploitative altogether rather than addressing the exploitative circumstances, such as through bolstering rights to unionization and collective bargaining or protecting fair living wages. This logic has also been applied to organ donation: Due to the lack of available organs, policymakers worry that a market in organ selling will target certain communities more willing to sell their organs than others out of financial need (Albertsen, 2020). To protect their bodily integrity, we then enact barriers, such as bans, to this.

[1] We now know this to be untrue in some cases—sex workers as well as surrogate mothers often give reasons including satisfaction, enjoyment, and desire to bring joy and pleasure to others as motivations as well (see Cattapan, 2014; Jadva et al., 2015; Ragone, 1994). This is not so dissimilar from other industries. Nevertheless, this is generally how the exploitation worry goes.

In a similar formulation of exploitation within reproductive ethics more broadly, the exploited are depicted as being used as a means to an end. In their discussion of preimplantation genetic diagnoses and screening to create "savior siblings" (children created purposefully to have specific genetic attributes crucial to saving the life of their sibling, most often used for the purpose of a bone marrow donation in cases of leukemia), Nandor Gabor Than and Zoltan Papp (2017) argue, "One of the major ethical arguments against the use of this technology is the possible exploitation of the child, such as the potential adverse psychologic effects on a child born not for itself but to save another" (p. 40). This concern also arises in anti-commodification worries surrounding surrogacy, that when the surrogate's body is objectified, it is seen merely as a conduit for others' benefit and happiness (Scott, 2009). This, for many, is a problem in and of itself, but for others it is wrong insofar as it can be degrading (Arneson, 1992). Surrogates may experience a loss of sense of self when paid for their reproductive capacity and thus alienated from the fruits of their labor (the child; Anderson, 1990).

In genetics, worries of exploitation feature prominently in discussions of research involving Black and Indigenous populations, as well as other vulnerable groups that historically have suffered in exploitative relationships with the medical establishment (Roberts, 2012). The infamous Tuskegee syphilis study and Henrietta Lacks cases, as well as myriad others before and after them, feature members of the medical community knowingly using bodies of vulnerable populations to advance their own agendas, almost always lacking consent (Sullivan, 2020). In the Havasupai case, tribal blood, something they hold sacred, was used without their permission to trace their ancestry (Berman, 2018). In this version of exploitation, the exploited have diminished autonomy and ability to make choices due to falsities and deceit. Further, this experience culminated in degrading and dehumanizing ends, entrenching distrust in the medical establishment (Sullivan, 2020). Failing to attain proper consent was not the only explanation of the moral depravity; it was that the research was done on a group of people that historically had been marginalized in part by their ends being regarded as secondary only to others' (Jaiswal & Halkitis, 2019).

One of the goals of All of Us (a U.S. government-led DNA database collection program) has been to recruit minority populations (Mancera et al., 2021). The dominant presence of European ancestry data has proved a disservice to research generally into diseases and specifically into those that affect minority populations more widely (Saey, 2021). But due to said historical exploitation of these groups, these populations have (understandably) been reticent to consent to provide their DNA (Fox, 2020). One of the goals of All of Us's messaging campaigns, as a result, has been to convey how the research will benefit these groups in ways crucial to their own welfare and benefit, as opposed to the researchers' or a broader political project of moral hierarchy (National Institutes of Health, 2017). This framing presents the research as one of achieving equal power insofar as both parties benefit equally. In other words, exploitation is thought to be reduced, or at least compensated, when the vulnerable population benefits. However, the fact of benefit by itself does not prove nonexploitation. Indeed, the element of benefit is partly what makes tracking exploitation a difficult task insofar as exploitation necessarily confers a benefit, either through payment or health, as we will explore more in the next section. The moral concern of exploitation becomes more worrisome when the *promised* benefit does not actualize—that is, individuals enter a contract to benefit them, only to discover the benefit was diminished.

In genetics clinical drug trials (including domestic ones), questions of payment for participation have long plagued many an Institutional Review Boards (IRBs; bodies charged with determining the ethical acceptance of clinical research trials; Largent & Lynch 2017). The worry here again is that payment compels a behavior the participant would not otherwise have agreed to (not unlike in the surrogacy case) and thus limits their individual autonomy and ability to fully consent. This worry may also manifest in pediatric cases wherein parents receive payments for their children's participation in research trials. Similarly, in international clinical trials, many have advanced the importance of distributing the fruits of pharmaceutical research when conducted particularly in poorer countries. If research is to be conducted on populations where benefit is sorely needed, and their bargaining power is therefore weaker, then mitigating exploitation requires that the benefit be increased and distributed equally, such as through free provision of drugs. Some think of this as a kind of offsetting of potential harms, others as a positive duty to provide a deserved benefit in exchange for participation.

Lastly, "exploitation of consumers" has been listed as an important moral consideration in the world of direct-to-consumer genetic testing (de Paor, 2018, p. 576). The fear is that direct-to-consumer testing promises valuable information when in fact it delivers significant uncertainty and lack of clarity, taking advantage of people's anxiety and curiosity to earn a profit. However, even in this domain, "exploitation" is mentioned in passing without much follow-through as to what the features of this exploitation look like.

Exploitation Literature

In the previous section, we explored the various uses of exploitation within domains adjacent to genetic counseling, such as reproductive technologies, clinical research trials, and direct-to-consumer technologies. In this section, we examine the literature on exploitation to provide greater clarity as to what exploitation is and what is morally concerning about it before then applying it to a genetic counseling context case analysis. In so doing, we will examine exploitation as alienation, as using another as a means to an end, and as unfairness. The role of vulnerability, loss of autonomy, and problems of consent will also be discussed throughout. Further, while much of the literature on exploitation understands an exploitative relationship as mostly existing between individuals of unequal power, systemic concerns of exploitation are also important to bear in mind. In other words, while A may exploit B, it is far more common and helpful to often talk about institutions and governance as perpetuating, if not thriving on, exploitative behavior. And thus, not unlike in the discourse on climate change and racial injustice, systemic solutions are emphasized more so than personal responsibility.

Alienation

To begin, we turn to Karl Marx, who in the 19th century identified exploitation as a technical explanation for where profit comes from in capitalist systems. Marx is a helpful starting point for discussions on exploitation not only because he is an early theorist on the subject but also because he helps us to better understand exploitation as a structural feature of unfair or unequal power relationships. Prior to Marx, others, such as John Locke and John Stuart Mill, had written about various kinds of unjust trade, unequal exchanges of goods that occurred when one party was in a position of ignorance or needed the trade more than the other, rendering them susceptible to being cheated or taken advantage of. While many of Marx's predecessors, particularly Adam Smith, praised the rise of commerce and exchange societies for aiding the growth of industry and liberating the worker, for Marx, capitalism does not actually create greater freedom but rather establishes a permanent class-based system that leads some (the laborers) to always be exploited and others (the capitalists) to always exploit (Marx, 1992).

Capitalism here refers to an economic–political–social system wherein one class owns private property and sells the "means of production" (the infrastructure and materials for creating commodities as well as the commodities themselves) and those that work for the capitalists to create the commodities. Exchanges primarily exist of two kinds: wage labor between the capitalist and the working class and payment for commodities. Alienation, for Marx, is the condition of being removed from the means of production, of not being able to own the private property through which one creates commodities that then get sold by someone else.

Exploitation is what happens when the laborers are forced to sell their labor power to the capitalists for less than the value of the commodities they produced with it. For the capitalist to profit, or accrue capital, they must "extract surplus labor." As such, exploitation, for Marx, is a definitional feature of a capitalist system. For example, when a laborer works to create a garment (such as on a factory assembly line), the value of their labor is the amount of time that is spent working on that item. In a nonexploitative and non-factory-based context, the laborer would buy the fabric and materials for the clothing, sew it, and sell it for the cost of their labor plus the parts. But in a capitalist system, a managerial class owns the parts of the car and the factory in which it is built. These are the means of production. For the capitalist to have money to purchase more parts and pay for the cost of the facility in which the jacket is made, the capitalist compensates the laborer for only part of the day that they spend working. In the other part of the day, the laborer produces surplus value for the capitalist. The greater the ratio of surplus value to total value, the greater the rate of exploitation. That is how, according to Marx, capitalist systems generate profit and why he takes exploitation to be an intrinsic feature of them (Marx & Engels 1970).

Marx's theory of exploitation has been scrutinized in a variety of ways. First, the theory of labor value has empirically been shown to be inaccurate in explaining where profit comes from, that it may not always be from exploiting the worker but rather come from different social forces that value different commodities at different times (think nonfungible tokens; Conti & Schmidt, 2021). Second, while Marx believes that the main class division is socioeconomic, we know that different racial and identity-based groups are more likely to be exploited than White or heteronormative groups (Davis, 1981). As such, the story is not as simple as one basic rate of exploitation for all in the laboring class. In other words, his story that everything can be understood through a class-based lens is incomplete. Third, some argue that exploitative systems are morally problematic, not because of alienation, but because they are *dominating*. John Roemer (1982), as well as others, examines exploitation as a problem of workplace power dynamics that create the conditions of domination, such as through inability to negotiate salary, rights, or fair treatment at work or to access alternative possibilities. The injustice therefore of substantial capital acquisition is that workers are *dominated* insofar as they are unable to quit and go to a job in which they will have more bargaining power. Consider, for example, the challenges that come with tying health insurance to employment—being unemployed (until the Affordable Care Act of 2010 made this less problematic) often entailed not only being out of a job but also being out of an affordable means of accessing healthcare, thus diminishing viable options.

In contemporary healthcare settings, many healthcare workers themselves are exploited by employers; Marx's analysis could be further helpful in understanding the production-like nature of for-profit medicine and the difficulty numerous Americans face in accessing affordable care (Ramesh et al., 2021). While Marx's framework is more helpful for thinking about employer–employee conditions rather than the counselor–client relationship, the concern of extracting excess and uncompensated labor to increase profit is pervasive in critiques of the American healthcare system and insurance markets.

Means to an end

When one is dominated in a system, one is subject to the arbitrary decisions of an overlord or boss. For some, the wrongness of exploitation in this case is not just tied to nonfreedom or consent worries, for one can quit and not have a job, but manifests as using others as a means to an end. In this account of exploitation, the exploited are only seen as instrumentally valuable to the company or corporation that employs them rather than as individuals with needs and goals of their own. For example, Allen Buchanan (1985) writes that exploitation is "the harmful, merely instrumental utilization of him or his capacities, for one's own advantage or for the sake of one's own needs" (p. 87). This, as we saw, is a common critique of commercial surrogate motherhood—the surrogate is exploited insofar as she is seen as and used merely as a conduit for others' benefit. We can see here how alienation and degradation may be similar, for they both create a feeling of loss of one's own sense of self.

Ruth Sample (2003) defines exploitation as "interacting with another being for the sake of advantage in a way that fails to respect the inherent value in that being" (p. 57). For Sample, exploitation as degradation is connected to vulnerability. When we exploit others, we "make use of their genuine need for the sake of advantage in ways that fail to respect them" (Sample, 2003, p. 75). Because exploitation occurs in vulnerable conditions and results in loss of respecting one's intrinsic worth, the wrongness is not necessarily in the consequential outcomes, but rather in understanding whether the person has been used (as a mere means). As Sample (2003) writes, an interaction can be beneficial while also not being "beneficial enough" (p. 60). This is why one can consent to being exploited and can even benefit materially, such as by having their basic needs met. Early in the COVID-19 pandemic, some people stockpiled significant amounts of hand sanitizer and sold it at higher rates. Not only were they charged with price gouging, but also they were taking advantage of the fact that other people desperately wanted (and perhaps needed) the supplies (Nicas, 2020). What is complicated about exploitation, again, is that even though these people sold each bottle for $1,000, they would still be benefiting the person who purchased the hand sanitizer insofar as they are creating the opportunity for others to be able to use hand sanitizer. It is exploitatively wrong because it denies these people as individuals with basic needs, not because it deprives them of something they need absolutely or even that it comes at a (steep) cost.

The wrongness of exploitation, then, is the erosion of the exploited's dignity. Because most exploitative transactions in a market economy occur at a macrolevel, they are often not felt at the micro level, leaving us in the strange predicament of realizing that many people who are exploited "*do not* feel exploited in a particular transaction when they *actually are* being exploited—largely because of a macrolevel system that is unjust in virtue of its exploitative features" (Sample, 2003, p. 61). Exploitation as degradation thus must take into account situations in which people consider themselves better off because of their ignorance of their own exploitation. Further,

> an exploitative system could be, all in all, the best system available to a given group of people. It may in fact be impossible to have any social system that is entirely free from exploitation. In our response to it, the badness of exploitation must be balanced against other moral evils. (Sample, 2003, p. 62)

Some of those moral evils may include barring someone from needed medical care, such as in the case of terminally ill patients with rare diseases who want to volunteer for pharmaceutical drug trials. In our attempts to save people from exploitation, we may bar them from the potential benefit they seek. For Sample (2003), then, intentionality is important: "Wrongful exploitation should be understood as pursuing a transaction or relationship with another *for the sake of* advantage in a way that is degrading to one's interaction" (p. 126, emphasis added).

Unfairness

Sample arrived at her critique of exploitation as rooted in a loss of respect for persons in response to claims that exploitation is wrong because it is unfair, or a kind of injustice. For these authors, Alan Wertheimer (1996) in particular, A exploits B when B could have benefited more from the transaction. Even if the transaction is mutually beneficial, if B is made worse off than they should have been, exploitation has occurred. Importantly, on this account, exploitation does not necessarily harm its victim. After all, the exchange may well be mutually beneficial. However, the transaction is still unfair given that the exploiter has gained a "cooperative surplus" to which the exploited is entitled (Feinberg, 1988, p. 178).

Hillel Steiner offers a helpful example of this: If a street sweeper was given a rag to wipe the streets on their hands and knees, this is clearly more exploitative than if they were given a functioning broom (Philosophy Bites, 2010). The Silicon Valley startup employee who works in a "safe" work environment and has all their services provided for, including even laundry and meals, is exploited insofar as they could be paid more and thus have the means to purchase something they truly valued, rather than given a ping-pong table. Further, their labor could be demanded more given the veneer of generous compensation in this environment.

Historical injustices, conditions of vulnerability, and systemic patterns of unfair exchanges all contribute to these kinds of exploitation as well. Examples from genetics are apt here—in recruiting patients to participate in database research, our concern of exploitation is greater for Indigenous and Black participants even if they are paid or compensated the same amount as White participants given the historical injustices done to these populations in the name of genetics research. And because the lack of participation in genetics research could harm Black communities due to exclusion from disease discoveries, the question may become, what kinds or levels of exploitation become acceptable in order to access health benefits?

How, then, should we do away with exploitation given that the exploited stand to benefit? From a policy perspective, is the alternative of *non*exploitation in moments of exploitation preferable given that this means that the exploited will not obtain the benefit they need? The utilitarian, whose aim is to maximize utility, could argue that it depends on whether the individual is overall worse off under exploitative exchanges. Scholars like Sample and Wertheimer may argue that even if the exploited benefits, there can still be injustices and harm done. The goal, then, for many who operate at the individual level, as opposed to at the systemic level where wages are set and research agendas are pursued, is to carve out spaces to be sensitive and aware of what it means to treat someone as a mere means, what historical injustices and vulnerabilities exist, and the way in which benefits should be distributed in maximizing ways.

Case Analysis and Discussion

Having explored three of the main formulations of exploitation and what is morally troublesome about them, I will now apply this analysis more directly to the realm of genetic counseling. Insofar as the job of a genetic counselor is to provide information and aid in testing decision making, information interpretation, and risk analysis, I look at these decisions in preconception, research trial moments, and educational endeavors. In so doing, I consider the macroenvironment in which the genetic counselor must struggle with understanding costs, payment, insurance coverage, and access to resources and information in ways that are often beyond their control. These cases emphasize the worry of data ownership and privacy as they are particularly ripe grounds for exploitation given the potential loss of self that can engender.

I argue that exploitation can emerge in many ways, including (a) treating the patient as a means to an end insofar as they are seen as a consumer of medical technology and products rather than as individuals or patients first and foremost; (b) creating unfair exchanges insofar as the clinical researcher has far more to gain than the participants and/or the participant could have benefited more than they did, such as through better privacy protection; and (c) by not fully understanding or taking into consideration the role of historical marginalization and exploitation of vulnerable populations in this context, particularly around group experiences of trauma by minorities, the disabled, and other eugenics-targeted or -affected populations. In examining the cases around these considerations, I ask: What should the genetic counselor advise? How should the counselor advise in such a way that avoids exploitation of parents while also ensuring maximal benefit to them and their child? What are some tools that a counselor could use to mitigate if not eliminate the problem of exploitation in these cases?

Parental carrier screening

Case: A couple is planning on conceiving a child. One member of the couple has a first cousin with cystic fibrosis (CF), and for this reason, the couple is interested in pursuing carrier testing for CF. This is in keeping with the American College of Obstetricians and Gynecologists' (ACOG's) recommendations that "Cystic fibrosis carrier screening should be offered to all women who are considering pregnancy or are currently pregnant" (ACOG, 2017, p. 2). *The couple conducts an online search and finds a direct-to-consumer genetic testing company that offers this screening. The female partner sends a sample and several weeks later receives the online result, which indicates she is a carrier of a pathogenic variant for CF. The couple is concerned by the result and seeks advice from the female partner's gynecologist, who recommends that the couple meet with a genetic counselor. During their appointment, the genetic counselor reviews the screening results, describes the importance of having the result confirmed by a clinical laboratory, and offers the option of carrier screening for the male partner. The male partner decides to have carrier screening for CF, which will involve panel testing for a core set of pathogenic variants. The genetic counselor explains that, given his family history, his risk for being a CF carrier is one in 25 and suggests that the couple check with insurance to see whether the cost will be covered. The couple learns during the session that should a pathogenic variant not be found, the risk for having a child with CF will be significantly reduced but will not be completely eliminated.*

In this situation, exploitation would most likely manifest as the direct-to-consumer company's capacity to take advantage of the couple's situation for their own benefit rather than primarily having the interests of the patients and/or the future child in mind. The couple may be vulnerable in a number of ways. They are interested in conceiving a child with unknown risks and therefore may harbor some anxiety and fear as well as willingness to engage in behavior (i.e., seek genetic screening) they would not otherwise have. Further, they may have difficulties in understanding the nuances and details of the direct-to-consumer market and the complexities of knowing the differences between online and clinically certified testing[2] (Moscarello et al., 2019). They may also be limited by what insurance enables them to afford in the screening, an often opaque and difficult process to navigate and to discover the extent of what one will pay and owe (Grant et al., 2021).

As a result, institutions, such as professional societies like ACOG, have a positive duty to provide as much clear and accessible information as possible to help patients make decisions about testing and screening options that are in their own interests rather than based merely on the enticing marketing of direct-to-consumer companies. Even when information is clear and patients seek to satisfy their own interests, there can remain ambiguity regarding what risk assessments for rarer diseases mean and to what extent screening or testing is necessary (Navon & Thomas, 2021).

The couple in this case is also suspectable to exploitation by the genetic counselor, who has more knowledge and familiarity of resources than the couple. This creates an unequal power dynamic in which the counselor is trusted with directing their procreative actions,

[2] Editors' note: In the United States clinical testing is certified through the Clinical Laboratory Improvement Amendments and the College of American Pathologists.

as well as their wallets. This dynamic is true when the couple is White, heterosexual, and wealthy. But if the couple are members of racial or minority groups that have experienced historical and chronic exploitation by medical institutions, and societal systems more generally, then this concern over exploitation deepens.

In this case, the genetic counselor should help to guide couples in finding out what insurance covers and should state early and clearly that they should have their testing done in a clinical lab rather than through a direct-to-consumer company. However, exploitation often exists due to institutional structures that make exchanges within or with it impossible. As such, the goals of workers within these exploitative institutions cannot always be to prevent vulnerable populations from making exchanges or decisions. In other words, while genetic counselors may have no control over what insurance does or does not cover, they should help to inform the patient about what is in the patient's interest, such as clinically certified testing, and which tests are worth taking.

Clinical trials, data ownership, and patient payment

> *Case: Clinical exome sequencing was recommended for a 5-year-old diagnosed with autism by the clinical genetics team; however, insurance will not cover the cost since exome sequencing is still regarded as experimental. A molecular diagnosis will assist the family in securing needed services/therapies for their child. The parents are presented with alternative options to pursue testing: industry-sponsored testing, a research program that offers sequencing and the potential of result with no promised turnaround time, or paying out of pocket for a small gene panel. Given the parents' desire for a molecular explanation, each option provides its own risks and benefits for the patient, parents, and test providers.*

Similar to the previous case, the first part of the exploitation analysis here concerns significant vulnerability given power, knowledge, and resource inequalities between the family and the clinical team, as well as the desired yet unknown benefit of this genetic information. Further, as the center of this case is a young pediatric patient with an autism diagnosis, consent to participate in clinical trials is limited to and reliant on the parents, who stand as surrogate decision makers tasked with making healthcare decisions that are in the patient's best interest. Additional concerns of data ownership, consent, and utilization arise with sponsored testing in clinical cases like these (Clayton et al., 2019). For example, a clinical exome will potentially lead to discovery of secondary findings that may have an impact on the patient's future care. Depending on where these results are stored and how they are shared, a child patient may be subjected to excessive or clinically nonindicated surveillance, or perhaps determined to be an unsuitable candidate for future interventions (Char et al., 2017).

Genetic information is an immensely important resource for companies to own, as it allows them to perform larger sets of data analysis, advance their own research programs, and thus create profitable pharmaceuticals. If both the company and the patient stand to benefit from improved information, how do we balance the ways in which these benefits are distributed? Inequality of benefit by itself is not the worry in exploitation; it is when the patient could have benefited more than they otherwise would have. Could they distribute the benefits of the research in ways that do not also return a profit for the company?

But are these factors that the *genetic counselor* can control? Or are these moral considerations better left to IRBs to evaluate, where it is their institutional role to evaluate whether payment will compel participation in ways that are exploitative by taking advantage of the patient's circumstances? Or perhaps they will rule that the payment is exploitative because it is not *enough*.

Another concern centers on treating a patient merely as a means to an end. Even if they are reimbursed fairly (i.e., enough), the family could still feel they were used as a means to an end, such as profit or institutional metrics, and that their well-being and care were not important to the medical system and the counselors.

So, while genetic counselors cannot directly control how the medical system operates or its inequality of power and drive for profit, or the historical injustices the genetics field has wrought, they can control their interactions with patients. A moral problem arising from a profit-driven system is that it can create circumstances in which those within it benefit far more than those outside of it, the decisions made are often based on profit, and, as a result, others should have benefited more and may experience alienation. What can mitigate this is explaining information clearly and with intentionality and treating the patient as a person rather than as a potential clinical trial data contributor or source of reimbursement.

Pediatric patient participation in extraclinical activities

> *Case: A 10-year-old biological male child presents to the genetics clinic with his parents. He was recently diagnosed with fibrodysplasia ossificans progressive (FOP), an ultra-rare autosomal dominant condition. Individuals with FOP develop heterotopic ossification in areas such as the muscles, tendons, and ligaments. The transformation of soft tissue into bone continues throughout life and can lead to difficulties with mobility, swallowing, speaking, and breathing. During the session, the family describes the emotional challenges of receiving the diagnosis given the prognosis of FOP and the lack of curative treatment. The geneticist and genetic counselor discuss the diagnosis, genetic testing options, management, and available resources with the family. Toward the end of the genetic counseling session, the geneticist and genetic counselor invite the family to share their experience with FOP at a monthly genetic case conference that is attended by medical students, genetic fellows, genetic counseling graduate students, and other genetic specialists in which different genetic conditions are presented for educational purposes. They explain to the parents that while their child is welcome to attend and participate, it is not viewed as necessary; his clinical information and medical images will be shared during the case conference. The geneticist and genetic counselor tell the family that the healthcare professionals would benefit from learning about an ultra-rare condition and the family's experience with the diagnosis. The family indicate their willingness to consider the invitation and that they would like to participate in efforts to educate healthcare professionals about FOP, but they express some hesitation since they have been devastated by the diagnosis.*

Similar to the last pediatric case, the greatest concerns of exploitation presented in this case are the family being used as a means to an end for the benefit of others and that this exchange may be unfair given the important services they will provide. First, there is a concern of exploitation as loss of dignity for both the patient and his family due to being used as a means to an end for the benefit of the clinical team and the medical or genetics field generally. While the conference provides an important opportunity for others to learn about this family's experiences, it is not for the benefit of the family that they are being asked to do this. It is for the benefit of those who attend and, perhaps ultimately, other patients and families with rare genetic conditions. Further, these conferences often are more clinical in nature, and the parents may feel distress at hearing their case presented in a more prognostic and clinical manner than they are prepared for. This by itself does not mean that their participation is exploitative—that would require participation that erodes their sense of self-worth and violates their personal boundaries and privacy in ways that make them feel bad or harm their dignity.

Thus, one role for a genetic counselor here could be to guide and process the decision making with them in terms of whether, how much, and when they will participate in the conference. The genetic counselor can thus act as a kind of mediator between the clinicians and the parents and help the parents prepare for what to expect at the conference and understand their role in it. This becomes especially important if the patient himself attends, as he is also vulnerable to harm from hearing clinical details about his disease.

Second, there is a concern of unfair exchange of benefits due to power inequalities. There are many vulnerabilities presented in this case. The pediatric patient is vulnerable due to his condition and age and, as such, his inability to fully consent to what happens in his life, particularly in his medical life. The parents are vulnerable due to the prestige of their genetics team and the weight of the diagnosis. They also may have limited emotional capacity given the circumstances, and asking them to be vulnerable in front of strangers who hold more power and knowledge than they do creates certain kinds of social and power inequalities. The genetic counselor can play a role in helping to prepare them for the conference if they choose to be present. In this situation, the genetic counselor is not necessarily in a position of power to exploit or to prevent exploitation but can mitigate any harms or inequalities that may present elsewhere by aiding the process and advocating for the patient.

Conclusion

I argue that the primary responsibilities of genetic counselors are to be fully aware of historical and chronic minority group exploitation and the tradeoffs inherent in exploitative exchanges. They may have other responsibilities, of course, including acting as thoughtful and careful engagers and interlocutors with those in power and speaking up insofar as is possible when injustices and alienation emerge.

There is much more to be said about exploitation, including what it is, when it happens, how morally wrong it is, and what harms may come from it. Systems-based critiques are crucial to this exercise through identifying ways that inequalities of power impacts patient vulnerability, access to information and resources, and how benefits are fairly distributed. The feeling of being treated as a means to an end can be circumvented more directly in individual one-on-one interactions. Even when structural problems persist, equipping one with the proper awareness of historical grievances, explaining information to and recruiting patients as people instead of as prospective data contributors, and understanding that many families are different in terms of their acceptability of risk and financial circumstances can help enormously in circumventing the worst of this feeling of alienation from medicine and general loss of self. If we are to take the NSGC Code of Ethics seriously, effecting meaningful change would involve addressing not just one-on-one instances of exploitation but overall exploitative practices within the industry writ large.

References

Albertsen, A. (2020). If the price is right: The ethics and efficiency of market solutions to the organ shortage. *Journal of Bioethical Inquiry, 17*, 357–367.

American College of Obstetricians and Gynecologists. (2017). *Carrier screening for genetic conditions.* https://www.acog.org/clinical/clinical-guidance/committee-opinion/articles/2017/03/carrier-screening-for-genetic-conditions

Anderson, E. S. (1990). Is women's labor a commodity? *Philosophy & Public Affairs, 19*(1), 71–92.

Arneson, R. J. (1992). Commodification and commercial surrogacy. *Philosophy & Public Affairs, 21*(2), 132–164.

Ballantyne, A. (2008). Benefits to research subject in international trials: Do they reduce exploitation or increase undue inducement? *Developing World Bioethics, 8*(3), 178–191.

Berliner, J. (Ed.). (2015). *Ethical dilemmas in genetics and genetic counseling: Principles through case scenarios.* Oxford University Press.

Berman, J. (2018). *Principles and practice of big data: Preparing, sharing, and analyzing complex information.* Academic Press.

Biesecker, B. B., Peters, K. F., & Resta, R. (2019). *Advanced genetic counseling: Theory and practice.* Oxford University Press.

Buchanan, A. (1985). *Ethics, efficiency, and the market.* Rowman and Allanheld.

Cattapan, A. (2014). Risky business: Surrogacy, egg donation, and the politics of exploitation. *Canadian Journal of Law and Society, 29*(3), 361–379.

Char, D. S., Lázaro-Muñoz, G., Barnes, A., Magnus, D., Deem, M. J., & Lantos, J. D. (2017). Genomic contraindications to heart transplantation. *Pediatrics, 139*(4), e20163471.

Clarke, A. J., & Wallgren-Pettersson, C. (2019). Ethics in genetic counselling. *Journal of Community Genetics, 10*(1), 3–33.

Clayton, E. W., Evans, B. J., Hazel, J. W., & Rothstein, M. A. (2019). The law of genetic privacy: Applications, implications, and limitations. *Journal of Law and the Biosciences, 6*(1), 1–36.

Conti, R., & Schmidt, J. (2021, May 14). What you need to know about non-fungible tokens (NFTs). *Forbes.* https://www.forbes.com/advisor/investing/nft-non-fungible-token/

Davis, A. (1981). *Women, race, and class.* Random House.

de Paor, A. (2018). Direct to consumer genetic testing—Law and policy concerns in Ireland. *Irish Journal of Medical Science, 187*, 575–584.

Emanuel, E. J., Joffe, S., Grady, C., Wendler, D., & Persad, G. (2015). Clinical research: Should patients pay to play? *Science Translational Medicine, 7*(298), 1–4.

Evans, C. R., Williams, D. R., Onnela, J.-P., & Subramanian, S. V. (2018). A multilevel approach to modeling health inequalities at the intersection of multiple social identities. *Social Science & Medicine, 203*, 64–73.

Feinberg, J. (1988). *Harmless wrongdoing.* Oxford University Press.

Fox, K. (2020). The illusion of inclusion—The "All of Us" Research Program and Indigenous Peoples' DNA. *New England Journal of Medicine, 383*(5), 411–413.

Goodyear-Smith, F., & Buetow, S. (2001). Power issues in the doctor-patient relationship. *Health Care Analysis, 9*, 449–462.

Grant, P., Langlois, S., Lynd, L. D., Study, G., Austin, J. C., & Elliott, A. M. (2021). Out-of-pocket and private pay in clinical genetic testing: A scoping review. *Clinical Genetics, 100*(5), 504–521.

Ikemoto, L. (2009). Reproductive tourism: Equality concerns in the global market for equality. *Law and Inequality, 27*(277), 295–298.

Jadva, V., Imrie, S., & Golombok, S. (2015). Surrogate mothers 10 years on: A longitudinal study of psychological well-being and relationships with the parents and child. *Human Reproduction, 30*(2), 373–379.

Jaiswal, J. & Halkitis, P. N. (2019). Toward a more inclusive and dynamic understanding of medical mistrust informed by science. *Behavioral Medicine, 45*(2), 79–85.

Largent, E. A., & Lynch, H. F. (2017). Paying research participants: The outsized influence of "undue influence." *IRB, 39*(4), 1–9.

MacFarlane, I., Veach, P. M., & LeRoy, B. (2014). *Genetic counseling research: A practical guide.* Oxford University Press.

Mancera, B. M., Sy, A., Williams, C. D., & Hargreaves, M. K. (2021). Utilizing a social-ecological health promotion framework to engage diverse populations for recruitment in the All of Us Research Program. *Journal of Community Engagement and Scholarship, 13*(2).

Marx, K. (1992). *Capital: Vol. 1. A critique of political economy.* Penguin Classics.

Marx, K., & Engels, F. (1970). *The German ideology.* International Publishers.

Moscarello, T., Murray, B., Reuter, C. M., & Demo, E. (2019). Direct-to-consumer raw genetic data and third-party interpretation services: More burden than bargain? *Genetics in Medicine, 21*, 539–541.

National Institutes of Health. (2017, July 25). *The All of Us Research Program announces first community partner awards.* https://allofus.nih.gov/news-events-and-media/announcements/all-us-research-program-announces-first-community-partner-awards

National Society of Genetic Counselors. (2017). *NSGC Code of Ethics.* https://www.nsgc.org/Policy-Research-and-Publications/Code-of-Ethics-Conflict-of-Interest/Code-of-Ethics

Navon, D., & Thomas, G. (2021). Screening before we know: Radical uncertainties in expanded prenatal genetics. *OBM Genetics, 5*(4), 12.

Nicas, J. (2020, March 14). He has 17,700 bottles of hand sanitizer and nowhere to sell them. *New York Times.* https://www.nytimes.com/2020/03/14/technology/coronavirus-purell-wipes-amazon-sellers.html

Panitch, V. (2013). Exploitation, justice, and parity in international clinical research. *Journal of Applied Philosophy, 30*(4), 304–318.

Philosophy Bites. (2010). *Hillel Steiner on exploitation.* https://philosophybites.com/2010/08/hillel-steiner-on-exploitation.html

President's Commission for the Study of Ethical Problems in Medicine and Biomedical and Behavioral Research. (1983). *Screening and counseling for genetic conditions: The ethical, social, and legal implications of genetic screening, counseling, and education programs.* https://repository.library.georgetown.edu/handle/10822/559349

Ragone, H. (1994). *Surrogate motherhood: Conception in the heart.* Routledge.

Ramesh, S., Su, K., & Haddad, T. (2021). A crisis of immeasurable proportions: Exploring issues in modern-day medical care through Marxist sociological theory. *Journal for Social Thought, 5*(1).

Rashkin, M. D., Bowes, J., Dunaway, K., Dhaliwal, J., Loomis, E., Riffle, S., Washington, N. L., Ziegler, C., Lu, J., & Levin, E. (2019). Genetic counseling, 2030: An on-demand service tailored to the needs of a price conscious, genetically literate, and busy world. *Journal of Genetic Counseling, 28*(2), 456–465.

Roberts, D. (2012). *Fatal invention: How science, politics, and big business re-create race in the twenty-first century*. New Press.

Roemer, J. (1982). Property relations vs. surplus value in Marxian exploitation. *Philosophy & Public Affairs, 11*(4), 281–313.

Rosenthal, E. (2017). *An American sickness: How healthcare became big business and how you can take it back*. Penguin Press.

Saey, T. H. (2021). DNA databases are too white, so genetics doesn't help everyone. How do we fix that? *Science News*. https://www.sciencenews.org/article/genetics-race-dna-databases-reference-genome-too-white

Sample, R. (2003). *Exploitation: What it is and why it's wrong*. Rowman & Littlefield.

Schupmann, W., Jamal, L., & Berkman, B. E. (2020). Re-examining the ethics of genetic counselling in the genomic era. *Journal of Bioethical Inquiry, 17*, 325–335.

Scott, E. S. (2009). Surrogacy and the politics of commodification. *Law and Contemporary Problems, 72*, 109–146.

Sinclair, L., & Griffiths, M. (1994). Medical genetics and mental handicaps. In A. Clarke (Ed.), *Genetic counselling: Practice and principles* (pp. 144–159). Routledge.

Sointu, E. (2016). "Good" patient/"bad" patient: Clinical learning and the entrenching of inequality. *Sociology of Health & Wellness, 39*(1), 63–77.

Southwick, S. V., Esch, R., Gasser, R., Cragun, D., Redlinger-Grosse, K., Marsalis, S., & Zierhut, H. A. (2020). Racial and ethnic differences in genetic counseling experiences and outcomes in the United States: A systematic review. *Journal of Genetic Counseling, 29*(2), 147–165.

Sullivan, L. S. (2020). Trust, risk, and race in American medicine. *Hastings Center Report, 50*(1), 18–26.

Than, N. G., & Papp, Z. (2017). Ethical issues in genetic counseling. *Best Practice and Research Clinical Obstetrics and Gynaecology, 43*, 32–49.

Veach, P. M., Bartels, D. M., & LeRoy, B. S. (2002). Ethical and professional challenges posed by patients with genetic concerns: A report of focus group discussions with genetic counselors, physicians, and nurses. *Journal of Genetic Counseling, 10*(2), 97–119.

Veach, P. M., LeRoy, B., & Callanan, N. P. (2018). *Facilitating the genetic counseling process* (2nd ed.). Springer.

Wertheimer, A. (1996). *Exploitation*. Princeton University Press.

Wheeler, A. M., & Bertram, B. (2015). *The counselor and the law: A guide to legal and ethical practice* (7th ed.). American Counseling Association.

CHAPTER 28

PRECISION MEDICINE'S ETHICAL CHALLENGES

Roles for Genetic Counselors

LISA S. PARKER

Introduction: Precision Medicine and the Roles of Genetic Counselors

Precision Medicine: What It Is and Should Be

During and since the later decades of the 20th century, study of the genetic contributions to disease intensified, with many referring to a dawning revolution or paradigm shift in the understanding, diagnosis, prevention, and treatment of disease (Chan & Ginsberg, 2011). With the mapping and sequencing of the human genome, there was talk of ushering in an era of "personalized medicine" or "genomic medicine," as well as criticism of each term and of the equation of personalized with genomic medicine (Horwitz et al., 2013; Pokorska-Bocci et al., 2014; Roden & Tyndale, 2013; Schleidgen et al., 2013). Physicians (and other clinicians), for example, argued that medical treatment has always been personalized and that medicine should be concerned with the whole person, not merely a disease (Ashley, 2015; Offit, 2011). Others expressed concern about how the terms—and the trends they denoted—could divert attention from both public health approaches (Burke et al., 2010) and environmental contributions to disease (Horwitz et al., 2013), while also exacerbating assignment of individual responsibility for ill health and raising hope for personal empowerment in healthcare that is especially unrealistic for those already facing healthcare disparities (Juengst et al., 2016; Rose, 2013).

By 2012, the term "personalized medicine" was giving way to "precision medicine" (PM), despite concerns that the term encouraged "an expectation of perfect outcomes that not only is unrealistic but runs the risk of overhyping the potential of the field to patients and their families" (Roden & Tyndale, 2013, p. 171). "Precision medicine" received a "decisive seal of approval" when President Obama announced the Precision Medicine Initiative in 2015 (Juengst et al., 2016, p. 22), and the term entered popular discourse with Obama characterizing it as "delivering the right treatments, at the right time, every time to the right person" (Obama, 2015). In the same year, however, scientific authorities such as Francis Collins and Harold Varmus noted that "the concept of PM—prevention and treatment strategies that take individual variability into account—is not new" (Collins & Varmus, 2015, p. 793) and cited not only blood typing used to guide transfusions for over a century but also the 2011 National Research Council's report, *Toward Precision Medicine*, which characterizes PM as

> the tailoring of medical treatment to the individual characteristics of each patient. It does not literally mean the creation of drugs or medical devices that are unique to a patient, but rather the ability to classify individuals into subpopulations that differ in their susceptibility to a particular disease or their response to a specific treatment. Preventive or therapeutic interventions can then be concentrated on those who will benefit, sparing expense and side effects for those who will not. (National Research Council Committee on a Framework for Developing a New Taxonomy of Disease, 2011; President's Council of Advisors on Science and Technology, 2008, p. 7)

Indeed, like the contemporary medical care that preceded and surrounds it, PM is evidence-based, epidemiologically based medicine. Despite rhetoric suggesting that PM involves personalization and tailoring of interventions to individuals, clinical trials in which participants' genotypes (and other particular features) figure in recruitment or data analysis still yield only average results for a given population. Clinical guidelines and interventions based on such studies still hold only a population-based probability of benefiting an individual patient who is relevantly similar to the studied population. Individual patients' experience with the resulting recommended intervention—drug, preventive or treatment regimen, behavior change—will still vary.

PM may also be thought of as stratification-based medicine: stratifying those who are likely to develop a disease or benefit from an intervention from those not likely to by first dividing people based on their genotype. Dividing people based on identified traits—particularly those that are stigmatized or deemed likely to require expenditure of social resources—has a long history of resulting in disparities and discrimination (Sabatello et al., 2021), disenfranchisement (Nelkin & Tancredi, 1989), and even death (genocide; e.g., Kimel et al., 2016). As Juengst et al. (2016) argue:

> On the surface, refining disease classifications does not seem like the same thing as stratifying patients into different subpopulations. But they amount to the same thing, to the extent that the science that associates particular molecular markers with different risks, outcomes, and clinical indications is population based to begin with. (p. 24)

Thus, societies, institutions, and healthcare professionals should take special care when embracing the stratification inherent in PM. They should carefully scrutinize the value-laden decisions that take place behind the scenes (or before the clinical scene), for example, in enrolling representative study populations, determining the characteristics and data used for stratification (Batten, 2018; Landry et al., 2018; Tranvåg et al., 2021), interpreting genetic variants (as benign, pathogenic, or of uncertain significance; Richards, 2015), judging evidence to be of sufficient quality as to be "actionable" or clinically relevant, or determining that a particular intervention has a sufficient prospect of benefit for a particular patient so that it should be prescribed or covered by health insurance (Aronson & Rehm, 2015).

Moreover, because PM encompasses, yet is broader than, genomic medicine, PM should take into account environmental, behavioral, and lifestyle factors, as well as genes, when identifying the best therapeutic or preventive intervention. However, in publicity surrounding PM—both research and early clinical practice (e.g., pharmacogenomics [PGx])—interest in the genetic/genomic contributions to treatment response and disease risk seems to eclipse concern for the other components of gene–environment interaction. Perhaps this is not surprising. Clinical medicine generally focuses its interventions at the level of individuals (Gostin, 2000). Upstream environmental causes of disease and disability are typically the province of public health, which focuses on population-level interventions and benefits. Sustaining change in individuals' health behaviors has long been a challenge, and results of studies evaluating whether genetic risk information motivates long-term behavior change are at best mixed (Hollands et al., 2016; Silarova et al., 2019; Smerecnik et al., 2012; Tan et al., 2018; Turnwald et al., 2019; Zoltick et al., 2019). Nevertheless, precisely tailored diagnosis and intervention based on newly discovered genetic knowledge may seem more promising than chipping away at environmental and behavioral contributions to ill health. In addition, those who explicitly call for the inclusion of social, environmental, and behavioral data in PM analyses—for both clinical care and research purposes—acknowledge that "biases in the collection and analysis of EHR-derived social and behavioral data can have ethical implications" and that these data, like genomic data, should be used in ways that "will not exacerbate existing injustices in health care" (Hollister & Bonham, 2018, pp. 877–878).

Roles for genetic counselors in achieving PM's promise

Genetic counselors may play an important role in reminding patients, the public, and researchers of the environmental component of the gene–environment interaction responsible for the vast majority of deleterious health conditions. They should promote both holistic care and holistic understanding of disease etiology and treatment, eschewing reductionistic understandings of people and their conditions. They are well suited to this role. Their education affords understanding not only of gene–environment interaction but also of the importance, for clinical decision making and positive health outcomes, of attending to culture (and culturally congruent care), psychology, communication, family dynamics, and social structures.

As genetics/genomics and PM enter all healthcare domains, genetic counselors will be called upon to use their particular knowledge and skills to make recommendations in light of the therapeutic goals of those domains and then to help patients make decisions about those recommendations in light of their own values and circumstances. Because of their specialized knowledge and communication skills, genetic counselors will not only be called upon within healthcare settings to benefit patients and their families but also be pressed to weigh in on a range of policies that may make the potential benefits of PM a reality for everyone no matter their geographic location, economic or insurance status, level of education, cultural or linguistic community, or continental ancestry. These evolving policies will include clinical practice guidelines, professional society recommendations (including about the classification, actionability, and reportability of genetic variants), hospital and clinic policies and practices, research protocols, industry standards, coverage/reimbursement policies of insurers and governmental agencies, and even legislation. Absent appropriate policies to shape and support its implementation, PM has the potential to exacerbate health and healthcare disparities and widen the wealth gap.

This chapter outlines some of the ethical considerations that genetic counselors and other clinicians should take into account when considering PM policies, practices, and even client/patient-level recommendations. In many ways, the ethical challenges of PM mirror those of traditional evidence-based medicine, coupled with the particular challenges presented by genetic screening and testing and -omic sequencing. Genetic counselors, other genetics specialists, and other clinicians will need to interpret the results of genetic testing and genomic sequencing for patients (and explain testing and sequencing to the media and public). Patients will need support to facilitate their sharing of relevant information with family members to benefit their health, and they will need access to relevant health-related information and services to reap the benefits of testing/sequencing results.

Thus, PM presents ethical issues on multiple levels: for individuals and families, within the professional–patient/client relationship and within healthcare institutions, and for society, social institutions, and commercial entities (including insurers, pharmaceutical companies, and direct-to-consumer [DTC] testing companies). This chapter addresses some of the issues that arise in domains where PM approaches are currently employed: PGx; cancer prediction, prevention, diagnosis, and treatment; resolving diagnostic odysseys and diagnosing, treating, and preventing rare diseases; predicting and preventing complex conditions through polygenic risk assessment; and research to develop the knowledge base for PM.

Pharmacogenomics

Clinical care

At first impression, PGx seems both a quintessential PM intervention and ethically unproblematic. As the study of inherited genetic variations that influence a person's metabolic response to a drug or class of drugs, thereby enabling prescription of the right drug to the right patient, PGx is an example of PM. Yet, pharmacogenomic testing arguably ignores many of the environmental and behavioral factors relevant to prescribing medication. Prescribing medication associated with increased rates of bleeding or clotting complications appropriately depends not only on drug metabolism but also on factors such as a patient's diet and activities, especially when these are not easily altered, as with value-based dietary commitments or an occupation requiring particular activities (like long-distance air travel). Factors such as drug cost and convenience influence whether patients actually take prescribed medications and thus are relevant to prescribing it. As long as such relevant factors are also taken into account when prescribing, what could be ethically problematic in using pharmacogenomic testing to pursue the goal of reducing adverse drug reactions (ADRs)—thereby reducing healthcare costs and patient suffering—while increasing the effectiveness of pharmacological treatment?

Though there is nothing particularly stigmatizing or psychosocially disruptive about being a slow or rapid drug metabolizer, pleiotropy in this context means that genetic variants associated with drug metabolism may also be associated with disease risk. While it may seem obvious that PGx test results should be shared with family members who may have the same inherited genetic variants, sharing information about inherited disease risk is more complicated and ethically fraught, including whether there is an obligation to inform one's family members, and if so, the ethical foundation for such an obligation (Buchanan, 1998; Dimond et al., 2022).[1]

The possibility of PGx testing yielding incidental findings of disease risk is one reason that specific informed consent for PGx testing may be considered appropriate. The potential familial relevance of such test results and incidental findings is one of the points to be disclosed during informed consent for PGx. Risks to privacy and of discrimination should also be disclosed. Though genetic discrimination in employment and health insurance is largely prohibited by the Genetic Information Nondiscrimination Act (GINA, 2008), increased genetic risk of disease may still be used in life, disability, and long-term care insurance underwriting. (Some of those who are not covered by GINA—federal and military employees, as well as people receiving their healthcare through the military, Veterans Administration, Indian Health Service, or Federal Employee Health Benefits Plan—have similar protections through other policies or by executive order, while employees in settings with fewer than 15 employees do not.) Learning of disease risk through PGx testing thus presents some economic and psychosocial risk, and this possibility should be disclosed in advance of testing.

Clinical use of PGx test results may seem deceptively straightforward. PGx test results sort people into categories vis-à-vis a drug or drug class. For those at low risk of ADRs and high likelihood of benefit, and those at high risk of ADRs and low likelihood of benefit, the course of action following testing seems fairly clear. The first group should be prescribed the drug; the second should not. But what if there is no safer alternative? In that case, prescribing the drug and carefully monitoring for ADRs may be appropriate. Especially because PGx testing stratifies patients according to probabilities of ADRs and benefits rather than identifying with certainty which individuals will/won't benefit or which will suffer adverse reactions, there may still be reasons to prescribe contrary to PGx test result indications. These reasons include patient circumstances and preferences, drug costs and convenience, and insurance coverage. As in other clinical medicine contexts where patients are permitted to make decisions in light of their values, circumstances, and degree of risk aversion or proneness, decisions to accept associated risks of treatment in hope of receiving benefits should be left to patients. Genetic counselors, with their training in risk communication and in explaining the complexities of probabilities, may contribute to the informed consent process to help ensure that such decisions are well informed and in keeping with the patients' values.

Where the results of PGx testing are used to determine the dosing regimen of specific drugs or to guide monitoring for ADRs, testing does not present peculiar ethical challenges. For example, the usual considerations for applying dosing guidelines for a particular patient still require clinical judgment to implement PGx-informed dosing guidelines for adults to pediatric patients (Wren & Park, 2018). As with the existence of clinical practice guidelines

[1] Editors' note: For discussion of family communication about genetic risk, see Chapter 24 by Samantha Leonard and Ainsley Newson in this volume.

and clinical decision support in general, the recommendations to use PGx to guide dosing may impose an obligation (ethical, legal, or both) on clinicians to make use of PGx testing, at least once such testing is considered part of standard care. Whether a patient should be permitted to refuse PGx testing to avoid learning disease risk information and still be prescribed the drug for which testing is recommended is an open—and likely a situation-specific—ethical question. The answer, from at least an ethical perspective, should depend on the specific risks involved, the challenges of monitoring for ADRs, the magnitude and probability of the treatment benefit being sought, and the patients' reasons, values, and circumstances.

How insurers will and should regard such indications and prescribing practices remains an open question. Health insurers typically cover only medically necessary treatments. While GINA prohibits health insurers from discriminating against people based on genetic information to deny them coverage or charge higher rates, insurers are permitted to use genetic information to determine medical need and, in turn, what is "medically necessary" treatment. A strong family history of breast cancer or positive *BRCA1/2* testing for a pathogenic variant, for example, may be used to establish a young woman's medical need and insurance coverage for mammography that would not otherwise be covered until a later age. Particularly as more drugs receive recommendations that PGx testing be performed, it remains an open question whether or under what conditions insurers may deny coverage for patients with "contraindicated" genotypes (i.e., those indicating an increased risk for ADRs or a lower probability of benefit); genetic counselors and bioethicists may contribute to the development of such coverage policies, including appeal procedures and criteria.

When institutions or national organizations develop clinical practice guidelines or insurers draft policies governing reimbursement/coverage, concern for patient well-being, just allocation of resources, and containing healthcare costs supports taking into account both patients' medical need and the growing body of PGx information (Caulfield & Zarzeczny, 2014). Nevertheless, because PGx yields results applicable with confidence to stratified patient groups but not with certainty to individual patients, concern for well-being and fairness suggests that an individual whose genotype indicates a relatively lower probability of positive treatment response should not be categorically denied access to (or coverage for) that intervention, so long as three conditions are met: (a) the intervention is otherwise available/covered, (b) no other intervention is available that is likely effective for patients with that genetic variation, and (c) the risk or burden of the intervention to the individual (i.e., the probability and magnitude of ADRs) is not unduly burdensome given the magnitude and probability of benefit. With regard to (c), some bioethicists have argued that an individual should be allowed to assume those risks and not be denied the opportunity to seek even remote benefit when no other good alternative exists and when others with a different genotype have access to the intervention (Parker & Satkoske, 2012). Genetic counselors may help to ensure that patients understand the risks they are accepting.

It is also unclear who will bear the liability for ADRs (and financial responsibility for treating sequelae of ADRs) if a drug is prescribed contrary to a PGx test result. In the absence of an alternative, or if alternatives are not affordable or are more cumbersome or otherwise unattractive to take, a patient may want to assume the risk of experiencing ADRs and receive the "contraindicated" drug. Especially if the intervention or drug with a remote (or relatively lower) prospect of benefit could be administered at the patient's own expense, it would seem quite reasonable to allow the patient to opt for a personally preferred drug over the one most recommended and to assume ADR-related risks—both risk of an adverse reaction eventuating and liability for the costs of treating the reaction. But most patients cannot afford to self-pay for medication or chemotherapy or for treatment of ADRs. Therefore, patients' requests for access to "genotype-contraindicated" drugs implicate the interests of institutions, insurers, and those in insurance pools whose rates are partially dependent on what insurers are required to pay out.

It is thus reasonable for institutions to consider these downstream costs when considering exceptions to clinical guidelines and for insurers to consider them when adjudicating appeals for coverage.

Nevertheless, decisions to deny an individual, on the basis of their genotype, an intervention that is available to others should not be made lightly or categorically. Appropriate appeals processes should be established, or existing appeals processes addressing coverage denials should be expanded, to address denials based on PGx results, just as they were for denials of coverage based on findings from comparative effectiveness research (Parker & Brody, 2011). In sum, the stratification intrinsic to PM should not be used to disadvantage people who would be afforded a chance to benefit from treatment in the absence of such stratification. Indeed, rather than allowing PGx testing to create a class of patients with a condition+genotype for whom there is no available treatment when there is a treatment for other patients with the same condition, it may be appropriate to afford patients a right to try a "genotype-contraindicated" drug. A request for such an opportunity might be modeled on "right to try" requests, though here the drugs would not be investigational but part of standard of care. In addition, the patient need not be in a life-threatening condition but instead be in a situation where a drug that is available to patients with other genotypes is "genotype contraindicated" for the patient making the appeal. Unlike the "right to try" in the context of investigational drugs, here there are no ethical concerns about this mechanism undermining the clinical trial process and production of generalizable knowledge (Joffe & Lynch, 2018). A parallel might be drawn from the "right to try" context, in which manufacturers are protected from liability, to develop measures to protect clinicians and institutions from liability for ADRs when prescribing a "genotype-contraindicated" drug.

Research

PGx testing presents advantages in research and drug development. It increases the likelihood of drug approvals yet raises some ethical questions, necessitating policy development (Kimmelman & Tannock, 2018). Drug developers may "rescue" and bring to market a drug that is ineffective for a study population as a whole if it proves to be effective for a subset of the study population. By characterizing that subset by genotype, enrolling study participants of that genotype in smaller follow-up studies, and then seeking approval and subsequently marketing the resulting drug for patients with that genotype, approvals may be faster, and the costs and risks of clinical trials and drug development may be reduced (Pregelj et al., 2018). However, policy or financial incentives may be necessary to ensure that patients with other condition+genotypes are not "orphaned" by the possibility of developing drugs that effectively treat subsets of study populations and subsequently ignoring other subsets of patients with the same condition. Genetic counselors may play a role in advocating that groups of patients not be left behind in the research and drug approval process.

Genetic counselors may also play a role in the research process, particularly to address the complex informational, psychological, and ethical challenges associated with enrolling participants in clinical studies based on their genotype (Michie et al., 2012). These challenges include determining whether and how to disclose results of a previous study, including genotype information, to explain the (re)contact of the specific individuals being recruited. They may also weigh in on debate about whether "genotype-driven recruitment [may] either attenuate or amplify obligations to return genetic research results" from the present study for which their participation is invited (Beskow et al., 2012, p. 1424).

Precision Oncology

Treatment

The appropriateness of the title of the National Research Council's report, *Toward Precision Medicine: Building a Knowledge Network for Biomedical Research and a New Taxonomy of Disease* (2011), becomes clear in the context of oncology. In light of genomic research, the taxonomy of cancers has been reconceptualized. It is no longer viewed as a single disease, with different cancers distinguished solely by their location (e.g., breast or bowel) and degrees of progression (stage) and cell abnormality (grade). Instead, as the report suggests, oncology is embracing "a disease taxonomy that describes and defines diseases based on their intrinsic biology in addition to traditional physical 'signs and symptoms'" (National Research Council Committee on a Framework for Developing a New Taxonomy of Disease, 2011, p. 41). Molecular profiling of tumors has led to new ways of categorizing cancers and new targeted treatment approaches. Defined as genomic testing to more precisely predict treatment response, precision oncology is developing rapidly and being applied to an increasing number of cancers (Schwartzberg et al., 2017). The goals of precision oncology are similar to those of PGx—namely, providing more effective treatment while avoiding adverse side effects (at least those associated with ineffective treatment). Tumor profiling that yields knowledge of actionable genomic alterations in an individual tumor may inform prognostication, treatment recommendations, and patients' personal decision making.

Precision oncology approaches and their mechanisms of action differ. Targeted therapies are trained on specific changes in a tumor's cells; they generally work by attacking deregulated proteins supporting cancer cell survival (Fernandez-Rozadilla et al., 2021; Lee et al., 2018). Among the earliest targeted therapies were hormone therapies that operate either by preventing production of hormones needed for cancer growth or by preventing the hormones from acting on cells. Some targeted therapies inhibit angiogenesis to starve blood supply to tumors and cause tumors to remain small or shrink. Immunotherapy utilizes stimulation of the patient's immune system to fight against cancer cells or seeks to block cell surface receptors specific to tumor cells (e.g., employing monoclonal antibodies to cause cell death). In some cases, monoclonal antibodies, combined with agents (chemotherapeutic agents or radiation), attach to cancer cells, delivering the agent to those cells and sparing noncancer cells. Pharmaco-diagnostics, clinical molecular pathology analysis examining tumor biology, predicts whether a tumor will respond to a particular therapy (Fernandez-Rozadilla et al., 2021).

Moreover, just as cancer cells can develop resistance to chemotherapy, resistance to targeted therapies may develop. Therefore, resampling and retesting of tumors may be necessary. Results of testing may differ between a recurring cancer and the original tumor. Liquid biopsy, a less invasive alternative to traditional tissue biopsy, may be used to test for biomarkers in some cases; through the collection of a body fluid sample to test for relevant biomarkers, for example, taking a peripheral blood sample to analyze cell-free circulating tumor DNA (Fernandez-Rozadilla et al., 2021; Schwartzberg et al., 2017). Liquid biopsy can also be informative about both primary and secondary tumors, is not affected by how skillfully a tumor biopsy is taken, and thus may provide an "unbiased overview of the tumor molecular features" (Fernandez-Rozadilla et al., 2021, p. 11). There are thus many points at which evidence-based interpretation and other human skills are critical for the effectiveness of precision cancer care.

The volume and complexity of information presented by precision oncology care may complicate both explanation of treatment options during informed consent and patients' decision making regarding those options at a time when they are facing a serious diagnosis. For clinicians, applying evidence from a research trial that employed one diagnostic technique to clinical decision making in a clinic that routinely uses a different technique introduces uncertainties, and the need to combine "different streams of evidence to prioritize their choice of treatment" places increased demands on their clinical judgment (Kimmelman & Tannock, 2018, p. 342).

The social and economic implications of increased use of precision cancer interventions are unclear and may differ substantially between the short and long term. The initial cost of developing each targeted therapy is very high, and research outcomes apply to a narrowly defined group of patients. But the potential to reduce healthcare spending by identifying therapy responders and nonresponders during clinical trials and eventually in clinical care is economically promising. Together with the promise of avoiding unnecessary suffering, such cost saving is obviously ethically attractive. If these targeted cancer treatments are proven cost effective, eventually insurers (both private and public) are more likely to cover them.

In the meantime, the high cost of these therapies will likely exacerbate disparities in both access to targeted cancer care and cancer-related morbidity and mortality. It should be noted that exceedingly high costs are associated not only with targeted cancer care but also with targeted therapies for other conditions (Wren & Park, 2018). Some worry that stratifying patients and targeting therapies will shrink therapeutics developers' market shares and result in their increasing pricing to offset reduced volume (Krzyszczyk et al., 2018), replicating economic issues associated with treatment for rare diseases and exacerbating healthcare disparities even in the long term. Moreover, currently, geographic, informational, and educational barriers prevent some patients from accessing these precision cancer treatments as they emerge in research-rich areas and more highly remunerative markets.

Finally, neither potential for profit nor the promise of effective targeted treatment should undermine investment in—and clinical advocacy of—public health interventions that reduce cancer risk (Gupta et al., 2017). Genetic counselors are well positioned to advocate for multiple pathways to cancer risk reduction and for attention to nongenetic factors in PM and public health approaches.

Eventually, nongenetic factors like a patient's disease presentation, environmental exposures, lifestyle, and specific behaviors could play a role in development of targeted cancer therapies. While each factor could represent an opportunity to increase effectiveness of treatment, focusing on these factors could again lead to some subsets of cancer patients benefiting and others being left behind in the development of ever more targeted therapies. Moreover, insofar as some of these factors (especially behavioral and lifestyle differences) may be considered a matter of choice and individual responsibility, some patients may be blamed for developing less treatable conditions, much like lung cancer patients being blamed for smoking and causing their cancer, even though it is likely that their genetics also plays a role in whether they develop cancer. Genetic counselors have experience in combatting self- and social blame for ill health, as well as advocating for appreciation of the multifactorial etiology of complex conditions, including cancer.

Research

When gene testing–guided individualized treatment is offered within clinical trials, the likelihood of patients experiencing therapeutic misconception would seem to be increased. Therapeutic misconception involves patient-participants mistakenly believing that the purpose of the research study is to provide treatment, that it will (or is designed to) benefit them, or that the intervention they receive will be chosen to benefit them individually (Appelbaum et al., 1987; Henderson et al., 2007). Labeling and advertising the study intervention as precise, individualized, tailored, personalized, and/or targeted may make it more difficult to appreciate the protocolized and uncertain nature of research to test such therapies. In short, it is challenging to explain the concept of *protocolized research* on *individualized treatment*, particularly in the context of a life-threatening condition that leads patients to experience time pressure, stress, desperation, and a mix of reasonable and unrealistic hope. Given their understanding of psychology and their highly developed communication skills, including facility with explaining probability, genetic counselors may help precision oncology patients accurately understand the purpose and procedures of the testing, as well as the protocol-based nature of, and uncertainties surrounding, study protocols.

In addition, the genomic sequencing required for study enrollment or for precision oncology care may reveal incidental findings. For some patients, learning this information may be particularly unwelcome while dealing with a cancer diagnosis. Employing sequencing technologies that only probe for variants of interest could reduce this problem of incidental findings but may be cost prohibitive or contrary to clinic, institutional, or health policies that embrace a practice of always seeking (at least clinically actionable) variants (Green et al., 2013; Miller et al., 2021).

The possibility of incidental findings must be discussed during the informed consent process, especially for studies involving genomic sequencing. Debate regarding the appropriate model and content of informed consent for sequencing continues (Appelbaum et al., 2014), with some suggesting that greater emphasis should be placed on governance than on informed consent in the context of research involving sequencing (Koenig, 2014). Among the models for informed consent and management of incidental findings is a "traditional consent model" whereby consent to return such findings is obtained at the time of study enrollment. A "staged consent model" involves disclosure of the possibility of incidental finding discovery during the consent process for participation; however, more detailed consent is to be obtained if such findings are discovered. The primary problems with this model are that participants may enroll without appreciating the decisions they may face in the future and that the future attempt to obtain consent for return of an incidental finding will necessarily disclose the finding to some degree. If participants do not consent to receiving full information about the incidental finding, they may misapprehend the information that is partially disclosed. Finally, obtaining consent to "mandatory return" of some set or class of incidental findings as a condition of study enrollment may be contrary to the voluntariness requirement of informed consent, may lead to a biased study population, and may not serve the interests of some participants.

In addition, the consent process for study participation must include discussion of alternatives to study participation, what is known and unknown regarding the pathophysiology of the disease condition, the function of the particular targeted therapy, and risks associated with the therapy (e.g., that immune checkpoint inhibitors trigger autoimmunity with immune-related adverse events; Kang, 2018). Sometimes, and perhaps especially for people with serious illness, it is important to recognize that some treatments and research opportunities may cause more harm than good. Genetic counselors may be even more attuned to quality-of-life considerations than some oncologists or cancer researchers and may advocate on behalf of patients so that they do not fall prey to the technological imperative that if something can be tried, it should be.

Prevention

Also ethically challenging are PM approaches to identifying those at increased cancer risk and implementing targeted prevention strategies, such as surveillance and prophylactic interventions, including behavioral and lifestyle changes. The magnitude of the psychosocial burdens and potential benefits of such precision prevention depends on personal values and circumstances. Qualitative research indicates both that there can be subtle psychological effects of learning individualized cancer risk information and, not surprisingly, that the timing of such information matters both for mitigating those effects and maximizing the potential to benefit from surveillance and prophylaxis (Grubs et al., 2014; Hamilton, 2012). Thus, the psychosocial burdens of sharing risk information within families to motivate relatives to undergo cancer risk assessment are relevant to analyzing whether people have a decisive ethical reason to "warn" their relatives.

Also relevant to analyzing whether that obligation obtains are considerations of general and specific (role-related) obligations to prevent harm, as well as the severity and probability of harm to be prevented, the probability of the harm being prevented if information about its potential is shared, and potential burdens to the informing and to-be-informed family members (Buchanan, 1998; Liao, 2009). Some have argued that there is a "duty to rescue" family members from the genetic risk of harm due to the familial nature of some genetic risks, the special nature of familial obligations, and/or a general duty to help those in need (e.g., Kilbride, 2018). Others respond that the magnitude and probability of such genetic risk rarely rise to the level generally thought to trigger a duty to "rescue," as when one passes a drowning child or can prevent someone from stepping into traffic (Liao & MacKenzie, 2018). They argue that potential benefit to the "rescuee" (a family member to be informed of familial risk) may appropriately be balanced against psychosocial and other costs to the "rescuer" (the family member who is to share genetic risk information). They also note that "rescuees" typically have alternate means of "rescue"—that is, unlike a drowning child who likely cannot rescue herself, individuals may seek genetic testing/screening (Liao & MacKenzie, 2018). Genetic counselors may help individuals make and implement these intrafamilial disclosure decisions.[2]

The question of whether people have the right not to know of their health risks has always accompanied discussion of whether there is a right and/or obligation to inform people of the genetic risks of disease. It is plausible to think that if preventive interventions become more effective, more accessible, and less onerous (i.e., less practically, economically, or psychically burdensome on ways of life), the benefit of receiving such risk information will outweigh the benefit of forgoing it, and assertion of the right not to know may dissipate. Nevertheless, risk-based medicine is likely to induce anxiety in some people: Those informed that they have (or may have) an increased risk of developing disease may join the "worried well" or become "previvors," survivors of an illness to which they are predisposed but that they have not yet developed (Mukherjee, 2018).

Clinicians also face challenges in utilizing available testing technologies to prevent cancer among their patients and patients' families. In light of low rates of genetic testing for cancer risk, it may be that clinicians—particularly those outside of oncology-focused specialties—lack the time or confidence to take three-generation family histories, recommend genetic testing, or interpret test results to ground prevention recommendations or referral to genetics specialists. A survey of gynecologic oncologists treating patients with epithelial ovarian cancer, however, indicates that oncologist-initiated genetic testing of diagnosed patients may be a model for increasing access to genetic testing for these patients and access to risk information for their families (Czekalsk et al., 2022). Clinical decision support and development of practice guidelines may help to increase utilization of risk assessment technologies. The American College of Clinical Oncology, for example, recommends that

> all women diagnosed with epithelial ovarian cancer should have germline genetic testing for BRCA1/2 and other ovarian cancer susceptibility genes. In women who do not carry a germline pathogenic or likely pathogenic BRCA1/2 variant, somatic tumor testing for BRCA1/2 pathogenic or likely pathogenic variants should be performed. (Konstantinopoulos et al., 2020, p. 1222)

In short, testing should not be performed solely to guide individual patients' current treatment but also to prevent their development of other cancers and to enable their family members to be informed of their own potential increased risk. Genetic counselors may facilitate such intrafamilial risk communication and may help upstream to develop clinic or institutional testing protocols to bridge between cancer treatment and cancer prevention.

[2] Editors' note: For a fuller discussion of the duty to warn/rescue in genetics, see Chapter 24 by Samantha Leonard and Ainsley Newson in this volume.

Rare Diseases: Diagnostic Odysseys and Quests for Treatment

For those with rare and often undiagnosed conditions, receiving information about the etiology of their symptoms is often the goal of serial clinical consultations and rounds of testing. Genomic sequencing can sometimes end this diagnostic odyssey—and inform the reproductive decisions of patients or their families—but often marks the beginning of a quest for effective treatment (Tabor & Goldenberg, 2018). The rhetoric promising that unlocking the genetic code of life would provide the key to treatment has thus far been disappointing for those with rare conditions, and indeed for many with more common conditions (Ball, 2010; Basel & McCarrier, 2017; Lazaridis et al., 2016; Michael, 2020; Nguyen & Charlebois, 2015; Pearson, 2009; Rosell et al., 2015; Thorp, 2022; Wu et al., 2020).

Defined in the United States as conditions affecting fewer than 200,000 people—and in Europe as those affecting fewer than 2,000 or in Canada fewer than 1,000—rare diseases present multiple challenges for research, diagnosis, and treatment development. The financial incentive for for-profit companies to invest in rare disease research and development is limited by the small markets for their successful innovation. The Orphan Drug Act (1983), along with the Food and Drug Administration's Office of Orphan Products Development, creates incentives to pursue effective interventions for rare diseases. The small number of affected individuals can nevertheless limit research: It is said that for many rare cancers there are as many slots in clinical trials as there are study-eligible patients (Albrecht et al., 2021), and as recently as 2017, 30% of children with a rare condition did not live beyond age 5 (National Organization for Rare Disorders, 2017). The challenges to enrolling a sufficient number of participants to conduct treatment trials provide cautionary lessons for PM and its tendency to create condition+genotype subgroups that may face similar challenges regarding research incentives and research design. Moreover, PM may actually create new healthcare disparities by identifying a rare genetic etiology for some patients' conditions: "For example, someone with lung cancer may be seen as ineligible for some kinds of treatment or research because she is part of the roughly 5% of non–small cell lung cancers with an ALK gene rearrangement" (Tabor & Goldenberg, 2018, p. 837).

When effective treatments are developed for rare conditions, they have often proved prohibitively expensive, costing hundreds of thousands of dollars each year, often for a patient's lifetime. Examples include Nusinersen for treatment of a rare recessive neuromuscular condition, spinal muscular atrophy, at an estimated $370,000 per year after the first year at $750,000 (Tabor & Goldenberg, 2018) and enzyme replacement therapy for mucopolysaccharidosis VI, a rare lysosomal storage disorder, that peaked at approximately $450,000 (Schlander & Beck, 2009). Canada regulates the prices of patented drugs to ensure their prices are not "excessive." Nevertheless, spending in Canada on drugs for treatment of rare diseases increased 11-fold from 2011 to 2020, reaching $3.1 billion, with drugs that cost more than $100,000 (USD) per year an increasingly large segment of the total expenditure (Rare Daily Staff, 2021).

As with precision oncology for the treatment of more common cancers, coupled with limitations presented by geography and education, the cost of treating rare diseases may limit access to either those with substantial wealth or those who qualify for company-provided treatment because of their lack of wealth or insurance coverage. Emerging treatments may create the need for clinicians to help patients and their families make difficult decisions about whether to incur astronomical costs of treatment, including helping parents of children with such expensive-to-treat conditions weigh the competing interests of their children. As they support families in making treatment decisions, genetic counselors' skills of nonjudgmental active listening may help clients/patients clarify their options and priorities.

Polygenic Risk Assessment and Complex Conditions

For common complex conditions resulting from multiple genomic variants and environmental influences, the use of polygenic risk assessment is a tool of precision prevention, which seeks to target the right preventive intervention (or set of interventions) to the right person at the right time to prevent the onset of disease. Again, genetic analysis is not the only tool; other assessments and interventions may focus on the environmental factors contributing to disease manifestation. Examples of nongenetic, environmental tests that can lead to both population-wide and targeted interventions and remediation abound: testing the lead level in a community's water supply or in the supply to one's home and the soil surrounding it, testing community or workplace air quality, testing food supply chains to ensure safety, housing-related health and safety hazard assessment, community-based mental health assessment, and reviewing diet and exercise regimens. Though genetic counselors should promote nongenetic risk assessments as a matter of policy and for clients who may benefit, their particular expertise will be called upon to explain, interpret, and make prevention plans based on a polygenic risk score (PRS). Further information on PRSs can be found in Chapter 20—"Common and Complex Traits: Considerations for Genetic Counseling" in this volume. The All of Us Research Program (National Institutes of Health, n.d.), for example, plans to offer participants research results, including PRSs, that are generated using its platform. It has contracted with Color, a population health technology company, to deliver the results and provide genetic counseling to All of Us participants (National Institutes of Health Office of the Director, 2019).

Though standard of care and clinical practice guidelines do not generally employ polygenic risk assessment, DTC genetic testing companies have embraced it and will report a PRS for a range of complex conditions, including cardiovascular conditions and diabetes (Regaldo, 2019). When a patient brings DTC test results, a clinician's first concern may be the accuracy of the results, as the quality of both laboratory testing and the reference genomes used for interpretation may vary (Tandy-Connor et al., 2018). At best, the risks predicted by PRSs are true of stratified groups and do not necessarily apply to a particular individual. Moreover, most PRSs are only "moderately predictive of group outcomes" (Matthews, 2020). Whatever the accuracy of the results, however, clients' beliefs and concerns about the results must be addressed. This is, of course, true of any DTC test results, but the current state of polygenic risk assessment makes both determining the accuracy of the results and helping clients interpret them particularly fraught.

Because a PRS is the product of statistical analysis, and because both clinicians and the public lack statistical literacy (Martyn, 2014), individuals may have a particularly difficult time understanding the PRS and the relevance of their relative risk for disease, which the PRS represents. For individual patients, it is their absolute risk of developing a condition—sometimes their lifetime risk and sometimes their risk of developing a condition during a particular time of life—that is typically of interest. There are also further complications. Over time, their absolute risk of developing disease may be affected by, for example, preventive interventions or environmental factors. Moreover, evolving science and additional information may alter their relative risk assessment, while a degree of "irreducible unpredictability" always remains (Spiegelhalter, 2008). Most importantly, there is increasing skepticism that supplying risk information leads to positive health behavior change, particularly the sustained change typically necessary to prevent disease (Resnicow & Page, 2008; Taylor-Robinson & Kee, 2019).

Perhaps most notable, as genomic studies have overwhelmingly examined genomes of people of European ancestry, there are generally insufficient data about genomic variants in populations of other ancestries to accurately calculate a PRS for individuals of those ancestral backgrounds (Mensah et al., 2020). The fact that currently polygenic risk assessment is generally only valid and useful for those of European ancestry exacerbates health and healthcare disparities. To address this unjust disparity, genomic research must include diverse and representative populations in research and employ unbiased genotyping and bias reduction methods in polygenic risk assessment (De La Vega & Bustamante, 2018). Further, for PM to alleviate, rather than exacerbate, health and healthcare disparities, "the *relative importance* of bias, racial discrimination, culture, socioeconomic status, access to care, environmental factors, and genetics to racial/ethnic differences in disease" must also be studied further (Borrell et al., 2021, pp. 478–479, emphasis added). Studies of polygenic risk factors must also be conducted for conditions that are particularly prevalent in underrepresented populations (Landry et al., 2018). Thus, for several reasons, use of PRSs may be premature for many people and with regard to many conditions. When contributing to policy discussions and providing clinical care with respect to complex conditions, genetic counselors can advance justice, anti-racism, and individual and population health by resisting indiscriminate embrace of a genomic turn in medicine, premature use of PRSs, and the individualization of health risk and risk mitigation.

Research

In the immediate future, as research pursues development of the knowledge base for PM, genetic counselors will be needed to help recruit research populations that reflect the diversity of the human population. Participants are needed who reflect not only diverse continental ancestries but also the full range of socioeconomic and environmental contexts, as well as behavioral factors and cultural commitments, that affect human health. The All of Us Research Program promises to be a valuable research platform for development of the knowledge base of PM. It seeks to enroll participants from diverse continental ancestries and to collect not only health history and genomic (and eventually other -omic) data but also a wide range of information about lifestyle, behaviors, and environmental exposures through self-reporting and wearable devices (Sankar & Parker, 2017). It is precisely because of the potential diversity of its million-American cohort that All of Us is considered distinctive and one of the most promising of all the global biobanking projects (Reardon, 2017).

Genetic counselors and their explanatory skills are needed to help enroll a diverse range of people in the All of Us Research Program and in genomic, environmental, and behavioral health studies and clinical trials—all of which will help to build the databases and biobanks that will help correct the current biases impacting genetic research tools and research results (De La Vega & Bustamante, 2018; Lachance & Tishkoff, 2013). To enroll, even overenroll, members of underrepresented populations, counselors need to be prepared to explain the apparent paradox in the fact that two individuals' DNA is 99.9% alike no matter their continental ancestry and that nevertheless a genetic variant may be reliably predictive with regard to a population of one ancestry but have uncertain significance in another. They will need to explain why studies need to enroll people of the full range of continental ancestries—and indeed environments and lifestyles—in order for results to be (more) generalizable. In the background is the ethical imperative that we must acknowledge these differences between individuals and populations "while insisting on their irrelevance for individual dignity and equality of right" (Edgar, 1992, p. 35). Continuing to make enrollment of representative study cohorts challenging is not only historically informed mistrust but also the fact that for some people genetics "is not important. And it is not important because there is *so much else wrong*" (Reardon, 2017, p. 64, quoting a prospective study participant).

To achieve some of the ethical goals suggested herein—reducing or at least avoiding exacerbation of health and healthcare disparities, avoiding blaming people for their ill health, mitigating the harms of acquiring health-relevant information, and maximizing its benefits—it is important for genetic counselors to emphasize the relevance of the environmental components of PM. They might also emphasize the importance of engaging in—and improving—behavioral research to inform health behavior change. Yet it will be critical not to focus primarily on individual-level interventions and changes in personal behavior, as there are multiple socioeconomic barriers to such change that require redress, as well as important changes in the physical and social environment that would improve individual and population health.

Conclusion

This chapter sketched multiple important roles for genetic counselors in helping to ensure that PM is implemented ethically and that its knowledge base is developed through ethically and scientifically sound research. In addition to addressing the usual issues of research design and informed consent, this means participating in efforts to enroll study populations from diverse ancestries and diverse socioeconomic and environmental backgrounds so that research findings are generalizable and the benefits and burdens of research are fairly distributed. In clinical care, it means supporting individual patient decision making and addressing issues of privacy, confidentiality, intrafamilial risk communication, and people's interests in knowing/not knowing risk information. It also means working to inform clinical practice guidelines, insurance reimbursement/coverage policies, and institutional and social policies to help ensure that PM will not exacerbate health and healthcare disparities.

Because of their expertise in psychology, probabilistic reasoning, and risk communication, as well as their understanding of genetics/genomics, disease etiology and treatment modalities, and healthcare structures and social service, genetic counselors are well equipped to contribute to PM's clinical implementation, research, and related policy development. They have the requisite knowledge—and a responsibility—to remind patients, colleagues, the public, and policymakers that genomic medicine is an important part but not the whole of PM. They should emphasize that environmental factors influence health and disease and may sometimes be a more appropriate focus for inquiry or intervention than genetic contributions.

Genetic counselors also tend to have strong interpersonal skills, including those of attentive listening and values clarification, as well as the ability to find common ground and to support those who are vulnerable or have difficulty asserting their own interests. They are thus well equipped to play an additional, critical role to ensure that use of genomic information does not create a new class of disparities in society.

New risks of genetic discrimination are emerging beyond the healthcare and employment contexts that are somewhat regulated by GINA (Martschenko & Trejo, 2022). Genetic counselors, along with others, will need to engage in debates regarding the relevance and use of genomics with regard to, for example, social traits, behavior, aptitudes, and responsibility. They will need to contribute to debates about how to study, understand, and weigh the components of gene × environment interaction. Given parental interest in testing their children for their genotype-related sports aptitude, commercial interests in genome-informed dating apps, and social interests in forensic uses of genetics, the possibility of new forms of genetic discrimination is not a matter of science fiction (Martschenko & Trejo, 2022).

It is beyond the scope of this chapter on PM to explore these debates; however, it is fitting to close this chapter by signaling the importance of genetic counselors' participation in them. These new means of discrimination threaten advances toward the effective and ethical implementation of PM because the genomic sequencing technology that is a key component and driver of PM can discover information believed to have relevance outside of the domains of health and healthcare. If people have reason to fear that they will suffer discrimination in other domains (e.g., in education or the justice system), they may be justifiably reluctant to participate in the research studies and genomic sequencing necessary for PM. Moreover, benefits from advances in genotype-guided preventive healthcare will be undercut if, for example, genetic profiling and "precision education" interventions limit people's prospects for achieving material well-being and personal fulfillment (Matthews et al., 2021).

But these potential effects on PM are not the only or primary reason that genetic counselors should help to illuminate and address concerns about genetic discrimination in other domains. Genetic counselors can bring a perspective informed by deep knowledge of past misuses of genetic information to help assess the degree to which these new risks of discrimination are really new. They can draw on their knowledge to explain and prevent or mitigate the risks. Equipped with specialized knowledge and skill, genetic counselors hold respected professional positions of authority with respect to genetics. They should use these assets to promote social well-being and justice by helping to ensure ethical use of genomic information within and beyond healthcare and public health. They should also encourage allocation of resources—intellectual and financial, public and private—toward scientific goals that are ethically desirable and attainable, through projects and programs that are well designed (Caulfield & Condit, 2012).

In this regard, genetic counselors should try to forestall premature use of genetic information in and beyond PM (Martschenko & Trejo, 2022). This means that genetic counselors should contribute to discussions about what "premature use" of genetic information means. Just as they have contributed to consideration of the return of either results that are not clinically actionable or variants of uncertain significance, they should consider whether the use of genomic information is premature when significant portions of the population cannot benefit from it, as is currently the case with polygenic risk assessment (Kaplan & Fullerton, 2022). They may contribute to discussion about whether offering vastly expensive individualized treatments is premature absent health policy plans to absorb the costs as more people access them. They may consider whether some risk assessment is premature absent a safety net to provide for long-term care or disability payments, or whether and when potential health benefits outweigh those economic risks. Some suggest that achieving consensus on these issues is neither possible nor desirable (Martschenko & Trejo, 2022). Nevertheless, the contributions that genetic counselors can make to their consideration is, however, beyond doubt.

References

Albrecht, B., Capra, E., Reichert, M., & Salazar, P. (2021, May 13). *Precision medicine in practice: Strategies for rare cancers*. McKinsey & Company. https://www.mckinsey.com/industries/life-sciences/our-insights/precision-medicine-in-practice-strategies-for-rare-cancers

Appelbaum, P. S., Parens, E., Waldman, C. R., Klitzman, R., Fyer, A., Martinez, J., Price, W. N., II, & Chung, W. K. (2014). Models of consent to return of incidental findings in genomic research. *Hastings Center Report*, *44*(4), 22–32. https://doi.org/10.1002/hast.328

Appelbaum, P. S., Roth, L. H., Lidz, C. W., Benson, P., & Winslade, W. (1987). False hopes and best data: Consent to research and the therapeutic misconception. *Hastings Center Report*, *17*(2), 20–24.

Aronson, S. J., & Rehm, H. L. (2015). Building the foundation for genomics in precision medicine. *Nature*, *526*(7573), 336–342. https://doi.org/10.1038/nature15816

Ashley, E. A. (2015). The precision medicine initiative: A new national effort. *JAMA*, *313*(21), 2119–2120. https://doi.org/10.1001/jama.2015.3595

Ball, P. (2010). Bursting the genomics bubble. *Nature*. https://doi.org/10.1038/news.2010.145

Basel, D., & McCarrier, J. (2017). Ending a diagnostic odyssey: Family education, counseling, and response to eventual diagnosis. *Pediatric Clinics of North America*, *64*(1), 265–272.

Batten, J. N. (2018). How stratification unites ethical issues in precision health. *AMA Journal of Ethics*, *20*(9), E798–E803. http://doi.org/10.1001/amajethics.2018.798

Beskow, L. M., Fullerton, S. M., Namey, E. E., Nelson, D. K., Davis, A. M., & Wilfond, B. S. (2012). Recommendations for ethical approaches to genotype-driven research recruitment. *Human Genetics*, *131*(9), 1423–1431. https://doi.org/10.1007/s00439-012-1177-z

Borrell, L. N., Elhawary, J. R., Fuentes-Afflick, E., Witonsky, J., Bhakta, N., Wu, A., Bibbins-Domingo, K., Rodríguez-Santana, J. R., Lenoir, M. A., Gavin, J. R., 3rd, Kittles, R. A., Zaitlen, N. A., Wilkes, D. S., Powe, N. R., Ziv, E., & Burchard, E. G. (2021). Race and genetic ancestry in medicine—A time for reckoning with racism. *New England Journal of Medicine*, *384*(5), 474–480. https://doi.org/10.1056/NEJMms2029562

Buchanan, A. (1998). Ethical responsibilities of patients and clinical geneticists. *Journal of Health Care Law & Policy*, *1*(2), 391–420. https://digitalcommons.law.umaryland.edu/jhclp/vol1/iss2/6

Burke, W., Burton, H., Hall, A. E., Karmali, M., Khoury, M. J., Knoppers, B., Meslin, E. M., Stanley, F., Wright, C. F., Zimmern, R. L., & Ickworth Group. (2010). Extending the reach of public health genomics: What should be the agenda for public health in an era of genome-based and "personalized" medicine? *Genetics in Medicine*, *12*(12), 785–791. https://doi.org/10.1097/GIM.0b013e3182011222

Caulfield, T., & Condit, C. (2012). Science and the sources of hype. *Community Genetics*, *15*(3/4), 209–217. https://doi.org/10.1159/000336533

Caulfield, T., & Zarzeczny, A. (2014). Defining "medical necessity" in an age of personalised medicine: A view from Canada. *BioEssays*, *36*(9), 813–817. https://doi.org/10.1002/bies.201400073

Chan, I. S., & Ginsburg, G. S. (2011). Personalized medicine: Progress and promise. *Annual Review of Genomics and Human Genetics*, *12*, 217–244. https://doi.org/10.1146/annurev-genom-082410-101446

Collins, F. S., & Varmus, H. (2015). A new initiative on precisions medicine. *New England Journal of Medicine*, *372*(9), 793–795. https://doi.org/10.1056/NEJMp1500523

Czekalski, M. A., Huziak, R. C., Durst, A. L., Taylor, S., & Mai, P. L. (2022). Mainstreaming genetic testing for epithelial ovarian cancer by oncology providers: A survey of current practice. *JCO Precision Oncology*, *6*(6), e2100409. https://doi.org/10.1200/PO.21.00409

De La Vega, F. M., & Bustamante, C. D. (2018). Polygenic risk scores: A biased prediction? *Genome Medicine*, *10*(1), 100. https://doi.org/10.1186/s13073-018-0610-x

Dimond, R., Doheny, S., Ballard, L., & Clarke, A. (2022). Genetic testing and family entanglements. *Social Science & Medicine (1982)*, *298*, 114857. https://doi.org/10.1016/j.socscimed.2022.114857

Edgar, H. (1992). Outside the community. *Hastings Center Report*, *22*(6), 32–35. https://doi.org/10.2307/3562947

Fernandez-Rozadilla, C., Simões, A. R., Lleonart, M. E., Carnero, A., & Carracedo, A. (2021). Tumor profiling at the service of cancer therapy. *Frontiers in Oncology*, *10*, 595613. https://doi.org/10.3389/fonc.2020.595613

Genetic Information Nondiscrimination Act of 2008, Pub.L. 110–233, 122 Stat. 881 (enacted May 21, 2008).

Gostin, L. O. (2000). A theory and definition of public health law. In L. O. Gostin (Ed.), *Public health law: Power duty, restraint* (pp. 3–22). University of California Press.

Green, R. C., Berg, J. S., Grody, W. W., Kalia, S. S., Korf, B. R., Martin, C. L., McGuire, A. L., Nussbaum, R. L., O'Daniel, J. M., Ormond, K. E., Rehm, H. L., Watson, M. S., Williams, M. S., Biesecker, L. G., & American College of Medical Genetics and Genomics. (2013). ACMG recommendations for reporting of incidental findings in clinical exome and genome sequencing. *Genetics in Medicine*, *15*(7), 565–574. https://doi.org/10.1038/gim.2013.73

Grubs, R. E., Parker, L. S., & Hamilton, R. (2014). Subtle psychosocial sequelae of genetic test results. *Current Genetic Medicine Reports*, *2*, 242–249. https://doi.org/10.1007/s40142-014-0053-7

Gupta, S., Smith, T. R., & Broekman, M. L. (2017). Ethical considerations of neuro-oncology trial design in the era of precision medicine. *Journal of Neuro-Oncology*, *134*(1), 1–7. https://doi.org/10.1007/s11060-017-2502-0

Hamilton, R. (2012). Being young, female, and BRCA positive. *American Journal of Nursing*, *112*(10), 26–32. https://doi.org/10.1097/01.NAJ.0000421021.62295.3b
Henderson, G. E., Churchill, L., Davis, A., Easter, M., Grady, C., Joffe, S., Kass, N., King, N., Lidz, C., Miller, F., Nelson, D., Peppercorn, J., Rothschild, B., Sankar, P., Wilfond, B., & Zimmer, C. (2007) Clinical trials and medical care: Defining the therapeutic misconception. *PLoS Medicine*, *4*, e324. https://doi.org/10.1371/journal.pmed.0040324
Hollands, G. J., French, D. P., Griffin, S. J., Prevost, A. T., Sutton, S., King, S., & Marteau, T. M. (2016). The impact of communicating genetic risks of disease on risk-reducing health behaviour: Systematic review with meta-analysis. *BMJ (Clinical Research Ed.)*, *352*, i1102. https://doi.org/10.1136/bmj.i1102
Hollister, B., & Bonham, V. L. (2018). Should electronic health record-derived social and behavioral data be used in precision medicine research? *AMA Journal of Ethics*, *20*(9), E873–E880. https://doi.org/10.1001/amajethics.2018.873
Horwitz, R. I., Cullen, M. R., Abell, J., & Christian, J. B. (2013). Medicine. (De)personalized medicine. *Science*, *339*(6124), 1155–1156. https://doi.org/10.1126/science.1234106
Joffe, S., & Lynch, H. F. (2018). Federal right-to-try legislation—Threatening the FDA's public health mission. *New England Journal of Medicine*, *378*(8), 695–697. https://doi.org/10.1056/NEJMp1714054
Juengst, E., McGowan, M. L., Fishman, J. R., & Settersten, R. A., Jr. (2016). From "personalized" to "precision" medicine: The ethical and social implications of rhetorical reform in genomic medicine. *Hastings Center Report*, *46*(5), 21–33. https://doi.org/10.1002/hast.614
Kang, J. S. (2018). Ethical ruminations of a rheumatologist: Autoimmunity is an important consideration for immunotherapy trials. *American Journal of Bioethics*, *18*(4), 75–76. https://doi.org/10.1080/15265161.2018.1444823
Kaplan, J. M., & Fullerton, S. M. (2022). Polygenic risk, population structure and ongoing difficulties with race in human genetics. *Philosophical Transactions of the Royal Society B*, *377* (1852), 20200427. https://doi.org/10.1098/rstb.2020.0427
Kilbride, M. K. (2018). Genetic privacy, disease prevention, and the principle of rescue. *Hastings Center Report*, *48*(3), 10–17. https://doi.org/10.1002/hast.849
Kimel, S. Y., Huesmann, R., Kunst, J. R., & Halperin, E. (2016). Living in a genetic world: How learning about interethnic genetic similarities and differences affects peace and conflict. *Personality and Social Psychology Bulletin*, *42*(5), 688–700. https://doi.org/10.1177/0146167216642196
Kimmelman, J., & Tannock, I. (2018). The paradox of precision medicine. *Nature Reviews Clinical Oncology*, *15*(6), 341–342. https://doi.org/10.1038/s41571-018-0016-0
Koenig, B. A. (2014). Have we asked too much of consent? *Hastings Center Report*, *44*(4), 33–34.
Konstantinopoulos, P. A., Norquist, B., Lacchetti, C., Armstrong, D., Grisham, R. N., Goodfellow, P. J., Kohn, E. C., Levine, D. A., Liu, J. F., Lu, K. H., Sparacio, D., & Annunziata, C. M. (2020). Germline and somatic tumor testing in epithelial ovarian cancer: ASCO Guideline. *Journal of Clinical Oncology*, *38*(11), 1222–1245. https://doi.org/10.1200/JCO.19.02960
Krzyszczyk, P., Acevedo, A., Davidoff, E. J., Timmins, L. M., Marrero-Berrios, I., Patel, M., White, C., Lowe, C., Sherba, J. J., Hartmanshenn, C., O'Neill, K. M., Balter, M. L., Fritz, Z. R., Androulakis, I. P., Schloss, R. S., & Yarmush, M. L. (2018). The growing role of precision and personalized medicine for cancer treatment. *Technology*, *6*(3–4), 79–100. https://doi.org/10.1142/S2339547818300020
Lachance, J., & Tishkoff, S. A. (2013). SNP ascertainment bias in population genetic analyses: Why it is important, and how to correct it. *Bioessays*, *35*(9), 780–786. https://doi.org/10.1002/bies.201300014

Landry, L. G., Ali, N., Williams, D. R., Rehm, H. L., & Bonham, V. L. (2018). Lack of diversity in genomic databases is a barrier to translating precision medicine research into practice. *Health Affairs*, *37*(5), 780–785. https://doi.org/10.1377/hlthaff.2017.1595

Lazaridis, K. N., Schahl, K. A., Cousin, M. A., Babovic-Vuksanovic, D., Riegert-Johnson, D. L., Gavrilova, R. H., McAllister, T. M., Lindor, N. M., Abraham, R. S., Ackerman, M. J., Pichurin, P. N., Deyle, D. R., Gavrilov, D. K., Hand, J. L., Klee, E. W., Stephens, M. C., Wick, M. J., Atkinson, E. J., Linden, D. R., Ferber, M. J., Wieben, E. D., & Farrugia, G. (2016). Outcome of whole exome sequencing for diagnostic odyssey cases of an individualized medicine clinic: The Mayo Clinic experience. *Mayo Clinic Proceedings*, *91*(3), 297–307. https://doi.org/10.1016/j.mayocp.2015.12.018

Lee, T. L., Tan, Y. J., & Oon, C. E. (2018). Molecular targeted therapy: Treating cancer with specificity. *European Journal of Pharmacology*, *834*, 188–196. https://doi.org/10.1016/j.ejphar.2018.07.034

Liao, S. M. (2009). Is there a duty to share genetic information? *Journal of Medical Ethics*, *35*(5), 306–309.

Liao, S. M., & MacKenzie, J. (2018). Genetic information, the principle of rescue, and special obligations. *Hastings Center Report*, *48*(3), 18–19. https://doi.org/10.1002/hast.850

Martschenko, D. O., & Trejo, S. (2022). Ethical, anticipatory genomics research on human behavior means celebrating disagreement. *Human Genetics and Genomics Advances*, *3*(1), 100080.

Martyn, C. (2014). Risky business: Doctors' understanding of statistics. *BMJ*, *349*, g5619. https://doi-org.pitt.idm.oclc.org/10.1136/bmj.g5619

Matthews, L. J. (2020). Precision (mis)education. *Hastings Center Report*, *50*(1), inside front cover. https://doi.org/10.1002/hast.1072

Matthews, L. J., Lebowitz, M. S., Ottman, R., & Appelbaum, P. S. (2021). Pygmalion in the genes? On the potentially negative impacts of polygenic scores for educational attainment. *Social Psychology of Education*, *24*(3), 789–808. https://doi.org/10.1007/s11218-021-09632-z

McConkie-Rosell, A., Pena, L. D. M., Schoch, K., Spillmann, R., Sullivan, J., Hooper, S. R., Jiang, Y.-H., Mathey-Andrews, N., Goldstein, D. B., & Shashi, V. (2016). Not the end of the odyssey: Parental perceptions of whole exome sequencing (WES) in pediatric undiagnosed disorders. *Journal of Genetic Counseling*, *25*(5), 1019–1031. https://doi.org/10.1007/s10897-016-9933-1

Mensah, G. A., Jaquish, C., Srinivas, P., Papanicolaou, G. J., Wei, G. S., Redmond, N., Roberts, M. C., Nelson, C., Aviles-Santa, L., Puggal, M., Green Parker, M. C., Minear, M. A., Barfield, W., Fenton, K. N., Boyce, C. A., Engelgau, M. M., & Khoury, M. J. (2019). Emerging concepts in precision medicine and cardiovascular diseases in racial and ethnic minority populations. *Circulation Research*, *125*(1), 7–13. https://doi.org/10.1161/CIRCRESAHA.119.314970

Michael, W. (2020). *Zebras do exist: The diagnostic odyssey of rare-disease patients*. https://rarepatientvoice.com/wp-content/uploads/2020/09/Zebras-Do-Exist-the-Diagnostic-Oddysey-of-Rare-Patients.pdf

Michie, M., Cadigan, R. J., Henderson, G., & Beskow, L. M. (2012). Am I a control?: Genotype-driven research recruitment and self-understandings of study participants. *Genetics in Medicine*, *14*(12), 983–989. https://doi.org/10.1038/gim.2012.88

Miller, D. T., Lee, K., Gordon, A. S., Amendola, L. M., Adelman, K., Bale, S. J., Chung, W. K., Gollob, M. H., Harrison, S. M., Herman, G. E., Hershberger, R. E., Klein, T. E., McKelvey, K., Richards, C. S., Vlangos, C. N., Stewart, D. R., Watson, M. S., Martin, C. L., & ACMG Secondary Findings Working Group. (2021). Recommendations for reporting of secondary findings in clinical exome and genome sequencing, 2021 update: A policy statement of

the American College of Medical Genetics and Genomics (ACMG). *Genetics in Medicine, 23*(8), 1391–1398. https://doi.org/10.1038/s41436-021-01171-4
Mukherjee, S. (2018). Cancer, our genes, and the anxiety of risk-based medicine. *Health Affairs, 37*(5), 817–820. https://doi.org/10.1377/hlthaff.2018.0344
National Institutes of Health. (n.d.). *All of Us Research Project*. U.S. Department of Health & Human Services. https://allofus.nih.gov/about/program-overview
National Institutes of Health Office of the Director. (2019, August 21). *NIH funds genetic counseling resource ahead of million-person sequencing effort*. https://www.nih.gov/news-events/news-releases/nih-funds-genetic-counseling-resource-ahead-million-person-sequencing-effort
National Organization for Rare Disorders. (2017, January 5). *Updated rare disease facts and figures*. https://rareundiagnosed.org/rare-disease-facts/
National Research Council Committee on a Framework for Developing a New Taxonomy of Disease. (2011). *Toward precision medicine: Building a knowledge network for biomedical research and a new taxonomy of disease*. National Academies Press.
Nelkin, D., & Tancredi, L. R. (1989). *Dangerous diagnostics: The social power of biological information*. Basic Books.
Nguyen, M. T., & Charlebois, K. (2015). The clinical utility of whole-exome sequencing in the context of rare diseases—The changing tides of medical practice. *Clinical Genetics, 88*(4), 313–319. https://doi.org/10.1111/cge.12546
Obama, B. (2015, January 30). *Remarks by the President on precision medicine*. https://obamawhitehouse.archives.gov/the-press-office/2015/01/30/remarks-president-precision-medicine
Offit, K. (2011). Personalized medicine: New genomics, old lessons. *Human Genetics, 130*(1), 3–14. https://doi.org/10.1007/s00439-011-1028-3
Orphan Drug Act of 1983, Pub.L. No. 97-414, 96 Stat. 2049-2057.
Parker, L. S., & Brody, H. (2011). Comparative effectiveness research: A threat to patient autonomy? *Health Progress, 92*(5), 64–71.
Parker, L. S., & Satkoske, V. B. (2012). Ethical dimensions of disparities in depression research and treatment in the pharmacogenomic era. *Journal of Law, Medicine and Ethics, 40*(4), 886–903. https://doi.org/10.1111/j.1748-720x.2012.00718.x
Pearson, H. (2009). Human genetics: One gene, twenty years. *Nature, 460*, 164–169. https://doi.org/10.1038/460164a
Pokorska-Bocci, A., Stewart, A., Sagoo, G. S., Hall, A., Kroese, M., & Burton, H. (2014). "Personalized medicine": What's in a name?. *Personalized Medicine, 11*(2), 197–210. https://doi.org/10.2217/pme.13.107
Pregelj, L., Hwang, T. J., Hine, D. C., Siegel, E. B., Barnard, R. T., Darrow, J. J., & Kesselheim, A. S. (2018). Precision medicines have faster approvals based on fewer and smaller trials than other medicines. *Health Affairs, 37*(5), 724–731. https://doi.org/10.1377/hlthaff.2017.1580
President's Council of Advisors on Science and Technology. (2008). *Priorities for personalized medicine*. https://bigdatawg.nist.gov/PCAST_Personalized_Medicine_Priorities.pdf
Rare Daily Staff. (2021, January 31). *Expensive rare disease drugs reflect growing portion of new approvals in Canada*. https://globalgenes.org/2022/01/31/expensive-rare-disease-drugs-reflect-growing-portion-of-new-approvals-in-canada/
Reardon, J. (2017). *The postgenomic condition*. University of Chicago Press.
Regaldo, A. (2019, March 8). 23andMe thinks polygenic risk scores are ready for the masses, but experts aren't so sure. *MIT Technology Review*. https://www.technologyreview.com/s/613095/23andme-thinks-polygenic-risk-scores-are-ready-for-the-masses-but-experts-arent-so-sure/

Resnicow, K., & Page, S. E. (2008). Embracing chaos and complexity: A quantum change for public health. *American Journal of Public Health, 98*(8), 1382–1389. https://doi.org/10.2105/AJPH.2007.129460

Richards, S., Aziz, N., Bale, S., Bick, D., Das, S., Gastier-Foster, J., Grody, W. W., Hegde, M., Lyon, E., Spector, E., Voelkerding, K., Rehm, H. L., & ACMG Laboratory Quality Assurance Committee. (2015). Standards and guidelines for the interpretation of sequence variants: A joint consensus recommendation of the American College of Medical Genetics and Genomics and the Association for Molecular Pathology. *Genetics in Medicine, 17*(5), 405–424. https://doi.org/10.1038/gim.2015.30

Roden, D. M., & Tyndale, R. F. (2013). Genomic medicine, precision medicine, personalized medicine: What's in a name? *Clinical Pharmacology and Therapeutics, 94*(2), 169–172. https://doi.org/10.1038/clpt.2013.101

Rose, N. (2013). Personalized medicine: Promises, problems and perils of a new paradigm for healthcare. *Procedia, Social and Behavioral Sciences, 77*, 341–352. https://doi.org/10.1016/j.sbspro.2013.03.092

Sabatello, M., Insel, B. J., Corbeil, T., Link, B. G., & Appelbaum, P. S. (2021). The double helix at school: Behavioral genetics, disability, and precision education. *Social Science & Medicine (1982), 278*, 113924. https://doi.org/10.1016/j.socscimed.2021.113924

Sankar, P. L., & Parker, L. S. (2017). The precision medicine initiative's All of Us Research Program: An agenda for research on its ethical, legal, and social issues. *Genetics in Medicine, 19*(7), 743–750. https://doi.org/10.1038/gim.2016.183

Schlander, M., & Beck, M. (2009). Expensive drugs for rare disorders: To treat or not to treat? The case of enzyme replacement therapy for mucopolysaccharidosis VI. *Current Medical Research and Opinion, 25*(5), 1285–1293. https://doi.org/10.1185/03007990902892633

Schleidgen, S., Klingler, C., Bertram, T., Rogowski, W. H., & Marckmann, G. (2013). What is personalized medicine: Sharpening a vague term based on a systematic literature review. *BMC Medical Ethics, 14*, 55. https://doi.org/10.1186/1472-6939-14-55

Schwartzberg, L., Kim, E. S., Liu, D., & Schrag, D. (2017). Precision oncology: Who, how, what, when, and when not? American Society of Clinical Oncology educational book. *American Society of Clinical Oncology, 37*, 160–169. https://doi.org/10.1200/EDBK_174176

Silarova, B., Sharp, S., Usher-Smith, J. A., Lucas, J., Payne, R. A., Shefer, G., Moore, C., Girling, C., Lawrence, K., Tolkien, Z., Walker, M., Butterworth, A., Di Angelantonio, E., Danesh, J., & Griffin, S. J. (2019). Effect of communicating phenotypic and genetic risk of coronary heart disease alongside web-based lifestyle advice: The INFORM Randomised Controlled Trial. *Heart (British Cardiac Society), 105*(13), 982–989. https://doi.org/10.1136/heartjnl-2018-314211

Smerecnik, C., Grispen, J. E., & Quaak, M. (2012). Effectiveness of testing for genetic susceptibility to smoking-related diseases on smoking cessation outcomes: A systematic review and meta-analysis. *Tobacco Control, 21*(3), 347–354. https://doi.org/10.1136/tc.2011.042739

Spiegelhalter, D. J. (2008). Understanding uncertainty. *Annals of Family Medicine, 6*(3), 196–197. https://doi.org/10.1370/afm.848

Tabor, H. K., & Goldenberg, A. (2018). What precision medicine can learn from rare genetic disease research and translation. *AMA Journal of Ethics, 20*(9), E834–E840. https://doi.org/10.1001/amajethics.2018.834

Tan, P. Y., Mitra, S. R., & Amini, F. (2018). Lifestyle interventions for weight control modified by genetic variation: A review of the evidence. *Public Health Genomics, 21*(5–6), 169–185. https://doi.org/10.1159/000499854

Tandy-Connor, S., Guiltinan, J., Krempely, K., LaDuca, H., Reineke, P., Sutierrez, S., Gray, P., & Tippin Davis, B. (2018). False-positive results released by direct-to-consumer genetic tests highlight the importance of clinical confirmation testing for appropriate patient care. *Genetics in Medicine*, *20*(12), 1515–1521. https://doi.org/10.1038/gim.2018.38

Taylor-Robinson, D., & Kee, F. (2019). Precision public health—The emperor's new clothes. *International Journal of Epidemiology*, *48*(1), 1–6. https://doi.org/10.1093/ije/dyy184

Thorp, E. (2022, March 22). The emotional odyssey of a rare disease diagnosis: Digging deeper, to do better. *Journal of Health*. https://thejournalofmhealth.com/the-emotional-odyssey-of-a-rare-disease-diagnosis-digging-deeper-to-do-better/

Tranvåg, E. J., Strand, R., Ottersen, T., & Norheim, O. F. (2021). Precision medicine and the principle of equal treatment: A conjoint analysis. *BMC Medical Ethics*, *22*(1), 55. https://doi.org/10.1186/s12910-021-00625-3

Turnwald, B. P., Goyer, J. P., Boles, D. Z., Silder, A., Delp, S. L., & Crum, A. J. (2019). Learning one's genetic risk changes physiology independent of actual genetic risk. *Nature Human Behaviour*, *3*(1), 48–56. https://doi.org/10.1038/s41562-018-0483-4

Wren, A. A., & Park, K. T. (2018). Targeted dosing as a precision health approach to pharmacotherapy in children with inflammatory bowel disease. *AMA Journal of Ethics*, *20*(9), E841. https://doi.org/10.1001/amajethics.2018.841

Wu, A. C., McMahon, P., & Lu, C. (2020). Ending the diagnostic odyssey—Is whole-genome sequencing the answer? *JAMA Pediatrics*, *174*(9), 821–822. https://doi.org/10.1001/jamapediatrics.2020.1522

Zoltick, E. S., Linderman, M. D., McGinniss, M. A., Ramos, E., Ball, M. P., Church, G. M., Leonard, D., Pereira, S., McGuire, A. L., Caskey, C. T., Sanderson, S. C., Schadt, E. E., Nielsen, D. E., Crawford, S. D., Green, R. C., & PeopleSeq Consortium. (2019). Predispositional genome sequencing in healthy adults: Design, participant characteristics, and early outcomes of the PeopleSeq Consortium. *Genome Medicine*, *11*(1), 10. https://doi.org/10.1186/s13073-019-0619-9

PART VI

CULTURE, DISABILITY, AND THE SOCIAL EFFECTS OF GENETIC COUNSELING

CHAPTER 29

CULTURAL RESPONSIVENESS AND LINGUISTIC COMPETENCE IN GENETIC COUNSELING

Taking Responsibility

NANCY STEINBERG WARREN

Introduction, Definitions, and Concepts

Genetic counseling is applicable to everyone; no cultural groups are exempt from genetic changes that lead to diseases, birth defects, or cancers. Yet, genetic counseling and testing services are underutilized by racial and ethnic minorities due to lack of awareness, reduced access, mistrust, fears of stigma or discrimination, and cultural/communication barriers (Aiyar et al., 2020; Glenn et al., 2012; Halbert & Harrison, 2018; Sheppard et al., 2013; Sussner et al., 2011). The genetic counseling profession is a distinct culture, with core principles, beliefs, and practices that are embodied by members and taught to students, including client-centeredness, nondirectiveness, and informed decision making. However, as a result of workforce homogeneity, blind spots can infiltrate standard genetic counseling professional practices and policies. According to the 2020 Professional Status Survey (PSS), 90% of genetic counselors identified as White or Caucasian and 95% identified as female. In contrast, according to the 2010 United States Census, 61% of the general population was reported as White non-Hispanic alone and one-third of the population reported their race and ethnicity as something other than non-Hispanic White alone. The latter group, referred to as the "minority" population, grew by 29% from 2000 to 2010. These trends in the nation's changing racial and ethnic diversity are expected to continue over time, with increasing numbers of states reporting "majority-minority" population profiles (Humes et al., 2011).

Individual and organizational cultural responsiveness

Cultural responsiveness pertains to individuals (genetic counselors and genetic counseling students) as well as organizations and environments in which genetics services are offered (staff, policies, procedures, practices, and activities of clinics, hospitals, labs, industry settings, and training programs) and to the professional associations of the field (National Society of Genetic Counselors [NSGC], the American Board of Genetic Counseling [ABGC], and the Accreditation Counsel for Genetic Counseling [ACGC]). Reducing health disparities (inequalities among racial, ethnic, or other population groups with respect to presence of disease, healthcare access, services, and/or outcomes) requires action by providers, training programs, institutions, and organizations. Applying strategies in multiple sectors is more effective than using a "siloed" approach to complicated issues (Mittman & Downs, 2008). Each sector of the profession has a role and responsibility to incorporate strategies promoting cultural responsiveness and linguistic competence to facilitate patient respect, trust, and satisfaction.

The Merriam-Webster (n.d.) definitions of *culture* apply broadly to individuals, communities, and organizations:

- the customary beliefs, social forms, and traits of a racial, religious, or social group
- the characteristic features of everyday existence (such as diversions or a way of life) shared by people in a place or time
- the set of shared attitudes, values, goals, and practices that characterizes an institution or organization
- the set of values, conventions, or social practices associated with a particular field, activity, or societal characteristic
- the integrated pattern of human knowledge, belief, and behavior that depends on the capacity for learning and transmitting knowledge to succeeding generations

At the provider level, the term "cultural competence" remains common in healthcare discourse. However, providers should not understand themselves to be capable of attaining, or striving to gain, mastery or achievement of an end result, but rather undertaking a process of self-awareness and learning, holding genuine respect and open attitudes toward individuals, having knowledge of cultural and religious/spiritual beliefs and values, and having effective communication skills. Hence, discourse about patients' cultural identities and values within healthcare has begun to shift away from the term "cultural competence" and toward terms that do not connote the presumption that one understands or "knows" to some appreciative degree another's cultural identities, values, and traditions.[1] This ongoing endeavor is fueled by *cultural desire*: providers' eager engagement to increase their awareness, knowledge, and

[1] Because the term "cultural competence" has been used historically and continues to be used occasionally in the literature, some references in this chapter reproduce that term. Nonetheless, there are clear trends in the healthcare literature that qualify or shift away altogether from the term "cultural competence." Terms such as "cultural humility," "cultural congruence," and "cultural responsiveness" are increasingly utilized, since they do not connote knowledge-based mastery of other individuals' cultural identities and values (e.g., Campinha-Bacote, 2018; Isaacson, 2014; Kirmayer, 2012).

skills to meet the needs of culturally multifaceted clients (Campinha-Bacote, 2015). Cultural humility also describes the provider's developmental journey throughout a professional career. Cross-cultural interactions help providers explore their own and others' cultures and engage in ongoing self-reflection and self-critique, leading to improved knowledge and skills (Tervalon & Murray-Garcia, 1998).

Linguistic competence is "providing readily available, culturally appropriate oral and written language services to limited English proficiency (LEP) members through such means as bilingual/bicultural staff, trained medical interpreters, and qualified translators," according to the Agency for Healthcare Research and Policy (2019) . Collectively, cultural and linguistic competence can be understood as the "ability of health care providers and health care organizations to understand and respond effectively to the cultural and linguistic needs brought by the patient to the health care encounter" (Agency for Healthcare Research and Policy, 2019) . Good communication facilitates effective cross-cultural interactions, but there are growing gaps between the languages spoken by healthcare providers and clients with LEP. Fully one-fifth of the U.S. population speaks a language other than English at home, and among this group, almost half self-report that they speak English less than "very well" (Ryan, 2013). Language barriers to genetic services are a structural constraint due to the workforce's lack of trained bilingual/bicultural genetic counselors (Joseph & Guerra, 2015; Vanneste et al., 2013). Only approximately 14% of genetic counselors are fluent in a language other than English (National Society of Genetic Counselors, 2020). Yet, non-English-speaking clients have been found to prefer communicating directly with bilingual healthcare providers without the need for interpreters (Barragan et al., 2011). It is unknown how many genetic counselors have achieved language certification or had formal assessment of their language proficiency, but it is likely very few. Most counselors rely on language interpreters, which may create more challenging dynamics around communication, building trust, and ensuring understanding in cross-cultural encounters.

Diversity encompasses characteristics of identity including race, gender, religion, sexual orientation, language, and dis/abilities. These and other parameters influence healthcare discussions. *When counseling a 50-year-old patient about a diagnosis of Lynch syndrome, how might approaches change if he was an immigrant from Mexico, or from Taiwan? What if he is a veteran? What if he has experienced age discrimination at work? Perhaps he has been a victim of trauma. What if several of these things are true? How does a genetic counselor determine which aspects of identity and personal experiences are most relevant to a particular session?*

People are multifaceted cultural beings. No one sees the world the way anyone else does, and genetic counselors should explore a client's individuality in the context of the session. Individual, family, and community fears of genetics are relevant. Clients who are immigrants, or descendants of slaves, or skeptical about anything around genetics and public health due to the legacy of Tuskegee deserve respect and understanding to accept (on their own terms) or reject genetic services. As a profession made up of mostly White women under the age of 40 (National Society of Genetic Counselors, 2020), genetic counselors must find empathy and respect for clients' perspectives. To reduce disparities, counselors must be proactive to break down long-standing barriers by spending time building trust, working with established community partners, and listening more than speaking.

All genetic counseling can be thought of as involving cross-cultural dynamics, although the impact of cultural differences can be difficult to predict. If the client is a practicing

Baptist, the client may prefer more (or less) attention be directed to spiritual issues. Rather than make assumptions around cultural identity and worldviews, however, the counselor should explore each client's needs related to the session. Parameters of identity should always be self-described, and inquiries about identity should be limited to those that pertain to the session (VandenLangenberg et al., 2012). For example, the counselor should ask about sexual orientation when it is relevant, such as in prenatal counseling. Inquiries into identity should be prefaced by establishing a respectful and supportive relationship so the client has a sense of safety. Valued approaches to building positive relationships by individuals who identify as gay, lesbian, or bisexual, for example, include eye contact, visual acceptance, gender-neutral language, and accepting designated partners in their family roles, especially in providing support and participating in decision making (VandenLangenberg et al., 2012).

Anderson et al. (2001) suggest that self-identified race should not be a proxy for genetic variation or social class. Genetic conditions often associated with race, such as sickle cell disease in individuals whose ancestors are from Africa, can also be found in families from Sicily, Puerto Rico, India, and other locations. Self-identified race forms part of the social history, as a complement to other clinically useful information such as education level, occupation, language, cultural beliefs, birthplace, area of residence, and type of health insurance (Anderson et al., 2001). Instead of starting a clinical presentation with: "The patient is a 30-year-old Black male with sickle cell disease who wants to learn whether stem cell therapy is an option," place race in the social history:

> This is a 30-year-old with sickle cell disease who wants to discuss stem cell therapy. Family history: The patient is married with no children. He is not aware of other family members with the disease. He states that his ancestors on both sides were from West Africa. Social history: The patient was born in Georgia; the family moved when he was a young child to New York City, where he currently resides. The patient self-identifies as male and Black. He works as an accountant and states his family lives comfortably; his wife has a flexible job as a part-time nurse. He believes their quality of family life would be much improved if he could remove the burden of sickle cell disease by undergoing stem cell therapy.

Generalizations emerge from one's worldview and previous experiences, forming a starting point for interpersonal interactions (Galanti, 2014). The genetic counselor can use a generalization (e.g., some Indian couples are consanguineous) to consider that an Indian client and her husband *might* be related. Articulating a generalization without evidence to support it becomes a stereotype that could be wrong, offensive, or, as characterized by Galanti (2014), an end for interpersonal interactions. The counselor should explore the family history without *assuming* the generalization necessarily applies. If consanguinity is present in this case, it will emerge in the assessment process. The counselor could say: "You told me that you know a lot about your families. Let's draw out your family history. Due to the form of inheritance of the baby's condition, it is important to identify your blood relationships, as far back as possible."

Explicit and implicit bias

Federal laws prohibit discrimination (a form of explicit bias) in treating an individual differently based on national origin, race, gender, color, disability, religion, or familial status. People cannot be denied opportunities or be discriminated against in housing, education, lending, employment, law enforcement, voting, and public accommodations (hotels, restaurants, places of entertainment) due to their name, national origin, race, culture, or accent. The Genetic Information Nondiscrimination Act (U.S. Equal Employment Opportunity Commission, 2014) provides limited protection by prohibiting genetic discrimination in the workplace and in obtaining health insurance in the United States. (GINA protections pertain only to companies with more than 15 individuals, do not extend to life/disability insurance, and do not regulate pricing.) Despite these legislative protections, challenges remain around providing equitable (fair and impartial) healthcare to all people. Racism and xenophobia, forms of explicit bias, remain prevalent in society.

Racism can be rooted at multiple levels: institutionalized (organizations), personally mediated (providers), and internalized (clients). One must examine all three levels to expect meaningful change.

- Institutionalized racism manifests in differential access to goods, services, and opportunities offered by the organization due to race.
- Personally mediated racism manifests in prejudice and discrimination, lack of respect, providing inferior or no service, failure to communicate options, suspicion, devaluation, and dehumanization (hate crimes) toward minorities by providers and members of majority groups.
- Internalized racism manifests in acceptance of negative messages by members of the stigmatized race, resulting in devalued personal abilities and intrinsic worth manifesting as resignation, helplessness, and hopelessness.

Jones's (2000) gardener's tale characterizes challenges around race and the role of providers, systems, and clients in a gardening metaphor. A garden requires healthy seeds, rich soil, ample water and sun, and careful tending to bear beautiful flowers from generation to generation. Say a gardener sows seeds in one garden with rich soil that gets abundant rain and sunlight, and also sows more seeds in a second garden with dry, rocky soil that gets little sunlight. The gardener tends the first garden carefully but neglects the second garden. We can predict marked differences in the flowers produced from the two gardens, even though the inherent potential of the seeds was identical. Try as it might, a seed cannot grow in certain environments. Applying this metaphor to race, if the gardener (society) confers more privileges and attention to one garden (White people), different outcomes can be expected (disparities). Poorer outcomes for nonprivileged groups (Black people) become a self-fulfilling prophesy unrelated to inherent potential.

Unearned privileges are enjoyed by individuals who are members of majority groups. Defined by the dominant group, unearned privileges result from simply belonging to the majority group. In contrast, minorities generally have to work for the privileges they enjoy, and even then, they may face barriers due to assumptions. For example, such an assumption might be to question how a Black student came to attend an Ivy League school in the United States, without considering that intelligence, hard work, goal setting, and planning created her pathway. A White student may not be subject to the same scrutiny. When people are treated unfairly, negative emotions and stress ensue. By acknowledging privileges and recognizing when people are treated unfairly, members of the majority can facilitate change.

Health disparities are numerous and well documented (U.S. Department of Health and Human Services, 2020). Health disparities include the influence of race, ethnicity, sex, sexual identity, age, disability status, income, and geography on a person's ability to achieve good health. Life expectancy, infant mortality, prevalence of chronic disease, and general perception of health and well-being are highly influenced by social factors. Lower income levels are associated with barriers to healthcare access and utilization due to unavailable or unaffordable transportation and childcare expenses, inflexible work schedules, and housing and food insecurity.

Although health disparities research in genetic counseling is limited, barriers to services have been identified. Knowledge and awareness about genetic testing are correlated with degree of education and income status. In one national sample, less than 50% of the U.S. adult population was aware of cancer genetic testing, with disparities for racial/ethnic minorities and individuals with limited healthcare access or income (Mai et al., 2014). Underutilization of clinical genetic testing and services by racial and ethnic minorities has been attributed to reduced awareness and referrals, general mistrust of the medical community, and particular fears of genetic discrimination, providers' inability to assess and address cultural and religious factors, financial and transportation limitations, and lack of diversity among genetic counselors and other healthcare professionals (Carroll et al., 2019; Cragun et al., 2015; Mittman & Downs, 2008; Sayani, 2019; Sharif et al., 2019). Shame, worry about other family members, misinformation, and concern about moral threats can also dampen interest in genetic testing (Chalela et al., 2012). Yet, low-income women from ethnic minority groups may have positive attitudes and strong interest in the concept of genetic testing, independent of understanding the risks, benefits, and limitations of testing (Chalela et al., 2012). Culturally adapted information about the risks and benefits of testing promotes informed testing decisions (Chalela et al., 2012).

Everyone has implicit (subconscious) biases around characteristics of identity, including race, religion, gender, and sexual orientation. Implicit biases are dangerous because they introduce feelings and thoughts that are not based on facts or reason. In an online study of genetic counselors, Schaa et al. (2015) showed a moderate to strong pro-White racial bias, which was correlated with using less emotionally responsive communication, both verbal and nonverbal, when counseling minority simulated clients. The consequences of implicit racial biases are significant; they may generate feelings of distance between the client and counselor, undermine trust, and ultimately contribute to disparities in service provision (Schaa et al., 2015). Genetic counselors and students have been shown to demonstrate greater implicit bias for heterosexual over homosexual people (Nathan et al., 2018). While participants were generally aware of the existence of biases, they were unaware of the extent of their biases, presenting a "near universal opportunity for bias reduction among North American genetic counselors and genetic counseling students" (Nathan et al., 2018, p. 97). Genetic counselors can use peer supervision to identify, explore, and reflect on specific and potential biases.

Microaggressions are subtle acts of discrimination based on perceived "otherness" due to race, skin color, or other characteristics. Examples of microaggressions include consistently asking the only woman in a meeting to take minutes, assuming a Hispanic person in the grocery is an employee, or asking the Black person in a group to speak for Black people in general. Talking over another person or not including their comments in meeting minutes reinforces power dynamics, often associated with gender differences. Using offensive or outdated words or slurs and making incorrect assumptions about identity are microaggressions that must be eliminated from everyday conversations in workplaces and personal interactions. Microaggressions can be more challenging than overt racism, since they cause people to question themselves or feel unfounded guilt, shame, or internalized stigma.

In situations where it is safe to do so, the person who is targeted with a microaggression can speak up using an "I" statement. For example: "I felt you were blaming me when you said you hope nobody travels to Asia so we don't get any more pandemics. My extended family lives in China. Like you, I also don't want another pandemic." Speaking up is important since people may not be aware of how their words are interpreted by others. However, when it is not safe to directly challenge a person due to power dynamics (student–supervisor interaction), it may be helpful to speak to someone else to validate the experience and strategize how policies can be changed. The genetic counselor should be an agent for change. If one personally makes a mistake, apologize and do not use the offending word again. If a colleague makes a mistake, call it out by stating that you find that wording offensive and ask that it not be used moving forward. If a patient uses racist or xenophobic language, the provider should proceed by modeling the appropriate language. Microaggressions introduce stress that can negatively impact health (Lui & Quexada, 2019; Nadal, 2014; Nadal et al., 2014; Sue et al., 2007). Until we deeply understand the historical realities of what people have endured over decades and generations and how hurt and feelings of "otherness" and oppression are reinforced today, true trust will be difficult to achieve. Identifying and addressing microaggressions in training settings, workplaces, and general society helps reduce disparities.

Cross-cultural genetic counseling is based on practicing client-centered counseling and the fundamental triad of empathy, genuineness, and unconditional positive regard. Genetic counselors explore clients' background, language, and health literacy level; determine what clients know and what they want to know; determine the relevant content and an approach for communicating information; evaluate learning; and assist in decision making. This complex and individualized process of assessment and counseling is what genetic counselors do every day. The skills for working with clients from a range of identities are largely the same, with some enhancements. Genetic counselors show genuine interest in the client as a unique individual by using open body language and culturally appropriate attending skills and by asking appropriate questions, listening, and using reflection to reinforce what is heard. Learning prevalent cultural customs (regarding touching and eye contact, for example) is respectful and informative (Online MSW Programs, 2020). Providers also show respect by learning the proper pronunciation of names and asking about preferred pronouns. Normalizing the concept of preferred pronouns shows acceptance of difference (Online MS Programs, 2020). Genetic counselors must self-monitor for potential biases between themselves and the client. Many clients come to genetics for similar indications, but it is essential not to make assumptions or use inflexible routines.

Strategies that work in all cross-cultural genetic counseling situations include asking questions, being ready to fully listen ("tell me more . . ."), communicating clearly, and determining what the client understands and what it means to them. At regular intervals, the counselor should check on the client's emotions ("How do you feel about this?") and ask what further information is needed. "Accepting responses" (not judging what the client says, acknowledging the client's own views and feelings, and validating their contribution) reinforce the reciprocal nature of the genetic counseling relationship (Back et al., 2005). Counselors should be tentative when attempting to characterize a client's emotions or responses: "I might be wrong, but I wonder if you feel (emotion) about this? Some people in this situation would feel (emotion)." Engage in an iterative discussion with a client to explain concepts and assess understanding. Give the client adequate time to respond so the session is not a lecture. Listen and use reflection to show the client you heard and respect their words. Determine who/what are sources of support for the client, including faith-based community resources, and encourage the client to engage with these resources when appropriate.

The Components of Cultural Responsiveness

Self-awareness, humility, and knowledge

Self-awareness and humility lie at the core of culturally competent genetic counseling. The **COUNSELING** mnemonic may be useful as a self-awareness and evaluation checklist for genetic counselors working in any setting, including telegenetics (Warren & Wilson, 2013; Warren et al., 2019).

- Client-centered counseling. Genetic counselors are concerned for each client as a unique person, who is also a member of a family and one or more communities, religions, and cultures. In the ongoing process of contracting, counselors ask questions to learn about the person and use client responses to inform the counseling.
- Open. Genetic counselors are willing to learn about diverse health beliefs and complementary medicine; they integrate these concepts into the discussion as appropriate.
- Unconditional positive regard. Genetic counselors do not judge clients for their actions or behaviors.
- Nondirectiveness. Genetic counselors strive to meet the client's agenda. This includes summarizing the pros and cons of all the options and reflecting back what the client said (or implied) about the best course of action.
- Self-awareness. Genetic counselors identify personal strengths and weaknesses. They resolve to continuously expand understanding of, and interest in, interacting with people from different background and experiences. This process improves professional expertise and makes us better people.
- Empathy. Genetic counselors use empathy to understand the client's experiences, emotions, perceptions of the world, behaviors, and decisions.
- Listen. Genetic counselors listen for what the client wants from the session. Counselors ask open- and closed-ended questions, using responses to develop and modify the agenda.
- Inclusive. Genetic counselors provide respectful and state-of-the-art counseling and information. Using people-first language, principles of health literacy, and interpreters and translators supports communicating information in a value-neutral manner.

- Nonverbals. Genetic counselors use nonverbal and verbal cues to fully appreciate a client's perspectives, feelings, and understanding. Counselors check their interpretations with the client to verify and modify their approaches.
- Genuine. Growing their knowledge and experience is a goal, and genetic counselors genuinely admit to their limitations as an opportunity to connect more deeply with clients.

Building cultural knowledge, another component of cultural responsiveness, requires expanding one's knowledge of cultures and using assessment strategies to gain insight into diverse beliefs and values and formulate responses that are consistent with a client's cultural framework (Fortier, 2011). Growth in cultural knowledge leads to greater self-awareness and skills. The genetic counseling literature, government and public health organizations, hospitals, and advocacy groups offer useful and accessible information and suggestions for working with individuals from specific cultures, religions, and populations (Cleveland Clinic, 2017; Galanti, 2014; Halbert & Harrison, 2018; Hunt & deVoogd, 2005; Mittman et al., 1998). The genetic counselor should curiously and respectfully explore the complexity of individuals from a multicultural, not a monocultural, perspective (Weil & Mittman, 1993). While counselors learn from listening to clients' personal cultural practices and beliefs in the context of a session, it is *not* clients' responsibility to educate providers about their culture(s). Clients should not be treated as a token representative of an entire culture or minority group. Similarly, minority students and colleagues should not be expected to educate majority members of training programs or worksites. Sharing should be a choice. Discussions about culture in genetic counseling should focus on the clients' beliefs, values, and affiliations and how these relate to the specific encounter.

Genetic counselors can use resources developed by local and regional health or advocacy organizations that provide insight into how to build respect with local community groups (Champlain Valley Area Health Education Center, 2013). Such resources can assist counselors and institutional staff to learn basic etiquette and greetings for interacting with clients from regional language and culture-diverse communities. While learning specific facts and trends can be interesting and educational, it is critical to treat clients as individuals and not make assumptions. Genetic counselors can invite community members to teach about common health beliefs or culturally based beliefs that do not align with Western science. For example, some people of Hispanic background hold stock in the health belief that a cleft lip is caused by the mother watching a lunar eclipse during her pregnancy (this belief is based on an ancient Aztec myth that an eclipse is a "bite" on the face of the moon; some believe that for protection, a pregnant woman should carry something metallic, like a safety pin [Centers for Disease Control and Prevention, n.d.]) or having used scissors during the pregnancy. Listening to community members broadens and deepens counselors' understanding of the range of beliefs and practices they may encounter and makes them less likely to fall back on stereotypes. By reaching out to local community, advocacy, and faith groups, genetic counselors build trust.

Research by Barragan et al. (2011) and others warns genetic counselors not to make assumptions about cultural beliefs and practices. Belief in Western medical care and adherence to cultural health practices are not necessarily mutually exclusive. Patients may believe/practice *both* Western medicine and traditional cultural health, to varying degrees, not necessarily related to acculturation. The genetic counselor can work *with* a patient's health beliefs. Counselors can "gently and respectfully inquire about their patients' cultural health practices, in order to understand how to be helpful" (Barragan et al., 2011, p. 622). It is important to acknowledge and explore the belief, while listening closely. *How strongly does the client hold this belief? What about the family members or the client's community? For the patient, does this belief interfere with or does it coexist with scientific/genetic causes or explanations?*

The genetic counselor can emphasize the synergy between cultural and Western medical approaches, if doing so poses no risks: "Thank you for sharing that some people in your culture, including your grandmother, believe that watching an eclipse causes cleft lip. In our research, often we cannot explain why cleft lip happens. Cleft lip often occurs to babies whose mothers take excellent care of themselves in the pregnancy, like you. If staying inside during an eclipse is something you can do in a future pregnancy, and that pleases your grandmother, then maybe that is what you should do. While there is no guarantee that a cleft lip will not happen again in another baby, no matter how well you take care of yourself, the chance is low, about one out of 20 babies." Discussing surgical and other healthcare treatments for the child would be done as usual. When there is no harm and all explanations and options are discussed, the genetic counselor can build trust by being respectful about cultural health beliefs and cover the usual information content and options.

Skills, strategies, and assessment tools for cultural responsiveness

Cultural responsiveness skills are not unique to cross-cultural counseling. Skills/techniques for cross-cultural communication (teach-back; using cultural and spiritual assessment tools) are applicable to any healthcare session. However, using a culturally appropriate approach is essential. For example, in focus groups conducted with Mexican American Latinas, Chalela et al. (2012) explored attitudes regarding breast cancer testing. The women generally preferred active guidance in decision making (in deference to the respect and trust placed in healthcare providers as authority figures), valued framing decision making and goals of testing in light of the benefits and implications for other family members, and preferred the use of words to percentages. Mismatch between the patients' information needs and preferences and the information provided by counselors must be avoided (Joseph & Guerra, 2015). Delivering information that patients do not need (biology of inheritance) to understand the concept of risk can confuse and "crowd out the communication of other critical information" (Joseph & Guerra, 2015, p. 73). Of note is that uptake of nonclinical genetic testing for ancestry- or health-related outcomes, when compared with uptake of clinical genetic testing, was found to be more approachable, desirable, accessible, and available to individuals across races and ethnicities (Carroll et al., 2019). Understanding why certain types of testing are perceived more positively can help inform culturally tailored genetic counseling.

Assessment skills are vital to the cultural responsiveness process. Cultural assessment in genetic counseling often begins with obtaining information from intake forms, medical records, and test results. Counselors should be deliberate about the information that is requested on forms. Each center should review existing forms and determine why each question or field is relevant. *What will be done with that information? Is there benefit to the patient from the genetic counselor knowing that information? Will the counseling be more definitive or specific with this information? What information is for clinic or institutional statistical tracking purposes only?* For example, is race and ethnicity information collected because it contributes to risk assessment, because it provides perspective on client self-identification, or primarily for institutional purposes, or all of these reasons? Whenever possible, explain the rationale for questions asked on forms to the client. *Are there prevalent cultural or religious groups in the area? Do intake questions align accordingly?* Examples of intake questions and forms from county and local health departments may assist in developing forms that reflect diverse local demographics.

Cultural and spiritual assessment tools can enhance genetic counseling. Kleinman et al. (1978) suggested incorporating several simple questions into healthcare interactions to facilitate a provider's understanding of what a patient wants, and why. Kleinman and colleagues' (at the time, radical) insight was that doctors should not assume patients and healthcare providers want or value the same things. The objective of each assessment tool varies, but in general, they help providers treat each client as an individual. Suggested questions can identify clients' specific cultural or religious beliefs and values and elucidate how those beliefs relate to the reason for the visit and related decision making. The insights gained should be considered tentative until they have been further explored with the client.

Genetic counseling is influenced by the provider's personal style and comfort. It has been shown that genetic counselors are particularly uncomfortable asking and discussing the relevance of religion and spirituality in their sessions (Reis et al., 2007). Cultural differences and biases may inhibit the counselor from exploring clients' health beliefs and practices. Genetic counselors enrich their practice by using particular assessment questions to facilitate intake and discourse. Two examples follow:

BATHE (Stuart & Lieberman, 1993) can be a useful device to discover the core issue or problem. A foundation of trust and rapport is built by using these steps, allowing the patient to feel comfortable sharing pertinent information.

Background: Asking a simple open-ended question, "What is going on in your life?" elicits the context of the patient's visit.

Affect: Asking, "How do you feel about it?" or "What is your mood?" allows the patient to report and label their current feeling state.

Trouble: Asking, "What troubles you most about the situation?" helps the physician and patient focus, and may elucidate the symbolic significance of the illness or event.

Handle: Asking, "What helps you handle the situation?" gives an assessment of functioning and provides direction for an intervention.

Empathy: Saying, "This must be very difficult for you" or "Anybody would feel as you do" legitimizes the patient's feelings and provides psychological support.

FICA (Puchalski & Romer, 2000) questions may assist the provider in taking a patient's spiritual history and facilitate discussion of the role of spirituality and religion in their well-being. The goal is to establish an environment of intimacy and trust where the patient feels more comfortable revealing fundamental information about their worldviews and sources of personal meaning.

Faith or beliefs: *What is your faith or belief? Do you consider yourself spiritual or religious? What things do you believe give meaning to your life?*

Importance and Influence: *What influence do your faith or beliefs have on how you take care of yourself? How have your beliefs influenced your behavior during this illness? What role do your beliefs play in regaining your health?*

Community: *Are you part of a spiritual or religious community? Is this a support to you, and how? Is there a person or group of people you really love or who are really important to you?*

Address: *How would you like me, your healthcare provider, to address and include these issues in our discussion?*

Social determinants of health should be part of the assessment process. Social determinants of health are contextual environmental factors that give rise to health inequity, including poverty, lack of health insurance, educational inequality, food insecurity, poor access to transportation, unaffordable housing, unemployment, uncertain maintenance of basic utilities, violence, and questionable domestic or public safety (Sherin et al., 2019). Social determinants of health influence who is more/less likely to receive genetic counseling and provide context for each client. Social determinants also influence how a client perceives the burden and options around a genetic condition, including risks and treatment and testing options. Health literacy, LEP, and mistrust of healthcare are important factors. About 15% of the U.S. population lives in poverty; 20% of individuals live below the poverty level if a language other than English is spoken at home; 10% of individuals under 65 years of age have no health insurance. In terms of highest level of educational attainment, 6% of the population reported completing less than ninth grade, and 30% report "less than HS graduate" as highest level of education. These percentages increase when languages other than English are spoken at home. While full screening for social determinants of health falls more to primary care providers, genetic counselors should be proactive about exploring needs when specific concerns emerge from history taking (Krist et al., 2019). When social determinants are recognized as affecting a client's health, counselors should communicate with institutional social workers and primary care providers and/or make referrals. Genetics clinics, hospitals, and healthcare systems should have formal affiliations and working relationships with community service, education, and advocacy organizations. Working with interdisciplinary providers and community liaisons can promote change in vulnerable populations.

Cultural and social identity, and myriad other factors, contribute to behaviors and decisions around health and wellness. The culture of genetic counseling, grounded in Western healthcare principles and guided by assumptions about the importance of autonomy and prevention, may mask conflicting patient priorities. For example, "noncompliant" is often used to describe patients who do not take medicine properly or do not follow through with appointments or recommendations. It should be considered that these outcomes may be due to a variety of challenges, including not understanding instructions, making mistakes, having inadequate time or transportation, forgetting, not understanding the seriousness or urgency of a follow-up test or referral, not appreciating the role of preventative care, and/or financial, family, social, or mental health challenges. In reality, noncompliance or lack of follow-through is rarely the patient's goal. Identifying, exploring, and assisting the client with these other life challenges is prudent and often requires collaboration with trusted members of the healthcare, social service, faith, and other local community agencies (Centers for Medicare and Medicaid Services, 2021).

Health literacy is another consideration within assessment. Health literacy is defined by the Centers for Disease Control and Prevention (CDC, 2024) and Healthy People 2020 as "the degree to which individuals have the capacity to obtain, process, and understand basic health information and services needed to make appropriate health decisions." The National Assessment of Adult Literacy ("Health Literacy of American Adults," 2006) summarized the results of assessment tasks designed specifically to measure the health literacy of adults living in the United States. One-third of U.S. adults were found to have limited health literacy (Joseph et al., 2019). These adults functioned at basic (22%) and below basic (14%) levels. Individuals with basic skills cannot consistently use a bus schedule, identify information from a bar graph, or write a brief letter of complaint. Individuals functioning at the below basic level cannot consistently understand or summarize an article or enter information on a social security application.

Limited ability to effectively understand and apply health-related information translates into poorer health outcomes. Studies have demonstrated that health literacy is a stronger predictor of health status than income, employment status, education level, or racial or ethnic group (Weiss, 2007). However, there are correlations among these factors. In the United States, 75% of welfare recipients, 57% of the Black population, and 79% of the Hispanic population read at the basic or below basic level. People with LEP are more likely to have lower health literacy (Joseph et al., 2019). People with limited health literacy underuse preventive health services and report poorer health. Factors that contribute to health literacy include general literacy, experience with the health system, complexity of information and how it is communicated, cultural and language factors, aging, and emotional burden of the information. Health literacy is situation dependent. Familiarity, motivation, and context of the messaging influence comprehension, and emotional factors can impair a person's ability to absorb and use health information to make decisions. A person's health literacy is influenced by the demands and complexities of the healthcare system itself (Joseph et al., 2019).

Health literacy skills are essential for finding needed information and services, communicating with professionals, processing information and understanding choices to make decisions, and reaching outcomes that align with a client's needs and preferences. Genetic counseling involves discussing personal and family health information that may be unexpected or unwanted or that impacts patients' emotions. All of these factors can impair clients' ability to listen, process, and understand information. Joseph et al. (2017) have described the "information mismatch" of cancer risk genetic counseling with diverse underserved patients. When counselors share more information than wanted or perceived to be relevant by patients, use terminology that is too complex, or discuss issues such as screening and prevention too vaguely, patients tend to disengage. Providers should be intentional about the amount and depth of information communicated. That is, rather than assume what patients want to know, ask and explore a patient's information needs and preferences, and engage often to determine if the information shared is meeting the patient's needs. Genetic counseling that does not consider the evidence-based principles of health literacy in both verbal and written communications contributes to health disparities (Joseph et al., 2017).

In the course of casual conversation, it can be difficult to determine whether someone has limited health literacy, but providers can look for clues. Patients who miss appointments, leave forms incomplete, or do not engage fully in conversation may have limited health literacy. The counselor or a staff member can be a surrogate reader if a patient seems reluctant to complete forms on site or if someone claims to have forgotten their glasses. When possible, suggest that forms be completed at home (allowing more time and/or assistance from a friend or family member) and returned by mail or at another visit. Suggest that the patient invite a support person or family member to future visits. As with verbal interactions, genetic counselors should verify patients' understanding of written materials. Written follow-up instructions or letters should be individualized and match in-person messaging. Given the complexity of genetics terminology, genetic counselors must intentionally simplify the words used to speak and write whenever possible to ensure that the genetic counseling environment is patient-friendly and shame-free for all. Even everyday language can be simplified by using words like "enough" instead of "adequate," "choice" instead of "option," "another thing" instead of "factor," "too much" instead of "excessive," and "work together" instead of "collaborate." Simplicity is best for communicating with patients of all backgrounds and educational levels. Evidence-based principles and strategies for effective verbal communication with patients with limited health literacy include using plain language and teach-back. An extensive list of vetted principles, strategies, and techniques for effective communication has been compiled by Joseph et al. (2019).

Health literacy pertains to the spoken and written word, and best communication practices are similar: Use simple, commonly used words; use active voice; determine what the patient already knows as a starting point and then cover the three to five most important points; and chunk information into discrete areas. Principles of health literacy should be considered when developing and evaluating written materials, including intake forms, patient letters, research forms, and so forth, and the materials should reflect the words used in person. While it is common for a genetics center to use generic materials (an efficient strategy for the institution), this approach does not accommodate a range of client reading and comprehension levels. Reading level is often used as a proxy for health literacy. Most adults in the United States read at an eighth-grade level, and 20% of the population reads at or below a fifth-grade level. Yet, most healthcare materials are written at a 10th-grade level (Safeer & Keenan, 2005). About three-quarters of people in populations at risk read at an eighth-grade level or below, and half of them read below a fifth-grade level. Therefore, genetic counseling patient education materials should be written at a sixth-grade or lower reading level, preferably including pictures and illustrations (Safeer & Keenan, 2005).

While they are crude methods, readability formulas can quickly assess written materials using two basic measures: vocabulary difficulty and sentence length. Two commonly used formulas in healthcare include SMOG and FRY. SMOG measures materials written between the fourth-grade and college level, and FRY measures materials between the first-grade and college level:

SMOG testing: https://readabilityformulas.com/free-readability-formula-tests.php
FRY Readability Graph: https://readabilityformulas.com/free-fry-graph-test.php

Using these measures, one can assess the reading level of commonly used written documents in genetic counseling practice. This exercise should be done with the following caveats: Readability tests cannot measure whether the material is written clearly, accurately, and grammatically correctly; whether the ideas are too complex; whether the content is presented logically using vocabulary that is appropriate for the patient; and whether the design is attractive and facilitates communication of the key points. More difficult is the task of adapting existing materials and writing new materials designed to increase readability and comprehension by more patients. The layout and illustrations of written materials should be simple; major points should be limited and presented logically; a conversational, friendly tone in active voice with pronouns when appropriate should be used; and bulleted lists should be used to highlight key points, take-home messages, and follow-up tasks.

Teach-back is an evidence-based assessment and counseling technique to check patient understanding. Teach-back can be used throughout a genetic counseling session, especially to check understanding of discrete chunks of information and key take-home messages. Using teach-back also helps counselors learn what the client thinks is most important. A client is asked to share in their own words what they understood about a particular concept or decision: "Who will you tell about this visit when you get home? To make sure I did a good job explaining (concept or option) to you, can you tell me what you are going to tell (named person[s]) about (concept or option)?" If/when a patient's response indicates confusion or misunderstanding, the provider should rephrase the information. The counselor should promote further discussion to reinforce or modify the client's understanding as appropriate, mirroring the client's words when possible. This simple technique provides insight into client understanding and encourages participation. The complexity of genetics terminology and concepts suggests that teach-back should be integrated at multiple times during genetic counseling sessions.

Working with language-diverse clients requires the ability to work with medical interpreters and translators. Medical interpreters are certified professionals who communicate the spoken word from one language to another. They undergo specific training, show proficiency in English, pass a board exam in each specific language area, and meet continuing education requirements. Partnering with trained medical interpreters in healthcare settings is preferable to providing services on an ad hoc basis (Locatis et al., 2009). It is not advised to ask or allow family members, hospital staff, or others to interpret in genetic counseling due to concerns with accuracy, privacy, and power dynamics (e.g., asking a child to interpret for a parent). Working with an interpreter *may* take more time, but advance planning can expedite a smooth and efficient process. The institutional staff at front-desk or registration stations should begin the language access process by determining patient language needs. Using downloadable *I Speak* cards (available from various public health and government agencies), staff should ask clients to self-identify their preferred language of communication and note this in the electronic medical record and other clinic documents. In the United States, agencies and institutions receiving federal and/or state funds are required to provide clients who speak limited or no English with free interpretation services in any language.

Interpretation can be done in person, by phone, or by video interpreting. Many institutions do not have on-site interpreters available at all times, but supplemental telephonic and video conference interpretation services can ensure language access, even for emergency visits. Clients do not show a strong preference for method of interpretation, although healthcare providers and interpreters have been shown to prefer in-person interpretation (Locatis et al., 2009). Whenever possible, genetic counselors should try to work with the same interpreter when there are multiple sessions with the same client. Clients value consistency in language support.

In the client's preferred language and using as close to a word-for-word interpretation as possible, the interpreter communicates to the client what the genetic counselor says and then proceeds to listen to the client and transmit this response back to the counselor in English. While recognizing that constraints of some clinical settings may impact implementation, ideally genetic counselors should strive for the following practices in interpretation:

- Schedule extra time.
- Communicate with the interpreter (in person or by phone) before a session to share plans and explain any technical terms that will be used. Encourage the interpreter to share any important cultural points that might be relevant.
- Greet the client warmly, and explore who is in the room and their relationship to the client and/or their role(s).
- Use simple terms and keep the content covered succinct. Deliver information in complete thoughts and in small chunks.
- Speak directly to the client, slowly and clearly (not louder).
- Ask the client for feedback regularly.
- When word-for-word interpretation is not possible in the preferred language, the interpreter should explain to the counselor any necessary modifications.

Throughout the process, the genetic counselor should pay careful attention to the pattern of communication and nonverbal clues. *Are you speaking too much? Does the client suddenly seem agitated? Who is answering your questions? Is the client looking at you? Have you gauged the client's understanding? Does the communication mediated by the interpreter seem to flow as you would expect? Are there side conversations that do not seem to be interpreted? What are you doing to keep the communications focused? Are you in control of the session?*

When the interpreter is present in person or via videoconference, both verbal and nonverbal clues can contribute to communication dynamics. Increasingly, however, telephone interpretation services are provided remotely by interpreters based at national or regional call centers (Kelly, 2008), especially for less commonly requested languages and dialects. The quality of the phone connection is critical to all parties being able to hear the others clearly. While visual cues are not available to the telephone interpreter, nonverbal information can be reflected in tone of voice, breath patterns, inflection, vocal volume, and other auditory cues (Kelly, 2008). Concerns about the accuracy and completeness of telephone interpretations have been raised due to their commonly being of shorter duration than other methods (Locatis et al., 2009). Sessions involving high levels of emotional stress or crises, or with patients who have hearing challenges, are best interpreted in person if possible.

Translators are credentialed and certified professionals who express the written word in documents, letters, consent forms, and so forth from one language to another. Translators may be hospital or agency based or hired on a consulting basis. Translating documents focused on topics in genetics and genetic counseling is particularly challenging due to conceptual complexity and lack of corresponding words in some languages. Because translating documents takes time (weeks to months), genetics centers should identify commonly used materials and have them translated into prevalent languages. Counselors can also identify existing appropriate online materials that have been translated into specific languages. Multilingual healthcare resources abound, although targeted resources for genetic counseling are limited. By collaborating with translation experts, genetic counselors can build a body of translated materials on specific topics.

Genetic counselors should determine what interpretation and translation resources are available at their institution. Building relationships with these professionals is critical in serving non-English-speaking clients. Counselors should take time to educate interpreters and translators about the common issues addressed and share medical and genetic terms often used in the clinic. Interpreters and translators can be a rich source of cultural and community information to help genetic counselors learn about language-diverse communities. In a *cultural broker* role, these professionals can provide insights and facilitate understanding of specific cultures and communities. Typically, a cultural broker is a member of the group and therefore can speak authentically about practices and beliefs the genetic counselor might encounter. The cultural broker can explain fears or experiences communities might have/have had around genetics.

Organizational Cultural Responsiveness

The genetic counseling workforce

The genetic counseling workforce is among the least diverse allied healthcare professions when compared to racial and ethnic and gender demographics of the U.S. population (Channaoui, Bui, & Mittman, 2020). It is well documented that the percentage of minority genetic counselors has remained virtually flat over time (Channaoui, Bui, & Mittman, 2020; Mittman & Downs, 2008; National Society of Genetic Counselors, 2020; Smith et al., 1993). Recommendations for increasing diversity in medicine (Garcia et al., 2004) can be applied to genetic counseling, including demonstrating institutional commitment to diversity through strong and active leadership, developing mission statements that reflect institutional commitment to diversity, ensuring careful assessment of personal qualities of applicants, appointing admissions committee members who reflect the diversity that is sought in the student body, and establishing and maintaining outreach programs.

Disparities between institutional staffing and community demographics represent a mandate for actively extending the reach of healthcare and genetics services to underserved communities. Recent advances in telemedicine and phone genetic counseling might provide greater accessibility for some individuals. Using their communication skills, genetic counselors can listen to community leaders and laypersons to understand specific needs, myths, requests, and/or concerns about genetics services and outreach. *What relationships are currently in place with community groups? What new community relationships should be formed?*

Health agencies, hospitals, and clinical environments

Agencies and hospitals offering genetic counseling services provide context that may help or hinder the efforts of providers to provide culturally competent care. Cultural responsiveness for organizations relates to broad domains including leadership, data collection and performance management, workforce diversity and training, community engagement, patient–provider communication, and care delivery (Weech-Maldonado, Dreachslin, et al., 2012). These domains can be measured against best practices, such as those cited in the National Standards for Culturally and Linguistically Appropriate Services in Health and Health Care (Weech-Maldonado, Dreachslin, et al., 2012). It is essential to determine how various areas of a healthcare system contribute positively and negatively to the patients' experiences and influence the dynamics of individual patient–provider relationships.

Multiple factors in the healthcare environment contribute to patients' experiences. Strategies for improving organizational cultural responsiveness in genetics clinics and hospitals overlap. Many strategies relate to increasing accessibility of services, including the following:

- The institution's mission statement and values should reflect the value of diversity.
- Provide access to medical interpreters and translators by contracting with credentialed professionals (on-site and/or remotely) for clients with LEP and with American Sign Language interpreters for hearing-impaired and Deaf clients.
- Post multilingual and/or universal signs throughout the institution. Appropriate signage should consider sensory and physical challenges as well as language diversity to help people navigate unfamiliar corridors and departments. Displaying welcome signs in different languages or a map of the world conveys the message that the institution values and respects clients from all countries and backgrounds.
- Review patient registration and intake forms for eliciting language, cultural, and religious information. Hospital registrars should be knowledgeable about variations in the region and able to help specify client needs.
- Hospitals and genetic counseling clinics should use medically inclusive forms and display LGBTQ+-friendly symbols (VandenLangenberg et al., 2012).
- An Office of Disabilities should be in place to provide advocacy and targeted services to meet the needs of disabled clients, visitors, staff, and students. The hospital or organization should have ample wheelchairs and escorts available.
- Institutional social workers and chaplains are essential partners. These professionals enhance genetic counseling practice by participating in case management, psychosocial counseling, support, and referrals.
- Institutional funds to waive or defray the costs of clinic visits and tests can enhance accessibility of genetics services for some clients.
- Providing vouchers or rideshare services may be essential for clients without ready access to a car or convenient public transportation.
- Days/times genetic counseling services are offered can influence accessibility. Is it possible to offer evening and/or weekend appointments?
- Are there alternative methods for providing services? Offering group counseling may be helpful as some clients prefer this method of service provision. Can some genetic counseling services be offered by telemedicine?
- Are there alternative locations for providing services? Can services expand to a trusted local setting such as a health department or community center? Genetic counselors may be able to train community health workers or nurses to manage some genetics intake, support, and follow-up tasks in local settings.

- Send appointment reminders by text. They are generally well accepted. Clients may not own a computer, but most own a phone.

At times, it is unknown why members of certain community groups are less likely to access genetics services. To further understand local needs, hospitals and agencies providing genetic services should seek ongoing community representation and input from local cultural groups. Diversity awareness training for institutional staff at all levels should include opportunities to identify biases and practice skills for treating people as unique individuals.

Genetic counseling training programs

Genetic counseling graduate training programs play a critical role in diversifying the workforce. Although the process of developing cultural responsiveness is never complete (it's about the journey, not the destination), graduate training is a crucial aspect of the journey (Bancroft, 2014). Similar to programs in psychology, each genetic counseling program will "create a somewhat different culturally supportive milieu, but they will all share a common need—faculty and students must take ownership of the holistic plan and process for the plan to be optimally effective" (Hansen et al., 2000, p. 659). Genetic counseling program recruitment strategies have not been the subject of rigorous examination for evidence of bias. Recruiting events and materials should highlight how the learning environment is supportive and capable of training diverse students (Hansen et al., 2000). Recruitment of bilingual students is another strategy for diversification of the profession (Vanneste et al., 2013). Consulting expertise and funding streams from a program's home institution can facilitate organizational cultural responsiveness assessment. Preparing students in cultural responsiveness that is infused throughout the program design includes review and modification as needed of the mission statement, the curriculum, research and clinical work, and evaluation measures. The program leadership should set feasible goals, take actions, reevaluate, and expand the process at least annually. Programs should consider: *What are the diversity goals for student enrollment and faculty? What is the composition of our program faculty? What institutional resources and support services are available to promote diversity? Who are the members of the recruitment/admissions committee? Are there institutional and/or community representatives who can enhance our admissions committee's membership and practices? Are program policies and procedures fair and equitable to all students?*

Programs are tasked with providing an environment and resources where student learning flourishes (Taylor & Hamdy, 2013) using best practices in adult and developmental learning. Adult learners are considered partners who bring past experiences and personal needs to the learning process. They plan their learning goals and participate in evaluating their results (Clement, 2018). They thrive in an environment where it feels safe to learn and make mistakes. Acquiring cultural knowledge is perhaps the easiest aspect of facilitating learning for trainees. Providing a learning environment that supports attitudinal growth and introspection is more difficult, but essential, to achieve goals in lifelong education, communication skills, empathy, and professionalism (Taylor & Hamdy, 2013). While cultural responsiveness is personal, learning can come from interactions with peers, clients, and faculty. Students can share experiences and perspectives, ask questions, reflect on new information, identify gaps in knowledge, and use reflection to assess learning and modify goals (Taylor & Hamdy, 2013). The training environment helps students become aware of their strengths, weaknesses, and possible blind spots in cultural knowledge, skills, and self-awareness.

Weil and Mittman (1993) state that providing culturally sensitive and appropriate genetic counseling should be a "central" tenet of the graduate training, to be integrated into psychosocial, medical, and testing areas of didactic and clinical training. Beneficial approaches to cultural responsiveness training include enhancing traditional coursework with cultural awareness and self-reflection activities that are integrated seamlessly into students' training and patient encounters (McGinnis et al., 2018; Warren, 2011). Diversity and cultural responsiveness goals should be part of curriculum materials (objectives, skills, examples, activities, reflective exercises), clinical practices, research projects, and recruitment practices. Training faculty and supervisors in cultural responsiveness is essential. Supervisors in other counseling fields who have engaged in multicultural training are perceived as more multiculturally competent by their supervisees (Lee at al., 2009).

Curriculum and experiential interventions of varying length and content have been effective for training providers in cultural responsiveness while not promoting stereotyping (Beach et al., 2005). Programs need to be cautious not to rely on categorical constructs that group patients of similar cultures with "characteristic" values, customs, and beliefs (Carrillo et al., 1999). Providing basic information about the range of communication styles, attitudes such as toward authority, healthcare beliefs, historical events, and experience with discrimination can be individualized by inviting community members to share personal stories. Students can be encouraged to continue learning through literary works, films, and visits to local community events and meeting places (Weil & Mittman, 1993). Training programs can use varied in-person and online instructional formats beginning with modifying or enhancing existing assignments and materials and expanded to incorporate online resources (videos, cases, slides), inviting speakers, conducting workshops, and offering short courses.

Programs can adapt elements of cultural responsiveness instruction developed for other healthcare trainees (Expert Panel on Cultural Competence Education for Students in Medicine and Public Health, 2012). Carrillo et al. (1999) proposed the content of a patient-based cross-cultural curriculum for residents and medical students that could be adapted for genetic counseling. The curriculum is grounded in empathy, curiosity, and respect as fundamental tenets of successful encounters in five 2-hour modules that cover basic concepts, core cultural issues, explanatory models of illness, determining social context, and negotiating across cultures. The Georgetown University National Center for Cultural Competence offers individual and organizational self-assessment checklists for providers and content that can be modified to meet program needs (https://nccc.georgetown.edu/index.php). Think Cultural Health offers a variety of instructional resources for healthcare providers (https://thinkculturalhealth.hhs.gov/).

The program must create a safe space for discussion, disagreement, and learning. Students may feel worried or vulnerable or have other fears talking about cultural diversity, religion and spirituality, and race. When emotionally charged content is not handled well, it will interfere with student learning. Tatum (1992) notes that powerful emotional responses such as anger, guilt, shame, and despair may be evoked by issues of oppression due to racism, classism, sexism, homophobia and heterosexism, anti-Semitism, ageism, and so forth. However, avoiding discussion of stereotypes and feelings is counterproductive to learning. Allowing individuals to use quick, funny comments for comic relief in tense situations or avoid self-reflection is also counterproductive to creating a trusting environment that encourages personal growth. Tatum (1992) suggests that individuals should speak from their own experience ("I think . . . ") rather than use generalizations ("People say . . . "). Clearly, there is no place for the use of ethnic slurs in the training program environment. However, if outdated terms are used, such as "Orientals" or "mentally retarded," this is a teachable moment. Faculty should assume no ill intent and provide correct terms. In clinic, genetic counselors and students should model use of appropriate terminology for clients.

The program environment should be welcoming and equitable for all students. Placing extra burden on minority students by expecting them to be spokespersons for a particular race or social identity is not appropriate. The conscripted curriculum (when issues of race or ethnicity are taught in a small group discussion format that relies on students sharing their individual experiences to educate their classmates) occurs in genetic counseling training (Carmichael et al., 2020). Carmichael et al. (2020) report that when minority students feel obliged (by their program, instructor, or peers) to contribute their unique perspectives to educate others, and the same obligations are not imposed on all students, feelings of frustration and exhaustion may result. All students possess culture, and requirements for all students should be equitable. Opportunities to explore parameters of personal identity and potential biases in working with clients must be flexible to accommodate a range of student backgrounds and experiences.

Programs should recruit a diverse pool of faculty instructors and/or ensure that all instructors are trained to facilitate difficult discussions about race and racism (Carmichael et al., 2020). Faculty and students should engage in honest discourse by discussing these and other prompts:

- Characterize trust in the program learning environment (classrooms, clinics).
- How does the program create a learning environment where it feels safe to learn, make mistakes, and share vulnerabilities? What could be improved?
- How do faculty members build trust with students?
- In what specific ways can cultural learning, practice, and reflection be enhanced in the program?

Students should be required to document and assess personal achievements and growth in cultural responsiveness in terms of knowledge, skills, and self-awareness. To evaluate their students' cultural responsiveness, programs can use a developmental framework model as may be used to evaluate achievement of other competences and skills in course and clinical evaluations (Guy, 2016). Gradual expectations of early, typical, and advanced knowledge, skills, and (critical) personal insights and growth are consistent with treating cultural responsiveness as an ongoing process without a specific endpoint. While tools for measuring skills in cultural responsiveness have not been rigorously evaluated (Gozu et al., 2007), clinical supervisors have proposed areas of student feedback to promote engagement in multiculturally sensitive genetic counseling: (a) assess and set goals, (b) be aware of cultural and family concepts, (c) respect patient autonomy, (d) provide empathy and support, (e) avoid assumptions, and (f) provide information and resources (Lee et al., 2009). Learning to become a genetic counselor and developing cultural responsiveness are formidable adult learning goals. Both must be done thoughtfully, gradually, and continually.

Program leaders are in a position of power to impact the workforce trajectory of the profession. Bao et al. (2020) encourage program leaders to practice inclusive teaching (faculty should share their own stories of identity development and vulnerabilities), listen to students, engage in holistic application review, offer continuing education opportunities for faculty and clinical supervisors, and recruit community organizers and experts to assist and guide. Minority genetic counseling students may have no minority role models or faculty to turn to when experiencing isolation or pressure attributed to race or ethnicity. Program leaders should identify academic role models and mentors related to identity for students. All genetic counseling students should participate in the NSGC Mentor Match to build relationships with counselors on the national level who can uniquely listen, share, and guide. And all members of the profession should use cultural responsiveness skills in daily interactions to create equitable learning and work environments (Channaoui, Khan, et al., 2020).

Professional organizations

The professional organizations of genetic counseling (ACGC, ABGC, NSGC) establish standards of training and practice. However, guidance to date from these organizations regarding cultural responsiveness has been limited. In "Efforts of Diversity and Inclusion, Cultural Responsiveness, and Equity in the Genetic Counseling Profession," Channaoui, Bui, and Mittman (2020) conclude that many valuable activities lacked impact and replicability due to a lack of coordination, recognition, and/or funding. Outside consultants/experts can expand an organization's perspectives and identify systemic bias. In 2020, such efforts were just beginning within genetic counseling professional organizations.

The ACGC defines 22 minimum practice-based competencies (PBCs) for an entry-level genetic counselor (ACGC, 2019b). The PBCs also define general content areas that must be covered in the training program curricula and assessed by the board certification examination (ACGC, 2019b, 2019c). The PBC most relevant to cultural responsiveness (#13) is "Apply genetic counseling skills in a culturally responsive and respectful manner to all clients" (ACGC, 2019c, p. 2). However, the ACGC offers limited further guidance: "The ACGC supports increasing diversity," and "programs are expected to develop strategies to promote applications from underrepresented populations and to summarize their efforts and progress in the accreditation application" (ACGC, 2019c, p. 16). When accreditation expectations are limited and vague, they can be achieved with minimal effort. While these standards give flexibility around recruitment of underrepresented students into the training programs, programs are not required to set firm recruitment goals. The ACGC provides no further guidance on admissions policies, procedures, committees, accountability, or evaluation around minority recruitment into genetic counseling training programs. Recently, the ACGC formulated a Diversity Taskforce to explore the theory and concepts of intersectionality in genetic counseling (ACGC, 2019a). The expected outcomes include producing revised language and measures around intersectionality that can be incorporated into a future version of the standards of accreditation and annual program reporting. The taskforce will also characterize current efforts/practices and measures of success in incorporating intersectionality into program curricula and recruitment pathways (ACGC, 2019a).

The ABGC, host of the genetic counseling board examination in the United States, sets expectations for examinees around psychosocial assessment, support, and counseling (ABGC, 2018). Examinees are expected to be able to assess client and/or family cultural/religious beliefs, traditions, and values; socioeconomic background, experiences, and lifestyles; health literacy; and health beliefs and attitudes. Further, the exam content for psychosocial support and counseling of all clients includes the ability to use an array of techniques to address client emotions and/or behavior. Acquisition and application of fundamental cultural knowledge, assessment, and counseling skills must therefore be achieved by the time a student graduates from training and begins working in the field. The ABGC sets no continuing education requirements around cultural responsiveness. Future efforts should include specifying cultural responsiveness continuing education unit learning in recertification requirements, as is expected of physicians and other healthcare providers in some states. In 2020, the ABGC committed to seeking outside consulting to review the exam development process and items for implicit bias.

The NSGC defines the core principles that guide the professional and personal ethics of genetic counselors. In the latest Code of Ethics (NSGC, 2018), cultural responsiveness is implicitly included among the values expected of genetic counseling providers and organizations. In 2020 the NSGC initiated efforts with outside consultants to develop a plan to support diversity, equity, and inclusion. Their strategic planning process includes goal setting and optimization of the organization "to promote a culture of inclusivity that supports visible and invisible diversity and leverage that culture to expand the perspectives represented in our field, build community and foster equity in genetic services" (Channaoui, Khan, et al., 2020, p. 194).

While these are notable efforts, they are recent, and the profession lags behind other fields in setting expectations around training and practice that support cultural responsiveness. Still needed is development of genetic counseling multicultural competencies to establish uniform definitions, standards, and goals to guide the activities of individuals, institutions, and training programs around cultural responsiveness, diversity, recruitment, and equity (Kessler & Love, 2020; Warren, 2011). Prioritizing the resolve and timeline for developing these competencies is essential. Insight on content for such an initiative can be gleaned from the National Standards for Culturally and Linguistically Appropriate Services in Health and Health Care (Office of Minority Health Resource Center, 2018), which "aim to promote health equity through providing clear plans and strategies to guide collaborative efforts that address racial and ethnic health disparities across the country." Guidelines on multicultural responsiveness developed by other fields may be helpful (American Psychological Association, 2017; National Association of Social Workers, 2015). A useful example offers 12 competencies for psychology that emphasize determining "what is useful or meaningful to the client as a person, not simply as a representative of certain cultural groups" by analyzing cases that promote understanding of within-group differences rather than stereotyping based on membership in a group (Ridley et al., 1994, p. 242). Interdisciplinary approaches have been used in other fields. For example, the Association of American Medical Colleges and the Association of Schools of Public Health collaborated to develop extensive competencies for the disciplines of medicine and public health to prepare culturally competent practitioners (Expert Panel on Cultural Competence Education for Students in Medicine and Public Health, 2012). These interdisciplinary competencies were enhanced with illustrative case examples, short video clips, and reflective exercises for trainees in either discipline. Once developed, guidelines on multicultural competencies in genetic counseling will need regular evaluation/modification by stakeholders including representatives of the professional organizations and training programs, underrepresented organizations/groups, and experts from other fields. The genetic counseling community can also champion broader efforts such as those proposed by Sharif et al. (2019), who noted that healthcare providers should be held to standards of genomic competence, cultural responsiveness, and research competence. Such collaborative efforts among healthcare provider organizations and systems are needed to facilitate equitable access to genomic clinical and research testing and services (Sharif et al., 2019).

Conclusion: Importance of Cultural Responsiveness in Genetic Counseling

Studies evaluating the effectiveness of interventions have shown that training professionals in cultural responsiveness increases knowledge and enhances the attitudes and skills of healthcare providers, as well as positively impacting patient satisfaction and follow-through with medical recommendations (Beach et al., 2005; Carrillo et al., 1999; Govere & Govere, 2016; Gozu et al., 2007). Honing patient-centered communication skills appears to be the most effective focus for provider training interventions (Raffoul & Lin, 2015). Evaluating providers' cultural learning and skill building with self-assessment questionnaires is a common approach, although there is a paucity of reliable, valid methods for assessment of cultural responsiveness (Gozu et al., 2007; Jongen et al., 2017). Further, self-assessment is subjective and may be biased (Truong et al., 2014). Cultural responsiveness training for providers is insufficient to improve patient outcomes without concurrent organizational efforts. Organizational cultural responsiveness assessment (usually by outside experts) includes review (and revision as needed) of documents, position statements, strategic plans, commitment of leadership, and workforce and leadership goals, followed by planning, implementation, and assessment of incremental organizational changes (Truong et al., 2014). A variety of online self- and organizational cultural responsiveness assessment resources and tools can help identify which areas of an organization are most in need of change (Campinha-Bacote, 2015; National Center for Cultural Competence, n.d.).

Patient satisfaction is influenced by numerous factors in the healthcare environment such as interactions with providers and other staff and physical aspects such as privacy and quietness of rooms, signage, and so forth. These and other important factors should be part of the process of organizational cultural responsiveness assessment. A provider's level of multicultural responsiveness has a significant effect on the satisfaction of minority patients in healthcare (Fuertes & Brobst, 2002). Counselors have considerable control over their attitudes, communication skills, technical skills, and responsiveness to the patient's needs, which all contribute to the patient experience (Ahmad et al., 2011). A provider's cultural responsiveness is, essentially, in the eye of the patient beholder. Patients' feelings of trust and satisfaction should be assessed early and often. In addition, given the prevalence of lack of trust in healthcare institutions and providers, it is appropriate to make general inquiries about prior experiences and expectations. To set a proactive tone for a session, genetic counselors can ask (in forms or in the intake process): "In general, how satisfied have you been with your past experiences in healthcare? Is there anything you want to share about your past experiences in healthcare that relates to our session?"

Genetic counselors and genetics centers can also assess patient trust and satisfaction by integrating questions into postcounseling surveys, such as in the example given in Table 29.1.

Satisfaction questions provide insight into the individual patient experience. When collected over time, the results may reveal trends about patients' perspectives on professionals' knowledge, skills, and attitudes. Patients' satisfaction with their interactions with providers is the most important aspect of the degree of cultural responsiveness of healthcare organizations (Weech-Maldonado, Elliott, et al., 2012). Patients consider friendliness, courtesy and respect, showing concern, spending enough time, promptness in receiving care/appointment, making the patient feel comfortable, answering questions, listening, using words that the patient can understand, and affordability/convenience of care to be important (Morales et al., 2003). These behaviors are also good practice. Effectively incorporating the skills of medical interpreters, using multilingual written and video resources, using teach-back, matching patient information needs to the information provided, offering additional appointments to gather more family history information and enhance rapport, and being flexible about the role of and implications for other family members regarding decision making and testing have been shown to be useful (Joseph & Guerra, 2015). Patients are more satisfied with culturally adapted genetic counseling sessions (Joseph & Guerra, 2015).

More research is needed to explore the impact of race and ethnicity on awareness, knowledge, and perceptions of genetic counseling, barriers and facilitators to participation, and outcomes (Southwick et al., 2020). Intersectionality challenges researchers and providers to understand the persistence of inequalities due to the complex and cumulative factors of racism, sexism, classism, and other experiences of discrimination, marginalization, and microaggressions in healthcare and society. It is essential to deeply explore the interactions of the social determinants of health and numerous social identities in determining interest in, use of, and satisfaction with genetic counseling services.

Minority patients benefit most by interacting with culturally competent providers working in a culturally competent milieu; both facilitate the goal of reducing racial/ethnic disparities in healthcare (Weech-Maldonado, Elliott, et al., 2012). Recruitment of diverse

Table 29.1 Example Post–Genetic Counseling Survey

	Mostly	Neutral	Rarely	Comments
I believe my genetic counselor was concerned about my well-being.				
My genetic counselor treated me with respect.				
My race and/or ethnicity did not affect the quality of care I received in genetic counseling.				
When I didn't understand what my genetic counselor said, I felt comfortable asking questions.				

students and providers adds valuable perspectives and approaches. Genetic counselors, graduate training programs, provider institutions, and professional organizations must all take responsibility. When the value of diversity is evident in standard clinical practice skills, program curricula, and institutions' and organizations' mission statements and policies, the field will be on track to provide culturally competent services to a multiracial/ethnic/religious/cultural society.

References

Accreditation Council for Genetic Counseling. (2019a). *Diversity task force.* https://www.gceducation.org/wp-content/uploads/2019/05/ACGC-Diversity-TF-charge-2019.pdf

Accreditation Council for Genetic Counseling. (2019b). *Practice-based competencies for genetic counselors.* https://www.gceducation.org/wp-content/uploads/2019/06/ACGC-Core-Competencies-Brochure_15_Web_REV-6-2019.pdf

Accreditation Council for Genetic Counseling. (2019c). *Standards of accreditation for graduate programs in genetic counseling.* file:///C:/Users/Warren/AppData/Local/Packages/Microsoft.MicrosoftEdge_8wekyb3d8bbwe/TempState/Downloads/Revised-Standards-of-Accreditation_Final_Effective-10.1.19%20(2).pdf

Agency for Healthcare Research and Quality. (2019). *What is cultural and linguistic competence?* https://www.ahrq.gov/ncepcr/tools/cultural-competence/definition.html

Ahmad, I., Nawaz, A., Khan, H., Rashid, M. A., & Khan, M. H. (2011). Predictors of patient satisfaction. *Gomal Journal of Medical Sciences, 9*(2), 183–188.

Aiyar, L., Channaoui, N., & Wang, V. O. (2020). Introduction: The state of minority and health disparities in research and practice in genetic counseling and genomic medicine. *Journal of Genetic Counseling, 29*(2), 142–146.

American Board of Genetic Counseling. (2018, August 1). *Examination specifications.* https://www.abgc.net/ABGC/media/Documents/ABGC-Exam-Specs-PUBLIC-effective-08-01-2018.pdf

American Psychological Association. (2017). *Multicultural guidelines. An ecological approach to context, identity, and intersectionality.* https://www.apa.org/about/policy/multicultural-guidelines.pdf

Anderson, M. R., Moscou, S., Fulchon, C., & Neuspiel, D. R. (2001). The role of race in the clinical presentation. *Family Medicine, 3*(6), 430–434.

Back, A. L., Arnold, R. M., Baile, W. F., Tulsky, J. A., & Fryer-Edwards, K. (2005). Approaching difficult communication tasks in oncology. *CA: A Cancer Journal for Clinicians, 55*(3), 164–177.

Bancroft, M. A. (2014). *Cultural competence in health and human services: A trainer's guide.* Culture and Language Press.

Bao, A. K., Bergner, A. L., Chan-Smutko, G., & Villiers, J. (2020). Reflections on diversity, equity, and inclusion in genetic counseling education. *Journal of Genetic Counseling, 29*(2), 315–323.

Barragan, D. I., Ormond, K. E., Strecker, M. N., & Weil, J. (2011). Concurrent use of cultural health practices and Western medicine during pregnancy: Exploring the Mexican experience in the United States. *Journal of Genetic Counseling, 20*(6), 609–624.

Beach, M. C., Price, E. G., Gray, T. L., Robinson, K. A., Gozu, A., Palacio, A., Smarth, C., Jenckes, M. W., Feuerstein, C., Bass, E. B., Powe, N. R., & Cooper, L. A. (2005). Cultural competence: A systematic review of health care provider educational interventions. *Medical Care, 43*(4), 356–373.

Campinha-Bacote, J. (2015). *Transcultural C.A.R.E. Associates.* http://transculturalcare.net/the-process-of-cultural-competence-in-the-delivery-of-healthcare-services/

Campinha-Bacote, J. (2018). Cultural competemility: A paradigm shift in the cultural competence versus cultural humility debate—Part I. *Online Journal of Issues in Nursing, 24*(1).

Carmichael, N., Redlinger-Grosse, K., & Birnbaum, S. (2020). Conscripted curriculum: The experiences of minority genetic counseling students. *Journal of Genetic Counseling, 29*(2), 303–314.

Carrillo, J. E., Green, A. R., & Betancourt, J. R. (1999). Cross-cultural primary care: A patient-based approach. *Annals of Internal Medicine, 130*(10), 829–834.

Carroll, N. M., Blum-Barnett, E., Madrid, S. D., Jonas, C., Janes, K., Alvarado, M., Bedoy, R., Paolino, V., Aziz, N., McGlynn, E. A., & Burnett-Hartman, A. N. (2020). Demographic differences in the utilization of clinical and direct-to-consumer genetic testing. *Journal of Genetic Counseling, 29*, 634–643. https://doi.org/10.1002/jgc4.1193

Centers for Disease Control and Prevention. (n.d.). *Building our understanding: Culture insights communicating with Hispanic/Latinos.* CDC's Healthy Communities Program. https://www.cdc.gov/nccdphp/dch/programs/healthycommunitiesprogram/tools/pdf/hispanic_latinos_insight.pdf

Centers for Disease Control and Prevention. (2024). *What is health literacy?* https://www.cdc.gov/health-literacy/php/about/index.html

Centers for Medicare and Medicaid Services. (2021). *Guide to developing a language access plan.* https://www.cms.gov/About-CMS/Agency-Information/OMH/Downloads/Language-Access-Plan-508.pdf

Chalela, P., Pagan, J. A., Su, D., Munoz, E., & Ramirez, A. G. (2012). Breast cancer genetic testing awareness, attitudes and intentions of Latinas living along the U.S.-Mexico border: A qualitative study. *Journal of Community Medicine and Health Education, 2*, 1000152. https://doi.org/10.4172/2161-0711.1000152

Champlain Valley Area Health Education Center. (2013). *Culturally competent care for providers.* https://www.researchgate.net/profile/Mohamed_Hammad11/post/How_do_you_develop_philosophical_competence_in_health_services/attachment/5bf0212a3843b00675456bd9/AS%3A693957570879489%401542463786117/download/Cultural+Competency+for+Healthcare+Providers13.pdf

Channaoui, N., Bui, K., & Mittman, I. (2020). Efforts of diversity and inclusion, cultural competency, and equity in the genetic counseling profession: A snapshot and reflection. *Journal of Genetic Counseling, 29*(2), 166–181.

Channaoui, N., Khan, A., Wiesman, C., Bui, K., Cunningham, M., Brown, K., Schneider, K. M., Platt, K., Delgado-Hodges, P., Thompson, N., Haas, B., Strang, K., Carey, M., Ramos, E., Arjunan, A., & Platt, J. (2020). Summary report of the 2019 Diversity and Inclusion Task Force of the National Society of Genetic Counselors. *Journal of Genetic Counseling, 29*(2), 192–201.

Clement, M. (2018, July 9). Six things that make college teachers successful. *Faculty Focus.*

Cleveland Clinic. (2017). *Diversity toolkit.* https://my.clevelandclinic.org/-/scassets/files/org/about/diversity/2016-diversity-toolkit.ashx

Cragun, D., Bonner, D., Kim, J., Akbari, M. R., Narod, S. A., Gomez-Fuego, M., Garcia, J. D., Vadaparampil, S. T., & Pal, T. (2015). Factors associated with genetic counseling and BRCA testing in a population-based sample of young Black women with breast cancer. *Breast Cancer Research and Treatment, 151*(1), 169–176.

Expert Panel on Cultural Competence Education for Students in Medicine and Public Health. (2012). *Cultural competence education for students in medicine and public health: Report of an expert panel.* Association of American Medical Colleges and Association of Schools of Public Health. https://www.pcpcc.org/sites/default/files/resources/Cultural%20Competence%20Education%20for%20Students%20in%20Medicine%20%26%20Public%20Health.pdf

Fortier, J. P. (2011). *Diversity training vs. cultural competency training.* http://www.diversityrx.org/blog/qa/diversity-training-v-cultural-competency-training

Fuertes, J. N., & Brobst, K. (2002). Clients' ratings of counselor multicultural competency. *Cultural Diversity and Ethnic Minority Psychology, 8*(3), 214–223.

Galanti, G.-A. (2008). *Caring for patients from different cultures* (4th ed.). University of Pennsylvania Press.

Garcia, G., Nation, C. L., & Parker, N. H. (2004). Paper contribution A. Increasing diversity in the health professions: A look at best practices in admissions. In B. D. Smedley, A. Stith Butler, & L. R. Bristow (Eds.), *In the nation's compelling interest: Ensuring diversity in the health-care workforce.* Institute of Medicine Committee on Institutional and Policy-Level Strategies for Increasing the Diversity of the U.S. Healthcare Workforce. National Academies Press.

Glenn, B. A., Chawla, N., & Bastani, R. (2012). Barriers to genetic testing for breast cancer risk among ethnic minority women: An exploratory study. *Ethnicity and Disease, 22*(3), 267–273.

Govere, L., & Govere, E. M. (2016). How effective is cultural competence training of healthcare providers on improving patient satisfaction of minority groups? A systematic review of literature. *Worldviews on Evidence-Based Nursing, 13*(6), 402–410.

Gozu, A., Beach, M. C., Price, E. G., Gary, T. L., Robinson, K., Palacio, A., Smarth, C., Jenckes, M., Feuerstein, C., Bass, E. B., Powe, N. R., & Cooper, L. A. (2007). Self-administered instruments to measure cultural competence of health professionals: A systematic review. *Teaching and Learning in Medicine, 19*(2), 180–190.

Guy, C. (2016). Genetic counseling milestones: A framework for student competency evaluation. *Journal of Genetic Counseling, 25*(4), 635–643.

Halbert, C. H., & Harrison, B. W. (2018). Genetic counseling among minority populations in the era of precision medicine. *American Journal of Medical Genetics, 178*(1), 68–74.

Hansen, N. D., Pepitone-Arreola-Rockwell, F., & Greene, A. F. (2000). Multicultural competence: Criteria and case examples. *Professional Psychology: Research and Practice, 31*(6), 652–660.

Humes, K. R., Jones, N. A., & Ramirez, R. R. (2011, March). *Overview of race and Hispanic origin: 2010. 2010 Census Briefs.* U.S. Census Bureau. https://www.census.gov/library/publications/2011/dec/c2010br-02.html

Hunt, L. M., & deVoogd, K. B. (2005). Clinical myths of the cultural "other": Implications for Latino patient care. *Academic Medicine, 80*(10), 918–924.

Isaacson, M. (2014). Clarifying concepts: Cultural humility or competency. *Journal of Professional Nursing, 30*(3), 251–258.

Jones, C. P. (2000). Levels of racism: A theoretical framework and a gardener's tale. *American Journal of Public Health, 20*(8), 1212–1215.

Jongen, C., McCalman, J., & Bainbridge, R. (2018). Health workforce cultural competency interventions: A systematic scoping review. *BMC Health Services Research, 18*(1), 232.

Joseph, G., & Guerra, C. (2015). To worry or not to worry: Breast cancer genetic counseling communication with low-income Latina immigrants. *Journal of Community Genetics, 6*(1), 63–76.

Joseph, G., Lee, R., Pasick, R. J., Guerra, C., Schillinger, D., & Rubin, S. (2019). Effective communication in the ear of precision medicine: A pilot intervention with low health literacy patients to improve genetic counseling. *European Journal of Medical Genetics, 62*(5), 357–367.

Joseph, G., Pasick, R. J., Schillinger, D., Luce, J., Guerra, C., & Cheng, J. K. Y. (2017). Information mismatch: Cancer risk counseling with diverse underserved patients. *Journal of Genetic Counseling, 26*(5), 1090–1104.

Kelly, N. (2008). *A medical interpreter's guide to telephone interpreting*. International Medical Interpreters Association. https://www.imiaweb.org/uploads/pages/307_2.pdf

Kessler, L. J., & Love, R. (2020). It's not wrong, it's just different. *Journal of Genetic Counseling, 29*(2), 324–328.

Kirmayer, L. J. (2012). Rethinking cultural competence. *Transcultural Psychiatry, 49*(2), 149–164.

Kleinman, A., Eisenberg, L., & Good, B. (1978). Culture, illness, and care: Clinical lessons from anthropologic and cross-cultural research. *Annals of Internal Medicine, 88*(2), 251–258.

Krist, A. H., Davidson, K. W., & Ngo-Metzger, Q. (2019). What evidence do we need before recommending routine screening for social determinants of health? *American Family Physician, 99*(10), 602–605.

Kutner, M., Greenberg, E., Jin, Y., Paulsen, C., Institute of Education Sciences, & National Center for Education Statistics. (2006). *Health literacy of America's adults: Results from the 2003 National Assessment of Adult Literacy*. https://nces.ed.gov/pubsearch/pubsinfo.asp?pubid=2006483

Lee, H. K., Veach, P. M., & LeRoy, B. S. (2009). An investigation of relationships among genetic counselors' supervision skills and multicultural counseling competence. *Journal of Genetic Counseling, 18*(3), 287–299.

Locatis, C., Williamson, D., Gould-Kabler, C., Zone-Smith, L., Detzler, I., Roberson, J., Maisiak, R., & Ackerman, M. (2009). Comparing in-person, video, and telephonic medical interpretation. *Journal of General Internal Medicine, 25*(4), 345–350.

Lui, P. P., & Quezada, L. (2019). Associations between microaggression and adjustment outcomes: A meta-analytic and narrative review. *Psychological Bulletin, 145*(1), 45–78.

Mai, P. L., Vadaparampil, S. T., Breen, N., McNeel, T. S., Wideroff, L., & Graubard, P. I. (2014). Awareness of cancer susceptibility genetic testing: the 2000, 2005, and 2010 National Health Interview Surveys. *American Journal of Preventative Medicine, 46*(5), 440–448.

McGinnis, M. A., Tahmassi, A. G., & Ramos, E. (2018). Towards cultural competence in the genomic age: A review of current health care provider educational trainings and interventions. *Current Genetic Medicine Reports, 6*(4), 187–198.

Merriam-Webster. (n.d.). *Culture*. https://www.merriam-webster.com/dictionary/culture

Mittman, I., Crombleholme, W. R., Green, J. R., & Golbus, M. S. (1998). Reproductive genetic counseling to Asian Pacific and Latin American Immigrants. *Journal of Genetic Counseling, 7*(1), 49–70.

Mittman, I. S., & Downs, K. (2008). Diversity in genetic counseling: Past, present and future. *Journal of Genetic Counseling, 17*(4), 301–313.

Morales, L. S., Puyol, J. A., & Hays, R. D. (2003). *Improving patient satisfaction surveys to assess cultural competence in health care*. California HealthCare Foundation, University of California at Los Angeles. https://www.chcf.org/wp-content/uploads/2017/12/PDF-PatientSurveysCulturalCompetence.pdf

Nadal, K. L. (2014). A guide to responding to microaggressions. *CUNY Forum*, *2*(1), 71–76.

Nadal, K. L., Griffin, K. E., Wong, Y., Hamit, S., & Rasmus, M. (2014). Racial microaggressions and mental health: Counseling clients of color. *Journal of Counseling and Development*, *92*(1), 57–66.

Nathan, M. L., Ormond, K. E., Dial, C. M., Gamma, A., & Lunn, M. R. (2018). Genetic counselors' and genetic counseling students' implicit and explicit attitudes towards homosexuality. *Journal of Genetic Counseling*, *28*(1), 91–101.

National Association of Social Workers. (2015). *Standards and indicators for cultural competence in social work practice*. https://www.socialworkers.org/LinkClick.aspx?fileticket=PonPTDEBrn4%3d&portalid=0

National Center for Cultural Competence. (n.d.). *Self-assessments*. Georgetown University, Thrive Center for Children, Families and Communities, Washington, DC. https://nccc.georgetown.edu/index.php

National Society of Genetic Counselors. (2018). Code of ethics. *Journal of Genetic Counseling*, *27*(1), 6–8.

National Society of Genetic Counselors. (2020). *PSS: Professional status survey*.

Office of Minority Health Resource Center. (2018). *National Standards for Culturally and Linguistically Appropriate Services in Health and Health Care (The National CLAS Standards)*. U.S. Department of Health and Human Services. https://minorityhealth.hhs.gov/omh/browse.aspx?lvl=2&lvlid=53

Online MSW Programs. (2020). *How to be culturally sensitive working with clients with a range of identities*. https://www.onlinemswprograms.com/resources/social-issues/how-to-be-culturally-sensitive/

Puchalski, C., & Romer, A. L. (2000). Taking a spiritual history allows clinicians to understand patients more fully. *Journal of Palliative Medicine*, *3*, 129–138.

Raffoul, M., & Lin, K. W. (2015). Cultural competence education for health care professionals. *American Family Physician*, *91*(8), 523–524.

Reis, L. M., Baumiller, R., Scrivener, W., Yager, G., & Warren, N. S. (2007). Spiritual assessment in genetic counseling. *Journal of Genetic Counseling*, *16*(1), 41–52.

Ridley, C. R., Mendoza, D. W., & Kanitz, B. G. (1994). Multicultural training: Reexamination, operationalization, and integration. *The Counseling Psychologist*, *22*, 227–289.

Ryan, C. (2013). *Language use in the United States: 2011* (American Community Survey Reports, ACS-22). U.S. Census Bureau. https://www.census.gov/library/publications/2013/acs/acs-22.html

Safeer, R. S., & Keenan, J. (2005). Health literacy: The gap between physicians and patients. *American Family Physician*, *72*(3), 463–468.

Sayani, A. (2019). Inequities in genetic testing for hereditary breast cancer: Implications for public health practice. *Journal of Community Genetics*, *10*(1), 35–39.

Schaa, K. L., Roter, D. L., Beisecker, B. B., Cooper, L. A., & Erby, L. H. (2015). Genetic counselors' implicit racial attitudes and their relationship to communication. *Health Psychology*, *34*(2), 111–119.

Sharif, S. M., Blyth, M., Admed, M., Sheridan, E., Saltus, R., Tonkin, E., & Kirk, M. (2019). Enhancing inclusion of diverse populations in genomics: A competence framework. *Journal of Genetic Counseling*, *29*(2), 282–292.

Sheppard, V. B., Mays, D., Tercyak, K. P., & LaVeist, T. (2013). Medical mistrust influences black women's level of engagement in BRCA1/2 genetic counseling and testing. *Journal of National Medical Association, 105*(1), 17–22.

Sherin, K., Adebanjo, T., & Jani, A. (2019). Social determinants of health: Family physicians' leadership role. *American Family Physician, 99*(8), 476–477.

Smith, S. C., Warren, N. S., & Misra, L. (1993). Minority recruitment into the genetic counseling profession. *Journal of Genetic Counseling, 2*(3), 171–181.

Southwick, S. V., Esch, R., Gasser, R., Cragun, D., Redlinger-Grosse, K., Marsalis, S., & Zierhut, H. A. (2020). Racial and ethnic differences in genetic counseling experiences and outcomes in the United States: A systematic review. *Journal of Genetic Counseling, 29*(2), 147–165.

Stuart, M. R., & Lieberman, J. A. (1993). *The fifteen-minute hour: Applied psychotherapy for the primary care physician* (2nd ed.). Praeger.

Sue, D. W., Capodilupo, C. M., Torino, G. C., Bucceri, J. M., Holder, A. M., Nadal, K. L., & Esquilin, M. (2007). Racial microaggressions in everyday life: Implications for clinical practice. *American Psychologist, 62*(4), 271–286.

Sussner, K., Edwards, T., Thompson, H., Jandorf, L., Kwate, N. O., Forman, A., Brown, K., Kapil-Pair, N., Bovbjerg, D., & Schwartz, M. (2011). Ethnic, racial and cultural identity and perceived benefits and barriers related to genetic testing for breast cancer among at-risk women of African descent in New York City. *Public Health Genomics, 14*(6), 356–370.

Tatum, B. D. (1992). Talking about race, learning about racism: The application of racial identity development theory in the classroom. *Harvard Educational Review, 62*(1), 1–25.

Taylor, M., & Hamdy, H. (2013). Adult learning theories: Implications for learning and teaching in medical education: AMEE Guide No. 83. *Medical Teacher, 35*(11), e1561–e1562. https://doi.org/10.3109/0142159X.2013.828153

Tervalon, M., & Murray-Garcia, J. (1998). Cultural humility versus cultural competence: A critical distinction in defining physician training outcomes in multicultural education. *Journal of Health Care for the Poor and Underserved, 9*(2), 117–125.

Truong, M., Paradies, Y., & Priest, N. (2014). Interventions to improve cultural competency in health care: A systematic review of reviews. *BMC Health Services Research, 14*, 99.

U.S. Equal Employment Opportunity Commission. (2014). *Fact sheet: Genetic Information Nondiscrimination Act*. https://www.eeoc.gov/laws/guidance/fact-sheet-genetic-information-nondiscrimination-act

U.S. Department of Health and Human Services. (2020). *Healthy People 2020*. https://www.healthypeople.gov/2020/about/foundation-health-measures/Disparities

VandenLangenberg, E., Veach, P. M., LeRoy, B. S., & Glessner, H. D. (2012). Gay, lesbian, and bisexual patients' recommendations for genetic counselors: A qualitative investigation. *Journal of Genetic Counseling, 21*(5), 741–747.

Vanneste, R., Chiu, S. M., Russell, L., & Fitzpatrick, J. (2013). Effects of second language usage on genetic counseling training and supervision. *Journal of Genetic Counseling, 22*(1), 58–75.

Warren, N. S. (2011). Introduction to the special issue: Toward diversity and cultural competence in genetic counseling. *Journal of Genetic Counseling, 20*(6), 543–546.

Warren, N. S., Parmar, S., & Wilson, P. L. (2019). COUNSELING and telegenetic encounters. *Perspectives in Genetic Counseling, 4*, 8–9.

Warren, N. S., & Wilson, P. L. (2013). COUNSELING: A 10-point approach to cultural competence in genetic counseling. *Perspectives in Genetic Counseling, 3*, 6–7.

Weech-Maldonado, R., Dreachslin, J. L., Brown, J., Pradhan, R., Rubin, K. L., Schiller, C., & Hays, R. D. (2012). Cultural competency assessment tool for hospitals: Evaluating hospitals' adherence to the culturally and linguistically appropriate service standards. *Health Care Management Review*, *37*(1), 54–66.

Weech-Maldonado, R., Elliott, M. N., Pradhan, R., Schiller, C., Hall, A., & Hays, R. D. (2012). Can hospital cultural competency reduce disparities in patient experiences with care? *Medical Care*, *50*(0), S48–S55.

Weil, J., & Mittman, I. (1993). A teaching framework for cross-cultural genetic counseling. *Journal of Genetic Counseling*, *2*(3), 159–169.

Weiss, B. D. (2007). *Health literacy and patient safety: Help patients understand. Manual for clinicians* (2nd ed.). AMA Foundation.

CHAPTER 30

GENETIC COUNSELING OUTCOMES, PATIENT EMPOWERMENT, AND THE GENETIC COUNSELING OUTCOME SCALE

MARION MCALLISTER

Introduction and Historical Context

Historically, what outcomes have been measured to evaluate genetic counseling and clinical genetics services?

It has long been recognized that measuring outcomes from genetic counseling is challenging. Traditional measures of outcomes used in other areas of healthcare (e.g., mortality and morbidity) are unlikely to be useful in genetic counseling due to the nature of the practice and intervention. In contrast to mortality and morbidity, outcome domains measured in studies assessing genetic counseling interventions include knowledge, information recall, reproductive intentions, decisions made, decisional conflict, psychological distress, patient satisfaction, perceived risk, perceived personal control, and subsequent health behaviors (Madlensky et al., 2017; Payne et al., 2008). Genetic counseling has been shown to increase patients' knowledge, perceived personal control, accuracy of perceived risk (but see the two following paragraphs), and positive health behaviors and to decrease psychological distress and decisional conflict. There is also evidence that patients are usually satisfied with genetic counseling (Madlensky et al., 2017).

Early studies aimed to assess genetic counseling patients' knowledge about genetic risks, testing, and inheritance. While some studies demonstrated good evidence of information recall (Somer et al., 1988), there is also published evidence that genetic counseling patients do not always accurately recall the precise recurrence risk figures given (Evans et al., 1994; Evers-Kieboons & van den Berghe, 1979). There is also evidence that educational interventions do not significantly improve subjective cancer risk perception among individuals from high-risk cancer families and that the best predictor of postintervention risk perception is individuals' baseline perceived risk (Dieng et al., 2014). Use of knowledge and recall of risk figures as outcome measures has been criticized, since these can be seen as tests of memory rather than measures of patient benefit. Edwards et al. (2008) found that addressing emotional issues (e.g., loss and grief) provided more benefit to patients than the educational aspects of genetic counseling.

In the context of genetic testing for autosomal dominant conditions, patient anxiety, depression, and worry have been assessed as outcomes. Similar patterns have been seen across a range of conditions (e.g., Huntington's disease, Alzheimer's disease, hereditary cancer syndromes), indicating that distress tends to increase in the short term after a test result noting pathogenic variant carrier status but that distress levels return to pretesting levels over the longer term. For individuals found not to be pathogenic variant carriers, distress tends to decrease over time (Almqvist et al., 2003; Butow et al., 2003; Duisterhof et al., 2001; Green et al., 2009; Hamilton et al., 2009; Meiser & Dunn, 2000; O'Neill et al., 2009; Timman et al., 2004). While these findings demonstrate that genetic testing does not cause significant long-term psychological harm to most people tested, small numbers of people tested do experience posttest distress, often those who have baseline levels of psychological distress (Almqvist et al., 2003; Meiser & Dunn, 2000). However, use of psychological distress as an outcome measure does not demonstrate positive change for individuals found to be pathogenic variant carriers, only that they tend not to experience increased distress over the long term.

What is the quality of outcome measures that have been used to evaluate genetic counseling and clinical genetics services?

A 2008 systematic review of outcome measures used to evaluate clinical genetics/genetic counseling identified 67 validated outcome measures that captured a total of 19 different outcome domains ranging from psychological distress and coping to decision-making knowledge, risk perception, and health status. Of those 67 measures, 37 were generic measures (e.g., health status, quality of life, psychological distress), and 30 measures had been developed for use in clinical genetics/genetic counseling (Payne et al., 2008). Forty-six of the identified measures had been used in just one study each. The wide range of outcome domains identified and the diversity of measures that had been used prior to 2008 to capture these domains as genetic counseling outcomes together demonstrate how much confusion there was at that time about which outcomes are most appropriate to measure in clinical genetics/genetic counseling.

For a psychometric measure to be fully validated, it should be assessed for certain properties including internal consistency, test–retest reliability, content validity, structural validity, construct validity, interpretability, and responsiveness (sensitivity to change over time; Mokkink et al., 2010; Terwee et al., 2012). As part of Payne and colleagues' (2008) systematic review, the extent of psychometric validation of the included measures was found to be limited, as shown in Table 30.1. While 63 of the 67 measures had been assessed for internal consistency, only 25 had been assessed for test–retest reliability, and only five for responsiveness.

Table 30.1 Extent of Psychometric Validation Was Limited

Validation	Number of studies
Validity	
Face	9
Content	23
Construct	26
Criterion	15
Reliability	
Internal consistency	63
Test–retest	25
Sensitivity to change	5
Interpretability	2

Internal consistency measures the correlations between items on the same test (Mokkink et al., 2010; Terwee et al., 2012) and is relatively straightforward to assess, requiring only a single administration of the questionnaire with a sample of the target population. The more items used to measure the relevant domain, the higher the internal consistency will be. A measure with many similar items will have a high internal consistency score, whereas a shorter measure with fewer items capturing the same domain is likely to have lower internal consistency. It is arguable whether internal consistency is a truly useful property for an outcome measure.

Test–retest reliability is not as straightforward to assess as internal consistency, because it requires two administrations of the questionnaire with the same sample of the target population, separated by a time interval during which the underlying construct is not expected to change but sufficiently long that participants will not remember their first set of responses (usually 2 to 4 weeks). Test–retest reliability is arguably a more useful property than internal consistency, as it assesses the likelihood that the questionnaire will provide, on average, a sufficiently similar score if the underlying construct measured (e.g., depression) has not changed (Mokkink et al., 2010; Terwee et al., 2012).

Assessment of responsiveness also requires two separate administrations of the questionnaire with the same sample of the target population, but this time an intervention is required between the two administrations that is expected to change the underlying construct (Mokkink et al., 2010; Terwee et al., 2012). Responsiveness is a very important property of any questionnaire intended for use as an outcome measure, because an outcome measure must be sensitive to change over time in the underlying construct measured; otherwise, postintervention benefits may not be detected. It is notable that only five of 67 measures identified by Payne et al. (2008) had been assessed for responsiveness.

Interpretability assesses whether a specific score change on the questionnaire matters to patients (versus statistically significant change), and it is assessed by establishing the minimal clinically important difference in a sample from the target population (McGlothlin & Lewis, 2014). Again, it is worth noting that only two of 67 outcome measures identified by Payne et al. (2008) had been assessed for interpretability.

Payne and colleagues' (2008) systematic review concluded that, at the time, there was considerable confusion about which outcomes are important for assessment of quality in clinical genetics/genetic counseling services and that the psychometric quality of available outcome measures was limited. The review also concluded that there are some aspects of the potential patient benefits that were not captured by the measures available at that time. However, the authors were unable to recommend which outcome measures were most appropriate to evaluate patient benefits.

Patient empowerment and the Genetic Counseling Outcome Scale

Patient-reported outcome measures and patient-reported experience measures

The terms "patient-reported outcome measures" (PROMs) and "patient-reported experience measures" (PREMs) have gained prominence in the last decade, alongside greater emphasis on gathering clinical data directly from patients regarding their perceptions of the outcomes they have gained from, as well as their experiences of clinical care. While these terms are relatively new and were not yet in widespread use in 2008, some of the outcome measures identified by Payne et al. (2008) would now be termed PROMs (e.g., the Perceived Personal Control [PPC] questionnaire; Berkenstadt et al., 1999) or PREMs (e.g., the Genetic Counseling Satisfaction Scale; Tercyak et al., 2001). PROMs are instruments, usually self-completion questionnaires, that measure patient-reported outcomes (PROs; Weldring & Smith, 2013). A PRO is "directly reported by the patient without interpretation of the patient's response by a clinician or anyone else and pertains to the patient's health, quality of life, or functional status associated with health care or treatment" (Weldring & Smith, 2013, p. 62). Examples of PROs include health-related quality of life, pain, and fatigue. In genetic counseling, an example is the perceived personal control construct, comprising cognitive, decisional, and behavioral control (Berkenstadt et al., 1999). PROMs can be generic (e.g., PROMs that measure health status such as the Euroqual (EQ-5D), which includes one item each capturing mobility, self-care, usual activity, pain/discomfort, and anxiety/depression) or disease or condition specific (e.g., PROMs that measure "asthma control"; Herdman et al., 2011; Weldring & Smith, 2013). A good-quality PROM will have evidence of reliability, validity, responsiveness, and interpretability (Mokkink et al., 2010). PREMs are "tools and instruments that report patient satisfaction scores with a health service and are generic tools that are often used to capture the overall patient experience of health care" (Weldring & Smith, 2013, p. 65). PROMs and PREMs are increasingly being used to evaluate healthcare delivered in practice, and there are moves toward using these data in making decisions about allocating funding resources in healthcare.

To address the issue identified by Payne et al (2008)—namely, that there are some aspects of the potential patient benefits from using clinical genetics/genetic counseling services that were not captured by available measures—a team at the North West Genetics Knowledge Park, Manchester, United Kingdom (Nowgen), embarked upon research to develop a valid, reliable, and responsive PROM.

Exploring patient outcomes from genetic counseling and clinical genetics services

Extensive qualitative research was conducted by the Nowgen team to explore patient benefits among those using clinical genetics/genetic counseling services. Participants in focus groups and interviews included patients and providers of those services, as well as representatives from a range of different patient support groups.

Focus group and interview transcripts were analyzed using grounded theory, a method for generating a theory or model of a (psycho)social concern or process using a qualitative approach (Glaser & Strauss, 1967; Strauss & Corbin, 2015). Analysis led to identification of an overarching construct labeled "empowerment," which summarized the patient outcomes valued by participants (McAllister et al., 2008; McAllister, Dunn, & Todd, 2011). Empowerment comprises five dimensions: cognitive, decisional, and behavioral control (which together make up the construct "perceived personal control") and two additional dimensions: emotional regulation and hope. *Cognitive control* refers to patients feeling that they have enough knowledge about a condition including risks to specified relatives and/or a satisfactory explanation for the sometimes tragic events that have occurred in their family relating to the condition. *Decisional control* refers to patients feeling able to make important life decisions relating to the family condition (e.g., whether and how to have children, whether or not to have a genetic test). *Behavioral control* refers to feeling able to use the health and social care systems for the benefit of the family. *Emotional regulation* refers to feeling able to manage one's feelings about having a genetic condition in the family. *Hope* refers to feeling hopeful about either one's own future or the future of one's children and other relatives and descendants. Interestingly, no differences emerged in this study between outcomes valued by different categories of patient (e.g., parents of a child affected by a genetic condition, adult patients affected by a genetic condition, individuals at genetic risk for developing a genetic condition or transmitting one to their children; McAllister et al., 2008; McAllister, Dunn, & Todd, 2011). However, this may have been due to the fact that the sample size was small, though it was relatively large for a qualitative study ($n = 52$).

The qualitative research also identified a series of emotional effects of genetic conditions among members of families affected by genetic conditions: anxiety, worry about risks to children, guilt, anger, uncertainty, depression, sadness, and grief (McAllister et al., 2007). Analysis identified the variability of genetic diseases and how the availability of early diagnosis and appropriate care can mitigate these emotional effects. Despite the many challenging emotional effects that genetic conditions can present to families, findings in this study also indicated that redemptive adjustment is possible, with some family members finding unexpected fulfillment and hope from rising to these challenges or by focusing their energy in new directions, such as involvement in or contributing to the work of patient support groups. The authors recommended that awareness among genetic counselors may support them to develop interventions to adjust the modifying conditions and support patients to manage the emotional challenges, thereby enabling them to better facilitate patient adjustment and improve patient outcomes (McAllister et al., 2007). While measures of psychological distress used as outcome measures from genetic counseling in the past have demonstrated that genetic counseling and testing do not cause significantly increased psychological distress, they may not be sufficiently sensitive to detect other changes in emotional effects that matter to patients, such as those relating to sadness, guilt, grief, and uncertainty.

Operationalizing "empowerment" to create a new PROM

At this point, it seemed opportune to consider whether the construct "empowerment" could be operationalized to create a PROM for use in evaluating genetic counseling and/or testing that could measure this novel outcome. Standard methods for questionnaire design were used, which involved creating a large item pool of 84 items with content validity ensured by comprehensively sampling from the qualitative data and supplementing this with the items from the PPC questionnaire (Berkenstadt et al., 1999) and those from the "emotional representations" subscale of the Revised Illness Perceptions questionnaire (Moss-Morris et al., 2002). Face validity was assessed in one focus group and four interviews with members of patient support groups for genetic conditions, which resulted in rewording of some items to improve clarity and understanding (McAllister, Wood, et al., 2011).

Exploratory factor analysis followed by oblique (promax) rotation was then performed on responses from a sample of 527 members of patient support groups for genetic conditions, with the aim of (a) informing item selection for the final (shorter) questionnaire and (2) assessing structural validity. Seven factors were extracted. Higher order factor analysis demonstrated that the seven factors exist under a single higher order construct, "empowerment." To create a more parsimonious measure, three to five items were selected from each of the seven factors based on factor loadings, but also based on issues identified in the qualitative data to be most troubling for participants, such as guilt and family communication, and on clinical judgment about which items might best inform interventions to improve patient outcomes. The final questionnaire is shown in Figure 30.1, containing 24 items and named the Genetic Counseling Outcome Scale (GCOS-24; McAllister, Wood, et al., 2011).

Psychometric properties of GCOS-24

Regarding structural validity of the GCOS-24, it is important to note that in the exploratory factor analysis, while the factor structure was stable as the sample size grew over 450, the rank order of items within factors was subject to sampling variation (McAllister, Wood, et al., 2011). The same factor structure has not been replicated in other studies (e.g., Costal Tirado et al., 2017), and we have recommended that the GCOS-24 be used as a unidimensional scale, providing one overall scale score, because the higher order factor analysis demonstrated that "empowerment" is a single higher order construct (McAllister, Wood, et al., 2011).

Internal consistency reliability (Cronbach's alpha = 0.87) and test–retest reliability of the GCOS-24 (intraclass correlation = 0.86) were assessed with samples of patient support group members (McAllister, Wood, et al., 2011). These reliability statistics are good, as reliabilities ideally should be between 0.7 and 0.9 (Mokkink et al., 2010). Responsiveness was assessed with a sample of patients attending a clinical genetics service in Manchester,

The Genetic Counseling Outcome Scale (GCOS-24)

Using the scale below, circle a number next to each statement to indicate how much you agree with the statement. Please answer all the questions. For questions that are not applicable to you, please choose option 4 (neither agree nor disagree).

1 = strongly disagree
2 = disagree
3 = slightly disagree
4 = neither disagree nor agree
5 = slightly agree
6 = agree
7 = strongly agree

		strongly disagree	disagree	slightly disagree	neither agree nor disagree	slightly agree	agree	strongly agree
1	I am clear in my own mind why I am attending the clinical genetics service.	1	2	3	4	5	6	7
2	I can explain what the condition means to people in my family who may need to know.	1	2	3	4	5	6	7
3	I understand the impact of the condition on my child(ren)/any child I may have.	1	2	3	4	5	6	7
4	When I think about the condition in my family, I get upset.	1	2	3	4	5	6	7
5	I don't know where to go to get the medical help I / my family need(s).	1	2	3	4	5	6	7
6	I can see that good things have come from having this condition in my family.	1	2	3	4	5	6	7
7	I can control how this condition affects my family.	1	2	3	4	5	6	7
8	I feel positive about the future.	1	2	3	4	5	6	7
9	I am able to cope with having this condition in my family.	1	2	3	4	5	6	7
10	I don't know what could be gained from each of the options available to me.	1	2	3	4	5	6	7
11	Having this condition in my family makes me feel anxious.	1	2	3	4	5	6	7
12	I don't know if this condition could affect my other relatives (brothers, sisters, aunts, uncles, cousins).	1	2	3	4	5	6	7
13	In relation to the condition in my family, nothing I decide will change the future for my children / any children I might have.	1	2	3	4	5	6	7
14	I understand the reasons why my doctor referred me to the clinical genetics service.	1	2	3	4	5	6	7
15	I know how to get the non-medical help I / my family needs(e.g. educational, financial, social support).	1	2	3	4	5	6	7
16	I can explain what the condition means to people outside my family who may need to know (e.g. teachers, social workers).	1	2	3	4	5	6	7
17	I don't know what I can do to change how this condition affects me / my children.	1	2	3	4	5	6	7
18	I don't know who else in my family might be at risk for this condition.	1	2	3	4	5	6	7
19	I am hopeful that my children can look forward to are warding family life.	1	2	3	4	5	6	7
20	I am able to make plans for the future.	1	2	3	4	5	6	7
21	I feel guilty because I (might have) passed this condition on to my children.	1	2	3	4	5	6	7
22	I am powerless to do anything about this condition in my family.	1	2	3	4	5	6	7
23	I understand what concerns brought me to the clinical genetics service.	1	2	3	4	5	6	7
24	I can make decisions about the condition that may change my child(ren)'s future / the future of any child(ren) I may have.	1	2	3	4	5	6	7

McAllister M, Wood A, Dunn G, Shiloh S,Todd C. (2011) The Genetic Counseling Outcome Scale: a new patient-reported outcome measure for clinical genetics services. *Clinical Genetics*, 79, 413–424.

FIGURE 30.1 The Genomics Counseling Outcome Scale (GCOS-24).

(From McAllister, Wood, et al., 2011)

United Kingdom. Two hundred and forty-one patients completed the GCOS-24 before, and 2 to 4 weeks after, their first appointment at the service. Mean GCOS-24 scores were statistically significantly higher following clinic attendance, with a medium-to-large effect size (Cohen's $d = 0.7$; McAllister, Wood, et al., 2011).

Construct validity of the GCOS-24 was assessed by testing some hypotheses regarding how GCOS-24 scores were theoretically expected to correlate or not correlate with scores on other related and unrelated measures (McAllister, Wood, et al., 2011). We expected GCOS-24 scores to be significantly positively correlated with internal health locus of control, PPC, authenticity, and satisfaction with life, with the highest correlation being with PPC. This is what we found, demonstrating good convergent validity. We predicted GCOS-24 scores to have no significant correlation with chance health locus of control and powerful others health locus of control, and this is what we found, demonstrating good divergent validity. We expected GCOS-24 scores to be significantly negatively correlated with depression and anxiety. We found that empowerment was significantly negatively correlated with depression, but we found a small positive but not significant correlation with anxiety (McAllister, Wood, et al., 2011). The lack of significant correlation with anxiety was unexpected, but this may reflect predictions of the helplessness/hopelessness model of depression, which postulates that the causes of depression are related to perceptions of lack of control over stressful life events (Abrahamson et al., 1978; Alloy et al., 1990). It is plausible that the GCOS-24, which contains a number of items relating to personal control, would correlate more significantly with depression than with anxiety.

A follow-up study published in 2019 established that the minimum clinically important difference for the GCOS-24 was a score increase of 10.3 points after using a clinical genetics service (Thomas & McAllister, 2019). This is the smallest change in genetic counseling outcome that matters to patients. However, the sample size in this study was quite small, and it will be important to replicate these findings in a larger study.

Together with the qualitative research, these findings demonstrate that the GCOS-24 is valid, reliable, interpretable, and responsive to change over time and that it measures an outcome domain (empowerment) that is valued by patients and by providers of genetic counseling and testing services. The GCOS-24 therefore has potential as a PROM for use in research to evaluate new interventions in, for example, randomized controlled trails, as well as in clinical practice to generate evidence that genetic counseling and testing provide benefits to patients; it may also potentially be useful in comparing the performance of different services.

Expanded Uses of GCOS-24

Since publication in 2011, the GCOS-24 has been used to evaluate genetic counseling and testing in clinical practice in a number of national and international contexts. In 2012–2013, the GCOS-24 was used in a pilot study evaluating the performance of five clinical genetics centers in the United Kingdom. Patients were asked to complete the GCOS-24 before and 2 to 4 weeks after their first appointment at the service. Each center was shown to demonstrate statistically significant improvement in mean GCOS-24 scores, even with small samples of patients (n = 42 to 74; McAllister, 2016). This was the first time that clinical genetics services delivered by the UK National Health Service were shown to demonstrate delivery of measurable patient benefits.

The GCOS-24 has also been used to evaluate a novel psychiatric genetic counseling service for individuals with nonsyndromic psychiatric disorders and their relatives in Vancouver, Canada. Seventy-five patients completed the GCOS-24 before and 1 month after clinic attendance, and again, a statistically significant improvement in mean GCOS-24 scores was observed, with a large effect size (Cohen's $d = 1$; Inglis et al., 2015). It is interesting that a higher effect size was achieved by a service that offers genetic counseling but no genetic testing. Large effect sizes have also been reported using the GCOS-24 in other contexts too (e.g., cardiovascular genetics; Ison et al., 2019).

A more recent study by the Vancouver group demonstrated that patients who derive the most benefit from psychiatric genetic counseling (greatest change scores on GCOS-24 after psychiatric genetic counseling) are the patients who score lowest before genetic counseling (Gerrard et al., 2020). The authors suggested that there may be some value in considering the use of baseline GCOS-24 scores to identify patients to prioritize (e.g., by providing earlier appointments to patients with the lowest GCOS-24 scores). The Vancouver group has also used the GCOS-24 to identify, prior to genetic counseling, where genetic counselors can best focus their genetic counseling, by addressing issues indicated by individual GCOS-24 items where patients score particularly low.

The GCOS-24 was used in a study in Wales exploring whether PROM data could be useful for quality improvement in clinical genetics (Costal Tirado et al., 2017). Ninety-six patients completed the GCOS-24 before and 2 to 4 weeks after clinic attendance. Once again, statistically significant improvements in GCOS-24 scores were observed following clinic attendance, with a medium-to-large effect size (Cohen's $d = 0.64$), demonstrating that patient benefits were delivered. However, a microanalysis indicated that there were some areas where the data demonstrated patients were deriving less benefit than other areas. For example, it was clear that patients were deriving less benefit in the area of emotional regulation than other aspects of empowerment captured by the GCOS-24, potentially signaling a need for additional counseling to address deeper levels of emotional distress. As data collection and analysis proceeded, meetings were held with the clinical team to monitor patient response rates and to discuss how the PROM data might be useful. Genetic counsellors ($n = 4$) and clinical geneticists ($n = 2$) were interviewed to explore their views. Qualitative analysis of the interview data demonstrated commitment among the clinical staff for use of PROM data for quality improvement, as well as strong support for the GCOS-24 in particular. Staff were in support of regular collection and analysis of GCOS-24 data, with a commitment to take steps to address areas where the data indicate that patients may not be benefiting as much as they could be (Costal Tirado et al., 2017). A study in Singapore evaluating a cancer genetics service using the GCOS-24 also found greater improvement in cognitive domains captured by the GCOS-24 than emotional domains (Yuen et al., 2020). This may reflect that emotional domains are particularly intractable among individuals from families affected by a range of genetic conditions, highlighting that a greater emphasis on using counseling skills in genetic counseling practice may improve patient outcomes.

Together, these studies demonstrate clearly that in many varied clinical and international contexts, the GCOS-24 can be used to measure patient outcomes effectively and demonstrate that services are providing measurable benefits to the patients they serve.

Translations of GCOS-24

Danish (Diness et al., 2017), Spanish (Munoz-Caballo et al., 2018), Brazilian Portuguese (Segundo-Ribeiro et al., 2020), and Dutch (Voorwinden et al., 2019) translations of the GCOS-24 have been published. The Danish, Spanish, and Brazilian Portuguese translations were developed using international guidelines on methods for translation and cross-cultural adaptation of measurement scales (Beaton et al., 2000; Wild et al., 2005). This involves two independent forward translations by native target-language speakers, two independent backward translations by native English-language speakers, cognitive interviews with 10 to 15 members of the target population to assess whether the questionnaire items retain the intended "meaning" in the target language, and oversight by an expert panel (Beaton et al., 2000; Wild et al., 2005). One issue that arose in adapting the GCOS-24 for use in both Spain and Denmark was translation of the term "genetic condition," which has no direct equivalent in either Spanish or Danish. In English, the term "genetic condition" was used to emphasize that some genetic conditions (e.g., deafness) are not necessarily considered disorders or diseases by members of affected families. For the Spanish GCOS-24, the Spanish term equivalent to "genetic disorder," *trastorno genético*, was used, which is the term commonly used by genetics health professionals in Spain. For the Danish GCOS-24, the word *tilstand* was the closest equivalent.

The Danish, Spanish, and Brazilian Portuguese translations retained all 24 items, but the Dutch version retained only 18 of the original items as following factor analysis, items 13, 15, 22, and 24 were found to have low factor loadings and low interitem correlations with other items in the scale (Voorwinden et al., 2019). The groups who developed the Danish, Spanish, and Brazilian Portuguese translations did not conduct any factor analysis, but the Dutch group conducted both exploratory and confirmatory factor analysis and proposed a main scale capturing empowerment with six subscales suggested: uncertainty about heredity, hope, negative emotions, knowledge about the condition, knowledge about genetic services, and uncertainty about the treatment (Voorwinden et al., 2019).

The Dutch GCOS-18 and the Spanish, Danish, and Brazilian Portuguese GCOS-24 all have good internal consistency (Diness et al., 2017; Munoz-Caballo et al., 2018; Segundo-Ribeiro et al., 2020; Voorwinden et al., 2019). Test–retest reliability has not yet been assessed for the Danish and Spanish GCOS-24, but the Dutch GCOS-18 has very good test–retest reliability (intraclass correlation = 0.92), and the Brazilian Portuguese GCOS-24 has moderate test–retest reliability (intraclass correlation = 0.52). The Danish GCOS-24 has not been assessed for responsiveness, but the Dutch GCOS-18 shows responsiveness to change with a small effect size (Cohen's $d = 0.3$), though the authors attribute this to the sample as effect sizes using other questionnaires with the same sample also showed small effect sizes (Voorwinden et al., 2019). The Spanish GCOS-24 also demonstrated responsiveness to change over time with a medium-to-large effect size (Cohen's $d = 0.7$; Munoz-Caballo et al., 2018).

Other translations of the GCOS-24 currently under development include Japanese (Sayako Takahashi, personal communication) and Swedish (Rebecka Pestoff, personal communication). The English-language GCOS-24 has also been adapted for use in Singapore (Yuen et al., 2020).

Development of a short form—the Genomics Outcome Scale

With 24 items, each with seven response options, the GCOS-24 produces a large number of possible response permutations (1.92×10^{20}). Furthermore, it is unclear how to interpret differences in score and between items. Attaching "preference weights" to the measure to reflect the value or priority placed on each item by the target population would make it clear how to interpret differences in score (Sinnott et al., 2007). A shorter version of the questionnaire would make it feasible to design a study to elicit preference weights and facilitate use of the measure in economic evaluations of genetic and genomic testing with and without genetic counseling. Another emerging issue with the GCOS-24 is that items 1, 14, and 23 refer specifically to clinical genetics services, which makes the measure unsuitable for use where genetic testing/counseling is done outside clinical genetics services. With the growth of "mainstreaming genetic testing," where genetic testing is offered in, for example, oncology, pediatrics, and neurology (Lo et al., 2014; Rahman et al., 2014; Velente et al., 2008), it would be helpful to have a valid and reliable PROM suitable for use in evaluating genetic counseling and/or testing in other contexts. A shorter measure would also reduce respondent burden.

For these reasons, we began a study in 2017 to develop a short form of the GCOS-24 for use both within and beyond clinical genetics services, which would maintain the ability of the GCOS-24 to capture empowerment, using both qualitative methods and modern psychometric methods (item response theory [IRT]; Alonso et al., 2013; Nguyen et al., 2014). IRT methods enable item comparison without loss of scale precision or content validity.

The study began with cognitive interviews (Irwin et al., 2009) with 10 members of UK-based patient support groups for genetic conditions to explore interpretability of GCOS-24 items and which GCOS-24 items were most highly valued by the target population. The interview identified 12 of the 24 GCOS items that were strong candidates for retention: items 2, 4, 5, 8, 9, 12, 15, 16, 17, 18, 20, and 24. The interviews also identified that participants experienced confusion when answering items beginning with "I don't know." Seven of the 10 participants selected a response option contrary to what they meant when thinking aloud about such an item. A decision was therefore made that any items retained in the shorter scale containing "I don't know" would be reworded to "I know" (Grant et al., 2019).

Items 1, 14, and 23 were not considered for retention because they specifically refer to "clinical genetics services." Items with poor discriminative properties were also not selected for retention. Item characteristic curves and item information curves were generated using the graded response model (Samejima, 1969) to assess the likelihood of respondents selecting a certain response option at various levels of "empowerment." Individual scale items that are good discriminators show clear peaks on item characteristic curves ordered from "strongly disagree" at low levels of "empowerment" to "strongly agree" at high levels of "empowerment," whereas items that are poor discriminators show that just one or two response options are the primary choice across a wide range of "empowerment." To avoid redundancy in the shorter scale, items that capture a similar domain were also not retained together. The item information curves as well as the findings from the cognitive interview were used to identify superior items. Following this, 10 GCOS-24 items remained under consideration: 4, 8, 9, 12, 15, 16, 17, 18, 20, and 24.

Rasch analysis was then performed to assess various combinations of these 10 items, ensuring that each dimension of empowerment was represented in every combination under consideration. This enabled identification of an optimal six-item scale containing GCOS-24 items 4, 16, 17, 18, 20, and 24. GCOS-24 items 16 and 17, which contained "I don't know," were reworded to "I know." GCOS-24 item 24 was reworded to "I can make decisions about the condition that may change my future or my child(ren)'s future" since the qualitative data indicated that participants without children found items only applicable to those with children to be problematic. The six-item scale correlates highly with the GCOS-24 (Pearson's $r = 0.838$, 99% confidence), demonstrating that the shorter scale retains the ability to capture "empowerment." Examination of the rating scale characteristic curves and the rating scale statistics for the items in the shorter scale showed only five peaks, indicating that the "slightly disagree" and "slightly agree" response options could be collapsed with "disagree" and "agree," respectively, without compromising scale quality.

As shown in Figure 30.2, the final six-item scale has five response options and was named the Genomics Outcome Scale (GOS) to facilitate its use where nongenetics healthcare professionals, outside the context of clinical genetics services, discuss genetic risks and/or genetic tests with patients.

The GOS provides a less burdensome scale for patients to complete yet still appropriately captures "empowerment." The GOS is applicable both within clinical genetics and genetic counseling services and in other healthcare contexts where genetic risks and/or genetic

The Genomics Outcome Scale (GOS)

Using the scale below, circle a number next to each statement to indicate how much you agree with the statement. Please answer all the questions.

1 = strongly disagree
2 = disagree
3 = neither disagree nor agree
4 = agree
5 = strongly agree

		strongly disagree	disagree	neither agree nor disagree	agree	strongly agree
1	I can explain what the condition means to people outside my family who may need to know (e.g. teachers, social workers).	1	2	3	4	5
2	I know who else in my family might be at risk for this condition.	1	2	3	4	5
3	When I think about the condition in my family, Iget upset.	1	2	3	4	5
4	I know what I can do to change how this condition affects me / my children.	1	2	3	4	5
5	I am able to make plans for thefuture.	1	2	3	4	5
6	I can make decisions about the condition that may change my future or my child(ren)'s future	1	2	3	4	5

Grant P, Pampaka M, Payne K, Clarke A, McAllister M. Developing a short-form of the Genetic Counselling Outcome Scale: The Genomics Outcome Scale. *Eur J Med Genet* EPub 26 November 2018. https://doi.org/10.1016/j.ejmg.2018.11.015

FIGURE 30.2 The Genomics Outcome Scale (GOS).

(From Grant et al., 2019)

tests are offered and generates a significantly smaller number of response permutations (1.56×10^4) compared to the GCOS-24 (1.92×10^{20}).

Current limitations of GOS

While the GOS has potential for use as a PROM, it has not yet been assessed for test–retest reliability, responsiveness, or interpretability (e.g., by establishing the minimum clinically important difference). Assessment of these important psychometric properties is needed before widespread use. Data are currently being collected across five clinical genetics centers in the United Kingdom for assessment of responsiveness of the GOS. Data analysis from these exercises will also be fed back to the relevant centers as these data may provide useful feedback for the centers regarding their performance in terms of delivering empowerment benefits for their patients.

The Future

The National Society of Genetic Counselors' Outcomes Committee is currently exploring whether the GCOS-24 can be endorsed by the National Quality Form (NQF). The NQF is a not-for-profit organization that aims to catalyze improvements in healthcare. The NQF endorsement is a quality mark, and NQF-endorsed measures are used across many federal, private, and state programs in the United States. NQF endorsement involves assessment of the psychometric properties of the instrument as well as development of a performance measure known as a PRO-PM (NQF, 2013). PRO-PMs are organization-level measures that enable measurement and comparison of the performance of different healthcare organizations. PROM-PMs can be used in quality improvement and accountability activities, including public reporting and performance-based payment. Key components of a PRO-PM include the instrument that measures the health concept of interest (in this case, the GCOS-24), the calculation of the performance score (PRO-PM), specification of the target population as well as inclusion and exclusion criteria, and a risk adjustment methodology.

Regarding the GOS, the authors commented that there is some scope to further develop this measure (Grant et al., 2019). An item of the GCOS-24 ("I can make decisions about the condition that may change my child[ren]'s future/the future of any child[ren] I may have") will only be relevant to patients who have or plan to have children. The item was reworded to include a reference to the patient's own future (e.g., "I can make decisions about the condition that may change my future, or my child[ren]'s future"). The authors also commented that the elimination of GCOS-24 item 2 ("I can explain what the condition means to people in my family who may need to know"), with GCOS-24 item 16 retained instead ("I can explain what the condition means to people outside my family who may need to know"), resulted in some loss of information that may be of value to patients and their healthcare providers (Grant et al., 2019). Another development that might be beneficial could be to merge these two items to create a new item that retains more valuable information (e.g., "I can explain what the condition means to people who may need to know"). These changes were beyond the scope of the GOS development study, because any newly worded items would result in a new and different scale that would require validation.

Conclusion

Following a period of confusion regarding how to best evaluate outcomes from genetic counseling, development of both the GCOS-24 and GOS has enabled clinical genetics and genetic counseling services to measure "empowerment," a patient-reported outcome shown to be valued by both patients and service providers. Both the GCOS-24 and GOS show good psychometric properties, with the GCOS-24 more fully validated to date than the GOS. Furthermore, the GCOS-24 has been translated and adapted for use in Denmark, Spain, Brazil, and the Netherlands with good psychometric properties to date. International clinical genetics/genetic counseling services consistently demonstrate delivery of empowerment benefits to their patients using English, Danish, Spanish, and Dutch versions of the GCOS-24.

References

Abrahamson, L. Y., Seligman, M. E. P., & Teasdale, J. D. (1978). Learned helplessness in humans: Critique and reformulation. *Journal of Abnormal Psychology*, *87*, 49–74.

Alloy, L. B., Kelly, K. A., Mineka, S., & Clements, C. M. (1990). Comorbidity of anxiety and depressive disorders: A helplessness–hopelessness perspective. In J. D. Master & C. R. Cloninger (Ed.), *Comorbidity of mood and anxiety disorders* (pp. 499–543). American Psychiatric Press.

Almqvist, E. W., Brinkman, R. R., Wiggins, S., Hayden, M. R., & Canadian Collaborative Study of Predictive Testing. (2003). Psychological consequences and predictors of adverse events in the first 5 years after predictive testing for Huntington's disease. *Clinical Genetics*, *64*, 300–309.

Alonso, J., Bartlett, S. J., Rose, M., Aaronson, N. K., Chaplin, J. E., Efficace, F., Lepglege, A., Lu, A., Tulsky, D. S., Raat, H., Ravens-Sieberer, U., Revicki, D., Terwee, C. B., Valderas, J. M., Cella, D., & Forrest, C. B. (2013). The case for an international patient-reported outcomes measurement information system (PROMIS®) initiative. *Health and Quality of Life Outcomes*, *11*, 210.

Beaton, D. E., Bombardier, C., Guillemin, F., & Ferraz, M. B. (2000). Guidelines for the process of cross-cultural adaptation of self-report measures. *Spine*, *25*, 3186–3191.

Berkenstadt, M., Shiloh, S., Barkai, G., Nat-Mariam Katznelson, M., & Goldman, B. (1999). Perceived personal control (PPC): A new concept in measuring outcome of genetic counseling. *American Journal of Medical Genetics*, *82*, 53–59.

Butow, P. N., Lobb, E. A., Meiser, B., Barratt, A., & Tucker, K. M. (2003). Psychological outcomes and risk perception after genetic testing and counselling in breast cancer: A systematic review. *Medical Journal of Australia*, *178*, 77–81.

Costal Tirado, A., McDermott, A. M., Thomas, C., Ferrick, D., Harris, J., Edwards, A., & McAllister, M. (2017). Using patient-reported outcome measures for quality improvement in clinical genetics: An exploratory study. *Journal of Genetic Counseling*, *26*, 1017–1028.

Dieng, M., Watts, C. G., Kasparian, N. A., Morton, R. L., Mann, G. J., & Cust, A. E. (2014). Improving subjective perception of personal cancer risk: Systematic review and meta-analysis of educational interventions for people with cancer or at high risk of cancer. *Psycho-Oncology, 23*, 613–625.

Diness, B. R., Overbeck, G., Hortshoj, T. D., Hammer, T. B., Timshel, S., Sorensen, E., & McAllister, M. (2017). Translation and adaptation of the Genetic Counselling Outcome Scale (GCOS-24) for use in Denmark. *Journal of Genetic Counseling, 26*(5), 1080.

Duisterhof, M., Trijsburg, R. W., Niermeijer, M. F., Roos, R. A., & Tibben, A. (2001). Psychological studies in Huntington's disease: Making up the balance. *Journal of Medical Genetics, 38*, 852–861.

Edwards, A., Gray, J., Clarke, A., Dundon, J., Elwyn, G., Gaff, C., Hood, K., Iredale, R., Sivell, S., Shaw, C., & Thornton, H. (2008). Interventions to improve risk communication in clinical genetics: Systematic review. *Patient Education and Counseling, 71*, 4–25.

Evans, D. G. R., Blair, V., Greenhalgh, R., Hopwood, P., & Howell, A. (1994). The impact of genetic counselling on risk perception in women with a family history of breast cancer. *British Journal of Cancer, 70*, 934–938.

Evers-Kiebooms, G., & van den Berghe, H. (1979). Impact of genetic counseling: A review of published follow-up studies. *Clinical Genetics, 15*, 465–474.

Gerrard, S., Inglis, A., Morris, E., & Austin, J. (2020). Relationships between patient- and session-related variables and outcomes of psychiatric genetic counseling. *European Journal of Human Genetics, 28*, 907–914.

Glaser, B., & Strauss, A. (1967). *The discovery of grounded theory: Strategies for qualitative research*. Aldine Publishing Company.

Grant, P., Pampaka, M., Payne, K., Clarke, A., & McAllister, M. (2019). Developing a short-form of the Genetic Counselling Outcome Scale: The Genomics Outcome Scale. *European Journal of Human Genetics, 62*, 324–334.

Green, R. C., Roberts, J. S., Cupples, L. A., Relkin, N. R., Whitehouse, P. J., Brown, T., Eckert, S. L., Butson, M., Sadovnick, A. D., Quaid, K. A., Chen, C., Cook-Deegan, R., & Farrer, L. A. (2009). Disclosure of *APOE* genotype for risk of Alzheimer's disease. *New England Journal of Medicine, 361*, 245–254.

Hamilton, J. G., Lobel, M., & Moyer, A. (2009). Emotional distress following genetic testing for hereditary breast and ovarian cancer: A meta-analytic review. *Health Psychology, 28*, 510–518.

Herdman, M., Gudex, C., Lloyd, A., Janssen, M. F., Kind, P., Parkin, D., Bonsel, G., & Badia, X. (2011). Development and preliminary testing of the new five-level version of EQ-5D (EQ-5D-5 L). *Quality of Life Research, 20*, 1727–1736.

Inglis, A., Koehn, D., McGillivray, B., Stewart, S. E., & Austin, J. (2015). Evaluating a unique, specialist psychiatric genetic counseling clinic: Uptake and impact. *Clinical Genetics, 87*, 218–224.

Irwin, D., Varni, J., Yeatts, K., & DeWalt, D. (2009). Cognitive interviewing methodology in the development of a pediatric item bank. *Health and Quality of Life Outcomes, 7*, 3.

Ison, H. E., Ware, S. M., Schwantes-An, T-H., Freeze, S., Elmore, L., & Spoonamore, K. G. (2019). The impact of cardiovascular genetic counseling on patient empowerment. *Journal of Genetic Counseling, 28*, 570–577.

Lo, C., Martindale, J., Hadjivassiliou, M., Martin, P., Dalton, A., & Bandmann, O. (2014). The documentation of consent and disclosure of neurogenetic testing outside clinical genetics. *Neurogenetics, 15*, 19–21.

Madlensky, L., Trepanier, A. M., Cragun, D., Lerner, B., Shannon, K. M., & Zierhut, H. (2017). A rapid systematic review of outcomes studies in genetic counseling. *Journal of Genetic Counseling, 26*, 361–378.

McAllister, M. (2016). Genomics and patient empowerment. In D. Kumar & R. Chadwick (Eds.), *Genomics and society* (pp. 39–68). Elsevier.

McAllister, M., Dunn, G., & Todd, C. (2011). Empowerment: Qualitative underpinning of a new patient reported outcome for clinical genetics services. *European Journal of Human Genetics, 19*, 125–130.

McAllister, M., Payne, K., Nicholls, S., Donnai, D., Davies, L., & MacLeod, R. (2007). The emotional effects of genetic disease: Implications for clinical genetics. *American Journal of Medical Genetics Part A, 143A*, 2651–2661.

McAllister, M., Payne, K., Nicholls, S., MacLeod, R., Donnai, D., & Davies, L. (2008). Patient empowerment in clinical genetics services. *Journal of Health Psychology, 13*, 887–897.

McAllister, M., Wood, A., Dunn, G., Shiloh, S., & Todd, C. (2011). The Genetic Counseling Outcome Scale: A new patient-reported outcome measure for clinical genetics services. *Clinical Genetics, 79*, 413–424.

McGlothlin, A. E., & Lewis, R. J. (2014). Minimal clinically important difference: Defining what really matters to patients. *JAMA, 312*, 1342–1343.

Meiser, B., & Dunn, S. (2000). Psychological impact of genetic testing for Huntington's disease: An update of the literature. *Journal of Neurology, Neurosurgery, and Psychiatry, 69*, 574–578.

Mokkink, L. B., Terwee, C. B., Patrick, D. L., Alonso, J., Stratford, P. W., Knol, D. L., Bouter, L M, & de Vet, H. C. W. (2010). The COSMIN checklist for assessing the methodological quality of studies on measurement properties of health status measurement instruments: An international Delphi study. *Quality of Life Research, 19*, 539–549.

Moss-Morris, R., Weinman, J., Petrie, K. J., Horne, R., Cameron, L. D., & Buick, D. (2002). The Revised Illness Perception Questionnaire (IPQ-R). *Psychology and Health, 17*, 1–16.

Munoz-Caballo, P., Garcia-Minaur, S., Espinell-Vallejo, M. E., Fernandez-Franco, L., Stephens, A., Santos-Simarro, F., Lapunzina-Badia, P., & McAllister, M. (2018). Translation and cross-cultural adaptation with preliminary validation of GCOS-24 for use in Spain. *Journal of Genetic Counseling, 27*(3), 732–743.

National Quality Forum. (2013). *Patient-reported outcomes in performance measurement*. https://www.qualityforum.org/Publications/2012/12/Patient-Reported_Outcomes_in_Performance_Measurement.aspx

Nguyen, T., Han, H., Kim, M., & Chan, K. (2014). An introduction to item response theory for patient-reported outcome measurement. *The Patient, 7*, 23–35.

O'Neill, S. C., Rini, C., & Schwartz, M. D. (2009). Distress among women receiving uninformative *BRCA1/2* results: 12-month outcomes. *Psycho-Oncology, 18*, 1088–1096.

Payne, K., Nicholls, S., McAllister, M., MacLeod, R., Donnai, D., & Davies, L. (2008). Outcome measurement in clinical genetics services: A systematic review of validated measures. *Value in Health, 11*, 497–508.

Rahman, N. (2014). Realizing the promise of cancer predisposition genes. *Nature, 505*, 302–308.

Samejima, F. (1969). Estimation of latent ability using a response pattern of graded scores. *Psychological Monographs, 34*, 386–415.

Segundo-Ribeiro, M., Tavares Bacala, B., de Andrade Alvarenga, W., Castanheria Nascimento, L., McAllister, M., & Floria-Santos, M. (2020). Adaptation and preliminary validation of the genetic counseling outcome scale (GCOS-24) in a Brazilian genetic counseling setting. *European Journal of Medical Genetics, 63*, 104018.

Sinnott, P., Joyce, V., & Barnett, P. (2007). *Preference measurement in economic analysis. Guidebook*. Health Economics Resource Center.

Somer, M., Mustonen, H., & Norio, R. (1988). Evaluation of genetic counselling: Recall of information, post-counselling reproduction, and attitude of the counsellees. *Clinical Genetics*, *34*, 352–365.

Strauss, J. M., & Corbin, A. L. (2015). *Basics of qualitative research: Techniques and procedures for developing grounded theory*. Sage.

Tercyak, K. P., Johnson, S. B., Roberts, S. F., & Cruz, A. C. (2001). Psychological response to prenatal genetic counseling and amniocentesis. *Patient Education and Counseling*, *43*, 73–84.

Terwee, C. B., Mokkink, L. B., Knol, D. L., Ostelo, R. W. J. G., Bouter L. M., & de Vet, H. C. W. (2012). Rating the methodological quality in systematic reviews of studies on measurement properties: A scoring system for the COSMIN checklist. *Quality of Life Research*, *21*, 651–657.

Thomas, C., & McAllister, M. (2019). Establishing the minimum clinically important difference for the Genetic Counseling Outcome Scale (GCOS-24). *Journal of Genetic Counseling*, *28*, 1003–1010.

Timman, R., Roos, R., Maat-Kievit, A., & Tibben, A. (2004). Adverse effects of predictive testing for Huntington disease underestimated: Long-term effects 7–10 years after the test. *Health and Psychology*, *23*, 189–197.

Valente, E., Ferraris, A., & Dallapiccola, B. (2008). Genetic testing for paediatric neurological disorders. *Lancet Neurology*, *7*, 1113–1126.

Voorwinden, J. S., Plantinga, M., Krijnen, W., Ausems, M., Knoers, N., Velthuizen, M., Birnie, E., Lucassen, A., van Langen, I., & Ranchor, A. V. (2019). A validated PROM in genetic counselling: The psychometric properties of the Dutch version of the Genetic Counselling Outcome Scale. *European Journal of Human Genetics*, *27*, 681–690.

Weldring, T., & Smith, S. M. S. (2013). Patient-reported outcomes (PROs) and patient-reported outcome measures (PROMs). *Health Services Insights*, *6*, 61–68.

Wild, D., Grove, A., Martin, M., Eremenco, S., McElroy, S., Varjee-Lorenz, A., & Erikson, P. (2005). Principles of good practice for the translation and cultural adaptation process for patient-reported outcomes (PRO) measures: Report of the ISPOR Task Force for Translation and Cultural Adaptation. *Value in Health*, *8*, 94–104.

Yuen, J., Ying Lee, S., Courtney, E., Lim, J., Tzu Li, S., Soh, H., Chen, Y., McAllister, M., Fenwick, E. K., & Ngeow, J. (2020). Evaluating empowerment in genetic counselling using patient reported outcomes. *Clinical Genetics*, *97*, 246–256.

CHAPTER 31

REFORMING INFORMED CONSENT

On Disability and Genetic Counseling

ELIZABETH DIETZ AND JOEL MICHAEL REYNOLDS

INTRODUCTION

DISABILITY rights activists and scholars have long posed critiques of and challenges to prenatal genetic testing (Parens & Asch, 2003). These include, for example, arguments that the practice of prenatal testing invariably judges certain disabled lives to be not worthy or less worthy of living or that its effect, regardless of such judgment, is the prevention of certain people with disabilities from otherwise coming into being. Importantly, calls for greater attention to the complexity of disability as well as calls for greater incorporation of the experiential testimony of various disability communities have for many years now also become increasingly common from inside the practice of prenatal genetic counseling (Boardman, 2020; Farrelly et al., 2012; Gould et al., 2019; Madeo et al., 2011; Sanborn & Patterson, 2014). Whether coming from inside or outside, these calls often assume that genetic counselors' responsibilities to disability communities revolve around dialogue, understanding, and representation. It is further assumed that remedying these communicative and symbolic issues will satisfy long-standing needs for improvement, especially with respect to communication practices designed to secure informed consent. In this chapter, we hope to build upon the profession of genetic counseling's laudable engagement with disability critiques by showing why informed consent is not enough and how this issue might be fixed.[1]

In short, we argue that informed consent, while undoubtedly crucial to the provision of just care, can in fact reinforce unjust epistemic frameworks—patterns of thinking—when treated as an endpoint instead of a starting point.[2] We suggest that what we call

[1] That is to say, while significant strides have been made by genetic counselors to better understand disability experiences, disability history, and disability activism, we hope to show that even an ideal form of such understanding, though important and laudable, will not go far enough.

[2] Patterns of thinking can involve several different features: concepts, ideas, principles, assumptions, biases (implicit and explicit), and so forth.

critically informed consent is needed for such unjust epistemic frameworks to be meaningfully addressed. Our focus in this chapter will be upon epistemic frameworks rooted in ableism. Ableism is a prejudice (analogous to but distinct from prejudices involved in sexism, racism, or homophobia) that presumes the "normal" abled body is better than an "abnormal" disabled body. This prejudice leads to a wide range of social ramifications, from employment discrimination to hate crimes to poor patient–provider communication to social oppressions that include such basic things as barring entry to a building because one uses a wheelchair for mobility or failing to provide closed captioning. In what follows, we discuss critically informed consent as a tool for *anti-ableist genetic counseling*, an approach to genetic counseling that is committed not just to informedness but also to the idea that genetic counselors and their clients must mutually acknowledge how the dominant epistemic frameworks that shape healthcare decision making in the first place can perpetuate ableism.[3] To be anti-ableist, genetic counselors must work not merely toward increases in information but toward *epistemic transformation*.

In the first section, we provide a brief overview of disability theory. We discuss long-standing debates over what disability is, why and how these debates matter for genetic counselors, and the roots of historical tensions between disability communities and genetic counselors (Madeo et al., 2011). This discussion will involve an overview of disability rights critiques of prenatal testing, the import of social and postsocial models of disability, and long-standing disagreements between disability rights and abortion rights/feminist choice theory more generally (Asch, 1999; Hodgson & Weil, 2021; Parens & Asch, 2003; Shakespeare, 2014).

In the second section, we turn to the concept of informed consent. We begin by discussing the history of informed consent in biomedicine as reaction to Tuskegee and other events of blatant medical injustice, explaining how and why "fully informed consent" has come to be invoked as an explicit goal of genetic counseling (Johnston, 2017). Informed consent is often framed as an output of nondirective counseling, whereby a client becomes informed in dialogue with a counselor. Informedness is a constituent part of nondirective counseling, because a client sufficiently informed in collaboration with a counselor is thought to have sufficient tools to make informed, legitimate decisions. We build on existing critiques of nondirectiveness to complicate the role of informed consent, arguing that being fully informed is impossible and, even if it were possible, it is insufficient to achieve anti-ableist aims in the context of genetic counseling (Caplan, 2017; Clarke, 1991).

In the third section, we move from critical analysis to practical recommendations. We show how critically informed consent (a) avoids communication practices that treat obtaining informed consent as an endpoint, (b) instead embeds consent within transformative dialogue, and (c) challenges ableist epistemic frameworks that unreflectively place absolute value in "individual abilities" or "capacities" (Weil, 2003).[4]

[3] By focusing on what it means to be "anti-ableist" as opposed to merely *not* ableist, we follow in the footsteps of scholars of racialization like Ibram X. Kendi, for whom the point is not whether or not one is racist but rather what one is doing and how one acts to actively combat racism (cf. Kendi, 2019).

[4] An initial qualification is in order: There are some in disability studies and other domains that take the practice of genetic counseling to be inherently and irremediably problematic. We take no position on those claims in this chapter. On the contrary, we assume that we are operating in a world in which genetic counseling is a staple service for those who can access it and a world in which many (though

Disability Theory: A Brief History

Prenatal genetic counseling is primarily about disability. To counsel about genetic variation, genetic mutations, or any other such concepts is to counsel about genetic differences, the many expressions of which we ultimately describe as *disabilities*. But what, precisely, does that term mean? Thanks to nearly 70 years of disability activism across parts of the globe and 50 years of academic work in the interdisciplinary field of disability studies, a significant body of theoretical work and on-the-ground organizing offers tools to answer this question. In what follows, we offer a brief overview of disability studies with an eye to its relevance for genetic counselors.

The concept of "disability" is not decided by dictionaries or other practices of description. On the contrary, there is no uncontroversial definition, because the concept of disability involves what Adrianne Asch calls a "boundary problem," a problem the defining stakes of which are sociopolitical and which cannot be determined by mere appeals to authority, whether dictionaries, experts, or what have you (Asch, 1999). This is unsurprising once one recognizes that debates over disability cut to the heart of how we understand what it means to be human and how we distinguish between differing ways of being so—hardly uncontroversial matters. This is part of the reason arguments concerning the meaning of disability show no sign of disappearing in the many academic and policy-related fields that engage with it (Garland-Thomson, 2020; Nadelhoffer, 2022; Parens, 2017; Timpe, 2022).

Yet, this presents a problem for genetic counselors. A sense of what disability means is essential for counselor–client communication. What are genetic counselors who are sensitive to the complexity of disability and sensitive to the responsibilities they have to disability communities to do, given disagreements over what disability means in the first place? To answer this question requires a brief dive into both disability theory and the more specific history of disability critiques of genetic counseling.

Disability rights critiques of prenatal testing—whether with respect to maternal blood screening, conventional genetic testing, or noninvasive prenatal genetic tests—have taken many forms over the years (Hodgson & Weil, 2012; Parens & Asch, 2000). One of the most basic yet most important distinctions is between *medical* and *social* models of disability. In short, on medical models of disability, disability is an individual misfortune or tragedy due to a genetic or environmental cause. Unsurprisingly, medical models tend to construe disability as overwhelmingly negative, and adherents of this view see disability as something that ought to be cured or otherwise fixed and as something that benefits from medical intervention through elimination, correction, or the like. On social models, this idea is in more than one way turned on its head, for a fundamental distinction is made between *impairments*, which refer to some atypicality of one's body and mind, and *disability*, which refers to the negative social ramifications of one's impairment.

However *impaired* someone might be, that does not explain how they are *disabled*, for disability is ultimately a question of how societies and bodies interact. If, for whatever

ideally all) genetic counselors aim to practice in a way that does justice to the experiences of various disability communities.

reason, my form of embodiment leads me to use a wheelchair as my primary form of mobility, what disadvantages me when I run into a staircase isn't my body as much as it is those who decided to build stairs and not a ramp. What impedes the fantastic student of classics who happens to be blind from becoming a professor is not their body as much as it is a world that does not make braille and/or audio versions of texts easily accessible.[5] There is a limit to this insight, of course, for one with neuropathic pain will not necessarily fare better with accessible architecture or reading materials. There are some impairments that very clearly call for a medical fix, as disability studies scholars like Susan Wendell and Tom Shakespeare have argued (Shakespeare, 2014; Wendell, 1996).

Still, the distinction between medical and social models of disability matters for genetic counseling and decision making concerning reproduction more generally because while such counseling aids individual decision making concerning the health and well-being of a developing fetus and potential person, that person's ability to flourish ought to be understood not merely as a function of the presence or absence of impairment but also in terms of the attitudes and design of the built and social world that they will come to inhabit. Consider one more example: Being deaf (or Deaf—which some capitalize to emphasize Deafness as an identity with a relationship to communities centered around the use of signing) is an impairment in the sense that one's hearing is not phenotypical. What makes someone who is deaf *disabled*, however, is a world in which most people do not know how to communicate in American Sign Language; social norms that uncritically assume the habits, needs, and cultural practices of hearing people as opposed to nonhearing people; and the many stigmas signers face in a predominantly hearing world. Where strict adherents to a medical model might find it obvious to advocate for cochlear implants or other interventions thought to advance the presumptive good of typical hearing, those adopting a social model might advocate for the normalization of captioning, more access to American Sign Language instruction, and a recognition of the richness of Deaf culture.[6]

There are many theories of disability, and the distinction between medical and social models is only the most basic. However basic, this distinction still illuminates the animating conflict between disability rights and genetic counseling. Prenatal genetic counseling tends toward medical model understandings of disability because the information gleaned in the course of prenatal testing is circumscribed within the medical and the genetic; it does not yet bear on a person living in a socially, culturally, and historically shaped world. The decisions formed in genetic counseling spheres are by their nature related in direct ways to traits about the body, while disability in fact has a great deal to do with the societies that promote or thwart the ability of people with a wide array of bodies to flourish. An appreciation of the social model makes the following observation salient: By default, the theoretical and practical orientation of genetic counseling encourages medical model–type thinking about genetics in terms of what can be predicted about the body and in turn how medicine can fix (or not fix) whatever testing uncovers.

[5] As one might imagine, the distinction between medical and social models of disability has been endlessly refined and debated over many decades. For the purposes at hand, we are merely offering the "Disability 101" version of this distinction.

[6] There is significant debate over the meaning of d/Deafness, and the discussion here is greatly simplified. Among many possible entry points for those wanting to learn more, see Mauldin (2016).

Let us return, then, to the heart of the issue: What are genetic counselors who wish to take seriously the complexity of disability and who also recognize a responsibility to disability communities to do? And, to make matters more complicated, what are they to do in light of ongoing disagreements concerning how to understand the concept and meaning of *disability* (whether in pockets of disability activism or disability studies)? The answer is more simple than it seems. Whatever model of disability is at play, *the upshot of disability theory as a whole is that we live in a world saturated by ableism, and a just world requires everyone to be actively anti-ableist*. That is to say, we live in a world where assumptions about ability and disability run rampant, assumptions that are overwhelmingly prejudicial toward disabled people of all sorts and stripes. Ableism is not just a question of people's opinions, beliefs, or presumptions. On the contrary, ableism is baked into the *way* that people think about themselves and others, as well as how they act—how, for example, political representation is configured, how labor laws are developed, how the built environment is constructed, and so forth. And, as we discuss at length below, it is exceedingly rare to change how people think by merely presenting information to them. On the contrary, to change the foundation of how one experiences a given phenomenon requires transformation of *how* one knows, not simply adding or subtracting various pieces of "information" about it. Having now given a very cursory overview of some points of disability theory, we will turn to show how the central concepts of *choice* and *consent* too easily lead to additive, not transformative, changes. After laying out that critique, we will then develop our account of critically informed consent.

Choice and Consent

Consent and choice are fundamental to the project of genetic counseling. By its nature, prenatal genetic counseling is an interpersonal exercise in informing and becoming informed. As Barbara Biesecker (2001) puts it, "The goal of reproductive genetic counseling is to promote the client's self-determination in exercising choices" (p. 328). Informed consent is both a formal procedure and a way of thinking. It is formal in that it has been codified such that clients must sign documents to indicate their understanding and choosing of procedures and clinical encounters. It is a way of thinking in that genetic counseling operates via the logic that there is a certain measure of knowledge—of informedness—that authorizes a person to make autonomous and trustable decisions, and counseling can help them get there. This logic is in line with other forms of healthcare decision making, where patients are furnished with information, and having information, demonstrated by signing informed consent paperwork, legitimizes consent and is understood to be a precondition for making independent healthcare choices. The nature of prenatal genetic testing, where the information gleaned about potential genetic abnormalities may be all that is known about the specific tested fetus, raises the stakes of this process of informed consent. That is to say, virtually all that is known about a tested fetus is the information that prenatal testing offers, and the parent(s), aided in understanding by genetic counselors, can use it as the predicate for significant choices. Informedness is taken as the condition sine qua non for making *good* significant choices, where what marks the "good" choice is the appreciation and uptake of relevant information, unconstrained by outside pressures.

Of course, unconstrained choice is impossible; societal norms and values that produce the meaning of disability for any given client are also present within reproductive decision making and the institutions that exist to support it. The history of genetic counseling bears this out. Since the mid-20th century, the field has operated, on the one hand, with the effect of elimination of genetic diseases leading to impairment and, on the other, with the aim of helping clients prepare and understand genetic conditions in a "neutral" manner (Biesecker, 2001). Many genetic counselors have long pushed back against the elimination of impairment as an explicit goal, and while their efforts have done important work to change attitudes and pedagogical models, tension between facilitation of reproductive autonomy and the promotion of anti-ableist aims means that the elimination of impairment is still a key outcome of much genetic testing and counseling (Hawkins et al., 2013; Mansfield et al., 1999).

The situation is even more complex than this, however, for the reasons that cause people to end up in a genetic counselor's office mediate the kinds of choices that will be available to them in the first place. These include the catalysts for testing, such as family history or previous miscarriage or advanced maternal age; whether or not testing occurs; the other providers involved in testing; the kinds of healthcare available to them thanks to wealth, income, and other vectors of their economic situation; and more. Economic resources beget more access to genetic testing, which on one hand represents greater access to the information upon which to base choices and on the other strongly predisposes one to making particular kinds of choices (Zhang, 2020). The social contexts in which decisions predicated on genetic information are made are also constrained by factors such as the healthcare, social, and school systems available and attitudes of family and community toward disability and care. These constraints are important because they provide context and motivation for reproductive decisions. But they also hint at how those decisions are profoundly shaped by factors well beyond individual clients. These factors include aspects of choice itself, such as the stories of choice and control told about genetic testing (Lippman, 1991) and the paradox of constraint that more choice can engender (Levitt, 2014). In other words, even when the purpose of genetic counseling is imagined by all parties to facilitate free and informed choice, choices are always mediated and always constrained in various ways.

Informed consent

The practice of informed consent results from an attempt to ensure that choice is as free as possible, but, of course, the mere provision of information cannot overcome the constraints imposed by the outside world. Even the information that generates informedness is not neutral; there are necessarily decisions to be made about what is included, what is left out, and what is unknowable. As will be discussed below, *critically* informed consent acknowledges that the provision of information is not without bias despite it being understood as a goal of the practice of genetic counseling. We argue that such biases must be deployed in the service of epistemic transformation, that is, to actively shift the profession of genetic counseling toward being an anti-ableist practice.

Genetic counselors are taught that informed consent is an important goal of their practice (Biesecker, 2001; Rantanen et al., 2008). This is understandable, for a key task of genetic counseling is indeed to generate informedness, that is, not only to furnish clients with information about the landscape of genetic knowing (what particular markers mean, how they are known, how to think about probabilistic risk, etc.) but also to offer bespoke information about clients' own genetic information. Nondirectiveness is thought to be key (albeit contested), because it is a method, if not *the* method, by which genetic counselors convey information without inflecting it via their own values. In this light, information is imagined to shape client decisions in ways that allow for the expression of their own autonomous values. Clients need to know enough about how genetic information works to understand what their own information means so that they can act on it.[7] This is the *consent* part of informed consent; consent is a kind of choice, and in genetic counseling and beyond, its legitimacy is authorized by virtue of it being sufficiently informed so that decisions can be trusted, both by clients and by other entities such as medical providers, family members, and the law.

Emphasis on choice, made manifest in informed consent, has an important history in genetic counseling. In biomedicine broadly, informed consent became codified as a way to prevent atrocities like those in the Tuskegee syphilis study from happening again. The commission investigating Tuskegee found that a key procedural injustice contributing to the suffering and unnecessary syphilis infection of thousands of Black men and their families was that those men were never asked for their consent to participate in the study. In the *Belmont Report*, authored in response to the study, the Belmont commission outlined a mandate for what they called "respect for persons." It requires that "subjects, to the degree that they are capable, be given the opportunity to choose what shall or shall not happen to them. This opportunity is provided when adequate standards for informed consent are satisfied" (National Commission for the Protection of Human Subjects of Biomedical and Behavioral Research, 1979, p. 6). This is a forceful expression of the value of individual autonomy, and the translation of a right to make decisions for oneself into medical practice.[8] In this chapter, we do not argue that such choosing is unimportant. Rather, we argue that it is more complicated—and less individual—than prevailing notions about informed consent suggest.

We offer this cursory gloss of the history of informed consent to point specifically to the problem of paternalism and how it historically gave rise to biomedicine's keen emphasis on individual autonomy as a solution. We understand paternalism in two senses: first, where "doctor knows best" and fails to furnish the patient with information necessary for making individual health decisions, and second, where "medicine knows best" and decides that, for example, the health of poor Black men in Tuskegee, Alabama, is an acceptable sacrifice in the name of population health and knowledge. Bioethics gained prominence in the United States, in particular, in large part due to public reaction to Tuskegee (Jonsen, 1997; Washington, 2008). Bioethics' emphasis on the protection of individual autonomy, through the informed consent mechanisms outlined in the *Belmont Report*, arose to gird against both sorts of paternalism. In this way, the emphasis on protecting autonomy is understandable and needed; clients and patients are important knowers and better suited to

[7] Editors' note: For a discussion of the historical understanding and uses of nondirectiveness in genetic counseling, see Chapter 23 by Michael J. Deem in this volume.

[8] The model of consent that initially developed in biomedicine was a research model. Importing this model into clinical care writ large (and genetic counseling, specifically) is perhaps one source of these troubles.

make decisions about their own well-being than doctors—particularly when doctors act maleficently.

At the same time, such a forceful expression of the need for choices to be free and individual disregards the ways that they often cannot be. Choices, particularly reproductive choices, do not exist in a vacuum and are rather conditioned by the reality of the world in which they sit. Attitudes about disability, the resources of available school systems and social programs, the quality of accessible healthcare, and the influence of racism all bear on such decisions. The fortification of individual autonomy and the mere provision of more information are inadequate responses to the inequitable milieu in which reproductive choices take place. In the case of Tuskegee, it is true that Black men were not asked for their consent to participate in trials that would leave them with untreated syphilis. But it is also the case that merely asking for their consent would not address the larger factors that rendered the trials unjust: the racism of the time and place of its occurrence, underresourcing of local healthcare systems, and a study design that presumed the biological difference and inferiority of Black people and justified harm in the name of confirming it. In other words, the presence of consent would not have transformed the trial, or the social systems in which it took place, into one that was ethical. Consent undertaken as an individual expression of choice is necessary, but it is insufficient for rendering the system in which it takes place just.

Informed consent is necessary, but also insufficient, as a mechanism to combat the paternalism that has caused long legacies of significant harm. As an individual matter and as a way that genetic counselors can facilitate and respect the reproductive autonomy of their clients, it is certainly a worthwhile aspiration. But it should be understood as the starting point, not the ending point. Informed consent itself also transforms the messiness and interdependence of the outside world into a decision where responsibility is placed on the individual. In this way, it is a tool of simplification and responsibility shifting and a way by which some liability is shifted away from providers; it is a bureaucratic tool that we find simultaneously important and insufficient for disability justice. In response, we encourage genetic counselors to think about underlying structural injustices to translate their responsibilities to individual clients into transformations of consciousness. Much like you aren't "racist or not racist" but rather racist or *anti*-racist, genetic counselors should be not merely "not ableist" but *anti*-ableist. In the following section, we elaborate the stakes of this critique and offer a way of thinking both about client autonomy and the impact of social structures within which decisions are made by thinking in terms of epistemic transformation rather than information provision. But first we will discuss the role that nondirectiveness has played in genetic counseling's understanding of client autonomy.

Nondirectiveness

Genetics in general, and genetic counseling more specifically, cannot but understand itself in relation to eugenics. Indeed, much writing on the subject begins with an explicit genealogical discussion of how and why nondirectiveness came to be a guiding principle for practice (Patterson & Sattz, 2002).[9] To understand a population at the level of the genome is

[9] Editors' note: For a discussion of the history of social eugenics programs and its relation to the genetic counseling profession, see Chapter 1 by Devon Stillwell in this volume.

to facilitate its management (on at least some level), which cannot escape deliberation over values and over who and what sorts of people ought to come into being, how they should be treated, and so forth. Nondirectiveness works to create an explicit separation between the "experts" and those making individual decisions about who comes to be and who does not. A key ethos of mainstream genetics researchers and genetic counselors is one that takes active steps to acknowledge the legacy of eugenics, implementing policies and practices that endeavor to render them impossible, outside the scope of practice, and a set of verboten and antiquated norms. Genetic counseling is motivated by the need to counter the legacy of paternalism so viciously embodied in various forms of egregiously immoral social engineering.[10] But in a field whose remit is to facilitate decisions about how to act on genetic information, the question of *how* to do that is one that requires critical vigilance and meaningful interrogation.

Nondirectiveness creates a separation between the production of genetic information and its deployment. Instead of locating knowledge about what genetic information is and means in the same hands as those who decide how to act on it—where "act" generally implies "decides what kinds of people should come into being"—nondirectiveness assigns genetic counselors to the role of information providers and clients to the role of decision makers. Nondirectiveness is, of course, complicated. It is "a principle, not a goal" (Biesecker, 2001, p. 325); it is "a technique by which genetics professionals explore whether clients can be trusted to make autonomous decisions within a climate of uncertainty" (Arribas-Ayllon & Sarangi, 2014, p. 171); it "has served as the central ethos for genetic counselling for the past decades and has provided both practical and ethical guidance to professionals" (Rantanen et al., 2008, p. 449). In other words, nondirectiveness exists not as an absolute or measurable goal but as a disposition, a way of thinking, an orientation. It is a general sense that to promote client autonomy and facilitate informed consent, counseling should be nondirective. It should furnish information, answer questions, acknowledge uncertainty and complexity (and in so doing, its own impossibility)—but remain a guiding force in the background, cautioning against the harms of genetic counselors making decisions for their clients.

The social factors that produce disability also generate a responsibility for genetic counselors to transform anti-ableist ways of thinking—not merely by providing more information (though that is certainly important) but also by helping clients to think differently about disability. To be sure, our interrogation of nondirectiveness is not novel.[11]

[10] The legacy of Nazi experimentation looms large in the establishment of nondirectiveness as a backstop against eugenics (Resta, 1997). Still, the most immediate foil is not in fact Nazi eugenics but instead late 19th- and early 20th-century social eugenics programs in the United States (e.g., the Eugenics Record Office in the United States and Margaret Sanger's overall goals in the founding of Planned Parenthood).

[11] Some assert the impossibility of nondirectiveness: The complexity of genetic information and the range of decisions that it potentiates couple with structural limitations on what genetic counselors can know and the inescapability of bias in human interactions to render true nondirectiveness impossible (Clarke, 2017). Others note that as a mechanism for promoting autonomy, it may also fall flat: One study found that clients of lower socioeconomic status or those judged to be "highly concerned" received more directive counseling (Michie et al., 1997). In a review of arguments against the nondirectiveness principle (NDP), Christoph Rehmann-Sutter (2009) summarizes them as follows: (a) "NDP can be against the best interests of the individuals concerned," (b) "NDP has ideological elements that do not adequately represent the counselling ethos," (c) "NDP was historically a defensive tool that protected the interests

On the contrary, we see this argument as building upon decades of work that has complicated, pushed back on, and otherwise transformed the centrality of nondirectiveness. Our aim here is to offer a translation of those critiques into something that can be concretely deployed in practice. We thus draw upon and expand such work by arguing that nondirectiveness is not only impossible but also *undesirable*.[12] To be anti-ableist requires being directive, at least with respect to how a client is pushed to think.[13] As our arguments here aim to make clear, there are ways to be directive in the practice of genetic counseling that are entirely defensible, morally, practically, and otherwise. One way that we suggest doing so is by aiming for transformation with respect to the epistemic framework within and through which a given client understands the meaning of disability.

Given their role in decisions that render judgments on the possibility and impossibility of disabled lives, genetic counselors must, we contend, take an active role in transforming their clients' larger epistemic relationship to ableism in making reproductive decisions, the communal (rather than individual) effects of those decisions, and how ableist thinking may not be a conscious facet of their analytical toolbox but is nevertheless a presence.

Critically Informed Consent

The concept of *critically informed consent* is premised upon work concerning how people filter information in the fields of social epistemology and psychology. A number of common cognitive biases and habits are well known today. For example, *implicit bias* refers to the way that people act on stereotypes and prejudices without realizing or intending to (Brownstein, 2019). *Confirmation bias* describes the way that people assimilate and act on information that is consistent, rather than inconsistent, with their prior conceptions (Khan et al., 2015). *Anchoring bias* refers to the way that people will too heavily focus on initial pieces of information provided to them at the expense of appropriately assessing forthcoming pieces of information (Wilson, 1996). Yet, these cognitive filters do not have to do with how we understand the world as such. That is to say, they are about *how* we think, not about the frameworks *through which* we think in general. Take the following example. If I hold implicit biases concerning engineers—that they have poor social skills, are exceptional at math, and dislike ambiguity—this will affect how I interact with engineers in a host of ways. So will the matrix of social factors that have (for instance) made engineering a male-dominated field and that have tended to devalue jobs typically held by women. But even if I overcome all of those biases, the larger background beliefs at play that make the

of geneticists against social criticism and against litigation," and (d) "NDP falsely assumes individual responsibility and hides the shared responsibility of other social actors" (pp. 117–118).

[12] That is to say, undesirable at least on traditional views of nondirectiveness. Consider Weil and Seymour's attempts to define nondirectiveness as a positive duty of genetic counselors, as well as Deem's argument that these attempts end up collapsing nondirectiveness into a broader principle of respect for autonomy (Deem, 2017; Kessler, 1997; Weil, 2003).

[13] That is to say, we are not endorsing being directive in the traditional sense within genetic counseling, that is, pushing a client toward a specific decision (much like a pediatrician would be recommending/pushing an option).

concept of an "engineer" something that is communicable remain. For example, the belief in modern scientific methods (as opposed to alternative systems of knowledge), the belief that abilities (like being good at math or "social skills") are properties of people, and the belief that knowledge exists on certain gradients (such as ranging from being clear to being opaque) might seem like *obvious* truths to most readers, but that is precisely the problem. The background or framing beliefs with which people typically operate strike them as obviously true. So what, you might be wondering, does this have to do with critically informed consent?

The problem of ableism is not, in the end, about a *lack of information* concerning disability, information that would include all the studies showing many people with disabilities to have similar quality of life as nondisabled people (Amundson, 2005) or information that demonstrates widespread stigma against disabled people that leads to hate crimes, underemployment, and high levels of interpersonal abuse (Sherry, 2010). The problem of ableism is, at its core, about the background organization of one's knowing, judging, and valuing in general (Reynolds & Peña-Guzmán, 2019). Put simply, the problem of ableism is about whether one's reflective relationship to the multifaceted phenomenon of disability is sufficiently *critical* or not.

Let us retrace our steps. As we discussed in the section on disability theory above, the dominant medical paradigm for conceptualizing embodied difference is between "ability" and "disability" or "normality" and "abnormality," conceptual pairs that often amount to the same in such contexts. On the medical model, to be able-bodied and normal is assumed to be both good and a goal; to be disabled and abnormal is assumed to be both bad and to be avoided/fixed/overcome. And given the larger sociocultural dynamics of our current epoch, this is also the dominant paradigm with which most genetic counseling *clients* operate. Yet, as we argued above, this paradigm is not simply empirically dubious—it is also morally problematic. To assume that all lives lived with disability are lives worse off is the most egregious form of "common sense" ableism.

Critically informed consent takes the medical model of disability head on. It aims not merely at what information clients have about disability but also at the framework clients use to make sense of the distinction between disability and ability in the first place. To echo above, the deeper challenge of ableism is not primarily a question of *exposure* to disability-positive information—whether it be in the form of social scientific studies demonstrating quality of life, anecdotes from families, or what have you. The deeper challenge of ableism is the framework in which broad value judgments can be assuredly inferred from claims about specific ability states such that responses like the following occur: "I never shared it [the results] with any family [members]. My dad would treat [the child] differently even though the results don't say anything definitive. If she drops a ball or says something really stupid, he would say, 'oh, there's something wrong with her; she's retarded, or she's autistic.' He would just go there" (Werner-Lin et al., 2016, p. 449; cf. Reynolds, 2020).

For example, one might consider oneself progressive on issues concerning disability and still think that a child with Down syndrome will live a less flourishing life and that one should not follow through with such a pregnancy. Such thinking is rooted in assumptions about what sort of well-being will follow from the "capacities" of a given individual in concert with the social reality in a given place. Disability theory, on the whole, has shown such assumptions to be more often misguided than not. For example, we know that most people with Down syndrome live happy, flourishing lives (Kaposy, 2018). While social contexts of course matter, they matter *for any child* regardless of their disability status, and they are profoundly impacted by how that child is treated and regarded as they develop (Stramondo, 2020). In other words, it is difficult to make an argument that social context will matter in categorically distinct ways between someone with Down syndrome and someone without Down syndrome—if, that is, one refuses to commit what Adrienne Asch calls the "sin of synecdoche," the practice of treating a part (like having an extra chromosome) for the whole (the varied phenotypical differences brought about *in relationship with* a given social, cultural, or historical context; Asch & Wasserman, 2005). Not being born with Down syndrome does *not* necessitate any guarantees about having or not having socially valuable intellectual or social skills, about developing or not developing drug dependencies that can run any life adrift, about living with or without severe depression or anxiety, or any number of other factors. *Not* being born with Down syndrome does not necessitate guarantees about living a happy life "on the whole." And if the primary concern of a parent is about the extent to which they are perceived to be "normal" and not the flourishing of their child, then we are outside of the moral sphere of reproductive ethics.[14]

This is why *critically informed consent* is a practice aimed at undermining ableism. The decision-making paradigms for much of the reproductive sphere are about "prevention," "information," and "intervention." We are suggesting that all of these can reinforce *injustice* against disabled people insofar as the conceptual framework that underwrites these terms is left to "common sense" about the meaning of ability and disability. To argue for critically informed consent is not to argue that the practice of genetic counseling should stop or that it necessarily contributes to injustices against disabled people. On the contrary, to argue for critically informed consent is to argue that *how* genetic differences are explained, understood, and communicated must take the problem of ableism and the epistemic frameworks underwriting it head on.

Conclusion

We have suggested that for genetic counselors to be aware of the problem of ableism is not enough. Genetic counseling as a practice must become actively anti-ableist. While informed consent is undoubtedly crucial to the provision of care that both meets client needs and is attentive to concerns about justice, we have argued that when treated as an endpoint rather than as a starting point, it can reinforce existing injustices at the level of how people think. To be sure, knowledge about the lived experiences of people with disabilities is vitally important, but that knowledge must be accompanied by an understanding of how ableism operates as a habit of thought, a habit all too often operating seamlessly in the background. We will not achieve a more just world through an uncritical belief that objective facts and informed consent will lead naturally toward just outcomes; on the contrary, justice requires an interrogation of how what we think of as "objective" facts are often in fact inflected with

[14] To want a child "like oneself" and use that as a defensible basis for one's reproductive choices is an especially egregious sort of narcissism, the analysis of which we simply set to the side here. See Rulli (2016).

biases that support the very unjust world in which we live. It is then not merely a matter of acknowledging these biases but working against the larger epistemic frameworks through which our values, judgments, and decision making are shaped. Practicing critically informed consent is one way for the profession of genetic counseling to more effectively work toward a just world. By doing so, it is our hope that genetic counseling will shift from being aware of the problem of ableism to being actively anti-ableist.

References

Amundson, R. (2005). Disability, ideology, and quality of life: A bias in biomedical ethics. In D. Wasserman, J. Bickenbach, & R. Wachbroit (Eds.), *Quality of life and human difference: Genetic testing, health care, and disability* (pp. 101–124). Cambridge University Press. https://doi.org/10.1017/CBO9780511614590.005

Arribas-Ayllon, M., & Sarangi, S. (2014). Counselling uncertainty: Genetics professionals' accounts of (non)directiveness and trust/distrust. *Health, Risk & Society*, *16*(2), 171–184. https://doi.org/10.1080/13698575.2014.884545

Asch, A. (1999). Prenatal diagnosis and selective abortion: A challenge to practice and policy. *American Journal of Public Health*, *89*(11), 1649–1657. https://doi.org/10/dv4cns

Asch, A., & Wasserman, D. (2005). Where is the sin in synecdoche? Prenatal testing and the parent-child relationship. In D. Wasserman, J. Bickenbach, & R. Wachbroit (Eds.), *Quality of life and human difference: Genetic testing, health care, and disability* (pp. 172–216). Cambridge University Press. https://doi.org/10.1017/CBO9780511614590.008

Biesecker, B. B. (2001). Goals of genetic counseling. *Clinical Genetics*, *60*(5), 323–330. https://doi.org/10.1034/j.1399-0004.2001.600501.x

Boardman, F. (2020). Human genome editing and the identity politics of genetic disability. *Journal of Community Genetics*, *11*(2), 125–127. https://doi.org/10/gjhgnd

Brownstein, M. (2019, Fall). Implicit bias. In E. N. Zalta (Ed.). *The Stanford encyclopedia of philosophy*. Metaphysics Research Lab, Stanford University. https://plato.stanford.edu/archives/fall2019/entries/implicit-bias/

Caplan, A. L. (2017). Neutrality is not morality: The ethics of genetic counseling: Ethical challenges and consequences. In D. M. Bartels, B. S. LeRoy, & A. L. Caplan (Eds.), *Prescribing our future: Ethical challenges in genetic counseling* (pp. 149–166). Aldine de Gruyter.

Clarke, A. (2017). The evolving concept of non-directiveness in genetic counselling. In H. I. Petermann, P. S. Harper, & S. Doetz (Eds.), *History of human genetics: Aspects of its development and global* (pp. 541–566). Springer Berlin Heidelberg.

Deem, M. (2017). Vulnerability in genetic counseling and the ground of nondirectiveness. In C. Straehle (Ed.), *Vulnerability, autonomy, and applied ethics* (pp. 144–162). Routledge. https://doi.org/10.4324/9781315647418-14

Farrelly, E., Cho, M. K., Erby, L., Roter, D., Stenzel, A., & Ormond, K. (2012). Genetic counseling for prenatal testing: Where is the discussion about disability? *Journal of Genetic Counseling*, *21*(6), 814–824. https://doi.org/10.1007/s10897-012-9484-z

Garland-Thomson, R. (2020). How we got to CRISPR: The dilemma of being human. *Perspectives in Biology and Medicine*, *63*(1), 28–43. https://doi.org/10/ggzfh3

Gould, H., Hashmi, S. S., Wagner, V. F., Stoll, K., Ostermaier, K., & Czerwinski, J. (2019). Examining genetic counselors' implicit attitudes toward disability. *Journal of Genetic Counseling*, *28*(6), 1098–1106. https://doi.org/10/fwwp

Hawkins, A., Stenzel, A., Taylor, J., Chock, V. Y., & Hudgins, L. (2013). Variables influencing pregnancy termination following prenatal diagnosis of fetal chromosome abnormalities. *Journal of Genetic Counseling*, *22*(2), 238–248. https://doi.org/10.1007/s10897-012-9539-1

Hodgson, J., & Weil, J. (2012). Talking about disability in prenatal genetic counseling: A report of two interactive workshops. *Journal of Genetic Counseling*, *21*, 17–23. https://doi.org/10/dwn3rf

Johnston, J., Farrell, R. M., & Parens, E. (2017). Supporting women's autonomy in prenatal testing. *New England Journal of Medicine*, *377*(6), 505–507. https://doi.org/10.1056/nejmp1703425

Jonsen, A. R. (1997). The birth of bioethics: The origins and evolution of a demi-discipline. *Medical Humanities Review*, *11*(1), 9–21.

Kaposy, C. (2018). *Choosing Down syndrome*. MIT Press.

Kendi, I. X. (2019). *How to be an antiracist*. Penguin Books.

Kessler, S. (1997). Psychological aspects of genetic counseling. XI. Nondirectiveness revisited. *American Journal of Medical Genetics*, *72*(October), 164–171. https://doi.org/10/dtqfdr

Khan, C. M., Rini, C., Bernhardt, B. A., Scott Roberts, J., Christensen, K. D., Evans, J. P., Brothers, K. B., Roche, M. I., Berg, J. S., & Henderson, G. E. (2015). How can psychological science inform research about genetic counseling for clinical genomic sequencing? *Journal of Genetic Counseling*, *24*(2), 193–204. https://doi.org/10.1007/s10897-014-9804-6

Levitt, M. (2014). Empowered by choice? In R. Chadwick, M. Levitt, & D. Shickle (Eds.), *The right to know and the right not to know: Genetic privacy and responsibility* (2 ed., pp. 85–99) (Cambridge Bioethics and Law). Cambridge University Press.

Lippman, A. (1991). Prenatal genetic testing and screening: Constructing needs and reinforcing inequities. *American Journal of Law & Medicine*, *17*(1–2), 15–50. https://doi.org/10.1017/S0098858800007917

Madeo, A. C., Biesecker, B. B., Brasington, C., Erby, L. H., & Peters, K. F. (2011). The relationship between the genetic counseling profession and the disability community: A commentary. *American Journal of Medical Genetics Part A*, *155*, 1777–1785. https://doi.org/10.1002/ajmg.a.34054

Mansfield, C., Hopfer, S., & Marteau, T. M. (1999). Termination rates after prenatal diagnosis of Down syndrome, spina bifida, anencephaly, and Turner and Klinefelter syndromes: A systematic literature review. *Prenatal Diagnosis*, *19*(9), 808–812. https://doi.org/10.1002/(SICI)1097-0223(199909)19:9<808::AID-PD637>3.0.CO;2-B

Mauldin, L. (2016). *Made to hear: Cochlear implants and raising deaf children*. University of Minnesota Press.

Michie, S., Bron, F., Bobrow, M., & Marteau, T. M. (1997). Nondirectiveness in genetic counseling: An empirical study. *American Journal of Human Genetics*, *60*(1), 40–47.

Nadelhoffer, T. (2022). Chronic pain, bad-differences, and disability variantism. *Journal of Philosophy of Disability*, *2*, 6–27. https://doi.org/10.5840/jpd20223110

National Commission for the Protection of Human Subjects of Biomedical and Behavioral Research. (1979). *The Belmont report*. Department of Health, Education, and Welfare. https://www.hhs.gov/ohrp/regulations-and-policy/belmont-report/read-the-belmont-report/index.html

Parens, E. (2017). Choosing flourishing: Toward a more "binocular" way of thinking about disability. *Kennedy Institute of Ethics Journal*, *27*(2), 135–150. https://doi.org/10/gf9gbc

Parens, E., & Asch, A. (2000). *Prenatal testing and disability rights*. Georgetown University Press.

Parens, E., & Asch, A. (2003). Disability rights critique of prenatal genetic testing: Reflections and recommendations. *Mental Retardation and Developmental Disabilities Research Reviews*, *9*, 40–47. https://doi.org/10.1002/mrdd.10056

Patterson, A. R., & Sattz, M. (2002). Genetic counseling and the disabled: Feminism examines the stance of those who stand at the gate. *Hypatia*, *17*, 118–142. https://doi.org/10.1111/j.1527-2001.2002.tb00944.x

Rantanen, E., Hietala, M., Kristoffersson, U., Nippert, I., Schmidtke, J., Sequeiros, J., & Kääriäinen, H. (2008). What is ideal genetic counselling? A survey of current international guidelines. *European Journal of Human Genetics*, *16*(4), 445–452. https://doi.org/10.1038/sj.ejhg.5201983

Rehmann-Sutter, C. (2009). Why non-directiveness is insufficient: Ethics of genetic decision making and a model of agency. *Medicine Studies*, *1*(2), 113–129. https://doi.org/10.1007/s12376-009-0023-7

Resta, R. G. (1997). Eugenics and nondirectiveness in genetic counseling. *Journal of Genetic Counseling*, *6*(2), 4.

Reynolds, J. M. (2020). "What if there's something wrong with her?" How biomedical technologies contribute to epistemic injustice in healthcare. *Southern Journal of Philosophy*, *58*(1), 161–185. https://doi.org/10/gh52z7

Reynolds, J. M., & Peña-Guzmán, D. M. (2019). The harm of ableism: Medical error and epistemic injustice. *Kennedy Institute of Ethics Journal*, *29*(3), 205–242. https://doi.org/10/ggdzqt

Rulli, T. (2016). Preferring a genetically-related child. *Journal of Moral Philosophy*, *13*(6), 669–698.

Sanborn, E., & Patterson, A. R. (2014). Disability training in the genetic counseling curricula: Bridging the gap between genetic counselors and the disability community. *American Journal of Medical Genetics Part A*, *164*, 1909–1915. https://doi.org/10.1002/ajmg.a.36613.

Shakespeare, T. (2014). *Disability rights and wrongs revisited* (2nd ed.). Routledge.

Sherry, M. (2010). *Disability hate crimes: Does anyone really hate disabled people?* Ashgate.

Stramondo, J. A. (2020). Disability and the damaging master narrative of an open future. *Hastings Center Report*, *50*(S1): S30–S36. https://doi.org/10/gg94m4

Timpe, K. (2022). Denying a unified concept of disability. *Journal of Philosophy and Medicine*, *47*(5), 583–596. https://doi.org/10.1093/jmp/jhac021

Washington, H. A. (2008). *Medical apartheid: The dark history of medical experimentation on Black Americans from colonial times to the present*. Anchor Books.

Weil, J. (2003). Psychosocial genetic counseling in the post-nondirective era: A point of view. *Journal of Genetic Counseling*, *12*, 199–211. https://doi.org/10.1023/a:1023234802124

Wendell, S. (1996). *The rejected body: Feminist philosophical reflections on disability*. Routledge.

Werner-Lin, A., Walser, S., Barg, F. K., & Bernhardt, B. A. (2016). "They can't find anything wrong with him, yet": Mothers' experiences of parenting an infant with a prenatally diagnosed copy number variant (CNV). *American Journal of Medical Genetics*, *173*(2), 444–451. https://doi.org/10/f9ptcp

Wilson, T. D. (1996). A new look at anchoring effects: Basic anchoring and its antecedents. *Journal of Experimental Psychology: General*, *125*(4), 387–402. https://doi.org/10/cxpc7n

Zhang, S. (2020). The last children of Down syndrome. *The Atlantic*. https://www.theatlantic.com/magazine/archive/2020/12/the-last-children-of-down-syndrome/616928/

CHAPTER 32

GENETICS AND DISADVANTAGE

Inequity, Stigma, and Expectation

ANGUS CLARKE

Introduction

The science of genetics, including new and powerful genomic technologies, has great potential to bring benefit to health and healthcare. It has much to offer patients affected by genetic disorders and their families, and it is also being applied fruitfully to understand and tackle diseases that are not thought of as primarily genetic or inherited.

The applications of genetics are still largely in the realm of diagnostics, explanation, and understanding rather than therapeutics, such as gene therapy and gene editing. However, there is an increasing role for precision medicine, including pharmacogenetic testing and the testing of tumors to identify indications for specific treatments. The better understanding of disease mechanisms opened up by genetic knowledge is also proving very useful in devising "conventional" (non-gene-based) treatments for rare diseases, as with the development of variant-specific therapies for cystic fibrosis. More broadly, the gene-based understanding of many rare disorders has a valuable role in identifying those affected by particular inherited conditions and guiding their management, especially for those at risk of serious disease complications.

Genomics is an immensely powerful development of genetic technologies. It greatly increases our ability to identify the principal genetic alteration responsible for Mendelian disease in a patient or family, thereby transforming the possibilities for achieving insight and understanding. It also allows us to make steps toward understanding more complex disorders that may be described as polygenic or multifactorial. Finding an explanation for a problem, however, does not in itself give the power to solve it. Attempts to intervene bring us up against more fundamental biological obstacles than our ability to establish associations between genotype and phenotype and, sometimes, to demonstrate causality. Association and explanation are much simpler to recognize than prediction and control are to achieve. Still, we must not underestimate the importance of the personal meaning of genetic information to patients and their families even when our capacity to intervene is limited.

These helpful applications of genetics are to be welcomed. In this chapter, however, I wish to view the genetic aspects of disease from a different perspective: to consider the ways in which genetic disease and genetic conditions cause problems for patients and families beyond the obvious clinical effects. I wish to look past the disturbances of developmental or physiological processes that they cause, and the resulting physical or mental impairments, to consider those burdens that are the result of how society, and sometimes health services, compound these problems. How can society's responses to genetic disorders add to the problems of those affected? In particular, in what ways may genetic services and genomic technologies be experienced as unhelpful, exacerbating the problems associated with genetic disease or genetic conditions, especially in the context of preexisting inequities in healthcare? This is an important exercise to undertake if the genetics community is to avoid amplifying the problems that we should be helping to mitigate or resolve.

I will approach this by considering the multiple ways in which society makes life more difficult for those affected by genetic conditions, through organizational processes and the micro-behaviors of individuals. While some problems arise from the biological facts of the matter and may be unavoidable, even these take place within a social setting that shapes the way events play out, both at the grand scale of policy and at the more local, "micro" level of interaction as a child plays in the schoolyard or an adult walks down the street. There is a need to bring this broader, societal perspective into the discussion. I will then turn to the delivery of genetics services and where this can "go wrong." I consider the impact of genetic information as it extends into the family. I attend to the differences between screening programs and the provision of the more usual, reactive healthcare services that respond to the problems and concerns presented by individual patients, and the ways in which the funding of healthcare shapes the care that is delivered. This allows us to focus on genetics services and their impact on equity, and to look toward the future.

Stigmatization and Discrimination

A key factor that enables a person—any person—to live a worthwhile life is being treated with decency and respect. Many of us can take this for granted much of the time, but those who look different, often in association with a genetic condition, have learned they cannot do this. There are aspects of living with a genetic condition that mark some people as "different" or "other" and that may lead to stigmatization and/or discrimination.

"Difference," in the playground and on the street, is itself a form of deviance. Every child learns that. There may be clear physical differences that mark a person as "different," and such attributes (Goffman, 1968), which result from nongenetic factors as well as genetics (Martindale & Fisher, 2019; Sabatello et al., 2015), are often deeply discrediting, even if they lead to little or no functional impairment. By way of contrast, however, those who look different serve to confirm other people as being unremarkable, usual, or "normal." This will bring pain to the stigmatized and comfort to those who appear "normal," especially perhaps even more so for those who feel insecure or threatened for other reasons. There is literature on genetic conditions that impact a person's physical features that may leave them exposed to stigmatization, as with those affected by neurofibromatosis type 1 (Ablon, 1996; Rozario, 2007), achondroplasia (Ablon, 1984), Marfan syndrome (Peters et al., 2005), and ectodermal dysplasia (Clarke, 2013, 2016). The way that people respond to stigmatization is enormously variable, and some can "carry it off" more successfully than others. However, the pain of being stigmatized can be grave, even life-threatening, as seen on the dedication page of Erving Goffman's monograph.[1] The gains to those who perform and enjoy the act of stigmatizing, and the medley of emotions experienced by those who merely observe it, are less widely discussed.

"Looking different" can be enough to deter people from having children who might be affected in the same way, as they reflect upon what they have suffered (Clarke, 2013). It can also lead other members of the family to make the decision that the quality of life led by their affected relatives is too badly impacted by stigma for them to risk having an affected child (Clarke, 2016). At the broader level of society, similarly difficult questions are raised by population antenatal screening for Down syndrome, for example, with a tension between respect for those affected by the condition and the wish to respect the decisions of pregnant women (Clarke, 1991; Parens & Ash, 2000; Shakespeare, 1998; Williams et al., 2002; Wilfond, 2017). How can society make such screening available without disrespecting those with the conditions for which screening is made available, and perhaps promoted? However, this "expressivist objection" to antenatal screening operates perhaps even more powerfully within particular families, where it is one or a few individuals whose lives are being assessed and perhaps found wanting by their close relatives (Clarke, 2016). Looking beyond physical appearance to questions of physical impairment and survival, studies of the making of reproductive decisions within families affected by spinal muscular atrophy show the complexity and sensitivity of the factors taken into account by prospective parents (Boardman, 2014, 2017).

Making judgments about the quality of life of close relatives—or of oneself—can be painful, especially when the factors to be weighed include the hurt arising from the lack of decency and respect experienced by those affected. There are important but systematic differences between diseases about who makes the reproductive decisions: Who is judging the quality of whose life? In autosomal recessive conditions, it is usually parents making decisions about the life of an older child, perhaps deceased, unless the condition is one for which population screening has been offered (see section on Population Screening). For dominant disorders, it will usually be an affected patient (or someone at risk of a late-onset disease) who is making a decision about their own quality of life as well as the quality of life of their affected relatives and how the family disorder has impacted them. In sex-linked disorders, it is often women—the carriers—who make their decisions about whether to become pregnant or about prenatal diagnosis and (perhaps) termination of a pregnancy on the basis of how the affected males in their family have coped with the condition (Clarke, 2016; Kay & Kingston, 2002). Who makes these judgments about life with a genetic condition takes a different shape in a society where marriage is usually arranged or at least heavily vetted by parents and/or when consanguinity is customary (Rozario, 2007).

[1] Goffman reproduces, as a frontispiece to his monograph *Stigma*, a letter from *Miss Lonelyhearts* by Nathaniel West (1962), pp. 14–15. Cited in Goffman (1968), p. 7.

Discreditable stigma

When the condition in question does not affect the physical appearance of the child but can nonetheless be severe, as with being at risk of neurodegenerative conditions or those that cause sudden cardiac death or malignancy, the stigmatization is triggered not so much by physical appearance but by the knowledge that a person will (or may) develop a serious condition in the future or that their children may be at risk of a serious condition. There is the potential that the person may become discredited if this information surfaces. This applies to nongenetic "episodic" conditions, as well as Mendelian disorders. Marriage into a family with known risks of an inherited condition or even simple social relationships may be impacted by judgments made about their reproductive undesirability (Mendes et al., 2017). In contrast to the overt (enacted) stigma of physical appearance, stigmatization on the basis of potential future illness or a risk of disease in a future child takes us into the world of discreditable information that one might know about someone else if they have disclosed it or if they are the subject of gossip and rumor.

Societal discrimination

We have so far considered the ways in which a genetic condition may, directly or indirectly, impact socially on those affected or those who may carry the condition without (yet) manifesting it in their appearance or their behavior. Such stigmatization occurs in social interaction at the "micro" level. In contrast, genetic information can impact a person at an altogether different level of society: at the level of institutional discrimination. Genetic information—whether this is a gene test result or simple information about family history—may be used to a person's disadvantage by the state or by insurance companies or, potentially, by an employer or an educational institution. We use the term "discrimination" to refer to this more general, higher level, societal disadvantaging and distinguish it from the micro-level disadvantaging of stigmatization in personal interactions.

Health and life insurance policies are important elements in today's society, enabling home purchases for many as well as confidence and solvency in the face of illness and injury. It is fortunate that many countries have established legal or regulatory constraints on the ability of insurers to access genetic information about their clients or to act (i.e., discriminate) on the basis of such information. However, concern about the potential for institutional discrimination remains a real phenomenon in contemporary societies (Bombard et al., 2012; Erwin et al., 2010; McCormack et al., 2016), especially if confidence in the insurance arrangements provided by the state or insurance corporations is low. In some jurisdictions that provide a degree of protection against specific types of discrimination, this may be narrow in scope and limited in financial worth (e.g., it may apply to health insurance only, or only for some conditions, and not to life insurance or disability insurance or employment).

Austerity

Another aspect of the contemporary experience of living with a genetic condition is the provision of support to those affected, in relation to their needs for health and social care and education. In the United Kingdom, the decade or so since 2010 has seen a fall in the quantity and quality of care provided for many of those with genetic conditions who present with multiple, complex problems. Individuals with very substantial needs and impairments have, in effect, been competing with each other for access to the diminishing resources available. In educational services, for example, being able to identify an underlying genetic diagnosis can make all the difference to the type of schooling that can be accessed. One child with precisely the same needs as another may be left without adequate support simply because, unlike the other, they have no molecular diagnosis. While the use of a confirmed diagnosis to strengthen the case for additional support for a child's schooling has been common practice for much longer, the recent increased competition between children for access to a more limited pool of resources has made this need for a diagnosis increasingly important since the financial crisis of 2008–2009. Of course, achieving a diagnosis can bring additional benefits—such as a sense of understanding, solidarity with other families, and the ability to make informed reproductive decisions—but access to basic care is now often also at stake. The decision to impose austerity on the public sector (cuts to local or central government spending on education, health, and social services) has had serious and often arbitrary consequences for many patients and families, varying with zone of residence. Comparable problems have arisen in countries with different healthcare systems.

An awareness of these problems creeps slowly through society, even in families with no experience of genetic disorders. As this has been in process for more than a decade in the United Kingdom, there is now rather less confidence that "society" would provide an effective safety net in the event of a child being born with complex needs. Acute healthcare would be provided, but there is less confidence in the quality of long-term social support or the ability of the education system to identify and deliver the appropriate input for children with special needs. These diminished expectations for support, if it were to be needed, shape the context within which people are now making decisions about the investigation and management of genetic conditions and decisions about reproduction. And this brings us to the genetics clinic.

Within the Consultation

Diagnosis and uncertainty

One common route into genetic services is the quest for a diagnosis. A patient or, more often, a child's parents wish to find a diagnosis to account for the condition affecting them. A unifying diagnosis—if the patient has more than one symptom or problem—can be very helpful not only because it provides some understanding and explanation but also practically; a diagnosis may give information about possible treatments, reproductive options, and the potential to anticipate future problems as well as allowing access to a family support group. As discussed above, this may also be used within a system where access to support is limited, to boost the strength of one's claim for educational, healthcare, or social services support. Those with a diagnosis that can be confirmed on genetic testing are at an advantage in seeking additional support, although such support should be rationed by an assessment of needs rather than the effectiveness otherwise of biomedical investigations. Rephrasing this, one could say that a child may be denied the support they need on the spurious and inappropriate grounds that a molecular diagnosis has not been identified that accounts for their difficulties. These problems in educational provision and social care have become important motivators for referral to clinical genetics services.

Only a decade ago, when precise genetic explanations for a child's neurodevelopmental problems were rather less likely to be found, the recognition of a syndrome as a unifying diagnosis often depended on clinical experience, skill, and intuition. Now, genome-wide investigations—chromosomal microarrays (CMAs) and high-throughput sequencing of exomes or genomes—make it more likely (closer to 50%) that a diagnosis will emerge. However, one form of uncertainty ("What is the explanation for these problems?") is often being replaced by others ("What difference does this label make?" "Does this mean you can treat my child more effectively?" "Is there anyone else in our country—or the world—whose child has precisely the same problem?" "What is the long-term outlook for someone with this genetic change you have identified?"). It is all too easy for us to gloss over the limitations of a precise molecular diagnosis in the excitement and enthusiasm at the hugely impressive scientific achievement, which it undoubtedly represents. And "in the long term" we can hope that there will be practical benefits for at least some of the patients, although the road to those benefits may be long and consume enormous effort and substantial resources.

For now, however, talking with families in clinics, we need to be realistic about what a diagnosis might bring and what it probably will not. As we will return to later, practitioners should not overpromise but must remain grounded in what are likely to be the outcomes of diagnostic efforts for their patients. To raise the expectations of patients and their families beyond what is realistic about the ability to treat some of the devastating rare diseases that we can now diagnose is desperately unfair, imposing huge emotional hurt.

We need to explain that there are at least four principal categories of results from genetic investigations, especially genome-wide investigations, that is, CMA and exome sequencing (ES) or genome sequencing (GS). This should be understood by practitioners and conveyed to their patients in the appropriate contexts:

1. A test may give clear results. It may provide a good explanation for the condition that has arisen, and this may sometimes be useful in terms of medical management, informing reproductive decisions, or indicating ways in which the patient may be monitored in case they develop disease complications. Distressing emotions may also surface—guilt and blame, stigmatization and the fear of discrimination—but it is difficult to reject efforts at a diagnosis so as to avoid such problems. These issues should be addressed head-on, not evaded by avoiding a diagnosis.
2. A test may fail to find an explanation for the condition. This does not necessarily mean that the condition in question is not genetic but rather that the investigation has simply failed to identify the genetic cause or explanation.
3. A test may find a genetic variant of uncertain significance (VUS). For example, a copy number variant may be found on CMA, indicating a deletion or duplication of a section of chromosome, or a change in DNA sequence may be found within a gene. However, it may be unclear whether the variant found is responsible for the signs or symptoms for which an explanation is being sought. This may greatly disappoint a patient or their family, and it may cause confusion. One approach might be to test other

individuals in the family; has the variant arisen as a de novo new event in a child, or is it also present in unaffected members of the family? Asking relatives to provide a blood sample to help is expecting a lot, when the results of testing might implicate them as being at risk of a problem, might reveal nonpaternity, or might simply draw them into the confusion. Another approach is to trust the accumulation of knowledge and experience over time, gathered in large, international databases, through which scientists share information about genetic variants. As more information is gathered, it becomes more feasible to make judgments about whether any specific variant is likely to be benign or pathogenic and, if pathogenic, to what problems it might contribute. Thus, when a patient is told that a genetic variant has been found, but it is classified as a VUS, there is usually no reason to doubt the DNA sequence itself. However, there is the potential hope that its interpretation may be changed and that it may be reclassified over the coming years. The result is thus provisional. It is also possible for results given as pathogenic or benign to be reinterpreted as more evidence accumulates, perhaps from benign to pathogenic or vice versa, or to become a VUS. While that type of reinterpretation does not happen often, and we can be highly confident of some results, any variant interpretation is in principle a provisional result. Adjusting to the uncertainty that surrounds such genomic information may be difficult for nonspecialist healthcare practitioners as well as patients and families, but it is important to keep this potential openness to new information if genomics is to be used to our patients' best advantage (Newson et al., 2016).

4. Finally, while looking for a possible genetic explanation for one problem, we might unexpectedly come across an indication of an altogether different problem or pathology. For example, CMA might fail to identify a likely cause for a young girl's developmental delay but might detect a deletion of one or more exons within *BRCA1* or *BRCA2*. Such a deletion would most likely be irrelevant in relation to the developmental delay but could indicate a substantially increased lifetime risk of cancer in the child and, very possibly, in one of her parents. Decisions will need to be made about how to manage this information, which might also be relevant to the wider family, not only to the girl and her parents.

Opportunistic genomic screening

This point in the discussion leads neatly into another question that may have to be raised with, and considered by, the family. This is whether any additional genetic information should be sought at the same time as carrying out the genetic testing suggested by the clinician and agreed to by the patient or their proxy to establish the molecular cause of the clinical diagnosis of an identified problem. If the investigation being performed is analysis of a large gene panel to identify the cause of a particular phenotype in the patient, the assay performed in the laboratory may have determined the exome or genome sequence and any variants in the genes of the panel that will then have been interpreted to assess their relevance to the presenting problem. Given that many other gene loci will have had their sequence determined too, the additional (marginal) cost of interpreting variants found in a selected set of additional loci and reporting the clinically important variants identified will be much less than the cost of establishing a genomic screening program from scratch to look at them across the whole population. It is argued by enthusiasts that such screening therefore need not meet the full, traditional Wilson and Jungner criteria for a standalone public health screening program (Wilson & Jungner, 1968; see also UK National Screening Committee, 2015); it may be feasible to regard this testing as an opportunistic form of genome screening for variants that are known to be pathogenic and where there are interventions proven to be useful to offer the patient alongside the unwelcome information about genetic risk (Mighton et al., 2025; Miller et al., 2021).

The term "opportunistic genomic screening" carries some negative connotations, at least in English, especially the suggestion that the test might in some way be unfairly taking advantage of the situation in which patients find themselves. Circumstances in which this may be true in relation to GS are certainly well recognized in the care of sick infants, with implications for the process of consent for testing as parents may be able to consent to a diagnostic assessment but not be in an appropriate emotional state to make judgments about opportunistic genomic screening and other issues with consequences for the long term. This is especially important when diagnostic findings on GS may be more likely to lead to the discontinuation of intensive care than to an improved prognosis (Char et al., 2018). However, such concerns are usually countered by the idea that the patient is—on the contrary—fortunate to gain some unlooked-for, additional insights into their profile of genetic susceptibilities. Surely this will be to their advantage? However, there are multiple difficulties with such active searching for additional genomic findings that are unrelated to the indication for carrying out the initial investigation. The patient or family may have other priorities in the face of serious illness (it depends on the full context), so their ability to make good decisions or adjust to additional unwelcome information may be limited. Furthermore, they will be expected to make decisions about a number of hypothetical scenarios, none of which is likely to arise. So, their engagement with the questions will be undermined for this reason too, and it may be difficult for professionals to feel confidence in abiding by these hypothetical advance decisions.

It is important that the patient is aware before having the investigation of the types of information that might emerge from it. This can complicate the patient's or family's decisions about testing and about communication, which have to be confronted despite the potential burden entailed in doing so. Thus, the reinterpretation of a test result or a finding that emerges later may have important implications for multiple members of a family, so the first in the family to be given such information will often be expected to pass it on to others. This process may be unwelcome and burdensome for the index case and may be unreliable from the perspective of others in the family who stand to benefit from the information.

Timing aside, this additional, sought information will sometimes prove helpful to the patient or others in the family, but sometimes it will not. Our ability to find the variant that explains or accounts for the disease in a family known to have a genetic problem (to travel in the direction "phenotype → genotype") is much greater than our ability to predict whether or not a novel genetic variant is likely to be pathogenic (to travel in the direction "genotype → phenotype") when the family is not known to have an inherited problem that could be accounted for by the variant identified. Our "genotype → phenotype" skills will improve, but they are far from robust; and it is likely that unhelpful inferences will sometimes be drawn.

The burden of knowledge and of decisions

The knowledge that a disorder is genetic, or has a predominantly genetic cause, can be burdensome. Not only is there the question of possible guilt or blame, but also simply knowing a problem is genetic raises questions that may be troubling. If you become aware that you may be at risk of a serious disease, that a genetic variant you have transmitted to a child is responsible for their severe neurodevelopmental problems, that the children you have already had are at risk of developing and manifesting a serious condition in the future, or that any future child you have may be affected, then that knowledge itself may bring sadness and perhaps grief (Evans, 2006; Kessler et al., 1984). This knowledge may then present you with decisions and choices to be made, which become additional burdens. You may have to decide whether, when, and how to share this information with other members of the family, with potential marriage partners, and with any children you may have. You may need to decide whether the risks involved should lead you to alter your plans for reproduction. Whatever decision you do or do not make, simply being aware of the problem is *per se* a burden. Indeed, even the much lower population risks that are addressed by antenatal screening programs impose a burden on many pregnant women (Lippman, 1991; Rapp, 2000; Rothman, 1988). From a detached and rational perspective, ignorance of familial risks may be worse than an accurate understanding of one's position; however, the human individual impacted by genetic test results may not experience it this way (Arribas-Ayllon et al., 2011; Weil, 1991). An accurate understanding of "the facts" is perfectly compatible with a range of beliefs about the underlying causes of the condition in question (Weil, 1991).

While any genetic counselor will wish to be "client led" and not to impose an agenda on their patients, it would be a professional failure for a patient to make unconsidered decisions by default, without having the potentially difficult consequences raised for discussion in advance. Striking the right balance is difficult.

The parents of a child born with a malformation or affected by a serious genetic disorder will often experience guilt and shame simply from being the parent of an affected child. If the child's problems have a clear genetic cause or were caused by exposure to antenatal infection, then the parent may assume "blame"—a sense of biological responsibility one could term "biological guilt," completely separate from any moral blameworthiness. The opportunities for such guilt and concerns about stigma and discrimination to be experienced are likely to increase as GS becomes more frequently used to make diagnoses in sick newborn infants (Deem, 2016), thereby adding to these emotional burdens for parents. Parental guilt can also become entangled with moral guilt if the child's problems may be the result of antenatal (*in utero*) exposure to alcohol or drugs. Genetic professionals will often seek to reduce the feelings of blameless, "biological guilt" felt by either or both parents. This is motivated by kindness and is generally to be commended. It is important, however, to take care about how this is done. Pointing out that "It was not your fault—you were not to know" or "There was nothing you could have done to prevent this" may well be true, but such statements carry with them a barbed judgment about future actions. While the relief of guilt at what has happened may be welcomed, the words spoken may be taken as a strong message not to let the same thing happen again. If the condition could be diagnosed early in a future pregnancy, the same simple reassurance would not be available a second time, so that form of reassurance could be experienced by the parents in the future as powerfully coercive.

Population Screening

Blame and antenatal screening

When antenatal screening for at least some genetic disorders and for major malformations is widely available, the birth of an affected infant may be regarded by the healthcare system as a failure of the screening program, if its goal is understood as being to reduce the population incidence of specific conditions, such as Down syndrome. This could then lead staff to want their patients to accept screening, which could lead to pressure on patients to do so. This pressure may be exerted or felt at multiple different levels. The drive to reduce the birth incidence of the condition may have been the reason for establishing the program, as in any disease prevention program driven by considerations of public health or health economics. Such considerations were certainly present as antenatal screening was introduced in the United Kingdom but have over time been more or less removed from policy documents and the information provided to pregnant women, with the explicit goal changing to the enabling of parental reproductive autonomy. The message that antenatal screening is designed to reduce or eliminate the birth incidence of infants affected by chromosomal disorders and malformation, however, may still be conveyed through the operation of the program. This may be regarded as a 'structural' form of directiveness (Clarke, 1991) because the routinization of participation in screening and, if an anomaly is found, a termination of pregnancy can be conveyed through the system of clinic organization as well as many subtle features of professional–patient interaction. And the scope for these implicit messages to impose responsibility on parents, conveyed through the availability of additional information, has expanded very substantially with the introduction of genomics into antenatal screening (Ravitsky et al., 2017).

Those who do not accept screening, or who continue a pregnancy despite its being identified as at increased risk of a disorder, may be regarded as irresponsible and therefore blameworthy. This can have a number of consequences that vary with the system of health care. In a fully private system, the family will have to meet the financial costs of caring for an infant who requires costly treatments, and the prospect of that financial burden may of course influence the family's decisions. If a family's access to healthcare depends on insurance arranged by an employer, there could be pressure from a company for employees to participate in antenatal screening, to terminate an affected pregnancy, and to not have a second child affected by the same condition if prenatal diagnosis can be offered. Even a system of national healthcare or a universal social insurance scheme could strongly encourage families to "take advantage of" antenatal screening and prenatal diagnosis and could fail to provide adequate support for women who decline to follow the "preferred" course of action, if they decide not to terminate a pregnancy when their fetus has been diagnosed with an autosomal trisomy or a major malformation.

While many developed countries now offer legal protection from (unfair) discrimination in health insurance, they cannot always counter the implicit (or even overt) pressure from professionals, as well as family, friends, and neighbors, to accept antenatal screening and prenatal diagnosis and to terminate an affected pregnancy (classic publications include Rothman, 1988, and Rapp, 2000). The strength of social expectations to comply with a national policy of screening that aims to prevent genetic disease—monitored by social networks as well as, perhaps, the state—could make screening difficult to resist. Antenatal screening can become effectively compulsory through a combination of routinization in the clinic and coercive social pressure in the outside world.

Carrier screening for beta-thalassemia (etc.)

Another type of reproductive genetic screening is screening to identify carriers of specific autosomal recessive disorders. This is currently promoted in two rather different contexts; it can be promoted by for-profit genetic testing corporations in developed countries, and it can be promoted by states as a way of reducing the birth incidence of genetic disorders, especially in developing countries (Dive et al., 2022; Molster et al., 2017). The corporate promotion of carrier screening now uses either chips to identify specific alleles at relevant single nucleotide polymorphisms (SNPs) or high-throughout DNA sequencing to look for variants in many (often hundreds of) recessive disease loci; this can be represented as either a matter of consumer choice (i.e., autonomy for those with the resources) or, by critics, as a consumer-driven eugenics (Duster, 1990).

The state promotion of carrier screening for recessive disorders—usually including beta-thalassemia and related haemoglobinopathies—is rather different (Cornel & Clarke, 2021; Modell, 2020). Such programs have often been established to enable the treatment of those already present in the population plus any additional affected infants born despite screening: Without screening, and the subsequent use by carrier couples of prenatal diagnosis, the treatment of those affected would rapidly become unaffordable for low-income countries as the number of treated survivors increased.

A program of carrier screening has been operating for some decades in Cyprus and other Mediterranean countries. This has more recently extended to Iran, Saudi Arabia, and a number of Gulf states. Pressure to comply with screening, often before marriage, may be considerable, with couples who are both carriers being led either to find different ("more compatible") marriage partners or to use prenatal diagnosis in any pregnancy, with a view to terminating the pregnancy if it is affected. The original motivation for these programs often related specifically to beta-thalassemia, as any attempt to treat this (eminently treatable) disorder would present a low-income country with immense difficulties. Treatment is either by blood transfusion and iron chelation treatment for life or by bone marrow transplantation (often needing lifelong immunosuppression). Without effective treatment, the life expectancy of those affected is only a few years, so if treatment were started, there would be a steadily growing population of affected children; the numbers to be treated would increase steadily and the costs would soon become unaffordable, as treatment could only be sustained if the birth incidence is low.

A somewhat intermediate form of screening has operated—again for decades—in Orthodox Jewish communities. Originally established to identify carriers of Tay-Sachs disease, these programs have adopted molecular genetic technologies to extend the screening to include other disorders common among the relevant community (especially Ashkenazi Jewish groups). Among specific groups, within which marriages are usually arranged, the individuals screened may not be given their results, but a marriage will be arranged that does not bring together a couple who are both carriers of the same condition.

Before long, comparable problems may arise even in wealthy countries if enormously expensive rational, gene-based therapies are devised for large numbers of rare disorders. The numbers to be treated for each rare disease alone would be very few, but the costs could become enormous if treatments for more and more diseases became possible. This is one reason gene editing holds out the tantalizing potential of a once-off (or at least very infrequent) genetic correction for many different disorders, while approaches such as enzyme replacement therapies for lysosomal storage disorders need to be lifelong and the treatments have distinct problems, such as unhelpful immune responses.

The question relevant to us here is that of personal control. In which of these programs is the individual able to make their own decisions about carrier screening? Where are they obliged or coerced to participate against their wishes? Are there ever circumstances in which the welfare of the community overrides the question of personal autonomy? It may be provocative to label this as "eugenics," as the word is often used as an insult comparable to the word "Nazi." However, there are some aspects of 19th-century eugenics that are unexceptionable and relate to nutritional support of pregnant women or the provision of health visitor services to families with young children. Where does the wish to reduce the birth incidence of some disorders, so as to enable the treatment of those affected children who are born, fit on the spectrum from effective antenatal care and community pediatric services ("good") to forcibly imposed terminations of pregnancy and involuntary sterilization ("bad")? This could well be regarded as an aspect of eugenics, and this is not intended here to be unhelpfully provocative: It is a real question, as the ability of a society to provide effective treatment for all its beta-thalassemia patients is of deep concern (Cornel & Clarke, 2021).

Some wealthy countries in North Africa and along the Red Sea and Persian Gulf are extending the range of disorders included in carrier screening. This ramps up the issues still further, especially where the society practices both customary consanguinity and arranged marriage. These societies often face a high incidence of severe childhood-onset recessive disease, and this strategy is a response that allows them to continue these social practices while reducing the otherwise high rates of infant and childhood mortality and the costs of healthcare. Different perspectives are possible on this use of genomic technologies to perpetuate the system of control over young women.

Antenatal screening again: Noninvasive prenatal genetic testing

An important development in antenatal screening has been noninvasive prenatal genetic testing (NIPT; Nuffield Council on Bioethics, 2017).[2] This technique examines short fragments of DNA present in maternal plasma; these are mostly derived from the mother's

[2] While the term "noninvasive prenatal screening" is used widely, there are reasons for preferring "NIPT." This is primarily because there are many uses of the same basic technology that spread across a spectrum of precision, from first-tier population screening to highly precise (i.e., diagnostic) applications in other contexts. It is preferable to use "NIPT" to cover the spectrum and then give an explanation as to the precise context and degree of precision in any particular application.

tissues, but from 9 to 10 weeks of gestation, some 5% to 10% will usually come from the chorion (i.e., the placenta). It is then possible to make inferences about the genetic constitution of the fetus, with varying levels of sensitivity and specificity and varying positive predictive values (PPVs) that depend on the precise circumstances. Some applications of NIPT are used as part of antenatal population genetic screening, while others are used in prenatal diagnosis.

The great advantage of NIPT in antenatal screening for Down syndrome, as compared to conventional biochemical and ultrasound screening, is its high sensitivity and lower rate of false-positive results. However, the PPV of a "screen positive" result for Down syndrome, when NIPT is used as a primary screening test, is still only ~80+%, and ~90+ % if used as a secondary screen. This means that the number of invasive tests that might be indicated from screening is much reduced, which reduces the anxiety of pregnant women and the number of procedure-related pregnancy losses. However, it is important to ensure that women understand the limitations of the test. An invasive test is still required to confirm a positive NIPT result (i.e., a result showing increased chance of an autosomal trisomy). It is crucial that neither the test providers nor the pregnant women think that the NIPT result is sufficiently reliable that they can dispense with an invasive diagnostic test.

There are four possible disadvantages of NIPT that we need now to mention, depending on the way in which it is made available: (a) the presentation of NIPT as highly "accurate" but often without any explanation of the PPV; (b) the ease with which NIPT can reveal fetal sex; (c) the marketing of the test with "add-on" dosage results, indicating chromosomal microdeletions or microduplications, as if this gives a bonus value; and (d) the possibility of NIPT exacerbating the damage that antenatal screening does to the well-being of those with Down syndrome, in particular, and intellectual disability more generally.

1. NIPT used as a screening test for fetal autosomal trisomy (especially Down syndrome) is indeed greater than 99% accurate. However, this is misleading, as the chance of such a chromosome anomaly is generally less than 1%, so one could say with greater than 99% accuracy that the fetus will have normal chromosomes without doing any test at all. The crucial information a woman needs to make her decision is the chance that a positive result is correct (or incorrect). If the test indicates an increased chance of Down syndrome, what is the chance that the fetus will indeed have Down syndrome (i.e., what is the test's PPV)? This depends on the circumstances but is often on the order of 80+% to 90+%, so there will often be a 15% to 20% or 5% to 10% chance that the fetus does not have Down syndrome (Taylor-Phillips et al., 2016). It is essential that the accuracy of such tests is set out in this fashion, and not as a global "accuracy" result, if the woman is to understand the test and appreciate what it is and is not able to do.
2. There are strong reasons to be wary of revealing fetal sex early in a pregnancy unless there are clinical, medical grounds for needing to know this. This is because it opens up the possibility that a female pregnancy may be interrupted because of a strong preference in some communities to have sons rather than daughters. This practice is unlawful in the United Kingdom (Patel, 2018) and also illegal in both India and China. Still, it is widely practiced in the latter two countries, to such an extent that the sex ratio at birth in parts of India is around 0.7 girls to 1.0 boy, with the ratio

overall being about 0.9:1 (Chao et al., 2019; Hesketh & Xing, 2011). Four factors have come together in a perfect storm, a collision of (a) a traditional patriarchal power structure; (b) a strong preference among men (and among women influenced by the patriarchal power structures) for male children; (c) the continuation of the illegal practice of dowry, at least in India; and (d) the recently developed ability to determine fetal sex in the first trimester by NIPT. This has exacerbated the practice, already widely established, of fetal sex selection making use of mobile ultrasound scanning to determine fetal sex in the second trimester. NIPT, however, has the "advantage" of allowing a result in the first trimester. The social and emotional consequences of the resulting distortion of the sex ratio were already grave but are likely to become much worse in the age of NIPT, even for those girls who survive to be born.

3. The commercial offer of NIPT screening for additional chromosomal anomalies, in addition to the autosomal trisomies, may appear to give the test more value. The technical performance of NIPT for these additional microdeletion syndromes has in general been less well established, and the PPVs in general are lower than for traditional trisomies (Blagowidow et al., 2023). Additional amniocenteses may then be triggered, so that the key advantage of using NIPT—many fewer invasive tests of unaffected pregnancies—could be lost.
4. Finally, there is the discrimination, experienced by many of those affected by Down syndrome, that society has chosen to implement antenatal screening "for" (i.e., against) them, with a realistic prospect of eliminating most Down syndrome births over the next few years in many countries. Whereas the practices of conventional (pre-NIPT) screening have had an emotional impact on those with Down syndrome, leading to sadness as a result of being stigmatized, NIPT is likely to reduce the birth incidence of the condition more effectively and may even threaten the very existence of the Down syndrome community (Alderson, 2001; Skotko et al., 2009; van den Heuvel et al., 2010). This, in turn, is likely to exacerbate the stigmatization of those individuals who are born with Down syndrome and of those parents who choose either not to be screened or to continue with an affected pregnancy. Stigmatization of those with Down syndrome is also likely to impact adversely on the experiences of those affected by many different forms of intellectual disability, and their families, and provoke further stigmatization.

Assumptions

Rather than deliberate attempts to persuade or coerce patients to behave against their values and wishes, professionals may implement such inappropriate directiveness either inadvertently through the systems within which they operate ("structural directiveness") or as individuals through the making of assumptions. This is especially true of screening programs, where a patient can be told what the next step will be or that "what everyone does now is . . ." (Pilnick, 2002).

Other assumptions that constrain the decisions of patients and families can be made. In the United Kingdom, some practitioners might imagine that Muslim women would never terminate a pregnancy on the grounds of fetal abnormality. They might, as a consequence of this mistake, decide not to offer them antenatal screening. This would compound the error—through making a further assumption, that termination of an affected pregnancy was the only purpose of antenatal screening—but would also serve to further remove agency from this patient (i.e., from patients who fit into this particular category in the mind of the practitioner). There is a fine line to be drawn between "cultural sensitivity" or "cultural competence" and inappropriate stereotyping, imposing a notional homogeneity on social groups that are in fact complex and diverse.[3] This represents a case of racial essentialism, one of the foundational steps underlying racism (Appiah, 2018).

Another common assumption is that everyone would want to terminate a pregnancy in which the fetus was found to be affected by an inevitably lethal malformation. This assumption leaves unsupported those women who wish to continue their pregnancy and to comfort and nurture their infant after birth, as the infant dies, and perhaps to enjoy the infant if they live for a few hours, days, or weeks. Such women may feel coerced to submit to a termination of pregnancy. If they wish not to do so, they may have to be repeatedly very assertive, over the course of the second half of the pregnancy, to resist being swept along toward a termination. The experience of a woman in such a situation can vary enormously, depending on the ethos of the particular unit or clinical team involved in providing her care (Hickerton et al., 2012).

Across the range of possible contexts and scenarios that arise in relation to genetic disorders, there are many other inappropriate assumptions that can be made about what a patient would or should wish to do or decide to do. While practitioners should of course be open to reading subtle cues from a patient's behaviors, from what they say and what they leave unsaid, they must not fall into the trap of making unwarranted assumptions but must reflect critically upon the inferences they are drawing.

Society

Promising too much: Exploitation through expectations

Some people expect a genetic diagnosis to lead promptly to a cure. Such a misapprehension can often be corrected without causing great distress, as it is usually based on a lack of knowledge and a simple explanation provides enough clarification. However, when patients or families think that scientists have promised them a cure, this can be much more problematic. If a patient or parent is clinging to falsely inflated expectations of deliverance and their hopes are dashed, it can cause immense distress. Not only do they now have to face the grim truth, but also they may feel foolish for having been deceived.

Family support groups, like physicians, have to walk a tightrope between maintaining hope and promoting realism, but it is an important balance for all of us to maintain. If the

[3] Editors' note: For a discussion of "cultural responsiveness" and the shift away from notions of "cultural competence" in the clinical literature, see Chapter 29 of this volume by Nancy Warren.

parents of children with profound developmental problems are persuaded that scientists have a cure for their child's condition almost within their grasp, they can be energized to raise funds for the science. This may advance understanding and might produce therapies that are effective in mice or that could in principle work in humans if the treatment was started in embryonic life or perhaps before the symptoms began. However, the chance that it would benefit the child now impacted by the condition (i.e., that it could reverse neurodevelopmental problems that began during early embryonic life) might be remote. Every disease is different, and for some conditions a postnatal treatment might lead to some benefit, although even that might depend on the class of disease-causing mutation. Treatments of benefit when the condition is caused by one type of mutational process might be of no value when the same disorder has been caused by a different class of mutation in the same gene. The enthusiastic researcher who wants to clarify the underlying mechanism of the disease, and thereby advance their career, has to take great care not to exploit the motivation—indeed, the desperation—of vulnerable families. Even when there are some prospects of benefit to the patients emerging from the research, great care, caution, and respect are needed to avoid exploitation (Clarke & Abdala Sheikh, 2018).

When a plausible treatment has been developed, there are still several ways in which practice can lose its way. Funding may be difficult to obtain, as the costs of research—and the costs of any potential treatment that emerges from it—may be exorbitant. Proof of the safety and efficacy of a treatment may be slow to arrive, and this problem and the high costs of a treatment arise in part because of the small number of patients who might be eligible for treatment, since the disease is likely to be rare. The number of patients who could be included in a trial will be very small, especially if they need to live close to a clinical team participating in the trial. Within a country, the families of those affected will often know each other and may be cared for by one principal team that combines care with research. Decisions about whether to participate in a trial may, as a result, be influenced by relationships and interpersonal dynamics within a support group or between a leading clinician and the various families. Every therapeutic trial has a potential for therapeutic misconception, but, in rare diseases, the scope for such problems in a trial may be much greater (Woods et al., 2014).

Genomic testing that is accessed through private and commercial systems, sometimes provided direct to consumer (DTC) without a physician mediating between the corporation and the patient/customer, is vulnerable to additional problems. While a state, social, or insurance-based healthcare system will usually aim to contain costs through only providing treatments of established efficacy and safety, this is not true in a fully private healthcare system. A genomic testing company can set out to promote its tests so as to maximize sales, without any concern for whether or how the information is applied. "Counseling" could be confused with marketing, and tests could be promoted even if the validity of their results or their clinical utility is poor. The Latin tag "*Caveat emptor*!" ("Buyer beware!") springs to mind.

The two areas of commercially sourced genome-wide testing that are most widely used in developed countries are those of "disease susceptibility screening," sometimes presented in the form of polygenic risk scores (PRSs), and NIPT, especially as it is used in antenatal population screening rather than its much more restricted use in some very specific, diagnostic applications. We have already considered the commercial programs of NIPT, and

I will turn here to disease susceptibility screening, based on genotyping individuals for very large numbers of SNPs.

It is very unusual for an SNP to be the direct cause of a serious disease, since there would then be strong selection against that allele. Rather, SNPs associated with a disease must be seen as sites in the genome where ancient variants either have been maintained passively through population history or are maintained actively through gene–environment or gene–gene interactions. Associations between an SNP and a disease may be highly significant statistically, but their magnitude is usually only very weak (a typical odds ratio for one allele compared to the other might be a 1.02:1 risk for developing the disease). By testing many SNPs, those associated with a disease can be identified and—making an assumption that they operate independently—the person's overall risk can be estimated by combining these risks multiplicatively. Problems with such SNP risk profiles—PRSs—include the assumptions on which they are based (e.g., that they operate independently) and their exclusion of the less common variants of much larger effect size. While it might be attractive to combine these with physiological measures (e.g., blood pressure or blood cholesterol, both of relevance in assessing a person's risk of stroke or myocardial infarction), that is difficult if the SNP risks are, or might be, mediated through the physiological variable as they would then not operate independently.

To summarize the field at present, it would be fair to say that PRSs developed from genome-wide SNP association studies have applications in research studies that seek insights into the pathogenesis of disease but currently have limited clinical utility in the investigation or medical management of patients (Janssens, 2019; Moorthie et al., 2021; Penders & Janssens, 2022).

The claim that a risk profile can help to motivate individuals to lead healthier lifestyles is supported by anecdote but not by evidence, which has given disappointing results (Hollands et al., 2016). Furthermore, the fact that the "healthy lifestyle" to be adopted is often much the same, whether an individual is at high risk or low risk of a specific disease, hardly supports the claim that the polygenic risk assessment of individuals is a valuable strategy for improving public health. The advice will be framed in terms of food, exercise, weight (body mass index), social networks, and occupational hazards and is hardly altered by the genetic testing. However, collective strategies are likely to be the simplest, cheapest, and most effective for tackling many of these risks. There are strong grounds for promoting "the public health" through collective approaches to the problems that confront us all in our communities, including food policy, air and water quality, town planning, efficient public transport, access to lifelong education, and "health and safety" at work. The genetic approach to tackling the common diseases of our time through the individualization of risk flies against the evidence and could be seen as a harmful distraction from what is important. Furthermore, if this process of individualized and privatized genetic risk assessment were (unexpectedly) to bring any substantial benefits, it would do so inequitably by benefiting only those who had opted to pay for such testing.

This leads us very naturally into a final consideration of the ways in which genomic medicine may function to exacerbate serious, preexisting inequities in health. The following section is therefore a pointer to areas of public health where we must strive to ensure that any benefits from genomic initiatives in medicine operate to the advantage of all sections of society.

Healthcare Funding and Healthcare Inequities

Funding

In several of the earlier sections of this chapter, we have seen how tests may be provided as a service despite being clinically inappropriate or even clearly harmful. Or they may be provided within a context that misleads the patient. Thus, NIPT antenatal screening tests may be provided without the patient appreciating the limitations of the test, either before having the test (and therefore agreeing to the test) or after a positive result (increased chance of fetal trisomy, leading to the patient seeking a termination of the pregnancy, despite a substantial chance that the test result did not reflect the chromosomal constitution of the fetus). Or a patient with a family history of breast cancer, coronary artery disease, or colon cancer may seek a "genome health check" and be given modestly reassuring PRSs for these conditions, which leads them not to seek proper advice about their family history, so that their greatly increased risk of disease because of their strong, Mendelian disease predisposition is not identified. Such unethical practices have been commonplace, sometimes arranged through regular clinical services (Nuffield Council of Bioethics, 2017) or through internet-based, DTC tests that provide an estimate of polygenic disease susceptibility of no clinical utility (as discussed earlier).

Even within a formally organized healthcare system, the way that genetics services are funded may shape the adequacy of the services delivered. Thus, if genetic counseling is seen as separable from testing in organizational and budgeting terms, then poor practice could easily be encouraged. If genetic counselors challenge clients, as they should at times, so that some of their patients decide not to be tested or at least to defer testing, then this element of the service may be seen as dysfunctional because the clinic is employing genetic counselors who reduce the earnings of the clinic instead of increasing them, as they discourage some "customers" from buying the test. As a result, the salaries of these genetic counselors may be seen as dispensable, unless genetic counselors function as marketing assistants who should promote testing uncritically and without reference to the circumstances of the patient and their considered view after carefully weighing their decision. This approach seeks to reduce genetics services to a market-based model that depends on maximizing the volume of testing. For this sort of reason, it is important that "counseling plus testing" is provided as a unified service, to avoid institutional pressures to minimize the "counseling" aspects of the service. Such problems have held back the recognition of genetic counseling within several European countries for years, in combination with ungrounded fears that genetic counselors would take over much of the workload of clinical geneticists.

Health inequity

In addition to the problems created by the operation of genetics services, there is real potential for genetic and especially genomic services to add to the preexisting health inequities within our societies, which will of course exacerbate the much more general problems of social inequity in access to healthcare on the basis of gender and age, occupation and education, social class, and wealth. Indeed, this final section of the chapter could be seen as an attempt to elucidate the way in which the inverse care law of Julian Tudor Hart applies in the context of genomics (Tudor Hart, 1971).

One process through which the practice of genomics can reinforce inequities is in our response to the recognition that the interpretation of variants, and of genome sequencing more broadly, is a rapidly developing field. If a variant is difficult to interpret and is reported as being of uncertain significance, then it would often be recommended that the patient should return to the clinic for a subsequent reassessment, including a reinterpretation of the VUS. This places an active obligation on the patient (or parent) to contact the clinic after an appropriate interval, perhaps 2 to 3 years. While that might initially appear reasonable, it is all too clear that there will be differential uptake of this not determined by clinical need but by access to the internet and often by access to a car. Those families who are worn down by unemployment and poverty or who experience physical disease, mental illness, disability, learning difficulties, or social chaos may find it more difficult to act proactively in the role of the compliant patient following these instructions.

Another important way in which genomics is exacerbating inequity is through the over-representation of genomic research and population databases on those of European ancestry, so that the benefits that accrue from genomic testing—especially the greater ease in interpreting genetic variants found in clinical diagnostics—occur predominantly for those of White European ancestry, who in any case generally receive more healthcare while suffering less disease than those from other population groups. Fortunately, the scientific community has recognized this problem and has already started work to mitigate it, although questions of access to the benefits of research on expanded databases may remain an issue for a long time. Just because more samples from those of African ancestry are included in research databases does not mean that residents of the African continent will suddenly gain ready access to the benefits of genomic medicine.

Related to this are other factors that shape the funding decisions that guide the future trajectory of genomics in healthcare. Into what type of diseases do states, corporations, and research charities choose to invest their resources? Corporations will certainly choose to invest in the development of diagnostics and therapeutics that relate to common diseases in wealthy countries, where healthcare systems can afford to purchase the companies' products. Such factors have long been at work in relation to the "orphan" status of treatments for rare diseases and the neglect of tropical disease research. Fortunately, there are some positive signs in these areas of concern. The European Union and the United States have both taken steps to facilitate the development and licensing of treatments for rare diseases. Tropical disease research has also been given support by the Wellcome Trust and the Bill and Melinda Gates Foundation, and we can hope that these initiatives lead to major and sustained improvement in the quality of life for those affected by such conditions.

Returning to consider those who are already disadvantaged, one must take stock of how their difficulties might be exacerbated by genomics. One area where this might happen is in the area of psychiatric genetic testing. If this were developed to the point where it entered psychiatric practice as a prognostic tool, it could lead to some most unhelpful consequences. Perhaps the area of greatest concern is that of "predictive" testing within a family, as if psychiatric disease were effectively Mendelian, when that appears to be an exceptional circumstance. However, even something weaker, such as susceptibility testing, could introduce an unfortunate element of self-fulfilling prophecy. This could arise in the setting of formal psychiatric care, if enthusiasm becomes stronger than understanding among certain practitioners, but also in DTC genetic testing. The psychiatrically vulnerable may very plausibly be especially susceptible to harmful effects from genetic testing for the risk of psychiatric disease.

Nonmedical applications of genomics that use the genetic dissection of multifactorial traits, to the extent that is possible with genome-wide association studies, could be applied to height, IQ, athleticism, and other socially valued traits. While it is difficult to see a valid and legitimate reason for doing this, such genetic assessments could all too easily be (mis) applied in educational and pre-employment assessments to determine the selection of trainees in various careers or the entry to courses in higher education. There are already signs of the abuse of research in IQ genetics, with selection on the basis of likely IQ being offered commercially at preimplantation genetic testing (Forzano et al., 2022). Further contentious research and its misapplication appear all too likely.

Conclusion

In this chapter, I have presented a survey of areas where the application of genetic knowledge and especially genomic testing can generate or amplify social disadvantage and where genomics has the potential to exacerbate the problems of those caught up in its applications. Some of these problems are inevitable, while others arise through the operation of social mechanisms that can be challenged and changed. It is important that the undoubted benefits of genomic technologies and clinical genetics services are made available to all in society while at the same time they are protected from exploitation. To achieve this, those professionally involved in genomics and in clinical genetics services must implement genomics with painstaking caution, so that we achieve the diagnostic and therapeutic benefits without exacerbating preexisting inequities and related, socially mediated difficulties.

Acknowledgments

I would like to thank several colleagues for helpful conversations and insights, including Pauline McCormack (Newcastle, England) and Carla van El (Amsterdam).

References

Ablon, J. (1984). *Little people in America: The social dimensions of dwarfism*. Praeger Publishers.

Ablon, J. (1996). Gender response to neurofibromatosis 1. *Social Science & Medicine*, *42*(1), 99–109.

Alderson, P. (2001). Down syndrome: Cost, quality and value of life. *Social Science & Medicine*, *53*, 627–638.

Appiah, K. A. (2018). *The lies that bind: Rethinking identity*. Profile Books.

Arribas-Ayllon, M., Sarangi, S., & Clarke, A. (2011). *Genetic testing: Accounts of autonomy, responsibility and blame*. Routledge.

Blagowidow, N., Nowakowska, B., Schindewolf, E., Grati, F. R., Putotto, C., Breckpot, J., Swillen, A., Crowley, T. B., Loo, J. C. Y., Lairson, L. A., Óskarsdóttir, S., Boot, E., Garcia-Minaur, S., Cristina Digilio, M., Marino, B., Coleman, B., Moldenhauer, J. S., Bassett, A. S., & McDonald-McGinn, D. M. (2023). Prenatal screening and diagnostic considerations for 22q11.2 microdeletions. *Genes, 14*(1), 160.

Boardman, F. (2014). The expressivist objection to prenatal testing: The experiences of families living with genetic disease. *Social Science & Medicine, 107*, 18–25.

Boardman, F. K. (2017). Experience as knowledge: Disability, distillation and (reprogenetic) decision-making. *Social Science & Medicine, 191*, 186–193.

Bombard, Y., Palin, J., Friedman, J. M., Veenstra, G., Creighton, S., Bottorff, J. L., & Hayden, M. R., & the Canadian Respond-HD Collaborative Research Group. (2012). Beyond the patient: The broader impact of genetic discrimination among individuals at risk of Huntington disease. *American Journal Medical Genetics Part B, 159B*, 217–226.

Chao, F., Gerland, P., Cook, A. R., & Alkema, L. (2019). Systematic assessment of the sex ratio at birth for all countries and estimation of national imbalances and regional reference levels. *Proceedings of the National Academy of Sciences of the USA, 116*(19), 9303–9311.

Char, D. S., Lee, S.S.-J., Magnus, D., & Cho, M. (2018). Anticipating uncertainty and irrevocable decisions: Provider perspectives on implementing whole-genome sequencing in critically ill children with heart disease. *Genetics in Medicine, 20*(11), 1455–1461.

Clarke, A. (1991). Is non-directive genetic counselling possible? *Lancet, 338*, 998–1001.

Clarke, A. (2013). Stigma, self-esteem and reproduction: Talking with men about life with hypohidrotic ectodermal dysplasia. *Sociology, 47*(5), 975–993.

Clarke, A. (2016). Anticipated stigma and blameless guilt: Mothers' evaluation of life with the sex-linked disorder, hypohidrotic ectodermal dysplasia (XHED). *Social Science & Medicine, 158*, 141–148.

Clarke, A. J., & Abdala Sheikh, A. P. (2018). A perspective on "cure" for Rett syndrome. *Orphanet Journal of Rare Diseases, 13*, 44.

Cornel, M. C., & Clarke, A. J. (2021). Costs, burdens and the prevention of genetic disorders: What role for professional influence? *Journal of Community Genetics, 12*, 503–505.

Deem, M. J. (2016). Whole-genome sequencing and disability in the NICU: Exploring practical and ethical challenges. *Pediatrics, 137*, S47–S55.

Dive, L., Archibald, A. D., & Newson, A. J. (2022). Ethical considerations in gene selection for reproductive carrier screening. *Human Genetics, 141*(5), 1003–1012. https://doi.org/10.1007/s00439-021-02341-9

Duster, T. (1990). *Backdoor to eugenics*. Routledge, Chapman and Hall.

Erwin, C., Williams, J. K., Juhl, A. R., Mengeling, M., Mills, J. A., Bombard, Y., Hayden, M. R., Quaid, K., Shoulson, I., Taylor, S., Paulsen, J. S., & the IRESPOND-HD Investigators of the Huntington Study Group. (2010). Perception, experience, and response to genetic discrimination in Huntington disease: The international RESPOND-HD study. *American Journal Medical Genetics Part B, 153B*, 1081–1093.

Evans, C. (2006). *Genetic counselling: A psychological approach*. Cambridge University Press.

Forzano, F., Antonova, O., Clarke, A., de Wert, G., Hentze, S., Jamshidi, Y., Moreau, Y., Perola, M., Prokopenko, I., Read, A., Reymond, A., Stefansdottir, V., van El, C., Genuardi, M., on behalf of the Executive Committee and the Public and Professional Policy Committee of the European Society of Human Genetics. (2022). The use of polygenic risk scores in pre-implantation genetic testing: An unproven, unethical practice. *European Journal of Human Genetics*, *30*(5), 493–495. https://doi.org/10.1038/s41431-021-01000-x

Goffman, E. (1968). *Stigma: Notes on the management of spoiled identity*. Penguin. (Original work published 1963)

Hesketh, T., & Xing, Z. W. (2011). The consequences of son preference and sex-selective abortion in China and other Asian countries. *Canadian Medical Association Journal*, *183*(12), 1374–1377.

Hickerton, C. L., Aitken, M. A., Hodgson, J., & Delatycki, M. B. (2012). "Did you find that out in time?": New life trajectories of parents who choose to continue a pregnancy where a genetic disorder is diagnosed or likely. *American Journal of Medical Genetics Part A*, *158A*, 373–383.

Hollands, G. J., French, D. P., Griffin, S. J., Prevost, A. T., Sutton, S., King, S., & Marteau, T. M. (2016). The impact of communicating genetic risks of disease on risk-reducing health behaviour: Systematic review with meta-analysis. *BMJ*, 352, i1102. https://doi.org/10.1136/bmj.i1102

Janssens, A. C. W. (2019). Validity of polygenic risk scores: Are we measuring what we think we are? *Human Molecular Genetics*, *28*(R2), R143–R150.

Kay, E., & Kingston, H. (2002). Feelings associated with being a carrier and characteristics of reproductive decision making in women known to be carriers of X-linked conditions. *Journal of Health Psychology*, *7*(2), 169–181.

Kessler, S., Kessler, H., & Ward, P. (1984). Psychological aspects of genetic counseling. III. Management of guilt and shame. *American Journal of Medical Genetics*, *17*(3), 673–697.

Lippman, A. (1991). Prenatal genetic testing and screening: Constructing needs and reinforcing inequities. *American Journal of Law and Medicine*, *17*, 15–50.

Martindale, A-M., & Fisher, P. (2019). Disrupted faces, disrupted identities? Embodiment, life stories and acquired facial "disfigurement." *Sociology of Health & Illness*, *41*(8), 1503–1519.

McCormack, P., Kole, A., Gainotti, S., Mascalzoni, D., Molster, C., Lochmüller, H., & Woods, S. (2016). "You should at least ask." The expectations, hopes and fears of rare disease patients on large-scale data and biomaterial sharing for genomics research. *European Journal of Human Genetics*, *24*, 1403–1408.

Mendes, A., Sousa, L., Sequeiros, J., & Clarke, A. (2017). Discredited legacy: Stigma and familial amyloid polyneuropathy in Northwestern Portugal. *Social Science & Medicine*, *182*, 73–80.

Mighton, C., Kodida, R., Shickh, S., Clausen, M., Reble, E., Sam, J., Grewal, S., Hirjikaka, D., Panchal, S., Piccinin, C., Aronson, M., Ward, T., Armel, S. R., Hofstedter, R., Graham, T., Mancuso, T., Forster, N., Capo-Chichi, J. M., Greenfeld, E., . . . Incidental Genomics Study Team. (2025). Opportunistic genomic screening has clinical utility: An interventional cohort study. *Genetics in Medicine*, *27*(2), 101323. https://doi.org/10.1016/j.gim.2024.101323

Miller, D. T., Lee, K., Chung, W. K., Gordon, A. S., Herman, G. E., Klein, T. E., Stewart, D. R., Amendola, L. M., Adelman, K., Bale, S. J., Gollob, M. H., Harrison, S. M., Hershberger, R. E., McKelvey, K., Richards, C. S., Vlangos, C. N., Watson, M. S., Martin, C. L., & ACMG Secondary Findings Working Group. (2021). ACMG SF v3.0 list for reporting of secondary findings in clinical exome and genome sequencing: A policy statement of the American College of Medical Genetics and Genomics (ACMG). *Genetics in Medicine*, *23*(8), 1381–1390. https://doi.org/10.1038/s41436-021-01172-3

Modell, B. (2020). Haemoglobin disorders—A point of entry for community genetics services in India? *Journal of Community Genetics*, *11*, 7–9.

Molster, C. M., Lister, K., Metternick-Jones, S., Baynam, G., Clarke, A. J., Straub, V., Dawkins, H. J. S., & Laing, N. (2017). Outcomes of an international workshop on preconception expanded carrier screening: Some considerations for governments. *Frontiers in Public Health*, *5*, 25. https://doi.org/10.3389/fpubh.2017.00025

Moorthie, S., Hall, A., Janus, J., Brigden, T., de Villier, C. B., Blackburn, L., Johnson, E., Kroese, M., for the Public Health Genomics Foundation. (2021). *Polygenic risk scores and clinical utility*. Public Health Genomics Foundation, Cambridge University.

Newson, A. J., Leonard, S. J., Hall, A., & Gaff, C. L. (2016). Known unknowns: Building an ethics of uncertainty into genomic medicine. *BMC Medical Genomics*, *9*, 57.

Nuffield Council on Bioethics. (2017). *Noninvasive prenatal genetic testing: Ethical issues*. Nuffield Council.

Parens, E., & Ash, A. (2000). The disability rights critique of prenatal genetic testing: Reflections and recommendations. In E. Parens & A. Asch (Eds.), *Prenatal testing and disability rights* (pp. 4–43). Georgetown University Press.

Patel, R. (2018, September 24). Prenatal tests are misused for sex-selection in the UK. *BioNews*, no. 968.

Penders, B., & Janssens, A. C. J. W. (2022). Do we measure or compute polygenic risk scores? Why language matters. *Human Genetics*, *141*(5), 1093–1097. https://doi.org/10.1007/s00439-021-02262-7

Peters, K., Apse, K., Blackford, A., McHugh, B., Michaelic, D., & Biesecker, B. (2005). Living with Marfan syndrome: Coping with stigma. *Clinical Genetics*, *68*, 6–14.

Pilnick, A. (2002). What "most people" do: Exploring the ethical implications of genetic counselling. *New Genetics and Society*, *21*, 339–350.

Rapp, R. (2000). *Testing women, testing the fetus: The social impact of amniocentesis in America*. Routledge.

Ravitsky, V., Rousseau, F., & Laberge, A-M. (2017). Providing unrestricted access to prenatal testing does not translate to enhanced autonomy. *American Journal of Bioethics*, *17*(1), 39–41.

Rothman, B. K. (1988). *The tentative pregnancy: Prenatal diagnosis and the future of motherhood*. Pandora.

Rozario, S. (2007). Growing up and living with neurofibromatosis1 (NF1): A British Bangladeshi case-study. *Journal of Genetic Counseling*, *16*, 551–560.

Sabatello, M., Phelan, J. C., Hesdorffer, D. C., Shostak, S., Goldsmith, J., Sorge, S. T., Winawer, M. R., Chung, W. K., & Ottman, R. (2015). Genetic causal attribution of epilepsy and its implications for felt stigma. *Epilepsia*, *56*(10), 1542–1550.

Shakespeare, T. (1998). Choices and rights: Eugenics, genetics and disability equality. *Disability & Society*, *13*, 665–681.

Skotko, B. G. (2009). With new prenatal testing, will babies with Down syndrome disappear? *Archives of Disease in Childhood*, *94*, 823–826.

Taylor-Phillips, S., Freeman, K., Geppert, J., Agbebiyi, A., Uthman, O., Madan, J., Clarke, A. J., Quenby, S., & Clarke, A. E. (2016). Accuracy of non-invasive prenatal testing using cell-free DNA for detection of Down, Edwards and Patau syndromes: A systematic review and meta-analysis. *BMJ Open*, *6*, e010002. https://doi.org/10.1136/bmjopen-2015-010002

Tudor Hart, J. (1971). The inverse care law. *Lancet*, *297*, 405–412.

UK National Screening Committee. (2015). *Criteria for appraising the viability, effectiveness and appropriateness of a screening programme*. https://www.gov.uk/government/publications/evidence-review-criteria-national-screening-programmes/criteria-for-appraising-the-viability-effectiveness-and-appropriateness-of-a-screening-programme van den Heuvel, A., Chitty, L., Dormandy, E., Newson, A., Deans, Z., Attwood, S., Haynes, S., & Marteau, T. M. (2010). Will the introduction of non-invasive prenatal diagnostic testing erode informed choices? *Patient Education and Counseling*, *78*, 24–28.

Weil, J. (1991). Mothers' postcounseling beliefs about the causes of their children's genetic disorders. *American Journal of Human Genetics*, *48*(1), 145–153.

West, N. (1962). *Miss Lonelyhearts*. New Directions Publishing.

Wilfond, B. S. (2017). Breaking the sounds of silence: Respecting people with disabilities and reproductive decision making. *American Journal of Bioethics*, *17*(1), 37–39.

Williams, C., Alderson, P., & Farsides, B. (2002). Is non-directiveness possible within the context of antenatal screening and testing? *Social Science & Medicine*, *54*, 339–347.

Wilson, J. M. G., & Jungner, G. (1968). *Principles and practice of screening for disease*. World Health Organization.

Woods, S., Hagger, L. E., & McCormack, P. (2014). Therapeutic misconception: Hope, trust and misconception in paediatric research. *Health Care Analysis: HCA: Journal of Health Philosophy and Policy*, *22*(1), 3–21.

PART VII

THE FUTURE OF GENETIC COUNSELING

CHAPTER 33

ANTICIPATING THE GROWTH OF GENETIC COUNSELING

MEGAN E. TRINKLE-TUCKER AND
BEVERLY M. YASHAR

Introduction

What does the future hold for genetic counselors and their practice? The ability of genetic counselors to rapidly pivot their practice by relying on core clinical skills, coupled with a deep base of cutting-edge knowledge in genetics and the capacity to identify emerging areas of practice in genetics-based care, has driven many phases in the evolution of the genetic counseling profession. Key to the success of these transitions is the fact that genetic counselors are able to leverage their knowledge and skills to build working alliances with novel groups of partners, including members of education institutions and healthcare providers who have limited knowledge of and/or training in genetics. A seminal example of this ability is the growth of cancer genetic counseling. Following the discovery that variants in the *BRCA1* and *BRCA2* genes increased the risk for hereditary breast and ovarian cancer in early 1990, Myriad Genetics began offering diagnostic genetic testing for pathogenic variants in these genes in 1996. By the late 1990s, cancer genetic counseling emerged as an expanding clinical specialty for genetic counselors. This growth was intertwined with novel partnerships with oncologists. The National Society of Genetic Counselors (NSGC) first identified cancer genetic counseling as a practice area for 34% of the membership (Parrott & Clark, 2004). By 2021 it represented 42% of genetic counseling practice and is a requirement, for some insurers, for coverage of cancer susceptibility genetic testing (NSGC, 2022a, p. 8; Reid et al., 2022). In addition, educational communities have been highly responsive by incorporating content such as novel cancer testing strategies and variant interpretation into the curriculum as well as adapting educational strategies to meet the needs of adult learners from diverse backgrounds to ensure trainees are adequately prepared to practice at the top of their scope after graduation.

This chapter attempts to predict how the genetic counseling profession may grow by exploring current innovations in genetic counseling practice and education. Our predictions arise from a scan of the relevant history in each area and evaluation of how current forces (referred to as "drivers" in this chapter) could interact to create future change. This "environmental scan" suggests opportunities for the profession moving forward. We recognize our predictions are based on current trends and our projections may only be partially realized. However, we encourage readers to use our predictions to envision ways in which genetic counseling practice and education could evolve moving forward and use these thought exercises as opportunities to challenge the status quo.

Growth in Genetic Counseling Practice

Predictions related to genetic counseling practice

Genomic-based medical care, also known as precision medicine, will impact the practice settings of a substantial proportion of the genetic counseling profession, including both newly minted and experienced genetic counselors (Denny & Collins, 2021). This will result in a movement away from direct patient care toward increased focus on using genetic counseling skills in nondirect patient care that both interfaces with and helps drive the future development of genomic-based medical care. We are already starting to see this shift. Among the 2,859 genetic counselors who completed the 2022 Professional Status Survey, 27% reported working in nondirect patient care with roles that included "variant interpretation and report writing, field support, utilization management, laboratory sales, and customer service" (NSGC, 2022b, p. 6). These services were provided to both academic labs and private companies offering varied products and services related to genetic testing, which is increasingly dependent on genome-based analyses that require fluency with multiple components of genome-focused medicine. These components include understanding the sequencing workflow from genomic DNA isolation through sequencing, genome assembly, and bioinformatic analysis. To appropriately utilize the results of genome-based analyses, both in providing genetic counseling and in educating members of the healthcare team, it is essential to have not only a global understanding of the process but also detailed knowledge of the limitations in this form of genetic testing. Acquiring this depth of understanding falls within a genetic counselor's skill set, and mastery will require acquiring novel educational content.

Similar shifts in professional practice have occurred previously as providers of genetic counseling have been able to leverage core genetic counseling skills and expertise to build and populate new areas of clinical practice (i.e., cancer and cardiology) and new roles for genetic counselors. We predict that the difference between historical growth and that in the future will be the pervasive reliance on genomics in nearly all areas of medicine and the general recognition by healthcare providers, private companies, patients, and the public of the value of genetic counseling expertise in navigating genomic-based medical care.

Drivers

A host of factors will support this growth and diversification, resulting in a positioning of genetic counseling professionals as both translators and decoders. Key among these drivers will be the continuing growth in techniques to identify and interpret novel genomic variations, as well as an increasing ability not only to map pathogenic variations across the genome but also to identify genomic modifications beyond those that impact the coding sequence (Cavalli & Heard, 2019; Kyono et al., 2019; Portela & Esteller, 2010; Shendure et al., 2019). These developments will increase the ability to identify genomic contributions to a broader set of disease states and susceptibilities and support further expansion of genetic testing. Currently, genetic testing is rapidly moving beyond the evaluation of Mendelian diseases in which a single pathogenic variant is sufficient to explain disease risk to include a wide variety of common complex conditions, such as varied types of cardiac and psychiatric diagnoses, and tailoring approaches to disease management in a wide variety of clinical specialties, including oncology and pharmacology (Denny & Collins, 2021; Shendure et al., 2019; Van Driest et al., 2014). Successful efforts by individual genetic counselors and the genetic counseling profession have enhanced recognition of genetic counselors' expertise in genetics, entrepreneurship, counseling, and education (Bamshad et al., 2018; Biesecker, 2020; Cho & Guy, 2020; NSGC, 2022b; Ramos, 2020) and increased the desire to hire genetic counselors in novel settings. Genetic testing laboratories are increasingly seeing the value of utilizing genetic counselors' expertise in molecular and clinical genetics and communication to support both clinical and commercial endeavors (Swanson et al., 2014; Zetzsche et al., 2014).[1] Simultaneously, non-genetics-trained healthcare providers who are now utilizing genetic testing as an essential clinical tool have recognized challenges in staying current in the knowledge and skills needed to effectively interpret genetic and genomic results and are seeking support from genetic counselors (Hsu et al., 2021; Mazzola et al., 2019; Weipert et al., 2018). Finally, there is the growing appeal of genomic information to the general public. In contrast to historical perceptions of genetics as eugenic, broader segments of the population see personal utility in having knowledge about how their genome impacts their health (Caulfield & McGuire, 2012; Majumder et al., 2021; Mukherjee et al., 2022; Yin et al., 2020; Zuckerman, 2021).[2]

Relevant history: Past to present to future

At the inception of the genetic counseling profession at Sarah Lawrence College in 1971, when eight students completed the first genetic counseling training program, many of the common genetic conditions that early practitioners were helping patients understand were chromosomally based, while those due to pathogenic variants in single genes were limited

[1] Editors' note: For more on the expansion of the genetic counseling workforce in industry settings, see Chapter 13 by Elissa Levin and Edgar MacBean in this volume.

[2] Editors' note: For more on the history of social eugenics programs, see Chapter 1 by Devon Stillwell in this volume.

in number (Rubinstein et al., 2013; Walker, 2009). The first edition of *Mendelian Inheritance in Man* in 1966 provided information on the phenotypes of 1,486 conditions that were thought to have a genetic basis. This resource was critical in supporting the genetic mastery of early genetic counselors. Their diagnostic tools included risk assessment based on family history and population frequencies, application of mathematical models like Bayesian analysis to help refine risk, and karyotypes to provide molecular insights (Stern, 2012; Walker, 2009). By 2023, a little more than 50 years after the graduation of Sarah Lawrence's first class, there were 26,756 Online Mendelian Inheritance in Man (OMIM) entries, and the molecular basis of 6,486 Mendelian conditions were known (OMIM, 2023). Genetic testing relies on expanding sets of technologies that allow geneticists, genetic counselors, and other healthcare professionals to interrogate the genome with increasing scope, sensitivity, and specificity (Claussnitzer et al., 2020). Increasing access to genetic testing has also occurred; this is supported by decreasing costs of genetic testing and expansion in both the number of companies that offer genetic testing and the types of clinical practice settings that rely on genomic knowledge and testing. The results from this expansion of genetic testing are being used in managing diagnoses, including tailoring medication prescription and dosing (pharmacogenomics), making predictions about prognosis (i.e., liquid tumor testing), and applying gene-targeted precision therapeutics and treatments for conditions such as sickle cell disease (Matte et al., 2019), cystic fibrosis (Joseph, 2019), spinal muscular atrophy (Schorling et al., 2020), Duchenne muscular dystrophy (Aartsma-Rus et al., 2016), and epidermolysis bullosa (Marinkovich & Tang, 2019).

The expanded diagnostic and prognostic tools also allow genetic counselors to make risk predictions with better precision for a greater variety of inherited conditions and in broader clinical settings. This includes improved screening and testing options in reproductive genetics (Bianchi & Chiu, 2018; Samura, 2020; Taylor-Phillips et al., 2016) and better diagnostic yields in determining the genetic basis of both pediatric and adult-onset conditions (Cirino et al., 2017; Mainali et al., 2022; Savatt & Myers, 2021). The broad range of this genetic information can be utilized by at-risk individuals and families to make life decisions that have always been at the bedrock of genetic counseling, including pregnancy management, family planning, and life choices. The more recent tools in risk prediction, which take advantage of computer algorithms and evaluate interactions between multiple genetic variants, such as polygenic risk scores,[3] are expanding the reach and personalization of genetic testing into established fields like oncology and cardiology and newer clinical specialties like psychiatry (Adeyemo et al., 2021; Wand et al., 2023). These tools have the potential to continue to improve decision making related to management. These developments have fostered enthusiasm by physicians in multiple specialties to utilize genetics and genomics as integral components of care but also have created challenges in staying abreast of the knowledge required to master this content (Snell & Helen, 2017). Several studies exploring the ways in which non-genetics-trained professionals utilize genetic and genomic results highlight limitations in their ability to accurately interpret and apply this information in clinical care (Hsu et al., 2021; Mazzola et al., 2019; Weipert et al., 2018).

While this growth brings several challenges, it also indicates the ways in which genomics has become central to genetic counseling practice. Some of the current dialogue

[3] Editors' note: For more on polygenic risk scores, see Chapter 20 by Eleanor Feingold in this volume.

surrounding variant interpretation in exome and genome sequencing test results has called attention to inconsistencies in defining the clinical significance of genetic testing results by laboratories and highlighted the important value added by genetic counselors in defining appropriate standards (Berrios et al., 2021; Wain et al., 2020). This growth has driven changes in training standards and motivated calls to add variant interpretation as a core genetic counseling skill (Accreditation Council for Genetic Counseling [ACGC], 2023b; Cho & Guy, 2020). The expanded focus on result interpretation in genetic research and genetic counseling practice has the potential to support increased specialization by genetic counselors of the future to fill these gaps and could lead to the development of new genetic counseling subspecialties focused on genomic test development, variant curation, bioinformatics, and genomics education. Some of these shifts have already started to occur; in the 2022 NSGC Professional Status Survey, 51% of genetic counselors who reported working in nondirect patient care worked for a commercial laboratory, and current professional special interest groups within the NSGC include Genomic Technologies, Health IT, Laboratory/Industry, and Precision Medicine (NSGC, 2022b, p. 22). Given the ways in which genetic counselors have shown the ability to adapt in the past, it is likely that the skill sets of genetic counselors of the future will include broader and deeper genomics focus.

Finally, the current growth of precision medicine is expanding possible consumers of genetic counseling services beyond medical settings to include the public (also previously known as the worried well), who are using this information to make decisions that impact their general well-being (Maio et al., 2013; Wand et al., 2023). The fact that the genetic counseling profession has solidified their reputation as the preferred experts to help the medical profession navigate the genomic revolution means that more and more individuals will likely seek genetic counseling as they try to make sense of their genome. One example of this type of driver is the proposed expansion of newborn screening to include genome-based analysis (Milko & Khoury, 2022; Minear et al., 2022; Roman et al., 2020). The ultimate result of this change in newborn screening methodology will be the availability of portable genome scans at birth.[4] Key challenges in determining the best ways to interrogate these genomes and subsequently use this knowledge to promote preventative genomic-based healthcare are educating the public about reasons to utilize genetic counselors (Pasca et al., 2022) and providing access to all who could benefit from their educational and counseling expertise (Hoskovec et al., 2018; Triebold et al., 2021).

What could this future practice look like?

The preceding discussion raises the following questions: What might genetic counselors of the future look like and how might they address the needs of the different populations they serve? Future expansion of genomics will likely include interrogation and interpretation of the transcriptome, the epigenome, and the proteome (Marwaha et al., 2022). Consequently, the core knowledge needed to be an effective genetic counselor will also need to change.

[4] Editors' note: For further discussion on ethical and practical considerations related to genomic sequencing in the newborn period, see Chapter 35 by Marsha Michie and Aaron J. Goldenberg in this volume.

To maintain the expertise of genetic counselors and individuate their practice from others with expertise in this domain, genetic counselors of the future will need to move beyond explaining the results of genetic testing technology and build deeper skills in evaluating its effectiveness and identifying the best ways to utilize this knowledge in clinical practice while staying true to the ethos of patient-centered care. In concordance with Section IV of the NSGC Code of Ethics (NSGC, 2017), genetic counselors have a duty to evaluate the utilization and application of the newest versions of genetic testing to promote the well-being of society and access to genetic services. To stay true to our training and have the ability to translate genetics into clinically useful tools for both patients and providers and to practice at the cutting edge of genetic discovery, larger segments of the genetic counseling workforce will need to engage with genetic/genomic testing technology beyond result interpretation (Ramos, 2020). This could result in a future in which larger numbers of genetic counselors serve as molecular genomics experts, bioinformaticians, consultants, and entrepreneurs. However, a number of factors could limit these developments, including the mismatch between the current size of the genetic workforce and the size needed to fulfill these roles (Hoskovec et al., 2018), challenges in billing and reimbursement for genetic counseling services (Boothe et al., 2021), and tensions about scope of practice between genetic counselors and others with relevant genetics and genomics expertise (American Medical Association, 2023).

Ultimately, as genomics-informed precision medicine continues to grow, there is the potential to alter the core definition of what it means to be a genetic counselor and further differentiate genetic counseling skills used in clinical settings from those used for genomic-focused work. The expertise of the segment of the genetic counseling workforce concentrated on generating (i.e., discovering and interpreting) genetics and genomics knowledge that will be used by clinical genetic counselors in providing patient care is expected to continue to grow. For the clinical genetic counselors of the future, their work will be concordant with our current definition of genetic counseling and emphasize helping "guide and support patients seeking more information about how inherited diseases and conditions might affect them or their families, and to interpret genetic test results based on your personal and family history" (NSGC, 2023, Who Are Genetic Counselors? section). For the segment of the genetic counseling workforce that is functioning as genomic experts who are interpreting the genome for clinical care, a broader definition of the central genetic counseling ethos will need to be developed that includes these newer skills alongside the ethos of providing patient- and family-centered care.

Growth of Genetic Counseling Education

Predictions related to genetic counseling education

The graduate training environment for prospective genetic counselors will adapt to incorporate education on the expanding skills and knowledge required to be a competent genetic counselor while meeting the needs of a diverse student population. This is likely to include more distance education, part-time training options, novel partnerships and collaborations, a focus on andragogy, and increased utilization of technology. In addition, the leadership teams of genetic counseling graduate programs will also change to include individuals with a broader scope of expertise and roles to meet these expanding educational needs. Finally, training programs will become more in tune with the needs of potential applicants by reducing barriers to training and increasing the diversity of students and therefore the face of the genetic profession as a whole.

Drivers

As the use of technology described in the previous section expands, so too must training in order for students to be prepared to enter the rapidly evolving genetic counseling field. As previously discussed, the clinical utility of genetic testing in the world of precision medicine is changing. Some of these new tests, including those that may be consumer initiated, may not have enough evidence to support clinical impact at this time. What do medical professionals do with knowing that someone may be more successful with endurance-style exercise? Is there enough data to support consumers changing their lifestyles? Genetic counselors are well suited to navigate the complexities of this kind of testing and, therefore, must be prepared to foster patient understanding and autonomous decision making related to testing for traits such as dietary needs, exercise, stress responses, alcohol preferences, nutrient supplements, sleep habits, and others that may or may not impact clinical care.

Genetic counseling practice will expand not only to include this new range of testing options but also to become more representative of the diverse patients who will utilize genetic services. To accommodate both of these drivers, genetic counselors will master increasingly complex technical and counseling skills to more adequately meet the needs of both students and patient populations.

Relevant history: Past to present to future

Genetic counseling training is in demand, and the number of applicants and the number of training programs have both increased in recent years. According to the Genetic Counselor Educators Association, the number of applicants increased by 60% (1,299 to 2,069) from 2017 to 2021 (Association of Genetic Counseling Program Directors, 2021).[5] Consequently, it is not surprising that some institutions would consider genetic counseling programs a worthwhile investment, since programs consistently have more applicants than available slots. In addition, the nearly 100% completion rate of genetic counseling programs is higher than most other STEM-related master's degree programs, which have completion rates closer to 60% to 70% (Allum et al., 2013; Baum & Stelle, 2017). Such high completion rates can help make genetic counseling programs a consistent success for the sponsoring institution. The number of training programs accredited by the ACGC has grown substantially in the

[5] Editors' note: The Genetic Counselor Educators Association was previously the Association of Genetic Counseling Program Directors but officially changed its name in 2023.

last 10 years. The number of accredited training programs in the United States and Canada increased by 6% from 2010 to 2014 (33 to 35 programs), followed by a 43% increase from 2015 to 2019 (35 to 50 programs), and as of 2024 there are 60 ACGC accredited programs in the United States and Canada (ACGC, 2024, Find an Accredited Program section).[6]

This increase in the number of programs and expansion in the size of training cohorts in both new and established graduate programs has resulted in a near tripling of the number of graduate slots available in only 15 years, from 190 in 2007 to 553 in 2021 (Association of Genetic Counseling Program Directors, 2021; Riconda et al., 2018). This growth has been accompanied by increasing diversity of the sponsoring institutions for these programs. Genetic counseling programs have primarily been sponsored by medical schools. However, we now see sponsoring entities in schools of public health, colleges of health and human services, colleges of arts and sciences, and schools of biomedical science, among others. With these expanding sponsoring institutions come increased collaborations with other healthcare fields that have allowed some programs to offer dual degrees in genetic counseling and master's degrees in public health at universities such as the University of Pittsburgh, the University of Michigan, and Boston University or dual doctoral degrees in genetics (or similar variations) at the University of Minnesota, Virginia Commonwealth University, and the University of Pittsburgh, to name a few.

Prior to 2007, programs were primarily administered face to face and required full-time attendance with fieldwork experiences typically taking place at local hospitals/clinics affiliated with the medical school. In 2007, the University of Arkansas initiated a unique model where students completed their fieldwork at satellite locations and joined synchronous educational classes via video. Prior to 2016, only 21 states in the United States had a genetic counseling training program. In 2017, two new and distinct models were established, one at Augustana-Sanford University and the other at Indiana State University. Augustana-Sanford University developed a program with two distinct campuses, with all students spending their first year in Sioux Falls, South Dakota, and half of the students spending their second year in San Diego, California, and the other half remaining in Sioux Falls; this is a distinct yet similar format to the University of Arkansas program. Indiana State University launched the first hybrid program resulting in a combination of traditional face-to-face synchronous courses during the first year and online asynchronous courses during the second year, allowing a broader array of fieldwork opportunities since students could be scattered across the United States. By 2018, the first two fully online programs were launched at Bay Path University and Boise State University. These online programs have the entirety of the students' academic training at a distance with a mix of asynchronous and synchronous sessions all completed entirely online, allowing students to complete their training from anywhere in the country.

Models such as these allow students to benefit from training with genetic counselors in novel geographic regions such as rural areas by tapping into previously unutilized sites while maintaining academic progress in their program. In addition, individual students within a cohort may have access to novel patient populations due to the geographic diversity

[6] Editors' note: Further information on the growth of genetic counseling programs and the development of education for genetic counselors can be found in Chapter 2 by Bonnie Jeanne Baty and Claire Davis in this volume.

of the group. These individuals are able to bring their unique experiences back to benefit the entire cohort, enhancing the overall learning and experience of the entire group. As more programs utilize models such as these, more extensive collaborations and coordination among everyone involved will be necessary. Since new programs and delivery models are being developed at a much more rapid pace than in the first three decades of the profession, it remains to be seen whether the professional resources necessary for sustaining these programs will keep up.

The skills and knowledge expected of practicing genetic counselors have also expanded. Multiple programs have already adopted various ways of utilizing distance delivery formats to incorporate some of these developing skills. For example, industry partners such as GeneDx developed an 8-week online module utilized by 17 programs in 2021 to educate students on the roles of genetic counselors in industry (T. Hart, personal communication, January 4, 2022). In addition, the Pharmacogenetics Working Group and the Precision Medicine Special Interest Group of the NSGC developed modules on pharmacogenetic testing, which were used by 27 training programs in 2021 (R. Mills, personal communication, January 5, 2022). More virtual options and collaborations such as these will be utilized in the future to help programs provide training that may not otherwise be available. Increased collaboration between the faculty, leadership, and students in different programs as well as collaborations with external entities will be valuable. These collaborations will enhance learning by offering students unique opportunities or experiences, thereby improving the accessibility of this educational content, which is an excellent mechanism for staying abreast of the field and incorporating new advances into training. These changes reflect newer roles and place additional demands/expectations on the graduate training environment. For example, the ACGC updated the accreditation standards in 2023 to state:

> Programs must demonstrate that participatory cases and other field experiences are conducted (1) across multiple specialties, including prenatal, pediatric, cancer, and other adult; (2) in a variety of diverse settings that may include clinical, laboratory, research, industry, and/or other environments; <u>and</u> (3) using more than one service delivery mode, such as telephone, group, in-person, and/or telemedicine. (ACGC, 2023b, p. 21)

The shift in language from "clinical" expectations to "fieldwork" expectations suggests recognition of the broadening roles of genetic counselors. Students are expected to learn about non-patient-facing roles by having an opportunity for fieldwork in industry or other settings.

In addition, the ACGC has recognized an increasing demand on program leadership to have skills beyond clinical supervision and teaching. This can be seen by the expanded qualifications for the program director (ACGC, 2023b). It is no longer enough to be a certified genetic counselor with 5 years of experience and to have knowledge and experience in teaching, clinical supervision, and relevant subjects as prior ACGC accreditation standards stated. The updated qualifications for the director are now more detailed. The qualifications include the ones previously mentioned and also require that the director have experience with postsecondary course instruction; 2 hours of continued training in curriculum design, assessment, evaluation, or educational andragogy annually; and documented training/experiences related to leadership, professional development, management, scholarly activities, mentoring, academic advising, andragogy, and diversity, equity, inclusion, and justice. These new qualifications reflect the expanding expectations of program leadership (ACGC, 2023b).

What could this future education look like?

Genetic counseling training in the future will be as adaptable as the profession itself. Some aspects are likely to stay consistent, such as a need for access to fieldwork experiences and providers, content experts in genetics and genomic healthcare, administrative assistance, research opportunities, financial stability/resources, and genetic counselors external to the graduate program. However, the strategies utilized will likely vary even more across programs. We will continue to see expanding diversity in the sponsoring entities of programs, which may include expanding beyond traditional academic settings to healthcare systems themselves or even industry-sponsored programs. This also opens the door for novel dual-degree programs in business, health administration, educational leadership, biotechnology, psychology, social work, and even law. Genetic counselors will continue to take on roles even beyond genomic testing as entrepreneurs by starting their own companies or as content experts for legislation or even legal teams related to genetics in healthcare. These expanding roles will stretch the ways in which the skills of genetic counselors are used. However, 94% (17 of 18) of program directors have identified access to fieldwork placement sites and supervisors as a primary barrier to growth, which will likely continue to be a concern (Pan et al., 2016). A shift from a one-to-one model of supervision may be necessary to accommodate the increasing number of trainees.

As healthcare continues to evolve and demand for genetic counseling services increases, the training models will likely shift from being exclusively a full-time and face-to-face format to including more options such as asynchronous delivery, distance delivery, and even part-time training. Many of the courses considered staples of a genetic counseling program including content related to genetics, medical decision making/testing, human development, cancer, and perinatal care can be readily taught in an asynchronous format. More advanced genetics/genomics content and counseling skills will also be obtained via distant learning and alternative formats such as standardized patients or patient simulations utilizing actors, peers, or others to serve as mock patients. This allows students to gain novice skills without access to a traditional fieldwork rotation. Other technology will likely be utilized to improve delivery of educational content in new ways, such as virtual reality to establish simulated experiences in clinical, industry, research, or other settings, which could be shared between programs. In addition, content areas that should be addressed in more depth in the future will include drug development, clinical trials/novel treatments for genetic disorders, business models, and the impact of legislation on healthcare offerings. Since every program has strengths and opportunities, this could be a mechanism for programs lacking resources to benefit from the strengths of other programs. If "Training Program A" does not have access to inpatient genetics services but has an excellent patient simulation center and "Training Program B" has limited access to simulated cases but a robust inpatient genetics service, an exchange of students could allow the students from both programs to mutually benefit. Therefore, in the future, collaborations like these will be crucial for ensuring students have access to a wide range of experiences without requiring every program to have the experience available at their own institution. In addition, external entities will be utilized to develop robust networks of supporting individuals that may contribute to multiple programs simultaneously. While this increases the complexity of organization and coordination needed for such collaborations, it also has the potential to utilize the expertise of a variety of individuals who may not otherwise be able to contribute to the training of genetic counselors. This will be useful as genetic counselors expand their skills and roles to provide genomics-informed precision medicine.

While expanding training delivery is critical to meeting the demand for genetic counselors, recent social movements focusing on equity, diversity, and inclusion highlight the need for more depth in genetic counseling training on social and ethical skills (NSGC, 2017). While patient autonomy and ensuring equal access to care have been staples of the profession, more guidance on incorporating these ethical principles into training will be valuable. The ACGC accreditation standards and practice-based competencies refer to the NSGC Code of Ethics, but they provide limited guidance (ACGC, 2023a, 2023b; NSGC, 2017). Therefore, the variations in how ethical principles are taught and learned in graduate training suggest there is an opportunity for the identification of effective approaches to incorporating these principles into training.

In addition to these changes in delivery and content, program personnel will also change. It will not be enough to have faculty and leadership with expertise in the core specialties such as prenatal, pediatric, and cancer clinical genetic counseling. Historically, programs often had a director and associate/assistant director along with a medical director. We now see programs with leadership teams including titles such as research coordinator/director and fieldwork coordinator/director. In the future, roles specific to admissions, curriculum design, external collaborations, and assessment among others may all be valuable. Since programs can differ in whether these individuals are full time or part time, it results in various combinations of roles from one program to the next. Program personnel will need to have a wider breadth of expertise to represent the growing profession and the ability to manage all the components such as administrative needs that are necessary for a successful program including budgeting, curriculum design, technology, hiring, and retaining talent. It will be critical to have this diversity in the faculty teaching in the programs and in the leadership.

Since a specific leadership pipeline for genetic counseling training programs has not existed historically, it will be helpful to consider where practicing genetic counselors gain the necessary skills to become a program leader. Recent efforts through the NSGC, ACGC, and Genetic Counselor Educators Association have begun to develop workshops and mentorship programs for those interested in developing leadership skills. Therefore, it will be likely that a clearer pipeline for gaining leadership skills to train future genetic counseling leaders and career ladders will be developed. This could be accomplished through structured mentorship programs, leadership certificates, or other mechanisms.

It will also be the responsibility of program leadership to identify ways to minimize barriers to the profession and increase diversity and inclusion within the field and program leadership itself. When considering racial/ethnic diversity alone, the pool of applicants applying to training programs is more diverse than the current practicing professionals but is not yet reflective of the general population. In 2020, 59% of individuals in the United States identified as White (non-Hispanic; U.S. Census Bureau, 2020). However, according to the 2022 Professional Status Survey, 89% of genetic counselors identified as White, while 70% of those applying to genetic counseling programs in 2022 identified as White (NSGC, 2022a, p. 8).

When considering ways to increase diversity, common components of the application review process will be reevaluated, including undergraduate academic performance, GRE scores, letters of reference, personal statement, advocacy experience, resume, and/or other components as determined by each individual program. These components have the potential to be a barrier to entering the profession, which will need to be addressed. The barriers discussed here are not all-encompassing, but a few for which alternatives may be beneficial are examined. One such barrier could be the utilization of GRE scores as part of the application evaluation process. Recent studies suggest that GRE scores may not be effective at predicting the future success of students in graduate programs and may have a negative impact on individuals from underrepresented populations (Myers et al., 2022). Similar to other fields, a recent study found that a better predictor of performance on the American Board of Genetic Counseling Certification Examination was grade point average (Myers et al., 2022). Therefore, it may be beneficial to remove the GRE from admissions requirements and replace it with something more meaningful. A shift away from utilizing the GRE has already begun, but it will be necessary to reassess in the future to determine if this has been beneficial or what alternatives will be identified to replace it. Other potential barriers for applicants could include specific prerequisite courses and possibly the lack of incorporation of work experience into qualifying undergraduate credits. While this has not been adopted by genetic counseling, some universities such as Southern New Hampshire University and Colorado State University already incorporate life experiences into college credits (Colorado State University, 2022; Southern New Hampshire University, 2022). This could be incorporated into genetic counseling through developing proficiency exams, creating academic portfolios, or other means of demonstrating skill proficiency. Incorporating these alternatives could replace certain admissions criteria, enhance accessibility for underrepresented applicants, and even serve as a means of customizing active student experiences. Therefore, more work will need to be done to eliminate barriers to entering the profession and enhance diversity in the applicant pool.

In addition to reducing barriers to the application itself, consideration of the applicant review process will also be critical. One option could be a horizontal applicant review process, which seemed to promote more fairness in one study among pharmacy residents (Hanson et al., 2012; Peeters et al., 2015). In a traditional vertical review process, a group of reviewers, such as program faculty, review only a certain percentage of the applications received. In this process, all or most of an individual applicant's materials are reviewed by the same individuals. However, in a horizontal review process, reviewers are blinded to the aspects of the application that they are not reviewing. For example, the same group of reviewers may review the essays from all applicants, while a different group of reviewers will evaluate the transcripts from all applicants. This style of review may be one of many options to consider in an attempt to reduce bias in the application evaluation process. To improve the diversity of the profession to better reflect our patients, we will continue to find ways to reduce barriers to the profession and support those from underrepresented groups. It will be critical to explore successful approaches used by other professions as the genetic counseling profession looks to promote diversity and inclusion.

A final barrier to admissions that will continue to change in the future will be the financial and time burden placed on applicants. This could be in the form of shadowing, crisis counseling, and even interviewing at programs. These experiences are often expected for an individual to be a competitive applicant. However, each of these may require applicants to take time off work and/or to be away from their families. While critical skills can be gained through these experiences, these expectations may also pose a significant financial burden on applicants. Applicants who do not have the financial means or time available for such experiences may be at a significant disadvantage compared to other applicants. As a result of the global pandemic in 2019, many programs shifted their onsite interviews to virtual interviews for applicants. While this was necessary to ensure the health and safety of everyone involved, it is possible that virtual interviews in the future could be an excellent opportunity to minimize at least one barrier for applicants while still meeting the needs of both applicants and programs in determining whether they are a good match for each other. This shift has already begun and is likely to continue to increase. It will be a challenge for program leadership to find ways to admit quality applicants while ensuring equity of access to genetic counseling education.

Conclusion

The current state of the genetic counseling profession was driven by the ability of practitioners to identify and evaluate emerging clinical opportunities and leverage core skills as experts in genetics and counseling to expand the status quo. Continuing this trend of growth and expansion in the future demands careful (re)evaluation of the didactic and experiential components of genetic counseling training curricula and the core competencies that are required for practice (ACGC, 2023b). To meet the needs of future trainees, training programs must reduce barriers to entering the profession and increase the diversity and inclusion of trainees. In addition, graduate programs of the future will need to provide more training in emerging technologies, tap into the unique expertise available through novel partnerships, and allow for greater geographic access to training. These expansions will increase the depth of knowledge incorporated into training programs and continue to support the ability of genetic counselors to stay abreast of new technologies and increase clinical and genomic specialization. By building these collaborations and allowing a wider array of geographic areas for training, the next generation of learners will be more familiar with providing services in a diverse manner, better equipped to collaborate with others, and more likely to return to underserved communities where they are from, thus expanding access to genetic counseling services overall. Growth in these areas will also ensure that genetic counselors of the future continue to remain on the cutting edge of genomics-based healthcare, both in providing direct patient care and in supporting the development and application of genomic discoveries that will result in more effective clinical tools. These changes will enable genetic counselors to remain adaptable, following historical precedents. Accordingly, they will continue to enjoy increased professional recognition, expansion of professional autonomy, and delivery of high-quality care that meets the needs of diverse constituencies.

References

Aartsma-Rus, A., Ginjaar, I. B., & Bushby, K. (2016). The importance of genetic diagnosis for Duchenne muscular dystrophy. *Journal of Medical Genetics*, 53, 145–151. https://doi.org/10.1136/jmedgenet-2015-103387

Accreditation Council for Genetic Counseling. (2023a). *Practice-based competencies for genetic counselors*. https://www.gceducation.org/forms-resources/

Accreditation Council for Genetic Counseling. (2023b). *Standards of accreditation for graduate programs in genetic counseling.* https://www.gceducation.org/forms-resources/

Accreditation Council for Genetic Counseling. (2024). *Find an accredited program.* https://www.gceducation.org/find-a-program/

Adeyemo, A., Balaconis, M. K., Darnes, D. R., Fatumo, S., Granados Moreno, P., Hodonsky, C. J., Inouye, M., Kanai, M., Kato, K., Knoppers, B. M., Lewis, A. C. F., Martin, A. R., McCarthy, M. I., Meyer, M. N., Okada, Y., Richards, J. B., Richter, L., Ripatti, S., Rotimi, C. N., . . . Zhou, A. (2021). Responsible use of polygenic risk scores in the clinic: Potential benefits, risks and gaps. *Nature Medicine, 27*(11), 1876–1884. https://doi.org/10.1038/s41591-021-01549-6

Allum, J., Nataraj Kirby, S., Sowell, R., Gonzales, L., & Council of Graduate Schools. (2013). *Completion and attrition in STEM master's programs: Pilot study findings.* https://prod.wp.cdn.aws.wfu.edu/sites/202/2021/04/EDITED_Completion_and_Attrition_in_STEM_Masters_Programs_2013-Copy.pdf

American Medical Association. (2023). *Fighting scope creep.* https://www.ama-assn.org/amaone/ama-recovery-plan-america-s-physicians-fighting-scope-creep?utm_effort=DAPSRH&utm_effort=DAPSRH&gclid=CjwKCAiA2rOeBhAsEiwA2Pl7Q_bJ6Mx70hK3-DsszhLboG3nospPspVwOuPmXErqtbHk2HX7FvCG2hoCTRwQAvD_BwE

Association of Genetic Counseling Program Directors. (2021). *The genetic counseling admissions match: Summary results of the match for positions beginning in 2021.* https://natmatch.com/

Bamshad, M. J., Magoulas, P. L., & Dent, K. M. (2018). Genetic counselors on the frontline of precision health. *American Journal of Medical Genetics Part C: Seminars in Medical Genetics, 178*, 5–9. https://doi.org/10.1002/ajmg.c.31610

Baum, S., & Stelle, P. (2017). *Who goes to graduate school and who succeeds?* Urban Institute. https://www.urban.org/research/publication/who-goes-graduate-school-and-who-succeeds

Berrios, C., Hurley, E. A., Willig, L., Thiffault, I., Saunders, C., Pastinen, T., Goggin, K., & Farrow, E. (2021). Challenges in genetic testing: Clinician variant interpretation processes and the impact on clinical care. *Genetics in Medicine, 23*(12), 2289–2299. https://doi.org/10.1038/s41436-021-01267-x

Bianchi, D. W., & Chiu, R. W. K. (2018). Sequencing of circulating cell-free DNA during pregnancy. *New England Journal of Medicine, 379*(8), 464–473. https://doi.org/10.1056/nejmra1705345

Biesecker, B. (2020). Genetic counseling and the central tenets of practice. *Cold Spring Harbor Perspectives in Medicine, 10*(3), a038968. https://doi.org/10.1101/cshperspect.a038968

Boothe, E., Greenberg, S., Delaney, C. L., & Cohen, S. A. (2021). Genetic counseling service delivery models: A study of genetic counselors' interests, needs, and barriers to implementation. *Journal of Genetic Counseling, 30*, 283–292. https://doi.org/10.1002/jgc4.1319

Caulfield, T., & McGuire, A. L. (2012). Direct-to-consumer genetic testing: Perceptions, problems, and policy responses. *Annual Review of Medicine, 63*, 23–33. https://doi.org/10.1146/annurev-med-062110-123753

Cavalli, G., & Heard, E. (2019). Advances in epigenetics link genetics to the environment and disease. *Nature, 571*, 489–499.

Cho, M. T., & Guy, C. (2020). Evolving roles of genetic counselors in the clinical laboratory. *Cold Spring Harbor Perspectives in Medicine, 10*, 1–12. https://doi.org/10.1101/cshperspect.a036574

Cirino, A. L., Harris, S., Lakdawala, N. K., Michels, M., Olivotto, I., Day, S. M., Abrams, D. J., Charron, P., Caleshu, C., Semsarian, C., Ingles, J., Rakowski, H., Judge, D. P., & Ho,

C. Y. (2017). Role of genetic testing in inherited cardiovascular disease: A review. *JAMA Cardiology, 2*(10), 1153–1160. https://doi.org/10.1001/jamacardio.2017.2352

Claussnitzer, M., Cho, J. H., Collins, R., Cox, N. J., Dermitzakis, E. T., Hurles, M. E., Kathiresan, S., Kenny, E. E., Lindgren, C. M., MacArthur, D. G., North, K. N., Plon, S. E., Rehm, H. L., Risch, N., Rotimi, C. N., Shendure, J., Soranzo, N., & McCarthy, M. I. (2020). A brief history of human disease genetics. *Nature, 577*, 179–189. https://doi.org/10.1038/s41586-019-1879-7

Colorado State University. (2022). Online Prior Learning Assessment (PLA) Programs. https://csuglobal.edu/admissions/transfer-students/alternative-credit-options/online-prior-learning-assessment-pla-programs

Denny, J., & Collins, F. (2021). Precision medicine in 2030—Seven ways to transform healthcare. *Cell, 184*, 1415–1419.

Hanson, M. D., Kulasegaram, K. M., Coombs, D. L., & Herold, J. (2012). Admissions file review: Applying the multiple independent sampling (MIS) methodology. *Academic Medicine, 87*(10), 1335–1340. https://doi.org/10.1097/ACM.0b013e3182674629

Hoskovec, J. M., Bennett, R. L., Carey, M. E., DaVanzo, J. E., Dougherty, M., Hahn, S. E., LeRoy, B. S., O'Neal, S., Richardson, J. G., & Wicklund, C. A. (2018). Projecting the supply and demand for certified genetic counselors: A workforce study. *Journal of Genetic Counseling, 27*(1), 16–20. https://doi.org/10.1007/s10897-017-0158-8

Hsu, R. L., Gutierrez, A. M., Schellhammer, S. K., Robinson, J. O., Scollon, S., Street, R. L., Salisbury, A. N., Pereira, S., Plon, S. E., Malek, J., Williams Parsons, D., & McGuire, A. L. (2021). Pediatric oncologists' experiences returning and incorporating genomic sequencing results into cancer care. *Journal of Personalized Medicine, 11*, Article No. 570. https://doi.org/10.3390/jpm11060570

Joseph, A. (2019). *New Vertex cystic fibrosis drug approved, extending treatments to 90% of patients*. StatNews. https://www.statnews.com/

Kyono, Y., Kitzman, J. O., & Parker, S. C. J. (2019). Genomic annotation of disease-associated variants reveals shared functional contexts. *Diebetologaa, 62*, 735–743. https://doi.org/10.1007/s00125-019-4823-3

Mainali, A., Athey, T., Bahl, S., Hung, C., Caluseriu, O., Chan, A., Eaton, A., Ghai, S. J., Kannu, P., MacPherson, M., Niederhoffer, K. Y., Siriwardena, K., & Mercimek-Andrews, S. (2022). Diagnostic yield of clinical exome sequencing in adulthood in medical genetics clinics. *American Journal of Medical Genetics Part A, 191*(2), 510–517. https://doi.org/10.1002/ajmg.a.63053

Maio, M., Carrion, P., Yaremco, E., & Austin, J. C. (2013). Awareness of genetic counseling and perceptions of its purpose: A survey of the Canadian public. *Journal of Genetic Counseling, 22*(6), 762–770. https://doi.org/10.1007/s10897-013-9633-z

Majumder, M. A., Guerrini, C. J., & McGuire, A. L. (2021). Direct-to-consumer genetic testing: Value and risk. *Annual of Review of Medicine, 72*, 151–166. https://doi.org/10.1146/annurev-med-070119

Marinkovich, M. P., & Tang, J. Y. (2019). Gene therapy for epidermolysis bullosa. *Journal of Investigative Dermatology, 139*(6), 1221–1226. https://doi.org/10.1016/j.jid.2018.11.036

Marwaha, S., Knowles, J. W., & Ashley, E. A. (2022). A guide for the diagnosis of rare and undiagnosed disease: Beyond the exome. *Genome Medicine, 14*(1), 23. https://doi.org/10.1186/s13073-022-01026-w

Matte, A., Zorzi, F., Mazzi, F., Federti, E., Olivieri, O., & De Franceschi, L. (2019). New therapeutic options for the treatment of sickle cell disease. *Mediterranean Journal of Hematology and Infectious Disease, 11*(1), e2019002. https://doi.org/10.4084/mjhid.2019.002

Mazzola, S. E., O'Connor, B., & Yashar, B. M. (2019). Primary care physicians' understanding and utilization of pediatric exome sequencing results. *Journal of Genetic Counseling, 28*, 1130–1138. https://doi.org/10.1002/jgc4.1163

Milko, L. V., & Khoury, M. J. (2022). Editorial: DNA-based population screening for precision public health. *Frontiers in Genetics, 13*, 1061329. https://doi.org/10.3389/fgene.2022.1061329

Minear, M. A., Phillips, M. N., Kau, A., & Parisi, M. A. (2022). Newborn screening research sponsored by the NIH: From diagnostic paradigms to precision therapeutics. *American Journal of Medical Genetics Part C: Seminars in Medical Genetics, 190*(2), 138–152. https://doi.org/10.1002/ajmg.c.31997

Mukherjee, M., Eby, M., Wang, S., Lara-Millán, A., & Earle, A. M. (2022). Medicalizing risk: How experts and consumers manage uncertainty in genetic health testing. *PLos One, 17*(8), e0270430. https://doi.org/10.1371/journal.pone.0270430

Myers, M. F., Bergner, A., Conway, L., Duquette, D., Durst, A. L., Yashar, B. M., Zhang, X., & Campion, M. (2022). A report of the AGCPD task force to evaluate associations between select admissions requirements, demographics, and performance on ABGC certification examination. *Journal of Genetic Counseling, 31*(2), 302–315. https://doi.org/10.1002/jgc4.1537

National Society of Genetic Counselors. (2017). *NSGC code of ethics*. https://www.nsgc.org/Policy-Research-and-Publications/Code-of-Ethics-Conflict-of-Interest/Code-of-Ethics

National Society of Genetic Counselors. (2022a). *Professional status survey 2022: Executive summary*. https://www.nsgc.org/Policy-Research-and-Publications/Professional-Status-Survey

National Society of Genetic Counselors. (2022b). *Professional status survey 2022: Work environment*. https://www.nsgc.org/Policy-Research-and-Publications/Professional-Status-Survey

National Society of Genetic Counselors. (2023). *Who are genetic counsellors*. https://www.aboutgeneticcounselors.org/Who-Are-Genetic-Counselors/Who-Are-Genetic-Counselors

Online Mendelian Inheritance in Man (OMIM). (2023). An Online Catalog of Human Genes and Genetic Disorders. https://www.omim.org/about

Pan, V., Yashar, B. M., Pothast, R., & Wicklund, C. (2016). Expanding the genetic counseling workforce: Program directors' views on increasing the size of genetic counseling graduate programs. *Journal of Genetic Counseling, 18*, 842–849. https://doi.org/10.1038/gim.2015.179

Parrott, S., & Clark, C. (2004). *National Society of Genetic Counselors: Membership trends 1980–2002*. https://www.nsgc.org/LinkClick.aspx?fileticket=ay_ZcQxXgKg%3d&portalid=0&timestamp=1673816621482

Pasca, C., Carroll, R., Cragun, R. T., & Cragun, D. L. (2022). Knowledge and perceptions of the genetic counseling profession among a national cross-sectional sample of U.S. adults. *Journal of Genetic Counseling, 31*, 206–217. https://doi.org/10.1002/jgc4.1473

Peeters, M., Gundram, T., & Murphy, J. (2015). Comparing vertical and horizontal screening methods for pharmacy resident candidates before interviews. *Innovations in Pharmacy, 6*(3), 1–5. https://doi.org/10.24926/iip.v6i3.388

Portela, A., & Esteller, M. (2010). Epigenetic modifications and human disease. *Nature Biotechnology, 28*, 1057–1068. https://doi.org/10.1038/nbt.1685

Ramos, E. (2020). Genetic counseling, personalized medicine, and precision health. *Cold Spring Harbor Perspectives in Medicine, 10*, 1–11. https://doi.org/10.1101/cshperspect.a036699

Reid, S., Spalluto, L. B., Lang, K., Weidner, A., & Pal, T. (2022). An overview of genetic services delivery for hereditary breast cancer. *Breast Cancer Research and Treatment, 191*, 491–500. https://doi.org/10.1007/s10549-021-06478-z

Riconda, D., Grubs, R. E., Campion, M. W., & Cragun, D. (2018). Genetic counselor training for the next generation: Where do we go from here? *American Journal of Medical Genetics Part C: Seminars in Medical Genetics, 178*(1), 38–45. https://doi.org/10.1002/ajmg.c.31598

Roman, T. S., Crowley, S. B., Roche, M. I., Foreman, A. K. M., O'Daniel, J. M., Seifert, B. A., Lee, K., Brandt, A., Gustafson, C., DeCristo, D. M., Strande, N. T., Ramkissoon, L., Milko, L. V., Owen, P., Roy, S., Xiong, M., Paquin, R. S., Butterfield, R. M., Lewis, M. A., . . . Berg, J. S. (2020). Genomic sequencing for newborn screening: Results of the NC NEXUS Project. *American Journal of Human Genetics, 107*(4), 596–611. https://doi.org/10.1016/j.ajhg.2020.08.001

Rubinstein, W. S., Maglott, D. R., Lee, J. M., Kattman, B. L., Malheiro, A. J., Ovetsky, M., Hem, V., Gorelenkov, V., Song, G., Wallin, C., Husain, N., Chitipiralla, S., Katz, K. S., Hoffman, D., Jang, W., Johnson, M., Karmanov, F., Ukrainchik, A., Denisenko, M., . . . Ostell, J. M. (2013). The NIH genetic testing registry: A new, centralized database of genetic tests to enable access to comprehensive information and improve transparency. *Nucleic Acids Research, 41*(Database issue), D925–D935. https://doi.org/10.1093/nar/gks1173

Samura, O. (2020). Update on noninvasive prenatal testing: A review based on current worldwide research. *Journal of Obstetric and Gynaecological Research, 46*(8), 1246–1254. https://doi.org/10.1111/jog.14268

Savatt, J. M., & Myers, S. M. (2021). Genetic testing in neurodevelopmental disorders. *Frontiers in Pediatrics, 9*, 526779. https://doi.org/10.3389/fped.2021.526779

Schorling, D. C., Pechmann, A., & Kirschner, J. (2020). Advances in treatment of spinal muscular atrophy—New phenotypes, new challenges, new implications for care. *Journal of Neuromuscular Diseases, 7*, 1–13. https://doi.org/10.3233/JND-190424

Shendure, J., Findlay, G. M., & Snyder, M. W. (2019). Genomic medicine—Progress, pitfalls, and promise. *Cell, 177*, 45–57. https://doi.org/10.1016/j.cell.2019.02.003

Snell, K., & Helen, I. (2017). Data systems, genomic data and expertise of doctors. *Duodecim, 133*(8), 801–807. https://www.ncbi.nlm.nih.gov/pubmed/29240350

Southern New Hampshire University. (2022). *Take credit for what you know*. https://www.snhu.edu/admission/transferring-credits/work-life-experience#/home

Stern, A. M. (2012). *Telling genes: The story of genetic counseling in America*. Johns Hopkins University Press.

Swanson, A., Ramos, E., & Snyder, H. (2014). Next generation sequencing is the impetus for the next generation of laboratory-based genetic counselors. *Cold Spring Harbor Perspectives in Medicine, 23*, 647–654. https://doi.org/10.1007/s10897-013-9684-1

Taylor-Phillips, S., Freeman, K., Geppert, J., Agbebiyi, A., Uthman, O. A., Madan, J., Clarke, A., Quenby, S., & Clarke, A. (2016). Accuracy of non-invasive prenatal testing using cell-free DNA for detection of Down, Edwards and Patau syndromes: A systematic review and meta-analysis. *BMJ Open, 6*(1), e010002. https://doi.org/10.1136/bmjopen-2015

Triebold, M., Skov, K., Erickson, L., Olimb, S., Puumala, S., Wallace, I., & Stein, Q. (2021). Geographical analysis of the distribution of certified genetic counselors in the United States. *Journal of Genetic Counseling, 30*(2), 448–456. https://doi.org/10.1002/jgc4.1331

U.S. Census Bureau. (2020). *Race and Hispanic origin*. https://www.census.gov/quickfacts/fact/table/US/PST045222

Van Driest, S., Shi, Y., Schildcrout, J., Peterson, J., Pulley, J., Denny, J., & Roden, D. (2014). Clinically actionable genotypes among 10,000 patients with preemptive pharmacogenomic testing. *Clinical Pharmacology and Therapeutics, 95*, 423–431.

Wain, K. E., Azzariti, D. R., Goldstein, J. L., Johnson, A. K., Krautscheid, P., Lepore, B., O'Daniel, J. M., Ritter, D., Savatt, J. M., Riggs, E. R., & Martin, C. L. (2020). Variant interpretation is a component of clinical practice among genetic counselors in multiple specialties. *Genetics in Medicine, 22*(4), 785–792. https://doi.org/10.1038/s41436-019-0705-9

Walker, A. (2009). *A guide to genetic counseling* (2nd ed., W. R. Uhlmann, J. L. Schuette, & B. M. Yahar, Eds.). Wiley-Blackwell.

Wand, H., Kalia, S. S., Helm, B. M., Suckiel, S. A., Brockman, D., Vriesen, N., Goudar, R. K., Austin, J., & Yanes, T. (2023). Clinical genetic counseling and translation considerations for polygenic scores in personalized risk assessments: A Practice Resource from the National Society of Genetic Counselors. *Journal of Genetic Counseling*. 32(3):558-575. https://doi.org/10.1002/jgc4.1668

Weipert, C. M., Ryan, K. A., Everett, J. N., Yashar, B. M., Chinnaiyan, A. M., Scott Roberts, J., De Vries, R., Zikmund-Fisher, B. J., & Raymond, V. M. (2018). Physician experiences and understanding of genomic sequencing in oncology. *Journal of Genetic Counseling, 27*, 187–196. https://doi.org/10.1007/s10897-017-0134-3

Yin, Z., Song, L., Clayton, E. W., & Malin, B. A. (2020). Health and kinship matter: Learning about direct-to-consumer genetic testing user experiences via online discussions. *PLoS One, 15*(9), e0238644. https://doi.org/10.1371/journal.pone.0238644

Zetzsche, L. H., Kotzer, K. E., & Wain, K. E. (2014). Looking back and moving forward: An historical perspective from laboratory genetic counselors. *Journal of Genetic Counseling, 23*, 363–370.

Zuckerman, S. (2021). The emergence of the "genetic counseling" profession as a counteraction to past eugenic concepts and practices. *Bioethics, 35*(6), 528–539. https://doi.org/10.1111/bioe.12861

CHAPTER 34

GLOBALIZATION OF GENETIC COUNSELING

MERCY YGOÑA LAURINO AND
AUSTIN EMANUEL BLAND

Introduction

"Globalization" is defined by the Oxford English Dictionary as the "process by which businesses or other organizations develop international influence or start operating on an international scale." As emphasized by the Global Advances in Health and Medicine, the goal of globalization is "not homogenization but rather to provide an opportunity for integration, convergence, and collaboration across cultures" (Mittelman & Hanaway, 2012, p. 5). This is important to keep in mind as the applications of genomics and genetic technology are increasingly incorporated in the global healthcare system—across diverse cultures, religions, and economies. Like other fields of medicine, the profession of genetic counseling is uniquely positioned to be shared worldwide, since the common desire for wellness and achieving an optimal quality of life is sought across individuals and communities.

The genetic counseling profession is spreading globally, with countries in various stages of development, implementation, and sustainability of genetic counseling training programs (Abacan et al., 2019; Ormond et al., 2018). In this chapter, we describe the global landscape of the genetic counseling field and highlight the availability of genetic counseling training programs and credentialing processes through government and professional bodies, while acknowledging healthcare system differences and cultural, social, ethical, and legal considerations. In some countries, the genetic counseling profession has been in existence for decades, where genetic counselors are increasingly recognized as an important and valued member of healthcare delivery. In other countries, the field is in the beginning stages of professional development. Approximately 7,000 genetic counselors were practicing worldwide in 2018 (Abacan et al., 2019), and training of genetic counselors remains highly variable in countries with practicing genetic counselors given national- and local-level factors (e.g., resource allocation for training, national policies).

The Global Landscape of Genetic Counseling

In describing the global landscape of the genetic counseling profession, we adapted the designation from the United Nations Department of Economic and Social Affairs, Population Division's (2022) published report wherein countries are grouped into continental regions. We used the following continental regions: *Africa*, *Asia*, *Europe*, *Latin America and the Caribbean*, *North America*, and *Oceania*. We also included the transcontinental region of the *Middle East*, as the professional landscape of genetic counseling in this region is unique from both Africa and Asia. Benchmarking the reported population trends in these regions is intended to provide the "international community with timely and accessible population data and analysis of population trends and development outcomes for all countries and areas of the world" (United Nations Department of Economic and Social Affairs, Population Division, 2002, p. ii) and thus allow for up-to-date insights into the emerging country-specific issues to help inform strategy for increasing implementation of genomics medicine, if applicable, and overall growth for genetic counseling services.

As we examine the globalization of genetic counseling services, the following are key trends for consideration: (a) the global population is estimated to grow to 8.5 billion by 2030, 9.7 billion by 2050, and 10.4 billion by 2100; (b) two-thirds of the projected global population increase through 2050 is attributed to the momentum of past growth, while acknowledging the youthful age structure of the current population; and (c) population growth rates vary significantly between countries and regions (United Nations Department of Economic and Social Affairs, Population Division, 2022). Figure 34.1 shows a timeline illustrating the birth of training programs for the genetic counseling profession in these regions.

Africa

In 1988, South Africa started its first master's degree training program in genetic counseling in the Division of Human Genetics of the National Health Laboratory Service at the University of the Witwatersrand in Johannesburg (Greenberg et al., 2012; Kromberg et al.,

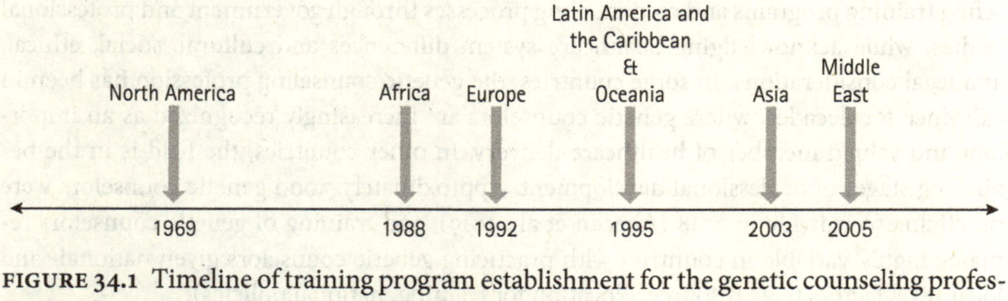

FIGURE 34.1 Timeline of training program establishment for the genetic counseling profession in the continental regions and Middle East.

2013). The program attracted prospective students from various postgraduate backgrounds (e.g., genetics, social work, psychology, and medicine). With a total population of 1.3 billion people, there are estimated to be fewer than 50 *formally* trained genetic counselors across the entire continent of Africa (Abacan et al., 2019). This number is incredibly striking, considering sub-Saharan Africa is currently projected to account for more than half of the growth of the world's population between 2022 and 2050 and is expected to almost double in that timeframe (more than 2 billion inhabitants by the late 2040s; United Nations Department of Economic and Social Affairs, Population Division, 2022). In South Africa, genetic counseling is primarily available in tertiary healthcare service centers in major cities. Patients in rural areas have limited access to these services, and most are provided by nongenetics healthcare providers (Greenberg et al., 2012).

Despite the increasing integration of genomic information into healthcare, the value of genetic counseling services, and the importance of genetic counseling to empowering patients, services continue to be underutilized in South Africa, and efforts are underway to elevate awareness of the profession's existence with other allied healthcare professionals (Thom & Haw, 2021). The Health Professions Council of South Africa governs the genetic counseling profession, while Genetic Counsellors South Africa (a subgroup of the Southern African Society for Human Genetics) develops standards of practice guidelines for the training and registration of genetic counselors. Kromberg et al. (2013) categorized the roles and responsibilities of genetic counselors in South Africa into five basic areas: counseling, teaching, research, marketing, and administration. In alignment with the commitment to increasing the availability of genetics services, training workshops on genetic counseling for nurses at St. Paul's Millennium Medical College in Addis Ababa, Ethiopia, were conducted in partnership with Michigan Medicine (Quinonez et al., 2021). Results of the workshops were promising as they noted high levels of satisfaction from the participants in terms of increasing their genetic counseling–specific knowledge. However, several barriers to learning were highlighted, which included logistical, financial, cultural, and system specific (i.e., nurses who completed the training workshops were rotated to work at other specialty areas in the hospital, which eventually impacted the full utilization of their gained genetics knowledge in their newly assigned work care environment). Feedback from participants highlighted the differences between "Western" genetic counseling practice and patient–provider communication practices in Ethiopia, along with patient autonomy and decision-making processes in the local culture. As an example, Alemayehu and Meskele (2017) published a study of the healthcare decision-making autonomy of over 900 women from rural districts of Southern Ethiopia, noting that 40.9% of decisions were exclusively made by the husbands of study participants. Thus, it is important to acknowledge and understand local cultural norms to strategically inform genetic counseling training education and overall healthcare provision to empower all individuals in the community. Results from a qualitative study conducted in Kenya of healthcare providers in genetics point to counseling challenges on how to explain genetics in nontechnical terms, along with addressing the social, cultural, and psychological implications of a genetic diagnosis (Zhong et al., 2021). In South Africa, efforts are underway by genetic counselors to increase outreach services, given that most of the patient population currently being served is living in metropolitan areas and the rural communities continue to be underserved (Greenberg et al., 2012). In South Africa, Kromberg and colleagues (2013) reported that genetic counselors take on roles specific to teaching, research, marketing, and administration, in addition to the provision of genetic counseling services. Since community providers had a lack of awareness and/or understanding on "who" and "what" genetic counselors do as partners in healthcare delivery, the authors argue that "Counselors also have a responsibility to market the genetic counseling service" (Greenberg et al., 2012, p. 540).

Asia

Eastern and South-Eastern Asia were reported in 2022 to have a population of 2.3 billion, and Central and Southern Asia were estimated to have a population of 2.1 billion, accounting for 29% and 26% of the global population, respectively. China and India, having populations of over 1.4 billion each, together account for most of the population in Asia. Although it is important to note that the development of genetic counseling training programs has been generally unregulated across this region, there are estimated to be more than 350 genetic counselors, with the first training program established in 2003 (see Figure 34.1; Abacan et al., 2019; Laurino et al., 2018; Ormond et al., 2018). Some countries offer 1- to 2-year master's programs in genetic counseling, while others offer 6-month tracks as part of existing master's program or genetics-focused clinical training of physicians and nurses (offered in the Philippines, Indonesia, and Taiwan, among others; Choi & Kim, 2009; Cutiongco-de la Paz et al., 2019, 2022; Laurino & Padilla, 2013). In 2022, Thailand established its genetic counseling certification program at Mahidol University, Bangkok, Thailand. India, Taiwan, and Japan have established a certification process with oversight by their respective national professional genetic counseling societies (Chien et al., 2013; Elackatt, 2013; Li, 2017). The Philippine Society of Genetic Counselors and the Genetic Counsellors Society Singapore were established in 2022 and 2023, respectively, to support professional development, while the Genetic Counselling Society of Malaysia was established in 2018.

Fostering partnerships among Asian countries, the Professional Society of Genetic Counselors in Asia (PSGCA) leadership convened meetings with representatives from the Board of Genetic Counseling in India, the Indonesian Society of Genetic Counselors, the Japanese Board of Genetic Counseling, and the Taiwan Association of Genetic Counseling to begin work on aligning core skill requirements and curricular standards for genetic counselor training in the region. Results from a survey conducted by the PSGCA of genetic counselors in the region acknowledged genetic counselors as a valuable "genetics-expert" resource to patients and families affected with genetic conditions. The genetic counselor's role in providing psychosocial counseling is highlighted as one of the main reasons for the profession's important contribution as a member of the healthcare team. As far as is possible, the provision of genetic counseling services respects local communities' religious, legal, and ethical norms (e.g., pregnancy termination being illegal in some countries; Laurino et al., 2018; Yoshida et al., 2020; Zayts et al., 2013). With respect to autonomous decision making, Cura (2015) emphasizes that in some cultures (e.g., Filipino communities), decisions may not necessarily be made by an individual but as a family, and genetic counselors should aim to actively engage with patients through an understanding of how the latter approach the decision-making process.

Middle East

Genetic counseling is a growing profession in the Middle East (Kennedy & Al-Saffar, 2010) with over 100 genetic counselors practicing in the region (Abacan et al., 2019), with approximately 40 of them located specifically in the Arab region. This equates to about 0.1 genetic counselor per million individuals in the Middle East (Abou Tayoun et al., 2021). Some countries (e.g., Qatar and Saudi Arabia) have established genetic counseling training programs in an effort to increase access to genetic counselors who are familiar with local cultural norms and practices. The first Middle Eastern training program was established in 2005 at the King Faisal Specialist Hospital and Research Center Division of Medical Genetics (Qari et al., 2013) in Riyadh, Saudi Arabia. In 2015, this program was recognized and accredited by the Saudi Commission for Health Specialties (Balobaid et al., 2016).

As genetic counseling is integrated into global health systems, it is important to recognize the influence of religion and cultural practices on the availability of healthcare services. In Saudi Arabia, challenges in the provision of genetic counseling include, but are not limited to, women's access to genetic services and other forms of healthcare; identifying, informing, and guiding carriers of recessive alleles; and understanding and managing complex molecular findings such as variants of uncertain significance (Balobaid et al., 2016).

Europe

The profession of genetic counseling in Europe started in the United Kingdom in the early 1990s (Ormond et al., 2018), with other countries (e.g., France) subsequently establishing their own training programs. As expected, the approach to the development and implementation of genetic counseling in European countries is heavily influenced by the country's healthcare system and existing national policies. At present, there are over 1,000 genetic counselors across Europe and the Middle East (Abacan et al., 2019), including, Belgium, Cyprus, Denmark, Finland, France, Ireland, Italy, the Netherlands, Norway, Qatar, Portugal, Romania, Saudi Arabia, Slovenia, Spain, Sweden, Switzerland, Turkey, and the United Kingdom (Abou Tayoun et al., 2021; Sagi & Uhlmann, 2013; Schwaninger et al., 2021).

Genetic counselor "registration" and "credentialing" have been important topics for several years as the avenue of work opportunities in various countries continues to expand (Ormond et al., 2018). In the United Kingdom, graduates from the master's-level genomic counseling degree apply for a Certificate of Attainment from the Academy for Healthcare Science, which allows registration as a clinical scientist (genomic counselor)[1] with the Health and Care Professions Council. Given the variability of curriculum for genetic counselor training in the region, the European Board of Medical Genetics eventually developed a core curriculum to support implementation of a standard practice (Paneque et al., 2017).

With increasing endeavors to "mainstream" genomics, the roles for genetic counselors in Europe have significantly expanded beyond the provision of clinical services to include

[1] We interchange the terms "genomic counselor" and "genetic counselor" to match region-specific conventions in language.

teaching, policy, research, and outreach (Middleton et al., 2017). To promote recognition of genetic counselors, the Associazione Italiana di Genetic Counsellors, established in 2019, is composed of a network of people appropriately trained and involved in genetic counseling services and/or projects that aim to increase awareness of genetic counselors as independent professionals (Crimi et al., 2020). In contrast, within Germany, Austria, and part of Switzerland, national legislatures allow the provision of genetic counseling solely by licensed medical physicians (Schwaninger et al., 2021). Nevertheless, current efforts are underway to establish training programs for genetic counselors in these countries while acknowledging the importance of a "clear definition of the professional role and scope of practice of genetic counselors in comparison to medical geneticists, in recognition of the special skill set of genetic counselors" (Schwaninger et al., 2021, p. 868).

Latin America and the Caribbean

The professional role of genetic counselors is not formally recognized as an allied healthcare provider in several Latin American countries. As such, medical doctors have mainly provided genetic counseling services. Recently, the Latin American Professional Society of Genetic Counseling was established to bring awareness to the importance of genetic counseling in the region. Their website provides a directory of available clinical genetics services. As of 2023, Cuba and Brazil are the only countries offering a master's in genetic counseling training in the region (Abacan et al., 2019), while a diploma course is offered in Chile (Simone et al., 2022).

Specifically, Cuba was reported to have approximately 900 genetic counselors in 2018 (Abacan et al., 2019), but the overall scope of genetic counseling practice in the country is unclear. Cruz (2013) provides an overview of genetic counseling training in Cuba and highlights two master's-level programs established between 1995 and 2000. Briefly, the development and establishment of the training program was overseen by professors in the Department of Medical Genetics, University of Medical Sciences of Havana. One training pathway in medical genetics was dedicated specifically for physicians, while the other was intended to train other professionals (e.g., nurses, social workers, etc.). From 2001 to 2003, a nationwide epidemiological screening was conducted to identify individuals with intellectual, visual, auditory, mental, and physical disabilities (Cruz, 2013), and findings led to the decision to increase access to genetic counseling services in all the municipalities in Cuba. Thus, the Cuban government rapidly implemented training positions that led to the graduation of 837 genetic counseling students who were specifically selected from specialized physicians and nursing graduates across the nation. To continue practicing as a genetic counselor, the Ministry of Public Health designates a tribunal wherein genetic counselors who are candidates for recertification (10 years postqualification) must demonstrate their competency. This is a legalized and obligatory recertification process.

In 2019, Bucio et al. (2019) conducted a needs assessment study to assess public awareness of genetic counseling in Mexico. Like the other countries in the region, medical doctors (i.e., medical geneticists) provide genetic counseling services in Mexico, and genetic counseling is yet to be recognized as a distinct and complementary profession to medical geneticists. Furthermore, Penchaszadeh (2015) reported the following barriers that lead to the inequitable provision of genetic services in Latin America:

> (a) lack of universal access to health care, with fragmented, inefficient and inequitable health systems; (b) the heavy burden of unmet needs in infectious diseases, malnutrition and basic primary health care, particularly in prenatal, newborn and infant care; (c) deficient understanding of genetics by health professionals and health officials; (d) discriminatory practices by for-profit health insurance leading to poor coverage for genetic conditions; and (e) weak governmental regulation of genetic testing. (p. 228)

Specifically in Chile, a country with more than 19 million people, there is only one formally trained genetic counselor and approximately 40 clinical geneticists. To address the increasing demand for genetic counseling services, the Faculty of Medicine and Nursing of Clínica Alemana Universidad del Desarrollo developed the first online certificate course in genetic counseling in Chile (Simone et al., 2022). Shortly after, the 2023 Human Genome (HUGO) Meeting was held in Rio de Janeiro in Brazil, and a genetic counseling workshop hosted by HUGO's Education subcommittee on genetic counseling further addressed this increased demand and aimed to define the core skills and competencies required of genetic counselors.

North America

The birth of the genetic counseling profession formally began in the United States in 1969 when the first master's-level training program at Sarah Lawrence College in New York was established (Stern, 2009). The American Board of Genetic Counseling (ABGC) was established in 1993 and is the main certifying professional body for genetic counselors. As of 2021, there is one certified genetic counselor for every 71,842 people in the United States, and the majority live and/or work in metropolitan areas (Berninger et al., 2021). The Accreditation Council for Genetic Counseling (ACGC) now has the responsibility to accredit training programs, which was previously part of the ABGC's role. As of 2025, there are 65 ACGC accredited training programs in the United States and Canada (ACGC, 2025).

In recent years, there has been much effort toward increasing diversity and equity in the genetic counselor workforce in the United States (Channaoui et al., 2020). Based on a recent Professional Status Survey (PSS) administered by the National Society of Genetic Counselors (NSGC), 93% of the respondents identified as women, 89% as White, and 89% as heterosexual/straight (NSGC, 2022). In 2017, the Minority Genetic Professionals Network was established for genetic counselors and other medical genetic professionals from racial and ethnic minority backgrounds to provide opportunities for community building, mentorship, and networking. Furthermore, a commitment to sex and gender inclusivity led the NSGC to revise its previously published pedigree nomenclature recommendations (Bennett et al., 2022), which were published to share this information with the global genetic counseling community.

In the mid-1980s, master's-level genetic counseling programs began to be established in Canada. In contrast to the United States, healthcare services in Canada are publicly funded, with the government setting healthcare standards through the Canada Health Act. Thus, each province has its own healthcare insurance plan and coverage of genetic testing is based on medical necessity. According to a recent PSS administered by the Canadian Association of Genetic Counsellors (CAGC), there are 635 genetic counselors who work in Canada to serve a population close to 40 million (United Nations Department of Economic and Social

Affairs, Population Division, 2022). Legal recognition of a profession in Canada is determined at the provincial or territorial rather than the federal level (Lambert et al., 2022). In 2021, the Canadian Board of Genetic Counselling assumed responsibility for certifying genetic counselors practicing in Canada, a role that had previously been held by the CAGC. Costa and colleagues (2021) recently published results from their study interviewing Canadian graduates of genetic counseling programs and employers of genetic counselors with patient-facing job responsibilities. Given increasing demand for genetics services and nonroutine available appointment wait times (which could be at least a year in some clinics in Canada), Costa and colleagues (2021) highlight the need for additional funding for training and employment of genetic counselors in Canada.

Oceania

In Australia, the first university-based training program in genetic counseling was established in 1995 at New South Wales, followed by programs in Victoria and Queensland (Sahhar et al., 2005) and, most recently, at the University of Technology Sydney in Sydney (McEwen & Jacobs, 2021). To date, there are 280 genetic counselors in Australia and New Zealand, with the Australasian Society of Genetic Counsellors (ASGC) serving as the professional body. This genetic counselor workforce serves approximately 44.8 million people living in this region (United Nations Department of Economic and Social Affairs, Population Division, 2022). McEwan and Jacobs (2021) highlighted professional regulation as an added benefit of practicing genetic counselors to shape genetic healthcare, with the Human Genetics Society of Australasia functioning as the regulatory body of genetic counselors in the region.

In Australia, genetics services are available through the public health system, and genetic testing is of no additional cost to the patient when medically necessary. The genetic counseling training programs in Australia have also established formal academic relationships with international programs to promote dialogue among students and faculty about curricular strategies and the ways in which local cultural, religious, healthcare, and psychosocial factors influence genetic counseling practice (Sahhar et al., 2005). In New Zealand, the Primary Health Organisations' stated aim is "to ensure general practitioner services are better linked with other primary health services (such as allied health services) to ensure a seamless continuum of care, in particular to better manage long-term conditions" (Sane et al., 2015, p. 790). To support this aim, collaboration with genetic counselors and primary care providers is necessary. Genetic counselors, who were ASGC members and had participated in the study conducted by Sane and colleagues (2015), reported their underlying vested interest for this type of working partnership in support of preparing primary care for genomic medicine.

Collaboration and Integration

Globally, the efforts to establish partnerships among genetic counseling professionals who share a commitment to increasing access to genetic counseling services continue to strengthen. The Transnational Alliance for Genetic Counseling (TAGC) has been actively promoting international networking and collaboration since 2006 (Edwards, 2013). In 2011, the TAGC formed an International Committee on Genetic Counseling Credentialing to document the diverse genetic counselor training modalities, along with the varying credentialing, registration, and licensure processes in countries with practicing genetic counselors (Ormond et al., 2018). In countries where the profession of genetic counseling has been established for several decades, professional societies often engage in activities to support other countries that are at the beginning stages of professional development. Specifically, partnerships via coaching and mentorship are needed in professional development areas pertaining to genetic counselor "registration" and "certification" (Ormond et al., 2018). Regional genetic counseling professional societies such as the PSGCA have been encouraging networking and clinical and research collaboration among local genetic counselors and across other professional bodies (Laurino et al., 2018). These endeavors are intended to support efforts to increase access and maintain the provision of quality genetic counseling services. Opportunities for genetic counseling student exchange rotation may arise, along with participation in policy and practice guideline development. Table 34.1 summarizes several professional societies in the continental regions and Middle East.

When considering reciprocity, or the equivalent exchange of ideas and agreement of requirements for a practicing genetic counselor across countries, it is imperative to consider the varying country-specific differences when providing "certification," since in some countries (e.g., the United States, Canada) this can be achieved via passing a national examination, while in others (e.g., Australia) it is through portfolio submissions of completed genetic counseling cases postgraduation. As mentioned above, the TAGC formed the International Committee on Genetic Counselor Credentialing, and one of its purposes is to promote dialogue between genetic counselors representing various countries and professional societies regarding their varying processes for certification, as different certification requirements can pose difficulties for workforce requests for "reciprocity" (Ormond et al., 2018). To date, there is no clear path forward on whether a solution is possible to meet the workforce reciprocity requests given the international variability in the training and certification of genetic counselors. Potentially, region-based reciprocity may be possible, as highlighted in current arrangements between Canada and U.S. trained genetic counselors. Genetic counselors across the globe typically work as members of a healthcare team. In some countries, however, genetic counselors have increased their autonomous role (in clinical and nonclinical positions), with more opportunities in diverse settings (Middleton et al., 2017). An important global difference influencing the practice of genetic counseling is the diverse types of healthcare delivery and insurance payment systems (private versus public, or hybrid) existing at a country-specific level.

In 2006, the World Health Organization requested that the various genetic counseling professional bodies develop international core competencies necessary for the provision of quality genetic counseling services given the diverse group of patients the field serves—within and across countries. In alignment with this endeavor, international exchange in genetic counseling training has been increasing (Ballantyne et al., 2006) but was halted due to the COVID-19 pandemic. Training programs have participated in international collaborations to increase their students' awareness of multicultural issues relevant to the delivery of genetic counseling services in the local setting. For example, the University of the Philippines-Manila and Stanford Genetic Counseling training programs hold joint virtual case conferences for genetic counseling students to present challenging cases, and the

Table 34.1 Genetic Counseling Professional Societies in the Continental Regions and Middle East

Region	Professional societies for genetic counselors
Africa	Genetic Counsellors South Africa (informal subgroup of the Southern African Society for Human Genetics; https://sashg.org)
Asia	Board of Genetic Counseling–India (https://www.geneticcounselingboardindia.com)
	Genetic Counseling Branch of the Chinese Genetics Society (https://www.cbgc.org.cn)
	Japanese Society for Genetic Counseling (https://www.jsgc.jp)
	Genetic Counselling Society of Malaysia (https://www.gcsocietymalaysia.org.my)
	Philippine Society of Genetic Counselors (https://www.facebook.com/PhilippineSocietyofGeneticCounselors/)
	Professional Society of Genetic Counselors in Asia (https://www.psgca.org)
	Taiwan Association of Genetic Counseling (https://www.taiwangc.org.tw)
	Genetic Counsellors Society Singapore (https://www.linkedin.com/in/genetic-counsellors-society-singapore-2aa2a429a)
Europe	Association Française des Conseillers en Génétique (https://www.af-cg.fr)
	Associazione Italiana Genetic Counsellors (https://www.facebook.com/aigeco.assitalianageneticcounselor/)
	Association of Genetic Nurses and Counsellors (https://www.agnc.org.uk)
Latin America and the Caribbean	Latin American Professional Society of Genetic Counseling (https://www.splagen.org)
Middle East	Arab Society of Genetic Counselors (https://www.asgcsociety.org/)
North America	National Society of Genetic Counselors (https://www.nsgc.org)
	Canadian Association of Genetic Counsellors (https://www.cagc-accg.ca)
	Minority Genetic Professionals Network (https://www.westernstatesgenetics.org/mgpn-resources/)
Oceania	Australasian Society of Genetic Counsellors (https://www.hgsa.org.au/asgc)

open forum discussions illuminated the differences in counseling approaches given existing local policies influencing clinical practices (Laurino & Padilla, 2013).

Importantly, culture, language, and religion influence the provision of genetic counseling services. Direct translation of genetic terms (e.g., "gene," "chromosome," "inheritance") may not be possible across all languages, thus making it challenging to implement the "Western" genetic counseling practice (Shaw & Ahmed, 2004). To improve understanding of how genetic counseling services can respect local culture, language, and religion, it is imperative to have more genetics-related projects honoring various Indigenous worldviews and participation of Indigenous researchers, such as the commitment of the New Zealand government's genomic initiative that aims to ensure that the Te Ao Māori (Māori worldview) is at its core (McEwen & Jacobs, 2021). The Te Ao Māori is an "interconnected worldview weaving spiritual and physical dimensions through stories and whakataukī [sayings]" (Hudson et al., 2016, p. 351). Active community engagement was emphasized by the study results of Gonzalez and colleagues (2020) wherein increased collaboration between Aboriginal health workers and genetic counselors was encouraged to enhance the provision of cancer genetic counseling services.

Together, genetic counselors from different regions can collaborate on endeavors to shape the future of the profession. As they share professional development experiences, they can incorporate best practices while remaining aware of the limitations pertaining to existing policies where implementation is desired. What works well in countries with established genetic counseling services may not necessarily work as well, if at all, in all countries given varying cultural and legal circumstances. To inform the integration of genetic counseling services into existing healthcare systems, several needs assessments from key stakeholders have been published from various countries across the globe. As an example, a qualitative study conducted in Romania with patients, family members, and healthcare professionals highlighted the importance of instilling hope primarily from their experience of receiving health information, specifically in genetics. In contrast, feelings of hopelessness were shared by participants who identified as cancer patients after getting information from unreliable sources or receiving medical information that they were unable to fully understand (Ciucă et al., 2021). Overall, study participants expressed the need for integrated healthcare, easier access to genetic counseling, personalized care, and "simple, plain language" when receiving medical information. These are highly relevant points to consider as the practice of genetic counseling expands to provide services to populations wherein local languages do not have direct translations of terms genetic counselors often use in their practice.

At present, there is a global shortage of healthcare providers trained in genetics, let alone genetic counseling. Several contextual factors influencing healthcare delivery, along with social, cultural, religious, and legal ramifications, contribute to the variability in training opportunities. Thus, the models for genetic counseling service delivery are highly variable and are country dependent. As the demand for quality genetic counseling services continues to grow in tandem with a growing global population, it is important to clearly define the core training requirements for healthcare providers to safely provide genetic counseling services and minimize patient and community harm. For example, in some countries, the training of nurses and social workers might be the best option given resource gaps (Barr et al., 2018; Cutiongco-de la Paz et al., 2022; Quinonez et al., 2021). Abad and Sur (2022), referring to developing countries like the Philippines, suggest that a strategic integration of genetics and genomics training in nursing practice would be feasible and beneficial. Currently, existing population-based genetics programs (e.g., newborn screening) are avenues to effectively introduce the genetics specialty field to nurses. Moreover, nurses constitute much of the healthcare workforce in several countries, and they have the front-line opportunity to provide genetics education and support (Barr et al., 2018). In partnership, and highly dependent on the local healthcare setting, genetic counselors and nurses play key roles in offering the much-needed support to an increasing number of patients with hereditary conditions and to their family members.

Conclusion

As the promise of precision medicine spreads across the globe, the need to access quality genetic counseling services simultaneously increases. It is thus important to be thoughtful, innovative, and strategic with the approach to expanding genetic counseling globally, recognizing and honoring the varying nation-specific healthcare delivery systems, as well as the religious, social, and cultural practices of the growing populations genetic counselors serve. Simultaneously, as genetic counseling services become routine and universally available, it is imperative that the prospect of cultural competency transforms into cultural humility. The first step in the process is to better grasp the global scope of the profession at present, which this chapter hoped to outline. The next step is continuing to diversify the perspectives within the field of genetic counseling in a way that reflects professionally the widely varying cultures and demographics of the world's diverse and growing population.

References

Abacan, M., Alsubaie, L., Barlow-Stewart, K., Caanen, B., Cordier, C., Courtney, E., Davoine, E., Edwards, J., Elackatt, N. J., & Gardiner, K. (2019). The global state of the genetic counseling profession. *European Journal of Human Genetics*, *27*(2), 183–197.

Abad, P. J. B., & Sur, A. L. D. (2022). Nursing engagement in genetics and genomics: A developing country's perspective. *International Nursing Review*, *69*(4), 559–565.

Abou Tayoun, A. N., Fakhro, K. A., Alsheikh-Ali, A., & Alkuraya, F. S. (2021). Genomic medicine in the Middle East. *Genome Medicine*, *13*(1), 1–3.

Accreditation Council for Genetic Counseling. (2025). *ACGC program directory* (pp. 1-7). March 12, 2025. https://www.gceducation.org/students-volunteers/#program

Alemayehu, M., & Meskele, M. (2017). Health care decision making autonomy of women from rural districts of Southern Ethiopia: A community based cross-sectional study. *International Journal of Women's Health*, *9*, 213.

Ballantyne, A., Goold, I., & Pearn, A. (2006). *Medical genetic services in developing countries: The ethical, legal, and social implications of genetic testing and screening* (pp. 1–114). World Health Organization. https://iris.who.int/handle/10665/43288

Balobaid, A., Qari, A., & Al-Zaidan, H. (2016). Genetic counselors' scope of practice and challenges in genetic counseling services in Saudi Arabia. *International Journal of Pediatrics and Adolescent Medicine*, *3*(1), 1–6.

Barr, J. A., Tsai, L. P., Welch, A., Faradz, S. M., Lane-Krebs, K., Howie, V., & Hillman, W. (2018). Current practice for genetic counselling by nurses: An integrative review. *International Journal of Nursing Practice*, *24*(2), e12629.

Bennett, R. L., French, K. S., Resta, R. G., & Austin, J. (2022). Practice resource-focused revision: Standardized pedigree nomenclature update centered on sex and gender inclusivity: A practice resource of the National Society of Genetic Counselors. *Journal of Genetic Counseling*, *31*(6), 1238–1248.

Berninger, T., Nusbaum, R., Redlinger-Grosse, K., Davis, C., & Reiser, C. (2021). A narrative literature review: Growing the workforce through increased fieldwork capacity in genetic counseling training programs. *Journal of Genetic Counseling*, *30*(2), 574–587.

Bucio, D., Ormond, K. E., Hernandez, D., Bustamante, C. D., & Lopez Pineda, A. (2019). A genetic counseling needs assessment of Mexico. *Molecular Genetics & Genomic Medicine*, *7*(5), e668.

Channaoui, N., Bui, K., & Mittman, I. (2020). Efforts of diversity and inclusion, cultural competency, and equity in the genetic counseling profession: A snapshot and reflection. *Journal of Genetic Counseling*, *29*(2), 166–181.

Chien, S., Su, P.-H., & Chen, S.-J. (2013). Development of genetic counseling services in Taiwan. *Journal of Genetic Counseling, 22*(6), 839–843.

Choi, J.-Y., & Kim, H.-J. (2009). A study on genetic counseling curriculum, accreditation of the training program, and the certification process of genetic counselors in Korea. *Journal of Genetic Medicine, 6*(1), 38–55.

Ciucă, A., Moldovan, R., & Băban, A. (2021). Developing genetic counselling services in an underdeveloped healthcare setting. *Journal of Community Genetics, 12*(4), 539–548. https://doi.org/10.1007/s12687-021-00546-z

Costa, T., Gillies, B., Oh, T., & Scott, J. (2021). The Canadian genetic counseling workforce: Perspectives from employers and recent graduates. *Journal of Genetic Counseling, 30*(2), 406–417.

Crimi, M., Mineri, R., Godino, L., Bertonazzi, B., Bruzzone, C., Pivetta, B., Cordier, C., Coviello, D. A., & Feroce, I. (2020). Building awareness on genetic counselling: The launch of Italian Association of Genetic Counsellors (AIGeCo). *Journal of Community Genetics, 11*(4), 495–496.

Cruz, A. L. (2013). An overview of genetic counseling in Cuba. *Journal of Genetic Counseling, 22*(6), 849–853.

Cura, J. D. (2015). Respecting autonomous decision making among Filipinos: A re-emphasis in genetic counseling. *Journal of Genetic Counseling, 24*(2), 213–224.

Cutiongco-de la Paz, E. M. C., Abadingo, M. E., Maceda, E. B. G., & Padilla, C. D. (2022). Genetics and genomics education and training in developing countries. In D. Kumar (Ed.), *Genomic and precision medicine in clinical practice, genomic medicine skills and competencies* (1st ed., pp. 17–30). Academic Press.

Cutiongco-de la Paz, E. M. C., Chung, B. H., Faradz, S. M. H., Thong, M. K., David-Padilla, C., Lai, P. S., Lin, S. P., Chen, Y. H., Sura, T., & Laurino, M. (2019). Training in clinical genetics and genetic counseling in Asia. *American Journal of Medical Genetics. Part C, Seminars in Medical Genetics, 181*(2), 177–186. https://doi.org/10.1002/ajmg.c.31703

Edwards, J. G. (2013). The transnational alliance for genetic counseling: Promoting international communication and collaboration. *Journal of Genetic Counseling, 22*(6), 688–689.

Elackatt, N. J. (2013). Genetic counseling: A transnational perspective. *Journal of Genetic Counseling, 22*(6), 854–857.

Oxford English Dictionary. (2023, July). Globalization [Noun]. Oxford University Press. https://doi.org/10.1093/OED/1404426084

Gonzalez, T., Harris, R., Williams, R., Wadwell, R., Barlow-Stewart, K., Fleming, J., & Buckman, M. (2020). Exploring the barriers preventing Indigenous Australians from accessing cancer genetic counseling. *Journal of Genetic Counseling, 29*(4), 542–552.

Greenberg, J., Kromberg, J., Loggenberg, K., & Wessels, T.-M. (2012). Genetic counseling in South Africa. In D. Kumar (Ed.), *Genomics and health in the developing world* (pp. 531–546). Oxford University Press.

Hudson, M., Russell, K., Uerata, L., Milne, M., Wilcox, P., Port, R. V., Smith, B., Toki, V., & Beaton, A. (2016). Te Mata Ira—Faces of the gene: Developing a cultural foundation for biobanking and genomic research involving Māori. *AlterNative: An International Journal of Indigenous Peoples, 12*(4), 341–355.

Kennedy, S. J., & Al-Saffar, M. (2010). Genetic counseling in the Middle East. In A. Teebi (Ed.), *Genetic disorders among Arab populations* (pp. 725–740). Springer.

Kromberg, J. G., Wessels, T.-M., & Krause, A. (2013). Roles of genetic counselors in South Africa. *Journal of Genetic Counseling, 22*(6), 753–761.

Lambert, D. M., Patrinos, D., Knoppers, B. M., Study, G., & Zawati, M. n. H. (2022). Genetic counselors and legal recognition: A made-for-Canada approach. *Journal of Genetic Counseling*, *31*(1), 49–58.

Laurino, M. Y., Leppig, K. A., Abad, P. J., Cham, B., Chu, Y. W. Y., Kejriwal, S., Lee, J. M., Sternen, D. L., Thompson, J. K., & Burgess, M. J. (2018). A report on ten Asia Pacific countries on current status and future directions of the genetic counseling profession: The establishment of the Professional Society of Genetic Counselors in Asia. *Journal of Genetic Counseling*, *27*(1), 21–32.

Laurino, M. Y., & Padilla, C. D. (2013). Genetic counseling training in the Philippines. *Journal of Genetic Counseling*, *22*(6), 865–868.

Li, M.-H. (2017). AB100. Current status, challenges, and future prospective of genetic counseling in Taiwan. *Annals of Translational Medicine*, 5(Suppl 2). https://doi.org/10.21037/atm.2017.s100

McEwen, A., & Jacobs, C. (2021). Preparing the genetic counseling workforce for the future in Australasia. *Journal of Genetic Counseling*, *30*(1), 55–60.

Middleton, A., Mendes, Á., Benjamin, C. M., & Howard, H. C. (2017). Direct-to-consumer genetic testing: Where and how does genetic counseling fit? *Personalized Medicine*, *14*(3), 249–257.

Mittelman, M., & Hanaway, P. (2012). *Globalization of healthcare* (Vol. 1). Sage Publications.

National Society of Genetic Counselors. (2022). *Professional status survey 2022: Executive summary*. https://www.nsgc.org/Portals/0/Executive%20Summary%20Final%2005-03-22.pdf

Ormond, K. E., Laurino, M. Y., Barlow-Stewart, K., Wessels, T. M., Macaulay, S., Austin, J., & Middleton, A. (2018). Genetic counseling globally: Where are we now?. *American Journal of Medical Genetics. Part C, Seminars in Medical Genetics*, *178*(1), 98–107. https://doi.org/10.1002/ajmg.c.31607

Paneque, M., Moldovan, R., Cordier, C., Serra-Juhé, C., Feroce, I., Pasalodos, S., Haquet, E., Lambert, D., Bjørnevoll, I., & Skirton, H. (2017). The perceived impact of the European registration system for genetic counsellors and nurses. *European Journal of Human Genetics*, *25*(9), 1075–1077.

Penchaszadeh, V. B. (2015). Ethical issues in genetics and public health in Latin America with a focus on Argentina. *Journal of Community Genetics*, *6*(3), 223–230.

Qari, A. A., Balobaid, A. S., Rawashdeh, R. R., & Al-Sayed, M. D. (2013). The development of genetic counseling services and training program in Saudi Arabia. *Journal of Genetic Counseling*, *22*(6), 835–838.

Quinonez, S. C., O'Connor, B. C., Jacobs, M. F., Mekonnen Tekleab, A., Marye, A., Bekele, D., Yashar, B. M., Hanson, E., Yeshidinber, A., & Wedaje, G. (2021). The introduction of genetic counseling in Ethiopia: Results of a training workshop and lessons learned. *PloS One*, *16*(7), e0255278.

Sagi, M., & Uhlmann, W. R. (2013). Genetic counseling services and training of genetic counselors in Israel: An overview. *Journal of Genetic Counseling*, *22*(6), 890–896. https://doi.org/10.1007/s10897-013-9576-4

Sahhar, M. A., Young, M. A., Sheffield, L. J., & Aitken, M. (2005). Educating genetic counselors in Australia: Developing an international perspective. *Journal of Genetic Counseling*, *14*(4), 283–294. https://doi.org/10.1007/s10897-005-0572-1

Sane, V., Humphreys, L., & Peterson, M. (2015). Are Australasian genetic counselors interested in private practice at the primary care level of health service? *Journal of Genetic Counseling*, *24*(5), 783–796.

Schwaninger, G., Benjamin, C., Rudnik-Schöneborn, S., & Zschocke, J. (2021). The genetic counseling profession in Austria: Stakeholders' perspectives. *Journal of Genetic Counseling, 30*(3), 861–871.

Shaw, A., & Ahmed, M. (2004). Translating genetics leaflets into languages other than English: Lessons from an assessment of Urdu materials. *Journal of Genetic Counseling, 13*(4), 321–342.

Simone, A., de Leon, A., Diaz Caro, D., & Margarit, S. (2022). *Creating a Genetic Counseling Professional Society in Latin America*. https://perspectives.nsgc.org/

Stern, A. M. (2009). A quiet revolution: The birth of the genetic counselor at Sarah Lawrence College, 1969. *Journal of Genetic Counseling, 18*(1), 1–11.

Thom, J., & Haw, T. (2021). Awareness of genetic counseling services among allied healthcare professionals in South Africa. *Journal of Genetic Counseling, 30*(6), 1649–1657.

United Nations Department of Economic and Social Affairs, Population Division. (2022). *World population prospects 2022: Summary of results*.

Yoshida, A., Nakada, H., Inaba, A., & Takahashi, M. (2020). Ethical and professional challenges encountered by Japanese healthcare professionals who provide genetic counseling services. *Journal of Genetic Counseling, 29*(6), 1004–1014.

Zayts, O., Sarangi, S., Thong, M. K., Chung, B. H. y., Lo, I. F. m., Kan, A. S. y., Lee, J. M. H., Padilla, C. D., Cutiongco-de la Paz, E. M., & Faradz, S. M. (2013). Genetic counseling/consultation in South-East Asia: A report from the workshop at the 10th Asia Pacific conference on human genetics. *Journal of Genetic Counseling, 22*(6), 917–924.

Zhong, A., Xia, K., Hadjis, Z., Lifman, G., Njambi, L., & Dimaras, H. (2021). Opportunities and barriers for genetic service delivery in Kenya from a health personnel perspective. *Journal of Community Genetics, 12*(4), 525–538.

CHAPTER 35

GROWING UP WITH GENOMES

Ethical and Practical Considerations of Prenatal and Postnatal Genomic Sequencing

MARSHA MICHIE AND AARON J. GOLDENBERG

Introduction

Genomic sequencing has entered clinical care in the prenatal and postnatal settings perhaps more quickly and forcefully than in any other clinical context. This is due primarily to scientific and medical advances, programmatic changes in research and clinical care, and policy changes at the federal, state, and local levels. Scientific advances in sequencing technologies, bioinformatics, and variant interpretation have propelled rapid changes in clinical implementation of genomic sequencing. Across the perinatal continuum, these shifts have been accompanied by a growing recognition of the overlapping practical and ethical concerns during this crucial period (Allyse et al., 2017; Berg et al., 2017; Farrell & Allyse, 2018; Holm et al., 2018; Johnston et al., 2018; National Human Genome Research Institute [NHGRI], n.d.; Parham et al., 2017; Vora & Wapner, 2018; Vora et al., 2017).

In the prenatal context, where karyotypes on samples from amniocentesis and chorionic villus sampling (CVS) long offered parents genetic information about their fetus, sequencing is expanding both the amount of available information and the ways of obtaining this information (Minear et al., 2015). Noninvasively obtained cell-free DNA in maternal serum now enables accurate and informative screening information about the fetus, thanks to sophisticated bioinformatics that extract information about the fetal genome from a mix of maternal and fetal DNA fragments (Chiu et al., 2008; Fan et al., 2008; Kitzman et al., 2012). These cell-free DNA screens, often called noninvasive prenatal testing (NIPT), have greatly expanded the number of women and couples who receive prenatal genetic information, since they require only a maternal blood sample (avoiding the need for a highly skilled amniocentesis or CVS procedure) and avoid the discomfort and risk to the fetus imposed by these more invasive procedures. Pregnant individuals and couples who may have categorically refused prenatal diagnosis to avoid any iatrogenic risk can now receive genetic screening with only a blood draw, often at little or no cost due to increasing coverage of NIPT by public and private insurance (American College of Obstetrics and Gynecology, n.d.; Norton et al., 2014; Norton & Rink, 2016).

Diagnostic sequencing in the prenatal setting still relies on invasively obtained samples, and while both exome and genome fetal sequencing are still available mostly in research contexts, they are finding their way into clinical care, especially for pregnancies with challenging ultrasound findings (Vora et al., 2020). After birth, rapid genome sequencing can now provide answers and treatment options "at the bedside" for critically ill neonates, and genomic sequencing is increasingly available for screening newborns for a host of possible conditions (Johnston et al., 2018). Many state newborn screening (NBS) programs have started to add genetic/genomic secondary or adjunct tests as a supplemental test to give more accurate genotypic information on condition severity and age of onset (Schimmenti et al., 2011). Additionally, some programs have started to consider adding conditions that require molecular testing, moving further away from the biochemical marker tests that have been the norm for NBS since the 1960s (Goldenberg et al., 2022). These new conditions and tests rely on genetic markers and sequencing technologies as the primary screening tool. These changes in screening platforms, combined with increased interest in screening for conditions with more genotypic and phenotypic variability, have pushed NBS programs toward even more sequencing. This movement, along with a desire to utilize genomic information to help diagnose and treat a wider set of childhood conditions, has raised interest and questions about whether genome or exome sequencing may be a goal for all babies born in the United States. Francis Collins, the former director of the National Institutes of Health and former head of the National Human Genome Research Institute, predicted in 2014 that

> Over the course of the next few decades, the availability of cheap, efficient DNA sequencing technology will lead to a medical landscape in which each baby's genome is sequenced, and that information is used to shape a lifetime of personalized strategies for disease prevention, detection and treatment. (Collins, 2014, n.p.)

In 2010, the National Institute for Child Health and Development (NICHD) held a symposium to develop a research agenda for the "application of new genomics concepts and technologies to newborn screening and child health" (Eunice Kennedy Shriver NICHD et al., 2010, n.p.). This meeting led to the development of the Newborn Sequencing in Genomic Medicine and Public Health (NSIGHT) program, aimed at assessing the potential impact, benefits, and challenges of integrating genomic sequencing technology into the newborn period (NHGRI, n.d.). These grants were aimed at exploring the possible uses of genomic information in both healthy and sick neonates in NBS, neonatal intensive care units, and other healthcare settings. The funded projects, along with a number of other studies to assess the potential use of genomics as a replacement technology for traditional state NBS testing platforms, have now increased programmatic interest in and likelihood of more genomic screening being utilized in perinatal settings.

As genomic technologies become more integrated into medical and public health settings in both the prenatal and postnatal contexts, genetic counselors will be on the front lines for this new perinatal genomic era. Genetic counselors are already deeply involved with patient care regarding prenatal and other genetic testing modalities. While genetic counselors are typically less involved in the return of results from NBS, they are becoming increasingly involved in NBS diagnostic and treatment decisions and will undoubtedly be called upon as sequencing gains wider use in the newborn settings.

Programmatic and Ethical Challenges of Perinatal Genomic Sequencing

Programmatic changes in research and clinical care have progressively incorporated genomic sequencing. The ability to learn about particular, easily detectable, and well-understood genetic conditions in the fetus transformed prenatal care and the experience of pregnancy and was one of the important developments that helped establish genetic counseling as a profession (Resta, 2019). However, in recent years, advances in both genome sequencing and noninvasive detection of circulating cell-free DNA have meant that increasing amounts of complex genetic information about a fetus are now available during pregnancy (Allyse et al., 2017; Norton & Rink, 2016; Rink & Norton, 2016; Vora et al., 2017). Fetal exome and genome sequencing are already obtainable for amniotic samples, with exome sequencing widely available clinically, though genome sequencing is largely still available only under research protocols (Vora et al., 2020). However, both are likely to see increasing clinical use soon, and noninvasive fetal genome sequencing, proven in concept, is on the clinical horizon (Kitzman et al., 2012; Norton, 2016). These newer developments do not always raise entirely new ethical issues, but they undoubtedly exacerbate long-recognized ethical concerns that have been raised since the early days of amniocentesis and fetal ultrasound (Donley et al., 2012; Michie & Allyse, 2015; Rapp, 1999).

While many common ethical issues permeate genetics and genomics in the period from preconception through early childhood, genomics in the prenatal period is unique in its inextricable linkage to elective termination. As amniocentesis gained popularity due to its enabling of fetal termination for Down syndrome and other genetic conditions, Barbara Katz Rothman (1986) noted with dismay that many women experienced a "tentative pregnancy" in which they did not feel able to bond with their future child until genetic test results had ruled out the need for a termination decision. After fetal screening and more sophisticated diagnostic techniques (including chromosomal microarray [CMA]) became increasingly common, Katz Rothman (1993) revisited the "tentative pregnancy" and lamented that not only had this phenomenon not been resolved but also complex and uncertain information had made this issue thornier than ever. She imagined scenarios in which clinicians will tell patients: "I see an increased probability, on the order of 12%, of cardiovascular disease in your child when he reaches middle age. Make of it what you will" (Rothman, 1993, p. 63). Rayna Rapp (1999), in her landmark ethnography of the amniocentesis experience, concluded that women and couples were forced into the role of "moral pioneers" by the availability of fetal genetic information without a clear roadmap for how to act on it (p. 307). Said one of Rapp's interviewees, "[T]hey all told me I'd feel more in control. But I guess I feel less in control. It's still my baby, but only if it's good enough to be our baby, if you see what I mean" (Rapp, 1999, p. 126). Those "moral pioneers" will continue to forge into unknown futures as the genomic information available prenatally mushrooms in sheer numbers of variants, along with the genotypic and phenotypic uncertainty that necessarily accompanies this information (Rapp, 1987). Similarly, the disability critique of prenatal testing (that it reflects and entrenches negative views of the conditions being tested for, and it exacerbates discrimination toward people already living with these conditions) continues to resonate today, as prenatal genomic testing expands to include not only more information but also larger and more diverse populations who bring widely varying experiences of disability, being "at risk," and encountering medical institutions and providers (Asch & Wasserman, 2005; Kaposy, 2013; Parens & Asch, 1999; Roberts & Jesudason, 2013). In addition, sequencing will likely inform maternal–fetal interventions being designed to prevent developmental features of genomic conditions from progressing as the fetus grows or even to inhibit or alter the expression of certain genes (Boardman, 2020; Guedj & Bianchi, 2013). The interaction between potentially disabling genetic conditions and the social circumstances in which those conditions are understood (or not), treated (or not), and accommodated (or not) will become increasingly complex as families consider the uncertainties associated with conditions of variable penetrance and expression, polygenic risk scores for complex traits, and waiting for the possible onset of symptoms later in life.

After a baby is born, ethical issues typically center on phenotypic and symptom prevention. While public health NBS programs are highly successful in increasing access to information about serious, treatable early childhood conditions, access to follow-up testing and care is more uneven (Brosco et al., 2015; Goldenberg et al., 2016). As genomic sequencing increasingly enters the NBS arena, those issues of access expand, perhaps to the screening itself (if the cost of sequencing is not folded into governmental programs), and certainly to diagnostic testing and therapeutics. Newborn and early childhood genomic sequencing that is targeted to infants with undiagnosed conditions, rather than used as a population screening tool, may present fewer issues of justice in unequal access, as public and private coverage for sequencing in these contexts increases (Douglas et al., 2019; Lavelle et al., 2022; Phillips, 2018; Trosman et al., 2020). However, all pediatric genomic sequencing brings ethical concerns about the breadth and complexity of information and the challenges of interpreting and delivering this information (Clayton, 2010; Goldenberg & Sharp, 2012; Farrell & Allyse, 2018; Tarini & Goldenberg, 2012). Genetic conditions often have different phenotypic features in neonates and young children than in older children and adults, and this factor, combined with the inability of young children to communicate their symptoms, creates challenges for interpreting genomic information. In addition, as is true of sequencing at any stage in the life course, genomic information presents challenges related to the sheer complexity of information, the number of variants of uncertain significance (VUSs), and the difficulty in predicting penetrance and future expression of variants. These factors not only may be difficult to communicate to parents but also may cause anxiety for new parents, possibly inhibiting bonding with a new baby or creating lifelong alterations in the ways parents set expectations for and interact with their child. If genomic information related to later-onset conditions is shared with parents, then families must reckon with the uncertainty of this information throughout childhood, and children are unable to make autonomous decisions about whether they would have chosen to receive this information (Knoppers, 2014; Tarini & Goldenberg, 2012; Timmermans & Buchbinder, 2010). Finally, all genomic information may have implications for other family members, including undiagnosed conditions, misidentified paternity and other family relationships, and possible risks for later-onset conditions in other family members.

What Do Stakeholders Think About Genomics in Perinatal Settings?

Clinicians, patients, and families are all stakeholders in the clinical implementation of exome and genome sequencing, and their perspectives, along with those of the general public, can illuminate ethical and practical issues along the life course. In the prenatal context, 85% of genetics professionals in a recent survey said that exome sequencing could provide parents with useful information about fetal health (Brew et al., 2019). However, the vast majority anticipated potential harm to parents from uncertain sequencing results and misunderstood results (97% and 99%, respectively), and over three-quarters expected that some parents would terminate pregnancies based on uncertain results (Brew et al., 2019). Public and parental concerns about prenatal sequencing, like those about all fetal screening and testing, are closely tied to views about abortion (Kalynchuk et al., 2015; Steinbach, 2016). They are likely also influenced by a belief—tied to the long-standing "collective fiction" of prenatal screening, along with the cultural responsibilities placed on parents—that taking advantage of all available tests will improve the health of the future child (Michie & Allyse, 2022; Press & Browner, 1993, 1997). For instance, over two-thirds of a sample of pregnant couples surveyed in 2015 agreed they "would do any available genetic test," and a large majority said that prenatal exome sequencing should be offered (Kalynchuk et al., 2015, p. 1032). However, only one-third said they would want prenatal exome sequencing in the absence of a medical problem, and only 17% said they would be willing to have amniocentesis in order to have fetal exome sequencing. Nevertheless, a majority in that study wanted to know about all conditions in the fetus, even nontreatable, adult-onset conditions, despite over 70% acknowledging that this knowledge, along with any VUSs, would cause them anxiety (Kalynchuk et al., 2015).

That anxiety is not insignificant. Although prenatal genome sequencing is still rare in clinical practice, data from the clinical use of CMA illuminate many of the issues raised by uncertain results. The landmark study by Bernhardt et al. (2013) coined the phrase "toxic knowledge," uninterpretable or uncertain information that many women in their study wished they had never received. Even after giving birth and finding no apparent health conditions, many parents in that study reported lingering anxiety about the possibility of developmental issues; and when a parent shared the variant of concern, that anxiety expanded to encompass questions and self-doubt regarding the carrier's own health or cognitive ability. A 2018 study found that parents who had received a VUS result from a prenatal CMA rated their children as less competent on a validated scale and reported lower satisfaction with their prior decision to accept testing compared to parents who received benign results (Desai et al., 2018).

Literature on parental experiences of prenatal exome sequencing so far has emerged from studies in which patients were receiving exome sequencing after anomalous fetal ultrasound results; in these situations, sequencing may be less likely to generate the effect of feeling "blindsided" reported in Bernhardt et al. (2013), although such results may still be worrying. An interview study by Wou et al. (2018) found that although facing a possible genetic diagnosis caused stress and worry, parents were eager to get answers from exome sequencing; nevertheless, when asked about their desire to receive less-than-certain results, enthusiasm for this information decreased as certainty decreased. In a survey of mothers receiving trio exome sequencing for a fetal structural anomaly, those who received genomic results that could explain the fetal anomaly experienced higher distress and more uncertainty regarding future reproduction compared to women receiving negative results and even compared to those receiving secondary findings about themselves or their partners (Talati et al., 2021). The authors of both of these studies strongly recommended careful attention to pretest counseling for prenatal exome sequencing, with particular emphasis on diagnostic and prognostic uncertainty. However, research on parents receiving exome or genome sequencing without a prior fetal indication is ongoing and the results will be instructive for genetic counseling. A recent study of demographically diverse parents receiving prenatal or postnatal exome sequencing found that a strong majority (76% prenatal, 80% postnatal) agreed to receive secondary findings (Rego et al., 2022). However, when surveyed about hypothetical types of secondary findings, parents were less enthusiastic about uncertain findings. Concerningly, the researchers reported that parents often did not recall being counseled about secondary findings and were often confused about what kinds of information this entailed—suggesting that even after receiving significant education and counseling, parents may have difficulty understanding the breadth of information they may receive from sequencing (Rego et al., 2022).

In the context of NBS, one nationally representative survey of 1,539 parents asked about their interest in receiving genome sequencing for their newborn. Seventy-four percent of parents in that study reported being either definitely or somewhat interested in receiving genomic information through their state's NBS program, while 70% of parents expressed interest in receiving this type of information if offered through their pediatrician (Goldenberg et al., 2014). A similar study conducted at Brigham and Women's Hospital found that, of the 514 parents surveyed within 48 hours after birth, over 80% reported being somewhat, very, or extremely interested in genome sequencing through NBS (Waisbren et al., 2015). While these data indicate a high level of interest, other studies have shown a more complex picture. One cross-sectional representative study of Canadian parents found that parents may be less likely to participate in NBS using genome or exome sequencing as opposed to traditional screening technologies (Bombard et al., 2014). Further, a randomized trial of genome sequencing in well-baby and intensive care settings found extremely low actual uptake among parents (Genetti et al., 2019). However, lower participation in that study appeared to be related more to discomfort with research participation than to a lack of interest in the sequencing itself.

Beyond parental views, a number of studies have also explored professional stakeholder perspectives on genome sequencing in the newborn period. A survey of members of the American College of Medical Genetics and Genomics found that, while 85% of respondents felt that genome sequencing should not currently be used extensively in NBS, 76% did "foresee" that genome sequencing would be used in NBS programs in the future (Ulm et al., 2015). A survey of members of the National Society of Genetic Counselors (NSGC) found that 82% of respondents "did not feel prepared to counsel for WGS [whole genome sequencing] results from NBS" and concluded there was a need for more training of counselors on interpreting and returning newborn genomic results before genome sequencing is integrated into NBS programs (Nardini et al., 2014, p. 506ff).

In addition to these empirical studies, a number of multidisciplinary workgroup statements and articles have addressed the use of genomic technology in the newborn period. In one such published statement, the NSIGHT Ethics and Policy Advisory Board called for a more nuanced approach to integrating genomic technology into the newborn period, concluding:

> While we recognize considerable benefit in using targeted sequencing to screen for or detect specific conditions that meet the criteria for inclusion in newborn screening panels, use of genome-wide sequencing as a sole screening tool for newborns is at best premature. (Johnston et al., 2018, pp. S4–S5)

Nevertheless, while this workgroup and others like it have called for a cautioned approach to utilizing genomic screening in newborns, momentum is growing in the push to expand the uses of genomic screening platforms in perinatal settings. It is therefore crucial to examine the potential impact that the expanded use of these technologies may have on genetic counselors and other healthcare providers who may be called on to work with families receiving results from perinatal genomic sequencing.

Why Does This Matter for Genetic Counselors?

As interest in the possible adoption of widespread population-based genomic sequencing in prenatal or newborn settings grows, it will be crucial for genetics professionals, including genetic counselors, to assess and address the challenges of families receiving a deluge of genomic information about their pregnancies and newborns. For most families, expectations regarding the utility of such information will inevitably be shaped by the healthcare providers who will ultimately work with families to interpret and translate genomic results into healthcare decisions. However, doing so effectively will undoubtedly be limited by a number of key factors that individual providers and the field of genetic counseling will need to address through adaptations to counseling policies and practices. We have outlined a series of questions meant to highlight a number of these key factors. While this list is not meant to be exhaustive, we intend it to suggest areas for needed interprofessional dialogue, guidance, and training.

How might genetic counselors better prepare for the scope and complexity of genomic newborn sequencing?

The increased use of genomic sequencing in newborns would represent a dramatic shift in the amount and kinds of information parents will receive about their newborn's health. While genomic sequencing has been used more frequently in children with undiagnosed conditions, geneticists and genetic counselors have less experience interpreting and communicating results from sequencing of healthy newborns (Sharp, 2011). Counselors may need to balance disclosing actionable health information to families while also making decisions about how to present VUS results and possibly information regarding adult-onset conditions. Counselors will need more training and better resources to help work with families to ensure they can access and understand valuable health information derived from sequencing. At the same time, counselors will need support if they find themselves in the difficult situation of having to weigh parental rights to their children's genomic information with the suppression of results deemed inappropriate to disclose (Goldenberg & Sharp, 2012).

How can genetic counselors better address uncertain or unclear results from genomic newborn sequencing?

Genetic counselors will also need to consider approaches to returning uncertain newborn genomic screening findings to parents and how to address the potential harms that may be caused by these kinds of results (Chakraborty et al., 2021; Friedman et al., 2017; Tarini et al., 2012). For example, some have raised concerns that integration of genomic technology into NBS might create large numbers of "patients-in-waiting"—otherwise healthy children now labeled as diseased because of DNA sequences that are not normal but are not associated with disease. These children and their families are left waiting to find out whether disease symptoms will develop (Kwon & Steiner, 2011; Timmermans et al., 2010). States that have begun including conditions that require genomic follow-up testing, such as Krabbe disease, are already seeing higher frequency of both diagnostic and prognostic uncertainty, which may lead to increased parental stress or anxiety. Similarly, a number of concerns have been raised in the prenatal setting about the negative impact that potential "toxic knowledge," or simply stressful knowledge, may have on parents receiving uncertain or unclear prenatal testing results (Bernhardt et al., 2013; Talati et al., 2021).

What kinds of information will parents and families need to know when receiving newborn genomic sequencing results?

As genetic counselors are more frequently called upon to deliver complex and possibly uncertain newborn genomic testing or screening results to parents, they will need to develop innovative and culturally appropriate education and communication approaches. Proposed models of informed consent and communication have recently included the use of video-based education models, app-based interactive consent frameworks, and chatbots to inform and educate parents (Haas et al., 2021; Ireland et al., 2021; Riggs et al., 2019). These issues are further challenged by shifting notions of access and control over genomic data as newborns grow up and patients have increased capacity to voice their own perspectives on how their own genomic data is used within the context of their own healthcare. For example, counselors and other healthcare providers will need to determine at what age children should be permitted to participate in a shared decision-making or assent process regarding ongoing interpretation of their genomic data. Further, at what age and through what mechanism should children obtain full control over their own genomic data? These issues are further complicated by certain kinds of results that could be obtained through newborn genomic sequencing, such as predisposition to an adult-onset condition or carrier status that may impact their own reproductive decision making. Genetics professional organizations have generally discouraged testing minors for adult-onset conditions, on the basis of protecting the rights of children to decide for themselves whether they would want that information (Bredenoord et al., 2013; Davis, 1997, 2002; Garrett et al., 2019; Wilfond et al., 2015). However, this protection of a child's right to an "open future" is evolving as genomic testing and screening have become more integrated into wider healthcare settings. Increasingly, when the disclosure of adult-onset information may help a family make future prevention decisions or plan for future possible health needs, a child's best interest standard may outweigh the potential harms of disclosing results and possibility violating a child's "right not to know" (Goldenberg et al., 2014; Waisbren et al., 2015). For example, current policy guidance from the NSGC discourages predictive genetic testing of minors for adult-onset conditions when the results may "not impact childhood medical management or significantly benefit the child"; however, it also recognizes that any genetic testing decisions (including sequencing) that identify variants for adult-onset conditions should be made "cautiously," with "appropriate assent of the minor" when possible, and encourages genetic counselors to "discuss strategies" with parents for sharing results when the minor reaches "the age of majority" (NSGC, 2018, n.p.). With this policy guidance in mind, the genetic counseling community will need to develop further resources to support counselors when returning newborn sequencing results that may include a variety of findings with adult-onset information.

Genomics and the Need for Expanded Scope of Practice and Training

In addition to challenges for counseling practice, the wider use of genomic sequencing in newborns has the potential to fundamentally change genetic counseling practices and genetic counselors' roles within clinical public health settings. Today, as genetic medicine is integrated into a wider range of clinical spaces, the need for health professionals trained in the delivery and interpretation of genetic tests is increasing. Although this may ultimately lead to a wider scope of practice, in many settings genetic counseling centers on a narrower testing encounter or timeframe, such as prenatal screening or genetic testing associated with a cancer diagnosis. As a more comprehensive shift toward genome and exome sequencing in the newborn period materializes, the provision of longer term and ongoing genetic counseling may be necessary for individuals and families to effectively utilize their own genomic information for what Francis Collins (2014) calls a "lifetime of personalized strategies for disease prevention, detection and treatment" (n.p.). In other words, genetic counseling may need to shift toward a *lifecourse* approach to consulting and patient care in which patients and their families form more long-term relationships with counselors who help to guide ongoing analysis and interpretation of genomic data over time. An increased uptake of newborn genomic sequencing and the possible implementation of more long-term counseling approaches will necessitate changes to genetic counseling training programs and continuing professional education. Programs will need to better prepare counselors to deal with the complexity and uncertainty of genomic results in the newborn setting and how to counsel families in ways that maximize the potential utility of these data while minimizing possible psychosocial harms.

Additionally, a lifecourse approach may also require shifts and enhancement of the relationships between patients, genetic counselors, and other healthcare providers to better inform and shape prevention and health promotion activities as well as the long-term management of disease predisposition. In a post–newborn genomic era, genetic counselors may be inevitably called upon to direct and coordinate the integration of genetic information into the larger landscape of patient care. A team-based approach to long-term genetic care where a genetic counselor would act as a *genetic medical home*, coordinating and directing the integration of genetic information into various parts of a patient's healthcare, could support this changing role. Nevertheless, implementing team-based care while an increasing number of patients are receiving genome data about themselves or their newborns may be challenging given the amount and complexity of results one can expect to receive at birth. A number of studies have shown that many healthcare providers feel unqualified to provide genetic counseling or provide genetic management to their patients once they receive genetic test results, again pointing to the need for genetic counselors to play an essential role (Bayefsky et al., 2016; Boland et al., 2015; Christensen et al., 2016; Nardini et al., 2014). Subsequently, a team-based approach to interpretation and use of genomic results could increase the confidence of primary care physicians around incorporating genetic services and genetic information into patient care. Additionally, this approach requires addressing issues such as a lack of access to genetic counseling services for many underserved patients, the need to update genetic counseling curricula to support this new role, and the potential shortage of genetic counselors generally.

Conclusion

Whether it is coordinating care with other genetic professionals or working with other team members in primary care settings, these types of collaborative efforts may help to ensure that patients and their families receive a more coordinated approach to utilizing genomic results in their healthcare, may provide a more stable and trusting base from which genetic information can be discussed, and thus lead to more effective delivery of care. As genomics is increasingly integrated into the perinatal continuum of care, genetic counselors will play a crucial role in both direct patient care and larger policy and practice dialogue regarding the utility and benefits of genomics for children and families.

References

Allyse, M., Aypar, U., Bonhomme, N., Darilek, S., Dougherty, M., Farrell, R., Grody, W., Highsmith, W. E., Michie, M., Nunes, M., Otto, L., Pabst, R., Palomaki, G., Runke, C., Sharp, R. R., Skotko, B., Stoll, K., & Wick, M. (2017). Offering prenatal screening in the age of genomic medicine: A practical guide. *Journal of Women's Health (2002)*, *26*(7), 755–761. https://doi.org/10.1089/jwh.2016.6098

American College of Obstetrics and Gynecology. (n.d.) *Policy priorities: Non-invasive prenatal testing*. https://www.acog.org/advocacy/policy-priorities/non-invasive-prenatal-testing

Asch, A., & Wasserman, D. (2005). Where is the sin in synecdoche? Prenatal testing and the parent-child relationship. In D. Wasserman, J. Bickenbach, & R. Wachbroit (Eds.), *Quality of life and human difference: Genetic testing, health care, and disability* (pp. 172–216). Cambridge University Press. https://doi.org/10.1017/CBO9780511614590.008

Bayefsky, M. J., White, A., Wakim, P., Hull, S. C., Wasserman, D., Chen, S., & Berkman, B. E. (2016). Views of American OB/GYNs on the ethics of prenatal whole-genome sequencing. *Prenatal Diagnosis*, *36*(13), 1250–1256. https://doi.org/10.1002/pd.4968

Berg, J. S., Agrawal, P. B., Bailey, D. B., Jr., Beggs, A. H., Brenner, S. E., Brower, A. M., Cakici, J. A., Ceyhan-Birsoy, O., Chan, K., Chen, F., Currier, R. J., Dukhovny, D., Green, R. C., Harris-Wai, J., Holm, I. A., Iglesias, B., Joseph, G., Kingsmore, S. F., Koenig, B. A., . . . Wise, A. L. (2017). Newborn sequencing in genomic medicine and public health. *Pediatrics*, *139*(2), e20162252. https://doi.org/10.1542/peds.2016-2252

Bernhardt, B. A., Soucier, D., Hanson, K., Savage, M. S., Jackson, L., & Wapner, R. J. (2013). Women's experiences receiving abnormal prenatal chromosomal microarray testing results. *Genetics in Medicine*, *15*(2), 139–145. https://doi.org/10.1038/gim.2012.113

Boardman, F. (2020). Human genome editing and the identity politics of genetic disability. *Journal of Community Genetics*, *11*(2), 125–127. https://doi.org/10.1007/s12687-019-00437-4

Boland, P. M., Ruth, K., Matro, J. M., Rainey, K. L., Fang, C. Y., Wong, Y. N., Daly, M. B., & Hall, M. J. (2015). Genetic counselors' (GC) knowledge, awareness, understanding of clinical next-generation sequencing (NGS) genomic testing. *Clinical Genetics*, *88*(6), 565–572. https://doi.org/10.1111/cge.12555

Bombard, Y., Miller, F. A., Hayeems, R. Z., Barg, C., Cressman, C., Carroll, J. C., Wilson, B. J., Little, J., Avard, D., Painter-Main, M., Allanson, J., Giguere, Y., & Chakraborty, P. (2014). Public views on participating in newborn screening using genome sequencing. *European Journal of Human Genetics*, *22*(11), 1248–1254. https://doi.org/10.1038/ejhg.2014.22

Bredenoord, A. L., de Vries, M. C., & van Delden, J. J. (2013). Next-generation sequencing: Does the next generation still have a right to an open future? *Nature Reviews Genetics*, *14*(5), 306. https://doi.org/10.1038/nrg3459

Brew, C. E., Castro, B. A., Pan, V., Hart, A., Blumberg, B., & Wicklund, C. (2019). Genetics professionals' attitudes toward prenatal exome sequencing. *Journal of Genetic Counseling*, *28*(2), 229–239. https://doi.org/10.1002/jgc4.1112

Brosco, J. P., Grosse, S. D., & Ross, L. F. (2015). Universal state newborn screening programs can reduce health disparities. *JAMA Pediatrics*, *169*(1), 7–8. https://doi.org/10.1001/jamapediatrics.2014.2465

Chakraborty, P., Potter, B. K., & Hayeems, R. Z. (2021). Maximizing benefits and minimizing harms: Diagnostic uncertainty arising from newborn screening. *Pediatrics*, *148*(6), e2021052822. https://doi.org/10.1542/peds.2021-052822

Chiu, R. W., Chan, K. C., Gao, Y., Lau, V. Y., Zheng, W., Leung, T. Y., Foo, C. H., Xie, B., Tsui, N. B., Lun, F. M., Zee, B. C., Lau, T. K., Cantor, C. R., & Lo, Y. M. (2008). Noninvasive prenatal diagnosis of fetal chromosomal aneuploidy by massively parallel genomic sequencing of DNA in maternal plasma. *Proceedings of the National Academy of Sciences of the United States of America*, *105*(51), 20458–20463. https://doi.org/10.1073/pnas.0810641105

Christensen, K. D., Vassy, J. L., Jamal, L., Lehmann, L. S., Slashinski, M. J., Perry, D. L., Robinson, J. O., Blumenthal-Barby, J., Feuerman, L. Z., Murray, M. F., Green, R. C., McGuire, A. L., & MedSeq Project Team. (2016). Are physicians prepared for whole genome sequencing? A qualitative analysis. *Clinical Genetics*, *89*(2), 228–234. https://doi.org/10.1111/cge.12626

Clayton, E. W. (2010). Currents in contemporary ethics. State run newborn screening in the genomic era, or how to avoid drowning when drinking from a fire hose. *Journal of Law, Medicine & Ethics, 38*(3), 697–700. https://doi.org/10.1111/j.1748-720X.2010.00522.x

Collins, F. (2014, July 7). Francis Collins says medicine in the future will be tailored to your genes. *Wall Street Journal.* https://www.wsj.com/articles/francis-collins-says-medicine-in-the-future-will-be-tailored-to-your-genes-1404763139

Davis, D. S. (1997). Genetic dilemmas and the child's right to an open future. *Hastings Center Report, 27*(2), 7–15.

Davis, D. S. (2002). Child's right to an open future. *Hastings Center Report, 32*(5), 6.

Desai, P., Haber, H., Bulafka, J., Russell, A., Clifton, R., Zachary, J., Lee, S., Feng, T., Wapner, R., Monk, C., & Chung, W. K. (2018). Impacts of variants of uncertain significance on parental perceptions of children after prenatal chromosome microarray testing. *Prenatal Diagnosis, 38*(10), 740–747. https://doi.org/10.1002/pd.5323

Donley, G., Hull, S. C., & Berkman, B. E. (2012). Prenatal whole genome sequencing: Just because we can, should we? *Hastings Center Report, 42*(4), 28–40. https://doi.org/10.1002/hast.50

Douglas, M. P., Parker, S. L., Trosman, J. R., Slavotinek, A. M., & Phillips, K. A. (2019). Private payer coverage policies for exome sequencing (ES) in pediatric patients: Trends over time and analysis of evidence cited. *Genetics in Medicine, 21*(1), 152–160. https://doi.org/10.1038/s41436-018-0043-3

Eunice Kennedy Shriver National Institute of Child Health and Human Development (NICHD), National Human Genome Research Institute (NHGRI), & NIH Office of Rare Disease Research (ORDR). (2010, December 13–14). *Newborn screening in the genomic era: Setting a research agenda.* https://www.genome.gov/Pages/PolicyEthics/StaffArticles/Newborn_Screening_Meeting_Summary.pdf

Fan, H. C., Blumenfeld, Y. J., Chitkara, U., Hudgins, L., & Quake, S. R. (2008). Noninvasive diagnosis of fetal aneuploidy by shotgun sequencing DNA from maternal blood. *Proceedings of the National Academy of Sciences of the United States of America, 105*(42), 16266–16271. https://doi.org/10.1073/pnas.0808319105

Farrell, R. M., & Allyse, M. A. (2018). Key ethical issues in prenatal genetics: An overview. *Obstetrics and Gynecology Clinics of North America, 45*(1), 127–141. https://doi.org/10.1016/j.ogc.2017.10.006

Friedman, J. M., Cornel, M. C., Goldenberg, A. J., Lister, K. J., Sénécal, K., Vears, D. F., & Global Alliance for Genomics and Health Regulatory and Ethics Working Group Paediatric Task Team. (2017). Genomic newborn screening: Public health policy considerations and recommendations. *BMC Medical Genomics, 10*(1), 9. https://doi.org/10.1186/s12920-017-0247-4

Garrett, J. R., Lantos, J. D., Biesecker, L. G., Childerhose, J. E., Chung, W. K., Holm, I. A., Koenig, B. A., McEwen, J. E., Wilfond, B. S., Brothers, K., & Clinical Sequencing Exploratory Research (CSER) Consortium Pediatrics Working Group. (2019). Rethinking the "open future" argument against predictive genetic testing of children. *Genetics in Medicine, 21*(10), 2190–2198. https://doi.org/10.1038/s41436-019-0483-4

Genetti, C. A., Schwartz, T. S., Robinson, J. O., VanNoy, G. E., Petersen, D., Pereira, S., Fayer, S., Peoples, H. A., Agrawal, P. B., Betting, W. N., Holm, I. A., McGuire, A. L., Waisbren, S. E., Yu, T. W., Green, R. C., Beggs, A. H., Parad, R. B., & BabySeq Project Team. (2019). Parental interest in genomic sequencing of newborns: Enrollment experience from the BabySeq Project. *Genetics in Medicine, 21*(3), 622–630. https://doi.org/10.1038/s41436-018-0105-6

Goldenberg, A. J., Comeau, A. M., Grosse, S. D., Tanksley, S., Prosser, L. A., Ojodu, J., Botkin, J. R., Kemper, A. R., & Green, N. S. (2016). Evaluating harms in the assessment of net benefit: A framework for newborn screening condition review. *Maternal and Child Health Journal, 20*(3), 693–700. https://doi.org/10.1007/s10995-015-1869-9

Goldenberg, A. J., Dodson, D. S., Davis, M. M., & Tarini, B. A. (2014). Parents' interest in whole-genome sequencing of newborns. *Genetics in Medicine, 16*(1), 78–84. https://doi.org/10.1038/gim.2013.76

Goldenberg, A. J., Ponsaran, R., Gaviglio, A., Simancek, D., & Tarini, B. A. (2022). Genomics and newborn screening: Perspectives of public health programs. *International Journal of Neonatal Screening, 8*(1), 11. https://doi.org/10.3390/ijns8010011

Goldenberg, A. J., & Sharp, R. R. (2012). The ethical hazards and programmatic challenges of genomic newborn screening. *JAMA, 307*(5), 461–462. https://doi.org/10.1001/jama.2012.68

Guedj, F., & Bianchi, D. W. (2013). Noninvasive prenatal testing creates an opportunity for antenatal treatment of Down syndrome. *Prenatal Diagnosis, 33*(6), 614–618. https://doi.org/10.1002/pd.4134

Haas, M. A., Teare, H., Prictor, M., Ceregra, G., Vidgen, M. E., Bunker, D., Kaye, J., & Boughtwood, T. (2021). "CTRL": An online, dynamic consent and participant engagement platform working towards solving the complexities of consent in genomic research. *European Journal of Human Genetics, 29*(4), 687–698. https://doi.org/10.1038/s41431-020-00782-w

Holm, I. A., Agrawal, P. B., Ceyhan-Birsoy, O., Christensen, K. D., Fayer, S., Frankel, L. A., Genetti, C. A., Krier, J. B., LaMay, R. C., Levy, H. L., McGuire, A. L., Parad, R. B., Park, P. J., Pereira, S., Rehm, H. L., Schwartz, T. S., Waisbren, S. E., Yu, T. W., BabySeq Project Team, . . . Beggs, A. H. (2018). The BabySeq project: Implementing genomic sequencing in newborns. *BMC Pediatrics, 18*(1), 225. https://doi.org/10.1186/s12887-018-1200-1

Ireland, D., Bradford, D., Szepe, E., Lynch, E., Martyn, M., Hansen, D., & Gaff, C. (2021). Introducing Edna: A trainee chatbot designed to support communication about additional (secondary) genomic findings. *Patient Education and Counseling, 104*(4), 739–749. https://doi.org/10.1016/j.pec.2020.11.007

Johnston, J., Lantos, J. D., Goldenberg, A., Chen, F., Parens, E., Koenig, B. A., & Members of the NSIGHT Ethics and Policy Advisory Board. (2018). Sequencing newborns: A call for nuanced use of genomic technologies. *Hastings Center Report, 48*(Suppl. 2), S2–S6. https://doi.org/10.1002/hast.874

Kalynchuk, E. J., Althouse, A., Parker, L. S., Saller, D. N., Jr., & Rajkovic, A. (2015). Prenatal whole-exome sequencing: Parental attitudes. *Prenatal Diagnosis, 35*(10), 1030–1036. https://doi.org/10.1002/pd.4635

Kaposy, C. (2013). A disability critique of the new prenatal test for Down syndrome. *Kennedy Institute of Ethics Journal, 23*(4), 299–324. https://doi.org/10.1353/ken.2013.0017

Kitzman, J. O., Snyder, M. W., Ventura, M., Lewis, A. P., Qiu, R., Simmons, L. E., Gammill, H. S., Rubens, C. E., Santillan, D. A., Murray, J. C., Tabor, H. K., Bamshad, M. J., Eichler, E. E., & Shendure, J. (2012). Noninvasive whole-genome sequencing of a human fetus. *Science Translational Medicine, 4*(137), 137ra76. https://doi.org/10.1126/scitranslmed.3004323

Knoppers, B. M., Sénécal, K., Borry, P., & Avard, D. (2014). Whole-genome sequencing in newborn screening programs. *Science Translational Medicine, 6*(229), 229cm2. https://doi.org/10.1126/scitranslmed.3008494

Kwon, J. M., & Steiner, R. D. (2011). "I'm fine; I'm just waiting for my disease": The new and growing class of presymptomatic patients. *Neurology, 77*(6), 522–523. https://doi.org/10.1212/WNL.0b013e318228c15f

Lavelle, T. A., Feng, X., Keisler, M., Cohen, J. T., Neumann, P. J., Prichard, D., Schroeder, B. E., Salyakina, D., Espinal, P. S., Weidner, S. B., & Maron, J. L. (2022). Cost-effectiveness of exome and genome sequencing for children with rare and undiagnosed conditions. *Genetics in Medicine*, *24*(6), 1349–1361. https://doi.org/10.1016/j.gim.2022.03.005

Michie, M., & Allyse, M. (2015). Old questions, new paradigms: Ethical, legal, and social complications of noninvasive prenatal testing. *AJOB Empirical Bioethics*, *6*(1), 1–4. https://doi.org/10.1080/23294515.2014.993440

Michie, M. M., & Allyse, M. A. (2022). Pathways to affluence: Socioeconomic incentives in prenatal testing and abortion. In M. A. Allyse & M. M. Michie (Eds.), *Born well: Prenatal genetics and the future of having children* (pp. 105–122). International Library of Bioethics. https://doi.org/10.1007/978-3-030-82536-2_8

Minear, M. A., Alessi, S., Allyse, M., Michie, M., & Chandrasekharan, S. (2015). Noninvasive prenatal genetic testing: Current and emerging ethical, legal, and social issues. *Annual Review of Genomics and Human Genetics*, *16*, 369–398. https://doi.org/10.1146/annurev-genom-090314-050000

Nardini, M. D., Matthews, A. L., McCandless, S. E., Baumanis, L., & Goldenberg, A. J. (2014). Genomic counseling in the newborn period: Experiences and views of genetic counselors. *Journal of Genetic Counseling*, *23*(4), 506–515. https://doi.org/10.1007/s10897-014-9706-7

National Human Genome Research Institute. (n.d.). *Newborn Sequencing in Genomic Medicine and Public Health (NSIGHT)*. https://www.genome.gov/Funded-Programs-Projects/Newborn-Sequencing-in-Genomic-Medicine-and-Public-Health-NSIGHT

National Society of Genetic Counselors. (2018, April 12). *Genetic testing of minors for adult-onset conditions*. https://www.nsgc.org/Polic y-Research-and-Publications/Position-Statements/Position-Statements/Post/genetic-testing-of-minors-for-adult-onset-conditions

Norton, M. E. (2016). Noninvasive prenatal testing to analyze the fetal genome. *Proceedings of the National Academy of Sciences of the United States of America*, *113*(50), 14173–14175. https://doi.org/10.1073/pnas.1617112113

Norton, M. E., Nakagawa, S., & Kuppermann, M. (2014). Women's attitudes regarding prenatal testing for a range of congenital disorders of varying severity. *Journal of Clinical Medicine*, *3*(1), 144–152. https://doi.org/10.3390/jcm3010144

Norton, M. E., & Rink, B. D. (2016). Changing indications for invasive testing in an era of improved screening. *Seminars in Perinatology*, *40*(1), 56–66. https://doi.org/10.1053/j.semperi.2015.11.008

Parens, E., & Asch, A. (1999). The disability rights critique of prenatal genetic testing. Reflections and recommendations. *Hastings Center Report*, *29*(5), S1–S22.

Parham, L., Michie, M., & Allyse, M. (2017). Expanding use of cfDNA screening in pregnancy: Current and emerging ethical, legal, and social issues. *Current Genetic Medicine Reports*, *5*(1), 44–53. https://doi.org/10.1007/s40142-017-0113-x

Phillips, K. A. (2018). Evolving payer coverage policies on genomic sequencing tests: Beginning of the end or end of the beginning? *JAMA*, *319*(23), 2379–2380. https://doi.org/10.1001/jama.2018.4863

Press, N. A., & Browner, C. H. (1993). "Collective fictions": Similarities in reasons for accepting maternal serum alpha-fetoprotein screening among women of diverse ethnic and social class backgrounds. *Fetal Diagnosis and Therapy*, *8*(Suppl. 1), 97–106. https://doi.org/10.1159/000263878

Press, N., & Browner, C. H. (1997). Why women say yes to prenatal diagnosis. *Social Science & Medicine (1982)*, *45*(7), 979–989. https://doi.org/10.1016/s0277-9536(97)00011-7

Rapp, R. (1987). Moral pioneers: Women, men and fetuses on a frontier of reproductive technology. *Women & Health, 13*(1–2), 101–116.

Rapp, R. (1999). *Testing women, testing the fetus: The social impact of amniocentesis in America*. Routledge.

Rego, S., Hoban, H., Outram, S., Zamora, A. N., Chen, F., Sahin-Hodoglugil, N., Anguiano, B., Norstad, M., Yip, T., Lianoglou, B., Sparks, T. N., Norton, M. E., Koenig, B. A., Slavotinek, A. M., & Ackerman, S. L. (2022). Perspectives and preferences regarding genomic secondary findings in underrepresented prenatal and pediatric populations: A mixed-methods approach. *Genetics in Medicine, 24*(6), 1206–1216. https://doi.org/10.1016/j.gim.2022.02.004

Resta, R. G. (2019). What have we been trying to do and have we been any good at it? A history of measuring the success of genetic counseling. *European Journal of Medical Genetics, 62*(5), 300–307. https://doi.org/10.1016/j.ejmg.2018.11.003

Riggs, E. R., Azzariti, D. R., Niehaus, A., Goehringer, S. R., Ramos, E. M., Rodriguez, L. L., Knoppers, B., Rehm, H. L., Martin, C. L., & Clinical Genome Resource Education Working Group. (2019). Development of a consent resource for genomic data sharing in the clinical setting. *Genetics in Medicine, 21*(1), 81–88. https://doi.org/10.1038/s41436-018-0017-5

Rink, B. D., & Norton, M. E. (2016). Screening for fetal aneuploidy. *Seminars in Perinatology, 40*(1), 35–43. https://doi.org/10.1053/j.semperi.2015.11.006

Roberts, D., & Jesudason, S. (2013). Movement intersectionality: The case of race, gender, disability, and genetic technologies. *Du Bois Review: Social Science Research on Race, 10*(2), 313–328. https://doi.org/10.1017/S1742058X13000210

Rothman, B. K. (1986). *The tentative pregnancy: Prenatal diagnosis and the future of motherhood*. Viking.

Rothman, B. K. (1993). The tentative pregnancy: Then and now. *Fetal Diagnosis and Therapy, 8*(Suppl. 1), 60–63. https://doi.org/10.1159/000263873

Schimmenti, L. A., Warman, B., Schleiss, M. R., Daly, K. A., Ross, J. A., McCann, M., Jurek, A. M., & Berry, S. A. (2011). Evaluation of newborn screening bloodspot-based genetic testing as second tier screen for bedside newborn hearing screening. *Genetics in Medicine, 13*(12), 1006–1010. https://doi.org/10.1097/GIM.0b013e318226fc2e

Sharp, R. R. (2011). Downsizing genomic medicine: Approaching the ethical complexity of whole-genome sequencing by starting small. *Genetics in Medicine, 13*(3), 191–194. https://doi.org/10.1097/GIM.0b013e31820f603f

Steinbach, R. J., Allyse, M., Michie, M., Liu, E. Y., & Cho, M. K. (2016). "This lifetime commitment": Public conceptions of disability and noninvasive prenatal genetic screening. *American Journal of Medical Genetics Part A, 170A*(2), 363–374. https://doi.org/10.1002/ajmg.a.37459

Talati, A. N., Gilmore, K. L., Hardisty, E. E., Lyerly, A. D., Rini, C., & Vora, N. L. (2021). Impact of prenatal exome sequencing for fetal genetic diagnosis on maternal psychological outcomes and decisional conflict in a prospective cohort. *Genetics in Medicine, 23*(4), 713–719. https://doi.org/10.1038/s41436-020-01025-5

Tarini, B. A., & Goldenberg, A. J. (2012). Ethical issues with newborn screening in the genomics era. *Annual Review of Genomics and Human Genetics, 13*, 381–393. https://doi.org/10.1146/annurev-genom-090711-163741

Timmermans, S., & Buchbinder, M. (2010). Patients-in-waiting: Living between sickness and health in the genomics era. *Journal of Health and Social Behavior, 51*(4), 408–423. https://doi.org/10.1177/0022146510386794

Trosman, J. R., Weldon, C. B., Slavotinek, A., Norton, M. E., Douglas, M. P., & Phillips, K. A. (2020). Perspectives of US private payers on insurance coverage for pediatric and prenatal exome sequencing: Results of a study from the Program in Prenatal and Pediatric Genomic Sequencing (P3EGS). *Genetics in Medicine*, *22*(2), 283–291. https://doi.org/10.1038/s41436-019-0650-7

Ulm, E., Feero, W. G., Dineen, R., Charrow, J., & Wicklund, C. (2015). Genetics professionals' opinions of whole-genome sequencing in the newborn period. *Journal of Genetic Counseling*, *24*(3), 452–463. https://doi.org/10.1007/s10897-014-9779-3

Vora, N. L., Gilmore, K., Brandt, A., Gustafson, C., Strande, N., Ramkissoon, L., Hardisty, E., Foreman, A. K. M., Wilhelmsen, K., Owen, P., Weck, K. E., Berg, J. S., Powell, C. M., & Powell, B. C. (2020). An approach to integrating exome sequencing for fetal structural anomalies into clinical practice. *Genetics in Medicine*, *22*(5), 954–961. https://doi.org/10.1038/s41436-020-0750-4

Vora, N. L., Powell, B., Brandt, A., Strande, N., Hardisty, E., Gilmore, K., Foreman, A. K. M., Wilhelmsen, K., Bizon, C., Reilly, J., Owen, P., Powell, C. M., Skinner, D., Rini, C., Lyerly, A. D., Boggess, K. A., Weck, K., Berg, J. S., & Evans, J. P. (2017). Prenatal exome sequencing in anomalous fetuses: New opportunities and challenges. *Genetics in Medicine*, *19*(11), 1207–1216. https://doi.org/10.1038/gim.2017.33

Vora, N. L., & Wapner, R. J. (2018). Introducing new and emerging genetic tests into prenatal care. *Seminars in Perinatology*, *42*(5), 283–286. https://doi.org/10.1053/j.semperi.2018.07.004

Waisbren, S. E., Bäck, D. K., Liu, C., Kalia, S. S., Ringer, S. A., Holm, I. A., & Green, R. C. (2015). Parents are interested in newborn genomic testing during the early postpartum period. *Genetics in Medicine*, *17*(6), 501–504. https://doi.org/10.1038/gim.2014.139

Wilfond, B. S., Fernandez, C. V., & Green, R. C. (2015). Disclosing secondary findings from pediatric sequencing to families: Considering the "benefit to families." *Journal of Law, Medicine & Ethics*, *43*(3), 552–558. https://doi.org/10.1111/jlme.12298

Wou, K., Weitz, T., McCormack, C., Wynn, J., Spiegel, E., Giordano, J., Wapner, R. J., & Chung, W. K. (2018). Parental Perceptions of Prenatal Whole Exome Sequencing (PPPWES) study. *Prenatal Diagnosis*, *38*(11), 801–811. https://doi.org/10.1002/pd.5332

CHAPTER 36

CONSIDERING THE FUTURE OF GENETIC COUNSELING

DEBORAH CRAGUN, ROBERT RESTA, AND DANIEL LEE RICONDA

Introduction

PREDICTING the future is an undertaking usually doomed to failure. The few successes can be written off as lucky guesses. If you make enough predictions, then there is a reasonable chance that one of them will turn out to be correct. Still, speculating about the future can be a fruitful exercise because it forces us to thoughtfully consider the past and the present to better understand future possibilities. Such an endeavor can help the genetic counseling profession to plan for possible changes and to avoid pathways that lead to undesirable outcomes. As the writer Ray Bradbury is supposed to have said, "I don't write to predict the future. I write to prevent it."

In this chapter we examine how genetic counseling as a clinical practice and as a profession may change in response to factors such as evolving ethical norms, systemic social disparities, demographic changes in patient populations and in genetic counselors themselves, legislative and judicial trends, workforce demand, new technology and service delivery models, expanding professional roles, global expansion of genetic counseling, and educational training of genetic counselors and other healthcare providers.

Evolving Ethical Perspectives

Over time, ethical perspectives and social norms can change in unpredictable ways. These changes are to some extent driven by demographics (the age profile of a population, ethnic composition, fertility rates, religious preferences, etc.), but not exclusively so. What is considered acceptable in one historical period—denying women the right to vote, slavery, acceptable ways of dressing, colonialism, banning same-sex or interracial marriage—may be labeled oppressive, immoral, or backward within a generation or two with no apparent connection to demographic variables.

This changing ethical perspective is well illustrated by the history of eugenics in the United States, the United Kingdom, Australia, and other countries in the early 20th century. In the past, eugenic philosophies were supported by many across the political spectrum. Eugenics was initially viewed as a scientifically enlightened policy that fit well with liberal and progressive notions of social underclasses who were thought to benefit from the interventions of the self-proclaimed social and economic elite (Allen, 1989; Paul, 1984). Nowadays, being called a eugenicist can have a negative connotation to the point where it has become an aspersion (Paul, 1998).

Geneticists' ethical concern about eugenics was great enough that it contributed to the adoption of a nondirective approach to genetic counseling (Resta, 1997). Nondirective counseling—commonly conceived of as an attempt by the counselor to remain value neutral and avoid overtly or covertly influencing patient decisions—arose as a response to past eugenic abuses in the name of genetics. Recognizing the influence genetic counselors have on patients (whether they intend to or not), Kessler (1992) conceptualized nondirective counseling as an attempt to influence thinking processes and contrasted this with directive counseling—which attempts to influence behavior. Although Kessler argued over 30 years ago that there may be a need for both approaches, the profession has been relatively slow to move away from a strictly nondirective approach to consider other counseling models and techniques. Even Carl Rogers, whose work is generally credited as serving as the initial model for psychological genetic counseling, came to discourage the use of the term "nondirectiveness," preferring "client-centered therapy" as a more accurate description of his approach to counseling (Dealey & Evans, 2020).

Despite many calls to replace nondirective counseling with better counseling models, this misunderstood term is still part of the professional vocabulary (Weil, 2003) and may be constraining what genetic counselors do. For example, genetic counselors should never let their attempts to remain nondirective prevent them from providing patients the benefit of their expertise. Nor should a misconstrued conception of nondirectiveness prevent genetic counselors from being actively involved by helping patients weigh various alternatives as part of the decision-making process.

One model that has entered genetic counseling practice is shared decision making (SDM) (Birch et al., 2018). SDM is a collaborative approach in which clinicians educate and support patients in making informed decisions that align with the patient's own values. SDM remains consistent with the original intent of nondirectiveness because it lacks any elements of persuasion or directionality. SDM remains appropriate for value-based decisions in which there is no one right choice that is universally agreed upon, which is often the case in prenatal settings. On the other hand, an SDM approach can sometimes work at cross-purposes in other areas of practice such as hereditary cancer and cardiomyopathies where one of the goals may be to encourage patients to undertake strategies to reduce their chances of manifesting life-threatening illnesses or detecting them at an earlier and possibly more treatable stage (Jamal, 2020). In such cases, it may in fact be unethical to take a nondirective approach given that such an approach may fail to make it clear which action is most effective or advantageous from a medical perspective.[1]

[1] Editors' note: For further discussion on nondirectiveness, see Chapter 23 by Michael J. Deem in this volume.

Another example of evolving ethical perspectives can be found in newborn screening. Traditionally based on the phenylketonuria (PKU) screening model, disorders were considered eligible for newborn screening if they were diagnosable only by reliable laboratory means, prior to the onset of symptoms, and an effective treatment or intervention was available, following the Wilson and Jungner (1968) criteria for screening for medical conditions. The last decade has seen a significant increase in the number of conditions included in newborn screening panels, many of which do not meet Wilson and Jungner criteria (El-Hattab et al., 2018). Often, the stated aim of including rare untreatable diseases is to reduce the length of the "diagnostic odyssey," a family's often frustrating and long search for a diagnosis of their child's condition, and to allow the family to better adapt to the psychological and medical impact of raising a child with an identified syndrome (Boardman et al., 2019; Nicholls et al., 2014; Pruniski et al., 2018).

It seems likely that the number of conditions included in newborn screening programs will increase as a result of the dropping cost of genetic testing, improvements in the ability to identify and interpret genetic variants, competition among laboratories that drives Lab A to offer a larger testing panel than Lab B, and the influence of patient support groups to add specific genetic diseases (Bailey & Zimmerman, 2019; Rajabi, 2018; Save Babies Through Screening Foundation, n.d.). This expansion will benefit some families and patients medically or psychologically but will also have its downsides, such as the phenomenon of "patients-in-waiting," wherein a child has a positive genetic test but has not yet manifested symptoms of a disease or has a test result that is not clearly positive or negative (Pruniski et al., 2018; Timmermans & Buchbinder, 2010). As we look to the future, additional research is needed to examine the positive and negative impact exome or genome sequencing of newborns might have, should that come to pass (Johnston et al., 2018).

Demographic Changes in the Patient Population

Starting in the 1980s, most of the Westernized world experienced a steady and significant increase in the number of women who delayed childbearing, in part driven by increasing opportunities for women to have rewarding and successful careers outside of the home (of which genetic counselors themselves are a prime example). During the 1980s and 1990s, "eligibility" for prenatal diagnosis was based primarily on maternal age as well as analysis of maternal serum analytes and sonographic markers, both of which are age-dependent screens. This demand for prenatal screening vastly expanded employment opportunities for genetic counselors. Although the trend of delayed childbearing shows no signs of abating, prenatal screening is now typically performed by primary care providers and offered to pregnant women of all ages. With the much lower false-positive rates of maternal serum cell-free DNA screening for aneuploidy and other conditions leading to fewer referrals to specialist centers (although this varies with the maternal age distribution and condition for which screening is performed), it is possible that prenatal screening will play a less dominant role in the employment of genetic counselors in the future (Familiari et al., 2021).

Traditionally, the majority of patients seen in many—but by no means all—genetic counseling clinics were upper middle class, educated, and primarily of Northern and Western European ancestry, a profile reflected in genetic counselors themselves. As genetic testing and prenatal screening become more affordable and are made more available to wider swaths of the population, in combination with global migration patterns that can significantly influence the ethnocultural makeup of the population, the demographic profile of the patient population will continue to expand. Not only will this affect the types of genetic diseases that genetic counselors will encounter, but also patients may very well have ethical, personal, and religious values that might not fit well with the traditional genetic counseling model based on a heavy educational component and a largely nondirective philosophy (Jamal et al., 2020). This will require genetic counselors to develop improved cultural awareness, alternative counseling techniques, ethical principles, and educational strategies to meet the needs of a changing and heterogeneous population. The changing demographics of patient populations also highlight the need for increasing the diversity of the genetic counseling workforce.

The aging population of many countries (Population Reference Bureau, n.d.) will also impact genetic counseling. As people age, they become more susceptible to health problems, including patients who carry a pathogenic variant for an adult-onset condition. Changing demographics raise additional questions that genetic counselors may help answer. For example, should women who carry a pathogenic *BRCA* variant continue to undergo high-risk breast cancer screening in their 70s and beyond? At what age should risk-reducing surgeries such as salpingo-oophorectomy no longer be considered for *BRCA* pathogenic variant carriers? Does an asymptomatic 75-year-old patient who carries a pathogenic Lynch syndrome gene variant still need frequent colonoscopy? Studies of the disease risks associated with pathogenic variants such as *BRCA1/2* have typically had a small number of septuagenarians and octogenarians, which limits the statistical confidence of actuarial risk estimates. Future research should address the residual disease risks and special counseling needs of older patients.

Legislative and Judicial Trends

Legislative efforts are ongoing in the United States to add genetic counselors to the ranks of recognized providers within the Centers for Medicare and Medicaid Services. Such recognition would expand access to, and coverage of, genetic counseling services. In addition, the number of states that have passed genetic counseling licensure legislation is now over 30 and will likely continue to grow. These efforts may result in improved reimbursement and coverage of genetic counseling services in the future. We anticipate these legislative trends will contribute to further growth and recognition of the genetic counseling profession in the United States.

One of the most contentious judicial and legislative debates in many countries is the availability of safe and legal abortion. Some countries, especially the United States, are witnessing greater legislative restrictions on abortion, while others, such as Mexico and Ireland, have moved toward legalization of abortion. Given the U.S. Supreme Court's *Dobbs* decision overturning *Roe v. Wade*, access to legal abortion has been severely restricted. Access to abortion will now be greatly influenced by whether a woman lives in a state where abortion is legal. The *Dobbs* decision will limit the options available to women whose pregnancies are diagnosed with genetic conditions. This may lead to fewer women undergoing prenatal testing and potentially fewer jobs for prenatal genetic counselors. Such restrictions will further exacerbate socioeconomic disparities. As shown in Brazil, where abortion is illegal, women who are better off economically can still obtain a safe, if technically illegal, abortion (Löwy & Dias Villela Corrêa, 2020). The net result may be an increased incidence of children with disabilities among economically disadvantaged families who may have fewer external resources to care for children who have special medical, educational, and social needs.

Because of these restrictions on abortion, and because it is the humanistic and ethically appropriate thing to do, genetic counselors should engage in more research that investigates whether prenatal testing improves the medical, psychological, and adaptational outcomes of families and patients who have a fetus diagnosed with a condition prenatally that is carried to term rather than terminated (Resta, 2021).

Demand for Genetic Counseling and Genetic Counselors

Recent workforce projections by the Department of Labor and Statistics estimated a 10-year growth rate for genetic counseling positions between 2016 and 2026 of 29% for clinical positions (U.S. Bureau of Labor Statistics, n.d.). At the time of these projections, two-thirds of jobs were clinical patient facing in nature and the remaining one-third were in nonclinical positions, often in private laboratories.

The number of genetic counselors entering the workforce will continue to grow (National Society of Genetic Counselors [NSGC], 2022). However, with the current and anticipated demand for genetic counseling services, it is difficult to imagine a future where that demand can realistically be met solely by genetic counselors and medical geneticists. Some forms of genetic testing will likely be increasingly incorporated into the daily practice of medicine. Ordering the appropriate testing and interpreting normal, positive, and uncertain results does not fit into the skill set of most primary care providers (Menke et al., 2021; Sharma et al., 2022; Wakefield et al., 2018). This may lead to the expansion of fee-for-service certificate training opportunities for nongenetic counselors to acquire training in genetic counseling–related skills and test interpretation.

Internationally, genetic counseling is often provided by healthcare professionals who have not undergone formal training in genetic counseling, and how the "practice" of genetic counseling is defined varies by the local and regional service delivery models (Abacan et al., 2019; Ormond et al., 2018). Healthcare delivery models are often physician driven, and in some countries, there is currently no role for nonphysician genetic counselors or that role is only beginning to gain a foothold (Abacan, 2019; Laurino et al., 2018). See further discussion in Chapter 34—"Globalization of Genetic Counseling" in this volume.

How Technology May Change the Delivery of Genetic Counseling Services

The concerns of some about the ability of the genetic counseling workforce to handle the potential increased demand for genetic counseling (Patch & Middleton, 2018) has sparked interest in using technology to facilitate some aspects of genetic counseling (Kaphingst et al., 2021; Schmidlen et al., 2019). Many practitioners and researchers agree that the current model of individual pretest and posttest counseling for all genetic testing by a genetic counselor is neither practical nor desirable.

Genetic information is growing more complex as the fine details of the genome are delineated and incorporated into clinical practice. This complexity could lead to genetic counseling sessions resembling advanced biomedical lectures as genetic counselors try to explain the implications and results of genetic testing. This would not be in many patients' best interests as most adults do not learn well through lectures (Deslauriers et al., 2019; Smith et al., 2009), and it could diminish the critical psychological and psychotherapeutic components of genetic counseling.

Different service delivery models have been tried and suggested to scale genetic counseling services to a population level (Khan et al., 2021; McCuaig et al., 2018; Stoll et al., 2018; Terry et al., 2019). Time, research trials, cost, patient acceptance, and the unique needs of each setting will ultimately determine their usefulness and feasibility. The All of Us initiative, which aims to sequence approximately 1 million healthy people, will be working with a commercial laboratory to develop and evaluate different ways of delivering genetic test results to large numbers of people (National Institutes of Health, 2020). The results of this study will be an important step toward understanding how complex genetic information can be delivered to large numbers of people in an efficient, effective, and compassionate way.

One approach to scaling genetic counseling to a population is chatbots—computer programs or apps that try to simulate natural conversation between a computer and a person over the internet (Schmidlen et al., 2019). They have been utilized with surprising success in settings as varied as entertainment, marketing, customer support, hospitality, and insurance (Abd-Alrazaq et al., 2020; "Chatbots on Websites," n.d.; Gabrielli et al., 2021). Chatbots are also receiving attention for the delivery of medical services (Chaix et al., 2019).

The real question, though, is not whether chatbots or some technological equivalent will play a role in genetic counseling services. Undoubtedly some form of information-sharing technology will be incorporated into the genetic testing process. The bigger question is whether employers will look to replace genetic counselors with some form of artificial intelligence that provides patient education. This could initially happen in the genetic testing industry. Most genetic testing is performed by for-profit laboratories. To be sure, some genetic testing also takes place in medical centers and university-affiliated hospitals, but large-scale testing will likely remain beyond the capabilities of these typically smaller laboratories. As more laboratories bypass medical practitioners and offer their tests directly to patients and consumers, the genetic counselor "middle person" will likely increasingly be left out of the workflow. Labs may have genetic counselors available for posttest counseling, but so far consumer demand for posttest counseling is low (Koeller et al., 2017) and chatbots or some equivalent may be able to fill this role more cost-effectively. To paraphrase an oft-cited quote about screening, the most useful genetic counseling service delivery model is the one that gets utilized the most.

Potentially, then, genetic counseling employers like medical centers, universities, and health maintenance organizations may look to reduce the number of genetic counselors they employ if laboratories provide what employers see as an equivalent/noninferior service at no apparent cost to the employers. It could also mean that more medical centers and community hospitals outsource their genetic counseling to telehealth genetic counseling companies that can provide their services, in theory at least, anywhere around the globe. It is possible such trends may be counterbalanced by the requirements for pretest genetic counseling instituted by some third-party payers as a prerequisite to coverage of genetic testing (Stenehjem et al., 2018) as well as licensure requirements that now exist in multiple states.

In essence, chatbots or their equivalents could reshape genetic counseling employment settings as well as change the focus of the services genetic counselors provide to patients and consumers. Their counseling skills, educational abilities, and technical knowledge will need to be applied and modified to different work settings. Perhaps genetic counselors will spend more time learning information technology skills or work as part of an interdisciplinary team to ensure materials and decision aids are high quality, accurate, easy to understand, and up to date. How this will play out will be determined by market factors and the flexibility of genetic counselors in integrating into new working environments and different demands for their services.

This will also require training programs to continuously adapt their curricula to a changing employment environment (Riconda et al., 2018).[2] Even if technology might reduce the need for some aspects of genetic counseling and eliminate some genetic counseling positions, employment opportunities will likely continue to grow as genetic testing is increasingly being incorporated into many aspects of medical treatment and well-patient care and new tests continue to be developed. More tests equal more jobs, though those jobs and employers may look different than they do today. At the same time, the increasing reliance of genetic counseling employment on the availability of an ever-growing list of genetic tests could create conflicts of interest that subtly influence genetic counselors' willingness to incorporate new tests into clinical care and potentially affect the counseling process itself.

Service Delivery Shifts and Evidence-Based Practice

There are and will continue to be shifts in the delivery of clinical genetic services. As exome and genome sequencing become commonplace, it may become too inconvenient for patients to see multiple genetic counselors to address the multiple different types of

[2] Editors' note: For discussion regarding the growth of genetic counseling, see Chapter 33 by Megan E. Trinkle-Tucker and Beverly M. Yashar in this volume.

disorders that may be detected by genomic testing, and general practice genetic counselors may become more common again concurrent with increasing specialization for other genetic counselors. This generalization might occur if some genetic counselors become embedded in primary care, perhaps with the establishment of point-of-care testing, as some have advocated (Hyatt et al., 2019).

Genetic counselors may also continue to have or create opportunities to weave themselves into multiple specialty clinics. The increasing number of special interest groups (SIGs) in the NSGC attests to the expansion of specialization with several newer specialties such as inpatient, psychiatric, renal, ophthalmologic/hearing loss, cystic fibrosis, and so forth. It may even be possible that several genetic counselors who have subspecialized will form a multidisciplinary clinic where patients can be seen by more than one genetic counselor at a single visit to discuss the multiple implications of sequencing results that cross a variety of health-related domains. As shifts in practice occur, systematic evaluation of different approaches to identify advantages and limitations of these service delivery models will need to be conducted to determine how patient outcomes are impacted.

One major challenge in conducting comparative effectiveness studies of different service delivery models is that we still don't know for certain what patient outcomes genetic counselors improve. Much of the research has focused on how genetic counseling by genetic counselors increases knowledge, does not increase distress or anxiety, and reduces decisional conflict (Athens et al., 2017; Biesecker et al., 2018; Inglis et al., 2015; Madlensky et al., 2017; Robinson et al., 2016; Wong et al., 2021). Automated educational tools and decision aids can also increase knowledge and reduce decisional conflict (Cragun et al., 2020; Russo et al., 2021). Although it is reassuring that genetic counselors do not appear to do harm by increasing distress or anxiety, genetic counselors should focus more on what we do rather than what we don't do. Perhaps in the future we will (Bombard et al., 2020) focus more on identifying and working primarily with patients who have unmet psychosocial needs and/or those who are having difficulty deciding on testing or adapting to the information they obtain from testing. However, justifying this from an evidence-based healthcare system perspective would require demonstrating that genetic counselors are addressing psychosocial needs and that they are effective at helping patients cope and adapt to living with genetic conditions or the risk of developing a genetic condition. Studies have shown that genetic counselors may help empower patients in several settings and increase self-efficacy to cope with mental illness (Inglis et al., 2015; McAllister et al., 2011; Robinson et al., 2016).[3] However, some genetic counselors may not feel it is their role to impact patient health outcomes presumably because such outcomes are influenced by so many other factors (Redlinger-Grosse et al., 2021). Nonetheless, health outcomes are the focus of the healthcare system, and since genetic counselors are healthcare providers, it could be argued that genetic counselors should ultimately be contributing to better health and reduction of disease incidence such as ovarian cancer among *BRCA* pathogenic variant carriers or colon cancer in Lynch syndrome families (Hooker et al., 2017).

[3] Editors' note: For discussion of measuring patient empowerment after genetic counseling services, see Chapter 30 by Marion McAllister in this volume.

Expanding and Evolving Roles of Genetic Counselors

What roles genetic counselors may assume in the future is open to speculation, but it is likely that these roles will evolve. We are optimistic that genetic counselors will adapt to the changing environment. We anticipate genetic counselors will not become extinct but will continue to expand into new niches, as the history of the profession clearly demonstrates. Questions about how genetic counselors will or should adapt are already on the horizon, a few of which are discussed below.

New genetic testing technologies may bring new niches for genetic counselors

In July of 2019, a patient with sickle cell disease became the first patient in the United States with a genetic disease to be treated with a CRISPR (clustered regularly interspaced short palindromic repeats)–based therapy (Baffoe-Bonnie, 2019). In the future, we may look back on this moment as the advent of a new area of practice for genetic counselors. Even before the announcement of this sentinel event, the occasional forward-thinking patient would ask their genetic counselor about the promise of CRISPR in shepherding an era of genome editing. Genetic counselors have long dreamed of the day that effective therapies for a wide array of genetic diseases would become viable options. One can imagine genetic counselors working with researchers to help with patient recruitment into CRISPR therapeutic trials.

As the $1,000 Genome (Davies, 2010) comes to fruition, the ability to perform laboratory-developed tests that allow rapid sequencing at the bedside or in the primary care setting on the same day of service (point of care) will create a paradigm shift in potential genetic counseling service delivery models. We already live in an age where immediate access to information is not an unrealistic expectation. Thus, it is not inconceivable that genetic test results, through the use of nanopore technologies or other methodologies, will create a market for rapid access to genetic counselors. The expansion of genetic technologies may result in ongoing growth of genetic counselors who are employed by testing labs. In the mid-2000s, the first of several companies offering genetic counseling services provided by genetic counselors was founded. At around that same time, some insurers implemented policies requiring genetic counseling of patients in order to make decisions about coverage of genetic testing for hereditary cancers. This soon expanded to hereditary cardiac disorders and exome sequencing (Stenehjem et al., 2018).

Genetic counselors in oncology settings have become involved in somatic tumor sequencing, primarily with regard to germline implications (Forman & Sotelo, 2020). However, other types of providers, such as pharmacists and oncologists, have remained the key clinicians in using somatic genetic test results to identify possible targeted cancer treatment recommendations. Consequently, one might anticipate that it is unlikely genetic counselors will take the lead in the somatic cancer testing realm, but hopefully they will continue to be part of an interdisciplinary team working in this area, especially in deciding which tumor-detected variants are appropriate for referral for germline genetic testing as well as in evaluating the pathogenicity of variants detected on tumor DNA sequencing (Gregory et al., 2022; Lewis & Vassos, 2020; McGuinness et al., 2021; Yanes et al., 2021).

As a healthcare profession, genetic counselors will continue to focus primarily on genetic tests with clinical and diagnostic utility. However, some genetic counselors have begun seeing patients who undergo "recreational" genetic testing, and they play an important role to ensure that test results are validated in a clinical laboratory when possibly actionable results are found due to the high rates of false-positive results for rare variants (Tandy-Connor et al., 2018). Genetic counseling skills also may come into play in addressing the psychological and emotional turmoil in a family when such testing reveals incidental findings such as unsuspected or misattributed paternity or previously unknown siblings.[4]

Some laboratory-based genetic counselors serve as technical experts for variant interpretation (Wain et al., 2020). Laboratory counselors also advise other healthcare providers on which tests to order. The technical expertise of genetic counselors has led to opportunities to serve as members of utilization management teams (aka laboratory stewardship), essentially functioning as "genetic testing gatekeepers" for laboratories and hospital pathology departments determining which genetic tests are appropriate based on a patient's clinical presentation and/or avoiding unnecessary or redundant testing (Miller et al., 2014; Waltman et al., 2016). Whether or not the role of utilization management will continue to increase is uncertain. As genetic testing costs continue to fall, the cost savings of ensuring the right test for the right person can be expected to dwindle, potentially reducing some of the benefits of utilization management. Even if that is the case, genetic counselors will likely still play a role in identifying which genetic testing technologies are most appropriate for a given patient. For example, trisomies, gene deletions, variations in gene copy number, and triplet expansion repeats are not always reliably detected by exome testing. Even as technical expertise increases, this does not mean that training in counseling skills will become obsolete as genetic counselors in these laboratory and utilization management roles have indicated that their counseling skills are transferable when communicating with healthcare providers (Miller et al., 2014).

Changes in specialty roles

In the early days of the profession, genetic counselors were the "Jack (or Jill) of all trades, and expert at none (all!)." In the decades that have passed, the expansion of practice areas has led many genetic counselors to specialize. Genetic counselors began primarily in prenatal and pediatric settings and expanded to cancer settings in the late 1990s (Kenen, 1997; Uhlmann et al., 2020). In the early 1990s cancer genetic counseling was not a substantial part of routine practice or training, but cancer genetic counselors now make up the largest SIG in the NSGC (NSGC, 2022). Genetic counselors have since moved into additional specialties such as cardiology, neurology, ophthalmology, and psychiatry (Baty, 2018). As

[4] Editors' note: For further discussion on direct-to-consumer genetic testing, see Chapter 11 by Anne E. Greb in this volume.

specialization continues, there may come a time when certification of genetic counselors in specialty areas would be adopted. As more genetic counselors have now specialized, it is not uncommon for patients to be sent to more than one genetic counselor to discuss different risks (Christensen et al., 2021). We anticipate that much of what happens with regard to specialization will be influenced by shifts in service delivery. In other words, how patients receive genetic counseling, via telehealth, the development of decision aids, or through other modalities, will influence what specialty areas may develop and which may have the greatest growth. It is also possible—as mentioned above—that this could lead to a trend for some genetic counselors to become generalists who can cover a wide variety of conditions and specialties (prenatal, cancer, pediatric, etc.), while others may become even more specialized.

Changes from less of an educator role to more of a counseling role

The educator versus counselor roles have long been debated in the genetic counseling profession (Kessler, 1997), with genetic counselors typically assuming an educator role in which they dominate the conversation and focus most of the time on technical and medical information (Joseph et al., 2017; Roter et al., 2006), even if they profess otherwise. As noted above, the educational component of genetic counseling is, to some extent, being replaced by online educational modules and decision aids, and genetic counseling by a genetic counselor may become uncoupled from genetic testing. The uncoupling of testing and counseling can already be seen as genetic testing is becoming more routine and increasingly being used to guide medical treatments (Slade, 2020). Perhaps genetic counselors should embrace the notion that automated education is better than what has long been happening as nongenetics providers often order genetic tests without what genetic counselors would consider adequate pretest counseling (Cragun et al., 2015; Vadaparampil et al., 2015). At least with the automated education and decision aids, patients and providers may be more informed (Cragun et al., 2020; Russo et al., 2021).

Genetic counseling, of course, is not only about genetic testing. The other skills of genetic counselors may come into greater demand if pretest and posttest education becomes a less integral part of genetic counselors' duties. These might include providing psychological and emotional support as well as revisiting with patients over time to help patients and families adapt to living with a genetic disorder or the risk of developing one, communicating diagnoses and anticipatory medical guidance, serving as resources for other medical care providers, and consulting for genetically complex situations. Many genetic counselors are recognizing that perhaps not everyone needs to meet with a genetic counselor prior to testing, as evidenced by the NSGC's recent task force evaluating ways to determine who would benefit most from seeing a genetic counselor (Hoskovec et al., 2018).

Some genetic counseling will continue to be performed in emotionally challenging circumstances. It's one thing for a healthy consumer to find out from genetic testing that they might be more susceptible to cancer, Alzheimer's disease, or multiple sclerosis. It's another thing altogether to have to break a diagnosis of a severe genetic disorder to the parents of a child in a neonatal intensive care unit or in the middle of a pregnancy. The counseling and support skills of a live, in-person genetic counselor will likely continue to serve patients better in these situations.

Shifting roles to encourage adherence to health guidelines or recommendations

Although some genetic counselors may feel it is not their role to encourage adherence to health guidelines, a study found that involvement of a genetic counselor in general genetics clinics increased the chance that patients followed medical recommendations as compared to those without a genetic counselor involved (Rutherford et al., 2014). Although the reason for this could not be identified given study limitations, results suggest that genetic counselors may in fact contribute to health outcomes, assuming that following medical recommendations improves health outcomes. As discussed above in the section on Evidence-Based Practice, improved health outcomes is potentially one measure of genetic counseling outcomes.

To prepare genetic counselors with skills needed to encourage behavior change, some genetic counseling programs are now teaching motivational interviewing, an evidence-based and person-centered approach that has been shown to be effective in moving individuals toward healthier behaviors (Ash, 2017). Genetic counselors have historically taken a nondirective approach, but with the development of the Reciprocal-Engagement Model as a practice model of genetic counseling (Veach et al., 2007),[5] genetic counselors have come to accept that being directive and supporting patient autonomy are not diametrically opposed. Providing education and encouraging risk-appropriate screening are often goals in cancer genetic counseling. Motivational interviewing has been applied by other healthcare providers to encourage multiple types of health behavior change (Tahan & Sminkey, 2012), but it remains unclear whether the genetic counseling profession will adopt an approach that promotes healthy behaviors and whether they will counsel individuals at increased risk for common conditions that have strong links to lifestyle risk factors.

Global Expansion of Genetic Counseling and Adaptations in Service Delivery

From an international perspective, it is likely that local, regional, national, and cultural differences will require different service delivery models to be effective. A variety of internal and external factors will influence who provides genetic counseling and how such services are delivered. Thus, the future of genetic counseling and genetic counselors may play out very differently in different parts of the globe. The same internal and external

[5] Editors' note: The Reciprocal-Engagement Model is discussed in Chapter 5 by Patricia McCarthy Veach and Bonnie S. LeRoy in this volume.

factors will likely be important internationally, but, for example, the demographics of India's inhabitants will be very different than the demographics of Dutch citizens, and the judicial and legislative future of Saudi Arabia will likely look very different than that of the United States.

The first meeting of the Transnational Alliance for Genetic Counseling (TAGC) took place in Manchester, England, in 2006 (Edwards, 2013). Representatives from 18 countries and 45 training programs attended the meeting. A goal of that first meeting was to bring together educators who had adopted training practices that were tailored to the varied service delivery models that reflect their respective countries and regions of the world. At around that same time, the accrediting body of the United States and Canada, the American Board of Genetic Counseling (ABGC), was grappling with the question of whether or not the ABGC should accept invitations to accredit programs from other countries. Ultimately, the ABGC decided that differences in service delivery models and curriculum design would not be amenable to a unifying accrediting organization, but ongoing communication of best practices between training programs would continue. In the years since, three other TAGC meetings have taken place and additional meetings are anticipated in the future. Since January of 2013, accreditation-related activities have been under the auspices of the Accreditation Council for Genetic Counseling (ACGC), which has thus far reaffirmed the decision not to accredit programs from outside the United States or Canada.

Genetic counseling as a profession has continued to grow globally, and the tenets of genetic counseling practice are gradually being introduced into regions of the world that have not previously integrated genetic counseling into healthcare delivery. This is exemplified by the creation of professional societies such as the Professional Society of Genetic Counselors in Asia and the Taiwan Association of Genetic Counseling (Laurino et al., 2018). Representatives from North American training programs as well as other genetic counselors in the United States and other countries have engaged in teaching genetic counseling skills to a variety of providers internationally in locations that have included Hong Kong, Taiwan, and other countries. As an example, one of the authors (Riconda) has taught a one-credit certificate course on genetic counseling at the Chinese University at Hong Kong in 2017, 2019, 2021, and 2025, and provided training in other countries in Asia. The export of training expertise provided by genetic counselors is likely to expand to regions of the world that are now in the formative stages of creating a niche for genetic counseling and defining a role for genetic counselors. For additional discussion see Chapter 34—"Globalization of Genetic Counseling" in this volume.

Any attempts to globalize genetic counseling services will require increased sensitivity to and familiarity with the diversity of cultural norms and traditions that exist in other countries. In some countries, healthcare is provided through a government-sponsored system. In such countries, establishing a role for healthcare professionals who are not physicians will be difficult, although it has been achieved in the United Kingdom, Canada, and other countries that provide national health insurance. Alternatively, training the existing healthcare providers about genetic counseling may be the more practical opportunity for integrating genetic counseling into the delivery of genetics-related services. In countries like China where the typical visit with a provider may be as short as 5 minutes or less (Jin et al., 2015), it will be necessary to adapt counseling to the realities of time constraints that may hamper the delivery of services that follow the Western model of service delivery.

Demographic Changes in the Genetic Counseling Profession

Diversity is difficult to define precisely. Often it is tacitly assumed to mean ethnic diversity. But ethnicity is only one aspect of diversity. People also vary by age, gender identification, sexual orientation, socioeconomic status, and physical abilities, to name a few examples. These categories intersect and are not mutually exclusive. Someone could be Hispanic, female, lesbian, and a teenager, or a Black, cisgender, heterosexual, hearing-impaired, upper-middle-class 40-year-old male. Another way to approach the issue is to think about demographic diversity. In other words, ideally, the demographic profile of genetic counselors and the general population should be broadly similar (though see discussion in the last paragraph of this section). The NSGC's 2019 strategic plan included a focus on promoting a culture of inclusivity that supports visible and invisible diversity while leveraging that culture to expand the perspectives represented in our field, build community, and foster equity in genetic services.

The demographic profile of genetic counselors reflects the history of the profession and the employment opportunities readily available to women in the 1970s and 1980s. From its inception, genetic counseling was an upper socioeconomic "woman's" profession. Even today, over 90% of genetic counselors identify as female (NSGC, 2022). In addition to historical factors, the lack of diversity among genetic counselors is a function of the many sociocultural and economic barriers faced by minorities, a problem not unique to genetic counseling. The genetic counseling workforce will not become substantially more diverse until systemic barriers such as explicit and implicit racism, socioeconomic and educational disparities, and the lack of political parity in a multiethnic population are eliminated.

In 2021, the number of certified genetic counselors in the United States reached 5,629 (NSGC, 2022). Increasing the number of genetic counselors globally will require the development of training programs that tailor their curriculum to train such providers. According to the 2022 Professional Status Survey of the NSGC, which included genetic counselors from the United States and Canada, 89% of respondents identify as White, 9% identify as Asian, and 2% identify as other ethnicities or did not respond (NSGC, 2022). Approximately 70% of respondents were under age 40, a statistic that has not significantly varied since the survey was first administered in 1980. About 95% self-identify as female. About 2% identify as gay or lesbian, 4% identify as bisexual, and 2% self-describe their sexual orientation.

The demographic profiles of genetic counselors in other countries are likely similar to that of the United States, except in Asian countries such as Japan, China, and India, where genetic counselors are predominantly from their native countries. Thus, genetic counselors are primarily young, nondisabled, upper-middle-class, White, largely heterosexual cisgender, politically liberal females.

A demographically diverse workforce is important for several reasons. From a social justice standpoint, everyone should have equal access to career pathways. Anyone and everyone should be able to pursue a career as a genetic counselor. Clinically, demographic homogeneity is implicitly and subconsciously incorporated into genetic counseling theory, practice, and ethics. The goals of genetic counseling, ethical values such as nondirectiveness and reproductive rights, and involvement in practice specialties such as prenatal screening reflect the sociocultural perspective of its practitioners. For example, if genetic counselors were largely Evangelical Christians, then prenatal testing would not likely be widely practiced and a pro-choice stance on abortion would not likely be integrated into the NSGC Code of Ethics. It is difficult to see one's own biases and resulting unintended injustices when nearly everyone else in the profession looks and thinks just like you. In addition, patients are more likely to utilize medical care and to feel confident that they are receiving appropriate care when medical practitioners are not overwhelmingly from a narrowly defined demographic segment (Jang et al., 2021; Maina et al., 2018; Mitchell et al., 2019).

The genetic counseling profession itself cannot eliminate cultural and systemic barriers to career opportunities. Nonetheless, genetic counseling training programs and professional organizations need to create an environment that embraces, encourages, and supports demographic diversity. To that end, the NSGC made justice, diversity equity, and inclusiveness areas of focus in its Strategic Plan for 2022–2024 (NSGC, n.d.).

Expanding diversity is critical to the survival and growth of the genetic counseling profession and the delivery of medical genetics services. However, the goals of such initiatives may be difficult to achieve in the face of current political trends that promote "nativist" platforms, stigmatize people who are not heterosexual and heteronormative, and vilify immigrants and refugees. The loud and proud voice of the genetic counseling profession could be lost in the shouting and screaming that unfortunately often poses as political "discussion." A further barrier to diversity goals is that it is difficult to define inclusivity and diversity. While it is vital for the genetic counseling profession to expand diversity and promote inclusiveness, it is important to recognize that the profession is too small to adequately represent the demographic range of the larger population. Inevitably, some groups will be underrepresented, depending on which demographic characteristics are used to define diversity (e.g., gender, age, ethnicity, ancestry, sexual orientation, etc.).

Changes in Training of Genetic Counselors and Other Health Professions

If we accept the prediction that genetic counselors and other healthcare providers will work together to meet current and future demands for genetic counseling and genetic testing to be incorporated into routine medical care and across medical specialties, then adaptations to how we train, who we train, how we recruit, and how we deliver such training will be needed (Angelini, 2011). Some training programs have already incorporated distance education to extend their reach to a more diverse cohort of trainees, while others have utilized interprofessional education (IPE) to expose a variety of learners to skills commonly used by genetic counselors in their practice (Hoffman et al., 2020). By definition, IPE refers to occasions when students and/or professionals from two or more professions in health and social care learn together during all or part of their professional training with the object of cultivating collaborative practice (Hoffman et al., 2020). This type of training serves two purposes: teaching the next generations of genetic counseling providers (master's-prepared genetic counselors and others who would provide varying levels of genetic counseling–related services) and increasing the aptitude of providers with respect to the role, utility, and expertise of trained genetic counselors.

What is taught will also continue to evolve as the science and technology evolve. For example, teaching skills in variant interpretation and curation is a relatively recent addition to many training programs' curriculums, and the importance of such skills is likely to increase in the next 10 to 15 years. Program curriculums will likely continue to teach the relatively new and evolving tenets of the Reciprocal-Engagement Model as our practice no longer is married to nondirectiveness as a primary goal in all encounters (Veach et al., 2007).

We have also seen a debate within our profession about moving to a doctoral degree as the terminal degree. To do so could negatively impact the viability of some existing training programs due to increases in costs, time, and resource utilization. However, given the need for outcomes research (Athens et al., 2017; Madlensky et al., 2017; Redlinger-Grosse et al., 2021) on the effectiveness of genetic counseling and other areas in which genetic counseling research is needed, there is a role for genetic counselors with PhD degrees as well as a continuation of master's degree programs.

Traditionally, genetic counseling graduate programs have focused on the training of master's-prepared genetic counselors. Although this will continue to be a primary focus of training programs for the foreseeable future, training other providers in how to incorporate some of the skills that will prepare them to provide genetic counseling may also fall under the purview of some genetic counseling training programs in the United States and abroad. For some, the idea that genetic counselors will take on the task of training others to provide genetic counseling raises concerns that we may threaten our very own existence as an independent profession by "giving away the store" to other providers. Nonetheless, genetic counselors will not be able to provide genetic counseling to everyone, and the profession needs to adapt to this reality. Change is not always easy or easily accepted.

Changes in genetic counseling program requirements

Genetic counseling programs are tasked with training genetic counselors in a manner that is consistent with the practice-based competencies (PBCs) and the standards of accreditation established by the ACGC (ACGC, 2023a, 2023b). The PBCs and standards are reviewed and updated on a regular basis, and future revisions will be driven, in part, by changes in the roles and responsibilities that are dictated by the career opportunities that evolve over time. In response to revisions made, the ACGC provides a grace period for training programs to incorporate new requirements. Programs will continue to reconcile the already crowded curriculum content with the need to respond to changes in practice and changes in the standards (Roche & Greb, 2016). Programs do have discretionary authority over how they choose to train their students while meeting the standards. This has allowed programs to develop innovative teaching strategies and expand the ways in which training of competent practitioners will continue. Some programs have been able to utilize distant field placements with curriculum designs that do not require a trainee to be on campus at all times during their training. The role and extent of distance education in the training of future generations of genetic counselors is also likely to expand if we are going to increase our diversity and recruit individuals who may require greater flexibility in the timing and format of curriculum delivery than currently exists in many programs.[6]

Conclusion

Since its inception as a profession in the 1970s, genetic counselors have been at the forefront of integrating advances in genetic technology and medicine into daily clinical practice. The profession has expanded its clinical roles from seeing primarily pediatric and prenatal patients to include clients with or at risk for a wide range of conditions such as cancer, neurological diseases, cardiac diseases, and psychiatric conditions. About one-third of U.S. genetic counselors now work in nondirect patient contact positions as educators, laboratory specialists, administrators, researchers, and insurance consultants (Hoskovec et al., 2018).

The future of genetic counseling may or may not play out as we outlined above. No doubt we will be flat out wrong about many predictions, and unanticipated social and technological changes and advances will render some of our predictions meaningless. What is certain is that change will happen. But the history of genetic counseling has made clear that embracing change and uncertainty is, if you will, in the DNA of the profession. The only thing that will hold back genetic counselors and the practice of genetic counseling is genetic counselors themselves; they must continue their half-century tradition of adapting to change, being agents of change, and engaging in critical self-examination and assessment. The next generations of genetic counselors will be unlikely to resemble the current practitioners in terms of demographics, ethics, scope of practice, work settings, responsibilities, or training. And that is a good thing. Whatever the future looks like, it will be very different than today.

References

Abacan, M., Alsubaie, L., Barlow-Stewart, K., Caanen, B., Cordier, C., Courtney, E., Davoine, E., Edwards, J., Elackatt, N. J., Gardiner, K., Guan, Y., Huang, L.-H., Malmgren, C. I., Kejriwal, S., Kim, H. J., Lambert, D., Lantigua-Cruz, P. A., Lee, J. M. H., Lodahl, M., . . . Wicklund, C. (2019). The global state of the genetic counseling profession. *European Journal of Human Genetics*, *27*(2), 183–197. https://doi.org/10.1038/s41431-018-0252-x

Abd-Alrazaq, A. A., Rababeh, A., Alajlani, M., Bewick, B. M., & Househ, M. (2020). Effectiveness and safety of using chatbots to improve mental health: Systematic review and meta-analysis. *Journal of Medical Internet Research*, *22*(7), e16021. https://doi.org/10.2196/16021

Accreditation Council for Genetic Counseling. (2023a). *Practice-based competencies for genetic counselors*. https://www.gceducation.org/wp-content/uploads/2023/12/ACGC_PracticeBasedCompetencies_2023.pdf

[6] Editors' note: For further information on the relationship between changes in approaches to genetic counseling training and the growth of genetic counseling, see Chapter 33 by Megan E. Trinkle-Tucker and Beverly M. Yashar in this volume.

Accreditation Council for Genetic Counseling. (2023b). *Standards of accreditation for graduate programs in genetic counseling*. https://www.gceducation.org/wp-content/uploads/2023/11/ACGC_StandardsOfAccreditation_2023.pdf

Allen, G. E. (1989). Eugenics and American social history, 1880–1950. *Genome, 31*(2), 885–889. https://doi.org/10.1139/g89-156

Angelini, D. J. (2011). Interdisciplinary and interprofessional education: What are the key issues and considerations for the future? *Journal of Perinatal & Neonatal Nursing, 25*(2), 175–179. https://doi.org/10.1097/JPN.0b013e318212ee7a

Ash, E. (2017). Motivational interviewing in the reciprocal engagement model of genetic counseling: A method overview and case illustration. *Journal of Genetic Counseling, 26*(2), 300–311. https://doi.org/10.1007/s10897-016-0053-8

Athens, B. A., Caldwell, S. L., Umstead, K. L., Connors, P. D., Brenna, E., & Biesecker, B. B. (2017). A systematic review of randomized controlled trials to assess outcomes of genetic counseling. *Journal of Genetic Counseling, 26*(5), 902–933. https://doi.org/10.1007/s10897-017-0082-y

Baffoe-Bonnie, M. S. (2019). A justice-based argument for including sickle cell disease in CRISPR/Cas9 clinical research. *Bioethics, 33*(6), 661–668. https://doi.org/10.1111/bioe.12589

Bailey, D. B., & Zimmerman, S. J. (2019). The future of newborn screening: Why and how partnerships will be needed for success. *North Carolina Medical Journal, 80*(1), 28–31. https://doi.org/10.18043/ncm.80.1.28

Baty, B. J. (2018). Genetic counseling: Growth of the profession and the professional. *American Journal of Medical Genetics Part C: Seminars in Medical Genetics, 178*(1), 54–62. https://doi.org/10.1002/ajmg.c.31601

Biesecker, B. B., Lewis, K. L., Umstead, K. L., Johnston, J. J., Turbitt, E., Fishler, K. P., Patton, J. H., Miller, I. M., Heidlebaugh, A. R., & Biesecker, L. G. (2018). Web platform vs in-person genetic counselor for return of carrier results from exome sequencing. *JAMA Internal Medicine, 178*(3), 338–346. https://doi.org/10.1001/jamainternmed.2017.8049

Birch, P. H., Adam, S., Coe, R. R., Port, A. V., Vortel, M., Friedman, J. M., & Légaré, F. (2018). Assessing shared decision-making clinical behaviors among genetic counsellors. *Journal of Genetic Counseling, 28*(1), 40–49. https://doi.org/10.1007/s10897-018-0285-x

Boardman, F. K., Hale, R., & Young, P. J. (2019). Newborn screening for haemophilia: The views of families and adults living with haemophilia in the UK. *Haemophilia, 25*(2), 276–282. https://doi.org/10.1111/hae.13706

Bombard, Y., Clausen, M., Shickh, S., Mighton, C., Casalino, S., Kim, T. H. M., Muir, S. M., Carlsson, L., Baxter, N., Scheer, A., Elser, C., Eisen, A., Panchal, S., Graham, T., Aronson, M., Piccinin, C., Mancuso, T., Semotiuk, K., Evans, M., . . . Incidental Genomics Study Team. (2020). Effectiveness of the Genomics ADvISER decision aid for the selection of secondary findings from genomic sequencing: A randomized clinical trial. *Genetics in Medicine, 22*(4), 727–735. https://doi.org/10.1038/s41436-019-0702-z

Chaix, B., Bibault, J.-E., Pienkowski, A., Delamon, G., Guillemassé, A., Nectoux, P., & Brouard, B. (2019). When chatbots meet patients: One-year prospective study of conversations between patients with breast cancer and a chatbot. *JMIR Cancer, 5*(1), e12856. https://doi.org/10.2196/12856

Chatbots on websites: How effective are they? (n.d.). *Ottawa Business Journal*. https://obj.ca/article/chatbots-websites-how-effective-are-they

Christensen, K. D., Bell, M., Zawatsky, C. L. B., Galbraith, L. N., Green, R. C., Hutchinson, A. M., Jamal, L., LeBlanc, J. L., Leonhard, J. R., Moore, M., Mullineaux, L., Petry, N., Platt, D.

M., Shaaban, S., Schultz, A., Tucker, B. D., Van Heukelom, J., Wheeler, E., Zoltick, E. S., & Hajek, C. (2021). Precision population medicine in primary care: The Sanford Chip experience. *Frontiers in Genetics, 12*, 626845. https://doi.org/10.3389/fgene.2021.626845

Cragun, D., Camperlengo, L., Robinson, E., Caldwell, M., Kim, J., Phelan, C., Monteiro, A. N., Vadaparampil, S. T., Sellers, T. A., & Pal, T. (2015). Differences in BRCA counseling and testing practices based on ordering provider type. *Genetics in Medicine, 17*(1), 51–57. https://doi.org/10.1038/gim.2014.75

Cragun, D., Weidner, A., Tezak, A., Zuniga, B., Wiesner, G. L., & Pal, T. (2020). A web-based tool to automate portions of pretest genetic counseling for inherited cancer. *Journal of the National Comprehensive Cancer Network, 18*(7), 841–847. https://doi.org/10.6004/jnccn.2020.7546

Davies, K. (2010). *$1,000 Genome: The revolution in DNA sequencing and the new era of personalized medicine*. Free Press.

Dealey, R. P., & Evans, M. R. (2020). *Discovering theory in clinical practice: A casebook for clinical counseling and social work practice*. Springer Nature.

Deslauriers, L., McCarty, L. S., Miller, K., Callaghan, K., & Kestin, G. (2019). Measuring actual learning versus feeling of learning in response to being actively engaged in the classroom. *Proceedings of the National Academy of Sciences, 116*(39), 19251–19257. https://doi.org/10.1073/pnas.1821936116

Edwards, J. G. (2013). The transnational alliance for genetic counseling: Promoting international communication and collaboration. *Journal of Genetic Counseling, 22*(6), 688–689. https://doi.org/10.1007/s10897-013-9621-3

El-Hattab, A. W., Almannai, M., & Sutton, V. R. (2018). Newborn screening: History, current status, and future directions. *Pediatric Clinics of North America, 65*(2), 389–405. https://doi.org/10.1016/j.pcl.2017.11.013

Familiari, A., Boito, S., Rembouskos, G., Ischia, B., Accurti, V., Fabietti, I., Volpe, P., & Persico, N. (2021). Cell-free DNA analysis of maternal blood in prenatal screening for chromosomal microdeletions and microduplications: A systematic review. *Prenatal Diagnosis, 41*(10), 1324–1331. https://doi.org/10.1002/pd.5928

Forman, A., & Sotelo, J. (2020). Tumor-based genetic testing and familial cancer risk. *Cold Spring Harbor Perspectives in Medicine, 10*(8), a036590. https://doi.org/10.1101/cshperspect.a036590

Gabrielli, S., Rizzi, S., Bassi, G., Carbone, S., Maimone, R., Marchesoni, M., & Forti, S. (2021). Engagement and effectiveness of a healthy-coping intervention via chatbot for university students during the COVID-19 pandemic: Mixed methods proof-of-concept study. *JMIR MHealth and UHealth, 9*(5), e27965. https://doi.org/10.2196/27965

Gregory, G., Das Gupta, K., Meiser, B., Barlow-Stewart, K., Geelan-Small, P., Kaur, R., Scheepers-Joynt, M., McInerny, S., Taylor, S., Antill, Y., Salmon, L., Smyth, C., Young, M.-A., James, P. A., & Yanes, T. (2022). Polygenic risk in familial breast cancer: Changing the dynamics of communicating genetic risk. *Journal of Genetic Counseling, 31*(1), 120–129. https://doi.org/10.1002/jgc4.1458

Hoffman, J. D., Thompson, R., Swenson, K. B., & Dasgupta, S. (2020). Complexities of clinical genetics consultation: An interprofessional clinical skills workshop. *MedEdPORTAL, 16*, 10869. https://doi.org/10.15766/mep_2374-8265.10869

Hooker, G. W., Babu, D., Myers, M., Zierhut, H., & McAllister, M. (2017). Standards for the reporting of Genetic Counseling Interventions in Research and Other Studies (GCIRS): An NSGC task force report. *Journal of Genetic Counseling, 26*(3), 355–360. https://doi.org/10.1007/s10897-017-0076-9

Hoskovec, J. M., Bennett, R. L., Carey, M. E., DaVanzo, J. E., Dougherty, M., Hahn, S. E., LeRoy, B. S., O'Neal, S., Richardson, J. G., & Wicklund, C. A. (2018). Projecting the supply and demand for certified genetic counselors: A workforce study. *Journal of Genetic Counseling*, *27*(1), 16–20. https://doi.org/10.1007/s10897-017-0158-8

Hyatt, C., Russo, J., & McDougall, C. (2019). Genetic counseling perspective of engagement with urology and primary care. *Canadian Journal of Urology*, *26*(5 Suppl. 2), 52–53.

Inglis, A., Koehn, D., McGillivray, B., Stewart, S. E., & Austin, J. (2015). Evaluating a unique, specialist psychiatric genetic counseling clinic: Uptake and impact. *Clinical Genetics*, *87*(3), 218–224. https://doi.org/10.1111/cge.12415

Jamal, L., Schupmann, W., & Berkman, B. E. (2020). An ethical framework for genetic counseling in the genomic era. *Journal of Genetic Counseling*, *29*(5), 718–727. https://doi.org/10.1002/jgc4.1207

Jang, Y., Yoon, H., Kim, M. T., Park, N. S., & Chiriboga, D. A. (2021). Preference for patient-provider ethnic concordance in Asian Americans. *Ethnicity & Health*, *26*(3), 448–459. https://doi.org/10.1080/13557858.2018.1514457

Jin, G., Zhao, Y., Chen, C., Wang, W., Du, J., & Lu, X. (2015). The length and content of general practice consultation in two urban districts of Beijing: A preliminary observation study. *PloS One*, *10*(8), e0135121. https://doi.org/10.1371/journal.pone.0135121

Johnston, J., Lantos, J. D., Goldenberg, A., Chen, F., Parens, E., Koenig, B. A., & Members of the NSIGHT Ethics and Policy Advisory Board. (2018). Sequencing newborns: A call for nuanced use of genomic technologies. *Hastings Center Report*, *48*(Suppl. 2), S2–S6. https://doi.org/10.1002/hast.874.

Joseph, G., Pasick, R. J., Schillinger, D., Luce, J., Guerra, C., & Cheng, J. K. Y. (2017). Information mismatch: Cancer risk counseling with diverse underserved patients. *Journal of Genetic Counseling*, *26*(5), 1090–1104. https://doi.org/10.1007/s10897-017-0089-4

Kaphingst, K. A., Kohlmann, W., Chambers, R. L., Goodman, M. S., Bradshaw, R., Chan, P. A., Chavez-Yenter, D., Colonna, S. V., Espinel, W. F., Everett, J. N., Gammon, A., Goldberg, E. R., Gonzalez, J., Hagerty, K. J., Hess, R., Kehoe, K., Kessler, C., Kimball, K. E., Loomis, S., . . . Ginsburg, O. (2021). Comparing models of delivery for cancer genetics services among patients receiving primary care who meet criteria for genetic evaluation in two healthcare systems: BRIDGE randomized controlled trial. *BMC Health Services Research*, *21*, 542. https://doi.org/10.1186/s12913-021-06489-y

Kenen, R. H. (1997). Opportunities and impediments for a consolidating and expanding profession: Genetic counseling in the United States. *Social Science & Medicine (1982)*, *45*(9), 1377–1386. https://doi.org/10.1016/s0277-9536(97)00062-2

Kessler, S. (1992). Psychological aspects of genetic counseling. VII. Thoughts on directiveness. *Journal of Genetic Counseling*, *1*(1), 9–17. https://doi.org/10.1007/BF00960080

Kessler, S. (1997). Psychological aspects of genetic counseling. IX. Teaching and counseling. *Journal of Genetic Counseling*, *6*(3), 287–295. https://doi.org/10.1023/A:1025676205440

Khan, A., Cohen, S., Weir, C., & Greenberg, S. (2021). Implementing innovative service delivery models in genetic counseling: A qualitative analysis of facilitators and barriers. *Journal of Genetic Counseling*, *30*(1), 319–328. https://doi.org/10.1002/jgc4.1325

Koeller, D. R., Uhlmann, W. R., Carere, D. A., Green, R. C., Roberts, J. S., & PGen Study Group. (2017). Utilization of genetic counseling after direct-to-consumer genetic testing: Findings from the Impact of Personal Genomics (PGen) study. *Journal of Genetic Counseling*, *26*(6), 1270–1279. https://doi.org/10.1007/s10897-017-0106-7

Laurino, M. Y., Leppig, K. A., Abad, P. J., Cham, B., Chu, Y. W. Y., Kejriwal, S., Lee, J. M. H., Sternen, D. L., Thompson, J. K., Burgess, M. J., Chien, S., Elackatt, N., Lim, J. Y., Sura,

T., Faradz, S., Padilla, C., Paz, E. C. de-la, Nauphar, D., Nguyen, K. N., . . . Thong, M.-K. (2018). A report on ten Asia Pacific countries on current status and future directions of the genetic counseling profession: The establishment of the professional society of genetic counselors in Asia. *Journal of Genetic Counseling*, *27*(1), 21–32. https://doi.org/10.1007/s10897-017-0115-6

Lewis, C. M., & Vassos, E. (2020). Polygenic risk scores: From research tools to clinical instruments. *Genome Medicine*, *12*, 44. https://doi.org/10.1186/s13073-020-00742-5

Löwy, I., & Dias Villela Corrêa, M. C. (2020). The "abortion pill" misoprostol in Brazil: Women's empowerment in a conservative and repressive political environment. *American Journal of Public Health*, *110*(5), 677–684. https://doi.org/10.2105/AJPH.2019.305562

Madlensky, L., Trepanier, A. M., Cragun, D., Lerner, B., Shannon, K. M., & Zierhut, H. (2017). A rapid systematic review of outcomes studies in genetic counseling. *Journal of Genetic Counseling*, *26*(3), 361–378. https://doi.org/10.1007/s10897-017-0067-x

Maina, I. W., Belton, T. D., Ginzberg, S., Singh, A., & Johnson, T. J. (2018). A decade of studying implicit racial/ethnic bias in healthcare providers using the implicit association test. *Social Science & Medicine (1982)*, *199*, 219–229. https://doi.org/10.1016/j.socscimed.2017.05.009

McAllister, M., Wood, A. M., Dunn, G., Shiloh, S., & Todd, C. (2011). The Genetic Counseling Outcome Scale: A new patient-reported outcome measure for clinical genetics services. *Clinical Genetics*, *79*(5), 413–424. https://doi.org/10.1111/j.1399-0004.2011.01636.x

McCuaig, J. M., Stockley, T. L., Shaw, P., Fung-Kee-Fung, M., Altman, A. D., Bentley, J., Bernardini, M. Q., Cormier, B., Hirte, H., Kieser, K., MacMillan, A., Meschino, W. S., Panabaker, K., Perrier, R., Provencher, D., Schrader, K. A., Serfas, K., Tomiak, E., Wong, N., . . . Kim, R. H. (2018). Evolution of genetic assessment for BRCA-associated gynaecologic malignancies: A Canadian multisociety roadmap. *Journal of Medical Genetics*, *55*(9), 571–577. https://doi.org/10.1136/jmedgenet-2018-105472

McGuinness, M., Fassi, E., Wang, C., Hacking, C., & Ellis, V. (2021). Breast cancer polygenic risk scores in the clinical cancer genetic counseling setting: Current practices and impact on patient management. *Journal of Genetic Counseling*, *30*(2), 588–597. https://doi.org/10.1002/jgc4.1347

Menke, C., Nagaraj, C. B., Dawson, B., He, H., Tawde, S., & Wakefield, E. G. (2021). Understanding and interpretation of a variant of uncertain significance (VUS) genetic test result by pediatric providers who do not specialize in genetics. *Journal of Genetic Counseling*, *30*(6), 1559–1569. https://doi.org/10.1002/jgc4.1422

Miller, C. E., Krautscheid, P., Baldwin, E. E., Tvrdik, T., Openshaw, A. S., Hart, K., & Lagrave, D. (2014). Genetic counselor review of genetic test orders in a reference laboratory reduces unnecessary testing. *American Journal of Medical Genetics Part A*, *164A*(5), 1094–1101. https://doi.org/10.1002/ajmg.a.36453

Mitchell, J., Williams, E.-D. G., Perry, R., & Lobo, K. (2019). "You have to be part of the process": A qualitative analysis of older African American men's primary care communication and participation. *American Journal of Men's Health*, *13*(4), 1557988319861569. https://doi.org/10.1177/1557988319861569

National Institutes of Health. (2020, June 1). *All of us*. https://allofus.nih.gov/future-health-begins-all-us

National Society of Genetic Counselors. (n.d.). *2022–2024 Strategic plan*. https://www.nsgc.org/About/About-NSGC/NSGC-2022-2024-Strategic-Plan

National Society of Genetic Counselors. (2022). *2022 Professional status survey*. https://www.nsgc.org/Policy-Research-and-Publications/Professional-Status-Survey

Nicholls, S. G., Wilson, B. J., Etchegary, H., Brehaut, J. C., Potter, B. K., Hayeems, R., Chakraborty, P., Milburn, J., Pullman, D., Turner, L., & Carroll, J. C. (2014). Benefits and burdens of newborn screening: Public understanding and decision-making. *Personalized Medicine, 11*(6), 593–607. https://doi.org/10.2217/pme.14.46

Ormond, K. E., Laurino, M. Y., Barlow-Stewart, K., Wessels, T., Macaulay, S., Austin, J., & Middleton, A. (2018). Genetic counseling globally: Where are we now? *American Journal of Medical Genetics Part C: Seminars in Medical Genetics, 178*(1), 98–107. https://doi.org/10.1002/ajmg.c.31607

Patch, C., & Middleton, A. (2018). Genetic counselling in the era of genomic medicine. *British Medical Bulletin, 126*(1), 27–36. https://doi.org/10.1093/bmb/ldy008

Paul, D. (1984). Eugenics and the Left. *Journal of the History of Ideas, 45*(4), 567–590. https://doi.org/10.2307/2709374

Paul, D. B. (1998). Genetic services, economics, and eugenics. *Science in Context, 11*(3–4), 481–491. https://doi.org/10.1017/s0269889700003161

Population Reference Bureau. (n.d.). *PRB's 2021 world population data sheet*. https://interactives.prb.org/2021-wpds/

Pruniski, B., Lisi, E., & Ali, N. (2018). Newborn screening for Pompe disease: Impact on families. *Journal of Inherited Metabolic Disease, 41*(6), 1189–1203. https://doi.org/10.1007/s10545-018-0159-2

Rajabi, F. (2018). Updates in newborn screening. *Pediatric Annals, 47*(5), e187–e190. https://doi.org/10.3928/19382359-20180426-01

Redlinger-Grosse, K., MacFarlane, I. M., Cragun, D., & Zierhut, H. (2021). A Delphi study to prioritize genetic counseling outcomes: What matters most. *Journal of Genetic Counseling, 30*(3), 676–692. https://doi.org/10.1002/jgc4.1352

Resta, R. G. (1997). Eugenics and nondirectiveness in genetic counseling. *Journal of Genetic Counseling, 6*(2), 255–258. https://doi.org/10.1023/a:1025624505382

Resta, R. (2021). Prenatal testing—What is it good for? A review and critique. *OBM Genetics, 5*(3), 136. https://doi.org/10.21926/obm.genet.2103136

Riconda, D., Grubs, R. E., Campion, M. W., & Cragun, D. (2018). Genetic counselor training for the next generation: Where do we go from here? *American Journal of Medical Genetics Part C: Seminars in Medical Genetics, 178*(1), 38–45. https://doi.org/10.1002/ajmg.c.31598

Robinson, C. L., Jouni, H., Kruisselbrink, T. M., Austin, E. E., Christensen, K. D., Green, R. C., & Kullo, I. J. (2016). Disclosing genetic risk for coronary heart disease: Effects on perceived personal control and genetic counseling satisfaction. *Clinical Genetics, 89*(2), 251–257. https://doi.org/10.1111/cge.12577

Roche, M. I., & Greb, A. E. (2016). It's time to ramp up genetic counseling training. *Genetics in Medicine, 18*(8), 768–769. https://doi.org/10.1038/gim.2016.25

Roter, D., Ellington, L., Erby, L. H., Larson, S., & W, D. (2006). The Genetic Counseling Video Project (GCVP): Models of practice. *American Journal of Medical Genetics Part C: Seminars in Medical Genetics, 142C*(4), 209–220. https://doi.org/10.1002/ajmg.c.30094

Russo, J., McDougall, C., Bowler, N., Shimada, A., Gross, L., Hyatt, C., Kelly, W. K., Calvaresi, A., Handley, N. R., Hirsch, I. H., Izes, J. K., Lallas, C. D., Mann, M., Mark, J. R., Mille, P. J., Preate, D., Trabulsi, E. J., Tsang, M., Chandrasekar, T., . . . Giri, V. N. (2021). Pretest genetic education video versus genetic counseling for men considering prostate cancer germline testing: A patient-choice study to address urgent practice needs. *JCO Precision Oncology, 5*, PO.21.00238. https://doi.org/10.1200/PO.21.00238

Rutherford, S., Zhang, X., Atzinger, C., Ruschman, J., & Myers, M. F. (2014). Medical management adherence as an outcome of genetic counseling in a pediatric setting. *Genetics in Medicine*, *16*(2), 157–163. https://doi.org/10.1038/gim.2013.90

Save Babies Through Screening Foundation. (n.d.). *Newborn screening*. http://www.savebabies.org/

Schmidlen, T., Schwartz, M., DiLoreto, K., Kirchner, H. L., & Sturm, A. C. (2019). Patient assessment of chatbots for the scalable delivery of genetic counseling. *Journal of Genetic Counseling*, *28*(6), 1166–1177. https://doi.org/10.1002/jgc4.1169

Sharma, Y., Cox, L., Kruger, L., Channamsetty, V., & Haga, S. B. (2022). Evaluating primary care providers' readiness for delivering genetic and genomic services to underserved populations. *Public Health Genomics*, *25*, 12–21. https://doi.org/10.1159/000518415

Slade, D. (2020). PARP and PARG inhibitors in cancer treatment. *Genes & Development*, *34*(5–6), 360–394. https://doi.org/10.1101/gad.334516.119

Smith, M. K., Wood, W. B., Adams, W. K., Wieman, C., Knight, J. K., Guild, N., & Su, T. T. (2009). Why peer discussion improves student performance on in-class concept questions. *Science*, *323*(5910), 122–124. https://doi.org/10.1126/science.1165919

Stenehjem, D. D., Au, T., Sainski, A. M., Bauer, H., Brown, K., Lancaster, J., Stevens, V., & Brixner, D. I. (2018). Impact of a genetic counseling requirement prior to genetic testing. *BMC Health Services Research*, *18*(1), 165. https://doi.org/10.1186/s12913-018-2957-5

Stoll, K., Kubendran, S., & Cohen, S. A. (2018). The past, present and future of service delivery in genetic counseling: Keeping up in the era of precision medicine. *American Journal of Medical Genetics Part C: Seminars in Medical Genetics*, *178*(1), 24–37. https://doi.org/10.1002/ajmg.c.31602

Tahan, H. A., & Sminkey, P. V. (2012). Motivational interviewing: Building rapport with clients to encourage desirable behavioral and lifestyle changes. *Professional Case Management*, *17*(4), 164–172; quiz 173–174. https://doi.org/10.1097/NCM.0b013e318253f029

Tandy-Connor, S., Guiltinan, J., Krempely, K., LaDuca, H., Reineke, P., Gutierrez, S., Gray, P., & Tippin Davis, B. (2018). False-positive results released by direct-to-consumer genetic tests highlight the importance of clinical confirmation testing for appropriate patient care. *Genetics in Medicine*, *20*(12), 1515–1521. https://doi.org/10.1038/gim.2018.38

Terry, A. B., Wylie, A., Raspa, M., Vogel, B., Sanghavi, K., Djurdjinovic, L., Caggana, M., & Bodurtha, J. (2019). Clinical models of telehealth in genetics: A regional telegenetics landscape. *Journal of Genetic Counseling*, *28*(3), 673–691. https://doi.org/10.1002/jgc4.1088

Timmermans, S., & Buchbinder, M. (2010). Patients-in-waiting: Living between sickness and health in the genomics era. *Journal of Health and Social Behavior*, *51*(4), 408–423. https://doi.org/10.1177/0022146510386794

Uhlmann, W. R., Hoskovec, J., & Freivogel, M. (2020). 40 years and beyond for the National Society of Genetic Counselors: Reflections on genetic counseling practice. *Journal of Genetic Counseling*, *29*(6), 888–893. https://doi.org/10.1002/jgc4.1301

U.S. Bureau of Labor Statistics. (n.d.). *Genetic counselors: Occupational outlook handbook*. https://www.bls.gov/ooh/healthcare/genetic-counselors.htm

Vadaparampil, S. T., Scherr, C. L., Cragun, D., Malo, T. L., & Pal, T. (2015). Pretest genetic counseling services for hereditary breast and ovarian cancer delivered by non-genetics professionals in the state of Florida. *Clinical Genetics*, *87*(5), 473–477. https://doi.org/10.1111/cge.12405

Veach, P. M., Bartels, D. M., & Leroy, B. S. (2007). Coming full circle: A reciprocal-engagement model of genetic counseling practice. *Journal of Genetic Counseling, 16*(6), 713–728. https://doi.org/10.1007/s10897-007-9113-4

Wain, K. E., Azzariti, D. R., Goldstein, J. L., Johnson, A. K., Krautscheid, P., Lepore, B., O'Daniel, J. M., Ritter, D., Savatt, J. M., Riggs, E. R., & Martin, C. L. (2020). Variant interpretation is a component of clinical practice among genetic counselors in multiple specialties. *Genetics in Medicine, 22*(4), 785–792. https://doi.org/10.1038/s41436-019-0705-9

Wakefield, E., Keller, H., Mianzo, H., Nagaraj, C. B., Tawde, S., & Ulm, E. (2018). Reduction of health care costs and improved appropriateness of incoming test orders: The impact of genetic counselor review in an academic genetic testing laboratory. *Journal of Genetic Counseling, 27*(5), 1067–1073. https://doi.org/10.1007/s10897-018-0226-8

Waltman, L., Runke, C., Balcom, J., Riley, J. D., Lilley, M., Christian, S., Zetzsche, L., & Goodenberger, M. L. (2016). Further defining the role of the laboratory genetic counselor. *Journal of Genetic Counseling, 25*(4), 786–798. https://doi.org/10.1007/s10897-015-9927-4

Weil, J. (2003). Psychosocial genetic counseling in the post-nondirective era: A point of view. *Journal of Genetic Counseling, 12*(3), 199–211. https://doi.org/10.1023/A:1023234802124

Wilson, J. M., & Jungner, Y. G. (1968). Principles and practice of mass screening for disease. *Boletin De La Oficina Sanitaria Panamericana. Pan American Sanitary Bureau, 65*(4), 281–393.

Wong, B., Lucente, D., Krivensky, S., Krahn, E., Karlawish, J., & Dickerson, B. C. (2021). Knowledge assessment and psychological impact of genetic counseling in people at risk for familial FTD. *Alzheimer's & Dementia: Diagnosis, Assessment & Disease Monitoring, 13*(1), e12225. https://doi.org/10.1002/dad2.12225

Yanes, T., Meiser, B., Kaur, R., Young, M.-A., Mitchell, P. B., Scheepers-Joynt, M., McInerny, S., Taylor, S., Barlow-Stewart, K., Antill, Y., Salmon, L., Smyth, C., Betz-Stablein, B., & James, P. A. (2021). Breast cancer polygenic risk scores: A 12-month prospective study of patient reported outcomes and risk management behavior. *Genetics in Medicine, 23*(12), 2316–2323. https://doi.org/10.1038/s41436-021-01288-6

Index

For the benefit of digital users, indexed terms that span two pages (e.g., 52–53) may, on occasion, appear on only one of those pages.

Note: Tables, figures, and boxes are indicated by an italic *t*, *f*, and *b* following the page number